Clinical Anesthesiology

Third edition

G. Edward Morgan, Jr., MD
President and Chief Executive Officer
Excellence In Medicine, LLC
OrthoSource Medical Clinics, Inc
Pasadena, California

Maged S. Mikhail, MD
Attending Anesthesiologist
San Fernando Valley Heart Institute
Encino-Tarzana Regional Medical Center
Los Angeles, California

Michael J. Murray, MD, PhD
Dean, Mayo School of Health Sciences
Professor of Anesthesiology, Mayo Medical School
Chair, Department of Anesthesiology
Mayo Clinic Jacksonville
Jacksonville, Florida

GUEST EDITOR, PROFILES IN ANESTHETIC PRACTICE
C. Philip Larson Jr., MDCM, MA
Professor Emeritus, Anesthesia and Neurosurgery
Stanford University
Palo Alto, California
Professor of Clinical Anesthesiology
UCLA School of Medicine
Los Angeles, California

Lange Medical Books/McGraw-Hill
Medical Publishing Division
New York   Chicago   San Francisco   Lisbon   London
Madrid   Mexico City   Milan   Montreal   New Delhi   San Juan   Seoul
Singapore   Sydney   Toronto

McGraw-Hill

BS

A Division of The McGraw·Hill Companies

Notice

Medicine is an ever-changing science. As new research and clinical experience broaden our knowledge, changes in treatment and drug therapy are required. The authors and the publisher of this work have checked with sources believed to be reliable in their efforts to provide information that is complete and generally in accord with the standards accepted at the time of publication. However, in view of the possibility of human error or changes in medical sciences, neither the authors nor the publisher nor any other party who has been involved in the preparation or publication of this work warrants that the information contained herein is in every respect accurate or complete, and they disclaim all responsibility for any errors or omissions or for the results obtained from use of the information contained in this work. Readers are encouraged to confirm the information contained herein with other sources. For example and in particular, readers are advised to check the product information sheet included in the package of each drug they plan to administer to be certain that the information contained in this work is accurate and that changes have not been made in the recommended dose or in the contraindications for administration. This recommendation is of particular importance in connection with new or infrequently used drugs.

This book was set in Times Roman by Pine Tree Composition.
The editors were Janet Foltin, Harriet Lebowitz, and Peter J. Boyle.
The production supervisor was Philip Galea.
The art manager was Charissa Baker.
The text was designed by Eve Siegel.
The index was prepared by Katherine Pitcoff.
R. R. Donnelley and Sons Company was printer and binder.

This book is printed on acid-free paper.

INTERNATIONAL EDITION ISBN: 0-07-112441-1

10/29/03

Contents

Preface xiii

1. The Practice of Anesthesiology 1

   Case Discussion: Medical Malpractice 10

I. ANESTHESIC EQUIPMENT & MONITORS

2. The Operating Room: Medical Gas Systems, Environmental Factors, & Electrical Safety 15

   Case Discussion: Checking Out the Medical Gas System in a New Operating Room 25

3. Breathing Systems 27

   Case Discussion: Unexplained Light Anesthesia 37

4. The Anesthesia Machine 40

   Case Discussion: Detection of a Leak 56

5. Airway Management 59

   Profiles in Anesthetic Practice: Laryngospasm: A Continuing Problem 78
   C. Philip Larson, Jr., MDCM, MA

   Case Discussion: Evaluation & Management of a Difficult Airway 80

6. Patient Monitors 86

   Profiles in Anesthetic Practice: If There Were Only One Monitor 94
   Wendell C. Stevens, MD

   Profiles in Anesthetic Practice: Application of the Basic Physical Examination
   to Intraoperative Monitoring 118
   John R. Moyers, MD

   Case Discussion: Monitoring During Magnetic Resonance Imaging 123

II. CLINICAL PHARMACOLOGY

7. Inhalational Anesthetics 127

   Case Discussion: Closed-circuit Anesthesia 146

8. Nonvolatile Anesthetic Agents 151

Profiles in Anesthetic Practice: Rational Administration of Intravenous Anesthesia **162**
J. G. Reves, MD

Case Discussion: Premedication of the Surgical Patient **175**

9. Neuromuscular Blocking Agents **178**

Profiles in Anesthetic Practice: A Current Practice of Relaxation **192**
John J. Savarese, MD

Case Discussion: Delayed Recovery from General Anesthesia **197**

10. Cholinesterase Inhibitors 199

Case Discussion: Respiratory Failure in the Recovery Room **205**

11. Anticholinergic Drugs 207

Case Discussion: Central Anticholinergic Syndrome **210**

12. Adrenergic Agonists & Antagonists 212

Case Discussion: Pheochromocytoma **222**

13. Hypotensive Agents 224

Case Discussion: Controlled Hypotension **231**

14. Local Anesthetics 233

Case Discussion: Local Anesthetic Overdose **240**

15. Adjuncts to Anesthesia 242

Case Discussion: Management of Patients at Risk for Aspiration Pneumonia **250**

III. REGIONAL ANESTHESIA & PAIN MANAGEMENT

16. Spinal, Epidural, & Caudal Blocks 253
Wayne Kleinman, MD

Case Discussion: Neuraxial Anesthetia for Lithotripsy **280**

17. Peripheral Nerve Blocks 283

Case Discussion: Dyspnea Following Interscalene Block **308**

18. Pain Management 309

Profiles in Anesthetic Practice: Should Patients Suffer Because Physicians Are Afraid? **344**
Carl C. Hug, Jr., MD, PhD

Case Discussion: Analgesia Following Thoracoabdominal Surgery **356**

IV. PHYSIOLOGY, PATHOPHYSIOLOGY, & ANESTHETIC MANAGEMENT

19. Cardiovascular Physiology & Anesthesia **359**

    Case Discussion: A Patient with a Short P–R Interval **381**

20. Anesthesia for Patients with Cardiovascular Disease **386**

    Case Discussion: Hip Fracture in an Elderly Woman Who Fell **427**

21. Anesthesia for Cardiovascular Surgery **433**

    Case Discussion: A Patient for Cardioversion **472**

22. Respiratory Physiology & Anesthesia **475**

    Case Discussion: Unilaterally Diminished Breath Sounds during General Anesthesia **509**

23. Anesthesia for Patients with Respiratory Disease **511**

    Case Discussion: Laparscopic Surgery **522**

24. Anesthesia for Thoracic Surgery **525**

    Case Discussion: Mediastinal Adenopathy **550**

25. Neurophysiology & Anesthesia **552**

    Case Discussion: Postoperative Hemiplegia **564**

26. Anesthesia for Neurosurgery **567**

    Profiles in Anesthetic Practice: Anesthesia for Neuronavigation **570**
    Robert F. Bedford, MD

    Case Discussion: Resection of a Pituitary Tumor **581**

27. Anesthesia for Patients with Neurologic & Psychiatric Diseases **583**

    Case Discussion: Anesthesia for Electroconvulsive Therapy **594**

28. Management of Patients with Fluid & Electrolyte Disturbances **597**

    Case Discussion: Electrolyte Abnormalities Following Urinary Diversion **624**

29. Fluid Management & Transfusion **626**

    Case Discussion: A Patient with Sickle Cell Disease **640**

30. Acid-Base Balance 644

   Case Discussion: A Complex Acid-Base Disturbance 660

31. Renal Physiology & Anesthesia 662

   Case Discussion: Intraoperative Oliguria 677

32. Anesthesia for Patients with Renal Disease 679

   Case Discussion: A Patient with Uncontrolled Hypertension 689

33. Anesthesia for Genitourinary Surgery 692

   Case Discussion: Hypotension in the Recovery Room 705

34. Hepatic Physiology & Anesthesia 708

   Case Discussion: Coagulopathy in a Patient with Liver Disease 717

35. Anesthesia for Patients with Liver Disease 723

   Case Discussion: Liver Transplantation 732

36. Anesthesia for Patients with Endocrine Disease 736

   Case Discussion: Multiple Endocrine Neoplasia 750

37. Anesthesia for Patients with Neuromuscular Disease 752

   Case Discussion: Anesthesia for Muscle Biopsy 759

38. Anesthesia for Ophthalmic Surgery 761

   Case Discussion: An Approach to a Patient with an Open Eye & a Full Stomach 768

39. Anesthesia for Otorhinolaryngologic Surgery 771

   Case Discussion: Bleeding Following Sinus Surgery 779

40. Anesthesia for Orthopedic Surgery 782

   Case Discussion: Managing Blood Loss in Jehovah's Witnesses 790

41. Anesthesia for the Trauma Patient 793

   Case Discussion: Anesthetic Management of the Burn Patient 801

42. Maternal & Fetal Physiology & Anesthesia 804

   Case Discussion: Postpartum Tubal Ligation 816

43. Obstetric Anesthesia 819

Case Discussion: Appendicitis in a Pregnant Woman 846

44. Pediatric Anesthesia 849

Profiles in Anesthetic Practice: Heart Rate Response to Surgical Incision in Children 858
John F. Ryan, MD, MEd

Case Discussion: Masseter Spasm & Malignant Hyperthermia. 869

45. Geriatric Anesthesia 875

Case Discussion: The Elderly Patient with a Fractured Hip 880

46. Outpatient Anesthesia. 882
Stuart Ackerman, MD

Case Discussion: Monitored Anethesia Care for Eye Surgery 886

V. SPECIAL PROBLEMS

47. Anesthetic Complications 889
Joseph T. Nitti, MD, & Gary J. Nitti, MD

Profiles in Anesthetic Practice: The Seated Position—Gone Forever?. 894
M. Jane Matjasko, MD, & Douglas G. Martz, MD

Case Discussion: Unexplained Intraoperative Tachycardia & Hypertension 909

48. Cardiopulmonary Resuscitation 912

Profiles in Anesthetic Practice: Management of the Difficult Airway by Anesthesiologists. 914
David J. Cullen, MD, MS

Case Discussion: Intraoperative Hypotension & Cardiac Arrest. 925

49. Postanesthesia Care. 936

Profiles in Anesthetic Practice: Routine Postoperative Suctioning: A Bad Idea. 942
Frederic A. Berry, MD

Case Discussion: Fever & Tachycardia in a Young Adult Male. 947

50. Critical Care 951

Case Discussion: An Obtunded Young Woman. 990

Index. 993

Contributing Authors

Stuart Ackerman, MD
Attending Anesthesiologist
San Fernando Valley Heart Institute
Encino-Tarzana Regional Medical Center
Los Angeles, California

Wayne Kleinman, MD
Director of Obstetric Anesthesia
Encino-Tarzana Regional Medical Center
Los Angeles, California

Gary J. Nitti, MD
Chairman, Department of Anesthesiology
Director, Cardiac Anesthesia Services
San Fernando Valley Heart Institute
Encino-Tarzana Regional Medical Center
Los Angeles, California

Joseph T. Nitti, MD
Attending Anesthesiologist
San Fernando Valley Heart Institute
Encino-Tarzana Regional Medical Center
Los Angeles, California

Contributors to Profiles in Anesthetic Practice

Editor
C. Philip Larson Jr., MDCM, MA
Professor Emeritus, Anesthesia and Neurosurgery
Stanford University
Palo Alto, California
Professor of Clinical Anesthesiology
UCLA School of Medicine
Los Angeles, California

Robert F. Bedford, MD
Clinical Professor of Anesthesiology
University of South Florida, College of Medicine
Tampa, Florida

Frederic A. Berry, MD
Professor, Anesthesiology and Pediatrics
University of Virginia School of Medicine
Charlottesville, Virginia

David J. Cullen, MD, MS
Clinical Professor of Anesthesiology
Tufts University School of Medicine
Boston, Massachusetts

Carl C. Hug, Jr., MD, PhD
Professor of Anesthesiology and Pharmacology
Emory University School of Medicine
Atlanta, Georgia

Douglas G. Martz, MD
Assistant Professor
Department of Anesthesiology
University of Maryland School of Medicine
Baltimore, Maryland

M. Jane Matjasko, MD
Professor and Chair
Department of Anesthesiology
University of Maryland School of Medicine
Baltimore, Maryland

John R. Moyers, MD
Professor
Department of Anesthesia
University of Iowa College of Medicine
Iowa City, Iowa

J. G. Reves, MD
Professor and Chair
Department of Anesthesiology
Duke University Medical Center
Durham, North Carolina

John F. Ryan, MD, MEd
Associate Professor of Anesthesiology
Harvard Medical School
Boston, Massachusetts

John J. Savarese, MD
Professor and Chair
Department of Anesthesiology
Weill Medical College of Cornell University
New York, New York

Wendell C. Stevens, MD
Professor Emeritus
Department of Anesthesiology
Oregon Health Sciences University
Portland, Oregon

The authors dedicate this book to their families, especially to their children: Victoria Morgan; Lara Mikhail; and Karl, Elise, Tess, Jennie and Greg Murray.

Preface

Doctors Morgan and Mikhail welcome Dr. Michael Murray as a new author for the third edition of *Clinical Anesthesiology*. The addition of Dr. Murray brings a fresh viewpoint to the book, intended to prevent the provinciality that a coauthored book tends to develop.

This new edition contains several important improvements and refinements of the highly successful first and second editions:

Profiles in Anesthetic Practice are exciting, unique features introduced in this edition. These brief essays, written by 11 internationally recognized leaders in anesthesiology and coordinated by Dr. C. Philip Larson, Jr., present editorialized counterpoints to the usual textbook dogma. They involve the reader in the dynamics of thinking through anesthetic problems and controversies. Thus, each essay is a profile in the sense that it represents more of a side perspective as opposed to a straight-on view. The Profiles in Anesthetic Practice are easily identified by the use of color, icons, and a line drawing of each author's profile.

Key Concepts are listed in the front of each chapter and a corresponding numbered icon identifies the section(s) within the chapter in which each concept is discussed. These should help the reader focus on truly important themes that constitute the core of understanding anesthesiology.

Case Discussions deal with clinical problems of current interest and provide a methodology and framework to approach oral examinations. They have been given a new look that makes them easy to spot when thumbing through the text.

Key Terms are identified with color type. These highlighted words provide the reader with a quick guide to the subject matter upon which many written exam questions are based.

- All chapters have been thoroughly updated and revised.
- The suggested reading has been expanded and updated.
- Several new illustrations have been added.

Nonetheless, the goal of *Clinical Anesthesiology* remains unchanged from the first and second editions "to provide a concise, consistent presentation of the basic principles essential to the modern practice of anesthesia." To this end, the authors have strived to minimize redundancies, eliminate contradictions, and write in a highly readable style. The case discussions that conclude each chapter continue to address the whys of clinical medicine, serve as a self-examination tool for the reader, and instill a logical approach to clinical situations. The suggested reading includes relevant texts, chapters, and review articles, emphasizing material published since 1995.

The authors wish to express their gratitude to Deb Schmaling, Nicole' Rodriguez-George, Nelson Koe, MD, Duraiyah Thangathurai, MD, Zheng Wang, MD, Steven R. Holets, RRT, RCP, CCRA, Jeffrey J. Ward, MED, RRT, and Jasper R. Daube, MD for their help in the preparation of this book. We would also like to thank and acknowledge the invaluable assistance of Janet Foltin, Harriet Lebowitz, and Jennifer McConnon.

G. Edward Morgan, Jr., MD
Maged S. Mikhail, MD
Michael J. Murray, MD, PhD
Los Angeles
December 2001

The Practice of Anesthesiology

KEY CONCEPTS

 1 An anesthetic plan should be formulated that will optimally accommodate the patient's baseline physiologic state, including any medical and surgical illnesses, the planned procedure, drug sensitivities, previous anesthetic experiences, and psychological makeup.

 2 Inadequate preoperative planning and errors in patient preparation are the most common causes of anesthetic complications.

 3 Anesthesia and elective surgery should not proceed until the patient is in optimal medical condition.

 4 To be valuable, a preoperative test implies an increased perioperative risk when it is abnormal and a reduced risk when the abnormality is corrected.

 5 The usefulness of a screening test depends on its sensitivity and specificity. Sensitive tests have a low rate of false-negative results, while specific tests have a low rate of false-positive results.

 6 If any procedure is performed without the patient's consent, the physician may be liable for assault and battery.

 7 The intraoperative anesthesia record serves many purposes. It functions as a useful intraoperative monitor, a reference for future anesthetics for that patient, and a tool for quality assurance.

INTRODUCTION

The Greek philosopher Dioscorides first used the term *anesthesia* in the first century AD to describe the narcotic-like effects of the plant mandragora. The term subsequently was defined in Bailey's *An Universal Etymological English Dictionary* (1721) as "a defect of sensation" and again in the *Encyclopedia Britannica* (1771) as "privation of the senses." The present use of the term to denote the sleeplike state that makes possible painless surgery is credited to Oliver Wendell Holmes in 1846. In the United States, use of the term *anesthesiology* to denote the practice of anesthesia was first proposed in the second decade of the 20th century to emphasize the growing scientific basis of the specialty. Although the specialty now rests on a scientific foundation that rivals any other, anesthesia remains very much a mixture of both science and art. Moreover, the practice of anesthe-

siology has expanded well beyond rendering patients insensible to pain during surgery or obstetric delivery (Table 1–1). The specialty is unique in that it requires a working familiarity with most other specialties, including surgery and its subspecialties, internal medicine, pediatrics, and obstetrics as well as clinical pharmacology, applied physiology, and biomedical technology. The application of recent advances in biomedical technology in clinical anesthesia continues to make anesthesia an exciting and rapidly evolving specialty. A significant number of physicians applying for residency positions in anesthesiology already have training and certification in other specialties.

This chapter reviews the history of anesthesia, its British and American roots, and the current scope of the specialty and presents the general approach to the preoperative evaluation of patients and documentation of the patient's anesthetic experience. The Case Discus-

Table 1-1. Definition of the practice of anesthesiology.*

Assessing, consulting, and preparing patients for anesthesia
Rendering patients insensible to pain during surgical obstetric, therapeutic, and diagnostic procedures
Monitoring and restoring homeostasis in perioperative and critically ill patients
Diagnosing and treating painful syndromes
Managing and teaching of cardiac and pulmonary resuscitation
Evaluating respiratory function and applying respiratory therapy
Teaching, supervising, and evaluating the performance of medical and paramedical personnel involved in anesthesia, respiratory care, and critical care
Conducting research at the basic and clinical science levels to explain and improve the care of patients in terms of physiologic function and drug response
Involvement in the administration of hospitals, medical schools, and outpatient facilities as necessary to implement these responsibilities

*Adapted from the American Board of Anesthesiology Booklet of Information, January 2000.

sion at the end of the chapter considers medicolegal aspects of the specialty.

■ THE HISTORY OF ANESTHESIA

Anesthetic practices date from ancient times, yet the evolution of the specialty began in the mid-nineteenth century and only became firmly established less than six decades ago. Ancient civilizations had used opium poppy, coca leaves, mandrake root, alcohol, and even phlebotomy (to the point of unconsciousness) to allow surgeons to operate. It is interesting that the ancient Egyptians used the combination of opium poppy (morphine) and hyoscyamus (hyoscyamine and scopolamine); a similar combination, morphine and scopolamine, is still used parenterally for premedication. Regional anesthesia in ancient times consisted of compression of nerve trunks (nerve ischemia) or the application of cold (cryoanalgesia). The Incas may have practiced local anesthesia as their surgeons chewed coca leaves and spat saliva (presumably containing cocaine) into the operative wound. Surgical procedures were for the most part limited to caring for fractures, traumatic wounds, amputations, and the removal of bladder cal-

culi. Amazingly, some civilizations were also able to perform trephination of the skull. A major qualification for a successful surgeon was speed.

The evolution of modern surgery was hampered not only by a poor understanding of disease processes, anatomy, and surgical asepsis but also by the lack of reliable and safe anesthetic techniques. These techniques evolved first with inhalational anesthesia, followed by local and regional anesthesia, and finally intravenous anesthesia. The discovery of surgical anesthesia is considered one of the most important in human history.

INHALATIONAL ANESTHESIA

Because the invention of the hypodermic needle did not occur until later, the first general anesthetics were destined to be inhalational agents. **Ether** (really diethyl ether, known at the time as "sulfuric ether" because it was produced by a simple chemical reaction between ethyl alcohol and sulfuric acid) was originally prepared in 1540 by Valerius Cordus, a 25-year-old Prussian botanist. Ether was known to the medical community for frivolous purposes ("ether frolics"), but was not used as an anesthetic agent in humans until 1842, when Crawford W. Long and William E. Clark used it independently on patients. However, they did not publicize this discovery. Four years later, in Boston, on October 16, 1846, William T.G. Morton conducted the first publicized demonstration of general anesthesia using ether. The dramatic success of that exhibition led the operating surgeon to exclaim to a skeptical audience: "Gentlemen, this is no humbug!"

Chloroform was independently prepared by von Leibig, Guthrie, and Soubeiran in 1831. Although first used by Holmes Coote in 1847, chloroform was introduced into clinical practice by the Scottish obstetrician Sir James Simpson, who administered it to his patients to relieve the pain of labor. Ironically, Simpson had almost abandoned his medical practice after witnessing the terrible despair and agony of patients undergoing operations without anesthesia.

Joseph Priestley produced **nitrous oxide** in 1772, but Humphry Davy first noted its analgesic properties in 1800. Gardner Colton and Horace Wells are credited for having first used nitrous oxide as an anesthetic in humans in 1844. Nitrous oxide's lack of potency (an 80% nitrous oxide concentration results in analgesia but not surgical anesthesia) led to clinical demonstrations that were less convincing than those with ether.

Nitrous oxide was the least popular of the three early inhalational anesthetics because of its low potency and its tendency to cause asphyxia when used alone (see Chapter 7). Interest in nitrous oxide was revived in 1868 when Edmund Andrews administered it in 20%

oxygen; it was, however, overshadowed by the popularity of ether and chloroform. It is ironic that nitrous oxide is the only one of these agents still in common use today. Chloroform initially superseded ether in popularity in many areas (particularly in the United Kingdom), but reports of chloroform-related cardiac arrhythmias, respiratory depression, and hepatotoxicity eventually caused more and more practitioners to abandon it in favor of ether.

Even after the introduction of other inhalational anesthetics (ethyl chloride, ethylene, divinyl ether, cyclopropane, trichloroethylene, and fluroxene), ether remained the standard general anesthetic until the early 1960s. The only inhalational agent that rivaled ether's safety and popularity was cyclopropane (introduced in 1934). However, both are highly combustible and have since been replaced by the nonflammable potent fluorinated hydrocarbons: halothane (developed in 1951; released, 1956), methoxyflurane (developed in 1958; released, 1960), enflurane (developed in 1963; released, 1973), and isoflurane (developed in 1965; released, 1981).

New agents continue to be developed. One such agent, desflurane (released 1992), has many of the desirable properties of isoflurane as well as the rapid uptake and elimination characteristics of nitrous oxide. Sevoflurane also has low blood solubility, but concerns about potentially toxic degradation products delayed its release in the United States until 1995 (see Chapter 7).

LOCAL & REGIONAL ANESTHESIA

The origin of modern local anesthesia is credited to Carl Koller, an ophthalmologist, who demonstrated the use of topical cocaine for surgical anesthesia of the eye in 1884. Cocaine had been isolated from the coca plant in 1855 by Gaedicke and later purified in 1860 by Albert Neimann. The surgeon William Halsted demonstrated in 1884 the use of cocaine for intradermal infiltration and nerve blocks (including the facial nerve, the brachial plexus, the pudendal nerve, and the posterior tibial nerve). August Bier is credited with administering the first spinal anesthetic in 1898; he used 3 mL of 0.5% cocaine intrathecally. He was also the first to describe intravenous regional anesthesia (Bier block) in 1908. Procaine was synthesized in 1904 by Alfred Einhorn and within a year was used clinically as a local anesthetic by Heinrich Braun. Braun was also the first to add epinephrine to prolong the action of local anesthetics. Ferdinand Cathelin and Jean Sicard introduced caudal epidural anesthesia in 1901. Lumbar epidural anesthesia was described first in 1921 by Fidel Pages and again in 1931 by Achille Dogliotti. Additional local anesthetics subsequently introduced clinically include dibucaine (1930), tetracaine (1932), lidocaine (1947), chloroprocaine (1955), mepivacaine (1957), prilocaine (1960), bupivacaine (1963), and etidocaine (1972). Ropivacaine is a newer agent with the same duration of action as bupivacaine but less cardiac toxicity (see Chapter 14).

INTRAVENOUS ANESTHESIA

Induction Agents

Intravenous anesthesia followed the invention of the hypodermic syringe and needle by Alexander Wood in 1855. Early attempts at intravenous anesthesia included the use of chloral hydrate (by Oré in 1872), chloroform and ether (Burkhardt in 1909), and the combination of morphine and scopolamine (Bredenfeld in 1916). Barbiturates were synthesized in 1903 by Fischer and von Mering. The first barbiturate used for induction of anesthesia was diethylbarbituric acid (barbital), but it was not until the introduction of hexobarbital in 1927 that barbiturate induction became a popular technique. Thiopental, synthesized in 1932 by Volwiler and Tabern, was first used clinically by John Lundy and Ralph Waters in 1934 and remains the most common induction agent for anesthesia. Methohexital was first used clinically in 1957 by V.K. Stoelting and is the only other barbiturate currently used for induction. Since the synthesis of chlordiazepoxide in 1957, the benzodiazepines—diazepam (1959), lorazepam (1971), and midazolam (1976)—have been extensively used for premedication, induction, supplementation of anesthesia, and intravenous sedation. Ketamine was synthesized in 1962 by Stevens and first used clinically in 1965 by Corssen and Domino; it was released in 1970. Ketamine was the first intravenous agent associated with minimal cardiac and respiratory depression. Etomidate was synthesized in 1964 and released in 1972; initial enthusiasm over its relative lack of circulatory and respiratory effects was tempered by reports of adrenal suppression after even a single dose. The release of propofol, diisopropylphenol, in 1989 was a major advance in outpatient anesthesia because of its short duration of action (see Chapters 8 and 46).

Muscle Relaxants

The use of curare by Harold Griffith and Enid Johnson in 1942 was a milestone in anesthesia. Curare greatly facilitated endotracheal intubation and provided excellent abdominal relaxation for surgery. For the first time, surgery could be performed on patients without having to administer relatively large doses of anesthetic to produce muscle relaxation. These large doses often resulted in excessive circulatory and respiratory depression as well as prolonged emergence; moreover, they were often not tolerated by frail patients.

Other muscle relaxants (also known as neuromuscular blocking agents; see Chapter 9)—gallamine, decamethonium, metocurine, alcuronium, and pancuronium—were soon introduced clinically. Because these agents were often associated with significant side effects (see Chapter 9), the search for the ideal muscle relaxant continued. Recently introduced agents that come close to this goal include vecuronium, atracurium, pipecuronium, and doxacurium. Succinylcholine was synthesized by Bovet in 1949 and released in 1951; it has become a standard agent for facilitating endotracheal intubation. Until recently, succinylcholine remained unparalleled in its rapid onset of profound muscle relaxation, but its occasional side effects continued to fuel the search for a comparable substitute. Mivacurium, a newer short-acting nondepolarizing muscle relaxant, has minimal side effects, but it still has a slower onset and longer duration of action than succinylcholine. Rocuronium is an intermediate-acting relaxant with a rapid onset approaching that of succinylcholine. Rapacuronium, the most recently released muscle relaxant, finally achieved the combination of succinylcholine's rapid onset, short duration of action, and an improved safety profile. However, the manufacturer of rapacuronium voluntarily withdrew it from the market due to several reports of serious bronchospasm, including a few unexplained fatalities.

Opioids

Morphine was isolated from opium in 1805 by Sertürner and subsequently tried as an intravenous anesthetic (see above). The morbidity and mortality initially associated with high doses of opioids in early reports caused many anesthetists to avoid opioids and favor pure inhalational anesthesia. Interest in opioids in anesthesia returned following the synthesis of meperidine in 1939. The concept of *balanced anesthesia* was introduced by Lundy and others and evolved to consist of thiopental for induction, nitrous oxide for amnesia, meperidine (or any opioid) for analgesia, and curare for muscle relaxation. In 1969, Lowenstein rekindled interest in opioid anesthesia by reintroducing the concept of high doses of opioids as complete anesthetics. Morphine was initially employed, but fentanyl, sufentanil, and alfentanil were all subsequently used as sole agents. As experience grew with this technique, its limitations in reliably preventing patient awareness and suppressing autonomic responses during surgery were realized. Remifentanil is a new rapidly metabolized opioid that is broken down by nonspecific plasma and tissue esterases.

EVOLUTION OF THE SPECIALTY

British Origins

Following its first public demonstration in the United States, the use of ether quickly spread to England. John Snow, generally considered the father of anesthesia, became the first physician to take a full-time interest in this new anesthetic, for which he invented an inhaler. He was the first to scientifically investigate ether and the physiology of general anesthesia. (Snow was also a pioneer in epidemiology who helped stop a cholera epidemic in London by proving that the causative agent was transmitted by ingestion rather than inhalation.) In 1847, Snow published the first book on general anesthesia, *On the Inhalation of Ether.* When the anesthetic properties of chloroform were made known (see above), he quickly investigated and developed an inhaler for that agent as well. He believed that an inhaler should be used in administering these agents in order to control the dose of the anesthetic. His second book, *On Chloroform and Other Anaesthetics,* was published posthumously in 1858.

After Snow's death, Joseph T. Clover took his place as England's leading physician anesthetist. Clover emphasized continuously monitoring the patient's pulse during anesthesia, a practice that was not widely accepted at the time. He was the first to use the jaw-thrust maneuver for airway obstruction, first to have resuscitation equipment always available during anesthesia, and first to use a cricothyroid cannula (to save a patient with an oral tumor who developed complete airway obstruction). Sir Frederick Hewitt became England's foremost anesthetist at the turn of the century. He was responsible for many inventions, including the oral airway. Hewitt also wrote what many consider to be the first true textbook of anesthesia, which went through five editions. Snow, Clover, and Hewitt established a tradition of physician anesthetists that still exists in England. In 1893, the first organization of physician specialists in anesthesia, the Society of Anaesthetists, was formed in England by J.F. Silk.

American Origins

In the United States, few physicians had specialized in anesthesia by the turn of the century. The task of giving anesthesia was usually delegated to junior surgical house officers or medical students, who tended to be more interested in the surgical procedure than in monitoring the patient. Because of the shortage of physicians interested in the specialty in the United States and the relative safety of ether anesthesia, surgeons at both the Mayo Clinic and Cleveland Clinic trained and employed nurses as anesthetists. The first organization of physician anesthetists in the United States was the Long

Island Society of Anesthetists in 1911. That society was eventually renamed the New York Society of Anesthetists and became national in 1936. It was subsequently renamed the American Society of Anesthetists and later, in 1945, the American Society of Anesthesiologists (ASA).

Three physicians stand out in the early development of anesthesia in the United States after the turn of the century: Arthur E. Guedel, Ralph M. Waters, and John S. Lundy. Guedel was the first to elaborate on the signs of general anesthesia after Snow's original description. He advocated cuffed endotracheal tubes and introduced artificial ventilation during ether anesthesia (later called *controlled respiration* by Waters). Ralph Waters added a long list of contributions to the specialty in the United States; probably the most important of these was his insistence on the proper training of specialists in anesthesia.

The first elective endotracheal intubations during anesthesia were performed in the late nineteenth century by surgeons: Sir William MacEwen in Scotland, Joseph O'Dwyer in the United States, and Franz Kuhn in Germany. Endotracheal intubation during anesthesia was popularized in England by Sir Ivan Magill and Stanley Rowbotham in the 1920s.

Official Recognition

Widespread specialization in anesthesia did not take place until just before World War II. Ralph Waters was appointed the first professor of anesthesia in United States in 1933 at the University of Wisconsin; the American Board of Anesthesiology was established in 1937. In England, the first examination for the Diploma in Anaesthetics took place in 1935, and the first Chair in Anaesthetics was awarded to Sir Robert Macintosh in 1937 at Oxford University. Anesthesia became an officially recognized specialty in England only in 1947, when the Faculty of Anaesthetists of the Royal College of Surgeons was established.

■ THE SCOPE OF ANESTHESIA

The practice of anesthesia has changed dramatically since the days of John Snow. The modern anesthesiologist is now both a consultant and a primary care provider. The consultant role is appropriate because the primary goal of the anesthetist—to see the patient safely and comfortably through surgery—generally takes only a short time (minutes to hours). However, because anesthesiologists manage all "noncutting" aspects of the patient's care in the immediate periopera-

tive period, they are also primary care providers. The "captain of the ship" doctrine, which held the surgeon responsible for every aspect of the patient's perioperative care (including anesthesia), is no longer valid. The surgeon and anesthesiologist must function together effectively, but both are ultimately answerable to the patient rather than to each other. Patients can select their own anesthesiologists, but their choices are usually limited by who is on the medical staff at a particular hospital, the surgeon's preference (if any), or the on-call schedule for anesthesiologists on a given day.

The practice of anesthesia is no longer limited to the operating room nor even confined to rendering patients insensible to pain (Table 1–1). Anesthesiologists are now routinely asked to monitor, sedate, and provide general or regional anesthesia outside the operating room—for lithotripsy, magnetic resonance imaging, computed tomography, fluoroscopy, electroconvulsive therapy, and cardiac catheterization. Anesthesiologists have traditionally been pioneers in cardiopulmonary resuscitation and continue to be integral members of resuscitation teams. An increasing number of practitioners have subspecialized in cardiac anesthesia (see Chapter 21), critical care (see Chapter 50), neuroanesthesia (see Chapter 26), obstetric anesthesia (see Chapter 43), pediatric anesthesia (see Chapter 44), and pain management (see Chapter 18). Certification requirements for special competence in critical care and pain management already exist in the United States. Anesthesiologists are actively involved in the administration and medical direction of many operating rooms, intensive care units, and respiratory therapy departments. They have also assumed administrative and leadership positions on the medical staffs of many hospitals and ambulatory care facilities.

■ PREOPERATIVE EVALUATION OF PATIENTS

As will become clear in later chapters, there is no one standard anesthetic. Rather, an anesthetic plan 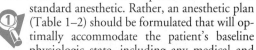 (Table 1–2) should be formulated that will optimally accommodate the patient's baseline physiologic state, including any medical and surgical illnesses, the planned procedure, drug sensitivities, previous anesthetic experiences, and psychological makeup. Inadequate preoperative 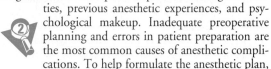 planning and errors in patient preparation are the most common causes of anesthetic complications. To help formulate the anesthetic plan, a general outline for assessing patients preoperatively is an important starting point (Table 1–3). This assess-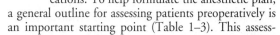

Table 1–2. The anesthetic plan.

Premedication
Type of anesthesia
  General
    Airway management
    Induction
    Maintenance
    Muscle relaxation
  Local or regional anesthesia
    Technique
    Agents
  Monitored anesthesia care
    Supplemental oxygen
    Sedation
Intraoperative management
  Monitoring
  Positioning
  Fluid management
  Special techniques
Postoperative management
  Pain control
  Intensive care
    Postoperative ventilation
    Hemodynamic monitoring

---

ment includes a pertinent history (including a review of medical records), a physical examination, and any indicated laboratory tests. (This book will present detailed discussions about evaluating patients with specific disorders and those undergoing unusual procedures.) Classifying the patient according to the ASA physical status scale completes the assessment. Assessing complicated patients may require consultations with other specialists to help determine whether the patient is optimally ready for the procedure and to have the specialist's assistance, if necessary, in perioperative care. Following the assessment, the anesthesiologist must discuss with the patient realistic options available for anesthetic management. The final anesthetic plan is based on that discussion and the patient's wishes (reflected in the informed consent; see below).

The Preoperative History

The preoperative history should clearly establish the patient's problems as well as the planned surgical, therapeutic, or diagnostic procedure. The presence and severity of known underlying medical problems must also be investigated as well as any prior and/or current treatments. Because of the potential for drug interactions with anesthesia, a complete medication history including any herbal therapeutics (Table 1–4) should be elicited from every patient. This should include the use of tobacco and alcohol as well as illicit drugs such as marijuana, cocaine, and heroin. An attempt must also be made to distinguish between true drug allergies (often manifested as dyspnea or skin rashes) and drug intolerances (usually gastrointestinal upset). Detailed questioning about previous operations and anesthetics may uncover prior anesthetic complications. A family history of anesthetic problems may suggest a familial problem such as malignant hyperthermia (see Case Discussion in Chapter 44). A general review of organ systems is important in identifying undiagnosed medical

Table 1–3. Routine preoperative anesthetic evaluation.

I. **History**
  1. Current problem
  2. Other known problems
  3. Medication history
    Allergies
    Drug intolerances
    Present therapy
      Prescription
      Nonprescription
    Nontherapeutic
      Alcohol
      Tobacco
      Illicit
  4. Previous anesthetics, surgery, and obstetric deliveries
  5. Family history
  6. Review of organ systems
    General (including activity level)
    Respiratory
    Cardiovascular
    Renal
    Gastrointestinal
    Hematologic
    Neurologic
    Endocrine
    Psychiatric
    Orthopedic
    Dematologic
  7. Last oral intake
II. **Physical examination**
  1. Vital signs
  2. Airway
  3. Heart
  4. Lungs
  5. Extremities
  6. Neurologic examination
III. **Laboratory evaluation: See Table 1–5.**
IV. **ASA classification: See Table 1–6.**

ASA = American Society of Anesthesiologists.

Table 1–4. Perioperative Effects of Common Herbal Medicines[1]

Name (other names)	Alleged Benefits	Perioperative Effects	Recommendations
Echinacea	Stimulates immune system	Allergic reactions; hepatotoxicity; interference with immune suppressive therapy (eg, organ transplants)	Discontinue as far in advance of surgery as possible
Ephedra (ma huang)	Promotes weight loss; increases energy	Ephedrine-like sympathetic stimulation with increased heart rate and blood pressure, dysrhythmias, myocardial infarction, stroke	Discontinue at least 24 hours prior to surgery; avoid monoamine oxidase inhibitors
Garlic (ajo)	Reduces blood pressure and cholesterol levels	Inhibition of platelet aggregation (irreversible)	Discontinue at least 7 days prior to surgery
Ginkgo (duck foot, maidenhair, silver apricot)	Improves cognitive performance (eg, dementia), increases peripheral perfusion (eg, impotence, macular degeneration)	Inhibition of platelet activating factor	Discontinue at least 36 hours prior to surgery
Ginseng	Protects against "stress" and maintains "homeostasis"	Hypoglycemia; inhibition of platelet aggregation and coagulation cascade	Discontinue at least 7 days prior to surgery
Kava (kawa, awa, intoxicating pepper)	Decreases anxiety	GABA-mediated hypnotic effects may decrease MAC (see chapter 7); possible risk of acute withdrawal	Discontinue at least 24 hours prior to surgery
St. John's wort (amber, goatweed, *Hypericum perforatum,* klamatheweed)	Reverses mild to moderate depression	Inhibits serotonin, norepinephrine, and dopamine reuptake by neurons; increases drug metabolism by induction of cytochrome P450	Discontinue at least 5 days prior to surgery
Valerian	Decreases anxiety	GABA-mediated hypnotic effects may decrease MAC; benzodiazepine-like withdrawal syndrome	Taper dose weeks before surgery if possible; treat withdrawal syndrome with benzodiazepines

[1]For more details, see Ang-Lee reference in Suggested Reading. GABA = γ-aminobutyric acid; MAC = minimum alveolar concentration.

problems. Questions should emphasize cardiovascular, pulmonary, endocrine, hepatic, renal, and neurologic function. A positive response to any of these questions should prompt more detailed inquiries to determine the extent of any organ impairment.

Physical Examination

The history and physical examination complement one another: The examination helps detect abnormalities not apparent from the history, while the history helps focus the examination on the organ systems that should be examined closely. Examination of healthy asymptomatic patients should minimally consist of measurement of vital signs (blood pressure, heart rate, respiratory rate, and temperature) and examination of the airway, heart, lungs, and extremities using standard techniques of inspection, eg, auscultation, palpation,

and percussion. An abbreviated neurologic examination is important when regional anesthesia is being considered and serves to document any subtle preexisting neurologic deficits. The patient's anatomy should be specifically evaluated when procedures such as a nerve block, regional anesthesia, or invasive monitoring procedure are planned; evidence of infection over or close to the site or significant anatomic abnormalities may contraindicate such procedures (see Chapters 6, 16, and 17).

The importance of examining the airway cannot be overemphasized. The patient's dentition should be inspected for loose or chipped teeth and the presence of caps, bridges, or dentures. A poor anesthesia mask fit should be expected in some edentulous patients and those with significant facial abnormalities. Micrognathia (a short distance between the chin and the hyoid bone), prominent upper incisors, a large tongue, limited range of motion of the temporomandibular joint or cervical spine, or a short neck suggests that difficulty may be encountered in endotracheal intubation (see Chapter 5).

Laboratory Evaluation

The usefulness of routine laboratory testing for healthy asymptomatic patients is doubtful when the history and physical examination fail to detect any abnormalities. Such routine testing is expensive and rarely alters perioperative management; moreover, abnormalities often are ignored—or result in unnecessary delays. Nonetheless, because of the current litigious environment in the United States, many physicians continue to order a hematocrit or hemoglobin concentration, urinalysis, serum electrolyte measurements, coagulation studies, an electrocardiogram, and a chest film for all patients.

To be valuable, a preoperative test implies an increased perioperative risk when it is abnormal and a reduced risk when the abnormality is corrected. The usefulness of a test in screening for disease depends on its sensitivity and specificity as well as the prevalence of the disease. Sensitive tests have a low rate of false-negative results, while specific tests have a low rate of false-positive results. The prevalence of a disease varies with the population tested and often depends on sex, age, genetic background, and lifestyle practices. Testing is therefore most effective when sensitive and specific tests are used in patients in whom the abnormality might be expected. Accordingly, laboratory testing should be based on the presence or absence of underlying diseases and drug therapy as suggested by the history and physical examination. The nature of the procedure should also be taken into consideration. Thus, a baseline hematocrit is desirable in any patient about to undergo a procedure that may result in extensive blood loss and require transfusion. General guidelines for preoperative testing of asymptomatic and seemingly healthy patients are given in Table 1–5.

Table 1–5. Routine preoperative laboratory evaluation of asymptomatic, apparently healthy patients.

Hematocrit or hemoglobin concentration:
    All menstruating women
    All patients over 60 years of age
    All patients who are likely to experience significant blood
      loss and may require transfusion
Serum glucose and creatinine (or blood urea nitrogen) concentration: all patients over 60 years of age
Electrocardiogram: all patients over 40 years of age
Chest radiograph: all patients over 60 years of age

Testing fertile women for an undiagnosed early pregnancy may be justified by the potentially teratogenic effects of anesthetic agents on the fetus; pregnancy testing involves detection of chorionic gonadotropin in urine or serum. Routine testing for AIDS (detection of the HIV antibody) is highly controversial. Routine coagulation studies and urinalysis are not cost-effective in asymptomatic healthy patients.

ASA Physical Status Classification

In 1961 the ASA adopted a five-category physical status classification system (Table 1–6) for use in assessing a patient preoperatively. A sixth category was later added to address the brain-dead organ donor. Although this system was not intended as such, the ASA physical status generally correlates with the perioperative mortality rate (Table 1–7). Because underlying disease is only one of many factors contributing to perioperative complications (see Chapter 47), it is not surprising that this correlation is not perfect. Nonetheless, the ASA physical status classification remains useful in planning anesthetic management, especially monitoring techniques (see Chapter 6).

Informed Consent

The preoperative assessment culminates in giving the patient a reasonable explanation of the options available for anesthetic management: general, regional, local, or topical anesthesia or intravenous sedation. The term *monitored anesthesia care* (previously referred to as *local standby*) is now commonly used and refers to monitoring the patient during a procedure performed with in-

Table 1–6. Preoperative physical status classification of patients according to the American Society of Anesthesiologists.

Class	Definition
1	A normal healthy patient.
2	A patient with mild systemic disease and no functional limitations.
3	A patient with moderate to severe systemic disease that results in some function limitation.
4	A patient with severe systemic disease that is a constant threat to life and functionally incapacitating.
5	A moribund patient who is not expected to survive 24 hours with or without surgery.
6	A brain-dead patient whose organs are being harvested.
E	If the procedure is an emergency, the physical status is followed by "E" (for example, "2E").

Table 1–7. American Society of Anesthesiologists classification and perioperative mortality rates.

Class	Mortality Rate
1	0.06–0.08%
2	0.27–0.4%
3	1.8–4.3%
4	7.8–23%
5	9.4–51%

travenous sedation or local anesthesia administered by the surgeon. Regardless of the technique chosen, consent must always be obtained for general anesthesia in case other techniques prove inadequate.

If any procedure is performed without the patient's consent, the physician may be liable for assault and battery. When the patient is a minor or otherwise not competent to consent, the consent must be obtained from someone legally authorized to give it, such as a parent, guardian, or close relative. Although oral consent may be sufficient, written consent is usually advisable for medicolegal purposes. Moreover, consent must be *informed* to ensure that the patient (or guardian) has sufficient information about the procedures and their risks to make a reasonable and prudent decision whether to consent. It is generally accepted that not all risks need be detailed but only those that are realistic risks in similar patients with similar problems. It is generally advisable to inform the patient that some complications may be life-threatening.

The purpose of the preoperative visit is not only to gather important information and obtain informed consent, it also helps establish a healthy doctor-patient relationship. Moreover, an empathically conducted interview that answers important questions and lets the patient know what to expect has been shown to be at least as effective in relieving anxiety as some premedication drug regimens (see Case Discussion in Chapter 8).

■ DOCUMENTATION

Documentation is important for both quality assurance and medicolegal purposes. Adequate documentation is essential for the defense of a malpractice action (see Case Discussion below).

The Preoperative Note

The preoperative note should be written in the patient's chart and should describe all aspects of the preoperative assessment, including the medical history, anesthetic his-

tory, medication history, the physical examination, laboratory results, ASA classification, and the recommendations of any consultants. It also describes the anesthetic plan and includes the informed consent. The plan should be as detailed as possible and should include the use of specific procedures such as endotracheal intubation, invasive monitoring, and regional or hypotensive techniques. Documentation of informed consent usually takes the form of a narrative in the chart indicating that the plan, alternative plans, their advantages and disadvantages (including the risk of complications) were presented, understood, and agreed to by the patient. Alternatively, the patient signs a special anesthesia consent form that contains the same information. A sample preanesthetic report form is illustrated in Figure 1–1. Although a completely handwritten note in the chart is acceptable, the use of a printed form lessens the likelihood of omitting important information.

The Intraoperative Anesthesia Record

The intraoperative anesthesia record (Figure 1–2) serves many purposes. It functions as a useful intraoperative monitor, a reference for future anesthetics for that patient, and a tool for quality assurance. This record should be as pertinent and accurate as possible. It should document all aspects of anesthetic care in the operating room, including the following:

- A preoperative check of the anesthesia machine and other equipment.
- A review or reevaluation of the patient immediately prior to induction of anesthesia.
- A review of the chart for new laboratory results or consultations.
- A review of the anesthesia and surgical consents.
- The time of administration, dosage, and route of intraoperative drugs.
- All intraoperative monitoring (including laboratory measurements, blood loss, and urinary output).
- Intravenous fluid administration and transfusion.
- All procedures (such as intubation, placement of a nasogastric tube, or placement of invasive monitors).
- Routine and special techniques such as mechanical ventilation, hypotensive anesthesia, one-lung ventilation, high-frequency jet ventilation, or cardiopulmonary bypass.
- The timing and course of important events such as induction, positioning, surgical incision, and extubation.
- Unusual events or complications.
- The condition of the patient at the end of the procedure.

ANESTHESIOLOGY PREOPERATIVE NOTE

DATE:　　　　　TIME:　　　　HT.　　　PREOP DIAGNOSIS:

AGE:　　　　　SEX:　M　F　WT.　　　PROPOSED OPERATION:

MEDICAL HISTORY　　　　　　　　　　**MEDICATIONS:**
ALLERGIES:
INTOLERANCES:
DRUG USE:　　　　　　　　TOBACCO:　　　　　　　ETOH:

PRESENT PROBLEM:

CARDIOVASCULAR

RESPIRATORY

DIABETES

NEUROLOGIC　　　　　　　　　　　RENAL

ARTHRITIS/MUSCULO-SKELETAL　　　　HEPATIC

　　　　　　　　　　　　　　　OTHER

PREVIOUS ANESTHETICS:

FAMILY HISTORY

LAST ORAL INTAKE

PHYSICAL EXAMINATION　　　BP　　　　P　　　R　　　T

　HEART　　　　　　　　　　　EXTREMITIES

　LUNGS　　　　　　　　　　　NEUROLOGIC

　AIRWAY　　　　　　　　　　OTHER

　TEETH

LABORATORY

　Hct/Hgb　　　　　ECG　　　　　　　　　CHEST X-RAY
　URINE
　LYTES:　Na　　　　Cl
　　　　K　　　　GLUCOSE　　　　　　OTHER
　　　　CO_2　　　BUN: CREATININE

PLAN　□ GENERAL　　　　　　INVASIVE MONITORS
　　　　□ REGIONAL
　　　　□ MONITORED ANESTHESIA CARE　SPECIAL TECHNIQUES

ASA CLASS　　　　　　SIGNATURE _____ M.D.
　　　　　　　　　　　　　　(RESIDENT)　　　　(STAFF)

PATIENT CONSENT
ANESTHETIC ALTERNATIVES AND RISKS RANGING FROM TOOTH DAMAGE
TO LIFE-THREATENING EVENTS HAVE BEEN EXPLAINED AND ACCEPTED.

PATIENT
NAME

PATIENT'S SIGNATURE

#

Figure 1–1. The preoperative note.

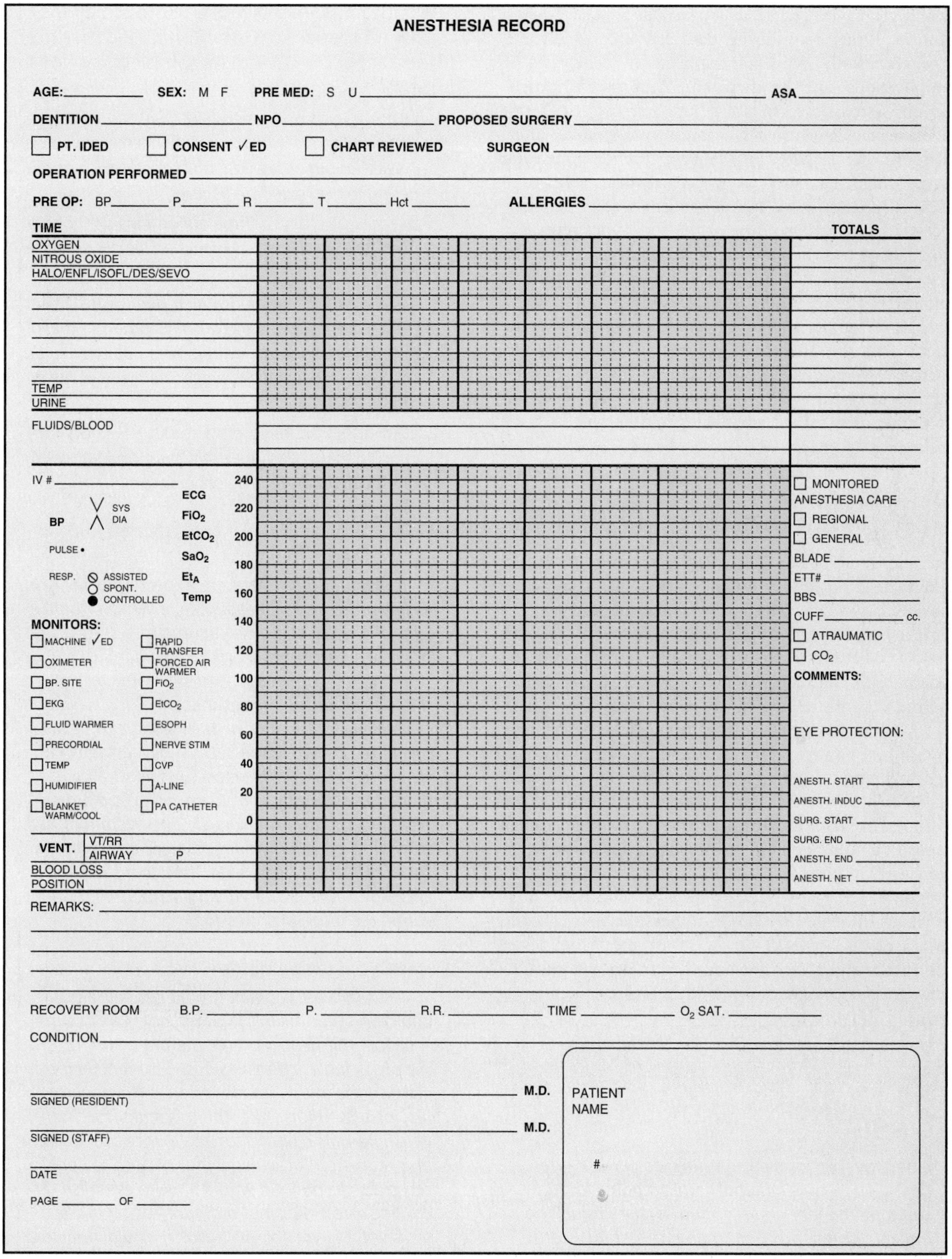

ANESTHESIA RECORD

AGE:_____ SEX: M F PRE MED: S U_____ ASA_____

DENTITION_____ NPO_____ PROPOSED SURGERY_____

☐ PT. IDED   ☐ CONSENT ✓ED   ☐ CHART REVIEWED   SURGEON_____

OPERATION PERFORMED_____

PRE OP: BP_____ P_____ R_____ T_____ Hct_____   ALLERGIES_____

TIME		TOTALS
OXYGEN		
NITROUS OXIDE		
HALO/ENFL/ISOFL/DES/SEVO		
TEMP		
URINE		
FLUIDS/BLOOD		

IV #_____

BP ∨ SYS / ∧ DIA

PULSE •

RESP. ⊘ ASSISTED
     ○ SPONT.
     ● CONTROLLED

ECG
FiO₂
EtCO₂
SaO₂
Et_A
Temp

240
220
200
180
160
140
120
100
80
60
40
20
0

MONITORS:

☐ MACHINE ✓ED   ☐ RAPID TRANSFER
☐ OXIMETER   ☐ FORCED AIR WARMER
☐ BP. SITE   ☐ FiO₂
☐ EKG   ☐ EtCO₂
☐ FLUID WARMER   ☐ ESOPH
☐ PRECORDIAL   ☐ NERVE STIM
☐ TEMP   ☐ CVP
☐ HUMIDIFIER   ☐ A-LINE
☐ BLANKET WARM/COOL ☐ PA CATHETER

VENT.	VT/RR	
	AIRWAY	P
BLOOD LOSS		
POSITION		

☐ MONITORED ANESTHESIA CARE
☐ REGIONAL
☐ GENERAL
BLADE_____
ETT#_____
BBS_____
CUFF_____ cc.
☐ ATRAUMATIC
☐ CO₂
COMMENTS:

EYE PROTECTION:

ANESTH. START_____
ANESTH. INDUC_____
SURG. START_____
SURG. END_____
ANESTH. END_____
ANESTH. NET_____

REMARKS:_____
_____
_____
_____

RECOVERY ROOM   B.P._____ P._____ R.R._____ TIME_____ O₂ SAT._____

CONDITION_____

SIGNED (RESIDENT)_____ M.D.

SIGNED (STAFF)_____ M.D.

PATIENT NAME

DATE_____

PAGE_____ OF_____

#

Figure 1–2. The intraoperative anesthesia record.

Vital signs are recorded graphically at least every 5 minutes. Other monitoring data are also usually entered graphically, while descriptions of techniques or complications are handwritten. Automated record-keeping systems are available, but their use is still not widespread. Unfortunately, the intraoperative anesthetic record is often inadequate for documenting critical incidents, such as a cardiac arrest. In such cases, a separate note in the patient's chart may be necessary. Careful recording of the course of events, actions taken, and their timing is necessary to avoid discrepancies between multiple simultaneous records (anesthesia record, nurses' notes, cardiopulmonary resuscitation record, and other physicians' entries in the medical record). Such discrepancies are frequently targeted as evidence of incompetence or dissembling by malpractice attorneys. Incomplete, inaccurate, or illegible records may subject physicians to otherwise unjustified legal liability.

The Postoperative Notes

The anesthesiologist's immediate responsibility to the patient does not end until the patient has completely recovered from the effects of the anesthetic. After accompanying the patient to the postanesthesia care unit (PACU), the anesthesiologist should remain with the patient until normal vital signs have been established and the patient's condition is deemed stable (see Chapter 49). Prior to discharge from the PACU, a discharge note should be written by the anesthesiologist to document the patient's recovery from anesthesia, any apparent anesthesia-related complications, the immediate postoperative condition of the patient, and the patient's disposition (discharge to an outpatient area, an inpatient ward, an intensive care unit, or home). Inpatients should be seen again at least once within 48 hours after discharge from the PACU. Postoperative notes should document the general condition of the patient, the presence or absence of any anesthesia-related complications, and any measures undertaken to treat such complications (Figure 1–3).

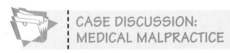

CASE DISCUSSION:
MEDICAL MALPRACTICE

A healthy 45-year-old man suffers a cardiac arrest during an elective inguinal hernia repair. Although cardiopulmonary resuscitation is successful, the patient is left with permanent mental status changes that preclude his return to work. One year later, the patient files a complaint against the anesthesiologist, surgeon, and hospital.

What four elements must be proved by the plaintiff (patient) to establish negligence on the part of the defendant (physician or hospital)?

1. **Duty:** *Once a physician establishes a professional relationship with a patient, the physician owes that patient certain obligations, such as adhering to the "standard of care."*

2. **Breach of Duty:** *If these obligations are not fulfilled, the physician has breached his duties to the patient.*

3. **Causation:** *The plaintiff must demonstrate that the breach of duty was causally related to the injury. This proximate cause does not have to be the most important or immediate cause of the injury.*

4. **Damages:** *An injury must result. The injury may cause general damages (eg, pain and suffering) or special damages (eg, loss of income).*

How is the standard of care defined and established?

Individual physicians are expected to perform as any prudent and reasonable physician would in light of the surrounding circumstances. As a specialist, the anesthesiologist is held to a higher standard of knowledge and skill with respect to the subject matter of that specialty than would be a general practitioner or a physician in another specialty. Expert witnesses usually establish the standard of care. While most jurisdictions have extended the "locality rule" to encompass a national standard of care, the specific circumstances pertaining to each individual case are taken into account. The law recognizes that there are differences of opinion and varying schools of thought within the medical profession.

How is causation determined?

It is usually the plaintiff who bears the burden of proving that the injury would not have occurred "but for" the negligence of the physician, or that the physician's action was a "substantial factor" in causing the injury. An exception is the doctrine of res ipsa loquitur ("the thing speaks for itself"), which permits a finding of negligence based solely on circumstantial evidence. For res ipsa to apply in this case, the plaintiff would have to establish that cardiac arrest does not ordinarily occur in the absence of negligence and that it could not have been due to something outside the control of the anesthesiologist. An important concept is that causation in civil cases need only be established by

ANESTHESIA POSTOP NOTES

IMMEDIATE POSTOP NOTE (BEFORE DISCHARGE FROM RECOVERY ROOM):

_____ NO COMPLICATIONS OF ANESTHESIA IMMEDIATELY APPARENT;
PATIENT HAS RECOVERED FROM IMMEDIATE EFFECTS OF
ANESTHESIA AND MAY BE TRANSFERRED TO WARD OR
OUTPATIENT DEPARTMENT.

_____ OTHER:

_____ M.D.   _____
                 SIGNED   DATE   TIME

FOLLOW-UP POSTOP NOTE (AFTER DISCHARGE FROM RECOVERY ROOM, BEFORE DISCHARGE
                              FROM HOSPITAL):

_____ NO APPARENT POSTANESTHETIC COMPLICATIONS.

_____ PATIENT DISCHARGED FROM HOSPITAL BY SURGEON PRIOR TO
POSTANESTHETIC VISIT.

_____ OTHER:

_____ M.D.   _____
                 SIGNED   DATE   TIME

PATIENT
NAME

#

CHART COPY

Figure 1–3. The postoperative note.

a preponderance of the evidence ("more likely than not")—as opposed to criminal cases, where all elements of a charged offense must be proved "beyond a reasonable doubt."

What factors influence the likelihood of a malpractice suit?

1. **The Physician-Patient Relationship:** *This is particularly important for the anesthesiologist, who usually does not meet the patient until the night before or on the morning of surgery. Another problem is that the patient is unconscious while under the anesthesiologist's care. Thus, the preoperative and postoperative visits with the patient assume vital importance. While anesthesiologists have less long-term contact with patients than other medical specialists do, it is possible and desirable to make this contact meaningful. Family members should also be considered during these meetings, particularly during the postoperative visit if there has been an intraoperative complication.*

2. **Adequacy of Informed Consent:** *Rendering care to a competent patient who does not consent constitutes assault and battery. Consent is not enough, however. The patient should be informed of the contemplated procedure, including its reasonably anticipated risks, its possible benefits, and the therapeutic alternatives. The physician may be liable for a complication—even if it is not due to the negligent performance of a procedure—if a jury is convinced that a reasonable person would have refused treatment if properly informed of the possibility of the complication. This does not mean, of course, that a documented consent relieves from liability physicians who violate the standard of care.*

3. **Quality of Documentation:** *Careful documentation of the perioperative visits, informed consent, consultation with other specialists, intraoperative events, and postoperative care is absolutely essential. The viewpoint of many courts and juries is that "if it isn't written, it wasn't done." It goes without saying that medical records should never be intentionally destroyed or altered.*

SUGGESTED READING

Abenstein JP, Warner MA: Anesthesia providers, patient outcomes, and costs. Anesth Analg 1996;82:1273. An interesting look at the relative safety of the anesthesia team concept.

Ang-Lee MK, Moss J, Yuan C: Herbal medicines and perioperative care. JAMA 2001;286:208. Herbal medications can negatively impact anesthetic management.

Byrne AJ, Sellen AJ, Jones JG: Errors on anaesthetic record charts as a measure of anaesthetic performance during simulated critical incidents. Br J Anaesth 1998;80:58. There is a high error rate in the charting of critical incidents.

Fischer SP: Development and effectiveness of an anesthesia preoperative evaluation clinic in a teaching hospital. Anesthesiology 1996;85:196. A preoperative clinic can increase efficiency by decreasing surgery cancellations and unnecessary lab tests.

Frost AM (editor): *Preanesthetic Assessment.* Anesthesiol Clin North Am 1990;8:No. 4. Anesthetic implications and preoperative management of patients with medical problems.

Kam PCA: Occupational stress in anaesthesia. Anaesth Intensive Care 1997;25:686. Highly recommended reading for anyone considering a career in anesthesia!

Little DM Jr: *Classical Anesthesia Files.* Wood Library—Museum of Anesthesiology 1985. Writings of historical interest.

Lyons AS, Petrucelli RJ: *Medicine: An Illustrated History.* Abrams, 1978.

Malviya S, D'Errico C, Reynolds P et al: Preoperative pregnancy testing in adolescent patients: A survey of current practice. Am J Anesthesiology 1997;24:23. Most clinicians ask about the possibility of pregnancy but only proceed with a pregnancy test if indicated by history.

Overdyk FJ, Harvey SC, Fishman RL: Successful strategies for improving operating room efficiency at academic institutions. Anesth Analg 1998;86:896.

Posner KL, Caplan RA, Cheney FW: Variation in expert opinion in medical malpractice review. Anesthesiology 1996;85:1049. This article points out one of the major injustices inherent in the current medical malpractice system in the United States.

Symposium on complications and medico-legal aspects of anaesthesia. Br J Anaesth 1987;59:813. British perspective on anesthetic complications and medical malpractice.

Waisel DB, Truog RD: The benefits of the explanation of the risks of anesthesia in the day surgery patient. J Clin Anesth 1995;7:200. Most parents want to be made aware of the risks of anesthesia.

Waisel DB, Truog RD: An introduction to ethics. Anesthesiology 1997;87:411.

Waisel DB, Truog RD: Informed consent. Anesthesiology 1997;87:968.

Warner MA, Caplan RA, Epstein BS et al: Practice guidelines for preoperative fasting and the use of pharmacologic agents to reduce the risk of pulmonary aspiration: Application to healthy patients undergoing elective procedures. Anesthesiology 1999;90:896. A review by the ASA Task Force on Preoperative Fasting that suggests these fasting guidelines for infants and adults: 2 hours for clear liquids, 4 hours for breast milk, 6 hours for infant formula or light solids.

SECTION I

Anesthetic Equipment & Monitors

The Operating Room: Medical Gas Systems, Environmental Factors, & Electrical Safety

2

KEY CONCEPTS

 Liquid oxygen must be stored well below its critical temperature of −119 °C since gases can be liquefied by pressure only if stored below their critical temperature.

 The only reliable way to determine residual volume of nitrous oxide is to weigh the cylinder.

 Because the critical temperature of air is −140.6 °C, it exists as a gas in cylinders whose pressures fall in proportion to their content.

 A pin index safety system has been adopted by cylinder manufacturers to discourage incorrect cylinder attachments.

 Body contact with two conductive materials at different voltage potentials may complete a circuit and result in an electrical shock.

 The magnitude of a leakage current is normally imperceptible to touch (less than 1 mA and well below the fibrillation threshold of 100 mA). If the current bypasses the high resistance offered by skin, however, and is applied directly to the heart (microshock), current as low as 100 μA (microamperes) may be fatal. The maximum leakage allowed in operating room equipment is 10 μA.

 Unlike the utility company's pole-top transformer, the secondary wiring of an isolation transformer is not grounded and provides two live ungrounded voltage lines for operating room equipment.

 Malfunction of the return electrode may result from disconnection from the electrosurgical unit, inadequate patient contact, or insufficient conductive gel. In these situations, the current will find another place to exit (eg, electrocardiogram pads or metal parts of the operating table), which may result in a burn.

 Since pacemaker and electrocardiogram interference is possible, pulse or heart sounds should be closely monitored when any electrosurgical unit is used.

Anesthesiologists, who spend more time in operating rooms than does any other group of physicians, are responsible for protecting unconscious patients against a multitude of possible dangers during surgery. Some of these threats are unique to the operating room. As a result, no medical specialist has a greater responsibility than the anesthesiologist for the proper functioning of the operating room's medical gases, environmental factors (eg, temperature, humidity, ventilation, noise), and electrical safety. This chapter describes the major features of operating rooms that are of special interest to anesthesiologists and the potential hazards associated with these systems. A case summary organizes some of this information into a protocol for testing a new operating room's medical gas pipeline system.

■ MEDICAL GAS SYSTEMS

The medical gases commonly used in operating rooms are oxygen, nitrous oxide, air, and nitrogen. While technically not a gas, vacuum exhaust for anesthetic waste gas disposal (scavenging) and surgical suction must also be provided and is considered an integral part of the medical gas system. Patients are endangered if medical gas systems, particularly oxygen, malfunction. The main features of such systems are the sources of the gases and the means of their delivery to the operating room. The anesthesiologist must understand both these elements to prevent and detect medical gas depletion or supply line misconnection. Estimates of a particular hospital's peak demand determine the type of medical gas supply system required.

SOURCES OF MEDICAL GASES

Oxygen

A reliable supply of oxygen is a critical requirement in any surgical area. Medical grade oxygen (99% or 99.5% pure) is manufactured by fractional distillation of liquefied air. Oxygen is stored as a compressed gas at room temperature or refrigerated as a liquid. Most small hospitals store oxygen in banks of H-cylinders connected by a manifold (Figure 2–1). The number of cylinders in each bank depends on anticipated daily demand. The manifold contains valves that reduce the cylinder pressure (approximately 2000 pounds per square inch [psig]) to line pressure (50 ± 5 psig) and automatically switch banks when one group of cylinders is exhausted.

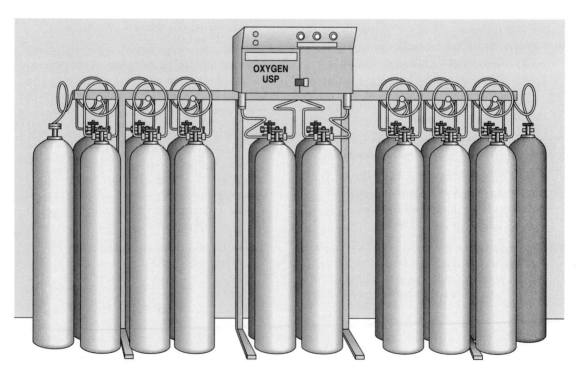

Figure 2–1. A bank of oxygen H-cylinders connected by a manifold.

A liquid oxygen storage system (Figure 2–2) is more economical for large hospitals. Liquid oxygen must be stored well below its critical temperature of −119 °C since gases can be liquefied by pressure *only* if stored below their **critical temperature.** A large hospital may have a smaller liquid oxygen supply or a bank of compressed gas cylinders that can provide one day's oxygen requirements as a reserve. To guard against a hospital gas-system failure, the anesthesiologist must always have an emergency supply of oxygen available in the operating room.

Most anesthesia machines accommodate one or two E-cylinders of oxygen (Table 2–1). As oxygen is expended, the cylinder's pressure falls in proportion to its content. A pressure of 1000 psig indicates an approximately half-full E-cylinder and represents 330 L of oxygen at atmospheric pressure and a temperature of 20 °C. If the oxygen is exhausted at a rate of 3 L/min, a half-full cylinder will be empty in 110 minutes. Oxygen cylinder pressure should be monitored before and periodically during use.

Nitrous Oxide

Nitrous oxide, the most commonly used anesthetic gas, is manufactured by heating ammonium nitrate (thermal decomposition). It is almost always stored by hospitals in large high-pressure cylinders (H-cylinders) connected by a manifold with an automatic crossover feature. Bulk liquid storage of nitrous oxide is economical only in very large institutions.

Since the critical temperature of nitrous oxide (36.5 °C) is above room temperature, it can be kept liquefied without an elaborate refrigeration system. If the liquefied nitrous oxide rises above its critical temperature, it will revert to its gaseous phase. Because nitrous oxide is not an ideal gas and is easily compressible, this transformation into a gaseous phase is not accompanied by a great rise in tank pressure. Nonetheless, all gas cylinders are equipped with an emergency pressure-relief valve (rupture disk) to prevent explosion under conditions of unexpectedly high gas pressure (eg, unintentional overfilling). The pressure-relief valve is designed to rupture at 3300 psig, well below the pressure E-cylinder walls should withstand (more than 5000 psig).

Although a disruption in supply is usually not catastrophic, most anesthesia machines have reserve nitrous oxide E-cylinders. Since these smaller cylinders also contain nitrous oxide in its liquid state, the volume remaining in a cylinder is **not** proportional to cylinder pressure. By the time the liquid nitrous oxide is expended and the tank pressure begins to fall, only about 400 L of nitrous oxide remains. If liquid nitrous oxide

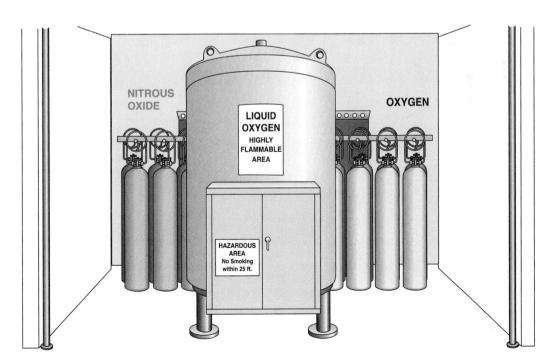

Figure 2–2. A liquid storage tank with reserve oxygen tanks in background.

Table 2–1. Characteristics of medical gas cylinders.

Gas	E-Cylinder Capacity* (L)	H-Cylinder Capacity* (L)	Pressure* (psig at 20 °C)	Color (USA)	Color (International)	Form
O_2	625–700	6000–8000	1800–2200	Green	White	Gas
Air	625–700	6000–8000	1800–2200	Yellow	White and back	Gas
N_2O	1590	15,900	745	Blue	Blue	Liquid
N_2	625–700	6000–8000	1800–2200	Black	Black	Gas

*Depending on the manufacturer.

is kept at a constant temperature (20 °C), it will vaporize at the same rate at which it is consumed and will maintain a constant pressure (745 psig) until the liquid is exhausted.

 The only reliable way to determine residual volume of nitrous oxide is to weigh the cylinder. For this reason, the tare weight (TW), or empty weight, of cylinders containing a liquefied compressed gas (eg, nitrous oxide) is often stamped on the shoulder of the cylinder. The pressure gauge of a nitrous oxide cylinder should not exceed 745 psig at 20 °C. A higher reading implies gauge malfunction, tank overfill (liquid fill), or a cylinder containing a gas other than nitrous oxide.

Since energy is consumed in the conversion of a liquid to a gas (the latent heat of vaporization), the liquid

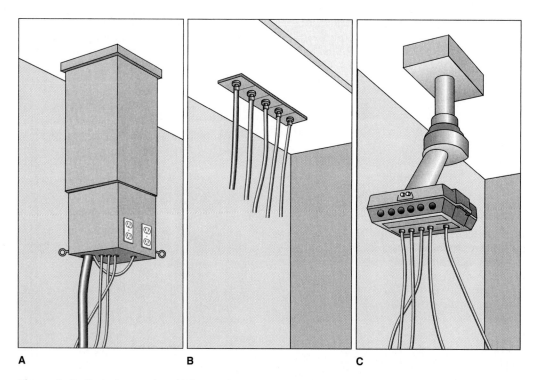

A   **B**   **C**

Figure 2–3. Typical examples of (***A***) gas columns, (***B***) ceiling hose drops, and (***C***) articulating arms. One end of a color-coded hose connects to the hospital medical gas supply system by way of a quick-coupler mechanism. The other end connects to the anesthesia machine through the diameter index safety system.

nitrous oxide cools. The drop in temperature results in a lower vapor pressure and lower cylinder pressure. The cooling is so pronounced at high flow rates that pressure regulators may freeze.

Air

The use of air is becoming more frequent in anesthesiology as the potential hazards of nitrous oxide and high concentrations of oxygen receive increasing attention. Cylinder air is medical grade and is obtained by blending oxygen and nitrogen. Dehumidified but unsterile air is provided to the hospital pipeline system by compression pumps. The inlets of these pumps must be distant from vacuum exhaust vents to minimize contamination. Because the critical temperature of air is −140.6 °C, it exists as a gas in cylinders whose pressures fall in proportion to their content.

Nitrogen

Although compressed nitrogen is not administered to patients, it provides power to many pieces of operating room equipment. It is most commonly stored in H-cylinders connected by a manifold.

Vacuum

A central hospital vacuum system usually consists of two independent suction pumps, each capable of handling peak requirements. Traps at every user location prevent contamination of the system with foreign matter.

DELIVERY OF MEDICAL GASES

Medical gases are delivered from their central supply source to the operating room through a piping network. Gas pipes are usually constructed of seamless copper tubing. Internal contamination of the pipelines with dust, grease, or water must be avoided. The hospital's gas delivery system appears in the operating room as hose drops, gas columns, or elaborate articulating arms (Figure 2–3). Operating room equipment, including the anesthesia machine, interfaces with these pipeline system outlets by color-coded hoses. Quick-coupler mechanisms, which vary in design with different manufacturers, connect one end of the hose to the appropriate gas outlet. The other end connects to the anesthesia machine through a noninterchangeable **diameter index safety system** fitting that prevents incorrect hose attachment.

 E-cylinders of oxygen, nitrous oxide, and air attach directly to the anesthesia machine. To discourage incorrect cylinder attachments, **a pin index safety system** has been adopted

by cylinder manufacturers. Each gas cylinder (sizes A–E) has two holes in its cylinder valve that mate with corresponding pins in the yoke of the anesthesia machine (Figure 2–4). The relative positioning of the pins and holes is unique for each gas. This system has been unintentionally defeated by multiple washers placed between the cylinder and yoke, which prevented proper engagement of the pins and holes. The pin index safety system is also ineffective if yoke pins are damaged or the cylinder is filled with the wrong gas.

The functioning of medical gas supply sources and pipeline systems is constantly monitored by central alarm systems. Indicator lights and audible signals warn of changeover to secondary gas sources and abnormally high (eg, pressure regulator malfunction) or low (eg, supply depletion) pipeline pressures (Figure 2–5).

Despite a multitude of safety devices, alarms, and detailed regulations (established by the National Fire Protection Association, the Compressed Gas Association, and the Department of Transportation), anesthetic catastrophes continue to result from malfunctioning medical gas systems. Mandatory periodic inspections of hospital gas delivery systems by independent agencies and increased involvement by anesthesiologists in gas-system design could ameliorate this problem.

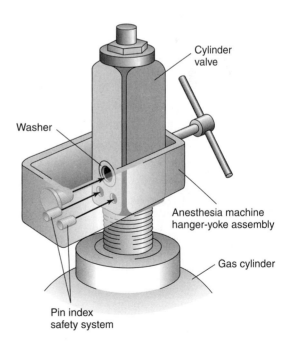

Figure 2–4. Pin index safety system interlink between the anesthesia machine and gas cylinder.

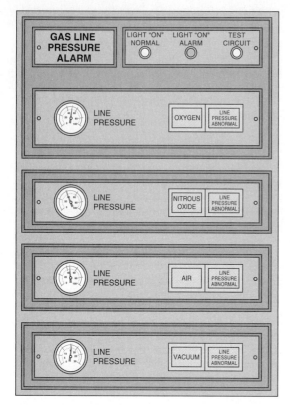

Figure 2–5. An example of a master alarm panel that monitors gas-line pressure. (Courtesy of Ohio Medical Products.)

■ ENVIRONMENTAL FACTORS IN THE OPERATING ROOM

TEMPERATURE

The temperature in most operating rooms seems uncomfortably cold to many conscious patients and, at times, to conscious anesthesiologists. On the other hand, standing in surgical garb for hours under operating room lights can be an endurance course for scrub nurses and surgeons. As a general principle, the comfort of operating room personnel must be reconciled with patient needs. For example, small children and patients with large exposed surfaces (eg, those with thermal burns) constitute specific indications for an operating room temperature of 24 °C or higher, since these patients lose heat rapidly and have a limited ability to compensate. Hypothermia has been associated with an increased incidence of wound infection, greater intra-

operative blood loss (impaired coagulation assessed by thromboelastography), and prolonged hospitalization (see Chapter 6). On the other hand, intraoperative hypothermia may offer a degree of neurologic protection during some intracranial or cardiopulmonary bypass surgeries.

HUMIDITY

In past decades, static discharges were a feared source of ignition in an operating room filled with flammable anesthetic vapors. Because increased humidity decreases the likelihood of static discharges, a relative humidity of at least 50% was recommended. Routine compliance with this requirement is no longer important in the modern era of nonflammable anesthetic agents. However, static sparks can still damage sensitive electrical equipment or lead to microshock (see below section on risk of electrocution).

VENTILATION

A high rate of operating room airflow decreases contamination of the surgical site. These flow rates are usually achieved by blending recirculated air with fresh air. Although recirculation conserves energy costs associated with heating and air conditioning, it is unsuitable for anesthetic waste gas disposal. Therefore, a separate anesthetic-gas scavenging system must always supplement operating room ventilation. Extreme rates of flow, such as those produced by a laminar air system, have been proposed for procedures with particularly high risks of infection (eg, total hip replacement).

NOISE

Multiple studies have demonstrated that exposure to noise can have a detrimental effect on multiple human cognitive functions. Operating room noise has been measured at 70–80 dB(A) with frequent sound peaks exceeding 80 dB, depending on which ventilation system (eg, laminar flow) and surgical instruments (eg, power drills and saws) were being used. One study demonstrated a reduction in mental efficiency and short-term memory in anesthesia residents exposed to operating room noise.

■ ELECTRICAL SAFETY

THE RISK OF ELECTROCUTION

The use of electronic medical equipment subjects patients and hospital personnel to the risk of electrocution. Anesthesiologists must have at least a basic understanding of electrical hazards and their prevention.

Body contact with two conductive materials at different voltage potentials may complete a circuit and result in an electrical shock. Usually, one point of exposure is a live 110 V or 240 V conductor, and the circuit is completed through a ground contact. For example, a grounded person need contact only one live conductor to complete a circuit and receive a shock. The live conductor could be the frame of a patient monitor that has developed a fault to the hot side of the power line. A circuit is now complete between the power line (which is earth-grounded at the utility's pole-top transformer) through the victim and back to the ground (Figure 2–6). The physiologic effect of electrical current depends on the location, duration, frequency, and magnitude (more accurately, current density) of the shock.

Leakage current is present in all electrical equipment as a result of capacitive coupling, induction between internal electrical components, or defective insulation. Current can flow as a result of capacitive coupling between two conductive bodies (eg, a circuit board and its casing) even though they are not physically connected. Some monitors are doubly insulated to decrease the effect of capacitive coupling. Other monitors are designed to be connected to a low-impedance ground (the safety ground wire) that should divert the current away from a person touching the instrument's case. The magnitude of such leaks is normally imperceptible to touch (less than 1 mA and well below the fibrillation threshold of 100 mA). If the current bypasses the high resistance offered by skin, however, and is applied directly to the heart (microshock), current as low as 100 μA (microamperes) may be fatal. The maximum leakage allowed in operating room equipment is 10 μA.

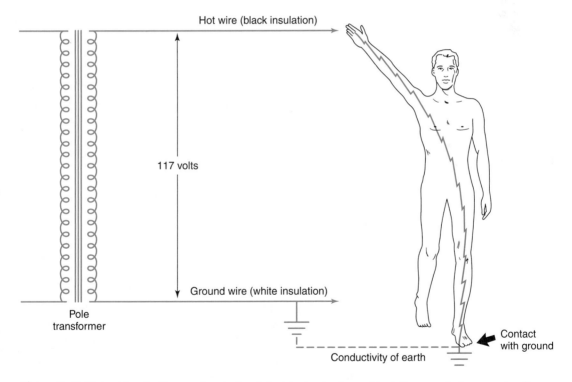

Figure 2–6. The setting for the great majority of electric shocks. An accidentally grounded person simultaneously contacts the hot wire of the electric service, usually via defective equipment that provides a pathway linking the hot wire to an exposed conductive surface. The complete electrical loop originates with the secondary of the pole transformer (the voltage source) and extends through the hot wire, the victim and the victim's contact with ground, the earth itself, the neutral ground rod at the service entrance, and back to the transformer via the neutral (or ground) wire. (Modified and reproduced, with permission, from Bruner J, Leonard PF: *Electricity, Safety, and the Patient.* Mosby Year Book, 1989.)

Cardiac pacing wires and invasive monitoring catheters provide a conductive pathway to the myocardial endothelium. In fact, blood and normal saline can serve as electrical conductors. The exact amount of current required to produce fibrillation depends on the timing of the shock relative to the vulnerable period of heart repolarization (the T wave on the electrocardiogram). Even small differences in potential between the earth connections of two electrical outlets in the same operating room might place a patient at risk for microelectrocution.

PROTECTION FROM ELECTRICAL SHOCK

Most patient electrocutions are caused by current flow from the live conductor of a grounded circuit through the body and back to a ground (Figure 2–6). This would be prevented if everything in the operating room were grounded except the patient. While direct patient grounds should be avoided, complete patient isolation is not feasible during surgery. Instead, the operating room power supply can be isolated from grounds by an isolation transformer (Figure 2–7).

Unlike the utility company's pole-top transformer, the secondary wiring of an isolation transformer is *not* grounded and provides two live ungrounded voltage lines for operating room equipment. Equipment casing—but not the electrical circuits—is grounded through the longest blade of a three-pronged plug (the safety ground). If a live wire is now unintentionally contacted by a grounded patient, current will not flow through the patient since no circuit back to the secondary coil has been completed (Figure 2–8).

Of course, if both power lines are contacted, a circuit is completed and a shock is possible. In addition, if either power line comes into contact with ground through a fault, contact with the other power line will complete a circuit through a grounded patient. To reduce the chance of two coexisting faults, a **line isolation monitor** measures the potential for current flow from the isolated power supply to ground (Figure 2–9). Basically, the line isolation monitor determines the degree of isolation between the two power wires and the ground and predicts the amount of current that *could* flow if a second short circuit were to develop. An alarm is activated if an unacceptably high current flow to ground becomes possible (usually 2 mA or 5 mA), but power is not interrupted unless a **ground-leakage circuit breaker** (also called a ground-fault circuit interrupter) is also activated. The latter is not usually installed in locations such as operating rooms, where discontinuation of life support systems is more hazardous than the risk of electrical shock. The alarm of the line isolation monitor merely indicates that the power supply has partially reverted to a grounded sys-

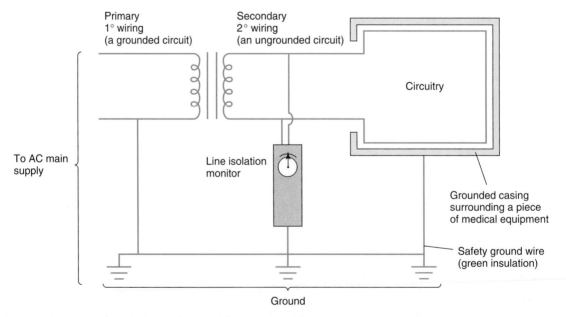

Figure 2–7. A circuit diagram of an isolation transformer and monitor.

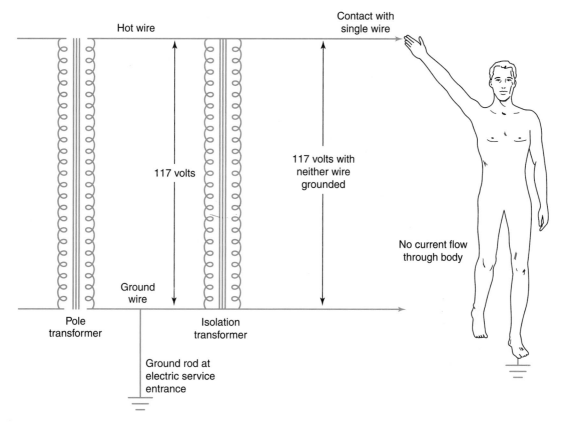

Figure 2–8. Even though a person is grounded, no shock results from contact with one wire of an isolated circuit. The individual is in simultaneous contact with two separate voltage sources but does not close a loop including either source. (Modified and reproduced, with permission, from Bruner J, Leonard PF: *Electricity, Safety, and the Patient.* Mosby Year Book, 1989.)

tem. In other words, while the line isolation monitor warns of the existence of a single fault (between a power line and ground), two faults are required for a shock to occur. If an alarm is activated, the last piece of equipment that was plugged in is suspect and should be removed from service until it is repaired.

Even isolated power circuits do not provide complete protection from the small currents capable of causing microshock fibrillation. Furthermore, the line isolation monitor cannot detect all faults, such as a broken safety ground wire within a piece of equipment. Despite their overall utility, the requirement for isolated power systems in operating rooms was deleted from the National Electrical Code in 1984, and newer or remodeled operating rooms may not offer this protection.

There are, however, modern equipment designs that decrease the possibility of microelectrocution. These in-

clude double insulation of the chassis and casing, ungrounded battery power supplies, and patient isolation from equipment-connected grounds by using optical coupling or transformers.

SURGICAL DIATHERMY

Electrosurgical units generate an ultra-high-frequency electrical current that passes from a small active electrode (the **cautery tip**) through the patient and exits by way of a large plate electrode (the **grounding pad,** or **return electrode**). The high current density at the cautery tip is capable of tissue coagulation or cutting, depending on the electrical waveform. Ventricular fibrillation is prevented by the use of ultrahigh electrical frequencies (0.1–3 million Hz) compared with line power (50–60 Hz). The large surface area of the low-

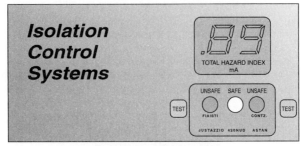

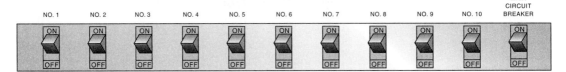

Figure 2–9. The panel of a line isolation monitor. (Courtesy of Ohio Medical Products.)

impedance return electrode avoids burns at the current's point of exit by providing a low current density (the concept of *exit* is technically incorrect, since the current is alternating rather than direct). The high power levels of electrosurgical units (up to 400 watts) can cause inductive coupling with monitor cables, leading to electrical interference.

Malfunction of the return electrode may result from disconnection from the electrosurgical unit, inadequate patient contact, or insufficient conductive gel. In these situations, the current will find another place to exit (eg, electrocardiogram pads or metal parts of the operating table), which may result in a burn (Figure 2–10). Precautions to prevent diathermy burns include proper return electrode placement that avoids bony protuberances and elimination of patient-to-ground contacts. Current flow through the heart may lead to pacemaker dysfunction. This can be minimized by placing the return electrode as close to the surgical field and as far away from the heart as practical.

Newer electrosurgical units are isolated from ground using the same principles as the isolated power supply (isolated output versus ground-referenced units). Because this second layer of protection provides these electrosurgical units with their own isolated power supply, the operating room's line isolation monitor may not detect an electrical fault. Although some electrosurgical units are capable of detecting poor contact between the return electrode and the patient by monitoring impedance, many older units trigger the alarm only if the return electrode is unplugged from the machine. Bipolar electrodes confine current propagation to a few

millimeters, eliminating the need for a return electrode. Since pacemaker and electrocardiogram interference is possible, pulse or heart sounds should be closely monitored when any electrosurgical unit is used.

■ FIRES & EXPLOSIONS

There are three requisites for a fire or explosion: a flammable agent (fuel), a gas that supports combustion, and a source of ignition. Flammable anesthetic agents (diethyl ether, divinyl ether, ethyl chloride, ethylene, and cyclopropane) are no longer used in the United States. The risk of fires or explosions has not been eliminated, however. Bowel gas, consisting of methane, hydrogen, and hydrogen sulfide, is highly flammable. Operating room supplies that may be combustible include endotracheal tubes, oxygen catheters, surgical drapes, benzoin aerosol, alcohol cleansing solutions, and even petroleum-based ointments (Lacri-Lube). If these substances ignite, they should be *immediately* removed from the patient and extinguished. Burning surgical drapes are particularly difficult to extinguish, since they are designed to be water-resistant.

Both oxygen and nitrous oxide are capable of vigorously supporting combustion; flammable agents that merely burn in air may explode in a mixture of nitrous oxide and oxygen. The accumulation of these agents under surgical drapes during head and neck surgery is particularly hazardous. With the routine use of pulse

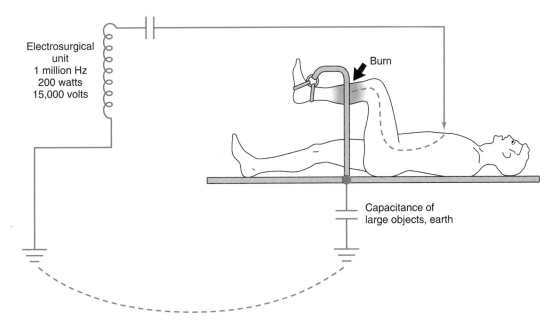

Electrosurgical
unit
1 million Hz
200 watts
15,000 volts

Burn

Capacitance of
large objects, earth

Figure 2–10. Electrosurgical burn. If the intended path is compromised, the circuit may be completed through other routes. Since the current is of high frequency, recognized conductors are not essential; capacitances can complete gaps in the circuit. Current passing through the patient to a contact of small area may produce a burn. (A leg drape would not offer protection in the situation depicted.) The isolated output electrosurgical (ESU) is much less likely than the ground-referenced ESU to provoke burns at ectopic sites. *Ground-referenced* in this context applies to the ESU output and has nothing to do with isolated versus grounded power systems. (Modified and reproduced, with permission, from Bruner J, Leonard PF: *Electricity, Safety, and the Patient.* Mosby Year Book, 1989.)

oximetry, there is no reason to indiscriminately insufflate oxygen under surgical drapes.

Historically, static electricity has been the most feared source of ignition. Numerous hospital regulations have attempted to minimize this cause of anesthetic explosions by prohibiting the use in operating rooms of materials apt to cause static discharge (eg, nylon, wool), by installing conductive breathing circuits and flooring, and by maintaining relative humidity above 50%. Most of these antiquated guidelines are now disregarded. In fact, conductive flooring increases the risk of electrical hazards. More contemporary sources of ignition include electrical equipment, such as the electrosurgical unit or laser. The use of diathermy near a distended bowel or the laser near combustible endotracheal tubes continues to provide proof that the danger of intraoperative explosion persists. Endotracheal tubes can be *partially* protected from the laser by wrapping them with foil or filling the cuff with saline. Special-purpose laser-resistant tubes are also available (see Chapter 39). The results of operating room fires are uniformly tragic.

CASE DISCUSSION: CHECKING OUT THE MEDICAL GAS SYSTEM IN A NEW OPERATING ROOM

A hospital has just dedicated its new obstetric wing, which includes two operating rooms. You are scheduled to deliver the first anesthetic.

Who is responsible for testing and certifying the medical gas delivery system?

No governmental or accreditation agency in the United States inspects hospital gas systems to enforce conformity with the National Fire Protection Association's 99–93 standard for health care facilities (the Canadian Standards Association certifies independent inspection firms in Canada). Ideally, third-party testing should certify that all aspects of the medical gas supply, piping, and outlet system comply with NFPA standards before use. Hospitals should have well-defined written policies for management, testing, and control of their medical gas systems and appropriate training of personnel. Although anesthesiologists are not responsible for hospital construction, they are responsible for intraoperative patient safety. In particular, the anesthesiologist is accountable for the portion of the medical gas system that extends from the wall outlet to the patient.

Which elements of the medical gas system need to be tested?

A 24-hour standing pressure test checks for system leaks and faulty pressure-relief valves. Cross-connection of pipelines is prevented by pressurizing each gas system separately and confirming that pressure is present only at corresponding gas outlets. The content purity of each pipeline is verified by analysis of samples collected from each outlet. Excessive contamination by volatile gases or water moisture can usually be removed by high-flow nitrogen purging of the system. The anesthesiologist should double-check each ceiling outlet to make certain that the correct color-coded hose and quick-connect device are present. Gas-line contents should be confirmed with an oxygen analyzer, gas chromatograph, or mass spectrometer. The vacuum system can be checked with a suction gauge capable of measuring negative pressure. Common problems include residual copper oxide particles inside the piping, improper joints, inadequate sizing, and component failure.

Can the new wing affect the preexisting operating room suites?

Whenever any new construction, remodeling, or expansion occurs near medical gas storage sites or pipelines, a high index of suspicion is justified regarding the use of medical gases throughout the hospital.

SUGGESTED READING

Dorsh JA, Dorsh SE: *Understanding Anesthesia Equipment,* 4th ed. Williams & Wilkins, 1999. A detailed discussion of compressed gases and medical gas delivery systems.

Greif R: Supplemental perioperative oxygen to reduce the incidence of surgical wound infection. N Engl J Med 2000;342:161. High levels (80% FiO_2) of intraoperative and postoperative (for 2 hours) oxygen supplementation decreased the incidence of surgical wound infection following colorectal surgery; a related study by the same author (Anesthesiology 1999;91:1246) found supplemental oxygen also reduced the incidence of postoperative nausea and vomiting.

Henderson KA, Matthews IP: An environmental survey of compliance with Occupational Exposure Standards (OES) for anesthetic gases. Anaesthesia 1999;54:941. Higher levels of nitrous oxide were found in areas without scavenging equipment (ie, radiology and delivery suites) than in operating rooms.

Kanmura Y, Sakai J, Yoshinaka H, Shirao K: Causes of nitrous oxide contamination in operating rooms. Anesthesiology 1999;90:693. Mask ventilation and faulty scavenging systems can lead to high levels of nitrous oxide.

Koch ME, Kain ZN, Ayoub C: The sedative and analgesic sparing effect of music. Anesthesiology 1998;89:300. Patients listening to their choice of music required less pharmacologic sedation and analgesia.

Macdonald MR, Wong A, Walker P, Crysdale WS: Electrocautery-induced ignition of tonsillar packing. J Otolaryngol 1994;23:426. A examination of factors that can decrease the risk of airway fire including lower oxygen concentration (using a cuffed endotracheal tube), completely soaked tonsil packs, and avoidance of contact between electrocautery and bismuth subgallate.

The National Fire Protection Association: Publications on fire hazards (NFPA 53M-1979) and electrical systems (NFPA 70-1984). Can be obtained by writing to Post Office Box 9146, Quincy, MA 02269, calling 1-800-735-0100, or visiting their Web site: www.NFPA.org.

Tobias JD: Helium: Applications in the practice of anesthesia and critical care. Am J Anesthesiol 1997;24:194. Helium has many useful properties including a high thermal conductivity (decreasing the risk of an airway fire) and a low density (decreasing turbulent flow through areas of airway obstruction).

Breathing Systems

KEY CONCEPTS

 Since insufflation avoids any direct patient contact, there is no rebreathing of exhaled gases. However, ventilation cannot be controlled with this technique, and the inspired gas contains unpredictable amounts of entrained atmospheric air.

 Long breathing tubes with high compliance increase the difference between the volume of gas delivered to a circuit by a breathing bag or ventilator and the volume actually delivered to the patient.

 The pressure-relief valve should be fully open during spontaneous ventilation so that circuit pressure remains negligible throughout inspiration and expiration.

 Because a fresh gas flow equal to minute ventilation is sufficient to prevent rebreathing, the Mapleson A design is the most efficient Mapleson circuit for spontaneous ventilation.

 The Mapleson D circuit is efficient during controlled ventilation, since fresh gas flow forces alveolar air away from the patient and toward the pressure-relief valve.

 The drier the soda lime, the more likely that it will absorb and degrade volatile anesthetics. Desflurane can be broken down to carbon monoxide by dry barium hydroxide lime to such a degree that it is capable of causing clinically significant carbon monoxide poisoning.

 Malfunction of either unidirectional valve in a circle system may allow rebreathing of carbon dioxide, resulting in hypercapnia.

 With an absorber, the circle system prevents rebreathing of carbon dioxide at fresh gas flows that are considered low-flow (fresh gas flow ≤ 1 L) or even fresh gas flows equal to the uptake of anesthetic gases and oxygen by the patient and the circuit itself (closed-system anesthesia).

 Because of the unidirectional valves, apparatus dead space in a circle system is limited to the area distal to the point of inspiratory and expiratory gas mixing at the Y-piece. Unlike Mapleson circuits, the breathing-tube length of a circle system does not directly affect dead space.

 Fraction of inspired oxygen (F_IO_2) delivered by a resuscitator breathing system to the patient is directly proportional to the oxygen concentration and flow rate of the gas mixture supplied to the resuscitator (usually 100% oxygen) and inversely proportional to the minute ventilation.

Breathing systems provide the final conduit for the delivery of anesthetic gases to the patient. In the modern practice of anesthesiology, breathing circuits link a patient to an anesthesia machine (Figure 3–1). Many modifications in circuit design have been developed, each with varying degrees of efficiency, convenience, and complexity. This chapter reviews the most important breathing systems: insufflation, open drop, Mapleson circuits, the circle system, and resuscitation systems.

Most traditional attempts to classify breathing systems artificially consolidate functional aspects (eg, the extent of rebreathing) with physical characteristics (eg, the presence of unidirectional valves). Because these

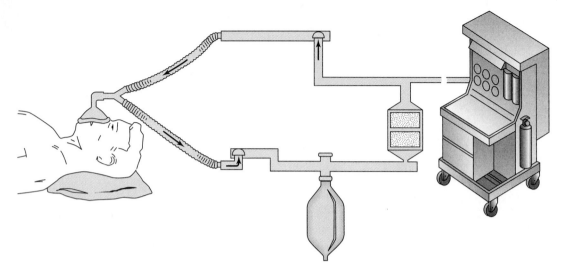

Figure 3–1. The relationship between the patient, the breathing system, and the anesthesia machine.

often-contradictory classifications (eg, open, closed, semiopen, semiclosed) tend to result in confusion rather than understanding, they are avoided in this discussion.

INSUFFLATION

The term **insufflation** usually denotes the blowing of anesthetic gases across a patient's face. Although insufflation is categorized as a breathing system, it is better considered a technique that avoids direct connection between a breathing circuit and a patient's airway. Because children resist the placement of a face mask or an intravenous line, insufflation is particularly valuable during pediatric inductions with inhalational anesthetics (Figure 3–2). It is useful in other situations as well. Carbon dioxide accumulation under head and neck draping is a hazard of ophthalmic surgery performed with local anesthesia. Insufflation of oxygen and air across the patient's face at a high flow rate (> 10 L/min) avoids this problem (Figure 3–3). Since insufflation avoids any direct patient contact, there is no rebreathing of exhaled gases. Ventilation cannot be controlled with this technique, however, and the inspired gas contains unpredictable amounts of entrained atmospheric air.

Insufflation can also be used to maintain arterial oxygenation during brief periods of apnea (eg, during bronchoscopy; see Chapter 39). Instead of blowing gases across the face, oxygen is directed into the lungs through a catheter placed in the trachea.

OPEN DROP ANESTHESIA

Although open drop anesthesia is not used in modern medicine, its historic significance and continued use in developing countries warrant a brief description here. A highly volatile anesthetic—most commonly ether or halothane—is dripped onto a gauze-covered mask

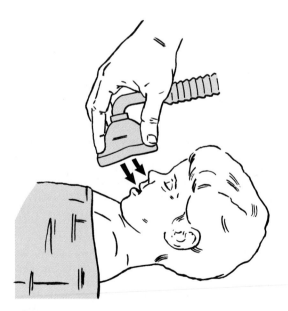

Figure 3–2. Insufflation of anesthetic agent across child's face during induction.

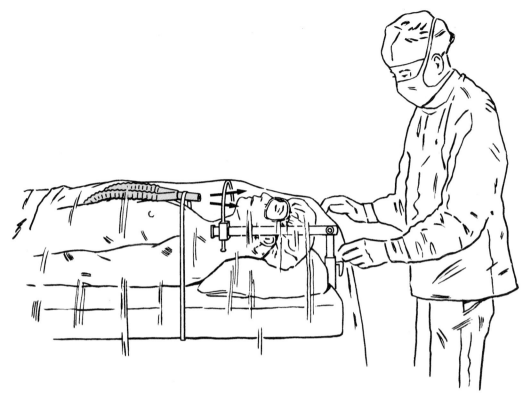

Figure 3–3. Insufflation of oxygen and air under head drape.

(Schimmelbusch mask) applied to the patient's face. As the patient inhales, air passes through the gauze, vaporizes the liquid agent, and carries high concentrations of anesthetic to the patient. The vaporization lowers mask temperature, resulting in moisture condensation and a drop in anesthetic vapor pressure (vapor pressure is proportional to temperature).

Deep levels of anesthesia will decrease minute ventilation and initiate a dangerous cycle of mask warming, increased vapor pressure, and higher concentrations of anesthetic. If sufficient CO_2 is trapped under the mask (apparatus dead space), rebreathing of anesthetic gases becomes significant. The anesthetic vapors further dilute inspired oxygen content, creating a potentially hypoxic mixture. To minimize dead space and increase inspired oxygen concentration, supplemental oxygen can be administered under the mask.

Another characteristic of the open drop technique is the uncontrollable pollution of the operating room environment with anesthetic—a serious disadvantage if a flammable agent such as ether is being administered.

A more modern derivative of open drop anesthesia utilizes draw-over vaporizers that depend on the patient's inspiratory efforts to draw ambient air through a vaporization chamber. This technique has a place in locations where compressed medical gases are unavailable (eg, developing countries and battlefields).

MAPLESON CIRCUITS

The insufflation and open drop systems have several disadvantages: poor control of inspired gas concentration and depth of anesthesia, inability to assist or control ventilation, no conservation of exhaled heat or humidity, difficult airway management during head and neck surgery, and pollution of the operating room with large volumes of waste gas. The **Mapleson systems** solve some of these problems by incorporating additional components (breathing tubes, fresh gas inlets, pressure-relief valves, and breathing bags) into the breathing circuit. The relative location of these components determines circuit performance and is the basis of the Mapleson classification (Table 3–1).

Table 3–1. Classification and characteristics of Mapleson circuits.

Mapleson Class	Other Names	Configuration	Required Fresh Gas Flows		Comments
			Spontaneous	Controlled	
A	Magill attachment		Equal to minute ventilation (≈ 80 mL/Kg/min)	Very high and difficult to predict	Poor choice during controlled ventilation. Enclosed Magill system is a modification that improves efficiency. Coaxial Mapleson A (Lack breathing system) provides waste-gas scavenging.
B			2 × minute ventilation	2–2½ × minute ventilation	
C	Waters' to-and-fro		2 × minute ventilation	2–2½ × minute ventilation	
D	Bain circuit		2–3 × minute ventilation	1–2 × minute ventilation	Bain coaxial modification: Fresh gas tube inside breathing tube (see Figure 3–6).
E	Ayre's T-piece		2–3 × minute ventilation	3 × minute ventilation (I:E = 1:2)	Exhalation tubing should provide a larger volume than tidal volume to prevent rebreathing. Scavenging is difficult.
F	Jackson-Rees' modification		2–3 × minute ventilation	2 × minute ventilation	A Mapleson E with a breathing bag connected to the end of the breathing tube to allow controlled ventilation and scavenging.

FGI = fresh gas inlet.

Components of Mapleson Circuits

A. BREATHING TUBES:

Corrugated breathing tubes—made of rubber (reusable) or plastic (disposable)—connect the components of the Mapleson circuit to the patient (Figure 3–4). The large diameter of the tubes (22 mm) creates a low-resistance pathway and a potential reservoir for anesthetic gases. In order to minimize fresh gas flow requirements, the volume of the breathing tube in most Mapleson circuits should be at least as great as the patient's tidal volume.

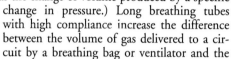 The compliance of the breathing tubes partially determines the compliance of the circuit. (Compliance is defined as the change of volume produced by a specific change in pressure.) Long breathing tubes with high compliance increase the difference between the volume of gas delivered to a circuit by a breathing bag or ventilator and the volume actually delivered to the patient. For example, if a breathing circuit with a compliance of 8 mL gas/cm H_2O is pressurized during delivery of a tidal volume to 20 cm H_2O, 160 mL of the tidal volume will be lost to the circuit. Specifically, the 160 mL represents a combination of gas compression and breathing-tube expansion. This is an important consideration in any circuit delivering positive pressure ventilation through breathing tubes (eg, circle systems).

B. FRESH GAS INLET:

Gases (anesthetics with oxygen or air) from the anesthesia machine continuously enter the circuit through the fresh gas inlet (a continuous-flow system). As discussed below, the relative position of this component is a key differentiating factor in Mapleson circuit performance.

C. PRESSURE-RELIEF VALVE (POP-OFF VALVE, ADJUSTABLE PRESSURE-LIMITING VALVE):

As anesthetic gases enter the breathing circuit, pressure will rise if the gas inflow is greater than the combined uptake of the patient and the circuit. Allowing gases to exit the circuit through a pressure-relief valve controls this pressure buildup. Exiting gases enter the operating room atmosphere or, preferably, a waste-gas scavenging system. All pressure-relief valves allow setting a variable pressure threshold for venting.

 The pressure-relief valve should be fully open during spontaneous ventilation so that circuit pressure remains negligible throughout inspiration and expiration. Assisted and controlled ventilation require positive pressure during inspiration to expand the lungs. Partial closure of the pressure-relief valve limits gas exit, permitting positive circuit pressures during breathing-bag compressions.

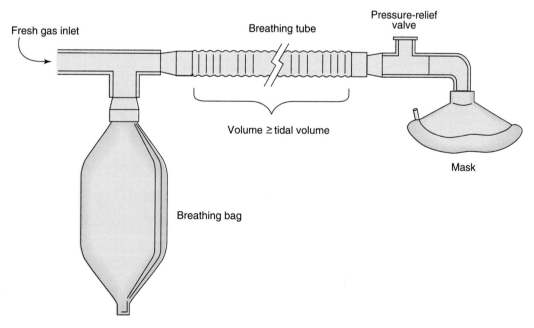

Figure 3–4. Components of a Mapleson circuit.

D. Breathing Bag (Reservoir Bag):

Breathing bags function as a reservoir of anesthetic gas and a method of generating positive pressure ventilation. They are designed to increase in compliance as their volume increases. Three distinct phases of breathing bag filling are recognizable (Figure 3–5). After the nominal 3-L capacity of an adult breathing bag is achieved (phase I), pressure rises rapidly to a peak (phase II). Further increases in volume result in a plateau or even a slight decrease in pressure (phase III). This ceiling effect helps to protect the patient's lungs against high airway pressures if the pressure-relief valve is unintentionally left in the closed position while fresh gas continues to flow into the circuit.

Performance Characteristics of Mapleson Circuits

Mapleson circuits are lightweight, inexpensive, and simple and do not require unidirectional valves. Breathing-circuit efficiency is measured by the fresh gas flow required to eliminate CO_2 rebreathing. Because there are no unidirectional valves or CO_2 absorption in Mapleson circuits, rebreathing is prevented by venting exhaled gas through the pressure-relief valve before inspiration. This usually requires high fresh gas flows.

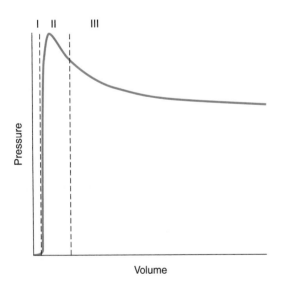

Figure 3–5. The increasing compliance and elasticity of breathing bags as demonstrated by three phases of filling. (Reproduced, with permission, from Johnstone RE, Smith TE: Rebreathing bags as pressure limiting devices. Anesthesiology 1973;38:192.)

Reexamine the drawing of a Mapleson A circuit in Figure 3–4. During spontaneous ventilation, alveolar gas containing CO_2 will be exhaled into the breathing tube or directly vented through an open pop-off valve. Before inhalation occurs, if the fresh gas flow exceeds alveolar minute ventilation, the inflow of fresh gas will force the alveolar gas remaining in the breathing tube to exit from the pressure release valve. If the breathing-tube volume is equal to or greater than the patient's tidal volume, the next inspiration will contain only fresh gas. Because a fresh gas flow equal to minute ventilation is sufficient to prevent rebreathing, the Mapleson A design is the most efficient Mapleson circuit for *spontaneous* ventilation.

Positive pressure during *controlled* ventilation, however, requires a partially closed pressure release valve. Although some alveolar and fresh gas exits through the valve during inspiration, no gas is vented during expiration. As a result, unpredictably high fresh gas flows (greater than three times minute ventilation) are required to prevent rebreathing with a Mapleson A circuit during controlled ventilation.

Interchanging the position of the pressure-relief valve and the fresh gas inlet transforms a Mapleson A into a **Mapleson D circuit** (Table 3–1). The latter system is efficient during controlled ventilation, since fresh gas flow now forces alveolar air *away* from the patient and *toward* the pressure-relief valve. Thus, simply moving components completely alters the fresh gas requirements of the Mapleson circuits.

The **Bain circuit** is a popular modification of the Mapleson D system that incorporates the fresh gas inlet tubing inside the breathing tube (Figure 3–6). This modification decreases the circuit's bulk and retains heat and humidity better than the Mapleson D as a result of partial warming of the inspiratory gas by countercurrent exchange with the warmer expired gases. A disadvantage of this coaxial circuit is the possibility of kinking or disconnection of the fresh gas inlet tubing. If unrecognized, either of these mishaps could result in significant rebreathing of exhaled gas.

THE CIRCLE SYSTEM

Although Mapleson circuits overcome some of the disadvantages of the insufflation and open drop systems, the high fresh gas flows required to prevent rebreathing result in waste of anesthetic agent, pollution of the operating room environment, and loss of patient heat and humidity (Table 3–2). In an attempt to avoid these problems, the **circle system** adds more components to the breathing system.

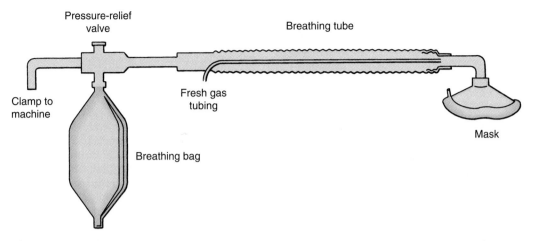

Figure 3–6. A Bain circuit is a Mapleson D design with the fresh gas tubing inside the corrugated breathing tube. (Redrawn and reproduced, with permission, from Bain JA, Spoerel WE: Flow requirements for a modified Mapleson D system during controlled ventilation. Can Anaesth Soc J 1973;20:629.)

Components of the Circle System

A. CARBON DIOXIDE ABSORBENT:

Rebreathing alveolar gas conserves heat and humidity. However, the CO_2 in exhaled gas must be eliminated to prevent hypercapnia. CO_2 chemically combines with water to form carbonic acid. CO_2 absorbents (eg, soda lime or barium hydroxide lime) contain hydroxide salts that are capable of neutralizing carbonic acid (Table 3–3). Reaction end products include heat (the heat of neutralization), water, and calcium carbonate. **Soda lime** is the more common absorbent and is capable of absorbing up to 23 L of CO_2 per 100 g of absorbent. Its reactions are as follows:

$$CO_2 + H_2O \rightarrow H_2CO_3$$

$$H_2CO_3 + 2NaOH \rightarrow Na_2CO_3 + 2H_2O + Heat$$
$$\text{(a fast reaction)}$$

Table 3–2. Characteristics of breathing circuits.

	Insufflation and Open Drop	Mapleson	Circle
Complexity	Very simple	Simple	Complex
Control of anesthetic depth	Poor	Variable	Good
Ability to scavenge	Very poor	Variable	Good
Conservation of heat and humidity	No	No	Yes*
Rebreathing of exhaled gases	No	No*	Yes*

*These properties depend on the rate of fresh gas flow.

Table 3–3. Comparison of soda lime and barium hydroxide lime.

	Soda Lime	Barium Hydroxide Lime
Mesh size*	4–8	4–8
Method of hardness	Silica added	Water of crystallization
Content	Calcium hydroxide Sodium hydroxide Potassium hydroxide	Barium hydroxide Calcium hydroxide
Usual indicator dye	Ethyl violet	Ethyl violet
Absorptive capacity (liters of CO_2/100 g granules)	14–23	9–18

*The number of openings per linear inch in a wire screen used to grade particle size.

Table 3–4. Indicator dye changes signaling absorbent exhaustion.

Indicator	Color when Fresh	Color when Exhausted
Ethyl violet	White	Purple
Phenolphthalein	White	Pink
Clayton yellow	Red	Yellow
Ethyl orange	Orange	Yellow
Mimosa 2	Red	White

$$Na_2CO_3 + Ca(OH)_2 \rightarrow CaCO_3 + 2NaOH$$
(a slow reaction)

Note that the water and sodium hydroxide initially required are regenerated.

Color conversion of a pH indicator dye by increasing hydrogen ion concentration signals absorbent exhaustion (Table 3–4). Absorbent should be replaced when 50–70% has changed color. Although exhausted granules may revert to their original color if rested, no significant recovery of absorptive capacity occurs. Granule size is a compromise between the higher absorptive surface area of small granules and the lower resistance to gas flow of larger granules. The hydroxide salts are irritating to skin and mucous membranes. Increasing the hardness of soda lime by adding silica minimizes the risk of sodium hydroxide dust inhalation. Since barium hydroxide lime incorporates water into its structure (the water of crystallization), it is sufficiently hard without silica. Additional water is added to both types of absorbent during packaging to provide optimal conditions for carbonic acid formation. Commercial soda lime has a water content of 14–19%.

Absorbent granules can absorb and later release significant amounts of volatile anesthetic. This property can be responsible for delayed induction or emergence. Trichloroethylene, an anesthetic no longer available in the United States, decomposes into neurotoxins (including phosgene gas) when exposed to soda lime and heat. Postoperative encephalitis and cranial nerve palsies have been traced to this toxic reaction. The drier the soda lime, the more likely that it will absorb and degrade volatile anesthetics. Desflurane can be broken down to carbon monoxide by dry barium hydroxide lime to such a degree that it is capable of causing clinically significant carbon monoxide poisoning.

A new carbon dioxide absorbent consisting of calcium hydroxide and calcium chloride (with calcium sulfate and polyvinylpyrrolidone added to increase hardness) has been developed. This absorbent (Amsorb) possesses greater inertness compared with soda lime or barium hydroxide lime, resulting in less degradation of volatile anesthetics (eg, sevoflurane into compound A or desflurane into carbon monoxide; see Chapter 7).

B. CARBON DIOXIDE ABSORBERS:

The granules of absorbent are contained within one or two canisters that fit snugly between a head and base plate. Together, this unit is called an **absorber** (Figure 3–7). Although bulky, double canisters permit more complete CO_2 absorption, less frequent absorbent changes, and lower gas flow resistance. To ensure complete absorption, a patient's tidal volume should not exceed the air space between absorbent granules, which is roughly equal to one-half the absorber's capacity. Indicator dye color is monitored through the absorber's transparent walls. Absorbent exhaustion typically occurs where exhaled gas enters the absorber and along the canister's smooth inner walls. Channeling through areas of loosely packed granules is minimized by a baffle system. A trap at the base of the absorber collects dust and moisture. Some older units have a bypass valve to

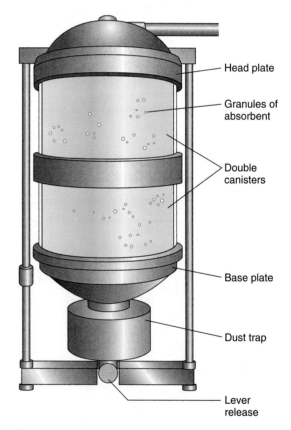

Figure 3–7. A carbon dioxide absorber.

— Head plate

— Granules of absorbent

— Double canisters

— Base plate

— Dust trap

— Lever release

allow absorbent change during ventilation. This bypass valve is easily overlooked and, if unintentionally left in the bypass position, may result in hypercapnia.

C. UNIDIRECTIONAL VALVES:

Unidirectional valves, which function as check valves, contain a rubber, plastic, or mica disk resting horizontally on an annular valve seat (Figure 3–8). Forward flow displaces the disk upward, permitting the gas to proceed through the circuit. Reverse flow pushes the disk against its seat, preventing reflux. Valve incompetence is usually due to warped disks or seat irregularities. The expiratory valve is especially vulnerable to damage since it is exposed to the humidity of alveolar gas.

Inhalation opens the inspiratory valve, allowing the patient to breath a mixture of fresh and exhaled gas that has passed through the CO_2 absorber. Simultaneously, the expiratory valve closes to prevent rebreathing of exhaled alveolar gas that still contains CO_2. The subsequent flow of gas away from the patient during exhalation opens the expiratory valve. This gas is vented through the pressure-relief valve or rebreathed by the patient after passing through the absorber. Closure of the inspiratory valve during exhalation prevents expiratory gas from mixing with fresh gas in the inspiratory limb. Malfunction of either valve may allow rebreathing of CO_2, resulting in hypercapnia.

Optimization of Circle System Design

Although the major components of the circle system (unidirectional valves, fresh gas inlet, pressure-relief valve, CO_2 absorber, and a breathing bag) can be placed in several configurations, the following arrangement is preferred (Figure 3–9):

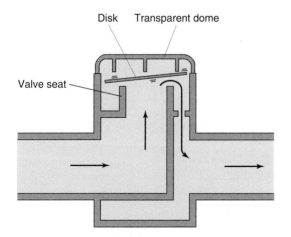

Figure 3–8. A unidirectional valve.

- **Unidirectional valves** should be close to the patient to prevent backflow into the inspiratory limb if a circuit leak develops. However, unidirectional valves should not be placed in the breathing tube Y-piece, since that makes it difficult to confirm proper orientation and intraoperative function.

- **The fresh gas inlet** is placed between the absorber and the inspiratory valve. Positioning it downstream from the inspiratory valve would allow fresh gas to bypass the patient during exhalation and be wasted. Fresh gas introduced between the expiration valve and the absorber would be diluted by recirculating gas. Furthermore, inhalational anesthetics may be absorbed or released by soda lime granules, thus slowing induction and emergence.

- **The pressure-relief valve** should be placed immediately before the absorber to conserve absorption capacity and to minimize venting of fresh gas.

- Resistance to exhalation is decreased by locating **the breathing bag** in the expiratory limb. Bag compression during controlled ventilation will vent alveolar gas through the pressure-relief valve, conserving absorbent.

Performance Characteristics of the Circle System

A. FRESH GAS REQUIREMENT:

With an absorber, the circle system prevents rebreathing of CO_2 at fresh gas flows that are considered low-flow (fresh gas flow ≤ 1 L) or even fresh gas flows equal to the uptake of anesthetic gases and oxygen by the patient and the circuit itself (closed-system anesthesia; see Case Discussion in Chapter 7). At fresh gas flows greater than 5 L/min, rebreathing is so minimal that a CO_2 absorber is usually unnecessary.

With low fresh gas flows, concentrations of oxygen and inhalational anesthetics can vary markedly between fresh gas (ie, gas in the fresh gas inlet) and inspired gas (ie, gas in the inspiratory limb of the breathing tubes). The latter is a mixture of fresh gas and exhaled gas that has passed through the absorber. The greater the fresh gas flow rate, the less time it will take for a change in fresh gas anesthetic concentration to be reflected in a change in inspired gas anesthetic concentration. Higher flows speed induction and recovery, compensate for leaks in the circuit, and decrease the risks of unanticipated gas mixtures.

B. DEAD SPACE:

That part of a tidal volume that does not undergo alveolar ventilation is referred to as dead space (see Chapter 22). Thus, any increase in dead space must be accom-

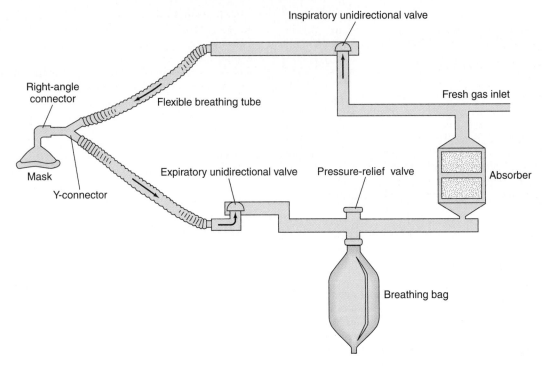

Figure 3–9. A circle system.

panied by a corresponding increase in tidal volume if alveolar ventilation is to remain unchanged. Because of the unidirectional valves, apparatus dead space in a circle system is limited to the area distal to the point of inspiratory and expiratory gas mixing at the Y-piece. Unlike Mapleson circuits, the breathing-tube length of a circle system does not directly affect dead space. Like Mapleson circuits, length does affect circuit compliance and thus the amount of tidal volume lost to the circuit during positive pressure ventilation. Pediatric circle systems have both a septum dividing the inspiratory and expiratory gas in the Y-piece and low-compliance breathing tubes to further reduce dead space.

C. RESISTANCE:

The unidirectional valves and absorber increase circle system resistance, especially at high respiratory rates and large tidal volumes. Nonetheless, even premature neonates can be successfully ventilated with circle systems.

D. HUMIDITY AND HEAT CONSERVATION:

Medical gas delivery systems supply dehumidified gases to the anesthesia circuit at room temperature. Exhaled gas, on the other hand, is saturated with water at body temperature. Therefore, the heat and humidity of inspired gas depends on the relative proportion of rebreathed gas to fresh gas. High flows are accompanied by low relative humidity, whereas low flows allow greater water saturation. Absorbent granules provide a significant source of heat and moisture in the circle system.

E. BACTERIAL CONTAMINATION:

There is a slight risk of microorganism retention in circle system components that could theoretically lead to respiratory infections in subsequent patients. For this reason, bacterial filters are sometimes incorporated into the inspiratory or expiratory breathing tubes.

Disadvantages of the Circle System

Although most of the problems of Mapleson circuits are solved by the circle system, the improvements have led to other disadvantages: greater size and less portability; increased complexity, resulting in a higher risk of disconnection or malfunction; increased resistance, dissuading some pediatric anesthesiologists from using the system; and the difficulty of predicting inspired gas concentrations during low fresh gas flows.

RESUSCITATION BREATHING SYSTEMS

Resuscitation bags (Ambu bags or bag-mask units) are commonly used for emergency ventilation because of their simplicity, portability, and ability to deliver almost 100% oxygen (Figure 3–10). These resuscitators are unlike a Mapleson circuit or a circle system because they contain **nonrebreathing valves.** (Remember that a Mapleson system is considered valveless although it contains a pressure-relief valve, while a circle system contains unidirectional valves that direct flow through an absorber but allow rebreathing of exhaled gases.)

High concentrations of oxygen can be delivered to a mask or endotracheal tube during spontaneous or controlled ventilation if a source of high fresh gas flow is connected to the inlet nipple. The **patient valve** opens during controlled or spontaneous inspiration to allow gas flow from the ventilation bag to the patient. Rebreathing is prevented by venting exhaled gas to the atmosphere through exhalation ports in this valve. The compressible, self-refilling ventilation bag also contains an **intake valve.** This valve closes during bag compression, permitting positive pressure ventilation. The bag is refilled by flow through the fresh gas inlet and across the intake valve. Connecting a reservoir to the intake valve helps prevent the entrainment of room air. The **reservoir valve assembly** is really two unidirectional valves: the inlet valve and the outlet valve. The **inlet valve** allows ambient air to enter the ventilation bag if fresh gas flow is inadequate to maintain reservoir filling. Positive pressure in the reservoir bag opens the **outlet valve,** which vents oxygen if fresh gas flow is excessive.

There are several disadvantages to resuscitator breathing systems. First, they require fairly high fresh gas flows to achieve a high inspired oxygen concentration (FIO_2). FIO_2 is directly proportional to the oxygen concentration and flow rate of the gas mixture supplied to the resuscitator (usually 100% oxygen) and inversely proportional to the minute ventilation delivered to the patient. For example, a Laerdal resuscitator equipped with a reservoir requires a flow of 10 L/min to achieve an inspired oxygen concentration approaching 100% if a patient with a tidal volume of 750 mL is ventilated at a respiratory rate of 12 breaths/min. The maximum achievable tidal volumes are less than with a system that uses a 3-L breathing bag. In fact, most adult resuscitators have a maximum tidal volume of 1000 mL. Finally, although a normally functioning patient valve has low resistance to inspiration and expiration, exhaled moisture can cause valve sticking.

CASE DISCUSSION: UNEXPLAINED LIGHT ANESTHESIA

A massively obese but otherwise healthy 5-year-old girl presents for inguinal hernia repair. After uneventful induction of general anesthesia and endotracheal intubation, the patient is placed on a ventilator set to deliver a tidal volume of 7 mL/kg at a rate of 16 breaths/min. Despite delivery of 2% halothane in 50% nitrous oxide, tachycardia (145 beats/min) and mild hypertension (140/90 mm Hg) are noted. In order to increase anesthetic depth, fentanyl (3 μg/kg) is administered. Heart rate and blood pressure continue to rise and are accompanied by frequent premature ventricular contractions.

What should be considered in the differential diagnosis of this patient's cardiovascular changes?

*The combination of tachycardia and hypertension during general anesthesia should always alert the anesthesiologist to the possibility of **hy-***

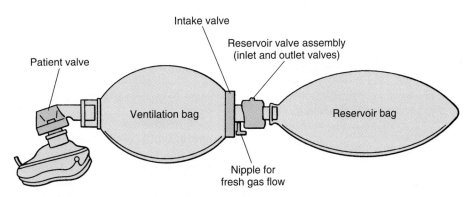

Figure 3–10. The Laerdal resuscitator. (Courtesy of Laerdal Medical Corp.)

percapnia or **hypoxia,** both of which produce signs of increased sympathetic activity. These life-threatening conditions should be quickly and immediately ruled out by end-tidal CO_2 monitoring, pulse oximetry, or arterial blood gas analysis.

A common cause of intraoperative tachycardia and hypertension is an **inadequate level of anesthesia.** Normally, this is confirmed by movement. If the patient is paralyzed, however, there are few reliable indicators of light anesthesia. The lack of a response to a dose of an opioid should alert the anesthesiologist to the possibility of other, perhaps more serious, causes.

Malignant hyperthermia is rare but must be considered in cases of unexplained tachycardia, especially if accompanied by premature contractions (see Case Discussion in Chapter 44). Certain **drugs** used in anesthesia (eg, pancuronium, ketamine, ephedrine) stimulate the sympathetic nervous system and can produce or exacerbate tachycardia and hypertension. Diabetic patients who become **hypoglycemic** from administration of insulin or long-acting oral hypoglycemic agents can have similar cardiovascular changes. Other **endocrine abnormalities** (eg, pheochromocytoma, toxic goiter, carcinoid) could also be considered.

Could any of these problems be related to an equipment malfunction?

On some older models of anesthesia machines, it is necessary to turn on a master control switch in addition to the vaporizer control knob to activate the vaporizers. This is often true of copper kettle vaporizers. Briefly sniffing the anesthetic gas being delivered to the patient is an easy—if not aesthetic—method of confirming the presence of a volatile agent. Nitrous oxide is more difficult to detect without sophisticated equipment, but an oxygen analyzer should provide a clue.

A misconnection of the ventilator could result in hypoxia or hypercapnia. In addition, a malfunctioning unidirectional valve will increase circuit dead space and allow rebreathing of expired CO_2. Soda lime exhaustion or activation of an absorber bypass valve could also lead to rebreathing in the presence of a low fresh gas flow. Rebreathing of CO_2 can be detected during the inspiratory phase on a capnograph or mass spectrometer (see Chapter 6). If rebreathing appears to be due to an equipment malfunction, the patient should be disconnected from the anesthesia machine and ventilated with a resuscitation bag until repairs are possible.

How are unidirectional valves checked before the anesthesia machine is used?

The incidence of incompetent unidirectional valves has been found to approach 15%. There is a quick procedure for testing the function of these valves:

(1) First, disconnect the breathing tubes from the anesthesia machine, close the pressure release valve, and turn off all gas flow.

(2) To check inspiratory valve function, connect one end of a section of breathing tube to the inhalation outlet and occlude the exhalation outlet. If a breathing bag that is connected to its usual site fills when air is blown into the breathing tube, the inspiratory valve is incompetent (Figure 3–11A).

(3) To check expiratory valve function, connect one end of a section of breathing tube to the usual breathing bag site and cover the inhalation outlet. If a breathing bag connected to the exhalation outlet fills when air is blown into the breathing tube, the expiratory valve is incompetent (Figure 3–11B).

What are some other consequences of hypercapnia?

Hypercapnia has a multitude of effects, most of them masked by general anesthesia. Cerebral blood flow increases proportionally with arterial CO_2. This effect is dangerous in patients with increased intracranial pressure (eg, from brain tumor). Extremely high levels of CO_2 (> 80 mm Hg) can cause unconsciousness related to a fall in cerebrospinal fluid pH. CO_2 depresses the myocardium, but this direct effect is usually overshadowed by activation of the sympathetic nervous system. During general anesthesia, hypercarbia usually results in an increased cardiac output, an elevation in arterial blood pressure, and a propensity toward dysrhythmias.

Elevated serum CO_2 concentrations can overwhelm the blood's buffering capacity, leading to respiratory acidosis. This causes other anions such as Ca^{2+} and K^+ to shift extracellularly. Acidosis also shifts the oxyhemoglobin dissociation curve to the right.

Carbon dioxide is a powerful respiratory stimulant. In fact, for each mm Hg rise of $PaCO_2$ above baseline, normal awake subjects increase their minute ventilation by about 2–3 L/min. General anesthesia markedly decreases this response, and paralysis would eliminate it. Finally, severe hyper-

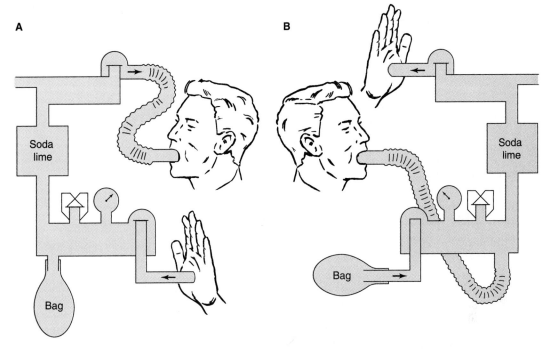

A

B

Figure 3–11. How to connect the reservoir bag and corrugated tube for the competence test of inhalation (**A**) and exhalation (**B**) unidirectional dome valves. Heavy arrows indicate direction of flow through valves. (From Kim J, Kovac AL, Mathewson HS: A method for detection of incompetent unidirectional dome valves: A prevalent malfunction. Anesth Analg 1985;64:745. Reprinted with permission of the International Anesthesia Research Society.)

capnia can produce hypoxia by displacement of oxygen from alveoli as the body attempts to rid itself of CO_2.

SUGGESTED READING

Dorsch JA, Dorsch SE: *Understanding Anesthesia Equipment,* 4th ed. Lippincott Williams & Wilkins, 1999. Detailed discussion of breathing systems.

Ehrenwerth J, Eisenkraft JB (editors): *Anesthesia Equipment—Principles and Applications.* Mosby Year Book, 1993. A review of anesthesia machines and monitoring equipment.

Healthcare Product Comparison System (HPCS), published by ECRI (a nonprofit agency), August 1999. This report compares several models of anesthesia machines and includes an excellent overview of breathing circuit components and potential problems.

Murray JM, Renfrew CW, Bedi A, et al: Amsorb: A new carbon dioxide absorbent for use in anesthetic breathing systems. Anesthesiology 1999;91:1342. Calcium hydroxide proves to be nonreactive with volatile anesthetic agents.

The Anesthesia Machine

4

KEY CONCEPTS

1. Preventable anesthetic mishaps are frequently traced to a lack of familiarity with anesthetic equipment and a failure to check machine function.

2. Only an oxygen pressure failure triggers a fail-safe valve and a gas whistle or electric alarm. These safety devices do not protect against other possible causes of hypoxic accidents.

3. Because oxygen is supplied at a line pressure of 45–55 psig, there is a real potential of lung barotrauma. For this reason, the oxygen flush valve must be used cautiously whenever a patient is connected to the breathing circuit.

4. Should a leak develop within or downstream from an oxygen flowmeter, a hypoxic gas mixture might be delivered to the patient. To reduce this risk, oxygen flowmeters should be positioned downstream (nearest the outlet) from the other medical gas flowmeters.

5. A rise in airway pressure may signal worsening pulmonary compliance, an increase in tidal volume, or an obstruction in the breathing circuit. A drop in pressure may indicate an improvement in compliance, a decrease in tidal volume, or a leak in the circuit.

6. Peak inspiratory pressure is the highest circuit pressure generated during an inspiratory cycle, and provides an indication of dynamic compliance. Plateau pressure is the pressure measured during an inspiratory pause (a time of no gas flow), and mirrors static compliance.

7. Modern vaporizers are agent-specific and filling them with the wrong anesthetic agent must be avoided.

8. There are two distinct circuits within the ventilator that are separated by the bellows wall: the external high-pressure oxygen circuit that powers the ventilator and an internal extension of the anesthesia breathing circuit.

9. Whenever a ventilator is used, a disconnect alarm must be activated. Breathing-circuit disconnection, a leading cause of anesthetic accidents, is detected by a drop in peak circuit pressure.

10. Whenever a ventilator is used, the circle system's pressure-relief valve should be closed or functionally removed from the circuit.

11. Because the ventilator's pressure-relief valve is closed during inspiration, the circuit's fresh gas flows contribute to the tidal volume delivered to the patient. The use of the oxygen flush valve during the inspiratory cycle of a ventilator must be avoided because the pressure-relief valve is closed and the surge of circuit pressure will be transferred to the patient's lungs.

12. General anesthesia should never be administered without an oxygen analyzer in the breathing circuit.

No piece of equipment is more intimately associated with the practice of anesthesiology than the anesthesia machine. In essence, the anesthesiologist uses the anesthesia machine to control the patient's inspired gas mixture and gas exchange. Proper functioning of the machine is crucial for patient safety. In an attempt to increase the safety of anesthesia, the American National Standards Institute has published a set of anesthesia machine requirements. Despite these and other efforts, preventable anesthetic mishaps are frequently traced to a lack of familiarity with anesthetic equipment and a failure to check machine function. In fact, the misuse and malfunction of anesthesia machines is a prominent cause of operative morbidity and death. This chapter is intended as an introduction to anesthesia machine design, function, and inspection.

OVERVIEW

Anesthesia machines have multiple functions that are performed by specific components (Figures 4–1 and 4–2), including the following:

- **Gas inlets** receive medical gases from attached cylinders or the hospital's gas delivery system.
- **Pressure regulators** reduce gas pressure.
- **Oxygen-pressure-failure devices** signal low oxygen pressure.
- **Flow-control valves and flowmeters** control the flow rate.
- **Vaporizers** blend gases with volatile anesthetic agents.
- A **fresh gas outlet** delivers the final gas composition to the breathing circuit.

All current anesthesia machines should be equipped with **spirometers** that measure respiratory volumes within the breathing circuit, **breathing-circuit pressure gauges, ventilators with disconnect alarms, waste-gas scavengers,** and **oxygen analyzers. Humidifiers** and **nebulizers** are available that connect between the anesthesia machine and the breathing circuit. Some newer models integrate a multitude of other vital patient monitors (eg, electrocardiographs, pulse oximeters, capnographs) that were traditionally considered separately (see Chapter 6), use new electronic technolo-

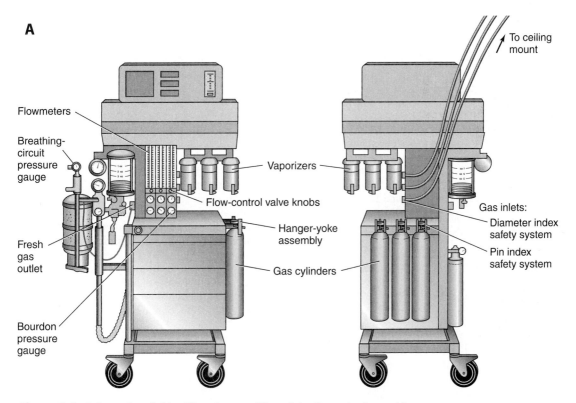

A

Flowmeters
Breathing-circuit pressure gauge
Vaporizers
Flow-control valve knobs
Hanger-yoke assembly
Fresh gas outlet
Gas cylinders
Bourdon pressure gauge
To ceiling mount
Gas inlets:
Diameter index safety system
Pin index safety system

Figure 4–1. Schematics of older (**A**) and newer (**B**) models of anesthesia machines.

(continued)

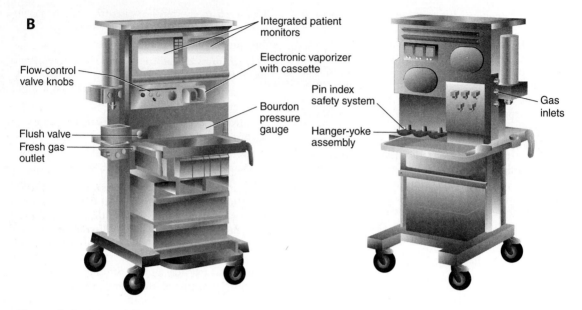

B

Integrated patient monitors

Electronic vaporizer with cassette

Flow-control valve knobs

Pin index safety system

Bourdon pressure gauge

Gas inlets

Flush valve

Fresh gas outlet

Hanger-yoke assembly

Figure 4–1. Continued

gies to measure gas flow and control anesthetic delivery, and perform automated machine checkouts.

GAS INLETS & PRESSURE REGULATORS

Cylinders attached to the anesthesia machine's **hanger-yoke assembly** are a high-pressure source of medical gases (Figure 4–1). The yoke assembly includes index pins (see the discussion of the pin index safety system in Chapter 2), a washer, a gas filter, and a check valve that prevents retrograde gas flow. Cylinder pressure is measured by a **Bourdon pressure gauge** (Figure 4–2). A flexible tube within this gauge straightens when exposed to gas pressure, causing a gear mechanism to move a needle pointer.

The high and variable gas pressure in a cylinder makes flow control difficult and potentially dangerous. To enhance safety and ensure optimal use of pipeline gases, a **pressure regulator** reduces the cylinder gas pressure to less than 50 psig. **Two-stage pressure regulators** (two one-stage regulators in series) further reduce any outlet pressure variations caused by fluctuations in cylinder pressure.

The hospital's medical gas delivery system connects to the anesthesia machine through the diameter index safety system (see Chapter 2). Because the pipeline gases are supplied at pressures between 45 psig and 55

psig, they do not need to be further reduced. After passing through Bourdon pressure gauges and check valves, the pipeline gases share a common pathway with the cylinder gases.

OXYGEN-PRESSURE-FAILURE DEVICES & OXYGEN FLUSH VALVES

While the nitrous oxide and air lines directly connect with the flowmeters, the oxygen line passes by pressure-failure devices, the oxygen flush valve, and the ventilator power outlet. If oxygen pressure falls below 25 psig (roughly 50% of normal), a fail-safe valve automatically closes the nitrous oxide and other gas lines to prevent accidental delivery of a hypoxic mixture to the patient (Figure 4–3). In addition, a gas whistle or electric alarm sounds. It must be stressed that only an oxygen pressure failure triggers these safety devices, ie, they do *not* protect against other possible causes of hypoxic accidents.

The oxygen flush valve provides a high flow (35–75 L/min) of oxygen directly to the common gas outlet, bypassing the flowmeters and vaporizers. Because oxygen is supplied at a line pressure of 45–55 psig, there is a real potential of lung barotrauma. For this reason, the flush valve must be used cautiously whenever a patient is

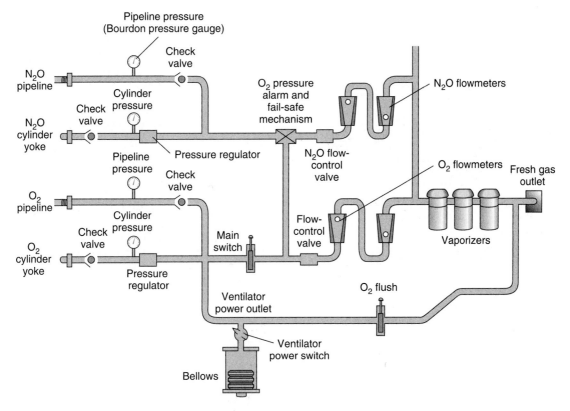

Figure 4–2. Simplified internal schematic of an anesthesia machine.

connected to the breathing circuit. A protective rim limits the possibility of unintentional activation.

FLOW-CONTROL VALVES, FLOWMETERS, & ELECTRONIC FLOW

Gas flows continuously from the anesthesia machine to the breathing circuit. The gas flow rate is determined by **flow-control valves** and is measured by **flowmeters.**

When the knob of the flow-control valve is turned counterclockwise, a pin is disengaged from its seat, allowing gas to flow through the valve (Figure 4–4). Stops in the full-off and full-on positions prevent valve damage. Touch- and color-coded control knobs make it harder to turn off or on the wrong gas (Figure 4–5).

The flowmeters on anesthesia machines are classified as constant-pressure variable-orifice flowmeters. An indicator ball, bobbin, or float is supported by the flow of gas through a tube (Thorpe tube) whose bore (orifice) is tapered. Near the bottom of the tube, where the diameter is small, a low flow of gas will create sufficient pressure under the bobbin to raise it in the tube. As the

bobbin rises, the orifice of the tube widens, allowing more gas to pass around the bobbin. The bobbin will stop rising when its weight is just supported by the difference in pressure between the top and the bottom of the bobbin. If flow is increased, the pressure under the bobbin increases, raising the bobbin higher in the tube until the pressure drop again just supports the bobbin's weight. This pressure drop is constant regardless of the flow rate or the position in the tube and depends on the weight of the bobbin and its cross-sectional area. Stated another way, the higher the bobbin rises in the tube, the larger the tube's orifice and the greater the gas flow required to maintain a constant pressure drop.

Flowmeters are calibrated for specific gases, since the flow rate across a constriction depends on the gas's viscosity at low laminar flows and its density at high turbulent flows. To minimize the effect of friction between the tube's wall and the bobbin, floats are designed to rotate constantly, which keeps them centered in the tube. The effect of static electricity is reduced by coating the tube's interior with a conductive substance that grounds the system. Causes of flowmeter

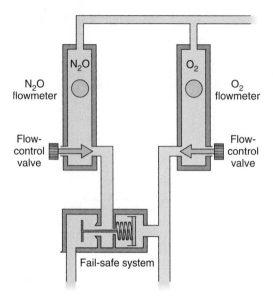

Figure 4–3. The fail-safe system controls the gas in its associated gas line in response to the pressure in the oxygen line. Its safety potential is limited. For example, it will permit the administration of hypoxic gas mixtures when the gas flow is erroneously composed so as not to contain a sufficient oxygen concentration, the oxygen flow control valve is accidentally adjusted downward, or the oxygen piping system contains a gas other than oxygen.

malfunction include dirt in the flow tube, less than perfectly vertical tube alignment, and sticking or concealment of a float at the top of a tube.

Should a leak develop within or downstream from an oxygen flowmeter, a hypoxic gas mixture might be delivered to the patient. To reduce this risk, oxygen flowmeters should be positioned downstream (nearest the outlet) from the other medical gas flowmeters. Not all flowmeters are constant-pressure devices. An adaptation of the Bourdon pressure gauge is commonly used to measure flow rates from free-standing gas cylinders. This device measures the pressure drop across a fixed orifice; it is proportional to the square of the flow rate. **Fixed-orifice flowmeters** are inaccurate if the flow is occluded or the flow rate is low.

Some newer anesthesia machines offer electronic gas delivery. The amount of pressure drop caused by a flow restrictor is the basis for measurement of gas flow rate in these systems. Oxygen and nitrous oxide (or air) each have an electrical flow measurement device in the flow control section before they are mixed together.

SPIROMETERS & BREATHING-CIRCUIT PRESSURE GAUGES

The tidal volume intermittently delivered to the patient from the breathing circuit is measured by a **spirometer,** or **respirometer.** The pneumotachograph is a type of fixed-orifice flowmeter that functions as a spirometer. A baffle chamber provides a slight resistance to airflow. The pressure drop across this resistance is sensed by a differential pressure transducer and is proportional to the flow rate. Tidal volumes are derived by integrating the flow rates. Inaccuracies due to water condensation and temperature changes limit the clinical usefulness of this device.

The **Wright respirometer,** located in the expiratory limb of the breathing tubes in front of the expiratory valve, also measures exhaled tidal volumes (Figure 4–6). The flow of gas across vanes or rotators within the respirometer causes their rotation, which is measured electronically, photoelectrically, or mechanically. Many

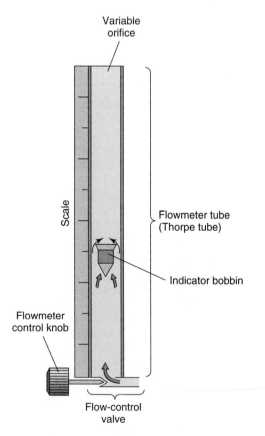

Figure 4–4. A constant-pressure variable orifice flowmeter (Thorpe type).

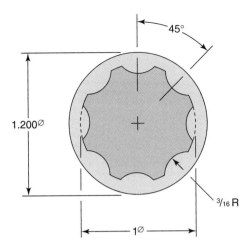

Figure 4–5. The touch-coded knob for the oxygen flow control valve reduces the possibility of operator error.

spirometers on anesthesia machines use this turbine principle to measure minute ventilation and tidal volume. Changes in exhaled tidal volumes usually represent changes in ventilator settings but can also be due to circuit leaks, disconnections, or ventilator malfunction. The Wright respirometer is prone to errors caused by inertia, friction, and water condensation. Furthermore, the measurement of exhaled tidal volumes includes gas that has been lost to the circuit in the form of gas compression and breathing tube expansion. This difference between the volume of gas delivered to the circuit and the volume of gas actually reaching the pa-

tient becomes significant with long compliant breathing tubes, rapid respiratory rates, and high airway pressures.

Newer spirometers address some of these inaccuracies with more sophisticated technologies. Some (eg, D-lite and Pedi-lite sensors) measure spirometry by using two Pitot tubes at the "y" connection. Gas flowing through the sensor creates a pressure difference between the Pitot tubes. This pressure differential is used to measure flow, direction (ie, inspiration versus expiration) and airway pressure. Respiratory gas is continuously sampled to correct the flow reading for changes in density and viscosity.

Other systems use two flow sensors. One sensor measures flow at the inspiratory port of the breathing system, and the other measures flow at the expiratory port. These sensors use a change in internal diameter to generate a pressure drop that is proportional to the flow through the sensor. Clear tubes connect the sensors to differential pressure transducers inside the anesthesia machine.

A **breathing-circuit pressure gauge** usually measures pressure somewhere between the expiratory and inspiratory unidirectional valves, the exact location depends on the model of anesthesia machine. Breathing-circuit pressure usually reflects airway pressure. A rise in airway pressure may signal worsening pulmonary compliance, an increase in tidal volume, or an obstruction in the breathing circuit. A drop in pressure may indicate an improvement in compliance, a decrease in tidal volume, or a leak in the circuit. If circuit pressure is being measured at the CO_2 absorber, however, it will not always mirror the pressure in the patient's airway. For exam-

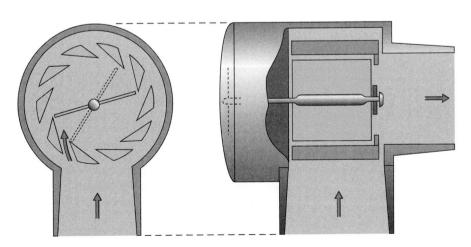

Figure 4–6. The Wright respirometer. (Reproduced, with permission, from Moshin WW et al: *Automatic Ventilation of the Lungs,* 2nd ed. Blackwell, 1969.)

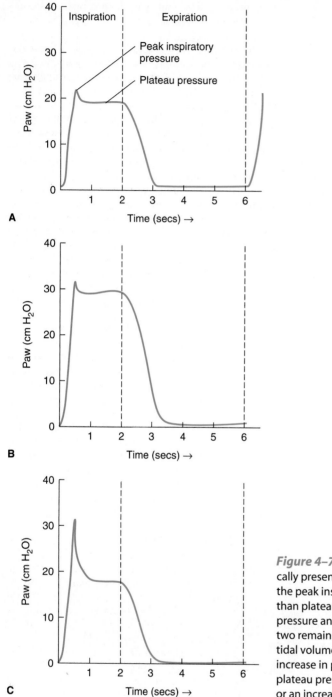

Figure 4–7. Airway pressures (Paw) can be diagrammatically presented as a function of time. **A:** In normal persons, the peak inspiratory pressure is equal to or slightly greater than plateau pressure. **B:** An increase in peak inspiratory pressure and plateau pressure (the difference between the two remains almost constant) can be due to an increase in tidal volume or decrease in pulmonary compliance. **C:** An increase in peak inspiratory pressure with little change in plateau pressure signals an increase in inspiratory flow rate or an increase in airway resistance.

ple, clamping the expiratory limb of the breathing tubes during exhalation will prevent the patient's breath from exiting the lungs. Despite this buildup in airway pressure, a pressure gauge at the absorber will read zero because of the intervening one-way valve.

Some anesthesia machines graphically display breathing-circuit pressure (Figure 4–7). **Peak inspiratory pressure** is the highest circuit pressure generated during an inspiratory cycle, and provides an indication of **dynamic compliance. Plateau pressure** is the pressure measured during an inspiratory pause (a time of no gas flow), and mirrors **static compliance.** During normal ventilation of a patient without lung disease, peak inspiratory pressure is equal to or only slightly greater than plateau pressure. An increase in both peak inspiratory pressure and plateau pressure implies an increase in tidal volume or a decrease in pulmonary compliance. An increase in peak inspiratory pressure without any change in plateau pressure signals an increase in airway resistance or inspiratory gas flow rate (Table 4–1). Thus, the shape of the breathing-circuit pressure waveform can provide important airway information. Airway secretions or kinking of the endotracheal tube can be easily ruled out with the use of a suction catheter. Flexible fiberoptic bronchoscopy will usually provide a definitive diagnosis.

Table 4–1. Causes of increased peak inspiratory pressure (PIP), with or without an increased plateau pressure (PP)

Increased PIP and PP
Increased tidal volume
Decreased pulmonary compliance
Pulmonary edema
Trendelenburg position
Pleural effusion
Ascites
Abdominal packing
Peritoneal gas insufflation
Tension pneumothorax
Endobronchial intubation
Increased PIP and Unchanged PP
Increased inspiratory gas flow rate
Increased airway resistance
Kinked endotracheal tube
Bronchospasm
Secretions
Foreign body aspiration
Airway compression
Endotracheal tube cuff herniation

VAPORIZERS

Volatile anesthetics (eg, halothane, isoflurane, enflurane, desflurane, sevoflurane) are vaporized before being delivered to the patient. At a given temperature, the molecules of a volatile agent in a closed container are distributed between the liquid and gaseous phases. The gas molecules bombard the walls of the container, creating the vapor pressure of that agent. The higher the temperature, the greater the tendency for the liquid molecules to escape into the gaseous phase and the higher the vapor pressure. Vaporization requires energy (the **heat of vaporization**), which is supplied as a loss of heat from the liquid. As vaporization proceeds, liquid temperature drops and vapor pressure decreases unless heat is readily available to enter the system.

Vaporizers contain a chamber in which a carrier gas becomes saturated with the volatile agent. Although many vaporizer models are available, only three representative models are examined in this chapter. In **copper kettle vaporizers,** the amount of carrier gas (oxygen) bubbled through the anesthetic is determined by a dedicated Thorpe tube flowmeter (Figure 4–8). A vaporizer-circuit flow-control valve separates the vaporizer circuit from the standard oxygen and nitrous oxide flowmeters. This valve should be off when the vaporizer circuit is not in use to prevent leakage and back-flushing of gas. Copper is used as the construction metal because its relatively high specific heat (the quantity of heat required to raise the temperature of 1 g of substance by 1 °C) and thermal conductivity (the speed of heat conductance through a substance) enhance the vaporizer's ability to maintain a constant temperature. Copper kettle vaporizers are rarely used in the United States today; they are principally used for veterinarian anesthesia. However, understanding how these vaporizers function provides a valuable insight into the delivery of volatile anesthetics.

All the gas entering the vaporizer passes through the anesthetic liquid and becomes saturated with vapor. One mL of liquid anesthetic is the equivalent of approximately 200 mL of anesthetic vapor. Because the vapor pressure of volatile anesthetics is greater than the partial pressure required for anesthesia, the saturated gas leaving a copper kettle must be diluted before it reaches the patient.

For example, the vapor pressure of halothane is 243 mm Hg at 20 °C, so the concentration of halothane exiting a copper kettle at 1 atmosphere is 243/760, or 32%. If 100 mL of oxygen enters the kettle, roughly 150 mL of gas will exit, one-third of which is halothane vapor. In contrast, a partial pressure of only 7 mm Hg—or less than 1% concentration (7/760) at 1 atm—may be required for anesthesia. To deliver a 1% con-

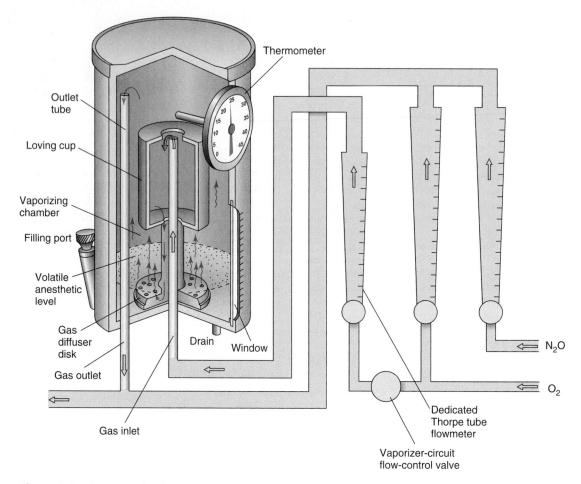

Figure 4–8. The copper kettle vaporizer. (Redrawn and reproduced, with permission, from Hill DW: *Physics Applied to Anaesthesia,* 4th ed. Butterworth, 1980.)

centration of halothane, the 50 mL of halothane vapor and 100 mL of carrier gas that are leaving the copper kettle would have to be diluted with another 4850 mL of gas (5000 − 150 = 4850). As can be seen from this example, every 100 mL of oxygen passing through a halothane vaporizer translates into a 1% increase in concentration if total gas flow into the breathing circuit is 5 L/min. Since flow through this vaporizer determines the ultimate concentration of anesthetic, the copper kettle is classified as a **measured-flow vaporizer** (or flowmeter-controlled vaporizer). Isoflurane has an almost identical vapor pressure, so the same relationship between copper kettle flow, total gas flow, and anesthetic concentration exists.

On the other hand, enflurane has a vapor pressure of 175 mm Hg at 20 °C. Saturated gas leaving a copper kettle filled with enflurane at sea level has a concentration of 175/760, or 23%. Stated another way, 100 mL of oxygen will pick up 30 mL of enflurane vapor (30/130 = 23%). Thus, every 100 mL of oxygen passing through a copper kettle vaporizer filled with enflurane translates into a 1% increase in concentration if total gas flow into the breathing circuit is 3 L/min (30/3000 = 1%).

In general, the amount of vapor leaving a copper kettle depends on the vapor pressure of the anesthetic agent (VP), the flow rate of the carrier gas to the vaporizer (CG), and the barometric pressure (BP):

$$\text{Vapor output} = \frac{CG \times VP}{BP - VP}$$

For the enflurane example:

$$\text{Vapor output} = \frac{(100 \text{ mL/min})(175 \text{ mm Hg})}{(760 \text{ mm Hg} - 175 \text{ mm Hg})} = 30 \text{ mL/min}$$

The percentage of anesthetic concentration is found by dividing vapor output by total gas flow into the circuit:

$$\text{Anesthetic concentration} = \frac{30 \text{ mL/min vapor output}}{3000 \text{ mL/min total gas flow}} = 1\%$$

If total gas flow falls unexpectedly (eg, exhaustion of a nitrous oxide cylinder), volatile anesthetic concentration will rise to potentially dangerous levels.

Because of the severe consequences of overdoses, it is essential to titrate the delivered concentration of anesthetic accurately. **Agent-specific vaporizers** are capable of delivering a constant concentration of agent regardless of temperature changes or flow through the vaporizer. Merely turning a single calibrated control knob counterclockwise (clockwise in some older units) to the desired percentage divides the total gas flow into carrier gas, which flows over liquid anesthetic in a vaporizing chamber, and the balance, which exits the vaporizer unchanged (Figure 4–9). Because some of the entering gas is never exposed to anesthetic liquid, the agent-specific vaporizer is also known as a **variable-bypass vaporizer.**

Temperature compensation is achieved by a strip composed of two different metals welded together. Altering flow rates within a wide range does not affect anesthetic concentration because the same proportion of gas is exposed to the liquid. Changing the gas composition, however, from 100% oxygen to 70% nitrous oxide may transiently decrease volatile anesthetic concentration owing to the greater solubility of nitrous oxide in volatile agents.

These vaporizers are agent-specific, and filling with the wrong anesthetic must be avoided. For example, unintentionally filling an enflurane-specific vaporizer with halothane could lead to an anesthetic overdose: First, halothane's higher vapor pressure (243 mm Hg versus 175 mm Hg) will cause a 40% greater amount of anesthetic vapor to be released. Second, halothane is more than twice as potent as enflurane (see Chapter 7). Conversely, filling

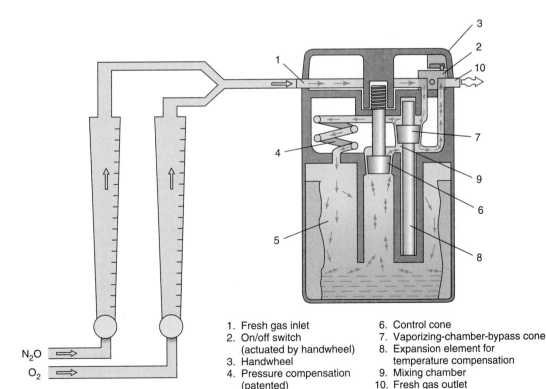

1. Fresh gas inlet
2. On/off switch (actuated by handwheel)
3. Handwheel
4. Pressure compensation (patented)
5. Vaporizing chamber
6. Control cone
7. Vaporizing-chamber-bypass cone
8. Expansion element for temperature compensation
9. Mixing chamber
10. Fresh gas outlet

N₂O

O₂

Figure 4–9. Agent-specific variable-bypass vaporizer.

a halothane vaporizer with enflurane will cause an anesthetic underdose.

Excessive tilting of the vaporizer may flood the bypass area and lead to dangerously high anesthetic concentrations. Fluctuations in pressure from positive pressure ventilation may cause a reversed flow through the vaporizer, unpredictably changing agent delivery. This "pumping effect" is more pronounced with low gas flows. Design modifications in newer units limit the possibility of some of these problems. These vaporizers automatically compensate for changes in ambient pressures (ie, altitude changes).

Desflurane's vapor pressure is so high that it almost boils at room temperature at sea level (see Table 7–3). This volatility, coupled with a potency only one-fifth that of other volatile agents, presents unique delivery problems. First, the vaporization required for general anesthesia produces a cooling effect that would overwhelm the ability of conventional vaporizers to maintain a constant temperature. Second, because it vaporizes so extensively, a tremendously high fresh gas flow would be necessary to dilute the carrier gas to clinically relevant concentrations. These problems have been addressed by the development of a special desflurane vaporizer, the Tec 6 (a heated blender vaporizer). The complexities inherent in this vaporizer's design resulted in the recall of some early models due to delivery of excessive desflurane concentrations. A reservoir containing desflurane (desflurane sump) is electrically heated to 39 °C creating a vapor pressure of 2 atmospheres. Unlike a variable-bypass vaporizer, no fresh gas flows through the desflurane sump. Rather, pure desflurane vapor joins the fresh gas mixture before exiting the vaporizer. The amount of desflurane vapor released from the sump depends on the concentration selected by turning the control dial and the fresh gas flow rate. Although the Tec 6 maintains a constant desflurane concentration over a wide range of fresh gas flow rates, it cannot automatically compensate for changes in elevation. Decreased ambient pressure does not affect the concentration of agent delivered, but decreases the partial pressure of the agent. Thus, at high elevations, the anesthesiologist must manually increase the concentration control dial to attain the desired anesthetic partial pressure.

Variable-bypass vaporizers should be located outside the circle system, between the flowmeters and the common gas outlet, to lessen the likelihood of concentration surges during use of the oxygen flush valve. An interlock or exclusion device prevents the concurrent use of more than one vaporizer. Older machines without this safety feature should have the vaporizers arranged in a specific order to lessen the risk of agent cross-contamination if two vaporizers are on simultaneously. Based on vapor pressures and potency, the following order (from upstream to downstream) is recommended: desflurane, methoxyflurane, enflurane, sevoflurane, isoflurane, halothane.

Electronically controlled vaporizers that can be integrated with an electronic flow-control (see above) are now available. Gas flow from the flow-control is divided into bypass flow and liquid chamber flow (Figure 4–10A). The latter is conducted into an agent-specific cassette (Aladin cassette) where the volatile anesthetic is vaporized. The cassette itself does not contain any bypass flow channels (Figure 4–10B). Therefore, unlike traditional vaporizers, liquid anesthetic cannot escape during handling and the cassette can be carried in any position. After leaving the cassette, the now anesthetic-saturated liquid chamber flow reunites with the bypass flow before exiting the fresh gas outlet. Adjusting the ratio between the bypass flow and liquid chamber flow changes the concentration of volatile anesthetic agent delivered to the patient. In practice, the clinician changes the concentration by turning the agent wheel, which operates a digital potentiometer. Software sets the desired fresh gas agent concentration according to the number of output pulses from the agent wheel. Sensors in the cassette measure pressure and temperature, thus determining agent concentration in the gas leaving the cassette. Correct liquid chamber flow is calculated based on desired fresh gas concentration and determined cassette gas concentration. Some electronically controlled vaporizers inject liquid anesthetic agent directly into the fresh gas flow (liquid-injector vaporizer).

VENTILATORS & DISCONNECT ALARMS

Ventilators function by creating a pressure gradient between the proximal airway and the alveoli. Older units relied on the generation of negative pressure in the thorax (eg, iron lungs), while modern ventilators develop positive pressure in the upper airway. The ventilatory cycle is divided into four phases: inspiration, the transition from inspiration to expiration, expiration, and the transition from expiration to inspiration. Ventilators are classified on the basis of their functioning during these phases.

During inspiration, mechanical ventilators generate tidal volumes by producing gas flow along a pressure gradient. Either pressure (**constant-pressure generators**) or flow rate (**constant-flow generators**) can remain constant throughout the cycle, regardless of changes in lung mechanics (Figure 4–11). **Nonconstant generators** produce pressures or flow rates that vary during the cycle but remain consistent from breath to breath. For instance, a ventilator that generates a flow pattern resembling a half cycle of a sine wave would be classified as a nonconstant flow generator

A

B

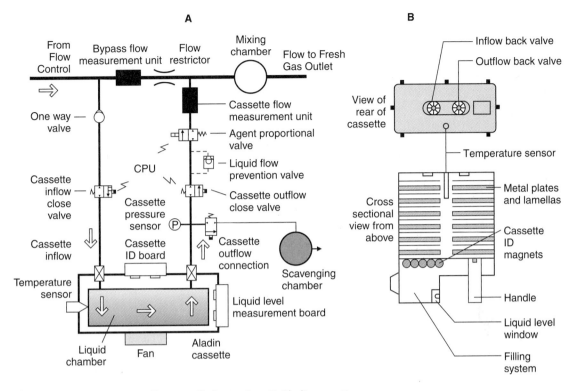

Figure 4–10. **A:** Electronically controlled vaporizer. **B:** Aladin cassette.

(Figure 4–11). An increase in airway resistance or a decrease in lung compliance would increase peak inspiratory pressure but would not alter the flow rate generated by this type of ventilator.

Termination of the inspiratory phase can be triggered by the attainment of a preset limit of time duration, inspiratory pressure, or tidal volume. **Time-cycled ventilators** allow tidal volume and peak inspiratory pressure to vary depending on lung compliance. Tidal volume is adjusted by setting inspiratory duration and inspiratory flow rate (eg, the Airshields ventilator). **Pressure-cycled ventilators** will not cycle from the inspiratory phase to the expiratory phase until a preset pressure is reached. If a large circuit leak decreases peak pressures significantly, a pressure-cycled ventilator may remain in the inspiratory phase indefinitely. On the other hand, a small leak may not markedly decrease tidal volume, because cycling will be delayed until the pressure limit is met. Because of their use of a Venturi jet, pressure-cycled ventilators increase flow at the expense of decreasing inspired oxygen content (eg, the small Bird ventilator models used to deliver intermittent positive pressure breathing [IPPB] therapy). **Volume-cycled ventilators** vary inspiratory duration and pressure in order to deliver a preset volume (there is

usually a safety pressure limit). **Pressure control ventilation** is a pressure-limited, time-cycled mode of positive pressure ventilation characterized by a rapid rise to peak pressure. In this mode, inspiratory flow and tidal volume are optimized for a given set pressure. The use of a decelerating inspiratory flow pattern can potentially improve distribution of gas within the lung. Pressure control ventilation may be delivered with an inverse inspiratory:expiratory ratio (I:E > 1:1). In some patients, this may allow recruitment of alveoli, improving oxygenation and ventilation (see Chapter 50).

The expiratory phase of most ventilators reduces airway pressure to atmospheric levels. Therefore, flow out of the lungs is passive and determined chiefly by airway resistance and lung compliance. Positive end-expiratory pressure can be created by retarding expiratory gas flow. A few older ventilator models were able to generate negative expiratory pressures. This feature is rarely used today because of the potential for premature airway closure.

The next inspiratory phase usually begins after a preset time interval (**controlled ventilation**), but in some machines it can be triggered by a negative pressure generated by the patient (**assisted ventilation). Intermittent mandatory ventilation (IMV)** allows patients to

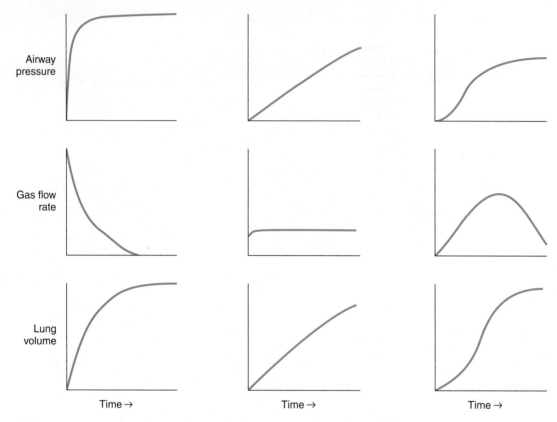

Airway pressure

Gas flow rate

Lung volume

Time →   Time →   Time →

Figure 4–11. Pressure, volume, and flow profiles of different types of ventilators.

breathe spontaneously between controlled breaths. In contrast to assisted and controlled ventilation, the patient receiving IMV does not necessarily receive the preset tidal volume during the spontaneous breaths. **Synchronized intermittent mandatory ventilation (SIMV)** helps prevent "fighting the ventilator" by providing mandatory breaths when the patient initiates spontaneous ventilation. Mechanical ventilation and modes of positive pressure ventilation (see Table 50–3 and Figure 50–1) are discussed in greater detail in Chapter 50.

There are structural similarities in many different types of ventilators used in anesthesiology. Tidal volume is delivered from a bellows assembly that consists of a rubber bellows and its clear plastic enclosure. A **standing (ascending) bellows** is preferred since it draws attention to a circuit disconnection by collapsing (Figure 4–12). In contrast, a **hanging (descending) bellows** continues to fill by gravity even though it is no longer connected to the breathing circuit (Figure 4–12).

The bellows takes the place of the breathing bag in the anesthesia circuit. Pressurized oxygen from the ven-

tilator power outlet (see Figure 4–2) is routed to the space between the inside wall of the enclosure and the outside wall of the bellows. The increased pressure compresses the pleated bellows, forcing the anesthetic gas it contains into the breathing circuit. Therefore, there are two distinct circuits within the ventilator that are separated by the bellows wall: the external high-pressure oxygen circuit that powers the ventilator and an internal extension of the anesthesia breathing circuit.

Oxygen is consumed to power the ventilator at a rate at least equal to minute ventilation. Thus, if oxygen fresh gas flow is 2 L/min and a ventilator is delivering 6 L/min to the circuit, a total of at least 8 L/min of oxygen is being consumed. This should be kept in mind if the hospital's medical gas system fails and cylinder oxygen is required.

An electronic control box enables modern anesthesia ventilators to deliver a wide range of tidal volumes, peak inspiratory pressures, respiratory rates, inspiratory pauses, inspiratory-to-expiratory ratios, intermittent sighs, and positive end-expiratory pressures. These ven-

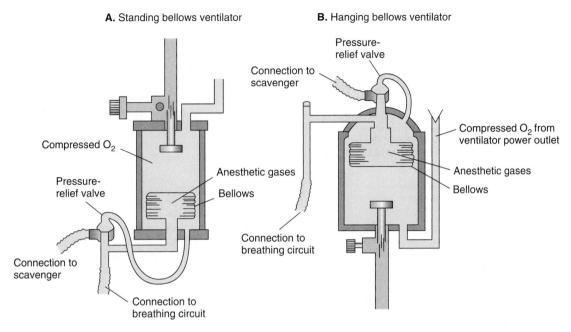

A. Standing bellows ventilator

B. Hanging bellows ventilator

Figure 4–12. Two types of bellows are available on anesthesia ventilators. Standing bellows (**A**) collapse if there is a leak greater than the fresh gas flow, while hanging bellows (**B**) refill and continue to cycle. Shading indicates the external high-pressure oxygen circuit that powers the ventilator and closes the pressure-relief valve during inspiration. The unshaded gases in the bellows are part of the anesthetic breathing circuit.

tilators require compressed oxygen to power the bellows and electricity (often with battery backup) to power the control box.

Alarms should be an integral part of all anesthesia ventilators. Whenever a ventilator is used, a **disconnect alarm** must be activated. Breathing-circuit disconnection, a leading cause of anesthetic accidents, is detected by a drop in peak circuit pressure. Other useful ventilator alarms signal excessive airway pressure, low oxygen-supply pressure, and the ventilator's inability to deliver the desired minute ventilation.

Whenever a ventilator is used, the circle system's pressure-relief valve should be closed or functionally removed from the circuit. Ventilators commonly used in anesthesia contain their own pressure-relief valves that remain closed during inspiration so that positive pressure can be generated. When the ventilator bellows are refilled during expiration, circuit pressure rises and the ventilator's pressure-relief valve opens. Sticking of this valve results in abnormally elevated airway pressure. In contrast, if the breathing circuit's pressure-relief valve is not fully closed or is not functionally removed from the system, airway pressures may be inadequate to ventilate the patient.

Because the ventilator's pressure-relief valve is closed during inspiration, the circuit's fresh gas flows contribute to the tidal volume delivered to the patient. For example, if the fresh gas flow is 6 L/min, the inspiratory-to-expiratory ratio is 1:2, and the respiratory rate is 10 breaths/min, each tidal volume will include 200 mL in addition to the ventilator's output:

$$\frac{(6000 \text{ mL/min}) (33\%)}{10 \text{ breaths/min}} \approx 200 \text{ mL/breath}$$

Thus, increasing fresh gas flow increases minute ventilation. Likewise, the use of the oxygen flush valve during the inspiratory cycle of a ventilator must be avoided because the pressure-relief valve is closed and the surge of circuit pressure will be transferred to the patient's lungs.

A leak in the bellows can transmit high oxygen pressure to the patient's airway, perhaps resulting in barotrauma. This may be detected by noticing a higher than expected inspired oxygen concentration. Misconnecting ventilator hoses on the anesthesia machine and the breathing circuit may cause hypoxic brain injury. Other potential problems include electrical failure, flow obstruction, electromagnetic interference, and valve malfunction.

WASTE-GAS SCAVENGERS

Waste-gas scavengers dispose of gases that have been vented from the breathing circuit by a pressure-release valve. Pollution of the operating room environment with anesthetic gases may pose a health hazard to surgical personnel (see Chapter 47). Although it is difficult to define safe levels of exposure, the **National Institute for Occupational Safety and Health (NIOSH)** recommends limiting the room concentration of nitrous oxide to 25 ppm and halogenated agents to 2 ppm (0.5 ppm if nitrous oxide is also being used). Reduction to these trace levels is possible only with properly functioning waste-gas scavenging systems.

To avoid the buildup of pressure, excess gas volume is vented through the pressure-relief valve in the breathing circuit or the ventilator. Both valves should be connected to hoses (transfer tubing) leading to the scavenging interface (Figure 4–13). The outlet of the scavenging system can be a direct line to the outside (**passive scavenging**), a line to the air conditioning system beyond any point of recirculation, or a connection to the hospital's vacuum system (**active scavenging**). The last method is the most reliable but also the most complex. Negative- and positive-pressure relief valves protect the patient from the negative pressure of the vacuum system or positive pressure from an obstruction in the disposal tubing. A reservoir bag accepts waste-gas overflow when the vacuum's capacity is exceeded.

The vacuum control valve should be adjusted to allow the evacuation of 10–15 L of waste gas per minute. This rate is adequate for periods of high fresh gas flow (ie, induction and emergence) yet minimizes the risk of transmitting negative pressure to the breathing circuit during lower flow conditions (maintenance).

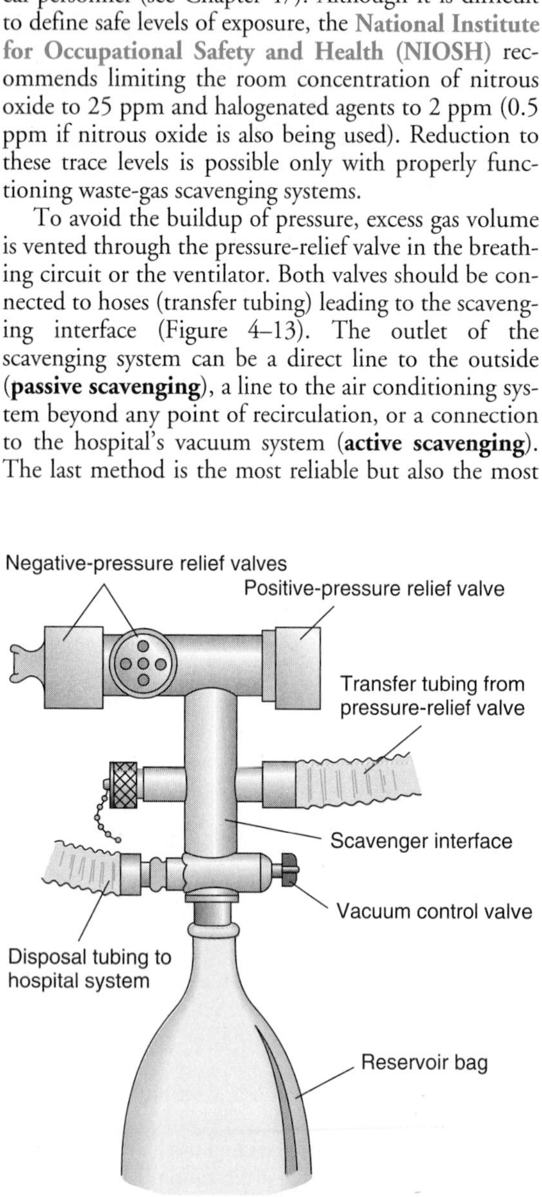

HUMIDIFIERS & NEBULIZERS

Relative humidity is the ratio of the mass of water present in a volume of gas (**absolute humidity**) to the maximum amount of water possible at a particular temperature. Inhaled gases are normally warmed to body temperature and saturated with water by the upper respiratory tract (100% relative humidity = 44 mg H_2O/L at 37 °C). Endotracheal intubation and high fresh gas flows bypass this normal humidification system and expose the lower airways to dry (< 10 mg H_2O/L), room temperature gases.

Humidification of gases by the lower respiratory tract leads to dehydration of mucosa, altered ciliary function, inspissation of secretions, and even ventilation/perfusion mismatching from atelectasis. Body heat is lost during ventilation in order to warm and, more important, to humidify dry gases. (The heat of vaporization of water = 560 cal/g of water vaporized.)

Humidifiers added to the breathing circuit minimize water and heat loss. The simplest designs are the **condenser humidifier** and the **heat and moisture exchanger** (Figure 4–14). These passive devices do not add heat or vapor but rather contain a hygroscopic material that traps exhaled humidification, which is released upon subsequent inhalation. Depending on the design, they may substantially increase apparatus dead space (more than 60 cc), which can cause significant rebreathing in pediatric patients. Likewise, by increasing breathing-circuit resistance, they increase the work of breathing and should be avoided during spontaneous respirations. Prolonged use has led to tracheostomy tube obstruction in patients with thick secretions. Some condenser humidifiers also act as effective filters that may protect the breathing circuit and anesthesia machine from bacterial or viral cross-contamination. This could be especially important when ventilating patients with respiratory infections or compromised immune systems.

Pass-over or **bubble-through humidifiers** expose gas to a cold or hot water bath. Because increasing temperature increases the capacity of a gas to hold water vapor, water baths heated by a thermostatically controlled element are more effective humidifiers. The haz-

Negative-pressure relief valves

Positive-pressure relief valve

Transfer tubing from pressure-relief valve

Scavenger interface

Vacuum control valve

Disposal tubing to hospital system

Reservoir bag

Figure 4–13. Waste-gas scavenging system.

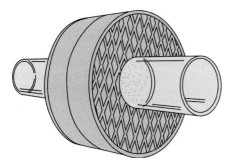

Figure 4–14. The condenser humidifier is an "artificial nose" that attaches between the endotracheal tube and the right-angle connector of the breathing circuit. (Courtesy of Terumo Corp.)

ards of active humidifiers include thermal lung injury (inhaled gas temperature should be monitored), nosocomial infection, increased airway resistance, and an increased likelihood of circuit disconnection. Nonetheless, in cases where the risk of intraoperative hypothermia is unacceptable, these humidifiers effectively provide heat and moisture. These humidifiers are particularly valuable with children since they help prevent both hypothermia and the plugging of small endotracheal tubes by dried secretions. Of course, any design that increases airway dead space should be avoided in pediatric patients. Unlike passive humidifiers, active humidifiers do not filter respiratory gases.

Nebulizers suspend (aerosolize) water particles into a spray. The size of the droplets depends on the method of nebulization: **high-pressure jet nebulizers** produce droplets 5–30 μm in diameter, while **ultrasonic nebulizers** create droplets of 1–10 μm. The former entrains a water stream by the Bernoulli effect (similar to the Venturi effect) and breaks it up with a high-velocity gas jet. Jet nebulizers are often used in recovery rooms to provide an aerosol at room temperature with high water content. Ultrasonic nebulizers are so efficient that they possess the potential for overhydration. Their primary usefulness is for the delivery of bronchodilator drugs to peripheral airways and the mobilization of secretions during respiratory therapy.

OXYGEN ANALYZERS

General anesthesia should never be administered without an oxygen analyzer in the breathing circuit. Oxygen concentration can be measured electrochemically, by paramagnetic analysis, or by mass spectrometry (see Chapter 6). Two electrochemical sensors are available: the **galvanic cell** (a fuel cell) and the **polarographic cell** (a Clark electrode). Both contain cathode and anode electrodes embedded in an electrolyte gel separated from the sample gas by an oxygen-permeable membrane. As oxygen reacts with the electrodes, a current is generated that is proportional to the oxygen partial pressure in the sample gas. The galvanic and polarographic sensors differ in the composition of their electrodes and electrolyte gels. The components of the galvanic cell are capable of providing enough chemical energy so that the reaction does not require an external power source. The differences between galvanic and polarographic sensors are summarized in Table 4–2.

Although the initial cost of the paramagnetic sensor is higher than that of the electrochemical sensors, paramagnetic devices are self-calibrating and have no consumable parts. In addition, their response time is fast enough to differentiate between inspired and expired oxygen concentrations.

All oxygen analyzers should have a low-level alarm that is automatically activated by turning on the analyzer. The sensor should be placed into the inspiratory or expiratory limb of the circle system's breathing circuit—but not into the fresh gas line. As a result of the patient's oxygen consumption, the expiratory limb has a slightly lower oxygen partial pressure than does the inspiratory limb, especially at low fresh gas flows. The increased humidity of expired gas does not significantly affect most modern sensors.

ANESTHESIA MACHINE CHECKOUT LIST

Machine malfunction is a significant cause of anesthesia accidents. A routine inspection of anesthesia equip-

Table 4–2. Comparison of galvanic and polarographic sensors

Property	Galvanic	Polarographic
Anodes	Lead	Silver
Cathodes	Silver or gold	Platinum or gold
Electrolyte solution	KOH	KCl
Cost	Expensive electrodes	Expensive initial cost
Response time	Slow	Fast
Warm-up time	None	A few minutes
Servicing requirements	Sensors	Electrolyte and membranes
Power source	Chemical reaction	Batteries

Table 4–3. Anesthesia Apparatus Checkout Recommendations

This checkout, or a reasonable equivalent, should be conducted before administration of anesthesia. These recommendations are valid only for an anesthesia system that conforms to current and relevant standards and includes an ascending bellows ventilator and at least the following monitors: capnograph, pulse oximeter, oxygen analyzer, respiratory volume monitor (spirometer), and breathing-system pressure monitor with high- and low-pressure alarms. Users are encouraged to modify this guideline to accommodate differences in equipment design and variations in local clinical practice. Such local modifications should have appropriate peer review. Users should refer to the appropriate operator manuals for specific procedures and precautions.

- -

Emergency Ventilation Equipment
*1. Verify backup ventilation equipment is available and functioning

High-Pressure System
*2. Check O_2 cylinder supply
    a. Open O_2 cylinder and verify at least half full (about 1000 psig).
    b. Close cylinder
*3. Check central pipeline supplies; check that hoses are connected and pipeline gauges read about 50 psig.

Low-Pressure System
*4. Check initial status of low-pressure system
    a. Close flow control valves and turn vaporizers off.
    b. Check fill level and tighten vaporizers' filler caps.
*5. Perform leak check of machine low-pressure system
    a. Verify that the machine master switch and flow control valves are off.
    b. Attach suction bulb to common (fresh) gas outlet.
    c. Squeeze bulb repeatedly until fully collapsed.
    d. Verify bulb stays *fully* collapsed for at least 10 seconds
    e. Open one vaporizer at a time and repeat c and d.
    f. Remove suction bulb, and reconnect fresh gas hose.
*6. Turn on machine master switch and all other necessary electrical equipment.
*7. Test flowmeters
    a. Adjust flow of all gases through their full range, checking for smooth operation of floats and undamaged flowtubes.

    b. Attempt to create a hypoxic O_2/N_2O mixture and verify correct changes in flow and/or alarm.

Scavenging System
*8. Adjust and check scavenging system
    a. Ensure proper connections between the scavenging system and both APL (pop-off) valve and ventilator relief valve.
    b. Adjust waste-gas vacuum (if possible).
    c. Fully open APL valve and occlude Y-piece.
    d. With minimum O_2 flow, allow scavenger reservoir bag to collapse completely and verify that absorber pressure gauge reads about zero.
    e. With the O_2 flush activated, allow scavenger reservoir bag to distend fully, and then verify that absorber pressure gauge reads < 10 cm H_2O.

Breathing System
*9. Calibrate O_2 monitor
    a. Ensure monitor reads 21% in room air.
    b. Verify low-O_2 alarm is enabled and functioning.
    c. Reinstall sensor in circuit and flush breathing system with O_2.
    d. Verify that monitor now reads greater than 90%.
10. Check initial status breathing system
    a. Set selector switch to Bag mode.
    b. Check that breathing circuit is complete, undamaged, and unobstructed.

(continued)

---

ment before each use increases operator familiarity and confirms proper functioning. The United States Food and Drug Administration has made available a generic checkout procedure for anesthesia gas machines and breathing systems (Table 4–3). This procedure should be modified as necessary, depending on the specific equipment being used. Note that although the entire checkout does not need to be repeated between cases on the same day, the conscientious use of a checkout list is mandatory before each anesthetic procedure. A mandatory check-off procedure has been demonstrated to increase the likelihood of detecting anesthesia machine faults. Some anesthesia machines provide an automated system check that requires a variable amount of human intervention. These system checks may include nitrous oxide delivery (hypoxic mixture prevention), agent delivery, mechanical and manual ventilation (leak detection), pipeline pressures, scavenging, breathing circuit.

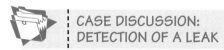

CASE DISCUSSION:
DETECTION OF A LEAK

After induction of general anesthesia and intubation of a 70-kg man for elective surgery, a standing bellows ventilator is set to deliver a tidal volume of 700 mL at a rate of 10 breaths/min. Within a few minutes, the anesthesiologist notices that the bel-

Table 4–3. Anesthesia Apparatus Checkout Recommendations (continued)

c. Verify that CO_2 absorbent is adequate.
d. Install breathing-circuit accessory equipment (eg, humidifier, PEEP valve) to be used during the case.
11. Perform leak check of the breathing system
   a. Set all gas flows to zero (or minimum).
   b. Close APL (pop-off) valve and occlude Y-piece.
   c. Pressurize breathing system to about 30 cm H_2O with O_2 flush.
   d. Ensure that pressure remains fixed for at least 10 seconds.
   e. Open APL (pop-off) valve and ensure that pressure decreases.
 	
Manual and Automatic Ventilation Systems
12. Test ventilation systems and unidirectional valves
   a. Place a second breathing bag on Y-piece.
   b. Set appropriate ventilator parameters for next patient.
   c. Switch to automatic-ventilation (ventilator) mode.
   d. Turn ventilator on and fill bellows and breathing bag with O_2 flush.
   e. Set O_2 flow to minimum, other gas flows to zero.
   f. Verify that during inspiration bellows delivers appropriate tidal volume and that during expiration bellows fills completely.
   g. Set fresh gas flow to about 5 L-min^{-1}.
   h. Verify that the ventilator bellows and simulated lungs fill and empty appropriately without sustained pressure at end expiration.
	i. *Check for proper action of unidirectional valves.*
	j. Exercise breathing circuit accessories to ensure proper function.
	k. Turn ventilator off and switch to manual ventilation (bag/APL) mode.
	l. Ventilate manually and assure inflation and deflation of artificial lungs and appropriate feel of system resistance and compliance.
	m. Remove second breathing bag from Y-piece.
	
	Monitors
	13. Check, calibrate and/or set alarm limits of all monitors: capnograph, pulse oximeter, O_2 analyzer, respiratory-volume monitor (spirometer), pressure monitor with high and low airway-pressure alarms.
	
	Final Position
	14. Check final status of machine
	   a. Vaporizers off
	   b. APL valve open
	   c. Selector switch to Bag mode
	   d. All flowmeters to zero (or minimum)
	   e. Patient suction level adequate
	   f. Breathing system ready to use

*If an anesthesia provider uses the same machine in successive cases, these steps need not be repeated, or they can be abbreviated after the initial checkout. Adapted from http://www.fda.gov/cdrh/humfac/anesckot.html

lows fails to rise to the top of its clear plastic enclosure during expiration. Shortly thereafter, the disconnect alarm is triggered.

Why has the ventilator bellows fallen and the disconnect alarm sounded?

Fresh gas flow into the breathing circuit is inadequate to maintain the circuit volume required for positive pressure ventilation. In a situation of no fresh gas flow, the volume in the breathing circuit will slowly fall because of the constant uptake of oxygen by the patient (metabolic oxygen consumption) and absorption of expired CO_2. An absence of fresh gas flow could be due to exhaustion of the hospital's oxygen supply (remember the function of the fail-safe valve) or failure to turn on the anesthesia machine's flow-control valves. These possibilities can be ruled out by examining the oxygen Bourdon pressure gauge and the flowmeters. A more likely explanation is a gas leak that exceeds the rate of fresh gas flow. Leaks are particularly important in closed-circuit anesthesia (see Case Discussion, Chapter 7).

How can the size of the leak be estimated?

When the rate of fresh gas inflow equals the rate of gas outflow, the circuit's volume will be maintained. Therefore, the size of the leak can be estimated by increasing fresh gas flows until there is no change in the height of the bellows from one expiration to the next. If the bellows collapses despite a high rate of fresh gas inflow, a complete circuit disconnection should be considered. The site of the disconnection must be determined immediately and repaired to prevent hypoxia and hypercapnia. A resuscitation bag can be used to ventilate the patient if there is a delay in correcting the situation.

Where are the most likely locations of a breathing-circuit disconnection or leak?

Frank disconnections occur most frequently between the right-angle connector and the endo-

tracheal tube, while leaks are most commonly traced to the base plate of the CO_2 absorber. In the intubated patient, leaks often occur in the trachea around an uncuffed endotracheal tube or an inadequately filled cuff. There are numerous potential sites of disconnection or leak within the anesthesia machine and the breathing circuit, however. Every addition to the breathing circuit, such as a humidifier, increases the likelihood of a leak.

How can these leaks be detected?

Leaks can be conceptualized as occurring before the fresh gas outlet (ie, within the anesthesia machine) or after the fresh gas inlet (ie, within the breathing circuit). Large leaks within the anesthesia machine are less common and can be ruled out by a simple test. Pinching the tubing that connects the machine's fresh gas outlet to the circuit's fresh gas inlet creates a back pressure that obstructs the forward flow of fresh gas from the anesthesia machine. This is indicated by a drop in the height of the flowmeter bobbins. When the fresh-gas tubing is released, the bobbins should briskly rebound and settle at their original height. If there is a substantial leak within the machine, obstructing the fresh gas tubing will not result in any back pressure, and the bobbins will not drop. A more sensitive test for small leaks occurring before the fresh gas outlet involves attaching a suction bulb at the outlet as described in step 5 of Table 4–3. Correcting a leak within the machine usually requires removing it from service.

Leaks within a breathing circuit not connected to a patient are readily detected by closing the pressure-relief valve, occluding the Y-piece, and activating the oxygen flush until the circuit reaches a pressure of 20–30 cm H_2O. A gradual decline in circuit pressure indicates a leak within the breathing circuit (Table 4–3, step 11).

How are leaks in the breathing circuit located?

Any connection within the breathing circuit is a potential site of a gas leak. A quick survey of the circuit may reveal a loosely attached breathing tube or a cracked oxygen analyzer adaptor. Less obvious causes include detachment of the tubing used by the disconnect alarm to monitor circuit pressures, an open pressure-relief valve, or an improperly adjusted scavenging unit. Leaks can usually be identified audibly or by applying a soap solution to suspect connections and looking for bubble formation.

Leaks within the anesthesia machine and breathing circuit are usually detectable if the machine and circuit have undergone an established checkout procedure. For example, steps 5 and 11 of the FDA recommendations (Table 4–3) will reveal most significant leaks.

SUGGESTED READING

Block FE, Schaff C: Auditory alarms during anesthesia monitoring with an integrated monitoring system. Int J Clin Monit Comput 1996;13:81.

Dorsch JA, Dorsch SE: *Understanding Anesthesia Equipment,* 4th ed. Lippincott Williams & Wilkins, 1999. The anesthesia machine is covered in many chapters of this classic reference.

Ehrenwerth J, Eisenkraft JB (editors): *Anesthesia Equipment—Principles and Applications.* Mosby Year Book, 1993. A review of anesthesia machines and monitoring equipment.

Eisenkraft JB, Leibowitz AB: Ventilators in the operating room. Int Anesthesiol Clin 1997;35:87.

Healthcare Product Comparison System (HPCS), published by ECRI (a nonprofit agency), August 1999, p1-24. This report compares several models of anesthesia machines and includes an excellent overview of machine components and reported problems (including recalls).

Groves J, Edwards N, Carr B: The use of a visual aid to check anaesthetic machines: Is performance improved? Anaesthesia 1994;49:122. This study demonstrates the advantages of a mandatory check-off procedure.

Klopfenstein CE, Van Gessel E, Forster A: Checking the anaesthetic machine: Self-reported assessment in a university hospital. Eur J Anaesthesiol 1998;15:314. Compliance with recommended safety checklists is low.

McMahon DJ: A synopsis of current anesthesia machine design. Biomed Instru Technol 1991;25:190.

Somprakit P, Soontranan P: Low pressure leakage in anaesthetic machines: Evaluation by positive and negative pressure tests. Anaesthesia 1996;51:461.

KEY CONCEPTS

 Improper face mask technique can result in continued deflation of the breathing bag when the pressure relief valve is closed, usually indicating a substantial leak around the mask. In contrast, the generation of high breathing-circuit pressures with minimal chest movement and breath sounds implies an obstructed airway.

 The laryngeal mask partially protects the larynx from pharyngeal secretions but not gastric regurgitation, and it should remain in place until the patient has regained airway reflexes.

 The Combitube should be avoided in patients with an intact gag reflex, esophageal pathology, or a history of caustic substance ingestion.

 After insertion of an endotracheal tube (ETT), the cuff is inflated with the least amount of air necessary to create a seal during positive pressure ventilation in order to minimize the pressure transmitted to the tracheal mucosa.

 Although the persistent detection of CO_2 by a capnograph is the best confirmation of tracheal placement of an ETT, it cannot exclude endobronchial intubation. The earliest manifestation of endobronchial intubation is an increase in peak inspiratory pressure.

 The cuff should not be felt above the level of the cricoid cartilage, because a prolonged intralaryngeal location may result in postoperative hoarseness and increases the risk of accidental extubation.

 Preventing unintentional esophageal intubation depends on direct visualization of the tip of the ETT passing through the vocal cords, careful auscultation for the presence of bilateral breath sounds and the absence of gastric gurgling, analysis of exhaled gas for the presence of CO_2 (the most reliable method), chest radiography, or use of fiberoptic bronchoscopy.

 Clues to the diagnosis of endobronchial intubation include unilateral breath sounds, unexpected hypoxia with pulse oximetry (unreliable with high inspired oxygen concentrations), inability to palpate the ETT cuff in the sternal notch during cuff inflation, and decreased breathing-bag compliance (high peak inspiratory pressures).

 Large negative intrathoracic pressures generated by a patient struggling in laryngospasm can result in development of pulmonary edema even in healthy young adults.

Adept airway management is an essential skill for an anesthesiologist. This chapter reviews the anatomy of the upper respiratory passages, describes the necessary equipment, presents techniques, and discusses complications of laryngoscopy, intubation, and extubation. Patient safety depends on a thorough understanding of each of these topics.

ANATOMY

Successful ventilation, intubation, cricothyrotomy, and regional anesthesia of the larynx require detailed knowledge of airway anatomy. There are two openings to the human airway: the nose, which leads to the **nasopharynx;** and the mouth, which leads to the **oropharynx.**

These passages are separated anteriorly by the palate, but they join posteriorly in the pharynx (Figure 5–1). The pharynx is a U-shaped fibromuscular structure that extends from the base of the skull to the cricoid cartilage at the entrance to the esophagus. It opens anteriorly into the nasal cavity, the mouth, and the larynx—the naso-, oro-, and laryngopharynx, respectively. At the base of the tongue, the **epiglottis** functionally separates the oropharynx from the laryngopharynx (or **hypopharynx**). The epiglottis prevents aspiration by covering the glottis—the opening of the larynx—during swallowing. The **larynx** is a cartilaginous skeleton held together by ligaments and muscle. The larynx is composed of nine cartilages (Figure 5–2): **thyroid, cricoid, epiglottic,** and (in pairs) **arytenoid, corniculate, and cuneiform.**

The sensory supply to the upper airway is derived from the cranial nerves (Figure 5–3). The mucous membranes of the nose are innervated by the ophthalmic division (V_1) of the trigeminal nerve anteriorly (**anterior ethmoidal nerve**) and by the maxillary division (V_2) posteriorly (**sphenopalatine nerves**). The **palatine nerves** provide sensory fibers from the trigeminal nerve (V) to the hard and soft palate. The **lingual nerve** (a branch of the mandibular division [V_3] of the trigeminal nerve) and the **glossopharyngeal nerve** (the ninth cranial nerve) provide general sensation to the anterior two-thirds and posterior third of the tongue, respectively. Branches of the **facial nerve** (VII) and **glossopharyngeal nerve** provide the sensation of taste to those areas, respectively. The **glossopharyngeal nerve** also innervates the roof of the pharynx, the tonsils, and the undersurface of the soft palate. The vagus nerve (the tenth cranial nerve) provides sensation to the airway below the epiglottis. The **superior laryngeal branch** of the vagus divides into an **external** (motor) nerve and an **internal** (sensory) **laryngeal nerve** that provides sensory supply to the larynx between the epiglottis and the vocal cords. Another branch of the vagus, the **recurrent laryngeal nerve,** innervates the larynx below the vocal cords and the trachea.

All the muscles confined to the larynx are innervated by the **recurrent laryngeal nerve** except the cricothyroid muscle, which is innervated by the **external (motor) laryngeal nerve.** The posterior cricoarytenoid muscles abduct the vocal cords, while the lateral cricoarytenoid muscles are the principal adductors.

Phonation involves complex simultaneous actions by several laryngeal muscles. Damage to the motor nerves innervating the larynx leads to a spectrum of speech disorders (Table 5–1). Because the superior laryngeal nerve provides only motor innervation to the cricothyroid muscle (by way of the external laryngeal nerve), unilateral denervation causes very subtle clinical findings. Bilateral palsy of the superior laryngeal nerve may result in hoarseness or easy tiring of the voice, but airway control is not jeopardized.

Unilateral paralysis of a recurrent laryngeal nerve results in paralysis of the ipsilateral vocal cord, causing a deterioration in voice quality. Assuming an intact superior laryngeal nerve, *acute* bilateral recurrent laryngeal nerve palsy can result in stridor and respiratory distress because of the remaining unopposed tension of the cricothyroid muscle. Airway problems are less frequent in *chronic* bilateral recurrent laryngeal nerve loss because of the development of various compensatory mechanisms (eg, atrophy of the laryngeal musculature).

Bilateral injury to the vagus nerve affects both the superior and the recurrent laryngeal nerves. Thus, bilateral vagal denervation produces flaccid, midpositioned vocal cords similar to those seen after succinylcholine administration. Although phonation is severely impaired in these patients, airway control is rarely a problem.

The blood supply of the larynx is derived from branches of the carotid arteries, especially the thyroid artery. The cricothyroid artery arises from the superior thyroid artery and crosses the upper cricothyroid membrane, which extends from the cricoid cartilage to

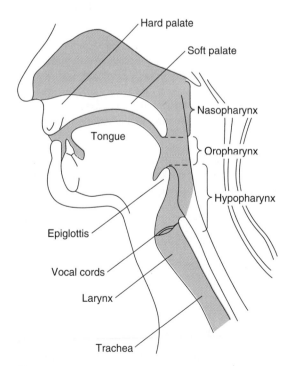

Figure 5–1. Anatomy of the airway.

Hard palate

Soft palate

Nasopharynx

Tongue

Oropharynx

Hypopharynx

Epiglottis

Vocal cords

Larynx

Trachea

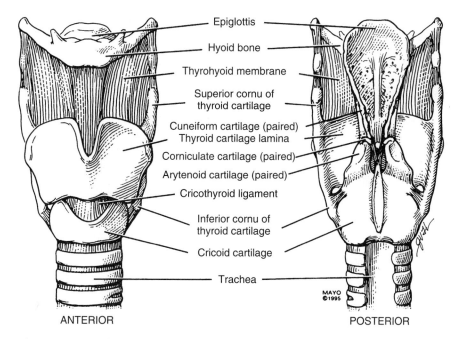

Figure 5–2. Cartilaginous structures comprising the larynx. (Modified and reproduced with permission from Mayo Clinic and Foundation from O'Connell F: Management of the airway and endotracheal intubation. In: Murray MJ, Coursin DB, Pearl RG, Prough DS (editors). *Critical Care Medicine: Perioperative Management.* Lippincott-Raven Publishers, 1997, p 58.)

the thyroid cartilage, in most persons. Oftentimes, the superior thyroid artery is found along the lateral edge of the cricothyroid membrane. When planning a cricothyrotomy, the anatomy of the cricothyroid artery and the thyroid artery should be considered but rarely should affect one's practice. One should stay in the midline, midway between the cricoid and thyroid cartilages.

EQUIPMENT

Oral & Nasal Airways

Loss of upper airway muscle tone (eg, genioglossus muscle) in anesthetized patients allows the tongue and epiglottis to fall back against the posterior wall of the pharynx (Figure 5–4). An artificial airway inserted through the mouth or nose creates an air passage between the tongue and the posterior pharyngeal wall (Figure 5–5). Awake or lightly anesthetized patients may cough or even develop laryngospasm during airway insertion if laryngeal reflexes are intact. Placement of an oral airway is sometimes facilitated by depressing the tongue with a tongue blade. Adult oral airways typically

come in small, 80 mm (Guedel No. 3); medium, 90 mm (Guedel No. 4); and large, 100 mm (Guedel No. 5) sizes.

The length of a nasal airway can be estimated as the distance from the nares to the meatus of the ear, and should be approximately 2 to 4 cm longer than oral airways. Because of the risk of epistaxis, nasal airways should not be used in anticoagulated patients or in children with prominent adenoids. Also, nasal airways should not be used in any patient who has a basilar skull fracture. Any tube inserted through the nose (eg, nasal airways, nasogastric catheters, nasotracheal tubes) should be lubricated and advanced at an angle perpendicular to the face to avoid traumatizing the turbinates or the roof of the nose. Nasal airways are usually better tolerated than oral airways in lightly anesthetized patients.

Face Mask Design & Technique

The use of a face mask can facilitate delivery of an anesthetic gas from a breathing circuit to a patient by creating an airtight seal with the patient's face (Figure 5–6).

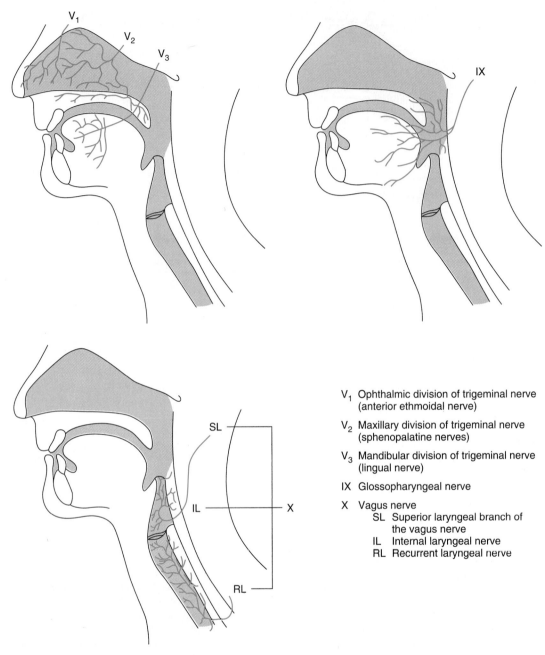

Figure 5–3. Sensory nerve supply of the airway.

The rim of the mask is contoured and conforms to a variety of facial features. The mask's 22-mm orifice attaches to the breathing circuit through a right-angle connector. Several mask designs are available. Transparent masks allow observation of exhaled humidified gas and immediate recognition of vomiting. Black rubber masks are pliable enough to adapt to uncommon facial structures. Retaining hooks surrounding the orifice attach to a head strap so that the mask does not have to be continually held in place by the anesthesiologist. Some pediatric masks are specially designed to minimize apparatus dead space (Figure 5–7).

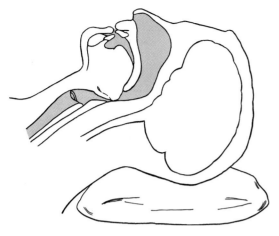

Figure 5–4. Loss of airway muscle tone in an anesthetized patient leads to obstruction.

Table 5–1. The effects of laryngeal nerve injury on the voice.

Nerve	Effect of Nerve Injury
Superior laryngeal nerve	
Unilateral	Minimal effects
Bilateral	Hoarseness, tiring of voice
Recurrent laryngeal nerve	
Unilateral	Hoarseness
Bilateral	
Acute	Stridor, respiratory distress
Chronic	Aphonia
Vagus nerve	
Unilateral	Hoarseness
Bilateral	Aphonia

Effective ventilation requires both a gas-tight mask fit and a patent airway. Continued deflation of the breathing bag when the pressure relief valve is closed usually indicates a substantial leak around the mask. In contrast, the generation of high breathing-circuit pressures with minimal chest movement and breath sounds implies an obstructed airway. Both these problems are usually resolved by proper mask technique.

By holding the mask with the left hand, one can use the right hand to generate positive pressure ventilation by squeezing the breathing bag. The mask is held against the face by downward pressure on the mask body exerted by the left thumb and index finger (Figure 5–8). The middle and ring finger grasp the mandible to facilitate extension of the atlanto-occipital joint. Finger pressure should be placed on the bony mandible and not on the soft tissues supporting the base of the tongue, which may obstruct the airway. The little finger slides under the angle of the jaw and thrusts it anteriorly.

In difficult situations, two hands may be needed to provide adequate jaw thrust and create a mask seal. Therefore, an assistant may be needed to squeeze the breathing bag. In such cases, the thumbs hold the mask down while the fingertips or knuckles displace the jaw forward (Figure 5–9). A ball-valve obstruction during expiration can usually be relieved by releasing the jaw thrust during this phase of the respiratory cycle. It is often difficult to form an adequate mask fit with the

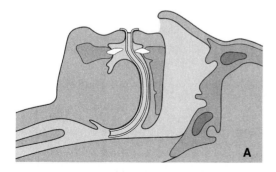
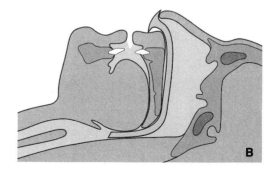

Figure 5–5. **A:** Oropharyngeal airway in place. The airway follows the curvature of the tongue, pulling it and the epiglottis away from the posterior pharyngeal wall and providing a channel for air passage. **B:** The nasopharyngeal airway in place. The airway passes through the nose and extends to just above the epiglottis. (Modified and reproduced with permission from: Face masks and airways. *In:* Dorsch JA, Dorsch SE (eds). *Understanding Anesthesia Equipment,* 4th ed. Williams & Wilkins, 1999, pp 441.)

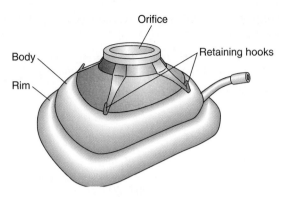

Figure 5–6. An adult face mask.

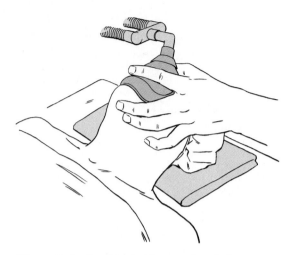

Figure 5–8. One-handed face mask technique.

cheeks of edentulous patients. Leaving dentures in place or packing the buccal cavities with gauze may help. Positive pressure ventilation should normally be limited to 20 cm H_2O to avoid stomach inflation.

Most patients' airways can be maintained with a face mask, an oral or nasal airway, and a face strap. Mask ventilation for long periods may result in pressure injury to branches of the trigeminal or facial nerves. Because of the absence of positive airway pressures during spontaneous ventilation, the latter requires only minimal downward force on the face mask to create an adequate seal. Face mask and face strap position should be regularly changed to prevent ischemic injury. Excessive pressure on the eye and corneal abrasions should be avoided.

Laryngeal Mask Design & Technique

The laryngeal mask airway (LMA) is being increasingly used in place of a face mask or endotracheal tube (ETT) during administration of an anesthetic; to facili-

tate ventilation and passage of an ETT in a patient with a difficult airway; and to aid in ventilation during fiberoptic bronchoscopy (FOB) as well as placement of the bronchoscope.

An LMA consists of a wide-bore tube whose proximal end connects to a breathing circuit with a standard 15-mm connector, and whose distal end is attached to an elliptical cuff that can be inflated through a pilot tube. The deflated cuff is lubricated and inserted

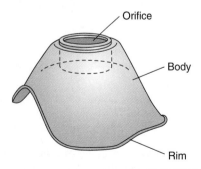

Figure 5–7. The Rendell-Baker-Soucek pediatric face mask has a shallow body and minimal dead space.

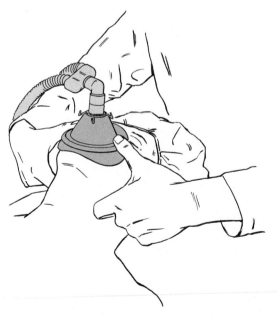

Figure 5–9. A difficult airway can often be managed with a two-handed technique.

blindly into the hypopharynx so that, once inflated, the cuff forms a low-pressure seal around the entrance into the larynx. This requires an anesthetic depth slightly greater than that required for the insertion of an oral airway. Although insertion is relatively simple, proper attention to detail will improve success rate (Table 5–2). An ideally positioned cuff is bordered by the base of the tongue superiorly, the pyriform sinuses laterally, and the upper esophageal sphincter inferiorly (Figure 5–10). Anatomic variations prevent adequate functioning in some patients. If the esophagus lies within the rim of the cuff, gastric distention and regurgitation become a distinct possibility. Because down-folding of the epiglottis or distal cuff account for most failures, LMA insertion under direct visualization with a laryngoscope or FOB may prove beneficial in difficult cases. Likewise, partial cuff inflation prior to insertion may be helpful in some patients. The shaft can be secured with tape, as an ETT would be. The LMA partially protects the larynx from pharyngeal secretions (but *not* gastric regurgitation), and it should remain in place until the patient has regained airway reflexes. This is usually signaled by coughing and mouth opening on command. The reusable LMA, which is autoclavable, is made of silicone rubber (ie, it is latex-free) and is available in many sizes (Table 5–3).

Table 5–2. Successful insertion of laryngeal mask depends upon attention to several details.

1. Choose the appropriate size (Table 5–3) and check for leaks before insertion.
2. The leading edge of the deflated cuff should be wrinkle-free and facing away from the aperture (Figure 5–10A).
3. Lubricate only the back side of the cuff.
4. Ensure adequate anesthesia (regional nerve block or general) before attempting insertion. Propofol with opioids provide superior conditions compared with thiopental.
5. Place patient's head in sniffing position (Figure 5–10B and Figure 5–17).
6. Use your index finger to guide the cuff along the hard palate and down into the hypopharynx until an increased resistance is felt (Figure 5–10C). The longitudinal black line should *always* be pointing directly cephalad (ie, facing the patient's upper lip).
7. Inflate with the correct amount of air (Table 5–3).
8. Ensure adequate anesthetic depth during patient positioning.
9. Obstruction after insertion is usually due to a down-folded epiglottis or transient laryngospasm.
10. Avoid pharyngeal suction, cuff deflation, or laryngeal mask removal until the patient is awake (eg, opening mouth on command).

Table 5–3. A variety of laryngeal masks with different cuff volumes are available for different-sized patients.

Mask Size	Patient Size	Weight (kg)	Cuff Volume (mL)
1	Infant	<6.5	2–4
2	Child	6.5–20	Up to 10
2½	Child	20–30	Up to 15
3	Small adult	>30	Up to 20
4–5	Normal and large adult		Up to 30

The LMA provides an alternative to ventilation through a face mask or ETT (Table 5–4). Contraindications for the LMA include patients with pharyngeal pathology (eg, abscess), pharyngeal obstruction, full stomachs (eg, pregnancy, hiatal hernia), or low pulmonary compliance (eg, obesity) requiring peak inspiratory pressures greater than 20 cm H_2O. Traditionally, the LMA has been avoided in patients with bronchospasm or high airway resistance, but new evidence suggests that because it is not placed in the trachea, use of an LMA is associated with less bronchospasm than an ETT. Although it is clearly not a substitute for endotracheal intubation, the LMA has proven particularly helpful as a temporizing measure in patients with difficult airways (those who cannot be ventilated or intubated) because of its ease of insertion and relatively high success rate (95% to 99%). It has been used as a conduit for an intubating stylet (eg, gum-elastic bougie), ventilating jet stylet, flexible FOB, or small diameter (6.0 mm) ETT. Several LMAs are available that have been modified to facilitate placement of a larger ETT with or without the use of a FOB. Insertion can be performed under topical anesthesia and bilateral superior laryngeal nerve blocks if the airway must be secured while the patient is awake.

Esophageal-Tracheal Combitube
Design & Technique

The esophageal-tracheal Combitube consists of two fused tubes, each with a 15-mm connector on its proximal end (Figure 5–11). The longer blue tube has an occluded distal tip that forces gas to exit through a series of side perforations. The shorter clear tube has an open tip and no side perforations. The Combitube is usually inserted blindly through the mouth and advanced until the two black rings on the shaft lie between the upper and lower teeth. The Combitube has two inflatable cuffs, a 100-cc proximal cuff and a 15-cc distal cuff,

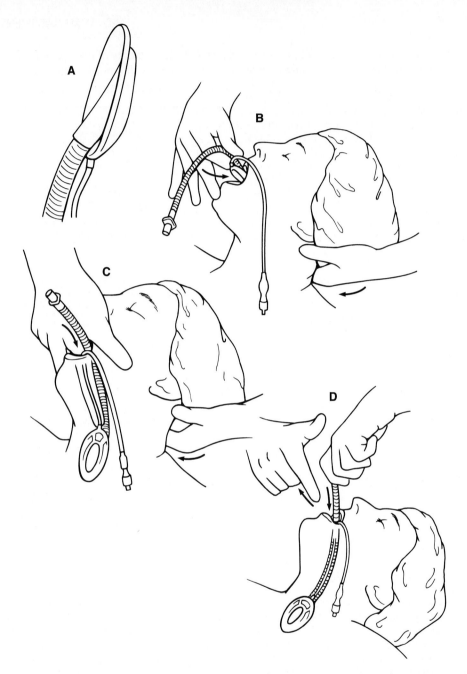

Figure 5–10. **A:** The laryngeal mask ready for insertion. The cuff should be deflated tightly with the rim facing away from the mask aperture. There should be no folds near the tip. **B:** Initial insertion of the laryngeal mask. Under direct vision, the mask tip is pressed upward against the hard palate. The middle finger may be used to push the lower jaw downward. The mask is pressed forward as it is advanced into the pharynx to ensure that the tip remains flattened and avoids the tongue. The jaw should not be held open once the mask is inside the mouth. The nonintubating hand can be used to stabilize the occiput. **C:** By withdrawing the other fingers and with a slight pronation of the forearm, it is usually possible to push the mask fully into position in one fluid movement. Note that the neck is kept flexed and the head extended. **D:** The laryngeal mask is grasped with the other hand and the index finger withdrawn. The hand holding the tube presses gently downward until resistance is encountered. (Reproduced with permission from Gensia Pharmaceuticals.)

Table 5–4. Advantages and disadvantages of the laryngeal mask compared with face mask ventilation or endotracheal intubation.

	Advantages	Disadvantages
Compared with face mask	Hands-free operation Better seal in bearded patients Less cumbersome in ENT surgery Often easier to maintain airway Protects against airway secretions Less facial nerve and eye trauma Less operating room pollution	More invasive More risk of airway trauma Requires new skill Deeper anesthesia required Requires some TMJ mobility N_2O diffusion into cuff Multiple contraindications
Compared with endotracheal intubation	Less invasive Less anesthetic depth required Useful in difficult intubations Less tooth and laryngeal trauma Less laryngospasm and bronchospasm Does not require muscle relaxation Does not require neck mobility Less effect on intraocular pressure Less risk of esophageal or endobronchial intubation	Increased risk of gastrointestinal aspiration Prone or jackknife positions Unsafe in morbidly obese Limits maximum PPV Less secure airway Greater risk of gas leak and pollution Can cause gastric distention

ENT = ear, nose, and throat; TMJ = temporomandibular joint; PPV = positive pressure ventilation.

both of which should be fully inflated after placement. The distal lumen of the Combitube usually comes to lie in the esophagus approximately 95% of the time so that ventilation through the longer blue tube will force gas out the side perforations and into the larynx. The shorter, clear tube can be used for gastric decompression. Alternatively, if the Combitube enters the trachea, ventilation through the clear tube will direct gas into the trachea. Occasionally, up to 160 cc may be needed to adequately seal the upper pharynx with the proximal cuff.

The Combitube has advantages and disadvantages compared with the LMA. The Combitube provides a better seal and better protection against gastric regurgitation and aspiration; however, it is available only in one disposable adult size (age > 15 years, height > 5 feet) and is expensive. The side perforations prevent the use of the Combitube as a guide for flexible FOB or intubation with a standard ETT. The Combitube should be avoided in patients with an intact gag reflex, esophageal pathology, or a history of caustic substance ingestion.

Endotracheal Tubes

ETTs can be used to deliver anesthetic gases directly into the trachea, and allow the most control of ventilation and oxygenation. Standards govern ETT manufacturing (American National Standard for Anesthetic Equipment; ANSI Z–79). ETTs are most commonly made from polyvinyl chloride. Tracheal tubes marked "I.T." or "Z–79" are implant-tested to ensure nontoxicity. The shape and rigidity of ETTs can be altered by inserting a stylet. The patient end of the tube is beveled to aid visualization and insertion through the vocal cords. Murphy tubes have a hole (the **Murphy eye**) to lessen the risk of occlusion should the distal tube opening abut the carina or trachea (Figure 5–12).

Resistance to airflow depends primarily on tube diameter, but is also affected by tube length and curvature. ETT size is usually designated in millimeters of internal diameter or, less commonly, in the French scale (external diameter in millimeters multiplied by 3). The choice of tube diameter is always a compromise between maximizing flow with a large size and minimizing airway trauma with a small size (Table 5–5).

Most adult ETTs have a cuff inflation system consisting of a valve, pilot balloon, inflating tube, and cuff (Figure 5–12). The valve prevents air loss after cuff inflation. The pilot balloon provides a gross indication of cuff inflation. The inflating tube connects the valve to the cuff and is incorporated into the tube's wall. By creating a seal, ETT cuffs permit positive pressure ventilation and reduce the likelihood of aspiration. Uncuffed tubes are usually used in children to minimize the risk of pressure injury and **postintubation croup** (see Chapter 44).

There are two major types of cuffs: high pressure (low volume) and low pressure (high volume). High-pressure cuffs are associated with more ischemic damage to the tracheal mucosa and are less suitable for intubations of long duration. Low-pressure cuffs may

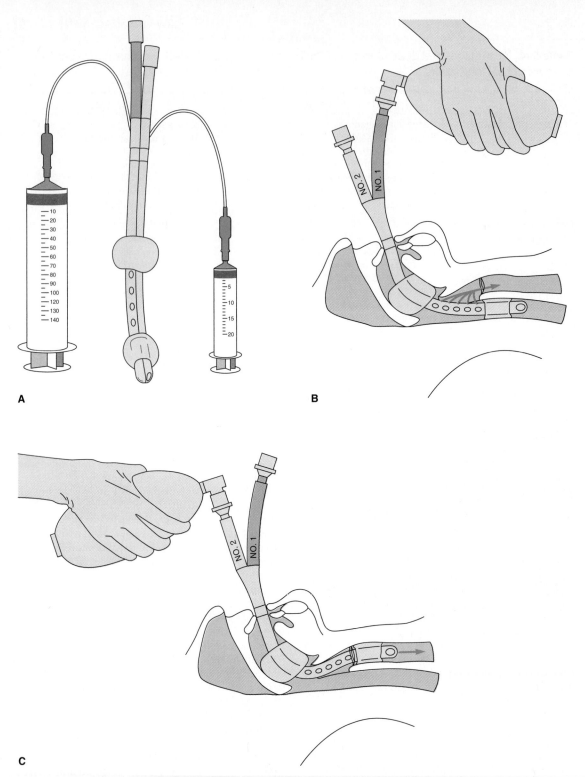

A

B

C

Figure 5–11. ***A:*** The esophageal-tracheal Combitube has two lumens and two cuffs. ***B:*** If placed in the esophagus, ventilation through the blind blue tube will force gas out the side perforations and into the larynx. ***C:*** If placed in the trachea, ventilation through the patient clear tube will direct gas into the trachea.

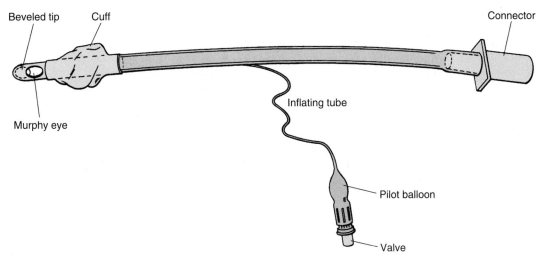

Figure 5–12. Murphy endotracheal tube.

increase the likelihood of sore throat (larger mucosal contact area), aspiration, spontaneous extubation, and difficult insertion (because of the floppy cuff). Nonetheless, because of their lower incidence of mucosal damage, low-pressure cuffs are more commonly recommended.

Cuff pressure depends on several factors: inflation volume, the diameter of the cuff in relation to the trachea, tracheal and cuff compliance, and intrathoracic pressure (cuff pressures increase with coughing). Cuff pressure may rise during general anesthesia as a result of the diffusion of nitrous oxide from the tracheal mucosa into the ETT cuff.

ETTs have been modified for a variety of specialized applications. Flexible, spiral-wound, wire-reinforced ETTs (armored tubes) resist kinking and may prove valuable in some head and neck surgical procedures or in the prone patient. If an armored tube becomes kinked from extreme pressure (eg, an awake patient bit-

Table 5–5. Oral endotracheal tube size guidelines.

Age	Internal Diameter (mm)	Cut Length (cm)
Full-term infant	3.5	12
Child	$4 + \dfrac{Age}{4}$	$14 + \dfrac{Age}{2}$
Adult		
Female	7.0–7.5	24
Male	7.5–9.0	24

ing it), however, the lumen will tend to remain occluded and the tube will need replacement. Other specialized tubes include microlaryngeal tubes (see Chapter 39), RAE preformed tubes (see Figures 39–1 and 39–3), and double-lumen ETTs (see Figure 24–8).

Rigid Laryngoscopes

A laryngoscope is an instrument used to examine the larynx and to facilitate intubation of the trachea. The handle usually contains batteries to light a bulb on the blade tip (Figure 5–13). The Macintosh and Miller blades are the most popular curved and straight designs, respectively, in the United States. The choice of blade depends on personal preference and patient anatomy. Because no blade is perfect for all situations, the clinician should become familiar and proficient with a variety of blade designs (Figure 5–14).

Flexible Fiberoptic Bronchoscopes

In some situations—eg, patients with unstable cervical spines or with poor range of motion of the temporomandibular joint or those with certain congenital upper airway anomalies—direct laryngoscopy with a rigid laryngoscope is undesirable or impossible. Flexible FOB allows indirect visualization of the larynx in such cases (Figure 5–15). This instrument is constructed of coated glass fibers that transmit light and images by internal reflection—ie, a light beam becomes trapped within a fiber and exits unchanged at the opposite end. The insertion tube contains two bundles of fibers, each consisting of 10,000 to 15,000 fibers. One bundle transmits light from the light source (light source bundle)

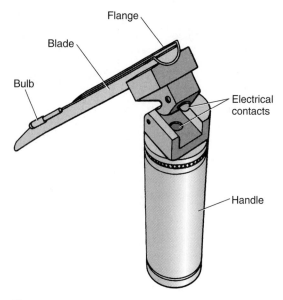

Figure 5–13. A rigid laryngoscope.

while the other provides a high-resolution image (image bundle). Directional manipulation of the insertion tube is accomplished with an angulation wire. Aspiration channels are convenient for suctioning secretions, insufflating oxygen, or instilling local anesthetic. Aspiration channels can be difficult to clean, however; they provide a nidus for infection and require a larger-diameter insertion tube.

TECHNIQUES OF DIRECT LARYNGOSCOPY & INTUBATION

Indications for Intubation

Inserting a tube into the trachea has become a routine part of delivering a general anesthetic. Intubation is not a risk-free procedure, however, and not all patients receiving general anesthesia require it. In general, intubation is indicated for patients who are at risk for aspiration and for those undergoing surgical procedures involving body cavities or the head and neck. Mask ventilation or ventilation with an LMA is usually satis-

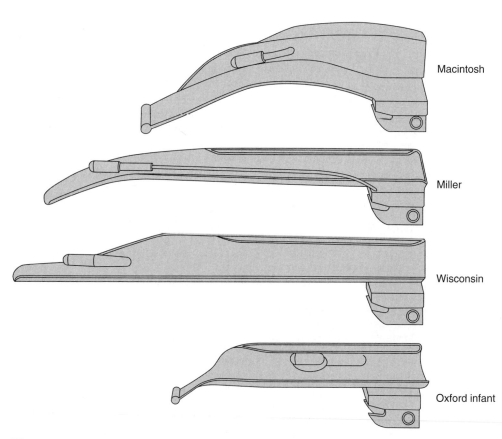

Figure 5–14. An assortment of laryngoscope blades.

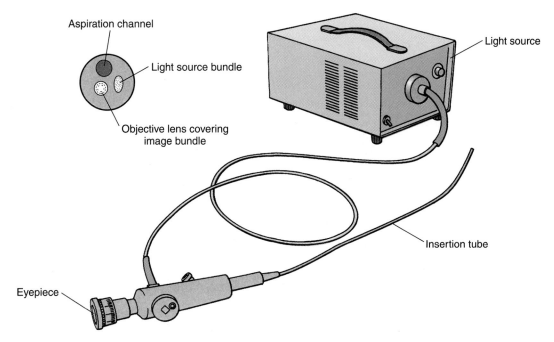

Aspiration channel

Light source bundle

Objective lens covering image bundle

Light source

Insertion tube

Eyepiece

Figure 5–15. A flexible fiberoptic bronchoscope.

factory for short minor procedures such as cystoscopy or eye examination under anesthesia.

Preparation for Rigid Laryngoscopy

Preparation for intubation includes checking equipment and properly positioning the patient. The ETT should be examined. The tube's cuff inflation system can be tested by inflating the cuff using a 10-mL syringe. Maintenance of cuff pressure *after detaching the syringe* ensures proper cuff and valve function. Some anesthesiologists cut the ETT to a preset length to lessen the risk of endobronchial intubation or occlusion from tube kinking (Table 5–5). The connector should be pushed into the tube as far as possible to lessen the likelihood of disconnection. If a stylet is used, it should be inserted into the ETT, which is then bent to resemble a hockey stick (Figure 5–16). This shape facilitates intubation of an anteriorly positioned larynx. The desired blade is locked onto the laryngoscope handle, and bulb function is tested. The light intensity should remain constant even if the bulb is slightly jiggled. A blinking light signals a poor electrical contact, while fading indicates low batteries. An extra handle, blade, ETT (one size smaller), and stylet should be immediately available. Ensure a functioning suction unit to clear the airway in case of unexpected secretions, blood, or emesis.

Successful intubation often depends on correct patient positioning. The patient's head should be level with the anesthesiologist's xiphoid process to prevent unnecessary back strain during laryngoscopy. Rigid laryngoscopy displaces pharyngeal soft tissues to create a direct line of vision from the mouth to the glottic opening. Moderate head elevation and extension of the atlanto-occipital joint places the patient in the desired **sniffing position** (Figure 5–17). The lower portion of the cervical spine is flexed by resting the head on a pillow.

Preparation for induction and intubation also involves the question of routine preoxygenation. Preoxy-

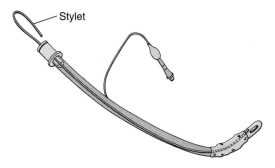

Stylet

Figure 5–16. An endotracheal tube with a stylet bent to resemble a hockey stick.

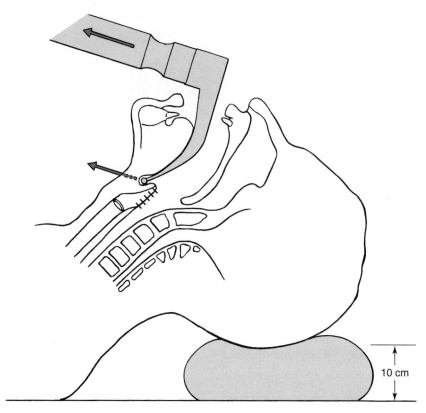

10 cm

Figure 5–17. The sniffing position and intubation with a Macintosh blade. (Modified and reproduced, with permission, from Dorsch JA, Dorsch SE: *Understanding Anesthesia Equipment: Construction, Care, and Complications.* Williams & Wilkins, 1991.)

genation with several (eight) deep breaths of 100% oxygen provides an extra margin of safety in case the patient is not easily ventilated after induction. Preoxygenation can be omitted in patients who object to the face mask, who are free of pulmonary disease, and who do not have a difficult airway.

After inducing general anesthesia, the anesthesiologist becomes the patient's guardian. Because general anesthesia abolishes the protective corneal reflex, care must be taken during this period not to injure the patient's eyes by unintentionally abrading the cornea. Thus, the eyes are routinely taped shut, often after applying a petroleum-based ophthalmic ointment.

Orotracheal Intubation

The laryngoscope is usually held in the nondominant (most frequently the left) hand. With the patient's mouth opened widely, the blade is introduced into the right side of the oropharynx—with care to avoid the teeth. The tongue is swept to the left and up into

the floor of the pharynx by the blade's flange. The tip of a curved blade is usually inserted into the vallecula, while the straight blade tip covers the epiglottis. With either blade, the handle is raised up and away from the patient in a plane perpendicular to the patient's mandible to expose the vocal cords (Figure 5–18). Trapping a lip between the teeth and the blade and leverage on the teeth are avoided. The ETT is taken with the right hand, and its tip is passed through the abducted vocal cords. The ETT cuff should lie in the upper trachea but beyond the larynx. The laryngoscope is withdrawn, again with care to avoid tooth damage. In order to minimize the pressure transmitted to the tracheal mucosa, the cuff is inflated with the least amount of air necessary to create a seal during positive pressure ventilation. Feeling the pilot balloon is *not* a reliable method of determining adequacy of cuff pressure.

After intubation, the chest and epigastrium are immediately auscultated and a capnographic tracing is monitored to ensure intratracheal location (Figures

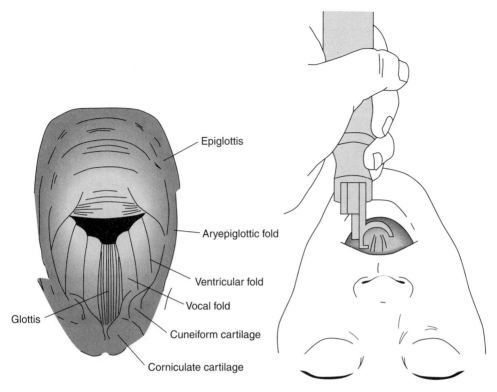

Figure 5–18. Typical view of the glottis during laryngoscopy with a curved blade. (Modified and reproduced with permission from Barash PG: *Clinical Anesthesia,* 2nd ed. Lippincott, 1992.)

Epiglottis

Aryepiglottic fold

Ventricular fold

Vocal fold

Glottis

Cuneiform cartilage

Corniculate cartilage

5–19 and 6–29). If there is doubt about whether the tube is in the esophagus or trachea, it is prudent to remove the tube and ventilate the patient with a mask. Otherwise, the tube is taped or tied in to secure its position (Figure 5–20). Although the persistent detection of CO_2 by a capnograph is the best confirmation of tracheal placement of an ETT, it cannot exclude endobronchial intubation. The earliest manifestation of endobronchial intubation is an increase in peak inspiratory pressure. Proper tube location can be reconfirmed by palpating the cuff in the sternal notch while compressing the pilot balloon with the other hand. The cuff should not be felt above the level of the cricoid cartilage, since a prolonged intralaryngeal location may result in postoperative hoarseness and increases the risk of accidental extubation. Tube position can be documented by chest radiography, but this is rarely required, except in an intensive care unit.

The description presented here assumes an unconscious patient. Oral intubation is usually poorly tolerated by patients who are awake. If necessary, in the latter case, intravenous sedation, application of local anesthetic spray in the oropharynx, regional nerve block, and constant reassurance will improve patient acceptance.

A failed intubation should not be followed by repeated attempts that are merely more of the same. Something must be changed to increase the likelihood of success, such as repositioning the patient, decreasing tube size, adding a stylet, selecting a different blade, attempting a nasal route, or requesting the assistance of another anesthesiologist. If the patient is also difficult to ventilate with a mask, alternative forms of airway management (eg, LMA, Combitube, cricothyrotomy with jet ventilation, tracheostomy) must be immediately pursued. The guidelines developed by the American Society of Anesthesiologists for the management of the difficult airway include a treatment-plan algorithm (Figure 5–21).

Nasotracheal Intubation

Nasal intubation is similar to oral intubation except that the ETT is advanced through the nose into the oropharynx before laryngoscopy. The nostril through

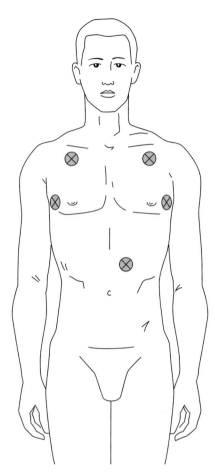

Figure 5–19. Sites for auscultation of breath sounds at the apices and over the stomach.

which the patient breathes most easily is selected in advance and prepared. Phenylephrine nose drops (0.5% or 0.25%) vasoconstrict vessels and shrink mucous membranes. If the patient is awake, local anesthetic drops and nerve blocks can also be utilized (see Case Discussion, later in this chapter).

An ETT lubricated with water-soluble jelly is introduced along the floor of the nose, below the inferior turbinate, *at an angle perpendicular to the face.* The tube's bevel should be directed laterally away from the turbinates. In order to make certain that the tube passes along the floor of the nasal cavity, the proximal end of the ETT should be pulled cephalad (Figure 5–22). The tube is gradually advanced until its tip can be visualized in the oropharynx. Laryngoscopy, as we have discussed, reveals the abducted vocal cords. Oftentimes the distal end of the ETT can be advanced into the trachea with-

out difficulty. If difficulty is encountered, passage of the tip of the tube through the vocal cords may be facilitated by manipulation with Magill forceps, being careful not to damage the cuff. Nasal passage of ETTs, airways, or nasogastric catheters is dangerous in patients with severe midfacial trauma because of the risk of intracranial placement (Figure 5–23).

Flexible Fiberoptic Nasal Intubation

Both nostrils are prepared with vasoconstrictive drops. The nostril through which the patient breathes more easily is identified. Oxygen can be insufflated through the suction port and down the aspiration channel of the bronchoscope to improve oxygenation and blow secretions away from the objective lens.

Alternately, a large nasal airway (eg, 36F) can be inserted in the contralateral nostril. The breathing circuit can be directly connected to the end of this nasal airway in order to administer 100% oxygen during laryngoscopy. If the patient is unconscious and not breath-

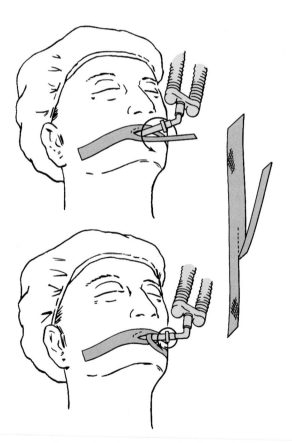

Figure 5–20. A method of securing the endotracheal tube with waterproof adhesive tape.

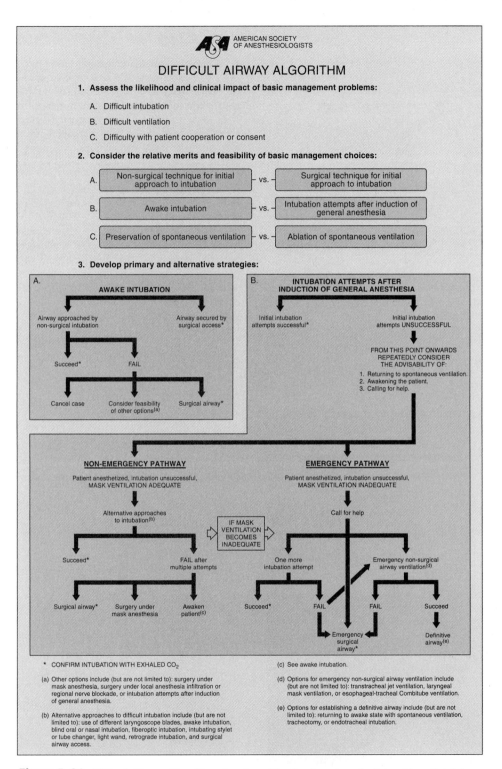

Figure 5–21. Difficult Airway Algorithm developed by the American Society of Anesthesiologists. (Reproduced with permission from Practice Guidelines for Management of the Difficult Airway: A report by the American Society of Anesthesiologists Task Force on Management of the Difficult Airway. Anesthesiology 1993;78:597.)

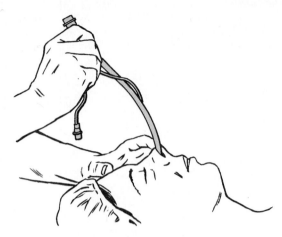

Figure 5–22. Cephalad traction on the tube will help direct its tip along the floor of the nasal cavity.

ing spontaneously, the mouth can be taped and respiration controlled through the single nasal airway. When this technique is used, adequacy of ventilation and oxygenation should be confirmed by capnography and pulse oximetry. An ETT is lubricated and inserted into the other nostril the length of a nasal airway. The lubricated shaft of the bronchoscope is introduced into the

ETT lumen. The single most important rule during endoscopy is to always advance the scope into a *lumen*—do not advance it if only the wall of the ETT or mucous membrane is seen. It is also important to keep the shaft of the FOB relatively straight (Figure 5–24) so that if the head of the bronchoscope is rotated in one direction, the distal end will move to a similar degree and in the same direction. As the tip of the fiberoptic instrument passes through the distal end of the ETT, the epiglottis or glottis should be visible. The tip of the bronchoscope is manipulated as needed to pass the abducted cords.

There is no need to hurry, since the patient's ventilation and oxygenation are being monitored. If either becomes inadequate, the bronchoscope is withdrawn in order to ventilate the patient with a mask. Having an assistant thrust the jaw forward or apply cricoid pressure may improve visualization in difficult cases. If the patient is breathing spontaneously, pulling the tongue forward with a clamp may also facilitate intubation.

Once in the trachea, the scope is advanced to within sight of the carina. The presence of tracheal rings and the

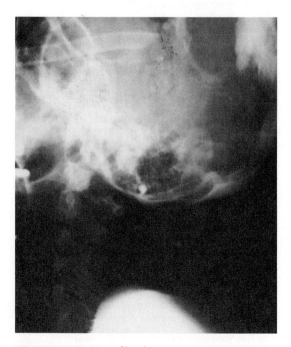

Figure 5–23. X-ray film demonstrating 7.0 mm endotracheal tube placed through cribiform plate into cranial vault in patient with basilar skull fracture.

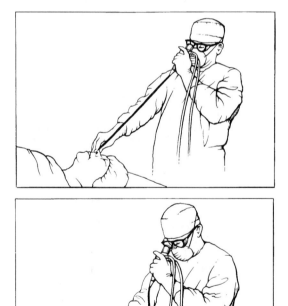

Figure 5–24. Correct technique for manipulating fiberoptic bronchoscope through endotracheal tube is shown in the top panel; avoid curvature in bronchoscope, which makes manipulation difficult.

carina is proof of proper positioning. The ETT is slipped over the bronchoscope. The acute angle around the arytenoid cartilage and epiglottis may prevent easy advancement of the tube. Use of an armored tube usually lessens this problem thanks to its greater lateral flexibility and more obtusely angled distal end. Proper ETT position is confirmed by viewing the tip of the tube above the carina before the fiberoptic scope is withdrawn.

TECHNIQUES OF EXTUBATION

Judging when to remove an ETT is part of the art of anesthesiology that develops with experience. In general, extubation is best performed when a patient is either deeply anesthetized or awake. In either case, adequate recovery from neuromuscular blocking agents should be established prior to extubation. Extubation during a light plane of anesthesia (ie, a state between deep and awake) is avoided because of the increased risk of laryngospasm. The distinction between deep and light anesthesia is usually apparent during pharyngeal suctioning: any reaction to suctioning (eg, breath holding, coughing) signals a light plane of anesthesia, while no reaction is characteristic of a deep plane. Similarly, eye opening or purposeful movements imply that the patient is awake.

Extubating an awake patient is usually associated with coughing (bucking) on the ETT. This reaction increases the heart rate, central venous pressure, arterial blood pressure, intracranial pressure, and intraocular pressure. It may also cause wound dehiscence and bleeding. The presence of an ETT in an awake asthmatic patient often triggers bronchospasm. While these consequences may be lessened by pretreatment with 1.5 mg/kg of intravenous lidocaine 1 to 2 minutes before suctioning and extubation, extubation during deep anesthesia may be preferable in patients who cannot tolerate these effects. On the other hand, such extubation would be contraindicated in a patient at risk for aspiration or one whose airway may be difficult to control after removal of the ETT.

Regardless of whether the tube is removed when the patient is deeply anesthetized or awake, the patient's pharynx should be thoroughly suctioned before extubation in order to lessen the risk of aspiration or laryngospasm. In addition, patients should be ventilated with 100% oxygen in case it becomes difficult to establish an airway after the ETT is removed. Just prior to extubation, the ETT is untaped and its cuff deflated. Applying a small degree of positive airway pressure on an anesthesia bag connected to the ETT may help blow secretions that have collected cephalad to the cuff, up out of the airway into the pharynx, which can then be suctioned. Whether the tube is removed when the patient is at end-expiration or end-inspiration is probably

not very important. The tube is withdrawn in a single, smooth motion, and a face mask is usually applied to deliver 100% oxygen until the patient is stable enough for transportation to the recovery room. In some institutions, oxygen delivery by face mask is maintained during the period of transportation.

COMPLICATIONS OF LARYNGOSCOPY & INTUBATION

The complications of laryngoscopy and intubation are usually due to airway trauma, tube malpositioning, physiologic responses to airway instrumentation, or tube malfunction. These complications can occur during laryngoscopy and intubation, while the tube is in place, or following extubation (Table 5–6).

Table 5–6. Complications of intubation.

During laryngoscopy and intubation
  Malpositioning
    Esophageal intubation
    Endobronchial intubation
    Laryngeal cuff position
  Airway trauma
    Tooth damage
    Lip, tongue, or mucosal laceration
    Sore throat
    Dislocated mandible
    Retropharyngeal dissection
  Physiologic reflexes
    Hypertension, tachycardia
    Intracranial hypertension
    Intraocular hypertension
    Laryngospasm
  Tube malfunction
    Cuff perforation
While the tube is in place
  Malpositioning
    Unintentional extubation
    Endobronchial intubation
    Laryngeal cuff position
  Airway trauma
    Mucosal inflammation and ulceration
    Excoriation of nose
  Tube malfunction
    Ignition
    Obstruction
Following extubation
  Airway trauma
    Edema and stenosis (glottic, subglottic, or tracheal)
    Hoarseness (vocal cord granuloma or paralysis)
    Laryngeal malfunction and aspiration
  Physiologic reflexes
    Laryngospasm

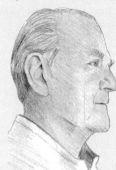

C. Philip Larson Jr., MDCM, MA

LARYNGOSPASM: A CONTINUING PROBLEM

Laryngospasm continues to be a problem for anesthesiologists and patients during induction or recovery from general anesthesia. Its incidence varies depending on several factors, the most important being patient health, anesthetic agents used, and the experience of the anesthesiologist. Patients with a history of smoking, asthma, bronchitis, bronchiectasis, or chronic obstructive lung disease are more susceptible than healthy patients to laryngospasm during induction of general anesthesia and after removal of an endotracheal tube at the conclusion of anesthesia. Laryngospasm occurs more commonly with certain anesthetic drugs (such as desflurane) than others (for example, sevoflurane). Finally, inexperience with induction or recovery and untimely

stimulation of the airway may precipitate laryngospasm. Generally laryngospasm does not result in serious sequelae if detected and treated promptly, although it can result in transient hypoxemia, negative-pressure pulmonary edema, and pulmonary hemorrhage.[1]

The classic treatment as recommended in virtually all of the standard textbooks, including this book, involves administering positive-pressure ventilation with 100% oxygen by bag and mask. If that fails to resolve the laryngospasm, most texts recommend administering succinylcholine, 0.25 to 1 mg/kg, to facilitate ventilation with oxygen.

I believe that there is a better method for resolving laryngospasm that works much more rapidly, is completely reliable if performed properly, and requires no special equipment or drugs. This method involves the application of digital pressure at the "laryngospasm notch".[2] This notch is located behind the lobule of the pinna of each ear. It is bounded anteriorly by the ascending ramus of the mandible adjacent to the condyle, posteriorly by the mastoid process of the temporal bone, and cephalad by the base of the skull (Figure 1). The therapist presses very firmly inwardly toward the base of the skull on each side using either the index or middle fingers while at the same time lifting the mandible at a right angle to the plane of the body (ie, forward displacement of the mandible or jaw thrust). Properly performed, it will convert laryngospasm within one or two breaths to laryngeal stridor, and in another breath or two to

Airway Trauma

Instrumentation with a metal laryngoscope blade and insertion of a stiff ETT often traumatizes delicate airway tissues. Although tooth damage is the most common cause of malpractice claims against anesthesiologists, laryngoscopy and intubation can lead to a range of complications from sore throat to tracheal stenosis. Most of these are due to prolonged external pressure on sensitive airway structures. When these pressures exceed the capillary-arteriolar blood pressure (approximately 30 mm Hg), tissue ischemia can lead to a sequence of inflammation, ulceration, granulation, and stenosis. Inflation of an ETT cuff to the minimum pressure that

creates a seal during routine positive pressure ventilation (usually at least 20 mm Hg) reduces tracheal blood flow by 75% at the cuff site. Further cuff inflation or induced hypotension can totally eliminate mucosal blood flow.

Postintubation croup caused by glottic, laryngeal, or tracheal edema is particularly serious in children. The efficacy of corticosteroids (eg, dexamethasone—0.2 mg/kg, up to a maximum of 12 mg) in preventing post-extubation airway edema remains controversial; however, they have been demonstrated to be efficacious in children with croup from other causes. Vocal cord paralysis from cuff compression or other trauma to the recurrent laryngeal nerve results in hoarseness and in-

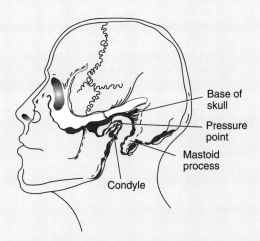

Figure 1. Schematic illustration of "laryngospasm notch" bounded anteriorly by the condyle of the mandible, posteriorly by the mastoid process, and superiorly by the base of the skull. Digital pressure is applied firmly inwardly and anteriorly on each side of the head at the apex of the notch (pressure point arrow), which is slightly cephalad to the plane of the earlobes (not shown) (Reproduced from Larson CP Jr: Laryngospasm, the best treatment. Anesthesiology 1998;89:1293. With permission from Lippincott Williams & Wilkins.)

unobstructed respirations. The technique works equally well in infants, children, and adults. One can simultaneously hold a mask over the face with the thumbs to augment the inspired oxygen concentration.

This technique should be used routinely as soon as an endotracheal tube or laryngeal-mask airway is removed unless it is clear that the patient is fully con-

scious, responsive, and able to maintain an airway. The procedure immediately and simultaneously corrects airway obstruction from either the tongue falling back against the posterior pharyngeal wall or laryngospasm and its routine use increases one's skill in applying it. Moreover, I have never observed any complications from it use. If all anesthesiologists would use the technique regularly during patients' emergence from general anesthesia, laryngospasm would virtually disappear as an important clinical entity during recovery. It would also eliminate the needless (and often wasted) daily precautionary preparation of a syringe of succinylcholine so common in clinical practice.

The obvious question is, Why does it work? Unfortunately, I cannot give a verified, scientific answer. It works in part by preventing airway obstruction from the tongue, but the more important aspect is the very painful stimulus that is elicited. Several nerves, including the facial nerves, are stimulated, and by pressure on the parotid gland the glossopharyngeal, vagus, and perhaps sympathetic nerves. The interconnections of the nerves at this location are complex, and specific functions are not completely understood.

1. Dolinski SY, MacGregor DA, Scuderi PE: Pulmonary hemorrhage associated with negative-pressure pulmonary edema. Anesthesiology 2000; 93:888.
2. Larson CP, Jr: Laryngospasm—the best treatment. Anesthesiology 1998; 89:1293.

creases the risk of aspiration. Some of these complications may be lessened by using an ETT shaped to conform to the anatomy of the airway (eg, Lindholm Anatomical Tracheal Tube). The incidence of postoperative hoarseness appears to increase with obesity, difficult intubations, and anesthetics of long duration. Applying water-soluble lubricant or an anesthetic-containing gel to the tip or cuff of the orotracheal tube does not decrease the incidence of postoperative sore throat or hoarseness. Smaller tubes (size 6.5 in women and size 7.0 in men) are associated with fewer complaints of postoperative sore throat. Repeated attempts at laryngoscopy during a difficult intubation may lead to **periglottic edema** and the inability to ventilate with

a face mask, thus turning a bad situation into a life-threatening one (see Figure 5–21).

Errors of Endotracheal Tube Positioning

Unintentional esophageal intubation can produce catastrophic results. Prevention of this complication depends on direct visualization of the tip of the ETT passing through the vocal cords, careful auscultation for the presence of bilateral breath sounds and the absence of gastric gurgling, analysis of exhaled gas for the presence of CO_2 (the most reliable method), chest radiography, or use of a bronchoscope.

Even though the tube is confirmed to be in the trachea, it may not be correctly positioned. Overinsertion usually results in intubation of the right main stem bronchus because of its less acute angle with the trachea. Clues to the diagnosis of endobronchial intubation include unilateral breath sounds, unexpected hypoxia with pulse oximetry (unreliable with high inspired oxygen concentrations), inability to palpate the ETT cuff in the sternal notch during cuff inflation, and decreased breathing-bag compliance (high peak inspiratory pressures).

In contrast, inadequate insertion depth will position the cuff in the larynx, predisposing the patient to laryngeal trauma. This can be detected by palpating the cuff over the thyroid cartilage or by radiography of the neck.

Since no single technique protects against all these possibilities for misplacing an ETT, it is suggested that minimal testing should include chest auscultation, cuff palpation, and routine capnography.

If the patient is repositioned, tube placement must be reconfirmed. Neck extension or lateral rotation moves an ETT away from the carina, while neck flexion moves the tube toward the carina.

Physiologic Responses to Airway Instrumentation

Laryngoscopy and tracheal intubation violate the patient's protective airway reflexes and predictably lead to hypertension and tachycardia. The insertion of an LMA is associated with significantly less hemodynamic changes. These hemodynamic changes can be attenuated by intravenous administration of drugs—lidocaine (1.5 mg/kg) 1 to 2 minutes, remifentanil (1.0 μg/kg) 1 minute, alfentanil (10–20 μg/kg) 2 to 3 minutes, or fentanyl (0.5–1.0 μg/kg) 4 to 5 minutes—before laryngoscopy. Hypotensive agents, including sodium nitroprusside, nitroglycerin, hydralazine, β-blockers, and calcium channel blockers, have also been shown to effectively attenuate the transient hypertensive response associated with laryngoscopy and intubation. Cardiac dysrhythmias—particularly ventricular bigeminy—are not uncommon during intubation and usually indicate light anesthesia.

Laryngospasm is a forceful involuntary spasm of the laryngeal musculature caused by sensory stimulation of the superior laryngeal nerve. Triggering stimuli include pharyngeal secretions or passing an ETT through the larynx during extubation. Laryngospasm is usually prevented by extubating patients either deeply asleep or fully awake, but it can occur—albeit rarely—in an awake patient. Treatment of laryngospasm includes providing gentle positive pressure ventilation with an anesthesia bag and mask using 100% oxygen or administering intravenous lidocaine (1–1.5 mg/kg).

If laryngospasm persists and hypoxia develops, succinylcholine (0.25–1 mg/kg) should be given in order to paralyze the laryngeal muscles and allow controlled ventilation. The large negative intrathoracic pressures generated by the struggling patient in laryngospasm can result in development of pulmonary edema even in healthy young adults.

While laryngospasm represents an abnormally sensitive reflex, aspiration can result from depression of laryngeal reflexes following prolonged intubation and general anesthesia.

Bronchospasm is another reflex response to intubation and is most common in asthmatic patients. Bronchospasm can sometimes be a clue to endobronchial intubation. Other pathophysiologic effects of intubation include increased intracranial and intraocular pressures.

Endotracheal Tube Malfunction

ETTs do not always function as intended. The risk of polyvinyl chloride tube ignition in an O_2/N_2O-enriched environment was mentioned in Chapter 2. Valve or cuff damage is not unusual and should be excluded prior to insertion. ETT obstruction can result from kinking, foreign body aspiration, or from thick or inspissated secretions in the lumen.

**CASE DISCUSSION:
EVALUATION & MANAGEMENT
OF A DIFFICULT AIRWAY**

A 17-year-old girl presents for emergency drainage of a submandibular abscess.

What are some important anesthetic considerations during the preoperative evaluation of a patient with an abnormal airway?

Induction of general anesthesia followed by direct laryngoscopy and oral intubation is dangerous, if not impossible, in several situations (Table 5–7). To determine the optimal intubation technique, the anesthesiologist must elicit an airway history and carefully examine the patient's head and neck. Any available prior anesthesia records should be reviewed for previous problems in airway management. If a facial deformity is severe enough to preclude a good mask seal, positive pressure ventilation may be impossible. Furthermore, patients with hypopharyngeal disease are more dependent on awake muscle tone to maintain airway patency. These two groups of patients should not be allowed to become apneic for any

Table 5–7. Conditions associated with difficult intubations.

Tumors
    Cystic hygroma
    Hemangioma
    Hematoma
Infections
    Submandibular abscess
    Peritonsillar abscess
    Epiglottitis
Congenital anomalies
    Pierre Robin syndrome
    Treacher Collins' syndrome
    Laryngeal atresia
    Goldenhar's syndrome
    Craniofacial dysostosis
Foreign body
Trauma
    Laryngeal fracture
    Mandibular or maxillary fracture
    Inhalation burn
    Cervical spine injury
Obesity
Inadequate neck extension
    Rheumatoid arthritis
    Ankylosing spondylitis
    Halo traction
Anatomic variations
    Micrognathia
    Prognathism
    Large tongue
    Arched palate
    Short neck
    Prominent upper incisors

---

reason—including induction of anesthesia, sedation, or muscle paralysis—until their airway is secured.

If there is an abnormal limitation of the temporomandibular joint that may not improve with muscle paralysis, a nasal approach should be considered. Infection confined to the floor of the mouth usually does not preclude nasal intubation. If the hypopharynx is involved to the level of the hyoid bone, however, any translaryngeal attempt will be difficult. Other clues to a potentially difficult laryngoscopy include limited neck extension (< 35 degrees), a distance between the tip of the patient's mandible and hyoid bone of less than 7 cm, a sternomental distance of less than 12.5 cm with the head fully extended and the mouth closed, and a poorly visualized uvula during voluntary tongue protrusion (Figure 5–25). It must be stressed that because no examination technique is foolproof and the signs of a difficult airway may be subtle, the anesthesiologist must always be prepared for unanticipated difficulties (see chapter 48, Profiles in Anesthetic Practice: Management of the Difficult Airway by Anesthesiologists).

The anesthesiologist should also evaluate the patient for signs of airway obstruction (eg, chest retraction, stridor) and hypoxia (agitation, restlessness, anxiety, lethargy). Aspiration pneumonia is more likely if the patient has recently eaten or if pus is draining from an abscess into the mouth. In either case, techniques that ablate laryngeal reflexes (eg, topical anesthesia) should be avoided.

In the case under discussion, physical examination reveals extensive facial edema that limits the mandible's range of motion. Mask fit does not appear to be impaired, however. Lateral radiographs of the head and neck suggest that the infection has spread over the larynx. Frank pus is observed in the mouth.

Which intubation technique is indicated?

Routine oral and nasal intubations have been described for anesthetized patients. Both of these can also be performed in awake patients. Whether the patient is awake or asleep or whether intubation is to be oral or nasal, it can be performed with rigid laryngoscopy, fiberoptic visualization, or a "blind" technique. Thus, there are at least 12 methods of translaryngeal intubation (eg, awake/ nasal/fiberoptic) possible with an ETT. Alternative techniques using an LMA or Combitube are available, and tracheostomy or cricothyrotomy can be lifesaving methods of airway preservation.

Intubation may be difficult in this patient; however, there is pus draining into the mouth, and positive pressure ventilation may be impossible. Induction of anesthesia should, therefore, be delayed until after the airway has been secured. The submandibular location of the abscess supports the choice of a nasal approach and probably excludes rigid laryngoscopy. Therefore, the alternatives are awake/nasal/fiberoptic intubation; and awake/nasal/blind intubation. The final decision depends on the availability of a bronchoscope and personnel experienced in its use.

Regardless of which alternative is chosen, an emergency tracheotomy may be necessary. Therefore, an experienced team including a surgeon should be in the operating room, all necessary equipment should be available and unwrapped, and the neck should be prepped and draped.

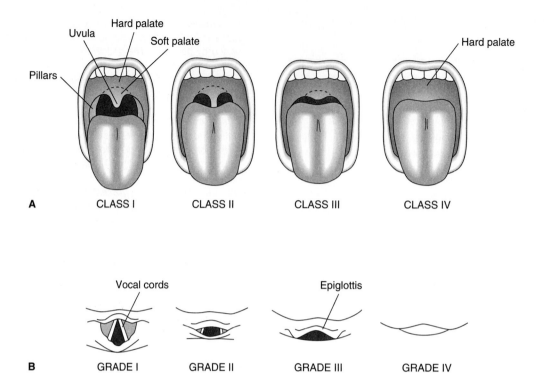

Figure 5–25. A difficult orotracheal intubation (grade III or IV) may be predicted by the inability to visualize certain pharyngeal structures (class III or IV) during the preoperative examination of a seated patient. (Reproduced with permission from Mallampati SR: Clinical signs to predict difficult tracheal intubation (hypothesis). Can Anaesth Soc J 1983;30:316.)

What premedication would be appropriate for this patient?

Any loss of consciousness or interference with airway reflexes could result in airway obstruction or aspiration. Glycopyrrolate would be a good choice of premedication since it minimizes upper airway secretions without crossing the blood-brain barrier (see Chapter 11). Parenteral sedatives should be very carefully titrated or omitted entirely. Psychological preparation of the patient, including explaining each step planned in securing the airway, may improve patient cooperation. Management of patients at risk for aspiration is the subject of the case discussion presented in Chapter 15.

Describe a "blind" nasotracheal intubation.

An ETT is lubricated with lidocaine jelly and deformed for a few minutes to exaggerate its curvature (Figure 5–26). The patient's head should be placed in the sniffing position. After preparation of the nares, the tip of the ETT is gently introduced into the naris at a plane perpendicular to the face. Air movement through the tube should be continually felt, heard, or monitored by capnography. The tube is incrementally advanced during inspiration. If the patient's respirations continue but no airflow is detected through the tube, the tip has passed the glottis and is in the esophagus. In that case, the tube must be withdrawn and advanced again. Breathholding and coughing signal close proximity to the larynx, and tube advancement should continue with each inspiration.

If the tube does not easily enter the trachea, several maneuvers may enhance success. After advancement to an area near the glottis, a stylet that has been bent to resemble a hockey stick can be inserted through the tube to direct its tip more anteriorly. Extension of the head will also tend to guide the tube more anteriorly, while head rotation will move the tip laterally. Laryngeal or cricoid pressure may beneficially change the relationship between the tip and the glottis. Inflation of the ETT

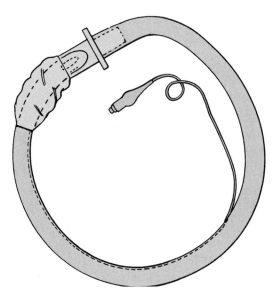

Figure 5–26. An endotracheal tube is bent to exaggerate its curvature so that it will pass anteriorly into the larynx during a blind nasal intubation.

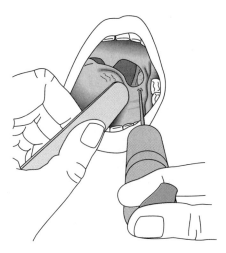

Figure 5–27. Nerve block. While the tongue is laterally retracted with a tongue blade, the base of the palatoglossal arch is infiltrated with local anesthetic to block the lingual and pharyngeal branches of the glossopharyngeal nerve. Note that the lingual branches of the glossopharyngeal nerve are not the same as the lingual nerve, which is a branch of the trigeminal nerve.

cuff in the hypopharynx may also force the tip anteriorly. If the tube persistently slips into the esophagus, voluntary tongue protrusion will inhibit swallowing and may move the tongue and the tube anteriorly.

After intubation is confirmed, intravenous induction may proceed. At the end of the procedure, the patient should be totally awake, with protective airway reflexes intact, before extubation is attempted. Necessary equipment and personnel should be available for unexpected reintubation.

What nerve blocks could be helpful during an awake intubation?

The lingual and some pharyngeal branches of the glossopharyngeal nerve that provide sensation to the posterior third of the tongue and oropharynx are easily blocked by bilateral injection of 2 mL of local anesthetic into the base of the palatoglossal arch (also known as the anterior tonsillar pillar) with a 25-gauge spinal needle (Figure 5–27).

Bilateral **superior laryngeal nerve blocks** and a transtracheal block would anesthetize the airway below the epiglottis (Figure 5–28). The hyoid bone is located, and 3 mL of 2% lidocaine is infiltrated 1 cm below each greater cornu where the internal branch of the superior laryngeal nerves penetrates the thyrohyoid membrane.

A transtracheal block is performed by identifying and penetrating the cricothyroid membrane while the neck is extended. After confirmation of an intratracheal position by aspiration of air, 4 mL of 4% lidocaine is injected into the trachea at end-expiration. A deep inhalation and cough immediately following injection distributes the anesthetic throughout the trachea. While these blocks may allow the awake patient to tolerate intubation better, they also obtund protective cough reflexes, depress the swallowing reflex, and may lead to aspiration. Topical anesthesia of the pharynx may induce a transient obstruction from the loss of reflex regulation of airway caliber at the level of the glottis.

Because of this patient's increased risk for aspiration, local anesthesia might best be limited to the nasal passages. Four percent cocaine has no advantages compared with a mixture of 4% lidocaine and 0.25% phenylephrine and can cause cardiovascular side effects. The maximum safe dose of local anesthetic should be calculated—and not exceeded (see Chapter 14). Local anesthetic is applied to the nasal mucosa with cotton-tipped applicators until a nasal airway that has

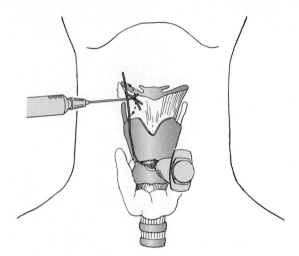

Figure 5–28. Superior laryngeal nerve block and transtracheal block.

been lubricated with lidocaine jelly can be placed into the naris with minimal discomfort.

Why is it necessary to be prepared for emergency tracheotomy?

Laryngospasm is always a possible complication of intubation in the nonparalyzed patient even if the patient remains awake. Laryngospasm may make positive pressure ventilation with a mask impossible. If succinylcholine is administered to break the spasm, the consequent relaxation of pharyngeal muscles may lead to upper airway obstruction and continued inability to ventilate. In this situation, emergency tracheotomy may be lifesaving.

What are some alternative techniques that might be successful?

Other possible strategies include the retrograde passage of a long guidewire or epidural catheter through a needle inserted across the cricothyroid membrane. The catheter is guided cephalad into the pharynx and out through the nose or mouth. An ETT is passed over the catheter, which is withdrawn after the tube has entered the larynx. Variations of this technique include passing the retrograde wire through the suction port of a flexible bronchoscope or the lumen of a reintubation stylet that has been preloaded with an ETT. These thicker shafts help the ETT negotiate the bend into the larynx more easily. Obviously, a vast array of specialized airway equipment exists and must be readily available for management of difficult airways (Table 5–8). Another possibility is

Table 5–8. Suggested contents of the portable storage unit for difficult airway management.

- Rigid laryngoscope blades of alternate design and size from those routinely used.
- Endotracheal tubes of assorted size.
- Endotracheal tube guides. Examples include (but are not limited to) semirigid stylets with or without a hollow core for jet ventilation, light wands, and forceps designed to manipulate the distal portion of the endotracheal tube.
- Fiberoptic intubation equipment.
- Retrograde intubation equipment.
- At least one device suitable for emergency nonsurgical airway ventilation. Examples include (but are not limited to) a transtracheal jet ventilator, a hollow jet ventilation stylet, the laryngeal mask, and a Combitube.
- Equipment suitable for emergency surgical airway access (eg, cricothyrotomy).
- An exhaled CO_2 detector.

The items listed in this table are suggestions. The contents of the portable storage unit should be customized to meet the specific needs, preferences, and skills of the practitioner and health-care facility.

(Modified and used, with permission, from American Society of Anesthesiologists: Practice guidelines for management of the difficult airway: A report by the American Society of Anesthesiologists Task Force on Management of the Difficult Airway. Anesthesiology 1993; 78:597).

cricothyrotomy, which is described in Chapter 48. Either of these techniques would have been difficult in the patient described in this case because of the swelling and anatomic distortion of the neck that can accompany a submandibular abscess.

SUGGESTED READING

Adams AP, Hewitt PB, Grande CM (editors): *Emergency Anaesthesia,* 2nd ed. Oxford University Press, 1998.

Benumof JL: Laryngeal mask airway and the ASA difficult airway algorithm. Anesthesiology 1996;84:686. An excellent review of the ASA algorithm and the use of the LMA.

Dorsch JA, Dorsch SE: *Understanding Anesthesia Equipment,* 4th ed. Williams & Wilkins, 1999. Endotracheal tubes, laryngoscopes, face masks, and airways.

Hurford WE: Orotracheal intubation outside the operating room: Anatomic considerations and techniques. Respir Care 1999; 44:615.

Jaeger JM, Durbin CG Jr: Special purpose endotracheal tubes. Respir Care 1999;44:661.

Kim ES, Bishop MJ: Endotracheal intubation, but not laryngeal mask airway insertion, produces reversible bronchoconstriction. Anesthesiology 1999;90:391.

Latto IP, Vaughan RS (editors): *Difficulties in Tracheal Intubation,* 2nd ed. WB Saunders and Company, 1997.

McIntyre JWR: Laryngoscope design and the difficult adult tracheal intubation. Can J Anaesth 1989;36:94. Relates choice of anesthetic blade (eg, Miller versus Macintosh) to the anatomic peculiarities of the individual patient.

Mercer MH, Gabbott DA: Insertion of the Combitube airway with the cervical spine immobilised in a rigid cervical collar. Anaesthesia 1998;53:971.

Ovassapian A (editor): *Fiberoptic Airway Endoscopy and the Difficult Airway.* Lippincott-Raven Press, 1996. Extensively illustrated.

Shelly MP, Nightingale P: ABC of intensive care. Respiratory support. BMJ 1999;318:1674.

Stauffer JL: Complications of endotracheal intubation and tracheostomy. Respir Care 1999;44:828.

Thompson AE: Issues in airway management in infants and children. Respir Care 1999;44:650.

Watson CB: Prediction of a difficult intubation: Methods for successful intubation. Respir Care 1999;44:777.

Patient Monitors

6

KEY CONCEPTS

 The possibility of carotid puncture during catheterization of the internal jugular vein can be ruled out by transducing the waveform or comparing the blood's color or PaO_2 with an arterial sample.

 The catheter's tip should not be allowed to migrate into the heart chambers.

 Relative contraindications to pulmonary artery catheterization include complete left bundle branch block (because of the risk of complete heart block), Wolff-Parkinson-White syndrome, and Ebstein's malformation (because of possible tachyarrhythmias).

 Pulmonary artery pressure should be continuously monitored to detect an overwedged position indicative of catheter migration.

 Accurate measurements of cardiac output depend on rapid and smooth injection, precisely known injectant temperature and volume, correct entry of the calibration factors for the specific type of pulmonary artery catheter into the cardiac output computer, and avoidance of measurements during electrocautery.

 Capnographs rapidly and reliably indicate esophageal intubation—a common cause of

anesthetic catastrophe—but do not detect endobronchial intubation.

 The electroencephalographic (EEG) changes that accompany ischemia, such as high-frequency activity, can be mimicked by hypothermia, anesthetic agents, electrolyte disturbances, and marked hypocapnia. Detection of EEG changes should lead to an immediate review of possible causes of cerebral ischemia before irreversible brain damage has a chance to occur.

 Because hypothermia reduces metabolic oxygen requirements, it has proved to be protective during times of cerebral or cardiac ischemia.

 Redistribution of heat from warm central compartments (eg, abdomen, thorax) to cooler peripheral tissues (eg, arms, legs) from anesthetic-induced vasodilation explains most of the initial drop in temperature, with heat loss being a minor contributor.

 During general anesthesia, however, the body cannot compensate for hypothermia because anesthetics inhibit central thermoregulation by interfering with hypothalamic function.

One of the primary responsibilities of an anesthesiologist is to act as a guardian for the anesthetized patient during surgery. In fact, "vigilance" is the motto of the American Society of Anesthesiologists (ASA). Because monitoring is implicit in maintaining effective vigilance, standards for intraoperative monitoring have been adopted by the ASA (the box delineates *minimum* standards—see pp 124–125). Optimal vigilance requires an understanding of the technology of sophisticated monitoring equipment—including cost-benefit considerations. This chapter reviews the indications, contraindications, techniques and complications, and clinical considerations relevant to the most important and widely used anesthetic monitors.

■ CARDIAC MONITORS

ARTERIAL BLOOD PRESSURE

The rhythmic contraction of the left ventricle, ejecting blood into the vascular system, results in pulsatile arterial pressures. The peak pressure generated during systolic contraction is the **systolic arterial blood pressure (SBP)**; the trough pressure during diastolic relaxation is the **diastolic arterial blood pressure (DBP). Pulse pressure** is the difference between the systolic and diastolic pressures. The time-weighted average of arterial pressures during a pulse cycle is the mean arterial pressure (MAP). MAP can be estimated by application of the following formula:

$$MAP = \frac{(SBP) + 2\,(DBP)}{3}$$

Measurements of arterial blood pressure are greatly affected by the sampling site. As a pulse moves peripherally through the arterial tree, wave reflection distorts the pressure waveform, leading to an exaggeration of systolic and pulse pressures (Figure 6–1). For example, radial artery systolic pressure is usually higher than aortic systolic pressure because of the former's more distal location. In contrast, radial artery systolic pressures are often lower than aortic pressures following hypothermic cardiopulmonary bypass because of a decrease in the hand's vascular resistance (Figure 6–2). Vasodilating drugs (eg, isoflurane, nitroglycerin) tend to accen-

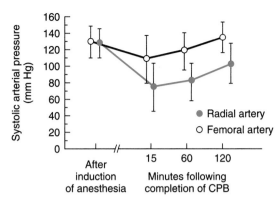

Figure 6–2. Systolic arterial pressures are higher in the radial artery than femoral artery at 15, 60, and 120 minutes following cardiopulmonary bypass (CPB). This gradient increases in patients receiving nitrates and calcium channel blockers. Mean arterial pressures do not differ during the same time-course. (Reproduced with permission from: Maruyama K et al: Effect of combined infusion of nitroglycerin and nicardipine on femoral-to-radial arterial pressure gradient after cardiopulmonary bypass. Anesth Analg 1990;70:431.)

tuate this discrepancy. The level of the sampling site relative to the heart will alter measurement of blood pressure because of the effect of gravity (Figure 6–3). Some patients with severe peripheral vascular disease may have a significant difference in blood pressure measurements between the right and left arms. The higher value should be used in these patients. Because nonin-

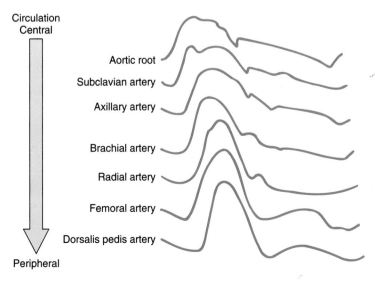

Figure 6–1. Changes in configuration as a waveform moves peripherally. (Reproduced with permission from Bedford RF: Invasive blood pressuring monitoring. In: Blitt CD (editor). *Monitoring in Anesthesia and Critical Care Medicine,* 2nd ed. Churchill Livingstone, New York, 1990, p 102).

$$(20 \text{ cm H}_2\text{O}) \left(\frac{0.74 \text{ mm Hg}}{\text{cm H}_2\text{O}} \right) = 14.7 \text{ mm Hg}$$

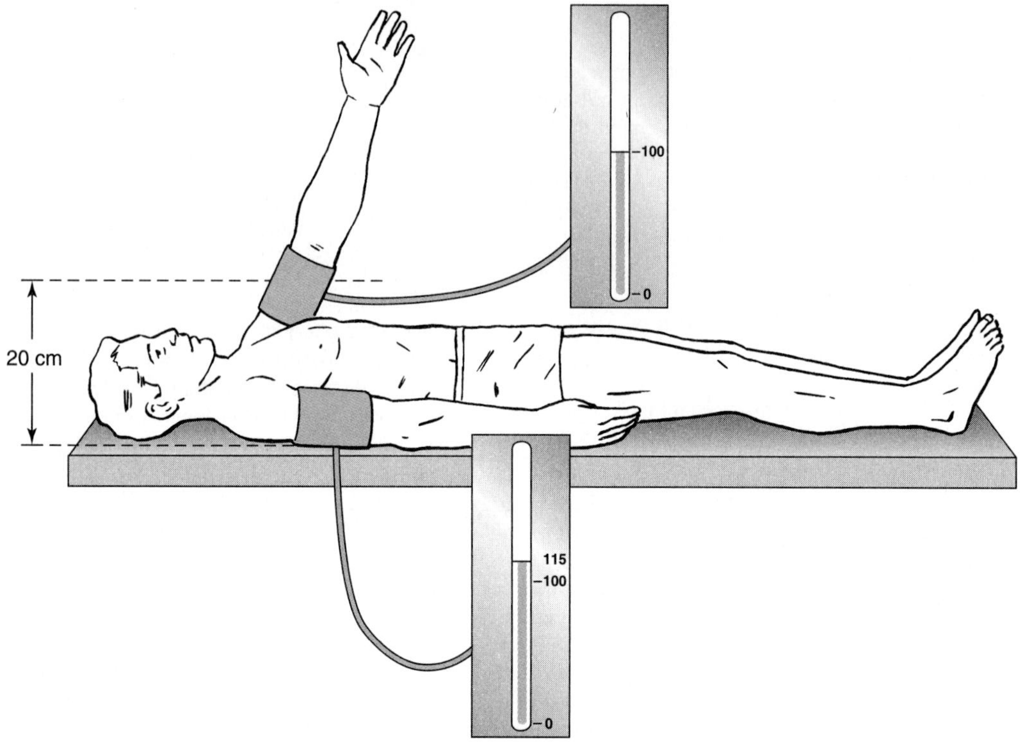

Figure 6–3. The difference in blood pressure (mm Hg) at two different sites of measurement equals the height of an interposed column of water (cm H_2O) multiplied by a conversion factor (1 cm H_2O = 0.74 mm Hg).

vasive (palpation, Doppler, auscultation, oscillometry, plethysmography) and invasive (arterial cannulation) methods of blood pressure determination differ greatly, they are discussed separately.

1. Noninvasive Arterial Blood Pressure Monitoring

Indications

General or regional anesthesia is an absolute indication for arterial blood pressure measurement. The techniques and frequency of pressure determination depend largely on the patient's condition and the type of surgical procedure. An auscultatory measurement every 3–5 minutes is adequate in most cases. Problems such as obesity may make auscultation unreliable, however; in such cases, a Doppler or oscillometric technique may be preferable.

Contraindications

Although some method of blood pressure measurement is mandatory, techniques that rely on a blood pressure cuff are best avoided in extremities with vascular abnormalities (eg, dialysis shunts) or with intravenous lines.

Techniques & Complications

A. PALPATION:

Systolic blood pressure can be determined by (1) locating a palpable peripheral pulse; (2) inflating a blood pressure cuff proximal to the pulse until flow is occluded; (3) releasing cuff pressure by 2 or 3 mm Hg per heartbeat; and (4) measuring the cuff pressure at which pulsations are again palpable. This method tends to underestimate systolic pressure, however, because of the insensitivity of touch and the delay between flow under the cuff and distal pulsations, and palpation does not provide a diastolic or mean arterial pressure. The equipment required is simple and inexpensive (Figure 6–4).

B. DOPPLER PROBE:

When a Doppler probe is substituted for the anesthesiologist's finger, arterial blood pressure measurement becomes sensitive enough to be useful in obese patients, pediatric patients, and those who are in shock (Figure 6–5). The **Doppler effect** is the apparent shift in the frequency of sound waves when their source moves relative to the observer. For example, the pitch of a train's whistle increases as a train approaches and decreases as it departs. The reflection of sound waves off a moving object similarly causes an apparent frequency shift. A Doppler probe transmits an ultrasonic signal that is reflected by underlying tissue. As red blood cells move through an artery, a Doppler frequency shift will be detected by the probe. The difference between transmitted and received frequency is represented by this monitor's characteristic swishing sound, which indicates blood flow. Because air reflects ultrasound, a coupling gel (but not corrosive electrode jelly) must be applied between the probe and the skin. Correct positioning of the probe directly above an artery is crucial, since the beam must pass through the vessel wall. Interference from probe movement or electrocautery is an annoying distraction. Note that only systolic pressures can be reliably determined with the Doppler technique.

A variation of Doppler technology uses a piezoelectric crystal to detect lateral arterial wall movement to the intermittent opening and closing of vessels between systolic and diastolic pressure. This instrument thus detects both systolic and diastolic pressures.

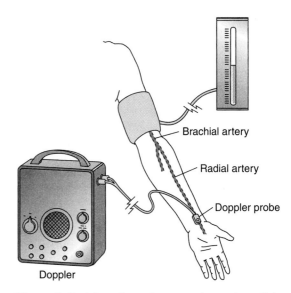

Figure 6–5. A Doppler probe secured over the radial artery will sense red blood cell movement as long as the blood pressure cuff is below systolic pressure. (Courtesy of Parks Medical Electronics.)

C. AUSCULTATION:

Inflation of a blood pressure cuff to a pressure between systolic and diastolic pressures will partially collapse an underlying artery, producing turbulent flow and the characteristic **Korotkoff sounds.** These sounds are audible through a stethoscope placed under—or just beyond—the distal third of an inflated blood pressure cuff. The Diasyst is a specially molded rubber stethoscope that is secured under the cuff with Velcro fasteners (Figure 6–6). Systolic blood pressure coincides with the onset of Korotkoff sounds; diastolic pressure is determined with their disappearance. Occasionally, Korotkoff sounds cannot be heard through part of the range from systolic to diastolic pressure. This **auscultatory gap** is most common in hypertensive patients and can lead to an inaccurate diastolic blood pressure measurement. Korotkoff sounds are often difficult to auscultate during episodes of hypotension or marked peripheral vasoconstriction. In these situations, the subsonic frequencies associated with the sounds can be detected by a microphone and amplified to indicate systolic and diastolic pressures. Motion artifact and electrocautery interference limit the usefulness of this method.

D. OSCILLOMETRY:

Arterial pulsations cause oscillations in cuff pressure. These oscillations are small if the cuff is inflated above

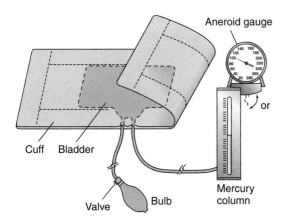

Figure 6–4. Equipment required for arterial blood pressure measurement by palpation.

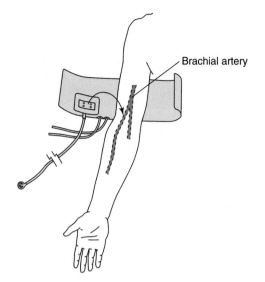

Brachial artery

Figure 6–6. The Diasyst—a type of stethoscope.

systolic pressure. When the cuff pressure decreases to systolic pressure, however, the pulsations are transmitted to the entire cuff and the oscillations markedly increase. Maximal oscillation occurs at the mean arterial pressure, after which oscillations decrease. Because some oscillations are present above and below arterial blood pressure, a mercury or aneroid manometer provides a gross and unreliable measurement. Automated

blood pressure monitors electronically measure the pressures at which the oscillation amplitudes change (Figure 6–7). A micro-processor derives systolic, mean, and diastolic pressures by using an algorithm. Machines that demand identical consecutive pulse waves for measurement confirmation may be unreliable during arrhythmias (eg, atrial fibrillation). Oscillometric monitors should not be used on patients on cardiopulmonary bypass. Nonetheless, the speed, accuracy, and versatility of oscillometric devices have greatly improved, and they have become the preferred noninvasive blood pressure monitors in the United States.

E. PLETHYSMOGRAPHY:

Arterial pulsations transiently increase the blood volume in an extremity. A finger photoplethysmograph, consisting of a light-emitting diode and a photoelectric cell, detects changes in finger volume. If the pressure in a proximally placed cuff exceeds systolic pressure, the pulsations and changes in volume cease. The Finapres (*fin*ger *a*rterial *pres*sure) plethysmograph continuously measures the minimum pressures required in a small finger cuff to maintain a constant finger volume. A solenoid-controlled air pump rapidly modulates cuff pressures, which are displayed as a beat-to-beat tracing. Although this monitor's measurements usually correspond to intra-arterial determinations, plethysmography has proved unreliable in patients with poor peripheral perfusion (eg, those with peripheral vascular disease or hypothermia) and is, therefore, not recommended for routine clinical use.

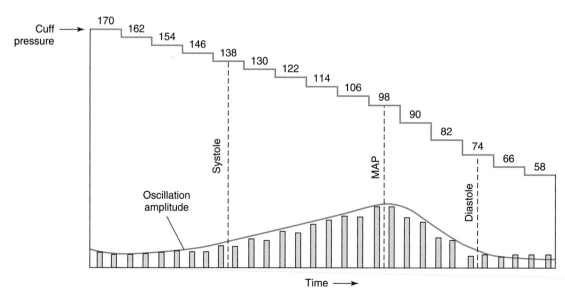

Figure 6–7. Oscillometric determination of blood pressure.

F. ARTERIAL TONOMETRY:

Arterial tonometry noninvasively measures beat-to-beat arterial blood pressure by sensing the pressure required to partially flatten a superficial artery that is supported by a bony structure (eg, radial artery). A tonometer consisting of several independent pressure transducers is applied to the skin overlying the artery (Figure 6–8). The contact stress between the pressure transducer directly over the artery and the skin reflects intraluminal pressure. Continuous pulse recordings produce a tracing very similar to an invasive arterial blood pressure waveform. Current limitations on this technology include sensitivity to movement artifact and the need for frequent calibration.

Clinical Considerations

Adequate oxygen delivery to vital organs must be maintained during anesthesia. Unfortunately, instruments to monitor specific organ perfusion and oxygenation are complex and expensive, and for that reason arterial blood pressure is assumed to reflect organ blood flow. Flow also depends on vascular resistance, however:

$$Flow = \frac{Pressure\ gradient}{Vascular\ resistance}$$

Even if pressure is high, if the resistance is also high, flow can be quite low. Thus, arterial blood pressure should be viewed as an indicator—but not a measure—of end-organ perfusion.

The accuracy of any method of blood pressure measurement that involves a blood pressure cuff depends on proper cuff size (Figure 6–9). The cuff's rubber bladder should extend at least halfway around the extremity, and the width of the cuff should be 20–50% greater than the diameter of the extremity (Figure 6–10).

Automated blood pressure monitors, using one or a combination of the methods described above, are frequently used in anesthesiology. A self-contained air pump inflates the cuff at predetermined intervals. Overzealous use of these automated devices has resulted in nerve palsies and extensive extravasation of intravenously administered fluids, however. In case of equipment failure, an alternative method of blood pressure determination must be immediately available.

2. Invasive Arterial Blood Pressure Monitoring

Indications

Indications for invasive arterial blood pressure monitoring by catheterization of an artery include elective hypotension, anticipation of wide intraoperative blood pressure swings, end-organ disease necessitating precise beat-to-beat blood pressure regulation, and the need for multiple analyses of arterial blood gases.

Contraindications

Catheterization should be avoided if possible in arteries without documented collateral blood flow or in extremities where there is a suspicion of preexisting vascular insufficiency (eg, Raynaud's phenomenon).

Techniques & Complications

A. SELECTION OF ARTERY FOR CANNULATION:

Several arteries are available for percutaneous catheterization.

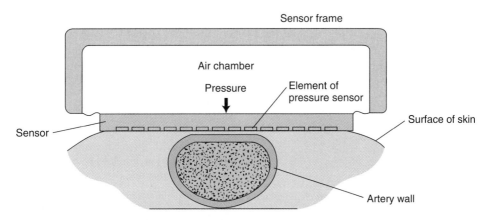

Figure 6–8. Tonometry is a method of continuous (beat-to-beat) arterial blood pressure determination. The sensors must be positioned directly over the artery.

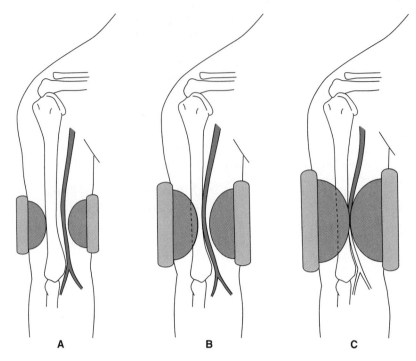

A **B** **C**

Figure 6–9. Blood pressure cuff width influences the pressure readings. Three cuffs, all inflated to the same pressure, are shown. The narrowest cuff (**A**) will require more pressure and the widest cuff (**C**) less pressure to occlude the brachial artery for determination of systolic pressure. Too narrow a cuff may produce a large overestimation of systolic pressure. While the wider cuff may underestimate the systolic pressure, the error with a cuff 20% too wide is not as significant as that with a cuff 20% too narrow. (Reproduced with permission from Gravenstein JS, Paulus DA: *Monitoring Practice in Clinical Anesthesia,* 2nd ed. Lippincott, Philadelphia, 1987, p 58.)

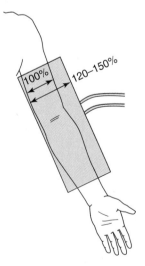

Figure 6–10. The width of the blood pressure cuff should be 20–50% greater than the diameter of the patient's extremity.

1. The radial artery is commonly cannulated because of its superficial location and collateral flow. Five percent of patients, however, have incomplete palmar arches and lack adequate collateral blood flow. **Allen's test** is a simple—but not completely reliable—method for determining the adequacy of ulnar collateral circulation in cases of radial artery thrombosis. To perform an Allen's test, have the patient exsanguinate his or her hand by making a fist. While the operator occludes the radial and ulnar arteries with fingertip pressure, the patient relaxes the blanched hand. Collateral flow through the hand's arterial arches is confirmed by flushing of the thumb within 5 seconds after pressure on the ulnar artery is released. Delayed return of normal color indicates an equivocal test (5–10 seconds) or insufficient collateral circulation (> 10 seconds). Alternatively, blood flow distal to the radial artery occlusion can be detected by palpation, Doppler probe, plethysmography, or pulse oximetry. Unlike Allen's test, these methods of determining the adequacy of collateral circulation do not require patient cooperation.

2. Ulnar artery catheterization is more difficult because of the artery's deeper and more tortuous course. Because of the risk of compromising blood flow to the hand, this should not be considered if the ipsilateral radial artery has been punctured but unsuccessfully cannulated.

3. The brachial artery is large and easily identifiable in the antecubital fossa. Its proximity to the aorta provides less waveform distortion. Being near the elbow predisposes brachial artery catheters to kinking.

4. The femoral artery is prone to pseudoaneurysm and atheroma formation but often provides an access of last resort in burn or trauma victims. This site has been associated with an increased incidence of infectious complications and with arterial thrombosis. Aseptic necrosis of the head of the femur is a rare but tragic complication of femoral artery cannulation in children.

5. The dorsalis pedis and posterior tibial arteries are at some distance from the aorta and therefore have distorted waveforms. Modified Allen's tests can be performed to document adequate collateral flow around these arteries.

6. The axillary artery is surrounded by the axillary plexus, and nerve damage can result from a hematoma or traumatic cannulation. Air or thrombi will quickly gain access to the cerebral circulation during retrograde flushing of the left axillary artery.

B. Technique of Radial Artery Cannulation:

One technique of radial artery cannulation is illustrated in Figure 6–11. Supination and extension of the wrist provide optimal exposure of the radial artery. The pressure-tubing-transducer system should be nearby and already flushed with heparinized saline (0.5–2.0 U of heparin per mL of saline) to ensure easy connection after cannulation. The radial pulse is palpated and the artery's course is determined by lightly pressing the *tips* of the index and middle fingers of the anesthesiologist's nondominant hand over the area of maximal impulse. After preparing the skin with a bactericidal agent, 0.5 mL of lidocaine is infiltrated directly above the artery with a 25- or 27-gauge needle. An 18-gauge needle can then be used as a skin punch, facilitating entry of an 18-, 20-, or 22-gauge Teflon catheter-over-needle through the skin at a 45-degree angle, directing it toward the point of palpation. Upon blood flashback, the needle is lowered to a 30-degree angle and advanced another 1 to 2 mm to make certain that the tip of the catheter is well into the vessel lumen. "Spinning" the catheter oftentimes aids advancement of the catheter off the needle, which is then withdrawn. Applying firm pressure over the artery, proximal to the catheter tip with the middle and ring fingertips prevents blood from spurting while the tubing is being firmly con-

nected. Waterproof tape or suture keeps the catheter in place.

C. Complications:

Complications of intra-arterial monitoring include **hematoma, bleeding** (if the transducer tubing is not tightly affixed and separates from the catheter hub), vasospasm, arterial **thrombosis,** embolization of air bubbles or thrombi, necrosis of skin overlying the catheter, nerve damage, **infection,** loss of digits, and unintentional intra-arterial drug injection. Factors associated with an increased rate of complications include prolonged cannulation, hyperlipidemia, repeated insertion attempts, female gender, extracorporeal circulation, and the use of vasopressors. The risks are minimized when the ratio of catheter to artery size is small, heparinized saline is continuously infused through the catheter at a rate of 2–3 mL/hour, flushing of the catheter is limited, and meticulous attention is paid to aseptic technique. Adequacy of perfusion can be continually monitored during radial artery cannulation by placing a pulse oximeter on an ipsilateral finger.

Clinical Considerations

Because intra-arterial cannulation allows continuous, beat-to-beat blood pressure measurement, it is considered the gold standard of blood pressure monitoring techniques. The quality of the transduced waveform, however, depends on the dynamic characteristics of the catheter-tubing-transducer system (Figure 6–12). False readings can lead to inappropriate therapeutic interventions.

A complex waveform, such as an arterial pulse wave, can be expressed as a summation of simple sine and cosine waves (**Fourier analysis**). For accurate measurement of pressure, the catheter-tubing-transducer system must be capable of responding adequately to the highest frequency of the arterial waveform (Figure 6–13). Stated another way, the natural frequency of the measuring system must exceed the natural frequency of the arterial pulse (approximately 16–24 Hz).

Most transducers have frequencies of several hundred Hz (> 200 Hz for disposable transducers); the addition of tubing and stopcocks, and air in the line, all decrease the frequency of the system. If the frequency response is too low, the system will be **overdamped** and will not faithfully reproduce the arterial waveform, underestimating the systolic pressure. **Underdamping** is also a serious problem, leading to overshoot and a falsely high systolic blood pressure.

Catheter-tubing-transducer systems must also prevent **hyperresonance** or artifact caused by reverberation of pressure waves within the system. A **damping co-efficient** (β) of 0.6–0.7 is optimal. The natural fre-

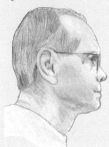

Wendell C. Stevens, MD

IF THERE WERE ONLY ONE MONITOR

This title begs for completion. If there were only one monitor, which one would I choose? Instructors sometimes use this type of inquiry as a pedagogical tool. If there were only one inhaled agent, one narcotic, one laryngoscope blade, one muscle relaxant, one local anesthetic, one intravenous solution, what would you choose?

In many parts of the world, the question is not a pedagogical exercise, but reality. There may be only one or at most a few choices of anesthetic drugs or monitors or other equipment. More than likely, the caregiver wishes, "If only there were a monitor..." or, the visiting doctor may be told, "That's all we have. Bring along what you need if you must have more."

Standard of care at this time in the more fully developed countries includes monitoring of oxygen concentration in the breathing system; a method or methods to assess oxygenation of the patient; mea-

surement of expired carbon dioxide; a method to detect disconnection of the breathing circuit from the patient; electrocardiography; measurement of arterial blood pressure, pulse rate, and additional circulatory variables in some circumstances; and finally, in most instances monitoring of body temperature.[1]

The reasons for each standard are clear enough. Their adoption was impelled by the desire for the greatest possible safety for patients. Additional monitors beyond those cited above are sometimes used, again, for purposes of safety, as well as to determine more precisely what is happening to a specific organ or system. The development has been encouraged by the desire to know more and to undertake safely more invasive and complex surgical procedures. The hope is that the information obtained can be used to alter anesthesia or surgical care to ensure the welfare of the patient. These special devices include electrocardiographic waveform analyses, real-time echocardiography, various kinds of sensory evoked responses, several types of electroencephalographic analyses, measures of regional cerebral perfusion, measurement of acid-base status in the gastrointestinal tract, and continuous determination of arterial or venous gases and acid-base values. A complete list would include many more. Another driving force for monitor development is the attempt to match depth and duration of anesthesia to the intensity and duration of surgery. The patient must be anesthetized but no more deeply than necessary, so the rationale goes. Thus, efforts are directed to develop monitors of anesthetic depth.

quency and damping coefficient can be determined by examining tracing oscillations after a high-pressure flush (Figure 6–14).

System dynamics are improved by minimizing tubing length, eliminating unnecessary stopcocks, removing air bubbles, and using low-compliance tubing. Although smaller diameter catheters lower natural frequency, they improve underdampened systems and are less apt to result in vascular complications. If a large catheter totally occludes an artery, reflected waves can distort pressure measurements.

Pressure transducers have evolved from bulky, reusable instruments to miniaturized, disposable chips. Transducers contain a diaphragm that is distorted by an

arterial pressure wave. The mechanical energy of a pressure wave is thereby converted into an electric signal. Most transducers are resistance types that are based on the **strain gauge** principle: stretching a wire or silicone crystal changes its electrical resistance. The sensing elements are arranged as a Wheatstone bridge circuit so that the voltage output is proportionate to the pressure applied to the diaphragm (Figure 6–15).

Transducer accuracy depends on correct calibration and zeroing procedures. A stopcock at the level of the desired point of measurement—usually the midaxillary line—is opened, and the zero switch on the monitor is activated. If the patient's position is altered by raising or lowering the operating table, the transducer must ei-

The array of available monitors and corresponding alarms have their problems. The inability to see them is one. Knowing which alarm applies to which variable is another. Recording all of the important data in a consistent, accurate manner is yet another. A still bigger problem is reliance on numerical data to the exclusion of feedback directly from the patient and from interaction with the surgeon. I do not intend to imply that anesthesia personnel are ignoring the patient or are inattentive. I do suggest that it is a mistake to have one's focus diverted from the patient and to fail to consider oneself always as part of the surgical team.

Being part of the surgical team can prevent over-reliance on monitors and allow one to provide good care with very few monitors. What I have in mind are such things as keeping an eye on the surgical field. The focus of attention for the greater part of the time should be on the patient and the operation, not on monitors. Is the patient making respiratory efforts and, if so, do they interfere with the operation? The respiratory dip on the end-tidal gas monitor does not always mean more relaxant is needed. Are the viscera protruding from the wound even as the twitch response to nerve stimulation is minimal? What can I do to make the operation easier? Will it soon be time for wound closure? When can awakening begin? It is appropriate for the surgeon to tell the anesthesiologist, "We're losing a lot of blood," or "The patient is moving," or "I only have a couple of stitches left to go." However, I am disappointed in my performance if alerts like these are my first inkling of the events.

All monitors that are effective for a particular operation can and perhaps should be used. Anesthesiologists must have the ability to apply monitors when they are indicated. More monitoring, however, does not necessarily lead to better care. For example, suppose an internal jugular catheter is to be inserted immediately after induction of anesthesia. The procedure will take place at a time of maximal instability—the anesthetic level will be changing rapidly, controlled ventilation may have just begun, the patient's position may need to be changed, and the patient may be fully draped. It is easy to recall the problems that have arisen under these circumstances: hypotension, hypertension, movement, arterial blood desaturation, all at a time when the patient is covered and those doing the procedure are gowned and gloved.

One of my professors and a former colleague, Dr. Jack Moyers, for many years a distinguished teacher and anesthesia clinician at the University of Iowa Hospitals, when speaking to anesthesia residents would say something like: You can be a much better anesthesiologist than I will ever be because you have learned how to apply all the new gadgets. You can know much more about your patients than I ever did. But I know you won't be better. What he had in mind, and stated in his inimitable way, was that rather than enhance what the resident learned from their patients, the monitors would divert the resident from hands-on and eyes-on care of the patient.

There is no reason to practice anesthesia with only one monitor, but there is reason to limit one's observation of monitors that may distract attention from the patient and the surgical procedure.

1. American Society of Anesthesiologists. *Standards for Basic Anesthetic Monitoring.* 1998.

---

ther be moved in tandem or zeroed to the new level of the midaxillary line. In a seated patient, the arterial pressure in the brain differs significantly from left ventricular pressure. In this circumstance, cerebral pressure is determined by setting the transducer to zero at the level of the ear, which approximates the circle of Willis. The transducer's zero should be regularly checked to eliminate any drift caused by temperature changes.

External calibration of a transducer compares the transducer's reading with a mercury column or a surrogate, but modern transducers rarely require external calibration.

Digital readouts of systolic and diastolic pressures are a running average of the highest and lowest measurements within a certain time interval. Since motion or cautery artifacts can result in some very misleading numbers, the arterial waveform should always be monitored. The shape of the arterial wave gives clues to several hemodynamic variables. The rate of upstroke indicates contractility, the rate of downstroke indicates peripheral vascular resistance, and exaggerated variations in size during the respiratory cycle suggest hypovolemia. Mean arterial pressure is calculated by integrating the area under the pressure curve.

Intra-arterial catheters also provide access for intermittent arterial blood gas sampling and analysis. The development of fiberoptic sensors that can be inserted through a 20-gauge arterial catheter enables continuous

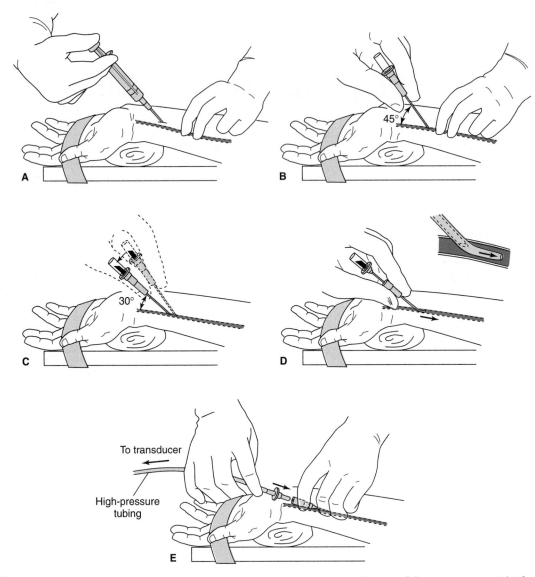

Figure 6–11. Cannulation of the radial artery. ***A:*** Proper positioning and palpation of the artery are crucial. After skin preparation, local anesthetic is infiltrated with a 25-gauge needle. ***B:*** A 20- or 22-gauge catheter is advanced through the skin at a 45-degree angle. ***C:*** Flashback of blood signals entry into the artery, and the catheter-needle assembly is lowered to a 30-degree angle and advanced 1–2 mm to ensure an intraluminal catheter position. ***D:*** The catheter is advanced over the needle, which is withdrawn. ***E:*** Proximal pressure with middle and ring fingers prevents blood loss, while the arterial tubing Luer-lock connector is secured to the intra-arterial catheter.

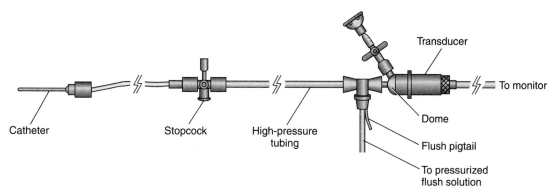

Figure 6–12. The catheter-tubing-transducer system.

blood gas monitoring. High-energy light is transmitted through the sensor to a tip containing fluorescent dyes. In response, the fluorescent dyes emit light of specific wavelengths and intensities, depending on pH, CO_2, and O_2 (**optical fluorescence**). The monitor detects changes in fluorescence and displays the corresponding blood gas values. Unfortunately, these sensors are quite expensive and are often inaccurate, so they are rarely used.

ELECTROCARDIOGRAPHY

Indications & Contraindications

All patients should have intraoperative monitoring of their electrocardiogram (ECG). There are no contraindications.

Techniques & Complications

Lead selection determines the diagnostic sensitivity of the ECG. The electrical axis of lead II parallels the atria, resulting in the greatest P wave voltages of any surface lead. This orientation enhances the diagnosis of dysrhythmias and detection of inferior wall ischemia. Lead V_5 lies over the fifth intercostal space at the anterior axillary line; this position is a good compromise for detecting anterior and lateral wall ischemia. A true V_5 lead is possible only on operating room electrocardiographs with at least five lead wires, but a modified V_5 can be monitored by rearranging the standard three-limb lead placement (Figure 6–16). Ideally, since each lead provides unique information, leads II and V_5 should be monitored simultaneously by an electrocardiograph with two channels. If only a single-channel

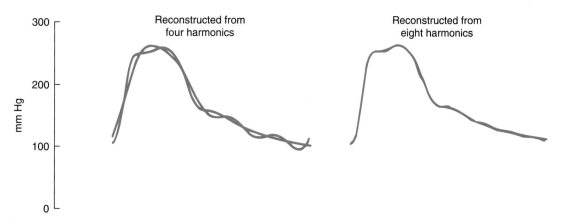

Figure 6–13. This illustration overlays an original waveform onto a four-harmonic reconstruction (***left***) and an eight-harmonic reconstruction (***right***). Note that the higher harmonic plot more closely resembles the original waveform. (Reproduced with permission from Saidman LS, Smith WT: *Monitoring in Anesthesia.* Butterworths, 1985, p 89.)

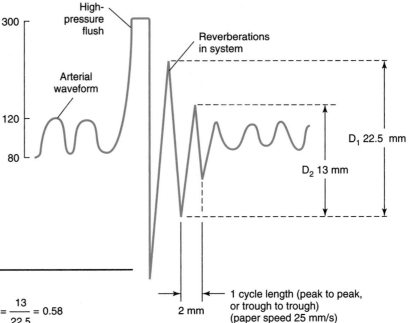

DAMPING

$$\text{Amplitude ratio} = \frac{D_2\ (mm)}{D_1\ (mm)} = \frac{13}{22.5} = 0.58$$

$$\text{Damping coefficient } \beta = \sqrt{\frac{\left(\ln\frac{D_2}{D_1}\right)^2}{\pi^2 + \left(\ln\frac{D_2}{D_1}\right)^2}} = 0.17$$

Amplitude ratio (D_2/D_1)	Damping coefficient
.9	.034
.8	.071
.7	.113
.6	.160
.5	.215
.4	.280
.3	.358
.2	.456
.1	.591

NATURAL FREQUENCY:

$$\text{Natural frequency} = f_n = \frac{1}{2\pi}\sqrt{\frac{\pi D^2\, \Delta P}{4\rho\, L\Delta V}} = \frac{\text{Paper speed (mm/sec)}}{\text{Length of 1 cycle (mm)}}$$

$$= \frac{25\ \text{mm/sec}}{2\ \text{mm}} = 12.5\ \text{Hz}$$

D = Internal diameter of tubing

ρ = Density of blood

L = Length of tubing

$\frac{\Delta P}{\Delta V}$ = Compliance (stiffness) of system

Figure 6–14. Damping and natural frequency of a transducer system can be determined by a high-pressure flush test. (Modified and reproduced with permission from Bedford RF: Invasive blood pressuring monitoring. In: Blitt CD (editor). *Monitoring in Anesthesia and Critical Care Medicine,* 2nd edition, Churchill Livingstone, New York, 1990, p 110.)

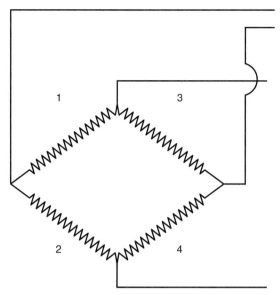

Figure 6–15. In the original strain gauge pressure transducers, a deformable diaphragm was connected to a Wheatstone bridge. When pressure was applied to the diaphragm, strain on two of the resistors (No. 2 and No. 3) increased, while strain on the other two (No.1 and No. 4) decreased. The change in total resistance across the bridge was proportional to the change in blood pressure allowing direct, accurate measurement of intravascular blood pressure.

machine is available, the preferred lead for monitoring depends on the location of any prior infarction or ischemia. Esophageal leads are even better than lead II for dysrhythmia diagnosis but have not yet gained general acceptance in the operating room.

Silver chloride electrodes are placed on the patient's body to monitor the ECG (Figure 6–17). Conductive gel lowers the skin's electrical resistance, which can be further decreased by cleansing the site of application with alcohol, a degreasing agent, or by mechanically exfoliating the superficial skin layer. Needle electrodes are used rarely and only if the silver chloride disks are unsuitable (eg, with an extensively burned patient).

Clinical Considerations

The ECG is a recording of the electrical potentials generated by myocardial cells. Its routine intraoperative use allows the detection of dysrhythmias, myocardial ischemia, conduction abnormalities, pacemaker malfunction, and electrolyte disturbances. Because of the small voltage potentials being measured, artifacts remain a major problem of electrocardiography. Patient or lead-wire movement,

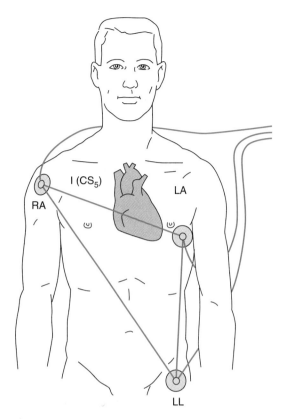

Figure 6–16. Rearranged three-limb lead placement. Anterior and lateral ischemia can be detected placing the left arm lead (LA) at the V_5 position. When lead I is selected on the monitor, a modified V_5 lead (CS$_5$) is displayed. Lead II allows detection of dysrhythmias and inferior wall ischemia. RA = right arm, LL = left leg.

electrocautery units, 60-cycle interference, and faulty electrodes can simulate dysrhythmias. Monitoring filters incorporated into the amplifier may lessen artifacts, but can lead to distortion of the ST segment and confuse the diagnosis of ischemia. Digital readout of heart rate may be

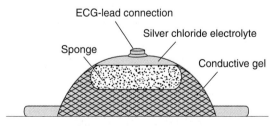

Figure 6–17. A cross-sectional view of a silver chloride electrode. ECG = electrocardiogram.

misleading because of the monitor's misinterpretation of artifacts or large T waves—often seen in pediatric patients—as QRS complexes.

Depending on equipment availability, a preinduction rhythm strip can be printed or frozen on the monitor's screen to compare with intraoperative tracings. To interpret ST-segment changes properly, the ECG must be standardized so that a 1-mV signal results in a deflection of 10 mm on a standard strip monitor. Newer units continuously analyze ST segments for early detection of myocardial ischemia. Automated ST-segment analysis increases the sensitivity of ECG ischemia detection, does not require much additional physician skill or vigilance, and may predict—if not prevent—adverse cardiac outcomes in some patients. Commonly accepted criteria for diagnosing myocardial ischemia include a flat or downsloping ST-segment depression exceeding 1 mm, 60 or 80 milliseconds after the J point (the end of the QRS complex), particularly in conjunction with T-wave inversion. ST-segment elevation with peaked T waves can also represent ischemia. Wolff-Parkinson-White syndrome, bundle branch blocks, extrinsic pacemaker capture, and digoxin therapy may preclude the use of ST-segment information. The audible beep associated with each QRS complex should be set loud enough for detection of rate and rhythm changes when the anesthesiologist's visual attention is directed to other responsibilities. Some ECGs are capable of storing aberrant QRS complexes for further analysis and some can even interpret and diagnose dysrhythmias. The interference caused by electrocautery units, however, has limited the usefulness of automated dysrhythmia analysis in the operating room.

CENTRAL VENOUS CATHETERIZATION

Indications

Central venous catheterization is indicated for monitoring central venous pressure for the fluid management of hypovolemia and shock, infusion of caustic drugs and total parenteral nutrition, aspiration of air emboli, insertion of transcutaneous pacing leads, and gaining venous access in patients with poor peripheral veins.

Contraindications

Contraindications include renal cell tumor extension into the right atrium or fungating tricuspid valve vegetations. Other contraindications relate to the cannulation site. For example, internal jugular vein cannulation is relatively contraindicated in patients who are receiving anticoagulants or who have had an ipsilateral carotid endarterectomy, because of the possibility of unintentional carotid artery puncture.

Techniques & Complications

Measurement of central venous pressure involves introducing a catheter into a vein so that the catheter's tip lies just above or at the junction of the superior vena cava and the right atrium. Because this location exposes the catheter tip to intrathoracic pressure, inspiration will increase or decrease central venous pressure, depending on whether ventilation is controlled or spontaneous. Measurement of central venous pressure is made with a water column (cm H_2O) or, preferably, an electronic transducer (mm Hg). Venous pressure should be measured during end-expiration.

Cannulation is possible at various sites. Long-term catheterization of the subclavian vein is associated with a significant risk of pneumothorax during insertion and with line-related infection the longer the catheter stays in place. The right internal jugular vein provides a combination of accessibility and safety (Table 6–1). Left-sided catheterization increases the risk of vascular erosion, pleural effusion, and chylothorax. There are at least three cannulation techniques: a catheter over a needle (similar to peripheral catheterization), a catheter through a needle (requiring a large-bore needle stick), and a catheter over a guidewire (Seldinger's technique). This last technique is illustrated in Figure 6–18 (A through D) and described below.

Table 6–1. Relative rating of central venous access.

	Basilic	External Jugular	Internal Jugular	Subclavian	Femoral
Ease of cannulation	1	3	2	5	3
Long-term use	4	3	2	1	5
Success rate (pulmonary artery catheter placement)	4	5	1	2	3
Complications (technique-related)	1	2	4	5	3

In each category, 1 = best, 5 = worst.

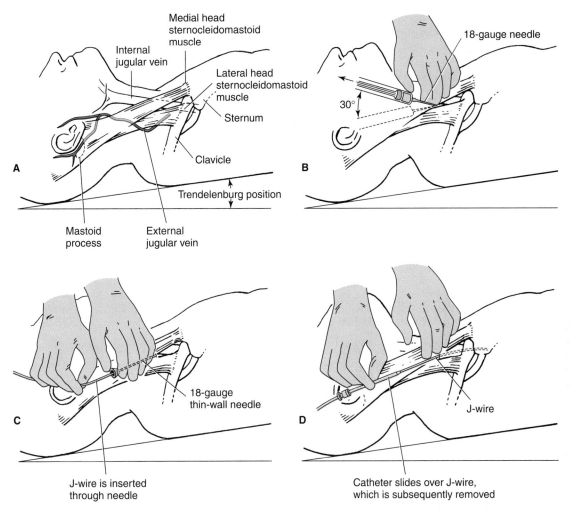

Figure 6–18. Right internal jugular cannulation with Seldinger's technique (see text).

The patient is placed in the Trendelenburg position to decrease the risk of air embolism and to distend the internal jugular vein. Venous catheterization requires full aseptic technique, including sterile gloves, mask, bactericidal skin preparation, and sterile drapes. The two heads of the sternocleidomastoid muscle and the clavicle form the three sides of a triangle (Figure 6–18A). A 25-gauge needle is used to infiltrate the apex of the triangle with local anesthetic. The internal jugular vein is found by advancing the 25-gauge needle—or a 23-gauge needle in heavier patients— along the medial border of the lateral head of the sternocleidomastoid, toward the ipsilateral nipple at an angle of 30 degrees to the skin. Alternatively, the vein can be located with the help of an ultrasound probe. Aspiration of

venous blood confirms the vein's location. The possibility of carotid puncture can be ruled out by transducing the waveform or comparing the blood's color or PaO_2 with an arterial sample. An 18-gauge thin-wall needle is advanced along the same path as the locator needle (Figure 6–18B). When free blood flow is achieved, a J-wire with a 3-mm-radius curvature is introduced (Figure 6–18C). The needle is removed, and a pliable catheter—Silastic, for example—is advanced over the wire (Figure 6–18D). The guidewire is removed, placing a thumb over the catheter hub to prevent aspiration of air until intravenous catheter tubing is connected to it. The catheter is then secured, and a sterile dressing is applied. Correct location is confirmed with a chest radiograph. The catheter's tip should not be allowed to migrate into the heart chambers. Fluid-administration sets should be changed every 72 hours.

The risks of central venous cannulation include **infection,** air or thrombus **embolism,** dysrhythmias (indicating that the catheter tip is in the right atrium or ventricle), hematoma, **pneumothorax,** hemothorax, hydrothorax, chylothorax, cardiac perforation, **cardiac tamponade,** trauma to nearby nerves and arteries, and thrombosis. Some of these complications can be attributed to poor technique.

Clinical Considerations

Normal cardiac function requires adequate ventricular filling by venous blood. Central venous pressure approximates right atrial pressure, which is a major determinant of right ventricular end-diastolic volume. In healthy hearts, right and left ventricular performance is parallel, so that left ventricular filling can also be judged by central venous pressure.

The shape of the central venous waveform corresponds to the events of cardiac contraction (Figure 6–19): *a* waves from *a*trial contraction are absent in atrial fibrillation and exaggerated in junctional rhythms (cannon waves); *c* waves are due to tricuspid valve elevation during early ventricular contraction; *v* waves reflect *v*enous return against a closed tricuspid valve; and the *x* and *y* descents are probably caused by the downward displacement of the ventricle during systole and tricuspid valve opening during diastole.

PULMONARY ARTERY CATHETERIZATION

Indications

As familiarization with pulmonary artery catheters (PAC) increases, so do the indications for their insertion (Table 6–2). The ASA has developed guidelines for pulmonary artery catheterization. Although the effectiveness of PAC monitoring remains largely unproven in many groups of surgical patients, the ASA concludes that the appropriateness of PAC use depends on the combination of risks associated with the patient, the operation, and the setting.

The ASA is participating in the Pulmonary Artery Catheter Clinical Outcome process, working to establish a Pulmonary Artery Catheter Educational Program (PACEP) for the use of the PAC and to examine the efficacy of the PAC. Monitoring pulmonary artery pressures and cardiac output has repeatedly been shown to provide more accurate cardiovascular information in critically ill patients than does clinical assessment. Basically, pulmonary artery catheterization should be considered whenever it is necessary to know cardiac indices, preload, volume status, or the degree of mixed venous blood oxygenation. These might prove particularly important in patients at high risk for hemodynamic instability (eg, recent myocardial infarction) or during surgical procedures associated with a high incidence of hemodynamic complications (eg, thoracic aortic aneurysm repair).

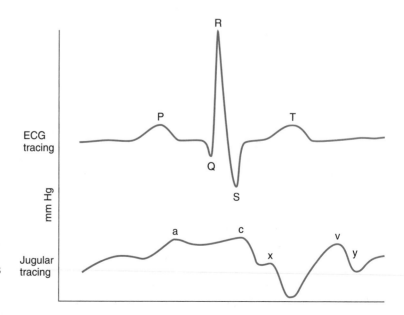

Figure 6–19. The upward waves (*a, c, v*) and the downward descents (*x, y*) of a central venous tracing in relation to the electrocardiogram.

Table 6–2. Indications for pulmonary artery catheterization.

Cardiac disease
  Coronary artery disease with left ventricular dysfunction or
    recent infarction
  Valvular heart disease
  Heart failure (eg, cardiomyopathy, pericardial tamponade,
    cor pulmonale)
Pulmonary disease
  Acute respiratory failure (eg, acute respiratory distress
    syndrome)
  Severe chronic obstructive pulmonary disease
Complex fluid management
  Shock
  Acute renal failure
  Acute burns
  Hemorrhagic pancreatitis
Specific surgical procedures
  Coronary artery bypass grafting
  Valve replacement
  Pericardiectomy
  Aortic cross-clamping (eg, aortic aneurysm repair)
  Sitting craniotomies
  Portal systemic shunts
High-risk obstetrics
  Severe toxemia
  Placental abruption

Contraindications

 Relative contraindications to pulmonary artery catheterization include complete left bundle branch block (because of the risk of complete heart block), Wolff-Parkinson-White syndrome, and Ebstein's malformation (because of possible tachyarrhythmias). A catheter with pacing capability is better suited to these situations. A PAC may serve as a nidus of infection in bacteremic patients or thrombus formation in those prone to hypercoagulation.

Techniques & Complications

Although various PACs are available, the most popular design integrates five lumens into a 7.5 catheter, 110 cm long, with a polyvinylchloride body (Figure 6–20). The lumens house the following features: wiring to connect the thermistor near the catheter tip to a thermodilution cardiac output computer; an air channel for inflation of the balloon; a proximal port 30 cm from the tip for infusions, cardiac output injections, and measurements of right atrial pressures; a ventricular port at 20 cm for infusion of drugs; and a distal port for aspiration of mixed venous blood samples and measurements of pulmonary artery pressure.

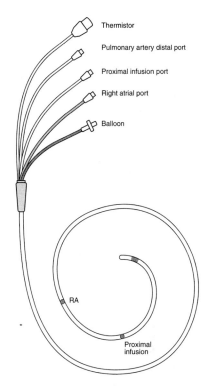

Figure 6–20. Balloon-tipped pulmonary artery flotation catheter (Swan-Ganz catheter). (Reproduced with permission from Catheter Reference Manual. Baxter Healthcare Corporation, Edwards Lifesciences LLC, 1993.)

Insertion of a PAC requires central venous access, which can be accomplished by Seldinger's technique, described above. Instead of a central venous catheter, a dilator and sheath are threaded over a guidewire. The sheath's lumen accommodates the PAC after removal of the dilator and guidewire (Figure 6–21).

Prior to insertion, the catheter is checked by inflating and deflating its balloon and irrigating all three intravascular lumens with heparinized saline. The distal port is connected to a transducer that is zeroed to the patient's midaxillary line.

The catheter is advanced through the sheath and into the internal jugular vein. At approximately 15 cm, the distal tip should enter the right atrium, and a central venous tracing that varies with respiration confirms an intrathoracic position. The balloon is inflated with air according to the manufacturer's recommendations (usually 1.5 mL) to protect the endocardium from the catheter tip and to allow the right ventricle's cardiac output to direct the catheter's forward migration. Con-

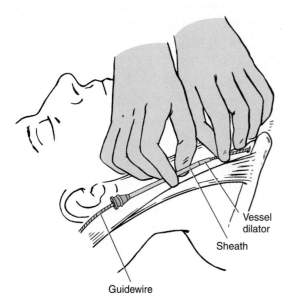

Figure 6–21. A percutaneous introducer consisting of a vessel dilator and sheath is passed over the guidewire.

treatment with intravenous lidocaine. A sudden increase in the *systolic* pressure on the distal tracing indicates a right ventricular location of the catheter tip (Figure 6–22). Entry into the pulmonary artery normally occurs by 35–45 cm and is heralded by a sudden increase in *diastolic* pressure.

To prevent catheter knotting, the balloon should be deflated and the catheter withdrawn if pressure changes do not occur at the expected distances. In particularly difficult cases (low cardiac output, pulmonary hypertension, or congenital heart anomalies), flotation of the catheter may be enhanced by having the patient inhale deeply; by positioning the patient in a head-up, right lateral tilt position; by injecting iced saline through the proximal lumen to stiffen the catheter (increasing the risk of perforation); or by administering a small dose of an inotropic agent to increase cardiac output.

After attaining a pulmonary artery position, minimal catheter advancement results in a pulmonary artery occlusion pressure (PAOP) waveform. The pulmonary artery tracing should reappear when the balloon is deflated. Wedging before maximal balloon inflation signals an overwedged position, and the catheter should be slightly withdrawn (with the balloon down, of course). Because **pulmonary artery rupture** carries a 50–70% mortality rate and can occur because of balloon overinflation, the frequency of wedge readings should be minimized. Pulmonary artery pressure should be continuously monitored to detect an overwedged position indicative of catheter migra-

versely, the balloon is always deflated during withdrawal. During the catheter's advancement, the ECG is monitored for dysrhythmias. Transient ectopy from irritation of the right ventricular endocardium by the balloon and catheter tip is common but rarely requires

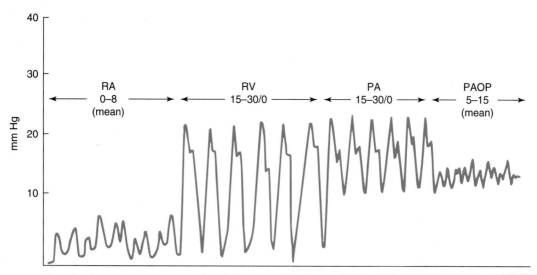

Figure 6–22. Normal pressure values and waveforms as a pulmonary artery catheter is advanced from the right atrium to a "wedged" position in a pulmonary artery. RA = right atrium; RV = right ventricle; PA = pulmonary artery; PAOP = pulmonary artery occlusion pressure.

tion. Furthermore, if the catheter has a right ventricular port 20 cm from the tip, distal migration will be detected by a change in the pressure tracing that indicates a pulmonary artery location.

Correct catheter position can be confirmed by a lateral chest radiograph. Although most catheters migrate caudally and to the right side, occasionally a catheter will wedge anterior to the vena cava. In this position, true pulmonary capillary pressures may be less than alveolar pressures, resulting in spuriously elevated measurements during positive pressure ventilation.

The numerous complications of pulmonary artery catheterization include those associated with central venous cannulation plus **bacteremia,** endocarditis, thrombogenesis, pulmonary infarction, **pulmonary artery rupture,** and hemorrhage (especially in patients who are taking anticoagulants, those who are elderly or female, or those who have pulmonary hypertension), catheter knotting, **dysrhythmias,** conduction abnormalities, and pulmonary valvular damage (Table 6–3). Even nominal hemoptysis should not be ignored, since it may herald pulmonary artery rupture. If the latter is suspected, prompt placement of a double-lumen endotracheal tube may maintain adequate oxygenation by the unaffected lung. The risk of complications increases with the duration of catheterization, which should not usually exceed 72 hours.

Clinical Considerations

The introduction of PACs into the operating room revolutionized the intraoperative management of critically ill patients. PACs allow more precise estimation of left ventricular preload than does central venous catheterization or physical examination. It also allows sampling of mixed venous blood and detection of air embolism and myocardial ischemia. Catheters with self-contained thermistors (discussed later in this chapter) can be used to measure cardiac output, from which a multitude of hemodynamic values can be derived (Table 6–4). Some catheter designs incorporate electrodes that allow intracavitary electrocardiography and pacing. Optional fiberoptic bundles allow continuous measurement of the oxygen saturation of mixed venous blood.

Starling demonstrated the relationship between left ventricular function and left ventricular end-diastolic muscle fiber length, which is usually proportionate to end-diastolic volume. If compliance is not abnormally decreased (eg, by myocardial ischemia, overload, ventricular hypertrophy, or pericardial tamponade), left ventricular end-diastolic pressure should reflect fiber length. In the presence of a normal mitral valve, left atrial pressure approaches left ventricular pressure dur-

Table 6–3. Reported incidence of adverse effects of pulmonary artery catheterization.

Complication	Reported Incidence (%)
Central Venous Access	
Arterial puncture	1.1–13
Bleeding at cut-down site	5.3
Postoperative neuropathy	0.3–1.1
Pneumothorax	0.3–4.5
Air embolism	0.5
Catheterization	
Minor dysrhythmias*	4.7–68.9
Severe dysrhythmias (ventricular tachycardia or fibrillation)*	0.3–62.7
Right bundle-branch block*	0.1–4.3
Complete heart block (in patients with prior LBBB)*	0–8.5
Catheter Residence	
Pulmonary artery rupture*	0.1–1.5
Positive catheter-tip cultures	1.4–34.8
Catheter-related sepsis	0.7–11.4
Thrombophlebitis	6.5
Venous thrombosis	0.5–66.7
Pulmonary infarction*	0.1–5.6
Mural thrombus	28–61
Valvular/endocardial vegetations or endocarditis*	2.2–100
Deaths*	0.02–1.5

*Complications thought to be more common (or exclusively associated) with pulmonary artery catheterization than with central venous catheterization. LBBB = left bundle branch block. (Reproduced with permission from: Practice guidelines for pulmonary artery catheterization: A report by the American Society of Anesthesiologists Task Force on pulmonary artery catheterization. Anesthesiology 1993;78:386).

ing diastolic filling. The left atrium connects with the right side of the heart through the pulmonary vasculature. The distal lumen of a correctly wedged PAC is isolated from right-sided pressures by balloon inflation. Its distal opening is exposed only to capillary pressure, which—in the absence of high airway pressures or pulmonary vascular disease—equals left atrial pressure. In fact, aspiration through the distal port during balloon inflation samples arterialized blood. This string of assumptions and relationships forms the rationale for monitoring PAOP—ie, it is an indirect method of measuring left ventricular fiber length and, therefore, ventricular function.

While central venous catheterization accurately reflects right ventricular function, a PAC is indicated if either ventricle is markedly depressed, causing disas-

Table 6–4. Hemodynamic variables derived from pulmonary artery catheterization data.

Variable	Formula	Normal	Units
Cardiac index	$\dfrac{\text{Cardiac output (L / min)}}{\text{Body surface area (m}^2\text{)}}$	2.2–4.2	L/min/m^2
Total peripheral resistance	$\dfrac{(\text{MAP} - \text{CVP}) \times 80}{\text{Cardiac output (L / min)}}$	1200–1500	dynes $\cdot$ sec $\cdot$ cm^{-5}
Pulmonary vascular resistance	$\dfrac{(\overline{\text{PA}} - \text{PAOP}) \times 80}{\text{Cardiac output (L / min)}}$	100–300	dynes $\cdot$ sec $\cdot$ cm^{-5}
Stroke volume	$\dfrac{\text{Cardiac output (L / min)} \times 1000}{\text{Heart rate (beats / min)}}$	60–90	mL/beat
Stroke index (SI)	$\dfrac{\text{Stroke volume (mL / beat)}}{\text{Body surface area (m}^2\text{)}}$	20–65	mL/beat/m^2
Right ventricular stroke-work index	0.0136 $(\overline{\text{PA}}-\text{CVP}) \times$ SI	30–65	g-m/beat/m^2
Left ventricular stroke-work index	0.0136 (MAP–PAOP) $\times$ SI	46–60	g-m/beat/m^2

g-m = gram meter, MAP = mean arterial pressure, CMP = central venous pressure, $\overline{\text{PA}}$ = mean pulmonary artery pressure, PAOP = pulmonary artery occlusion pressure.

sociation of right- and left-sided hemodynamics. Central venous pressures are not predictive of pulmonary capillary pressures in patients with ejection fractions less than 0.50. Even the PAOP does not always predict left ventricular end-diastolic pressure (Table 6–5). The relationship between left ventricular end-diastolic volume (actual preload) and PAOP (estimated preload) can become unreliable during conditions associated with changing left atrial or ventricular compliance, mitral valve function, or pulmonary vein resistance. These conditions are common immediately following major cardiac or vascular surgery and in critically ill patients who are on inotropic agents or in septic shock.

Table 6–5. Pulmonary artery occlusion pressure (PAOP) can wrongly estimate left ventricular end-diastolic pressure (LVEDP) in certain conditions.

PAOP > LVEDP
Mitral stenosis
Left atrial myxoma
Pulmonary venous obstruction
Elevated alveolar pressure
PAOP < LVEDP
Decreased left ventricular compliance (stiff ventricle or LVEDP > 25 mm Hg)
Aortic insufficiency

CARDIAC OUTPUT

Indications

Patients who benefit from measurements of pulmonary artery pressure also benefit from cardiac output determination. In fact, to use the information available from PACs most effectively, cardiac outputs must be obtained (see Table 6–4). Perfection of noninvasive techniques may eventually lead to routine intraoperative cardiac output monitoring.

Contraindications

There are no contraindications for cardiac output measurement by thermodilution other than those for pulmonary artery catheterization.

Techniques & Complications

A. THERMODILUTION:

The injection of a quantity (2.5, 5, or 10 mL) of fluid that is below body temperature (usually room temperature or iced) into the right atrium changes the temperature of blood in contact with the thermistor at the tip of the PAC. The degree of change is inversely proportionate to cardiac output: Temperature change is minimal if there is a high blood flow but pronounced if flow is low. Plotting the temperature change as a function of time produces a **thermodilution curve.** Cardiac output is determined by a computer program that integrates the area under the curve. Accurate measurements depend on rapid and smooth injection, precisely known injectant temperature and volume, correct entry of the calibration factors for the specific type of PAC into the cardiac output computer, and avoidance of measurements during electrocautery. Tricuspid regurgitation and cardiac shunts invalidate results because only right ventricular output is actually being measured. Rapid infusion of iced injectant has rarely resulted in cardiac dysrhythmias.

A modification of the thermodilution technique allows continuous cardiac output measurement with a special catheter and monitor system. The catheter contains a thermal filament that introduces small pulses of heat into the blood proximal to the pulmonic valve and a thermistor that measures changes in pulmonary artery blood temperature. A computer in the monitor determines cardiac output by cross-correlating the amount of heat input with the changes in blood temperature.

B. Dye Dilution:

If indocyanine green dye (or another indicator such as lithium) is injected through a central venous catheter, its appearance in the arterial circulation can be measured by analyzing arterial samples with an appropriate detector, a densitometer for indocyanine green, for example. The area under the resulting dye indicator curve is related to cardiac output. The dye-dilution technique, however, introduces the problems of indicator recirculation, arterial blood sampling, and background tracer buildup.

C. Ultrasonography:

A two-dimensional image of the heart can be obtained by passing a probe containing piezoelectric crystals into the esophagus. Oversized esophageal probes can cause aortic compression in infants or small children. **Transesophageal echocardiography** (TEE) assesses left ventricular filling (end-diastolic volume and end-systolic volume), ejection fraction, wall motion abnormalities, and contractility. Because ischemic myocardium does not exhibit normal inward movement or thickening during systole, TEE has proved to be a very sensitive indicator of intraoperative myocardial ischemia. In addition, air bubbles are easily recognized during air embolism (including paradoxic air embolism). Limitations include the need for the patient to be anesthetized before insertion (thus it is not useful during induction and intubation), difficulty distinguishing increased afterload from myocardial ischemia, and variability of interpretation.

Pulsed Doppler is a related technology that measures the velocity of aortic blood flow. Combined with TEE, which determines the aortic cross-sectional area,

this instrument can measure stroke volume and cardiac output. Further applications of ultrasonography include **transesophageal Doppler color-flow mapping,** which evaluates valvular function and intracardiac shunting. Blood flow information is represented by color (indicating flow direction) and intensity (indicating flow velocity). The major limitation of all of these systems is their expense.

Continuous-wave suprasternal Doppler also measures aortic blood velocity. Instead of requiring TEE, it uses a nomogram based on the patient's age, sex, and weight to estimate the aortic cross-sectional area for cardiac output calculations. While considerably less expensive, the use of a nomogram introduces the possibility of error, particularly in patients with aortic disease.

Transtracheal Doppler consists of a Doppler transducer attached to the distal end of an endotracheal tube. Cardiac output is derived from the ascending aorta diameter and blood velocity. Accurate results depend on a properly positioned probe.

D. Thoracic Bioimpedance:

Changes in thoracic volume cause changes in thoracic resistance (bioimpedance). If thoracic bioimpedance changes are measured following ventricular depolarization, stroke volume can be continuously determined. This noninvasive technique requires four pairs of electrocardiographic electrodes to inject microcurrents and to sense bioimpedance on both sides of the chest. Disadvantages of thoracic bioimpedance include susceptibility to electrical interference and reliance upon correct electrode positioning. As with both suprasternal and transtracheal Doppler, the accuracy of this technique is questionable in several groups of patients, including those with aortic valve disease or previous heart surgery.

E. Fick Principle:

The amount of oxygen consumed by an individual ($\dot{V}O_2$) equals the difference between arterial and venous (a-v) oxygen content (C) multiplied by cardiac output (CO). Therefore:

$$CO = \frac{\text{Oxygen consumption}}{\text{a-v } O_2 \text{ content difference}} = \frac{\dot{V}O_2}{C_aO_2 - C_vO_2}$$

Mixed venous and arterial oxygen content are easily determined if a PAC and an arterial line are in place. Oxygen consumption can also be calculated from the difference between the oxygen content in inspired and expired gas. Variations of the Fick principle are the basis of all indicator-dilution methods of cardiac output determination.

Clinical Considerations

Cardiac output measurements allow calculation of many indices that reflect the function of the entire circulatory system. Pulmonary artery pressures are difficult to interpret without knowing cardiac output. For instance, a patient with normal blood pressure and PAOP may have poor vital organ perfusion because of a low cardiac output and high systemic vascular resistance. Effective pharmacologic manipulation of preload, afterload, and contractility depends on accurate determination of cardiac output.

■ RESPIRATORY SYSTEM MONITORS

PRECORDIAL & ESOPHAGEAL STETHOSCOPES

Indications

Many anesthesiologists believe that all anesthetized patients should be monitored with a precordial or esophageal stethoscope.

Contraindications

Instrumentation of the esophagus should be avoided in patients with esophageal varices or strictures.

Techniques & Complications

A precordial stethoscope (Wenger chestpiece) is a heavy, bell-shaped piece of metal placed over the chest or suprasternal notch. Although its weight tends to maintain its position, double-sided adhesive disks provide an acoustic seal to the patient's skin (Figure 6–23). Various chestpieces are available, but the child size works well for most patients. The bell is connected to the anesthesiologist by extension tubing. A molded monaural earpiece allows simultaneous monitoring of the stethoscope and the operating room environment. Complications of precordial monitoring are extremely unlikely, though local allergic reactions, skin abrasion, and pain during removal of the adhesive disk rarely occur.

The esophageal stethoscope is a soft plastic catheter (8–24F) with balloon-covered distal openings (Figure 6–24). Although the quality of breath and heart sounds is much better with an esophageal stethoscope, its use is limited to intubated patients. Temperature probes, electrocardiographic leads, and even atrial pacemaker electrodes have been incorporated into esophageal

stethoscope design. Placement through the mouth or nose can occasionally cause mucosal irritation and bleeding. Rarely, the stethoscope slides into the trachea instead of the esophagus, resulting in a gas leak around the endotracheal tube cuff.

Clinical Considerations

The information provided by a precordial or esophageal stethoscope includes confirmation of ventilation, quality of breath sounds (eg, wheezing), regularity of heart rate, and quality of heart tones (muffled tones are associated with decreased cardiac output). The confirmation of bilateral breath sounds after endotracheal intubation, however, should be made with a more sensitive binaural stethoscope.

PULSE OXIMETRY

Indications & Contraindications

Pulse oximeters are mandatory intraoperative monitors. They are particularly useful when patient oxygenation must be measured frequently because of preexisting lung disease (eg, bleomycin toxicity), the nature of the surgical procedure (eg, hiatal hernia repair), or the requirements of special anesthetic technique (eg, one-lung anesthesia). Pulse oximeters are also helpful in monitoring neonates at risk for the retinopathy of prematurity. There are no contraindications.

Techniques & Complications

Pulse oximeters combine the principles of oximetry and plethysmography to noninvasively measure oxygen saturation in arterial blood. A sensor containing light sources (two or three light-emitting diodes) and a light detector (a photodiode) is placed across a finger, toe, ear-lobe, or any other perfused tissue that can be transilluminated.

Oximetry depends on the observation that oxygenated and reduced hemoglobin differ in their absorption of red and infrared light (**Lambert-Beer law**). Specifically, oxyhemoglobin (HbO_2) absorbs more infrared light (eg, 960 nm), while deoxyhemoglobin absorbs more red light (eg, 660 nm) and thus appears blue, or cyanotic, to the naked eye. Therefore, the change in light absorption during arterial pulsations is the basis of oximetry determinations (Figure 6–25). The ratio of the absorptions at the red and infrared wavelengths is analyzed by a microprocessor to give the oxygen saturation (SpO_2) of arterial pulsations. Arterial pulsations are identified by plethysmography, allowing corrections for light absorption by nonpulsating venous blood and tissue. Heat from the light source or sensor pressure may rarely result in tissue damage if the moni-

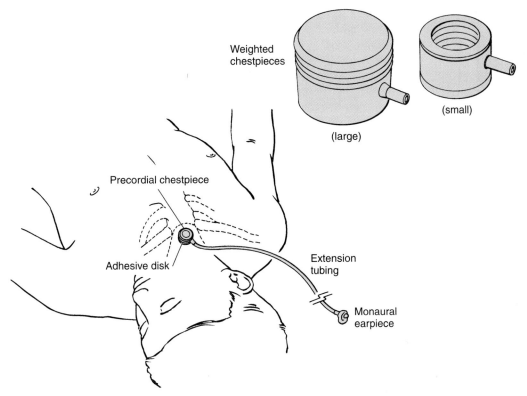

Figure 6–23. Precordial stethoscope.

tor is not periodically moved. No user calibration is required.

Clinical Considerations

In addition to SpO_2, pulse oximeters provide an indication of tissue perfusion (pulse amplitude) and measure heart rate. Because SpO_2 is normally close to 100%,

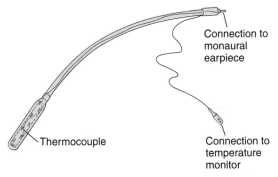

Figure 6–24. Esophageal stethoscope.

only gross abnormalities are detectable in most anesthetized patients. Depending on a particular patient's oxygen-hemoglobin dissociation curve, a 90% saturation may indicate a PaO_2 of less than 65 mm Hg. This compares with clinically detectable cyanosis, which requires 5 g of desaturated hemoglobin and usually corresponds to an SpO_2 of less than 80%. Endobronchial intubation will usually go undetected by pulse oximetry in the absence of lung disease or low inspired oxygen concentrations.

Because **carboxyhemoglobin (COHb)** and HbO_2 absorb light at 660 nm identically, pulse oximeters that only compare two wavelengths of light will register a falsely high reading in patients suffering from carbon monoxide poisoning. Methemoglobin has the same absorption coefficient at both red and infrared wavelengths. The resulting 1:1 absorption ratio corresponds to a saturation reading of 85%. Thus, **methemoglobinemia** causes a falsely low saturation reading when SaO_2 is actually greater than 85% and a falsely high reading if SaO_2 is actually less than 85%.

Most pulse oximeters have been found to be inaccurate at low SpO_2, and all demonstrate a delay between

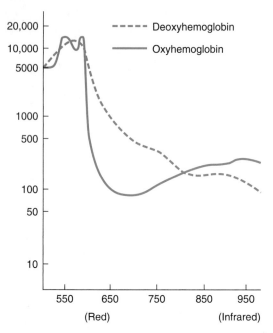

Figure 6–25. Oxyhemoglobin and deoxyhemoglobin differ in their absorption of red and infrared light.

changes in SaO_2 and SpO_2. Ear probes detect changes in saturation sooner than finger probes as a result of the shorter lung-to-ear circulation time. Loss of signal from peripheral vasoconstriction can be countered by performing a volar digital nerve block with plain local anesthetic solution. Other causes of pulse oximetry artifact include excessive **ambient light; motion; methylene blue dye;** venous pulsations in a dependent limb; low perfusion (eg, low cardiac output, very low hemoglobin, hypothermia, increased systemic vascular resistance); malpositioned sensor; and leakage of light from the light-emitting diode to the photodiode, bypassing the arterial bed (optical shunting). Nevertheless, pulse oximetry can be an invaluable aid to the rapid diagnosis of catastrophic hypoxia, which may occur in unrecognized esophageal intubation, and it furthers the goal of monitoring oxygen delivery to vital organs. In the recovery room, pulse oximetry helps identify postoperative respiratory problems such as severe hypoventilation, bronchospasm, and atelectasis.

Two extensions of pulse oximetry technology are **mixed venous blood oxygen saturation** ($S\bar{v}O_2$) and **noninvasive brain oximetry.** The former requires the placement of a special PAC containing fiberoptic sensors that continuously determine $S\bar{v}O_2$ in a manner analogous to pulse oximetry. Because $S\bar{v}O_2$ varies with

changes in hemoglobin concentration, cardiac output, arterial oxygen saturation, and whole-body oxygen consumption, its interpretation is somewhat complex (see Chapter 22). A variation of this technique involves placing the fiberoptic sensor in the internal jugular vein, which provides measurements of jugular bulb oxygen saturation in an attempt to assess the adequacy of cerebral oxygen delivery.

Noninvasive brain oximetry monitors regional oxygen saturation of hemoglobin in the brain (rSO_2). A sensor placed on the forehead emits light of specific wavelengths and measures the light reflected back to the sensor (near-infrared optical spectroscopy). Unlike pulse oximetry, brain oximetry measures venous and capillary blood oxygen saturation in addition to arterial blood saturation. Thus, its oxygen saturation readings represent the average oxygen saturation of all regional microvascular hemoglobin (approximately 70%). Cardiac arrest, cerebral embolization, deep hypothermia, or severe hypoxia causes a dramatic decrease in rSO_2.

END-TIDAL CARBON DIOXIDE ANALYSIS

Indications & Contraindications

Determination of end-tidal CO_2 ($ETCO_2$) concentration to confirm adequate ventilation is useful during all anesthetic procedures. Ventilator control of increased intracranial pressure by lowering $PaCO_2$ is easily monitored by analysis of $ETCO_2$. A rapid fall of $ETCO_2$ is a sensitive indicator of air embolism, a major complication of sitting craniotomies. There are no contraindications.

Techniques & Complications

Capnography is a valuable monitor of the respiratory, cardiac, and anesthetic breathing systems. Both types of capnographs in common use rely on the absorption of infrared light by CO_2 (Figure 6–26).

A. FLOW-THROUGH:

Flow-through (mainstream) capnographs measure CO_2 passing through an adaptor placed in the breathing circuit (Figure 6–27). Infrared light transmission through the gas is measured and CO_2 concentration determined by the monitor. Because of problems with drift, older flow-through models self-zeroed during inspiration. Thus, they were incapable of detecting inspired CO_2, such as would occur with a breathing circuit malfunction (eg, absorbent exhaustion, sticking unidirectional valves). The weight of the sensor causes traction on the endotracheal tube, and its radiant heat generation can cause skin burns. Newer designs address these problems.

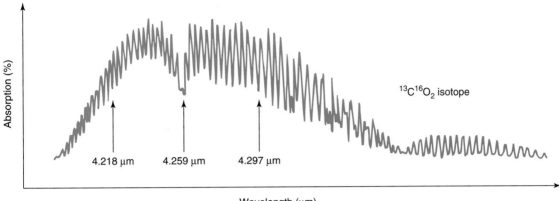

Figure 6–26. Absorption spectrum for CO_2. (Reproduced with permission from Hill DW: Methods of analysis in the gaseous and vapour phase. In: Scurr C, Feldman S (editors). *Scientific Foundations of Anesthesia.* Year Book, 1982, p 85.)

B. ASPIRATION:

Aspiration (sidestream) capnographs continuously suction gas from the breathing circuit into a sample cell within the monitor. CO_2 concentration is determined by comparing infrared light absorption in the sample cell with a chamber free of CO_2. Continuous aspiration of anesthetic gas essentially represents a leak in the breathing circuit that will contaminate the operating room unless it is scavenged or returned to the breathing

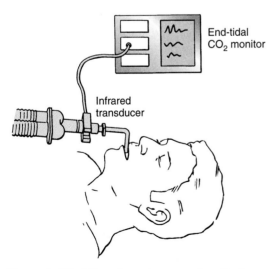

Figure 6–27. A flow-through sensor placed in-line analyzes CO_2 concentration at the sampling site.

system. High aspiration rates (up to 250 mL/min) and low-dead-space sampling tubing usually increase sensitivity and decrease lag time. If tidal volumes are small (eg, pediatric patients), however, a high rate of aspiration may entrain fresh gas from the circuit and dilute $ETCO_2$ measurement. Low aspiration rates (less than 50 mL/min) can retard $ETCO_2$ measurement and underestimate it during rapid respiratory ventilation. These units are zeroed to room air, but calibration requires a source of known CO_2 concentration (usually 5%). Expiratory valve malfunction is detected by the presence of CO_2 in inspired gas. Although inspiratory valve failure also results in rebreathing CO_2, this is not as readily apparent since part of the inspiratory volume will still be free of CO_2, causing the monitor to read zero during part of the inspiratory phase. Aspiration units are prone to water precipitation in the aspiration tube and sampling cell that can cause obstruction of the sampling line and erroneous readings.

Clinical Considerations

Other gases (eg, nitrous oxide) also absorb infrared light, leading to a **pressure-broadening** effect. To minimize the error introduced by nitrous oxide, various modifications and filters have been incorporated into monitor design. Capnographs rapidly and reliably indicate **esophageal intubation**—a common cause of anesthetic catastrophe—but do not reliably detect **endobronchial intubation.** While there may be some CO_2 in the stomach from swallowing expired air (< 10 mm Hg), this should be washed out within a few breaths. Sudden cessation of CO_2 during the expiratory phase may indicate a circuit disconnection. The increased metabolic rate caused by malignant hyperthermia causes a marked rise in $ETCO_2$.

The gradient between $ETCO_2$ and $PaCO_2$ (normally 2–5 mm Hg) reflects alveolar dead space (alveoli that are ventilated but not perfused). Any significant reduction in lung perfusion (eg, air embolism, upright positions, decreased cardiac output, or decreased blood pressure) increases alveolar dead space, dilutes expired CO_2, and lessens $ETCO_2$. True capnographs (as op-

posed to capnometers) display a waveform of CO_2 concentration that allows recognition of a variety of conditions (Figure 6–28).

TRANSCUTANEOUS OXYGEN & CARBON DIOXIDE MONITORS

Indications & Contraindications

Although useful in the management of many critically ill patients, transcutaneous gas monitors have gained

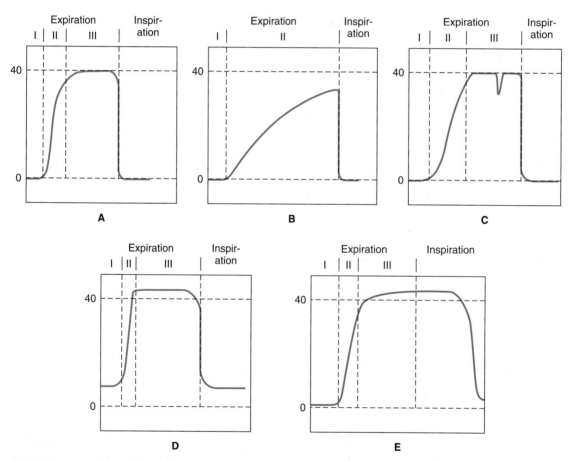

Figure 6–28. A: A normal capnograph demonstrating the three phases of expiration: Phase I-dead space; phase II-mixture of dead space and alveolar gas; phase III-alveolar gas plateau. **B:** Capnograph of a patient with severe chronic obstructive pulmonary disease. No plateau is reached before the next inspiration. The gradient between end-tidal CO_2 and arterial CO_2 is increased. **C:** Depression during phase III indicates spontaneous respiratory effort. **D:** Failure of the inspired CO_2 to return to zero may represent an incompetent expiratory valve or exhausted CO_2 absorbent. **E:** The persistence of exhaled gas during part of the inspiratory cycle signals the presence of an incompetent inspiratory valve.

widest acceptance in pediatric intensive care units. There are no contraindications.

Techniques & Complications

A sensor containing a CO_2 or oxygen (Clark) electrode—or both—and a heating element (skin heated to $\geq 41.5\ °C$ to arterialize the tissue bed) is attached to the skin. The oxygen electrode senses alterations in gas composition by changes in electrical conductivity of an electrolyte solution (polarography). Most CO_2 electrodes measure changes in pH:

$$pH = 0.97\ (log\ PCO_2)$$

The heating element vasodilates capillary vessels and increases gas diffusion by arterializing the stratum corneum. Dry standard gases and room air can be used for calibration and zeroing. Depending on blood flow, skin thickness, and heat settings, most sensors require 15–30 minutes to reach a stable plateau. Sensor location should be changed every 2 to 4 hours (every 8 hours if only CO_2 is being measured) to prevent skin burns, especially if perfusion is low.

Clinical Considerations

Transcutaneous sensors actually measure cutaneous partial pressures, which approach arterial values if cardiac output and perfusion are adequate. $PtcO_2$ (P_sO_2) is approximately 75% of PaO_2, and $PtcCO_2$ (P_sCO_2) is 130% of $PaCO_2$. A gradual drop in $PtcO_2$ may be due to a lower PaO_2 or a decrease in skin perfusion. The lack of consistent correlation between $PtcO_2$ and PaO_2 should not be viewed as a fault of this technology but rather as an early warning of inadequate tissue perfusion (eg, shock, hyperventilation, hypothermia). The $PtcO_2$ index is the ratio of $PtcO_2$ to PaO_2 and varies proportionately with cardiac output and peripheral blood flow. A rapid increase in $PtcO_2$ to 150 mm Hg indicates a displaced sensor that is exposed to room air.

Transcutaneous monitoring has not gained the popularity of pulse oximetry because of its warm-up time, difficulties of sensor maintenance, and complexities of interpretation. This is unfortunate, because it is a true indicator of tissue—albeit skin—oxygen delivery. Pulse oximetry and transcutaneous oxygen should be viewed as complimentary, not competing technologies. For example, a fall in $PtcO_2$ in the face of unchanging SpO_2 is a strong indication of poor tissue perfusion. Conjunctival oxygen sensors, which appear to be capable of non-invasively estimating arterial pH, are not commonly used clinically.

ANESTHETIC GAS ANALYSIS

Indications

Analysis of anesthetic gases could be useful during any procedure requiring inhalational anesthesia. There are no contraindications to analyzing these gases.

Techniques

The most common techniques for analyzing multiple anesthetic gases involve mass spectrometry, Raman spectroscopy, or infrared absorption.

A vacuum pump inside a **mass spectrometer** draws a gas sample from a side port in a breathing circuit elbow, through long tubing 1 mm in diameter, into the analyzer. Because of cost considerations, one mass spectrometer is usually shared by several operating rooms (a multiplexed system), and an inlet selector valve automatically switches sampling from one room to the next. The gas sample is ionized by an electron beam and passed through a magnetic field. The ions with the highest mass-to-charge ratio are least deflected and follow a curved path with the greatest radius (Figure 6–29). The spectrum of ion deflection forms the basis of analysis. Gases with identical molecular weights (CO_2 and N_2O) are differentiated by the deflection of

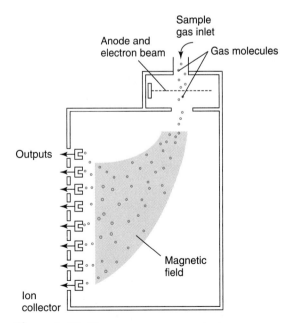

Figure 6–29. The mass spectrometer ionizes a gas sample and exposes it to a magnetic field. The degree of ion deflection determines its identity.

the fragments generated during electron-beam bombardment.

Raman spectroscopy identifies and measures gas concentrations by analyzing the intensity of light emitted when a gas sample returns to its unexcited state after being energized by a laser beam.

Infrared units use a variety of techniques similar to that described for capnography. Variations of infrared absorption include acoustic sensing, near-infrared optical sensing, and far-infrared optical sensing. Because oxygen molecules do not absorb infrared light, their concentration cannot be measured with monitors that rely on infrared technology.

Clinical Considerations

Although dedicated units are available, most mass spectrometers service more than one operating room. Therefore, gas samples are usually analyzed sequentially and results updated every 1–2 minutes. Newer units continuously measure CO_2 by infrared analysis and have the advantages of a separate capnograph. Other gases identified and quantified include nitrogen, oxygen, nitrous oxide, halothane, desflurane, sevoflurane, enflurane, and isoflurane. Rising end-tidal nitrogen quantitatively detects air embolism or leakage of air into the breathing system. Measurement of volatile agents guards against unintentional overdoses from vaporizer malfunction or unintentional vaporizer misfilling. For example, an isoflurane vaporizer partially filled with desflurane will deliver a much higher than expected, and dangerous, anesthetic dose because of the differences in vapor pressure of these agents.

One of mass spectrometry's disadvantages is that the constant aspiration of sample gas complicates the measurement of oxygen consumption during closed system techniques. In the presence of small tidal volumes or valveless Mapleson circuits, a high sampling rate may entrain fresh gas and dilute expired concentrations. In the future, mass spectrometry may include the capability of noninvasive lung volume and cardiac output measurement.

Mass spectrometers and Raman spectroscopy are equally accurate despite their basic technologic differences. Raman spectroscopy may have the advantages of a faster response time, self-calibration, and increased durability. Furthermore, the currently available Raman unit (the Rascal) is a stand-alone monitor that is not shared by multiple operating rooms.

Stand-alone units are also available that measure the concentration of volatile anesthetics by quartz oscillation or variations of infrared absorption instead of either mass or Raman spectroscopy. Although less expensive, many of these are unable to detect improperly filled vaporizers since they cannot distinguish between agents.

■ NEUROLOGIC SYSTEM MONITORS

ELECTROENCEPHALOGRAPHY

Indications & Contraindications

The electroencephalogram (EEG) is occasionally used during cerebrovascular surgery, cardiopulmonary bypass, and controlled hypotension to confirm the adequacy of cerebral oxygenation. Monitoring the depth of anesthesia with a full 16-lead, 8-channel EEG is not warranted, considering the availability of simpler techniques. There are no contraindications.

Techniques & Complications

The EEG is a recording of electrical potentials generated by cells in the cerebral cortex. Although standard ECG electrodes can be used, silver disks containing a conductive gel are preferred. Platinum or stainless steel needle electrodes traumatize the scalp and have high impedance (resistance); however, they can be sterilized and placed in a surgical field. Electrode position (**montage**) is governed by the international 10–20 system (Figure 6–30). Electric potential differences between

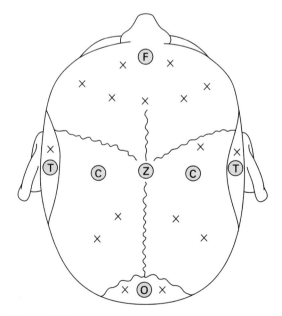

Figure 6–30. International 10–20 system. Montage letters refer to cranial location. F = frontal, C = coronal, T = temporal, O = occipital, Z = middle.

combinations of electrodes are filtered, amplified, and displayed by an oscilloscope or pen recorder.

A new two-channeled processed EEG device passes the EEG signal through a fast Fourier transform leading to a traditional power spectrum. The Bispectral Index (BIS) represents a numerical value that has been correlated with the patient's current hypnotic state (see below).

Clinical Considerations

Acceptance of intraoperative EEG monitoring has been limited by its space requirements, difficulty of interpretation, equivocal efficacy, and need to avoid high concentrations of anesthetic agents. Its accuracy has proved questionable in patients who have sustained prior brain damage (eg, stroke). The changes that accompany ischemia, such as high-frequency activity, can be mimicked by hypothermia, anesthetic agents, electrolyte disturbances, and marked hypocapnia. Nonetheless, detection of EEG changes should lead to an immediate review of possible causes of cerebral ischemia before irreversible brain damage has a chance to occur.

Bispectral analysis takes the data generated by electroencephalography, and through a number of steps (Figure 6–31), calculates a single number that, as mentioned, correlates with depth of anesthesia/hypnosis.

BIS values of 65 to 85 have been advocated as a measure of sedation, whereas values of 40 to 65 have been recommended for general anesthesia (Figure 6–32). It holds the potential to reduce patient awareness during anesthesia, an issue that is important in the public's eye. It has also been advocated to reduce resource utilization because less drug is required in order to ensure amnesia, facilitating a faster wake-up time and perhaps a shorter stay in the recovery room.

Many of the initial studies of its use were not prospective, randomized, controlled trials, but were primarily observational in nature. Artifacts can be a problem. There is also an additional cost per case. The monitor, in and of itself, costs several thousand dollars and the electrodes are approximately $10 to $15 per anesthetic and are unable to be reused.

Some cases with awareness have been identified as having a BIS less than 65. However, in other cases of awareness, either there were problems with the recordings or awareness could not be related to any specific time or BIS value. Whether this monitoring technique becomes a standard of care in the future remains to be seen.

EVOKED POTENTIALS

Indications

Indications for intraoperative monitoring of **evoked potentials** include surgical procedures associated with

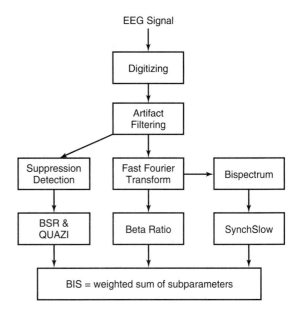

Figure 6–31. Calculation of the Bispectral Index. (Reproduced with permission from Rampil IJ: A primer for EEG signal processing in anesthesia. Anesthesiology 1998;89:980.) EEG = electroencephalogram; BSR = burst suppression ratio; BIS = Bispectral Index Scale.

possible neurologic injury: cardiopulmonary bypass, carotid endarterectomy, spinal fusion with Harrington rods, thoracoabdominal aortic aneurysm repair, and craniotomy. Global ischemia from hypoxia or anesthetic overdose is detectable. Evoked potential monitoring facilitates probe localization during stereotactic neurosurgery.

Contraindications

Although there are no specific contraindications, this modality is severely limited by the availability of monitoring sites, equipment, and trained personnel.

Techniques & Complications

Evoked potential monitoring noninvasively assesses neural function by measuring electrophysiologic responses to sensory stimulation. Commonly monitored evoked potentials are visual, auditory, somatosensory evoked potentials (SSEPs), and increasingly motor evoked potentials (MEPs) (Table 6–6).

For SSEPs, a brief electrical current is delivered to a sensory or mixed peripheral nerve by a pair of electrodes. If the intervening pathway is intact, an evoked potential will be transmitted to the contralateral sensory

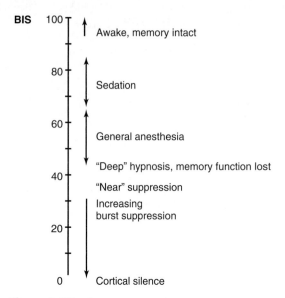

Figure 6–32. The Bispectral Index Scale (BIS versions 3.0 and higher) is a dimensionless scale from 0 (complete cortical electroencephalographic suppression) to 100 (awake). BIS values of 65–85 have been recommended for sedation, whereas values of 40–65 have been recommended for general anesthesia. At BIS values lower than 40, cortical suppression becomes discernible in raw electroencephalogram as a burst suppression pattern. (Reproduced with permission from Johansen JW et al: Development and clinical application of electroencephalographic Bispectrum monitoring. Anesthesiology 2000;93:1337.)

cortex. This potential is measured by scalp electrodes. To distinguish the cortical response to a specific stimulus, multiple responses are averaged and background noise is eliminated. Evoked potentials are represented by a plot of voltage versus time. The resulting waveforms are analyzed for their **poststimulus latency** (the time between stimulation and potential detection) and **peak amplitude.** These are compared with baseline

tracings. The significance of any change must be determined. Complications of evoked potential monitors are infrequent but include electrical shock, skin irritation, and pressure ischemia at the sites of electrode application.

Clinical Considerations

Evoked potentials are altered by many variables other than neural damage. The effect of anesthetics is complex and not easily summarized. In general, balanced anesthetic techniques (nitrous oxide, neuromuscular blocking agents [also called muscle relaxants], and opioids) cause minimal changes, while volatile agents (halothane, enflurane, sevoflurane, desflurane, and isoflurane) are best avoided. Early-occurring (specific) evoked potentials are less affected by anesthetics than are late-occurring (nonspecific) responses. In fact, changes in auditory evoked potentials may provide a measure of the depth of anesthesia. Physiologic (eg, blood pressure, temperature, and oxygen saturation) and pharmacologic factors should be kept as constant as possible.

Persistent obliteration of evoked potentials is predictive of postoperative neurologic deficiency. Unfortunately, because of their different anatomic pathways, *sensory* (dorsal spinal cord) evoked potential preservation does not guarantee normal *motor* (ventral spinal cord) function (false-negative). Furthermore, SSEPs elicited from posterior tibial nerve stimulation cannot distinguish between peripheral and central ischemia (false-positive). Investigational techniques that elicit MEPs by using transcranial magnetic stimulation or direct electrical stimulation by inserting needle electrodes in the cervical region are being used experimentally in a number of institutions. The advantage of using MEPs as opposed to SSEPs for spinal cord monitoring is that the MEPs monitor the ventral spinal cord, and if sensitive and specific enough, can be used to predict those patients who might develop a postoperative motor deficit. The same considerations for SSEPs are applicable to MEPs in that they are affected by volatile inhalational agents, by high-dose benzodiazepines, and by moderate hypothermia (temperatures less than 32 °C).

Table 6–6. Characteristics and uses of evoked potentials.

Type	Stimulus	Method of Delivering Stimulus	Surgical Procedure
Visual	Flashing lights	Light-emitting goggles	Pituitary tumor resection
Auditory	Clicks, tones	Ear transducer	Cerebellopontine angle tumor resection
Somatosensory	Electric current	Electrodes	Spinal cord injury
Motor	Electric current/magnetic field	Electrodes/magnet	Spinal cord injury

■ MISCELLANEOUS MONITORS

TEMPERATURE

Indications

The temperature of patients undergoing general anesthesia should be monitored. Very brief procedures (eg, less than 15 minutes) may be an exception to this guideline.

Contraindications

There are no contraindications, though a particular monitoring site may be unsuitable in certain patients.

Techniques & Complications

Intraoperatively, temperature is usually measured by a thermistor or thermocouple. **Thermistors** are semiconductors whose resistance decreases predictably with warming. A **thermocouple** is a circuit of two dissimilar metals joined so that a potential difference is generated when the metals are at different temperatures. Disposable thermocouple and thermistor probes are available for monitoring the temperature of the tympanic membrane, rectum, nasopharynx, esophagus, bladder, and skin.

Complications of temperature monitoring are usually related to trauma caused by the probe (eg, rectal or tympanic membrane perforation).

Clinical Considerations

Hypothermia, usually defined as a body temperature less than 36 °C, occurs frequently during anesthesia and surgery. Because hypothermia reduces metabolic oxygen requirements, it has proved to be protective during times of cerebral or cardiac ischemia. Unintentional hypothermia has several deleterious physiologic effects, however (Table 6–7). In fact, perioperative hypothermia has been associated with an increased mortality rate.

Table 6–7. Deleterious effects of hypothermia.

Cardiac dysrhythmias
Increased peripheral vascular resistance
Left shift of the hemoglobin-oxygen saturation curve
Reversible coagulopathy (platelet dysfunction)
Postoperative protein catabolism and stress response
Altered mental status
Impaired renal function
Decreased drug metabolism
Poor wound healing

Postoperative shivering increases oxygen consumption as much as 5-fold, decreases arterial oxygen saturation, and has been shown to correlate with an increased risk of **myocardial ischemia** and angina. Although postoperative shivering can be effectively treated with intravenous meperidine (25 mg), the best solution remains prevention by maintaining normothermia. The incidence of unintentional perioperative hypothermia increases with extremes of age, abdominal surgery, surgery of long duration, and cold ambient operating-room temperature.

Core temperature (central blood temperature) usually drops 1 or 2 °C during the first hour of general anesthesia (phase I), followed by a more gradual decline during the ensuing 3–4 hours (phase II), eventually reaching a point of steady-state or equilibrium (phase III). Redistribution of heat from warm central compartments (eg, abdomen, thorax) to cooler peripheral tissues (eg, arms, legs) from anesthetic-induced vasodilation explains most of the initial drop in temperature, with heat loss being a minor contributor. Nonetheless, continuous heat loss to the environment appears to be primarily responsible for the slower subsequent decline. During steady-state equilibrium, heat loss equals metabolic heat production (Figure 6–33).

Normally the hypothalamus maintains core body temperature within a very narrow range (the **interthreshold range**). Raising body temperature a fraction of a degree induces sweating and vasodilation, while lowering temperature triggers vasoconstriction and shivering. During general anesthesia, however,

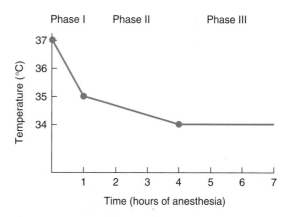

Figure 6–33. Unintentional hypothermia during general anesthesia follows a typical pattern: a steep drop in core temperature during the first hour (phase I redistribution), followed by a gradual decline during the next 3–4 hours (phase II heat loss), eventually reaching a steady state (phase III equilibrium).

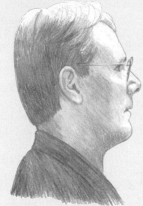

John R. Moyers, MD

APPLICATION OF THE BASIC PHYSICAL EXAMINATION TO INTRAOPERATIVE MONITORING

As an observer in today's operating rooms, one is struck by the devotion of the anesthesiologist to the complex array of sophisticated electronics that comprise the operating room monitoring system. Anesthesiologists sit with eyes fixed on the display screens, often with their backs to a patient whose head is completely covered, arms carefully tucked at the side, and eyelids meticulously taped closed.[1] The observer then witnesses at 5-minute intervals the careful, but unanalytic and uncritical recording on the anesthesia record, of every value displayed on each of the monitors. I submit that applying the basics of the physical examination learned in medical school to intraoperative monitoring enhances patient care and safety.

Several examples may lead to a better understanding of this premise. Basic monitoring variables include assessment of depth of anesthesia, ventilation, oxygenation, circulation, and temperature. Currently it is popular among some to rely upon the index derived from bispectral analysis of the electroencephalogram for assessing depth of anesthesia and prevention of awareness.[2] Nonetheless, the bispectral index does have its disadvantages. It is not as reliable as one would like with all anesthetic agents, and in many situations it may be neither sensitive nor specific enough to evaluate depth reliably. I once applied bispectral index electrodes to a serving of cherry gelatin with fruit cocktail from our cafeteria and recorded an index of 22. More appropriately and convincingly, a recent review by Drummond suggests that the peer-reviewed literature does not support the notion that such a device can serve to either monitor depth of anesthesia or prevent awareness.[3] With application of the physical examination, using pupillary response, ventilatory pattern, muscle tone, response to command, or movement, one can also assess depth of anesthesia. Clinical observation and judgment in concert with sophisticated monitoring provide a fuller and more accurate assessment of patient responsiveness to anesthesia than does monitoring alone.

After placement of a double-lumen endotracheal tube one often sees the anesthesiologist immediately inserting a fiberoptic bronchoscope through the lumen of the tube to assess proper placement. Alternatively, or prior to fiberoptic bronchoscopy, one can assess ventilation and tube placement (albeit with less precision) by inspection, palpation, and auscultation of the chest. With some experience

the body cannot compensate for hypothermia because anesthetics inhibit central thermoregulation by interfering with hypothalamic function. For example, isoflurane produces a dose-dependent decrease in the vasoconstrictive threshold (3 °C for each percentage of isoflurane).

Spinal and epidural anesthesia also lead to hypothermia by causing vasodilation and subsequent internal redistribution of heat (phase I). The accompanying thermoregulatory impairment from regional anesthesia that allows continued heat loss (phase II) appears to be due

to an altered perception of temperature in the blocked dermatomes by the hypothalamus—as opposed to a central drug effect as seen with general anesthetics. Thus, both general and regional anesthesia increase the interthreshold range, albeit by different mechanisms.

Prewarming for half an hour with convective forced-air warming blankets effectively prevents phase I hypothermia by eliminating the central-peripheral temperature gradient. Methods to minimize phase II hypothermia from heat loss include forced-air warming blankets, warm-water blankets, heated humidification one can detect ventilation of one hemithorax by each method. After this assessment of ventilation, there is time to proceed safely with bronchoscopy and to correct any difficulties with visualization or minor problems with tube placement that may have occurred. Also, using physical examination trains one to obtain a quick assessment of single-lung ventilation, or to recognize rapidly when a single-lumen tube has been inserted too deeply. In a similar fashion, assessment of capillary refill and palpation of a peripheral pulse can provide the anesthesiologist with a window into the circulatory status, and confirmation of more objective and sophisticated data gathered from monitoring devices. A finding of a warm and pink nose, good capillary refill, warm extremities, and bounding pulses provides a great deal of information about circulatory status. Conversely, a patient whose skin appears gray and mottled, has cold extremities, poor capillary refill, and a weak pulse needs some attention to circulatory status almost regardless of what the monitoring devices may display.

Indeed, sophisticated and complex monitoring techniques are necessary for good anesthesia practice. Simpler assessments are not always available or useful. Many patients are paralyzed with neuromuscular blocking agents necessitating controlled ventilation, which precludes the use of muscle tone or respiratory pattern to assess depth. It is difficult without sophisticated tools to monitor depth of anesthesia in a hypothermic patient in whom a cardiopulmonary bypass technique has been instituted. Adequacy of oxygenation does not lend itself very well to observation. A patient with a normal hemoglobin level will usually not appear cyanotic until the reading on the pulse oximeter is below 75%. For many procedures the anesthesiologist is remote from some or all of the patient's body, making direct contact difficult or impossible. Also, complex monitors free up time for other activities and allow objective measurement. Finally, other extremely important monitors measure parameters beyond our senses or quantitate otherwise inaccessible variables. For example, it is impossible to assess blood pH by physical examination.

Applying the physical examination to monitoring in the operating room adds no cost and leads to more patient contact and focus. There is no substitute for vigilance and common sense. Observation of the patient in the operating room can minimize recording of either incorrect or unnecessarily complex information and tends to eliminate a false sense of security that may result when viewing only the monitors. Judgment based upon both electronic monitors and aspects of the physical examination is usually a better assessment of patient status than either alone. There is comfort in assessing the same variable by more than one method and obtaining a similar answer. A local television weatherman once told me that he always looks out the window before he gives the weather report. Because human error plays a major role in most anesthesia disasters, applying the tenets of physical examination and common sense to monitoring may help to provide safer anesthetic care.

1. Hamilton WK: Do we monitor enough? We monitor too much. J Clin Monitoring 1986:2:246.

2. Kissin I: Ambulatory anesthesia: Depth of anesthesia and bispectral index monitoring. Anesth Analg 2000;90: 1114.

3. Drummond JC: Monitoring depth of anesthesia with emphasis on the application of the bispectral index and the middle latency auditory evoked response to the prevention of recall. Anesthesiology 2000;93:876.

of inspired gases, warming of intravenous fluids, and raising ambient operating room temperature. Passive insulators such as heated cotton blankets or so-called space blankets have little utility unless most of the body is covered.

Each monitoring site has advantages and disadvantages. The **tympanic membrane** theoretically reflects brain temperature because the auditory canal's blood supply is the external carotid artery. Trauma during insertion and cerumen insulation detract from the routine use of tympanic probes. **Rectal** temperatures have a slow response to changes in core temperature. **Nasopharyngeal** probes are prone to cause epistaxis but accurately measure core temperature if placed adjacent to the nasopharyngeal mucosa. The thermistor on a **pulmonary artery catheter** also measures core temperature. There is a variable correlation between **axillary** temperature and core temperature, depending on skin perfusion. Liquid crystal adhesive strips placed on the skin are inadequate indicators of core body temperature during surgery. **Esophageal** temperature sensors, often incorporated into esophageal stethoscopes, provide the best combination of economy, performance, and safety. To avoid measuring the temperature of tracheal gases, the temperature sensor should be positioned behind the heart in the lower third of the esophagus. Conveniently, heart sounds are most prominent at this location.

URINARY OUTPUT

Indications

Urinary bladder catheterization is the only reliable method of monitoring urinary output. Insertion of a urinary catheter is indicated in patients with congestive heart failure, renal failure, advanced hepatic disease, or shock. Catheterization is routine in some surgical procedures such as cardiac surgery, aortic or renal vascular surgery, craniotomy, major abdominal surgery, or procedures in which large fluid shifts are expected. Lengthy surgeries and intraoperative diuretic administration are other possible indications. Occasionally, postoperative bladder catheterization is indicated in patients having difficulty voiding in the recovery room after general or regional anesthesia.

Contraindications

Bladder catheterization should be done with utmost care in patients at high risk for **infection.**

Techniques & Complications

Bladder catheterization is usually performed by surgical or nursing personnel. To avoid unnecessary trauma, a urologist should catheterize patients suspected of having abnormal urethral anatomy. A soft rubber Foley catheter is inserted into the bladder transurethrally and connected to a disposable calibrated collection chamber. To avoid urine reflux, the chamber should remain at a level below the bladder. Complications of catheterization include urethral trauma and urinary tract infections. Rapid decompression of a distended bladder can cause hypotension. Suprapubic catheterization with plastic tubing inserted through a large-bore needle is an uncommon alternative.

Clinical Considerations

An additional advantage of placing a Foley catheter is the ability to include a thermistor in the catheter tip so that **bladder** or core temperature can be better monitored. As long as urinary output is high, bladder temperature accurately reflects core temperature. An added value with more widespread use of urometers is the ability to electronically monitor and record urinary output and core temperature.

Urinary output is a reflection of kidney perfusion and function. It is an indicator of renal, cardiovascular, and fluid volume status. Inadequate urinary output (**oliguria**) is often arbitrarily defined as urinary output of less than 0.5 mL/kg/hour, but actually is a function of the patient's concentrating ability and osmotic load. Urine electrolyte composition, osmolality, and specific gravity aid in the differential diagnosis of oliguria (see Chapter 50).

PERIPHERAL NERVE STIMULATION

Indications

Because of the variation in patient sensitivity to neuromuscular blocking agents, the neuromuscular function of all patients receiving intermediate- or long-acting neuromuscular blocking agents should be monitored. In addition, peripheral nerve stimulation is helpful in assessing paralysis during rapid-sequence inductions or during continuous infusions of short-acting agents. Furthermore, peripheral nerve stimulators can help to locate nerves to be blocked by regional anesthesia and determine the extent of sensory blockade.

Contraindications

There are no contraindications to neuromuscular monitoring, although certain sites may be precluded by the surgical procedure.

Techniques & Complications

A peripheral nerve stimulator delivers a current of variable frequency and amplitude to a pair of either electrocardiographic silver chloride pads or subcutaneous needles placed over a peripheral motor nerve. The evoked mechanical or electrical response of the innervated muscle is observed. Although electromyography provides a fast, accurate, and quantitative measure of neuromuscular transmission, visual or tactile observation of muscle contraction is usually relied upon in clinical practice. Ulnar nerve stimulation of the adductor pollicis muscle and facial nerve stimulation of the orbicularis oculi are most commonly monitored (Figure 6–34). Since it is the inhibition of the neuromuscular receptor that needs to be monitored, direct stimulation of muscle should be avoided by placing electrodes over the course of the nerve and not over the muscle itself. To deliver a supramaximal stimulation to the underlying nerve, peripheral nerve stimulators must be capable of generating at least a 50-mA current across a 1000-ohm load. This current is uncomfortable for a conscious patient. Complications of nerve stimulation are limited to skin irritation and abrasion at the site of electrode attachment.

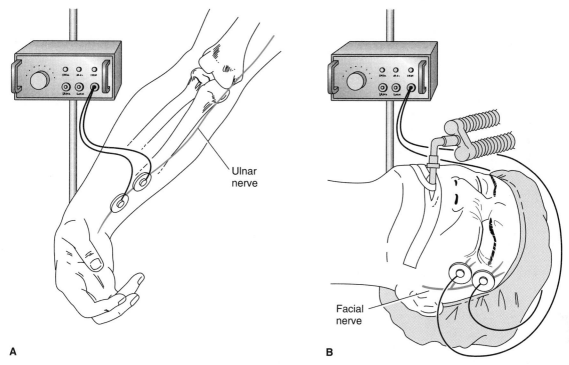

A   **B**

Figure 6–34. ***A:*** Stimulation of the ulnar nerve causes contraction of the adductor pollicis muscle. ***B:*** Stimulation of the facial nerve leads to orbicularis oculi contraction. The orbicularis oculi recovers from neuromuscular blockade before the adductor pollicis.

Clinical Considerations

The degree of neuromuscular blockade is monitored by applying various patterns of electrical stimulation (Figure 6–35). All stimuli are 200 μsec in duration, of square-wave pattern, and of equal current intensity. A **twitch** is a single pulse that is delivered from every second to every 10 seconds (1–0.1 Hz). Increasing block results in decreased evoked response to stimulation.

Train-of-four stimulation denotes four successive 200 μsec stimuli in 2 seconds (2 Hz). The twitches in a train-of-four pattern progressively fade as relaxation increases. The ratio of the responses to the first and fourth twitches is a sensitive indicator of nondepolarizing muscle relaxation. Because it is difficult to estimate the train-of-four ratio, it is more convenient to visually observe the sequential disappearance of the twitches, since this also correlates with the extent of blockade. Disappearance of the fourth twitch represents a 75% block, the third twitch an 80% block, and the second twitch a 90% block. Clinical relaxation usually requires 75–95% neuromuscular blockade.

Tetany at 50 or 100 Hz is a sensitive test of neuromuscular function. Sustained contraction for 5 seconds indicates adequate—but not necessarily complete—reversal from neuromuscular blockade. **Double-burst stimulation** (DBS) represents two variations of tetany that are less painful to the patient. The DBS$_{3,3}$ pattern of nerve stimulation consists of three short (200 μsec) high-frequency bursts separated by 20-msec intervals (50 Hz) and followed 750 msec later by another three bursts. DBS$_{3,2}$ consists of three 200-μsec impulses at 50 Hz followed 750 msec later by two such impulses. Double-burst stimulation is more sensitive than train-of-four stimulation for the clinical (ie, visual) evaluation of fade.

Since muscle groups differ in their sensitivity to neuromuscular blocking agents, use of the peripheral nerve stimulator cannot replace direct observation of the muscles (eg, the diaphragm) that need to be relaxed for a specific surgical procedure. Furthermore, recovery of adductor pollicis function does not exactly parallel recovery of muscles required to maintain an airway. The diaphragm, rectus abdominis, laryngeal adductors, and orbicularis oculi muscles recover from neuromus-

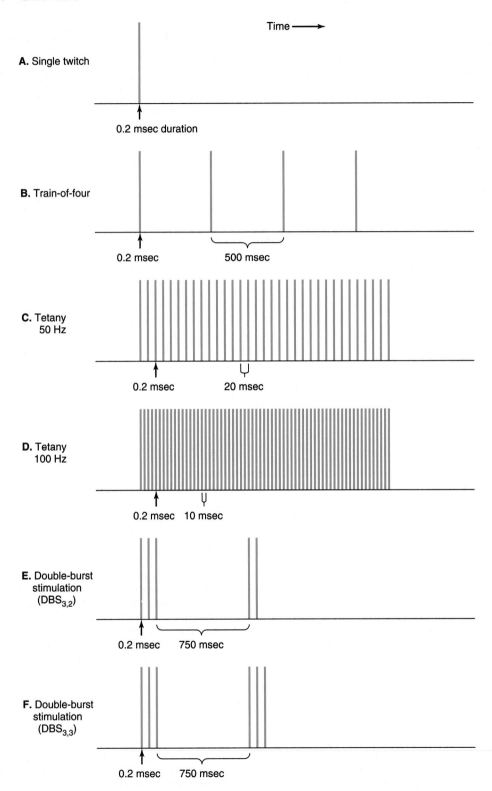

Figure 6–35. Peripheral nerve stimulators can generate various patterns of electrical impulses.

cular blockade sooner than does the adductor pollicis. Other indicators of adequate recovery include sustained head lift, an inspiratory effort of −25 cm H_2O, and a forceful hand grip. Twitch tension is reduced by hypothermia of the monitored muscle group (6% per degree C). Peripheral nerve stimulation is further considered in Chapter 9.

CASE DISCUSSION: MONITORING DURING MAGNETIC RESONANCE IMAGING

A 50-year-old man with recent onset of seizures is scheduled for magnetic resonance imaging (MRI). A prior MRI attempt was unsuccessful because of the patient's severe claustrophobic reaction. The radiologist requests your help in providing either sedation or general anesthesia.

Why does the MRI suite pose special problems for the patient and the anesthesiologist?

MRI studies tend to be long (often more than 1 hour) and most scanners totally surround the body, causing a high incidence of claustrophobia in patients already anxious about their health. Good imaging requires immobility, something that is difficult to achieve in many patients without sedation or general anesthesia.

Because the MRI uses a powerful magnet, no ferromagnetic objects can be placed near the scanner. This includes implanted prosthetic joints, artificial pacemakers, surgical clips, batteries, anesthesia machines, watches, pens, or credit cards. Ordinary metal lead wires for pulse oximeters or electrocardiographs act as antennas and may attract enough radiofrequency energy to distort the MRI image or even cause patient burns. In addition, the scanner's magnetic field causes severe monitor artifact. The more powerful the scanner's magnet as measured in Tesla units (1 Tesla = 10,000 gauss), the greater the potential problem. Other obstacles include poor access to the patient during the imaging (particularly the patient's airway), hypothermia in pediatric patients, dim lighting within the patient tunnel, and very loud noise (up to 100 decibels).

How have these monitoring and anesthesia machine problems been addressed?

Equipment manufacturers have developed monitor modifications that are compatible with the MRI environment. These include nonferro-magnetic electrocardiographic (ECG) electrodes, graphite and copper cables, extensive filtering and gating of signals, extra-long blood pressure cuff tubing, and use of fiberoptic technologies. Anesthesia machines with no ferromagnetic components (eg, aluminum gas cylinders) have been fitted with MRI-compatible ventilators and long circle systems or Mapleson D breathing circuits.

What factors influence the choice between general anesthesia and intravenous sedation?

Although most patients will tolerate an MRI study with sedation, head injury and pediatric patients present special problems and will often require general anesthesia. Because of machine and monitoring limitations, an argument could be made that sedation, when possible, would be a safer choice. On the other hand, loss of airway control from deep sedation could prove catastrophic because of poor patient access and delayed detection. Other important considerations include the monitoring modalities available at a particular facility and the general medical condition of the patient.

Which monitors should be considered mandatory in this case?

The patient should receive at least the same level of monitoring and care in the MRI suite as in the operating room for a similarly noninvasive procedure. Thus, the American Society of Anesthesiologists (ASA) Standards for Basic Anesthetic Monitoring would apply as they would to a healthy patient undergoing general anesthesia.

The MRI suite itself precludes some monitoring methods commonly used during intravenous sedation and requires modification of others. For example, because adequacy of oxygenation cannot be assessed by observing skin and nail bed color while the patient is in the scanner, pulse oximetry becomes even more necessary. Continuous auscultation of breath sounds with a plastic (not metal) precordial stethoscope could help identify airway obstruction caused by excessive sedation. Since palpation of a peripheral pulse or listening for Korotkoff sounds is impractical in this setting, ensuring adequacy of circulation depends more heavily on electrocardiography and oscillometric blood pressure monitoring. Although not mandatory, aspiration end-tidal carbon dioxide analyzers can be adapted to sedation cases by connecting the sampling line to a site near the patient's mouth or nose. Because room air entrainment

STANDARDS FOR BASIC ANESTHETIC MONITORING

(Approved by the ASA House of Delegates on October 21, 1986 and last amended on October 21, 1998)

These standards apply to all anesthesia care although, in emergency circumstances, appropriate life support measures take precedence. These standards may be exceeded at any time based on the judgment of the responsible anesthesiologist. They are intended to encourage quality patient care, but observing them cannot guarantee any specific patient outcome. They are subject to revision from time to time, as warranted by the evolution of technology and practice. They apply to all general anesthetics, regional anesthetics, and monitored care. This set of standards addresses only the issue of basic anesthetic monitoring, which is one component of anesthesia care. In certain rare or unusual circumstances, (1) some of these methods of monitoring may be clinically impractical, and (2) appropriate use of the described monitoring methods may fail to detect untoward clinical developments. Brief interruptions of continual[1] monitoring may be unavoidable. *Under extenuating circumstances, the responsible anesthesiologist may waive the requirements marked with an asterisk (*); it is recommended that when this is done, it should be so stated (including the reasons) in a note in the patient's medical record.* These standards are not intended for application to the care of the obstetric patient in labor or in the conduct of pain management.

STANDARD I

Qualified anesthesia personnel shall be present in the room throughout the conduct of all general anesthetics, regional anesthetics, and monitored anesthesia care.

Objective: Because of the rapid changes in patient status during anesthesia, qualified anesthesia personnel shall be continuously present to monitor the patient and provide anesthesia

care. In the event there is a direct known hazard, eg, radiation, to the anesthesia personnel that might require intermittent remote observation of the patient, some provision for monitoring the patient must be made. In the event that an emergency requires the temporary absence of the person primarily responsible for the anesthetic, the best judgment of the anesthesiologist will be exercised in comparing the emergency with the anesthetized patient's condition and in the selection of the person left responsible for the anesthetic during the temporary absence.

STANDARD II

During all anesthetics, the patient's oxygenation, ventilation, circulation, and temperature shall be continually evaluated.

OXYGENATION

Objective: To ensure adequate oxygen concentration in the inspired gas and the blood during all anesthetics.

Methods:

(1) Inspired gas: During every administration of general anesthesia using an anesthesia machine, the concentration of oxygen in the patient breathing system shall be measured by an oxygen analyzer with a low oxygen concentration limit alarm in use.*

(2) Blood oxygenation: During all anesthetics, a quantitative method of assessing oxygenation such as pulse oximetry shall be employed.* Adequate illumination and exposure of the patient are necessary to assess color.

precludes exact measurements, this technique provides a qualitative indicator of ventilation. Whenever sedation is planned, equipment for emergency conversion to general anesthesia (eg, endotracheal tubes, resuscitation bag) must be immediately available.

Is the continuous presence of anesthesia personnel required during standby cases?

*Absolutely yes. The term **standby anesthesia** is a misnomer; it has been replaced with **moni-***

***tored anesthesia care.** Sedated patients need to be continuously monitored to prevent a multitude of unforeseen complications, such as apnea or emesis.*

SUGGESTED READING

Bernard GR, Sopko G, Cerra F, et al: Pulmonary artery catheterization and clinical outcomes. National Heart, Lung, and Blood

VENTILATION

Objective: To ensure adequate ventilation of the patient during all anesthetics.

Methods:

(1) Every patient receiving general anesthesia shall have the adequacy of ventilation continually evaluated. Qualitative clinical signs such as chest excursion, observation of the reservoir breathing bag, and auscultation of breath sounds are useful. Continual monitoring for the presence of carbon dioxide shall be performed unless invalidated by the nature of the patient, procedure, or equipment. Quantitative monitoring of the volume of expired gas is strongly encouraged.*

(2) When an endotracheal tube or laryngeal mask is inserted, its correct positioning must be verified by clinical assessment and by identification of carbon dioxide in the expired gas. Continual end-tidal carbon dioxide analysis, in use from the time of endotracheal tube/laryngeal mask placement, until extubation/removal or initiating tranfer to a postoperative care location, shall be performed using a quantitative method such as capnography, capnometry, or mass spectroscopy.*

(3) When ventilation is controlled by a mechanical ventilator, there shall be in continuous use a device that is capable of detecting disconnection of components of the breathing system. The device must give an audible signal when its alarm threshold is exceeded.

(4) During regional anesthesia and monitored anesthesia care, the adequacy of ventilation shall be evaluated, at least, by continual observation of qualitative clinical signs.

CIRCULATION

Objective: To ensure the adequacy of the patient's circulatory function during all anesthetics.

Methods:

(1) Every patient receiving anesthesia shall have the electrocardiogram continuously displayed from the beginning of anesthesia until preparing to leave the anesthetizing location.*

(2) Every patient receiving anesthesia shall have arterial blood pressure and heart rate determined and evaluated at least every 5 minutes.*

(3) Every patient receiving general anesthesia shall have, in addition to the above, circulatory function continually evaluated by at least one of the following: palpation of a pulse, auscultation of heart sounds, monitoring of a tracing of intra-arterial pressure, ultrasound peripheral pulse monitoring, or pulse plethysmography or oximetry.

BODY TEMPERATURE

Objective: To aid in the maintenance of appropriate body temperature during all anesthetics.

Methods: Every patient receiving anesthesia shall have temperature monitored when clinically significant changes in body temperature are intended, anticipated or suspected.

---

[1] Note that "continual" is defined as "repeated regularly and frequently in steady rapid succession," whereas "continuous" means "prolonged without any interruption at any time."

Institute and Food and Drug Administration Workshop Report. JAMA 2000;19:2568.

Blitt CD, Hines RL (editors): *Monitoring in Anesthesia and Critical Care Medicine,* 3rd ed. Churchill Livingstone, 1995. All aspects of patient monitoring during anesthesia.

Brodsky JB: What intraoperative monitoring makes sense? Chest 1999;115:101S.

Dorsch JA, Dorsch SE: *Understanding Anesthesia Equipment,* 4th ed. Williams & Wilkins, 1999. Includes an excellent discussion on capnographs and mass spectrometers.

Ehrenwenh J, Eisenkraft JB (editors): *Anesthesia Equipment: Principles and Applications.* Mosby Year-Book, 1993. Very clearly written text that explains equipment design, standards, and hazards.

Fenelly M: Spinal cord monitoring. Anaesthesia 1998;53:41.

Jubran A: Advances in respiratory monitoring during mechanical ventilation. Chest 1999;116:1416.

Kawahito S, Kitahata H, Kimura H, et al: Recurrent laryngeal nerve palsy after cardiovascular surgery: Relationship to the placement of a transesophageal echocardiographic probe. J Cardiothorac Vasc Anesth 1999;13:528.

Keenan SP, Guyatt GH, Sibbald WJ, et al: How to use articles about diagnostic technology: Gastric tonometry. Crit Care Med 1999;27:1726.

Lake CL, Hines RL, Blitt CD: *Clinical Monitoring: Practical Implications for Anesthesia and Critical Care.* WB Saunders and Company, 2001.

Practice guidelines for pulmonary artery catheterization: A report by the American Society of Anesthesiologists task force on pulmonary artery catheterization. Anesthesiology 2002. In press.

Schell RM, Cole DJ: Cerebral monitoring: Jugular venous oximetry. Anesth Analg 2000;90:559.

Stump DA, Jones TJ, Rorie KD, et al: Neurophysiologic monitoring and outcomes in cardiovascular surgery. J Cardiothorac Vasc Anesth 1999;13:600.

Thornton C, Sharpe RM: Evoked responses in anaesthesia. Br J Anaesth 1998;81:771.

SECTION II
Clinical Pharmacology

Inhalational Anesthetics

KEY CONCEPTS

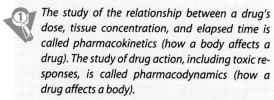

1 The study of the relationship between a drug's dose, tissue concentration, and elapsed time is called pharmacokinetics (how a body affects a drug). The study of drug action, including toxic responses, is called pharmacodynamics (how a drug affects a body).

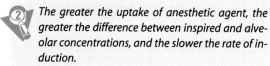

2 The greater the uptake of anesthetic agent, the greater the difference between inspired and alveolar concentrations, and the slower the rate of induction.

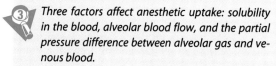

3 Three factors affect anesthetic uptake: solubility in the blood, alveolar blood flow, and the partial pressure difference between alveolar gas and venous blood.

4 Low-output states predispose patients to overdosage with soluble agents, since the rate of rise in alveolar concentrations will be markedly increased.

5 Many of the factors that speed induction also speed recovery: elimination of rebreathing, high fresh gas flows, low anesthetic-circuit volume, low absorption by the anesthetic circuit, decreased solubility, high cerebral blood flow, and increased ventilation.

6 General anesthesia is an altered physiologic state characterized by reversible loss of consciousness, analgesia of the entire body, amnesia, and some degree of muscle relaxation.

7 The unitary hypothesis proposes that all inhalational agents share a common mechanism of action at the molecular level. This is supported by the observation that the anesthetic potency of inhalational agents correlates directly with their lipid solubility (Meyer-Overton rule).

8 The alveolar concentration of an inhaled anesthetic that prevents movement in 50% of patients in response to a standardized stimulus (eg, surgical incision) is the minimum alveolar concentration (MAC).

9 Prolonged exposure to anesthetic concentrations of nitrous oxide can result in bone marrow depression (megaloblastic anemia) and even neurologic deficiencies (peripheral neuropathies and pernicious anemia).

(continued)

(continued)

 Halothane hepatitis is extremely rare (1 per 35,000 cases). Patients exposed to multiple halothane anesthetics at short intervals, middle-aged obese women, and persons with a familial predisposition to halothane toxicity or a personal history of toxicity are considered to be at increased risk.

 The cytochrome P-450 liver metabolism of methoxyflurane to free fluoride is responsible for vasopressin-resistant high-output renal failure.

 Isoflurane dilates coronary arteries but is not nearly as potent a dilator as nitroglycerin or adenosine. Dilation of normal coronary arteries could theoretically divert blood away from fixed stenotic lesions. There have been conflicting reports about whether the coronary steal syndrome causes regional myocardial ischemia during episodes of tachycardia or drops in perfusion pressure.

 The low solubility of desflurane in blood and body tissues causes a very rapid wash-in and wash-out of anesthetic.

Rapid increases in desflurane concentration lead to transient but sometimes worrisome elevations in heart rate, blood pressure, and catecholamine levels that are more pronounced than with isoflurane.

 Sevoflurane is an excellent choice for smooth and rapid inhalational inductions in pediatric and adult patients due to its nonpungency and rapid increases in alveolar anesthetic concentration.

Nitrous oxide, chloroform, and ether were the first universally accepted general anesthetics. Although chloroform and ether have long been abandoned in the United States (chiefly because of problems with toxicity and flammability), seven inhalational agents continue to be used in clinical anesthesiology: nitrous oxide, halothane, methoxyflurane, enflurane, isoflurane, desflurane and sevoflurane.

The course of general anesthesia can be divided into three phases: (1) induction, (2) maintenance, and (3) emergence. Inhalational anesthetics are particularly useful in the induction of pediatric patients unwilling to accept an intravenous line. In contrast, adults usually prefer rapid induction with intravenous agents, although the nonpungency and rapid onset of sevoflurane have made a single-breath induction practical for adults. Regardless of the patient's age, anesthesia is often maintained with inhalational agents. Emergence depends chiefly upon the pulmonary elimination of these agents.

Because of their unique route of administration, inhalational anesthetics have useful pharmacologic properties not shared by other anesthetic agents. For instance, exposure to the pulmonary circulation allows a more rapid appearance of drug in arterial blood than does intravenous administration. The study of the relationship between a drug's dose, tissue concentration, and elapsed time is called **pharmacokinetics (how a body affects a drug)**. The study of drug action, including toxic responses, is called **pharmacodynamics (how a drug affects a body)**.

After a general description of the pharmacokinetics and pharmacodynamics of inhalational anesthetics, this chapter presents the clinical pharmacology of individual agents.

■ PHARMACOKINETICS OF INHALATIONAL ANESTHETICS

Although the mechanism of action of inhalational anesthetics remains obscure, it is assumed that their ultimate effect depends on attainment of a therapeutic tissue concentration in the central nervous system. There are many steps, however, between the administration of an anesthetic from a vaporizer and its deposition in the brain (Figure 7–1).

FACTORS AFFECTING INSPIRATORY CONCENTRATION (Fi)

The fresh gas leaving the anesthesia machine mixes with gases in the breathing circuit before being inspired by the patient. Therefore, the patient is not necessarily receiving the concentration set on the vaporizer. The actual composition of the inspired gas mixture depends mainly on the fresh gas flow rate, the volume of the breathing system, and any absorption by the machine or breathing circuit. The higher the fresh gas flow rate, the smaller the breathing system volume, and the lower

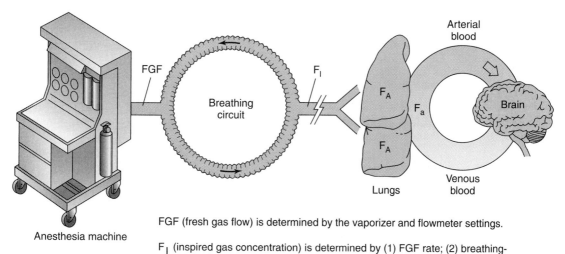

FGF (fresh gas flow) is determined by the vaporizer and flowmeter settings.

F_I (inspired gas concentration) is determined by (1) FGF rate; (2) breathing-circuit volume; and (3) circuit absorption.

F_A (alveolar gas concentration) is determined by (1) uptake (uptake = $\lambda_{b/g}$ x C(A-V) x Q); (2) ventilation; and (3) the concentration effect and second gas effect:
  a) concentrating effect
  b) augmented inflow effect

F_a (arterial gas concentration) is affected by ventilation/perfusion mismatching.

Figure 7–1. Inhalational anesthetic agents must pass through many barriers between the anesthesia machine and the brain.

the circuit absorption, the closer the inspired gas concentration will be to the fresh gas concentration. Clinically, these attributes translate into quicker induction and recovery times.

FACTORS AFFECTING ALVEOLAR CONCENTRATION (F_A)

Uptake

If there were no uptake of anesthetic agent by the body, the alveolar gas concentration (F_A) would rapidly approach the inspired gas concentration (F_I). Since anesthetic agent is taken up by the pulmonary circulation during induction, however, alveolar concentrations lag behind inspired concentrations ($F_A/F_I < 1.0$). The greater the uptake, the slower the rate of rise of the alveolar concentration and the lower the F_A:F_I ratio.

Because the concentration of a gas is directly proportional to its partial pressure, the alveolar partial pressure will also be slow to rise. The alveolar partial pressure is important because it determines the partial

pressure of anesthetic in the blood and, ultimately, in the brain. Similarly, the partial pressure of the anesthetic in the brain is directly proportional to its brain tissue concentration, which determines clinical effect.

 Therefore, the greater the uptake of anesthetic agent, the greater the difference between inspired and alveolar concentrations, and the slower the rate of induction.

 Three factors affect anesthetic uptake: solubility in the blood, alveolar blood flow, and the partial pressure difference between alveolar gas and venous blood.

Insoluble agents, such as nitrous oxide, are taken up by the blood less avidly than are soluble agents, such as halothane. As a consequence, the alveolar concentration of nitrous oxide rises faster than that of halothane, and induction is faster. The relative solubilities of an anesthetic in air, blood, and tissues are expressed as **partition coefficients** (Table 7–1). Each coefficient is the ratio of the concentrations of the anesthetic in two phases at equilibrium. Equilibrium is defined as equal partial pressures in the two phases. For instance, the

Table 7–1. Partition coefficients of volatile anesthetics at 37°C.*

Agent	Blood/Gas	Brain/Blood	Muscle/Blood	Fat/Blood
Nitrous oxide	0.47	1.1	1.2	2.3
Halothane	2.4	2.9	3.5	60
Methoxyflurane	12	2.0	1.3	49
Enflurane	1.9	1.5	1.7	36
Isoflurane	1.4	2.6	4.0	45
Desflurane	0.42	1.3	2.0	27
Sevoflurane	0.65	1.7	3.1	48

*These values are averages derived from multiple studies and should be used for comparison purposes, not as exact numbers.

blood/gas partition coefficient ($\lambda_{b/g}$) of nitrous oxide at 37 °C is 0.47. In other words, at equilibrium, 1 mL of blood contains 0.47 as much nitrous oxide as does 1 mL of alveolar gas, even though the partial pressures are the same. Stated another way, blood has 47% of the capacity for nitrous oxide as does gas. Nitrous oxide is much less soluble in blood than is halothane, which has a blood/gas partition coefficient at 37 °C of 2.4. Thus, almost five times more halothane than nitrous oxide must be dissolved to raise the partial pressure of blood. The higher the blood/gas coefficient, the greater the anesthetic's solubility and the greater its uptake by the pulmonary circulation. As a consequence of this high solubility, alveolar partial pressure rises more slowly, and induction is prolonged. Since fat/blood partition coefficients are greater than 1, it is not surprising that blood/gas solubility is increased by postprandial lipidemia and decreased by anemia.

The second factor that affects uptake is alveolar blood flow, which—in the absence of pulmonary shunting—is essentially equal to cardiac output. If the cardiac output drops to zero, so will anesthetic uptake. As cardiac output increases, anesthetic uptake increases, the rise in alveolar partial pressure slows, and induction is delayed. The effect of changing cardiac output is less pronounced for insoluble anesthetics, since so little is taken up regardless of alveolar blood flow. Low-output states predispose patients to overdosage with soluble agents, since the rate of rise in alveolar concentrations will be markedly increased. Higher than anticipated levels of a volatile anesthetic, which is also a myocardial depressant (eg, halothane), may create a positive feedback loop by lowering cardiac output even further.

The final factor affecting uptake of anesthetic by the pulmonary circulation is the partial pressure difference between alveolar gas and venous blood. This gradient depends on tissue uptake. If anesthetic did not pass into organs such as the brain, venous and alveolar partial pressures would become identical and there would be no pulmonary uptake. The transfer of anesthetic from blood to tissues is determined by three factors analogous to systemic uptake: tissue solubility of the agent (tissue/blood partition coefficient), tissue blood flow, and the partial pressure difference between arterial blood and the tissue.

Tissues can be assigned into four groups based on their solubility and blood flow (Table 7–2). The highly perfused **vessel-rich group** (brain, heart, liver, kidney, and endocrine organs) is the first to take up appreciable amounts of anesthetic. Moderate solubility and small volume limit the capacity of this group, however, so it is also the first to fill (ie, arterial and tissue partial pressures are equal). The **muscle group** (skin and muscle) is not as well perfused, so uptake is slower. In addi-

Table 7–2. Tissue groups based on perfusion and solubilities.

Characteristic	Vessel-Rich	Muscle	Fat	Vessel-Poor
Percentage of body weight	10	50	20	20
Percentage of cardiac output	75	19	6	0
Perfusion (mL/min/100 g)	75	3	3	0
Relative solubility	1	1	20	0

tion, it has a greater capacity owing to a larger volume, and uptake will be sustained for hours. Perfusion of the **fat group** nearly equals that of the muscle group, but the tremendous solubility of anesthetic in fat leads to a total capacity (tissue/blood solubility × tissue volume) that would take days to fill. The minimal perfusion of the **vessel-poor group** (bone, ligaments, teeth, hair, and cartilage) results in insignificant uptake.

Anesthetic uptake produces a characteristic curve that relates the rise in alveolar concentration to time (Figure 7–2). The shape of this graph is determined by the uptakes of individual tissue groups (Figure 7–3). The initial steep rate of uptake is due to unopposed filling of the alveoli by ventilation. The rate of rise slows as the vessel-rich group—and eventually the muscle group—reach their capacity.

Ventilation

The lowering of alveolar partial pressure by uptake can be countered by increasing alveolar ventilation. In other words, constantly replacing anesthetic taken up by the pulmonary bloodstream, maintains alveolar concentra-

tion better. The effect of increasing ventilation will be most obvious in raising the FA/FI for soluble anesthetics, since they are more subject to uptake. Since the FA/FI is already high for insoluble agents, increasing ventilation has minimal effect. In contrast to the effect of anesthetics on cardiac output, anesthetics that depress ventilation (eg, halothane) will decrease the rate of rise in alveolar concentration and create a negative feedback loop.

Concentration

The effects of uptake can also be lessened by increasing the inspired concentration. Interestingly, increasing the inspired concentration not only increases the alveolar concentration but also increases its rate of rise (ie, increases FA/FI). This has been termed the **concentration effect** (see Figure 7–1), which is really the result of two phenomena. The first is confusingly called the **concentrating effect.** If 50% of an anesthetic is taken up by the pulmonary circulation, an inspired concentration of 20% (20 parts of anesthetic per 100 parts of gas) will result in an alveolar concentration of 11% (10 parts of anesthetic remaining in a total volume of 90 parts of

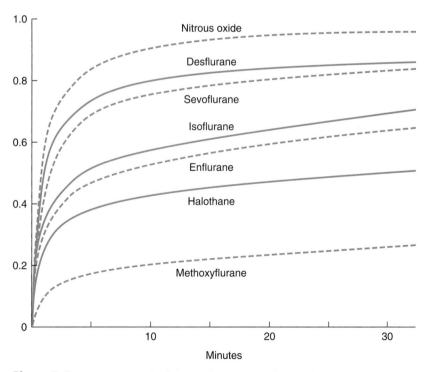

Figure 7–2. FA rises toward FI faster with nitrous oxide (an insoluble agent) than with methoxyflurane (a soluble agent). See Figure 7–1 for explanation of FA and FI. (Modified and reproduced, with permission, from Eger EL II: *Isoflurane [Forane]: A Reference and Compendium.* Ohio Medical Products, 1981.)

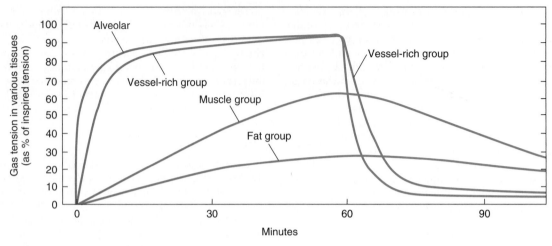

Figure 7–3. The rise and fall in alveolar partial pressure precedes that of other tissues. (Modified and reproduced, with permission, from Cowles AL et al: Uptake and distribution of inhalation anesthetic agents in clinical practice. Anesth Analg 1968;4:404.}

gas). On the other hand, if the inspired concentration is raised to 80% (80 parts per 100), the alveolar concentration will be 67% (40 parts of anesthetic remaining in a total volume of 60 parts). Thus, even though 50% of the anesthetic is taken up in both examples, a higher inspired concentration results in a disproportionately higher alveolar concentration. In this example, increasing the inspired concentration 4-fold results in a 6-fold increase in alveolar concentration. The extreme case is an inspired concentration of 100% (100 parts of 100), which, despite a 50% uptake, will result in an alveolar concentration of 100% (50 parts remaining in a total volume of 50 parts).

The second phenomenon responsible for the concentration effect is the **augmented inflow effect.** Using the example above, the 10 parts of absorbed gas must be replaced by an equal volume of the 20% mixture to prevent alveolar collapse. Thus, the alveolar concentration becomes 12% (10 plus 2 parts of anesthetic in a total of 100 parts of gas). In contrast, after absorption of half of the anesthetic in the 80% gas mixture, 40 parts of 80% gas must be inspired. This further increases the alveolar concentration from 67% to 72% (40 plus 32 in a volume of 100).

The concentration effect is more significant with nitrous oxide than with the volatile anesthetics, since the former can be used in much higher concentrations. Nonetheless, a high concentration of nitrous oxide will augment (by the same mechanism) not only its own uptake but theoretically that of a concurrently administered volatile anesthetic. The concentration effect of one gas upon another is called the **second gas effect.**

The second gas effect has been shown to be extremely weak and probably insignificant in the clinical practice of anesthesiology.

FACTORS AFFECTING ARTERIAL CONCENTRATION (Fa)

Ventilation/Perfusion Mismatch

Normally, alveolar and arterial anesthetic partial pressures are assumed to be equal, but in fact the arterial partial pressure is consistently less than end-expiratory gas would predict. Reasons for this may include venous admixture, alveolar dead space, and nonuniform alveolar gas distribution. Furthermore, the existence of ventilation/perfusion mismatching will increase the alveolar-arterial difference. Mismatch acts like a restriction to flow: It raises the pressure in front of the restriction, lowers the pressure beyond the restriction, and reduces the flow through the restriction. The overall effect is an increase in the alveolar partial pressure (especially for highly soluble agents) and a decrease in the arterial partial pressure (especially for poorly soluble agents). Thus, an endobronchial intubation or a right-to-left intracardiac shunt will slow the rate of induction with nitrous oxide more than with halothane.

FACTORS AFFECTING ELIMINATION

Recovery from anesthesia depends on lowering anesthetic concentration in brain tissue. Anesthetics can be eliminated by biotransformation, transcutaneous loss, or exhalation. Biotransformation usually accounts for a minimal increase in the rate of decline of alveolar partial pressure. Its greatest impact is on the elimination of soluble anesthetics that undergo extensive metabolism (eg, methoxyflurane). The greater biotransformation of halothane compared with enflurane accounts for halothane's faster elimination despite its being more soluble. The cytochrome P-450 group of isozymes (specifically CYP 2EI) appears to be important in the metabolism of some volatile anesthetics. Diffusion of anesthetic through the skin is insignificant.

 The most important route for elimination of inhalational anesthetics is the alveolus. Many of the factors that speed induction also speed recovery: elimination of rebreathing, high fresh gas flows, low anesthetic-circuit volume, low absorption by the anesthetic circuit, decreased solubility, high cerebral blood flow (CBF), and increased ventilation. Nitrous oxide elimination is so rapid that it dilutes alveolar oxygen and CO_2. The resulting **diffusion hypoxia** is prevented by administering 100% oxygen for 5–10 minutes after discontinuing nitrous oxide. Rate of recovery is usually faster than induction because tissues that have not reached equilibrium will continue to take up anesthetic until the alveolar partial pressure falls below tissue partial pressure. For instance, fat will continue to take up anesthetic and hasten recovery until its partial pressure exceeds alveolar partial pressure. This redistribution is not as available after prolonged anesthesia—thus, the speed of recovery also depends on the length of time the anesthetic has been administered.

PHARMACODYNAMICS OF INHALATIONAL ANESTHETICS

THEORIES OF ANESTHETIC ACTION

General anesthesia is an altered physiologic state characterized by reversible loss of consciousness, analgesia of the entire body, amnesia, and some degree of muscle relaxation. The multitude of substances capable of producing general anesthesia is remarkable: inert elements (xenon), simple inorganic compounds (nitrous oxide), halogenated hydrocarbons (halothane), and complex organic structures (barbiturates). A unifying theory explaining anesthetic action would have to accommodate this diversity of structure. In fact, the various agents probably produce anesthesia by different methods (**agent-specific theory**). For example, opioids are known to interact with stereospecific receptors, while inhalational agents do

not have a predominant structure-activity relationship (opiate receptors may mediate some minor inhalational anesthetic effects).

There does not appear to be a single macroscopic site of action that is shared by all inhalational agents. Specific brain areas affected by various anesthetics include the reticular activating system, the cerebral cortex, the cuneate nucleus, the olfactory cortex, and the hippocampus. Anesthetics have also been shown to depress excitatory transmission in the spinal cord, particularly at the level of the dorsal horn interneurons that are involved in pain transmission. Differing aspects of anesthesia may be related to different sites of anesthetic action. For example, unconsciousness and amnesia are probably mediated by cortical anesthetic action, while the suppression of purposeful withdrawal from pain may be related to subcortical structures such as the spinal cord or brainstem. One study in rats revealed that removal of the cerebral cortex did not alter the potency of the anesthetic!

At a microscopic level, synaptic transmission is much more sensitive to general anesthetic agents than axonal conduction, though small-diameter nerve axons may be vulnerable. Both presynaptic and postsynaptic mechanisms are plausible.

The **unitary hypothesis** proposes that all inhalational agents share a common mechanism of action at the molecular level. This is supported by the observation that the anesthetic potency of inhalational agents correlates directly with their lipid solubility (**Meyer-Overton rule**). The implication is that anesthesia results from molecules dissolving at specific hydrophobic sites. Of course, not all lipid-soluble molecules are anesthetics (some are actually convulsants), and the correlation between anesthetic potency and lipid solubility is only approximate (Figure 7–4).

Neuronal membranes contain a multitude of hydrophobic sites in their phospholipid bilayer. Anesthetic binding to these sites could expand the bilayer beyond a critical amount, altering membrane function (**critical volume hypothesis**). While this theory is probably an oversimplification, it explains an interesting phenomenon: the reversal of anesthesia by increased pressure. Laboratory animals exposed to elevated hydrostatic pressure develop a resistance to anesthetic effects. Perhaps the pressure is displacing a number of molecules from the membrane, increasing anesthetic requirements.

Anesthetic binding might significantly modify membrane structure. Two theories suggest disturbances in membrane form (the **fluidization theory of anesthesia** and the **lateral phase separation theory**), while another proposes decreases in membrane conductance. Altering membrane structure could produce anesthesia

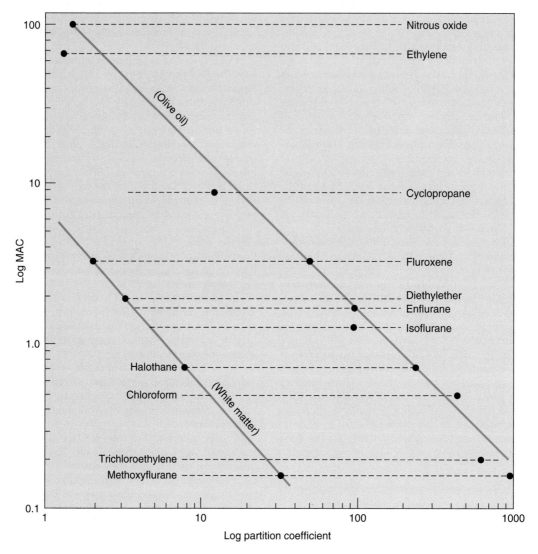

Figure 7–4. There is good but not perfect correlation between anesthetic potency and lipid solubility. MAC = minimum alveolar concentration. (Modified and reproduced, with permission, from Lowe HJ, Hagler K: *Gas Chromatography in Biology and Medicine.* Churchill, 1969.)

in a number of ways. For instance, electrolyte permeability could be changed by disrupting ion channels. Alternatively, hydrophobic membrane proteins might undergo conformational changes. In either event, synaptic function could be inhibited.

General anesthetic action could be due to alterations in any one of several cellular systems including ligand-gated ion channels, second messenger functions, or neurotransmitter receptors. For example, many anesthetics enhance γ-aminobutyric acid (GABA) inhibition of the central nervous system. Furthermore, GABA receptor agonists appear to enhance anesthesia, while GABA antagonists reverse some anesthetic effects. There appears to be a strong correlation between anesthetic potency and potentiation of GABA receptor activity. Thus, anesthetic action may relate to hydrophobic binding to channel proteins (GABA receptors). Modulation of GABA function may prove to be a principal mechanism of action for many anesthetic drugs. Other ligand-gated ion channels whose modulation may play a role in anesthetic action include nicotinic acetylcholine receptors (see Chapter 10) and N-methyl D-aspartate-receptors.

MINIMUM ALVEOLAR CONCENTRATION

 The alveolar concentration of an inhaled anesthetic that prevents movement in 50% of patients in response to a standardized stimulus (eg, surgical incision) is the **minimum alveolar concentration (MAC)**. MAC is a useful measure because it mirrors brain partial pressure, allows comparisons of potency between agents, and provides a standard for experimental evaluations (Table 7–3). Nonetheless, it should be considered a statistical average with limited value in managing individual patients, especially during times of rapidly changing alveolar concentrations (eg, induction).

The MAC values for different anesthetics are roughly additive. For example, a mixture of 0.5 MAC

Table 7–3. Properties of modern inhalation anesthetics.

Agent	Structure	MAC%[1]	Vapor Pressure (mm Hg @ 20°C)
Nitrous oxide	N=N \O/	105[2]	—
Halothane (Fluothane)	F—C—C—H (F, Cl, F, Br)	0.75	243
Methoxyflurane (Penthrane)	H—C—O—C—C—H (H, H, F, F, Cl, Cl)	0.16	22.5
Enflurane (Ethrane)	H—C—O—C—C—H (F, F, F, Cl, F)	1.7	175
Isoflurane (Forane)	H—C—O—C—C—F (F, F, H, Cl, F, F)	1.2	240
Desflurane (Suprane)	H—C—O—C—C—F (F, F, H, F, F, F)	6.0	681
Sevoflurane (Ultane)	H—C—O—C (F, H) with F—C—F above and F—C—F below, F	2.0	160

[1]These minimum alveolar concentration (MAC) values are for 30- to 55-year-old human subjects and are expressed as a percentage of 1 atm. High altitude requires a higher inspired concentration of anesthetic to achieve the same partial pressure.
[2]A concentration greater than 100% means that hyperbaric conditions are required to achieve 1.0 MAC.

Table 7–4. Factors affecting MAC.*

Variable	Effect on MAC	Comments
Temperature		
Hypothermia	↓	
Hyperthermia	↓	↑ if > 42 °C
Age		
Young	↑	
Elderly	↓	
Alcohol		
Acute intoxication	↓	
Chronic abuse	↑	
Anemia		
Hematocrit < 10%	↓	
PaO$_2$		
<40 mm Hg	↓	
PaCO$_2$		
>95 mm Hg	↓	Caused by < pH in CSF
Thyroid		
Hyperthyroid	No change	
Hypothyroid	No change	
Blood pressure		
MAP < 40 mm Hg	↓	
Electrolytes		
Hypercalcemia	↓	
Hypernatremia	↑	Caused by altered CSF
Hyponatremia	↓	Caused by altered CSF
Pregnancy	↓	MAC decreased by ⅓ at 8 wks gestation; normal by 72 hours postpartum
Drugs		
Local anesthetics	↓	Except cocaine
Opioids	↓	
Ketamine	↓	
Barbiturates	↓	
Benzodiazepines	↓	
Verapamil	↓	
Lithium	↓	
Sympatholytics		
Methyldopa	↓	
Reserpine	↓	
Clonidine	↓	
Dexmedetomidine	↓	
Sympathomimetics		
Amphetamine		
Chronic	↓	
Acute	↑	
Cocaine	↑	
Ephedrine	↑	

*These conclusions are based on human and animal studies.

of nitrous oxide (53%) and 0.5 MAC of halothane (0.37%) approximates the degree of central nervous depression of 1.0 MAC of enflurane (1.7%). In contrast to central nervous system depression, the degree of myocardial depression may not be equivalent at the same MAC: 0.5 MAC of halothane causes more myocardial depression than does 0.5 MAC of nitrous oxide. MAC represents only one point on the dose-response curve—it is the equivalent of an ED_{50}. MAC multiples are clinically useful if the dose-response curves of the anesthetics being compared are parallel, straight, and continuous for the effect being predicted. Roughly 1.3 MAC of any of the volatile anesthetics (eg, for halothane: $1.3 \times 0.74\% = 0.96\%$) has been found to prevent movement in about 95% of patients (an approximation of the ED_{95}); 0.3–0.4 MAC is associated with awakening from anesthesia (MAC awake).

MAC can be altered by several physiologic and pharmacologic variables (Table 7–4). One of the most striking of these is the 6% decrease in MAC per decade of age, regardless of volatile anesthetic. MAC is relatively unaffected by species, sex, or duration of anesthesia. Surprisingly, MAC is not altered after hypothermic spinal cord transection in rats, leading to the hypothesis that the site of anesthetic inhibition of motor responses lies in the spinal cord.

■ CLINICAL PHARMACOLOGY OF INHALATIONAL ANESTHETICS

NITROUS OXIDE

Physical Properties

Nitrous oxide (N_2O; laughing gas) is the only inorganic anesthetic gas in clinical use (see Table 7–3). It is colorless and essentially odorless. Although nonexplosive and nonflammable, nitrous oxide is as capable as oxygen of supporting combustion. Unlike the potent volatile agents, nitrous oxide is a gas at room temperature and ambient pressure. It can be kept as a liquid under pressure because its critical temperature lies above room temperature (see Chapter 2). Nitrous oxide is a relatively inexpensive anesthetic, however concerns regarding its safety have led to continued interest in alternatives such as xenon (Table 7–5).

Effects on Organ Systems

A. Cardiovascular:

The circulatory effects of nitrous oxide are explained by its tendency to stimulate the sympathetic nervous sys-

Table 7–5. Advantages and disadvantages of xenon (Xe) anesthesia.

Advantages
  Inert (probably nontoxic with no metabolism)
  Minimal cardiovascular effects
  Low blood solubility
  Rapid induction and recovery
  Does not trigger malignant hyperthermia
  Environmentally friendly
  Nonexplosive
Disadvantages
  High cost
  Low potency (MAC = 70%)
  No commercially available anesthesia equipment

MAC = minimum alveolar concentration.

tem. Even though nitrous oxide directly depresses myocardial contractility in vitro, arterial blood pressure, cardiac output, and heart rate are essentially unchanged or slightly elevated in vivo because of its stimulation of catecholamines (Table 7–6). Myocardial depression may be unmasked in patients with coronary artery disease or severe hypovolemia. The resulting drop in arterial blood pressure may occasionally lead to myocardial ischemia. Constriction of pulmonary vascular smooth muscle increases pulmonary vascular resistance, which results in an elevation of right atrial pressure. Despite vasoconstriction of cutaneous vessels, peripheral vascular resistance is not significantly altered. Because nitrous oxide increases endogenous catecholamine levels, it may be associated with a higher incidence of epinephrine-induced dysrhythmias.

B. Respiratory:

Nitrous oxide increases respiratory rate (tachypnea) and decreases tidal volume as a result of central nervous system stimulation and, perhaps, activation of pulmonary stretch receptors. The net effect is a minimal change in minute ventilation and resting arterial CO_2 levels. **Hypoxic drive,** the ventilatory response to arterial hypoxia that is mediated by peripheral chemoreceptors in the carotid bodies, is markedly depressed by even small amounts of nitrous oxide. This has serious implications in the recovery room, where patients with low arterial oxygen tensions may go unrecognized.

C. Cerebral:

By increasing CBF and cerebral blood volume, nitrous oxide produces a mild elevation of intracranial pressure. Nitrous oxide also increases cerebral oxygen consumption ($CMRO_2$). Levels of nitrous oxide below MAC provide analgesia in dental surgery and other minor procedures.

Table 7–6. Clinical pharmacology of inhalational anesthetics.

	Nitrous Oxide	Halothane	Methoxyflurane	Enflurane	Isoflurane	Desflurane	Sevoflurane
Cardiovascular							
Blood pressure	N/C	↓↓	↓↓	↓↓	↓↓	↓↓	↓
Heart rate	N/C	↓	↑	↑	↑	N/C or ↑	N/C
Systemic vascular resistance	N/C	N/C	N/C	↓	↓↓	↓↓	↓
Cardiac output[1]	N/C	↓	↓	↓↓	N/C	N/C or ↓	↓
Respiratory							
Tidal volume	↓	↓↓	↓↓	↓↓	↓↓	↓	↓
Respiratory rate	↑	↑↑	↑↑	↑↑	↑	↑	↑
PaCO₂							
Resting	N/C	↑	↑	↑↑	↑	↑↑	↑
Challenge	↑	↑	↑	↑↑	↑	↑↑	↑
Cerebral							
Blood flow	↑	↑↑	↑	↑	↑	↑	↑
Intracranial pressure	↑	↑↑	↑	↑↑	↑	↑	↑
Cerebral metabolic rate[2]	↑	↓	↓	↓	↓↓	↓↓	↓↓
Seizures	↓	↓	↓	↑	↓	↓	↓
Neuromuscular							
Nondepolarizing blockade[3]	↑	↑↑	↑↑	↑↑↑	↑↑↑	↑↑↑	↑↑
Renal							
Renal blood flow	↓↓	↓↓	↓↓	↓↓	↓↓	↓	↓
Glomerular filtration rate	↓↓	↓↓	↓↓	↓↓	↓↓	?	?
Urinary output	↓↓	↓↓	↓↓	↓↓	↓↓	?	?
Hepatic							
Blood flow	↓	↓↓	↓↓	↓↓	↓	↓	↓
Metabolism[4]	0.004%	15–20%	50%	2–5%	0.2%	<0.1%	2–3%

[1]Controlled ventilation.
[2]CMRO₂ would increase with enflurane-induced seizure.
[3]Depolarizing blockage is probably also prolonged by these agents, but this is usually not clinically significant.
[4]Percentage of absorbed anesthetic undergoing metabolism.
NC = no change; ? = uncertain.

D. NEUROMUSCULAR:

In contrast to other inhalational agents, nitrous oxide does not provide significant muscle relaxation. In fact, at high concentrations in hyperbaric chambers, nitrous oxide causes skeletal muscle rigidity. Nitrous oxide is probably not a triggering agent of malignant hyperthermia.

E. RENAL:

Nitrous oxide appears to decrease renal blood flow by increasing renal vascular resistance. This leads to a drop in glomerular filtration rate and urinary output.

F. HEPATIC:

Hepatic blood flow probably falls during nitrous oxide anesthesia, but to a lesser extent than with the volatile agents.

G. GASTROINTESTINAL:

Some studies have implicated nitrous oxide as a cause of postoperative nausea and vomiting, presumably as a result of activation of the chemoreceptor trigger zone and the vomiting center in the medulla. Other studies, particularly in children, have failed to demonstrate any association between nitrous oxide and emesis.

Biotransformation & Toxicity

During emergence, almost all nitrous oxide is eliminated by exhalation. A small amount diffuses out through the skin. Biotransformation is limited to the less than 0.01% that undergoes reductive metabolism in the gastrointestinal tract by anaerobic bacteria.

By irreversibly oxidizing the cobalt atom in vitamin B₁₂, nitrous oxide inhibits enzymes that are vitamin

B_{12}–dependent. These enzymes include methionine synthetase, which is necessary for myelin formation, and thymidylate synthetase, which is necessary for DNA synthesis. Prolonged exposure to anesthetic concentrations of nitrous oxide can result in bone marrow depression (megaloblastic anemia) and even neurologic deficiencies (peripheral neuropathies and pernicious anemia). However, administration of nitrous oxide for bone marrow harvest appears not to affect the viability of bone marrow mononuclear cells. Because of possible teratogenic effects, nitrous oxide is often avoided in pregnant patients. Nitrous oxide may also alter the immunologic response to infection by affecting chemotaxis and motility of polymorphonuclear leukocytes.

Contraindications

Although nitrous oxide is insoluble in comparison with other inhalational agents, it is 35 times more soluble than nitrogen in blood. Thus, it tends to diffuse into air-containing cavities more rapidly than nitrogen is absorbed by the bloodstream. For instance, if a patient with a 100-mL pneumothorax inhales 50% nitrous oxide, the gas content of the pneumothorax will tend to approach that of the bloodstream. Since nitrous oxide will diffuse into the cavity more rapidly than the air (principally nitrogen) diffuses out, the pneumothorax expands until it contains 100 mL of air and 100 mL of nitrous oxide. If the walls surrounding the cavity are rigid, pressure rises instead of volume. Examples of conditions where nitrous oxide might be hazardous include air embolism, pneumothorax, acute intestinal obstruction, intracranial air (tension pneumocephalus following dural closure or pneumoencephalography), pulmonary air cysts, intraocular air bubbles, and tympanic membrane grafting. Nitrous oxide will even diffuse into endotracheal tube cuffs, increasing the pressure against the tracheal mucosa.

Because of the effect of nitrous oxide on the pulmonary vasculature, it should be avoided in patients with pulmonary hypertension. Obviously, nitrous oxide is of limited value in patients requiring high inspired oxygen concentrations.

Drug Interactions

Because the relatively high MAC of nitrous oxide prevents its use as a complete general anesthetic, it is frequently used in combination with the more potent volatile agents. The addition of nitrous oxide decreases the requirements of these other agents (65% nitrous oxide decreases the MAC of the volatile anesthetics by approximately 50%). While nitrous oxide should not be considered a benign carrier gas, it does attenuate the circulatory and respiratory effects of volatile anesthetics in adults. Nitrous oxide potentiates neuromuscular blockade, but less so than the volatile agents (see Chapter 9). The concentration of nitrous oxide flowing through a vaporizer can influence the concentration of volatile anesthetic delivered. For example, decreasing nitrous oxide concentration (ie, increasing oxygen concentration) increases the concentration of volatile agent despite a constant vaporizer setting. This disparity is due to the relative solubilities of nitrous oxide and oxygen in liquid volatile anesthetics. The second gas effect was discussed earlier.

HALOTHANE

Physical Properties

Halothane is a halogenated alkane (see Table 7–3). The carbon-fluoride bonds are responsible for its nonflammable and nonexplosive nature. Thymol preservative and amber-colored bottles retard spontaneous oxidative decomposition. Halothane is the least expensive volatile anesthetic.

Effects on Organ Systems

A. CARDIOVASCULAR:

A dose-dependent reduction of arterial blood pressure is due to direct myocardial depression; 2.0 MAC of halothane results in a 50% decrease of blood pressure and cardiac output. Cardiac depression—from interference with sodium-calcium exchange and intracellular calcium utilization—causes an increase in right atrial pressure. Although halothane is a coronary artery vasodilator, coronary blood flow decreases, owing to the drop in systemic arterial pressure. Adequate myocardial perfusion is usually maintained, since oxygen demand also drops. Normally, hypotension inhibits baroreceptors in the aortic arch and carotid bifurcation, causing a decrease in vagal stimulation and a compensatory rise in heart rate. Halothane blunts this reflex. Slowing of sinoatrial node conduction may result in a junctional rhythm or bradycardia. In infants, halothane decreases cardiac output by a combination of decreased heart rate and depressed myocardial contractility. Halothane sensitizes the heart to the dysrhythmogenic effects of epinephrine, so that doses of epinephrine above 1.5 µg/kg should be avoided. This phenomenon may be a result of halothane interfering with slow calcium channel conductance. Although organ blood flow is redistributed, systemic vascular resistance is unchanged.

B. RESPIRATORY:

Halothane typically causes rapid, shallow breathing. The increased respiratory rate is not enough to counter the decreased tidal volume, so alveolar ventilation drops and resting $PaCO_2$ is elevated. **Apneic threshold,** the highest $PaCO_2$ at which a patient remains apneic, also rises because the difference between it and resting $PaCO_2$ is not altered by general anesthesia. Similarly, halothane limits the increase in minute ventilation that normally accompanies a rise in $PaCO_2$. Halothane's ventilatory effects are probably due to central (medullary depression) and peripheral (intercostal muscle dysfunction) mechanisms. These changes are exaggerated by preexisting lung disease and attenuated by surgical stimulation. The increase in $PaCO_2$ and the decrease in intrathoracic pressure that accompany spontaneous ventilation with halothane partially reverse the cardiac output, arterial blood pressure, and heart rate depression described above. Hypoxic drive is severely depressed by even low concentrations of halothane (0.1 MAC).

Halothane is considered a potent bronchodilator, since it often reverses asthma-induced bronchospasm. In fact, halothane may be the best bronchodilator among the currently available volatile anesthetics. This action is not inhibited by propranolol, a β-adrenergic blocking agent. Halothane attenuates airway reflexes and relaxes bronchial smooth muscle by inhibiting intracellular calcium mobilization. Halothane also depresses clearance of mucus from the respiratory tract (**mucociliary function**), promoting postoperative hypoxia and atelectasis.

C. CEREBRAL:

By dilating cerebral vessels, halothane lowers cerebral vascular resistance and increases CBF. **Autoregulation,** the maintenance of constant CBF during changes in arterial blood pressure, is blunted. Concomitant rises in intracranial pressure can be prevented by establishing hyperventilation *prior to* halothane administration. Cerebral activity is decreased, leading to electroencephalographic slowing and modest reductions in metabolic oxygen requirements.

D. NEUROMUSCULAR:

Halothane relaxes skeletal muscle and potentiates nondepolarizing neuromuscular blocking drugs. Like the other potent volatile anesthetics, it is a triggering agent of malignant hyperthermia.

E. RENAL:

Halothane reduces renal blood flow, glomerular filtration rate, and urinary output. Part of this decrease can be explained by a fall in arterial blood pressure and cardiac output. Because the reduction in renal blood flow is greater than the reduction in glomerular filtration rate, the filtration fraction is increased. Preoperative hydration limits these changes.

F. HEPATIC:

Halothane causes hepatic blood flow to decrease in proportion to the depression of cardiac output. Hepatic artery vasospasm has been reported during halothane anesthesia. The metabolism and clearance of some drugs (eg, fentanyl, phenytoin, verapamil) appear to be impaired by halothane. Other evidence of hepatic cellular dysfunction includes sulfobromophthalein (BSP) dye retention and minor liver transaminase elevations.

Biotransformation & Toxicity

Halothane is oxidized in the liver by a particular isozyme of cytochrome P-450 (2EI) to its principal metabolite, trifluoroacetic acid. This metabolism can be inhibited by pretreatment with disulfiram. Bromide, another oxidative metabolite, has been incriminated but is an improbable cause of postanesthetic changes in mental status. In the absence of oxygen, reductive metabolism may result in a small amount of hepatotoxic end products that covalently bind to tissue macromolecules. This is more apt to occur following enzyme induction by phenobarbital. Elevated fluoride levels signal significant anaerobic metabolism.

Postoperative hepatic dysfunction has several causes: viral hepatitis, impaired hepatic perfusion, preexisting liver disease, hepatocyte hypoxia, sepsis, hemolysis, benign postoperative intrahepatic cholestasis, and drug-induced hepatitis. **Halothane hepatitis** is extremely rare (1 per 35,000 cases). Patients exposed to multiple halothane anesthetics at short intervals, middle-aged obese women, and persons with a familial predisposition to halothane toxicity or a personal history of toxicity are considered to be at increased risk. Signs include increased serum alanine and aspartate transferase, elevated bilirubin (leading to jaundice), and encephalopathy.

The hepatic lesion seen in humans—**centrilobular necrosis**—also occurs in rats pretreated with an enzyme inducer (phenobarbital) and exposed to halothane under hypoxic conditions ($FiO_2 < 14\%$). This *halothane hypoxic model* implies hepatic damage from reductive metabolites or hypoxia.

More recent evidence points to an immune mechanism. For instance, some signs of the disease indicate an allergic reaction (eg, eosinophilia, rash, fever) and do not appear until a few days after exposure. Furthermore, an antibody that binds to hepatocytes previously exposed to halothane has been isolated from patients with halothane-induced hepatic dysfunction. This antibody response has implicated liver microsomal proteins that have been modified by trifluoroacetic acid as the triggering antigens (trifluoroacetylated liver proteins such as microsomal carboxylesterase).

Contraindications

It would seem prudent to withhold halothane from patients with unexplained liver dysfunction following previous exposure. Because halothane hepatitis appears to affect primarily adults and children past puberty, some anesthesiologists choose other volatile anesthetics in these patients. There is no compelling evidence associating halothane with worsening of preexisting liver disease.

Halothane should be used with great caution in patients with intracranial mass lesions because of the possibility of intracranial hypertension.

Hypovolemic patients and some patients with severe cardiac disease (aortic stenosis) may not tolerate halothane's negative inotropic effects. Sensitization of the heart to catecholamines limits the usefulness of halothane when exogenous epinephrine is administered or in patients with pheochromocytoma.

Drug Interactions

The myocardial depression seen with halothane is exacerbated by β-adrenergic blocking agents (eg, propranolol) and calcium channel-blocking agents (eg, verapamil). Tricyclic antidepressants and monoamine oxidase inhibitors have been associated with blood pressure fluctuations and dysrhythmias, although neither represents an absolute contraindication. The combination of halothane and aminophylline has resulted in serious ventricular dysrhythmias.

METHOXYFLURANE

Physical Properties

Methoxyflurane, a halogenated methylethyl ether, is a colorless anesthetic with a sweet, fruity odor. It is light-sensitive and stabilized with butylated hydroxytoluene. As with other modern volatile anesthetics, methoxyflurane is nonexplosive and nonflammable at clinical concentrations. It is the most potent of the inhalational agents, but its high solubility (leading to breathing circuit absorption) and low vapor pressure at room temperature (maximum inspired concentration of 3%) limit its rate of induction.

Effects on Organ Systems

A. CARDIOVASCULAR:

Methoxyflurane depresses cardiac contractility, lowering cardiac output and arterial blood pressure. Unlike halothane, methoxyflurane does not alter the carotid baroreflex, and the heart rate usually rises.

B. RESPIRATORY:

Despite an increased respiratory rate, methoxyflurane reduces minute ventilation by lowering tidal volume. Resting $PaCO_2$ is elevated. Methoxyflurane has mild bronchodilating properties. Mucociliary function is depressed.

C. CEREBRAL:

Methoxyflurane vasodilates the cerebral vasculature, increasing CBF and intracranial pressure. Cerebral metabolic requirements are reduced.

D. NEUROMUSCULAR:

Methoxyflurane relaxes skeletal muscle.

E. RENAL:

Methoxyflurane resembles other volatile anesthetics in that it causes a fall in renal blood flow and glomerular filtration rate. It is unclear whether these changes are entirely due to lower perfusion pressure or result in part from impaired autoregulation of renal blood flow. Postoperative high-output renal failure is an important distinguishing feature of methoxyflurane anesthesia (see Biotransformation & Toxicity).

F. HEPATIC:

Methoxyflurane depresses hepatic blood flow.

Biotransformation & Toxicity

The extensive metabolism of methoxyflurane is principally due to cytochrome P-450 liver microsomal enzyme activity. Oxidative metabolites include free fluoride (F^-) and oxalic acid. While both of these end products are nephrotoxic, fluoride is responsible for the **vasopressin-resistant high-output renal failure** that characterizes methoxyflurane toxicity. Toxicity is proportional to peak plasma fluoride levels and the duration of exposure. A fluoride level of 50 μmol/L, an approximate threshold for renal dysfunction associated with methoxyflurane but not necessarily other volatile anesthetics, is achievable after 2.5–3 MAC-hours of exposure (1 MAC-hour is 1 MAC sustained for 1 hour). Methoxyflurane metabolism is greater in obese and elderly patients and can be induced by a variety of drugs.

Fluoride directly inhibits tubular function (eg, chloride transport in the ascending loop of Henle), leading to a concentrating defect. Clinical signs of methoxyflurane nephrotoxicity include polyuria resistant to vasopressin; increased serum osmolality, sodium, creatinine, and BUN; decreased urinary clearance of creatinine and urea nitrogen; and urine hypo-osmolality.

Methoxyflurane has been rarely associated with postoperative hepatic dysfunction.

Contraindications

Nephrotoxicity has severely limited the usefulness of methoxyflurane, which is, in fact, presented here more as a model of nephrotoxicity than as a modern anesthetic agent. Patients with any degree of preexisting renal dysfunction represent a clear contraindication. Even in healthy patients, exposure should be limited to 2 MAC-hours.

Drug Interactions

Methoxyflurane should be avoided in patients receiving other nephrotoxic drugs (eg, aminoglycoside antibiotics). Several drugs, including phenobarbital, isoniazid, and ethanol, enhance methoxyflurane metabolism, resulting in higher than expected fluoride levels. Methoxyflurane potentiates nondepolarizing muscle relaxants.

ENFLURANE

Physical Properties

Enflurane is a halogenated ether. It has a mild, sweet, ethereal odor and is nonflammable at clinical concentrations.

Effects on Organ Systems

A. CARDIOVASCULAR:

Enflurane, like halothane, depresses myocardial contractility. This negative inotropic action appears to involve depression of calcium influx and sarcoplasmic reticulum release during myocardial membrane depolarization. Arterial blood pressure, cardiac output, and myocardial oxygen consumption are lowered. Unlike halothane, enflurane decreases systemic vascular resistance; the heart rate usually rises. Enflurane sensitizes the heart to the dysrhythmic effects of epinephrine, but doses up to 4.5 μg/kg are usually well tolerated.

B. RESPIRATORY:

Enflurane shares most of halothane's respiratory properties: decreased minute ventilation despite an increase in respiratory rate, increased resting $PaCO_2$, decreased response to hypercapnia, abolishment of hypoxic drive, depressed mucociliary function, and bronchodilatation.

Enflurane causes marked respiratory depression—at 1 MAC, resting $PaCO_2$ is 60 mm Hg. Even assisted ventilation (supplementing respiratory rate or tidal volume during spontaneous ventilation) will not lower the $PaCO_2$ much below 55 mm Hg because of the unchanged relationship between resting $PaCO_2$ and the apneic threshold.

C. CEREBRAL:

Enflurane increases CBF and intracranial pressure. Interestingly, enflurane has been shown to increase the secretion of cerebrospinal fluid and the resistance to cerebrospinal fluid outflow. During deep enflurane anesthesia, high-voltage high-frequency electroencephalographic changes can progress to a spike-and-wave pattern that culminates in frank tonic-clonic seizures. This epileptiform activity is exacerbated by high anesthetic concentrations and hypocapnia. Therefore, hyperventilation is not recommended to attenuate enflurane-induced intracranial hypertension. Cerebral metabolic requirements are decreased by enflurane unless seizure activity is initiated.

D. NEUROMUSCULAR:

Enflurane relaxes skeletal muscle.

E. RENAL:

Renal blood flow, glomerular filtration rate, and urinary output fall during enflurane anesthesia. A metabolite of enflurane is nephrotoxic (see Biotransformation & Toxicity).

F. HEPATIC:

The decrease in hepatic blood flow with enflurane is similar to that caused by equipotent doses of other volatile anesthetics.

Biotransformation & Toxicity

Although fluoride is an end product of enflurane metabolism, defluorination is much less than with methoxyflurane, and detectable renal dysfunction is unlikely. After almost 10 MAC-hours, fluoride concentrations in healthy patients average less than 40 μmol/L, causing a mild reduction in renal concentrating ability.

The evidence of postoperative hepatic damage following enflurane anesthesia is circumstantial at best.

Contraindications

Enflurane should probably be avoided in patients with preexisting kidney disease even though deterioration in renal function is unlikely. Similarly, another inhalational agent should probably be chosen for patients with seizure disorders. Precautions concerning intracranial hypertension, hemodynamic instability, and malignant hyperthermia are the same as those associated with halothane.

Drug Interactions

Isoniazid (but not phenobarbital, ethanol, or phenytoin) induces enflurane defluorination, perhaps by induction of cytochrome P-450 2EI. This may be clinically significant in so-called *rapid acetylators,* ie, patients with an autosomal dominant trait that increases the rate of hepatic acetylation.

Enflurane potentiates nondepolarizing blocking agents.

ISOFLURANE

Physical Properties

Isoflurane is a nonflammable volatile anesthetic with a pungent ethereal odor. Although it is a chemical isomer of enflurane, it has different physicochemical properties (see Table 7–3).

Effects on Organ Systems

A. CARDIOVASCULAR:

Isoflurane causes minimal cardiac depression in vivo. Cardiac output is maintained by a rise in heart rate due to partial preservation of carotid baroreflexes. Mild β-adrenergic stimulation increases skeletal muscle blood flow, decreases systemic vascular resistance, and lowers arterial blood pressure. Rapid increases in isoflurane concentration lead to transient increases in heart rate, arterial blood pressure, and plasma levels of norepinephrine. Isoflurane dilates coronary arteries, particularly if its concentration is abruptly increased, although it is not nearly as potent a dilator as nitroglycerin or adenosine. Dilation of normal coronary arteries could theoretically divert blood away from fixed stenotic lesions. There have been conflicting reports regarding whether this **coronary steal syndrome** causes regional myocardial ischemia during episodes of tachycardia or drops in perfusion pressure. Despite the negative results of several large outcome studies, some anesthesiologists still avoid isoflurane in patients with coronary artery disease.

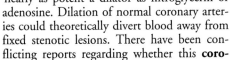

B. RESPIRATORY:

Respiratory depression during isoflurane anesthesia resembles that of other volatile anesthetics, except that tachypnea is less pronounced. The net effect is a more pronounced fall in minute ventilation. Even low levels of isoflurane (0.1 MAC) blunt the normal ventilatory response to hypoxia and hypercapnia. Despite a tendency to irritate upper airway reflexes, isoflurane is considered a good bronchodilator, but may not be as potent a bronchodilator as halothane.

C. CEREBRAL:

At concentrations greater than 1 MAC, isoflurane increases CBF and intracranial pressure. These effects are thought to be less pronounced than with halothane or enflurane and are reversed by hyperventilation. In contrast to halothane, the hyperventilation does not have to be instituted prior to the use of isoflurane in order to prevent intracranial hypertension. Isoflurane reduces cerebral metabolic oxygen requirements, and at 2 MAC it produces an electrically silent electroencephalogram. EEG suppression probably provides some degree of brain protection during episodes of cerebral ischemia.

D. NEUROMUSCULAR:

Isoflurane relaxes skeletal muscle.

E. RENAL:

Isoflurane decreases renal blood flow, glomerular filtration rate, and urinary output.

F. HEPATIC:

Total hepatic blood flow (hepatic artery and portal vein flow) is reduced during isoflurane anesthesia. Hepatic oxygen supply may be better maintained with isoflurane than halothane or enflurane, however, because hepatic artery perfusion and hepatic venous oxygen saturation are preserved. Liver function tests are minimally affected.

Biotransformation & Toxicity

Isoflurane is metabolized to one-tenth of the extent of enflurane. Trifluoroacetic acid is the principal end product. Although serum fluoride fluid levels may rise, nephrotoxicity is extremely unlikely even in the presence of enzyme inducers. Prolonged sedation (> 24 hours at 0.1–0.6% isoflurane) of critically ill patients has resulted in elevated plasma fluoride levels (15–50 μmol/L) without evidence of renal impairment. Similarly, up to 20 MAC-hours of isoflurane may lead to fluoride levels exceeding 50 μmol/L without detectable postoperative renal dysfunction. Its limited metabolism also minimizes any possible risk of significant hepatic dysfunction.

Contraindications

Isoflurane presents no unique contraindications other than the controversy concerning the possibility of coronary steal. Patients with severe hypovolemia may not tolerate its vasodilating effects.

Drug Interactions

Epinephrine can be safely administered in doses up to 4.5 μg/kg. Nondepolarizing muscle relaxants are potentiated by isoflurane.

DESFLURANE

Physical Properties

Desflurane's structure is very similar to that of isoflurane. In fact, the only difference is the substitution of a fluorine atom for isoflurane's chlorine atom. That "minor" change has profound effects on the physical properties of the drug, however. For instance, because the vapor pressure of desflurane at 20 °C is 681 mm Hg, it boils at room temperature at high altitudes (eg, Denver, Colorado). This problem has been dealt with by development of a special desflurane vaporizer (see Chapter 4). Furthermore, the low solubility of desflurane in blood and body tissues causes a very rapid wash-in and wash-out of anesthetic. Therefore, the alveolar concentration of desflurane will tend to approach the inspired concentration much more rapidly than the other volatile agents will, giving the anesthesiologist tighter control over anesthetic level. Wake-up times are approximately half as long as those observed following isoflurane. This is principally attributable to a blood/gas partition coefficient (0.42) that is even lower than that of nitrous oxide (0.47). While desflurane is roughly one-fourth as potent as the other volatile agents, it is 17 times more potent than nitrous oxide. A high vapor pressure, an ultrashort duration of action, and moderate potency are desflurane's most characteristic features.

Effects on Organ Systems

A. CARDIOVASCULAR:

The cardiovascular effects of desflurane appear to be similar to those of isoflurane. Increasing the dose is associated with a decline in systemic vascular resistance that leads to a fall in arterial blood pressure. Cardiac output remains relatively unchanged or slightly depressed at 1–2 MAC. There is a moderate rise in heart rate, central venous pressure, and pulmonary artery pressure that often does not become apparent at low doses. Rapid increases in desflurane concentration lead to transient but sometimes worrisome elevations in heart rate, blood pressure, and catecholamine levels that are more pronounced than with isoflurane. These cardiovascular responses to rapidly increasing desflurane concentration can be attenuated by fentanyl, esmolol, or clonidine. Unlike isoflurane, desflurane does not increase coronary artery blood flow.

B. RESPIRATORY:

Desflurane causes a decrease in tidal volume and an increase in respiratory rate. There is an overall decrease in alveolar ventilation that causes a rise in resting $PaCO_2$.

Like other modern volatile anesthetic agents, desflurane depresses the ventilatory response to increasing $PaCO_2$. Pungency and airway irritation during desflurane induction can be manifested by salivation, breath-holding, coughing, and laryngospasm. These problems make desflurane less than ideally suited for pediatric inhalation inductions.

C. CEREBRAL:

Like the other volatile anesthetics, desflurane directly vasodilates the cerebral vasculature, increasing CBF and intracranial pressure at normotension and normocapnia. Countering the decrease in cerebral vascular resistance is a marked decline in cerebral metabolic rate of oxygen ($CMRO_2$) that tends to cause cerebral vasoconstriction and moderate any increase in CBF. The cerebral vasculature remains responsive to changes in $PaCO_2$, however, so that intracranial pressure can be lowered by hyperventilation. Cerebral oxygen consumption is decreased during desflurane anesthesia. Thus, during periods of desflurane-induced hypotension (mean arterial pressure = 60 mm Hg), CBF is adequate to maintain aerobic metabolism despite a low cerebral perfusion pressure. The effect on the electroencephalogram is similar to that of isoflurane.

D. NEUROMUSCULAR:

Desflurane is associated with a dose-dependent decrease in the response to train-of-four and tetanic peripheral nerve stimulation.

E. RENAL:

There is no evidence of any nephrotoxic effects caused by exposure to desflurane.

F. HEPATIC:

Hepatic function tests are unaffected, and there is no evidence of hepatic injury following desflurane anesthesia.

Biotransformation & Toxicity

Desflurane undergoes minimal metabolism in humans. Serum and urine inorganic fluoride levels following desflurane anesthesia are essentially unchanged from preanesthetic levels. There is insignificant percutaneous loss. Desflurane, more than other volatile anesthetics, is degraded by desiccated carbon dioxide absorbent (particularly barium hydroxide lime, but also sodium and potassium hydroxide) into potentially clinically significant levels of carbon monoxide. Carbon monoxide poisoning is difficult to clinically diagnose under general anesthesia, but the presence of carboxyhemoglobin may be detectable by arterial blood gas analysis or lower than expected pulse oximetry readings (although still falsely high). Disposing of dried out absorbent or use of calcium hydroxide (see Chapter 3) can minimize the risk of carbon monoxide poisoning.

Contraindications

Desflurane shares many of the contraindications of other modern volatile anesthetics: severe hypovolemia, malignant hyperthermia, and intracranial hypertension.

Drug Interactions

Desflurane potentiates nondepolarizing muscle relaxants to the same extent as isoflurane. Epinephrine can be safely administered in doses up to 4.5 µg/kg since desflurane does not sensitize the myocardium to the dysrhythmogenic effects of epinephrine. Although emergence is more rapid following desflurane anesthesia than after isoflurane anesthesia, switching from isoflurane to desflurane toward the end of anesthesia does not significantly accelerate recovery nor does faster emergence usually translate into faster discharge times from a postanesthesia care unit. Desflurane emergence has been associated with delirium in some pediatric patients.

SEVOFLURANE

Physical Properties

Like desflurane, sevoflurane is halogenated with fluorine. Sevoflurane combines a solubility in blood slightly greater than desflurane ($\lambda_{b/g}$ 0.65 versus 0.42) with a potency slightly less than enflurane (see Table 7–3). Nonpungency and rapid increases in alveolar anesthetic concentration make sevoflurane an excellent choice for smooth and rapid inhalational inductions in pediatric or adult patients. In fact, single-breath induction with 4% to 8% sevoflurane in a 50% mixture of nitrous oxide and oxygen can be achieved in approximately 1 to 3 minutes. Likewise, its low blood solubility results in a rapid fall in alveolar anesthetic concentration upon discontinuation and a quicker emergence compared with isoflurane (although not necessarily quicker discharge from the postanesthesia care unit). As with desflurane, this faster emergence has been associated with a greater incidence of delirium in some pediatric populations, which can be successfully treated with 1.0 to 2.0 µg/kg of fentanyl. Sevoflurane's modest vapor pressure permits the use of a conventional variable bypass vaporizer. Although sevoflurane has been available in Japan for years, the US Food and Drug Administration delayed its release in the United States because of questions regarding biodegradability. Some of the following conclusions are based on animal studies and should therefore be viewed as tentative.

Effects on Organ Systems

A. CARDIOVASCULAR:

Sevoflurane mildly depresses myocardial contractility. Systemic vascular resistance and arterial blood pressure decline slightly less than with isoflurane or desflurane. Because sevoflurane causes little, if any, rise in heart rate, cardiac output is not as well maintained as with isoflurane or desflurane. There is no evidence associating sevoflurane with coronary steal syndrome. Sevoflurane may prolong the QT interval, the clinical significance of which is unknown.

B. RESPIRATORY:

Sevoflurane depresses respiration and reverses bronchospasm to an extent similar to that of isoflurane.

C. CEREBRAL:

Similar to isoflurane and desflurane, sevoflurane causes slight increases in CBF and intracranial pressure at normocarbia, although some studies show a decrease in cerebral blood flow. High concentrations of sevoflurane (> 1.5 MAC) may impair autoregulation of CBF, thus allowing a drop in CBF during hemorrhagic hypotension. This effect on CBF autoregulation appears to be less pronounced than with isoflurane. Cerebral metabolic oxygen requirements decrease, and seizure activity has not been reported.

D. NEUROMUSCULAR:

Sevoflurane produces adequate muscle relaxation for intubation of children following an inhalational induction.

E. RENAL:

Sevoflurane slightly decreases renal blood flow. Its metabolism to substances associated with impaired renal tubule function (eg, decreased concentrating ability) is discussed below.

F. HEPATIC:

Sevoflurane decreases portal vein blood flow, but increases hepatic artery blood flow, thereby maintaining total hepatic blood flow and oxygen delivery.

Biotransformation & Toxicity

The liver microsomal enzyme P-450 (specifically the 2E1 isoform) metabolizes sevoflurane at a rate similar to enflurane and may be induced with ethanol or phenobarbital pretreatment. The potential nephrotoxicity of the resulting rise in inorganic fluoride (F^-) was discussed earlier. The overall rate of sevoflurane metabolism is 5%, or ten times that of isoflurane. Nonetheless, there has been no association with peak fluoride levels following sevoflurane and any renal concentrating abnormality.

Alkali such as soda lime (but not calcium hydroxide—see Chapter 3) can degrade sevoflurane, producing another proven (at least in rats) nephrotoxic end product (*compound A,* fluoromethyl-2,2-difluoro-1-(trifluoromethyl) vinyl ether). Accumulation of compound A increases with increased respiratory gas temperature, low-flow anesthesia (see Case Discussion, following), dry barium hydroxide absorbent (Baralyme), high sevoflurane concentrations, and anesthetics of long duration.

Whether sevoflurane anesthesia can under any circumstances achieve toxic concentrations of compound A or inorganic fluoride is yet to be definitively determined. However, most studies have not associated sevoflurane with any detectable postoperative impairment of renal function that would indicate toxicity or injury. Nonetheless, some clinicians recommend against fresh gas flows less than 2 liters/min for anesthetics lasting more than a few hours and avoid sevoflurane in patients with preexisting renal dysfunction.

Sevoflurane can also be degraded into hydrogen fluoride by metal and environmental impurities present in manufacturing equipment, glass bottle packaging, and anesthesia equipment. Hydrogen fluoride can produce an acid burn on contact with respiratory mucosa. The risk of patient injury has been substantially reduced by inhibition of the degradation process by adding water to sevoflurane during the manufacturing process and packaging it in a special plastic container.

Contraindications

Contraindications include severe hypovolemia, susceptibility to malignant hyperthermia, and intracranial hypertension.

Drug Interactions

Like other volatile anesthetics, sevoflurane potentiates nondepolarizing muscle relaxants. It does not sensitize the heart to catecholamine-induced dysrhythmias.

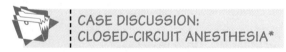

CASE DISCUSSION:
CLOSED-CIRCUIT ANESTHESIA*

A 22-year-old man weighing 70 kg is scheduled for shoulder reconstruction under general anesthesia. You are considering a closed-circuit anesthetic technique.

---

* The authors would like to thank Harry J. Lowe, MD, for his contribution to this Case Discussion.

Describe closed-circuit anesthesia and tell how it differs from other techniques.

Anesthesia systems can be classified as nonrebreathing, partial rebreathing, or total rebreathing systems. In nonrebreathing systems (open systems), the fresh gas flow into the breathing circuit exceeds the patient's minute ventilation. All gases not absorbed by the patient are exhausted through the pressure-relief valve; there is no flow through the CO_2 absorber; and no gas is rebreathed by the patient.

In partial rebreathing systems (semiopen or semiclosed), the fresh gas flow into the breathing circuit is less than the minute ventilation provided to the patient but greater than the rate of uptake of all gases by the patient. The difference between the fresh gas flow and patient uptake is equal to the exhaust volume from the pressure relief valve. Therefore, exhaled gas can take one of three courses: It can be evacuated by the pressure relief valve, absorbed by the CO_2 absorber, or rebreathed by the patient.

A total rebreathing system (closed system) does not evacuate any gas through the pressure relief valve. This has several implications: all exhaled gases except CO_2 are rebreathed; expired CO_2 must be eliminated by the CO_2 absorber to prevent hypercapnia; and the total amount of fresh gas delivered to the system must nearly equal the amount of gas taken up by the patient's lungs. The fresh gas flow required to maintain the desired alveolar partial pressure of anesthetic agent and oxygen depends upon anesthetic uptake and metabolic rate. This flow rate is achieved by maintaining both a constant circuit volume, as reflected in an unchanging end-expiratory breathing-bag volume or ventilator-bellows height, and a constant expired oxygen concentration.

What are the advantages and disadvantages of closed-circuit anesthesia?

Rebreathing anesthetic gases conserves heat and humidity, decreases anesthetic pollution, demonstrates the principles of anesthetic uptake, and allows early detection of circuit leaks and metabolic changes. Flow rates are a major determinant of volatile anesthetic cost. Some anesthesiologists, however, consider closed-circuit techniques to impose a greater risk of hypoxia, hypercapnia, and anesthetic overdose. Without question, closed-circuit anesthesia requires a high level of vigilance and a comprehensive understanding of pharmacokinetics. Some anesthetic machines cannot deliver low flows because they have mandatory oxygen flow rates greater than metabolic oxygen consumption or do not allow the administration of potentially hypoxic gas mixtures.

What factors determine the cost of delivering an inhalational anesthetic?

Fresh gas flow rates are only one factor that determines consumption of anesthetic agent. Other considerations include potency, blood and tissue solubility, and the amount of vapor produced per milliliter of liquid anesthetic. Obviously, the price charged to the pharmacy by the manufacturer plays an important role, as would any special equipment required for delivery (eg, Tec 6) or monitoring. Less obvious are the indirect factors that influence discharge from the recovery room or hospital: time to awakening, incidence of vomiting, and so on.

Is any special equipment necessary for closed-circuit anesthesia?

General anesthesia should never be performed without an oxygen analyzer in the breathing circuit. During low-flow anesthesia, the oxygen concentrations in the expiratory limb may be significantly lower than in the inspiratory limb owing to the patient's oxygen consumption. Therefore, some authorities suggest that expiratory oxygen concentration should be measured whenever the anesthesia system is closed. Gas leaks in the anesthetic system will interfere with estimates of nitrous oxide and oxygen consumption. These leaks are proportional to mean airway pressure and inspiratory time. Modern circle systems have more than 20 potential sites of leaks, including the absorber, tubing connections, unidirectional valves, rubber hoses, and breathing bag (see Case Discussion, Chapter 4). Vaporizers and flow meters must be accurate at low flows and varying circuit pressures. An alternative to a vaporizer is the direct injection of volatile agent into the expiratory limb of the breathing circuit.

How are oxygen requirements predicted during closed-circuit anesthesia?

Anesthesia establishes a basal metabolic rate that is dependent upon the patient's weight and body temperature. Basal metabolic oxygen consumption ($\dot{V}O_2$) equals 10 times a patient's weight in kilograms to the three-quarters power:

$$\dot{V}O_2 = 10 \text{ kg}^{3/4}$$

For a 70-kg patient, oxygen consumption is:

$$\dot{V}O_2 = 10 \times (24.2) = 242 \text{ mL } O_2/\text{min}$$

Oxygen requirements decrease by 10% for each degree below 37.6 °C:

$$\dot{V}O_2 \text{ at } 36.6 \,°C = 242 - 24 = 218 \text{ mL } O_2/\text{min}$$
$$\dot{V}O_2 \text{ at } 35.6 \,°C = 218 - 22 = 196 \text{ mL } O_2/\text{min}$$

This is only a model for prediction. Actual oxygen requirements vary, and must be determined for each patient. For example, hypovolemic shock, hypothyroidism, and aortic cross-clamping are associated with decreased metabolic oxygen consumption. In contrast, malignant hyperthermia, hyperthyroidism, thermal burns, and sepsis lead to greater than predicted oxygen requirements. Increasing depth of anesthesia does not significantly alter basal metabolic rate unless tissue perfusion is compromised.

What is the relationship between oxygen consumption and CO_2 production?

Carbon dioxide production is approximately 80% of oxygen consumption (ie, respiratory ratio = 0.8):

$$\dot{V}CO_2 = 8 \text{ kg}^{3/4} = 194 \text{ mL } CO_2/\text{min}$$

How much ventilation is required to maintain normocapnia?

Minute ventilation is the sum of alveolar ventilation and ventilation of anatomic dead space and equipment dead space. Normocapnia is approximately a 5.6% alveolar concentration of CO_2:

$$\frac{40 \text{ mm Hg}}{760 \text{ mm Hg} - 47 \text{ mm Hg}} = 5.6\%$$

Therefore, alveolar ventilation must be sufficient to dilute the 194 mL of expired CO_2 to a concentration of 5.6%:

$$\dot{V}_A = \frac{\dot{V}CO_2}{5.6\%} = \frac{194 \text{ mL}/\text{min}}{5.6\%} = 3393 \text{ mL}/\text{min}$$

Anatomic dead space is estimated as 1 mL/kg/breath:

$$\text{Anatomic dead space} = \text{Weight} \times 1 \text{ mL / kg}$$
$$= 70 \text{ mL / breath}$$

Equipment dead space consists primarily of the ventilation lost to expansion of the breathing circuit during positive-pressure ventilation. This can be estimated if the circuit compliance and peak airway pressure are known:

Equipment dead space
$$= \text{Compliance} \times \text{Pressure}$$
$$= (10 \text{ mL / cm H}_2\text{O}) \times (20 \text{ cm H}_2\text{O})$$
$$= 200 \text{ mL / breath}$$

Therefore, at a respiratory rate of 10 breaths/min, total ventilation as measured by a spirometer should be $\dot{V}_T = 3393 + 700 + 2000 = 6093$ mL/min, and tidal volume would equal 609 mL.

How is the uptake of a volatile anesthetic predicted?

Anesthetic uptake by the pulmonary circulation depends upon the agent's blood/gas partition coefficient ($\lambda_{b/g}$), the alveolar/venous difference ($C_A - v$), and the cardiac output ($\dot{Q}$):

$$\text{Uptake} = \lambda_{b/g} \times C_{(A-V)} \times (\dot{Q})$$

The blood/gas partition coefficients of anesthetic agents have been experimentally determined (see Table 7–1). At the beginning of an anesthetic procedure, the venous concentration of anesthetic is zero, so the alveolar-venous difference is equal to the alveolar concentration. The alveolar concentration required for surgical anesthesia is typically 1.3 MAC (see Table 7–3). Cardiac output (dL/min) is related to metabolic rate and oxygen consumption:

$$\dot{Q} = 2 \text{ kg}^{3/4}$$

Thus, the rate of halothane uptake ($\dot{Q}_{an}$) by the pulmonary circulation at the end of the first minute of anesthesia can be predicted:

$$\dot{Q}_{an} \text{ at 1 min} = (2.4) \times (1.3)(.75) \times (2)(24.2)$$
$$= 113 \text{ mL of vapor}$$

As organs fill with anesthetic, the rate of uptake declines. An empiric mathematical model that closely fits observed uptake demonstrates the fall in uptake as being inversely proportionate to the square root of time (the **square root of time model**). In other words, the uptake at 4 minutes is one-half that at 1 minute and twice that at 16 minutes. Thus, the rate of uptake in our example would be 112 mL/min (112 ÷ 1) at the end of the first minute, 56 mL/min (112 ÷ 2) at the end of the fourth minute, and 28 mL/min (112 ÷ 4) at the end of the 16th minute. In general, the rate of uptake at any time (t) is:

$$\dot{Q}_{an} \text{ at } t \text{ min} = (\dot{Q}_{an} \text{ at 1 min}) \times t^{-1/2}$$

How can the amount of anesthetic taken up be predicted from the rate of uptake?

The cumulative anesthetic dose at any time t can be determined by integrating the rate function (finding the area under the F_A/F_I curve):

$$\text{Cumulative uptake} = 2 \times (\dot{Q}_{an} \text{ at 1 min}) \times t^{+1/2}$$

Therefore, at 1 minute the total amount of anesthetic that has been taken up is 224 mL; a total of 448 mL is taken up by 4 minutes; and 672 mL is taken up by 9 minutes. Stated another way, 224 mL is required to maintain a constant alveolar concentration during each square-root-of-time interval. This quantity is called the **unit dose**.

What is a priming dose?

The breathing circuit, the patient's functional residual capacity, and the arterial circulation must be primed with anesthetic before tissue uptake can begin. The amount of anesthetic required to prime the breathing circuit and the functional residual capacity is equal to their combined volume (approximately 100 dL) multiplied by the desired alveolar concentration (1.3 MAC). Similarly, the amount of anesthetic required to prime the arterial circulation is equal to the blood volume—roughly equal to cardiac output—multiplied by the desired concentration and the blood/gas partition coefficient. For simplicity, these two priming doses are considered to be equal to one unit dose. Thus, during the first minute of anesthesia, two unit doses are administered: one as a priming dose and the other for tissue uptake.

By what methods can a unit dose of anesthetic be administered during a square-root-of-time interval?

The 224 mL of halothane vapor can be administered by a copper kettle vaporizer or an agent-specific variable bypass vaporizer, or it can be directly injected in liquid form into the expiratory limb of the anesthesia circuit. Because the vapor pressure of halothane is 243 mm Hg at 20 °C, the concentration of halothane exiting a copper kettle is 243 ÷ 760, or 32%. Therefore, 477 mL of oxygen must enter a copper kettle during one interval for 224 mL of halothane vapor to exit (see the vapor output equation in Chapter 4):

$$224 \text{ mL} \times \frac{760 - 243}{243} = 477 \text{ mL}$$

Modern agent-specific vaporizers deliver a constant concentration of agent regardless of flow. Therefore, if the total flow (nitrous oxide, oxygen, and anesthetic vapor) is 5 L during one time interval, a 4.5% concentration is required:

$$\frac{224 \text{ mL}}{5000 \text{ mL}} = 4.5\%$$

Direct injection into the circuit from a glass syringe with a metal stopcock is an easy way to administer volatile agents. Each milliliter of liquid halothane, methoxyflurane, isoflurane, enflurane, desflurane, or sevoflurane represents approximately 200 mL (±10%) of vapor. Therefore, a little more than 1 mL needs to be injected during one time interval:

$$\frac{224 \text{ mL vapor}}{200 \text{ mL vapor} / \text{mL liquid}} = 1.12 \text{ mL liquid}$$

Can nitrous oxide uptake be predicted in a similar manner?

Similar predictions can be made for nitrous oxide—with two qualifications. First, 1.3 MAC (approximately 137% N_2O) cannot be delivered at atmospheric pressure because of the certainty of hypoxia. Second, because 30% of the blood supply to highly perfused organs is shunted, only 70% of the predicted nitrous oxide is actually taken up by blood recirculating through the lungs. This introduces a shunt factor of 0.7 into the uptake equation:

$$\text{Uptake } N_2O = 0.7 \times 0.47 \times \%N_2O \times \dot{Q}$$

For a 70-kg patient at 65% nitrous oxide:

$$\dot{Q}_{an} \text{ at 1 min} = 0.7 \times 0.47 \times 65 \times (2)(24.2)$$
$$= 1035 \text{ mL} / \text{min}$$

The unit dose for nitrous oxide would be:

$$\text{Unit dose} = 2 \times \dot{Q}_{an} \text{ at 1 min} = 2070 \text{ mL}$$

A large priming dose is required:

$$\text{Circuit prime} = (\text{FRC} + \text{Circuit volume}) \times 65\%$$
$$= (100 \text{dL})(0.65) = 65 \text{ dL}$$
$$\text{Arterial prime} = \text{Blood volume} \times \lambda_{b/g} \times 65\%$$
$$= (50 \text{dL})(0.45)(0.65) = 15 \text{ dL}$$

$$\text{Total prime} = 80 \text{ dL} = 8 \text{L}$$

Therefore, in the first minute of a nitrous oxide anesthetic procedure, several liters of nitrous oxide would be administered. In clinical practice, nitrous oxide is empirically administered in amounts sufficient to maintain circuit volume as judged by constant breathing bag size or the height of a ventilator's standing bellows. If expired oxygen concentration falls below acceptable levels, the metabolic oxygen flow (242 mL/min) is increased. Sixty-five percent nitrous oxide anesthesia would be supplemented with intravenous or volatile agents. Since MAC is additive, 0.65 MAC of volatile anesthetic is required to attain a total of 1.3 MAC.

Briefly describe the first few minutes of a closed-circuit anesthetic procedure with nitrous oxide and halothane.

After preoxygenation, intravenous induction, and intubation, oxygen flow is set to the predicted metabolic oxygen requirement (242 mL/min). At the same time, nitrous oxide is administered at 6–8 L/min to prime the circuit and the patient's functional residual capacity. When expired oxygen drops to 40%, the nitrous oxide is reduced to match the calculated rate of uptake (2070 mL per square-root-of-time interval), and the pressure-relief valve is closed. If the ventilator bellows or breathing bag indicates an increasing or decreasing circuit volume, the nitrous oxide flowmeter is adjusted accordingly. If the expired oxygen con-

centration falls too low, the oxygen flow rate is increased. The priming and unit doses of volatile anesthetic can be administered by either of the methods described. Dosing intervals and amounts are only predictions. The correct dose for each patient is determined by the clinical signs of anesthetic depth: blood pressure, heart rate, respiratory rate, tearing, pupillary changes, diaphoresis, movement, and the like.

SUGGESTED READING

Bacher A, Burton AW, Uchida T, Zornow MH: Sevoflurane or halothane anesthesia: Can we tell the difference? Anesth Analg 1997;85:1203-1206. A group of anesthesiologists, consisting of residents and faculty, could not consistently differentiate halothane from the more expensive alternative sevoflurane in a series of pediatric cases.

Cittanova M-L, Lelongt B, Verpont M-C: "Fluoride ion toxicity in human kidney collecting duct cells." Anesthesiology 1996;84:428-435. A reexamination of the mechanism of methoxyflurane metabolism and nephrotoxicity.

Ebert TJ: Myocardial ischemia and adverse cardiac outcomes in cardiac patients undergoing noncardiac surgery with sevoflurane and isoflurane. Anesth Analg 1997;85:993-999. This article by the Sevoflurane Ischemia Study Group concludes there is no difference in the incidence of myocardial ischemia between sevoflurane and isoflurane.

Eger EI, Bowland T, Ionescu P: Recovery and kinetic characteristics of desflurane and sevoflurane in volunteers after 8-h exposure, including kinetics of degradation products. Anesthesiology 1997;87:527-526. An excellent overview of the pharmacokinetics of these agents.

Hans-Joachim P: Isoflurane and coronary hemodynamics. Anesthesiology 1989;71:960. An overview of the controversy of coronary steal.

Njoku D, Laster MJ, Gong DH: Biotransformation of halothane, enflurane, isoflurane, and desflurane to trifluoroacetylated liver proteins: Association between protein acylation and hepatic injury. Anesth Analg 1997;84:173-178. A review of the hepatotoxicity of several volatile anesthetic agents and its relationship to their metabolism.

Mazze RI, Callan CM, Galvez ST, Delgado-Herrera L, Mayer DB: The effects of sevoflurane on serum creatinine and blood urea nitrogen concentrations. A retrospective, twenty-two-center, comparative evaluation of renal function in adult surgical patients. Anesth Analg 2000;90:683-688. This large study could not find a relationship between sevoflurane administration and renal toxicity; it was accompanied by an editorial (Bedford RF, Ives HE: The renal safety of sevoflurane. Anesth Analg 2000;90:505-508).

Stoelting RK: *Pharmacology and Physiology in Anesthetic Practice,* 3rd ed. Lippincott, 1999. One of the best discussions of the clinical pharmacology of volatile anesthetic agents.

Summors AC, Gupta AK, Matta BF: Dynamic cerebral autoregulation during sevoflurane anesthesia: A comparison with isoflurane. Anesth Analg 1999;88:341-345. This study confirms the lesser effects of sevoflurane on cerebral autoregulation.

Sun X, Su F, Shi Y, Lee C: The "second gas effect" is not a valid concept. Anesth Analg 1999;88:188-192. This study failed to show any increase in volatile anesthetic concentration due to nitrous oxide administration.

Nonvolatile Anesthetic Agents

KEY CONCEPTS

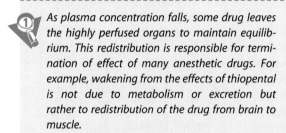

1. As plasma concentration falls, some drug leaves the highly perfused organs to maintain equilibrium. This redistribution is responsible for termination of effect of many anesthetic drugs. For example, wakening from the effects of thiopental is not due to metabolism or excretion but rather to redistribution of the drug from brain to muscle.

2. Non–protein-bound drugs freely cross from plasma into the glomerular filtrate. The nonionized fraction of drug is reabsorbed in the renal tubules, while the ionized portion is excreted in urine.

3. Elimination half-life of a drug is proportional to the volume of distribution and inversely proportional to the rate of clearance.

4. Drug plasma concentration is determined by six pharmacokinetic parameters and not just half-lives, as is often assumed.

5. Repetitive administration of barbiturates will saturate the peripheral compartments, so that redistribution cannot occur and the duration of action will become more dependent on elimination.

6. Barbiturates constrict the cerebral vasculature. This effect may provide some brain protection from transient episodes of focal ischemia (eg, cerebral embolism) but probably not from global ischemia (eg, cardiac arrest).

7. Although apnea may be less common after benzodiazepine induction than after barbiturate induction, even small intravenous doses of diazepam and midazolam have resulted in respiratory arrest. Ventilation must be monitored in all patients receiving intravenous benzodiazepines, and resuscitation equipment must be immediately available.

8. The accumulation of morphine metabolites (morphine 3-glucuronide and morphine 6-glucuronide) in patients with renal failure has been associated with narcosis and ventilatory depression lasting several days.

9. Opioids (particularly fentanyl, sufentanil, and alfentanil) can induce chest wall rigidity severe enough to prevent adequate ventilation.

10. The stress response to surgical stimulation is measured in terms of the secretion of specific hormones, including catecholamines, antidiuretic hormone, and cortisol. Opioids block the release of these hormones more completely than do volatile anesthetics.

11. In sharp contrast to other anesthetic agents, ketamine increases arterial blood pressure, heart rate, and cardiac output. These indirect cardiovascular effects are due to central stimulation of the sympathetic nervous system and inhibition of the reuptake of norepinephrine.

(continued)

Induction doses of etomidate transiently inhibit enzymes involved in cortisol and aldosterone synthesis. Long-term infusions lead to adrenocortical suppression that may be associated with an increased mortality rate in critically ill patients.

 Since propofol formulations can support the growth of bacteria, good sterile technique must be observed in preparation and handling; sepsis and death have been linked to contaminated propofol preparations.

 Droperidol is a potent antiemetic; however, delayed awakening limits its intraoperative use to low doses (0.05 mg/kg, to a maximum of 2.5 mg). Its antidopaminergic activity rarely precipitates extrapyramidal reactions (eg, oculogyric crises, torticollis, agitation), which can be treated with diphenhydramine. Nonetheless, droperidol should be avoided in patients with Parkinson's disease.

(continued)

General anesthesia is not limited to the use of inhalational agents. Numerous drugs that are administered orally, intramuscularly, and intravenously augment or produce an anesthetic state within their therapeutic dosage range. Preoperative sedation, the topic of this chapter's case study, is traditionally accomplished by way of oral or intramuscular routes. Induction of anesthesia in adult patients usually involves intravenous administration, and the development of EMLA (eutectic [easily melted] mixture of local anesthetic) cream (see Chapter 14) has significantly increased the popularity of intravenous inductions in children. Even maintenance of general anesthesia can be achieved with a total intravenous anesthesia technique (see Case Discussion, Chapter 46). This chapter begins with a review of the pharmacologic principles of pharmacokinetics and pharmacodynamics and how they apply to this class of drugs. The clinical pharmacology of several anesthetic agents is presented: barbiturates, benzodiazepines, opioids, ketamine, etomidate, propofol, and droperidol.

■ PHARMACOLOGIC PRINCIPLES

PHARMACOKINETICS

As explained in Chapter 7, pharmacokinetics is the study of the relationship between a drug's dose, tissue concentration, and time since administration. Simply stated, it describes how the body affects a drug. Pharmacokinetics is defined by four parameters: **absorption, distribution, biotransformation,** and **excretion. Elimination** implies drug removal by both biotransformation and excretion. **Clearance** is a measurement of the rate of elimination.

Absorption

There are many possible routes of systemic drug absorption: oral, sublingual, rectal, inhalational, transdermal, subcutaneous, intramuscular, and intravenous. Absorption, the process by which a drug leaves its site of administration to enter the bloodstream, is affected by the physical characteristics of the drug (solubility, pK_a, and concentration) and the site of absorption (circulation, pH, and surface area). Absorption differs from **bioavailability,** which is the fraction of unchanged drug that reaches the systemic circulation. For instance, nitroglycerin is well absorbed by the gastrointestinal tract. It has low bioavailability when administered orally, since it is extensively metabolized by the liver before it can reach the systemic circulation and the myocardium (**first-pass hepatic metabolism**).

Oral administration is convenient, economical, and relatively tolerant of dosage error. However, it is unreliable since it depends on patient cooperation, exposes the drug to first-pass hepatic metabolism, and allows interference by gastric pH, enzymes, motility, food, and other drugs.

The nonionized forms of drugs are preferentially absorbed. Therefore, an acidic environment favors the absorption of acidic drugs ($A^- + H^+ \rightarrow AH$), while an alkaline environment favors basic drugs ($BH^+ \rightarrow H^+ + B$). Regardless of ionization considerations, the large surface area of the small intestine provides a preferential site of absorption for most drugs compared with the stomach.

Because the veins of the mouth drain into the superior vena cava, **sublingual** or **buccal** drug absorption bypasses the liver and first-pass metabolism. **Rectal** administration is an alternative to oral medication in patients who are uncooperative (eg, pediatric patients) or unable to tolerate oral ingestion. Because the venous drainage of the rectum bypasses the liver, first-pass metabolism is less significant than with small intestinal absorption. Rectal absorption can be erratic, however, and many drugs cause irritation of the rectal mucosa. Absorption of **inhalational** agents is discussed in Chapter 7.

Transdermal drug administration has the advantage of prolonged and continuous absorption with a minimal total drug dose. The stratum corneum serves as an effective barrier to all but small, lipid-soluble drugs (eg, clonidine, nitroglycerin, scopolamine).

Parenteral injection includes **subcutaneous, intramuscular,** and **intravenous** routes of administration. Subcutaneous and intramuscular absorption depends on diffusion from the site of injection to the circulation. The rate of diffusion depends on the blood flow to the area and the carrier vehicle (solutions are absorbed faster than suspensions). Irritating preparations can cause pain and tissue necrosis. Intravenous injection completely bypasses the process of absorption, since the drug is placed directly into the bloodstream.

Distribution

Distribution plays a key role in clinical pharmacology since it is a major determinant of end-organ drug concentration. A drug's distribution depends primarily on organ perfusion, protein binding, and lipid solubility.

After absorption, a drug is distributed by the bloodstream throughout the body. Highly perfused organs (the **vessel-rich group**) take up a disproportionately large amount of drug compared with less perfused organs (the **muscle, fat,** and **vessel-poor groups**). Thus, even though the total mass of the vessel-rich group is small, it can account for substantial initial drug uptake (Table 8–1).

As long as a drug is bound to a plasma protein, it is unavailable for uptake by an organ regardless of the extent of perfusion to that organ. Albumin often binds acidic drugs (eg, barbiturates), while α_1-acid glycoprotein (AAG) binds basic drugs (local anesthetics). If these proteins are diminished or if the protein binding sites are occupied (eg, other drugs), the amount of free drug available for tissue uptake is increased. Renal disease, liver disease, chronic congestive heart failure, and malignancies decrease albumin production. Trauma (including surgery), infection, myocardial infarction, and chronic pain increase AAG levels.

Availability of a drug to a specific organ does not ensure uptake by that organ. For instance, the permeation by ionized drugs into the central nervous system is limited by pericapillary glial cells and endothelial-cell tight junctions, which constitute the **blood-brain barrier.** Lipid-soluble, nonionized molecules pass freely through lipid membranes. Other factors, such as molecular size and tissue binding—especially by the lung—can also influence drug distribution.

After the highly perfused organs are saturated during initial distribution, the greater mass of the less perfused organs will continue to take up drug from the bloodstream. As plasma concentration falls, some drug will leave the highly perfused organs to maintain equilibrium. This **redistribution** from the vessel-rich group is responsible for termination of effect of many anesthetic drugs. For example, wakening from the effects of thiopental is not due to metabolism or excretion but rather to redistribution of the drug from brain to muscle. As a corollary, if the less perfused organs are saturated from repeated doses of drug, redistribution cannot occur and awakening will depend to a greater extent on drug elimination. Thus, rapid-acting drugs such as thiopental and fentanyl will become longer acting after repeated administration or when a large single dose is given. The *apparent* volume into which a drug has been distributed is called its **volume of distribution (V_d)** and is determined by dividing the dose of drug administered by the resulting plasma concentration:

$$V_d = \frac{Dose}{Concentration}$$

This calculation is complicated by the need to adjust for the effects of drug elimination and continual redistribution. A small V_d implies relative confinement of the drug to the intravascular space, which leads to a high plasma concentration (eg, the V_d of pancuronium = 10 L in a 70-kg person). Causes for a small V_d include high protein binding or ionization. On the other hand, the apparent V_d may exceed total body water (approximately 40 L). Explanations for this include high solubility or binding of the drug in tissues other than plasma (eg, the V_d of fentanyl = 350 L). Therefore, the V_d does not represent a real volume but rather reflects

Table 8–1. Tissue group composition, relative body mass, and percentage of cardiac output.

Tissue Group	Composition	Body Mass (%)	Cardiac Output (%)
Vessel-rich	Brain, heart, liver, kidney, endocrine glands	10	75
Muscle	Muscle, skin	50	19
Fat	Fat	20	6
Vessel-poor	Bone, ligament, cartilage	20	0

the volume of plasma that would be necessary to account for the observed plasma concentration.

Biotransformation

Biotransformation is the alteration of a substance by metabolic processes. The end products of biotransformation are usually—but not necessarily—inactive and water-soluble. The latter property allows excretion by the kidney. The liver is the primary organ of biotransformation.

Metabolic biotransformation can be divided into phase I and phase II reactions. **Phase I reactions** convert a parent drug into more polar metabolites through oxidation, reduction, or hydrolysis. **Phase II reactions** couple (conjugate) a parent drug or a phase I metabolite with an endogenous substrate (eg, glucuronic acid) to form a highly polar end product that can be eliminated in the urine. Although this is usually a sequential process, phase I metabolites may be excreted without undergoing phase II biotransformation, and a phase II reaction can precede a phase I reaction.

Hepatic clearance is the rate of elimination of a drug as a result of liver biotransformation. More specifically, clearance is the volume of plasma cleared of drug per unit of time and is expressed as milliliters per minute. The hepatic clearance depends on the hepatic blood flow and the fraction of drug removed from the blood by the liver (**hepatic extraction ratio**). Drugs that are efficiently cleared by the liver have a high hepatic extraction ratio, and their clearance is proportionate to hepatic blood flow. On the other hand, drugs with a low hepatic extraction ratio are poorly cleared by the liver, and their clearance is limited by the capacity of the hepatic enzyme systems. Therefore, the effect of liver disease on drug pharmacokinetics depends on the drug's hepatic extraction ratio and the disease's propensity to alter hepatic blood flow or hepatocellular function.

Excretion

The kidney is the principal organ of excretion. Non–protein-bound drugs freely cross from plasma into the glomerular filtrate. The non-ionized fraction of drug is reabsorbed in the renal tubules, while the ionized portion is excreted. Thus, alterations in urine pH can alter renal excretion. The kidney also actively secretes some drugs. **Renal clearance** is the rate of elimination of a drug from kidney excretion. Renal failure changes the pharmacokinetics of many drugs by altering protein binding, volumes of distribution, and clearance rates.

Relatively few drugs depend on biliary excretion, since they are usually reabsorbed in the intestine and are consequently excreted in the urine. Delayed toxic effects from some drugs (eg, fentanyl) may be due to this **enterohepatic recirculation.**

The lungs are responsible for excretion of volatile agents, such as inhalational anesthetics (see Chapter 7).

Compartment Models

Compartment models offer a simple way to characterize the distribution and elimination of drugs in the body. A compartment can be conceptualized as a group of tissues that possess similar pharmacokinetics. For example, plasma and the vessel-rich group could represent the **central compartment,** while muscle, fat, and skin could represent the **peripheral compartment.** Having said this, it must be stressed that compartments are *conceptual* and do not represent actual tissues.

A **two-compartment model** correlates well with the distribution and elimination phases of many drugs (Figure 8–1). After an intravenous bolus, the plasma concentration of a drug will instantaneously rise. The initial rapid decline in plasma concentration, called the **distribution phase,** or **alpha (α) phase,** corresponds to the redistribution of drug from the plasma and the vessel-rich group of the central compartment to the less perfused tissues of the peripheral compartment. As dis-

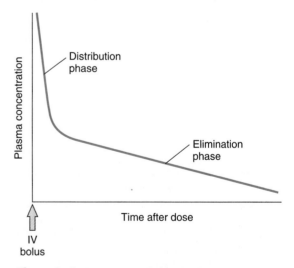

Figure 8–1. Two-compartment model demonstrates the distribution phase (α phase) and the elimination phase (β phase). During the distribution phase, the drug moves from the central compartment to the peripheral compartment. The elimination phase consists of metabolism and excretion.

tribution slows, elimination of drug from the central compartment is responsible for a continued—but less steep—decline in plasma concentration called the **elimination phase** or **beta (β) phase.** Elimination half-life 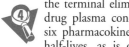 is proportional to the V_d and inversely proportional to the rate of clearance. The plasma concentration curves of many drugs are better characterized by a **three-compartment model** consisting of a central compartment and two peripheral compartments.

Plasma concentration following a bolus administration of a drug can be expressed by a triexponential equation:

$$Cp\,(t) = Ae^{-\alpha t} + Be^{-\beta t} + Ce^{-\gamma t}$$

where $Cp(t)$ equals plasma concentration at time t, and A, B, and C are fractional coefficients that denote the relative contributions of each of three hybrid rate constants (α corresponding to the rapid distribution half-life, β to the slow distribution half-life, and γ to the terminal elimination half-life). Therefore, drug plasma concentration is determined by six pharmacokinetic parameters and not just half-lives, as is often assumed. Because the fractional coefficients quantify the amount that each half-life contributes to the overall decline in drug concentration, they are as important as half-lives in predicting termination of drug action. For example, drug x may have longer distribution and elimination half-lives than does drug y, but its plasma concentration may fall more rapidly if its fractional coefficient of distribution (A) is greater. Stated another way, the plasma concentration of a drug with long half-lives may still fall rapidly if distribution accounts for the vast majority of the decline and elimination is a relatively insignificant contributor. Therefore, the rate of clinical recovery from a drug cannot be predicted by its half-lives alone.

Rates of distribution and biotransformation can usually be described in terms of **first-order kinetics.** In other words, a constant fraction or percentage of drug is distributed or metabolized per unit of time, regardless of plasma concentration. For instance, 10% of a drug may be biotransformed hourly whether the plasma concentration is 10 μg/mL or 100 μg/mL. If the concentration of drug exceeds the biotransformation capacity, however, then a constant amount of drug may be metabolized per unit of time (**zero-order kinetics**). Using a similar example, 500 μg of drug might be metabolized each hour regardless of whether the plasma concentration was 10 μg/mL or 100 μg/mL. Alcohol metabolism can be predicted by zero-order kinetics.

PHARMACODYNAMICS

Pharmacodynamics is the study of the therapeutic and toxic organ system effects of drugs (how a drug affects a body). The extent of these effects determines a drug's efficacy, potency, and therapeutic ratio. Pharmacodynamics also inquires into mechanisms of action, drug interactions, and structure-activity relationships. Understanding dose-response curves and drug receptors provides a framework to help explain these diverse parameters of pharmacodynamics.

Dose-Response Curves

Dose-response curves express the relationship between drug dose and pharmacologic effect. Drug dose or steady-state plasma concentration is plotted on the abscissa (x axis) and is represented in linear (Figure 8–2A) or logarithmic scale (Figure 8–2B). Pharmacologic effect is plotted on the ordinate (y axis) in terms of absolute units (Figure 8–2A) or as a fraction of maximal effect (Figure 8–2B). The position of the dose-response curve along the abscissa is an indication of drug **potency.** The maximal effect of the drug relates to its **efficacy.** The slope of the dose-response curve reflects receptor-binding characteristics. The influence of pharmacokinetics in dose-response curves can be minimized by studying the relationship of blood concentration to pharmacologic response.

The **median effective dose** (ED_{50}) is the dose of drug required to produce a given effect in 50% of the population. Note that the ED_{50} is *not* the dose required to produce one-half the maximal effect. The ED_{50} of inhalational anesthetics is the same as the minimum alveolar concentration (see Chapter 7). The **median lethal dose** (LD_{50}) is the dose that results in death in 50% of the population exposed to that dose. The **therapeutic index** is the ratio of the median lethal dose to the median effective dose ($LD_{50}:ED_{50}$).

Drug Receptors

Drug receptors are macromolecules—usually proteins embedded into cell membranes—that interact with a drug to mediate characteristic intracellular changes. The mechanism of action of several (not all) drugs depends on interaction with a receptor. Endogenous substances (eg, hormones) or exogenous substances (eg, drugs) that directly change cell function by binding to receptors are called **agonists. Antagonists** also bind to the receptors but without causing a direct effect on the cell. The pharmacologic effect of antagonist drugs depends on the subsequent inability of agonist substances to activate the receptors. **Competitive antagonists** bind reversibly to receptors and can be displaced by higher concentrations of agonists. **Noncompetitive (irreversible) antagonists**

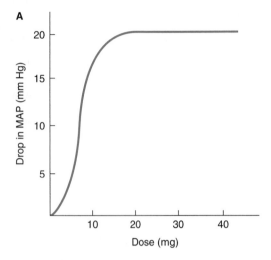

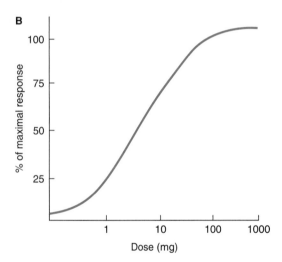

Figure 8–2. The shape of the dose-response curve depends on whether the dose or steady-state plasma concentration (C_{CPSS}) is plotted on a linear (**A**) or logarithmic (**B**) scale.

bind to the receptor with such affinity that even high concentrations of agonists cannot reverse the receptor blockade. Competition of two drugs for the same receptor is one source of drug interactions.

Receptors affect cell function either directly (eg, by changing transmembrane ion flux) or by controlling the production of another regulatory molecule (eg, the second-messenger cyclic adenosine monophosphate). Individual variability in response to receptor binding is a significant cause of inconsistency in drug responsiveness. Continued activation of a receptor often leads to **hyporeactivity,** while lack of stimulation results in

hyperreactivity. Chemical structure determines the degree of affinity between a drug and a receptor (**structure-activity relationship**). Minor changes in molecular configuration can have dramatic effects on clinical pharmacology.

■ SPECIFIC NONVOLATILE ANESTHETIC AGENTS

BARBITURATES

Mechanisms of Action

Barbiturates depress the reticular activating system—a complex polysynaptic network of neurons and regulatory centers—located in the brainstem that controls several vital functions, including consciousness. In clinical concentrations, barbiturates preferentially affect the function of nerve synapses rather than axons. They suppress transmission of excitatory neurotransmitters (eg, acetylcholine) and enhance transmission of inhibitory neurotransmitters (eg, γ-aminobutyric acid [GABA]). Specific mechanisms include interfering with transmitter release (presynaptic) and stereoselectively interacting with receptors (postsynaptic).

Structure-Activity Relationships

Barbiturates are barbituric acid derivatives (Figure 8–3). Substitution at the number 5 carbon (C_5) determines hypnotic potency and anticonvulsant activity. For example, a long-branched chain conveys more potency than does a short straight chain. Likewise, the **phenyl** group in *pheno*barbital is anticonvulsive, while the **methyl** group in *metho*hexital is not. Replacing the **oxygen** at C_2 (*oxy*barbiturates) with a **sulfur** atom (*thio*barbiturates) increases lipid solubility. As a result, thiopental and thiamylal have greater potency, more rapid onset of action, and shorter durations of action than do pentobarbital and secobarbital. The short duration of action of methohexital is related to the methyl substitution at N_1. The sodium salts of the barbiturates are water-soluble but markedly alkaline (pH of 2.5% thiopental > 10) and relatively unstable (2-week shelf-life for 2.5% thiopental solution). Concentrations higher than recommended cause an unacceptable incidence of both pain on injection and venous thrombosis.

Pharmacokinetics

A. ABSORPTION:

In clinical anesthesiology, barbiturates are most frequently administered intravenously for induction of

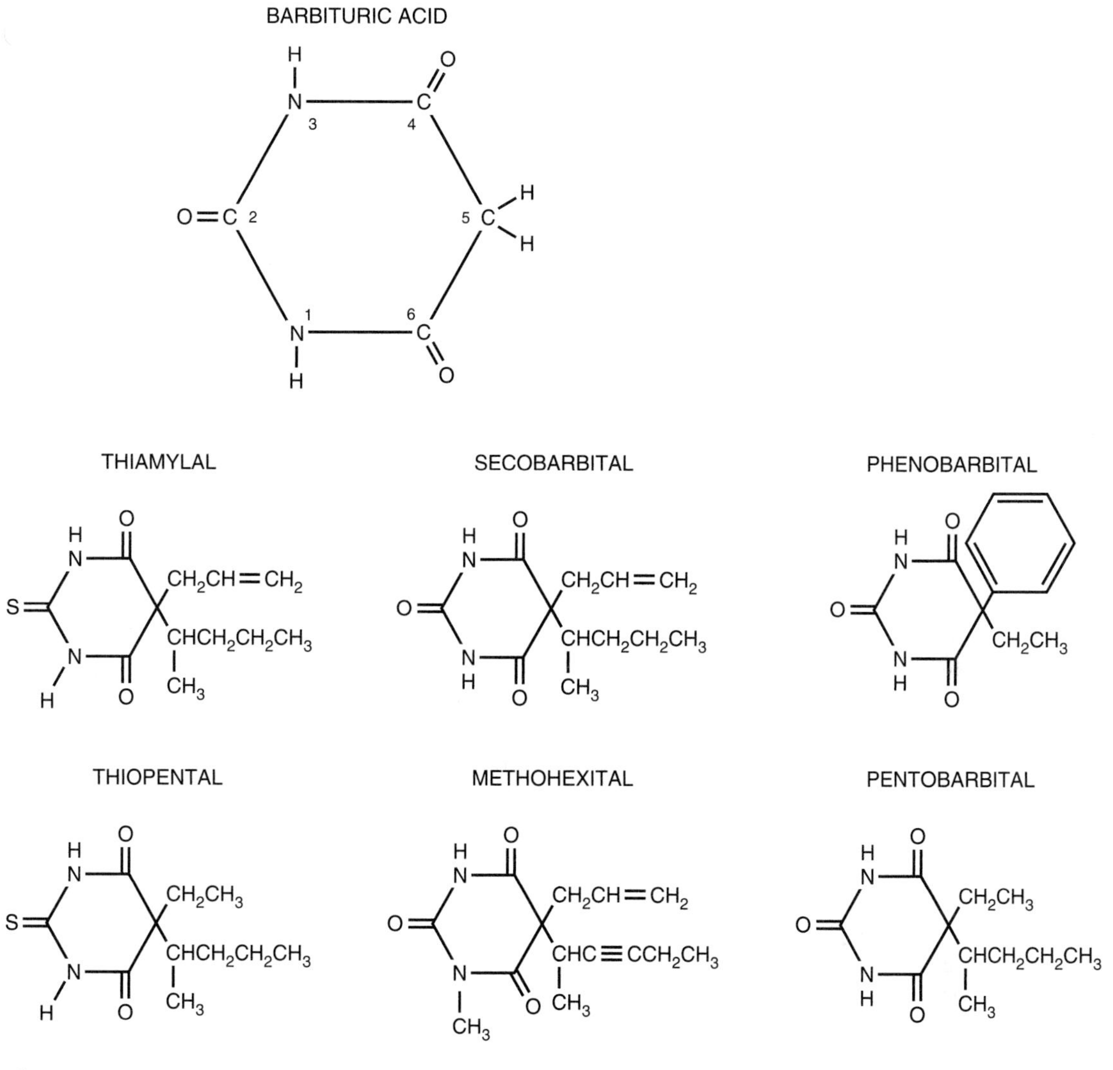

BARBITURIC ACID

Figure 8–3. Barbiturates share the structure of barbituric acid and differ in the C_2, C_3, and N_1 substitutions.

general anesthesia in adults and children with an intravenous line. Exceptions include rectal thiopental or methohexital for induction in children and intramuscular pentobarbital or secobarbital for premedication of all age groups.

B. DISTRIBUTION:

The duration of action of highly lipid-soluble barbiturates (thiopental, thiamylal, and methohexital) is determined by redistribution, not metabolism or elimination. For example, although thiopental is highly protein-bound (80%), its great lipid solubility and high nonionized fraction (60%) account for maximal brain uptake within 30 seconds. If the central compartment

is contracted (eg, hypovolemic shock), if the serum albumin is low (eg, severe liver disease), or if the nonionized fraction is increased (eg, acidosis), higher brain and heart concentrations will be achieved for a given dose. Subsequent redistribution to the peripheral compartment—specifically, the muscle group—lowers plasma and brain concentration to 10% of peak levels within 20–30 minutes (Figure 8–4). This pharmacokinetic profile correlates with clinical experience—patients typically lose consciousness within 30 seconds and awaken within 20 minutes. Induction doses of thiopental depend on body weight and age. Lower induction doses in elderly patients is a reflection of higher peak plasma levels because of slower redistribu-

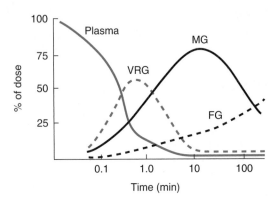

Figure 8–4. Distribution of thiopental from plasma to vessel-rich group (VRG), to muscle group (MG), and finally to fat group (FG). (Modified and reproduced, with permission, from Price HL et al: The uptake of thiopental by body tissues and its relation to the duration of narcosis. Clin Pharmacol Ther 1960;1:16.)

tion. In contrast to the rapid initial distribution half-life of a few minutes, the elimination half-life of thiopental ranges from 3 to 12 hours. Thiamylal and methohexital have similar distribution patterns, while less lipid-soluble barbiturates have much longer distribution half-lives and durations of action. Repetitive administration of barbiturates will saturate the peripheral compartments, so that redistribution cannot occur and the duration of action will become more dependent on elimination.

C. BIOTRANSFORMATION:

Biotransformation of barbiturates principally involves hepatic oxidation to inactive water-soluble metabolites. Because of greater hepatic extraction, methohexital is cleared by the liver three to four times more rapidly than thiopental or thiamylal. While redistribution is responsible for the awakening from a single dose of any of these lipid-soluble barbiturates, full recovery of psychomotor function is more rapid following methohexital owing to its enhanced metabolism.

D. EXCRETION:

High protein binding decreases barbiturate glomerular filtration, while high lipid solubility tends to increase renal tubular reabsorption. Except for the less protein-bound and less lipid-soluble agents such as phenobarbital, renal excretion is limited to water-soluble end products of hepatic biotransformation. Methohexital is excreted in the feces.

Effects on Organ Systems

A. CARDIOVASCULAR:

Induction doses of intravenously administered barbiturates cause a fall in blood pressure and an elevation in heart rate. Depression of the medullary vasomotor center vasodilates peripheral capacitance vessels, which increases peripheral pooling of blood and decreases venous return to the right atrium. The tachycardia is probably due to a central vagolytic effect. Cardiac output is often maintained by a rise in heart rate and increased myocardial contractility from compensatory baroreceptor reflexes. Sympathetically induced vasoconstriction of resistance vessels may actually increase peripheral vascular resistance. However, in the absence of an adequate baroreceptor response (eg, hypovolemia, congestive heart failure, β-adrenergic blockade), cardiac output and arterial blood pressure may fall dramatically owing to uncompensated peripheral pooling and unmasked direct myocardial depression. Patients with poorly controlled hypertension are particularly prone to wide swings in blood pressure during induction. The cardiovascular effects of barbiturates therefore vary markedly, depending on volume status, baseline autonomic tone, and preexisting cardiovascular disease. A slow rate of injection and adequate preoperative hydration attenuate these changes in most patients.

B. RESPIRATORY:

Barbiturate depression of the medullary ventilatory center decreases the ventilatory response to hypercapnia and hypoxia. Barbiturate sedation typically leads to upper airway obstruction; apnea usually follows an induction dose. During awakening, tidal volume and respiratory rate are decreased. Barbiturates do not completely depress noxious airway reflexes, and bronchospasm in asthmatic patients or laryngospasm in lightly anesthetized patients is not uncommon following airway instrumentation. Laryngospasm and hiccuping are more common after methohexital than after thiopental. Bronchospasm following induction with thiopental may be due to cholinergic nerve stimulation (which would be preventable by pretreatment with atropine), histamine release, or direct bronchial smooth muscle stimulation.

C. CEREBRAL:

 Barbiturates constrict the cerebral vasculature, causing a decrease in cerebral blood flow and intracranial pressure. The drop in intracranial pressure exceeds the decline in arterial blood pressure, so that **cerebral perfusion pressure (CPP)** is usually increased. (CPP equals cerebral artery pressure minus the greater of cerebral venous pressure or intracranial pressure.) The decrease in cerebral blood flow is not detrimental, since barbiturates induce an even greater decline in **cerebral oxygen consumption** (up to 50% of normal). Alterations in cerebral activity and oxygen requirements are reflected by changes in the electroencephalogram (EEG), which progresses from low-voltage fast activity with small doses to high-voltage slow activity and electrical silence (suppression) with very large doses of barbiturate (a bolus of 15–40 mg/kg of thiopental followed by an infusion of 0.5 mg/kg/min). This effect of barbiturates may provide some brain protection from transient episodes of focal ischemia (eg, cerebral embolism) but probably not from global ischemia (eg, cardiac arrest). Furthermore, doses required for EEG suppression have been associated with prolonged awakening, delayed extubation, and the need for inotropic support.

The degree of central nervous system depression induced by barbiturates ranges from mild sedation to unconsciousness, depending on the dose administered (Table 8–2). Some patients relate a taste sensation of garlic or onions during induction with thiopental. Unlike narcotics, barbiturates do not selectively impair the perception of pain. In fact, they sometimes appear to have an **antianalgesic effect** by lowering the pain threshold. Small doses occasionally cause a state of excitement and disorientation that can be disconcerting when sedation is the objective. Barbiturates do not produce muscle relaxation, and some induce involuntary skeletal muscle contractions (eg, methohexital). Relatively small doses of thiopental (50–100 mg intravenously) rapidly control most grand mal seizures. Unfortunately, acute tolerance and physiologic dependence on the sedative effect of barbiturates develop quickly.

D. RENAL:

Barbiturates reduce renal blood flow and glomerular-filtration rate in proportion to the fall in blood pressure.

E. HEPATIC:

Hepatic blood flow is decreased. Chronic exposure to barbiturates has opposing effects on drug biotransformation. Induction of hepatic enzymes increases the rate of metabolism of some drugs (eg, digitoxin), while combination with the cytochrome P-450 enzyme system interferes with the biotransformation of others (eg, tricyclic antidepressants). The induction of aminolevulinic acid synthetase stimulates the formation of **porphyrin** (an intermediary in heme synthesis), which may precipitate **acute intermittent porphyria** or **variegate porphyria** in susceptible individuals.

F. IMMUNOLOGIC:

Anaphylactic and anaphylactoid allergic reactions are rare. Sulfur-containing thiobarbiturates evoke mast cell histamine release in vitro, while oxybarbiturates do not. For this reason, some anesthesiologists prefer methohexital over thiopental or thiamylal in asthmatic or atopic patients.

Drug Interactions

Contrast media, sulfonamides, and other drugs that occupy the same protein-binding sites as thiopental will increase the amount of free drug available and potentiate the organ system effects of a given dose.

Ethanol, narcotics, antihistamines, and other central nervous system depressants potentiate the sedative effects of barbiturates. The common clinical impression that chronic alcohol abuse is associated with increased thiopental requirements lacks scientific proof.

Table 8–2. Uses and dosages of commonly used barbiturates.

Agent	Use	Route	Concentration (%)	Dose
Thiopental, thiamylal	Induction	IV	2.5	3–6 mg/kg
	Sedation	IV	2.5	0.5–1.5 mg/kg
Methohexital	Induction	IV	1	1–2 mg/kg
	Sedation	IV	1	0.2–0.4 mg/kg
	Induction	Rectal (children)	10	25 mg/kg
Secobarbital, pentobarbital	Premedication	Oral	5	2–4 mg/kg*
		IM		2–4 mg/kg*
		Rectal suppository		3 mg/kg

IV = intravenous; IM = intramuscular.
*Maximum dose is 150 mg.

BENZODIAZEPINES

Mechanisms of Action

Benzodiazepines interact with specific receptors in the central nervous system, particularly in the cerebral cortex. Benzodiazepine-receptor binding enhances the inhibitory effects of various neurotransmitters. For example, benzodiazepine-receptor binding facilitates GABA receptor binding, which increases the membrane conductance of chloride ions. This causes a change in membrane polarization that inhibits normal neuronal function. Flumazenil (an imidazobenzodiazepine) is a specific benzodiazepine-receptor antagonist that effec-tively reverses most of the central nervous system effect of benzodiazepines (see Chapter 15).

Structure-Activity Relationships

The chemical structure of benzodiazepines includes a benzene ring and a seven-member diazepine ring (Figure 8–5). Substitutions at various positions on these rings affect potency and biotransformation. The imidazole ring of midazolam contributes to its water solubility at low pH. The insolubility of diazepam and lorazepam in water requires parenteral preparations to contain propylene glycol, which has been associated with venous irritation.

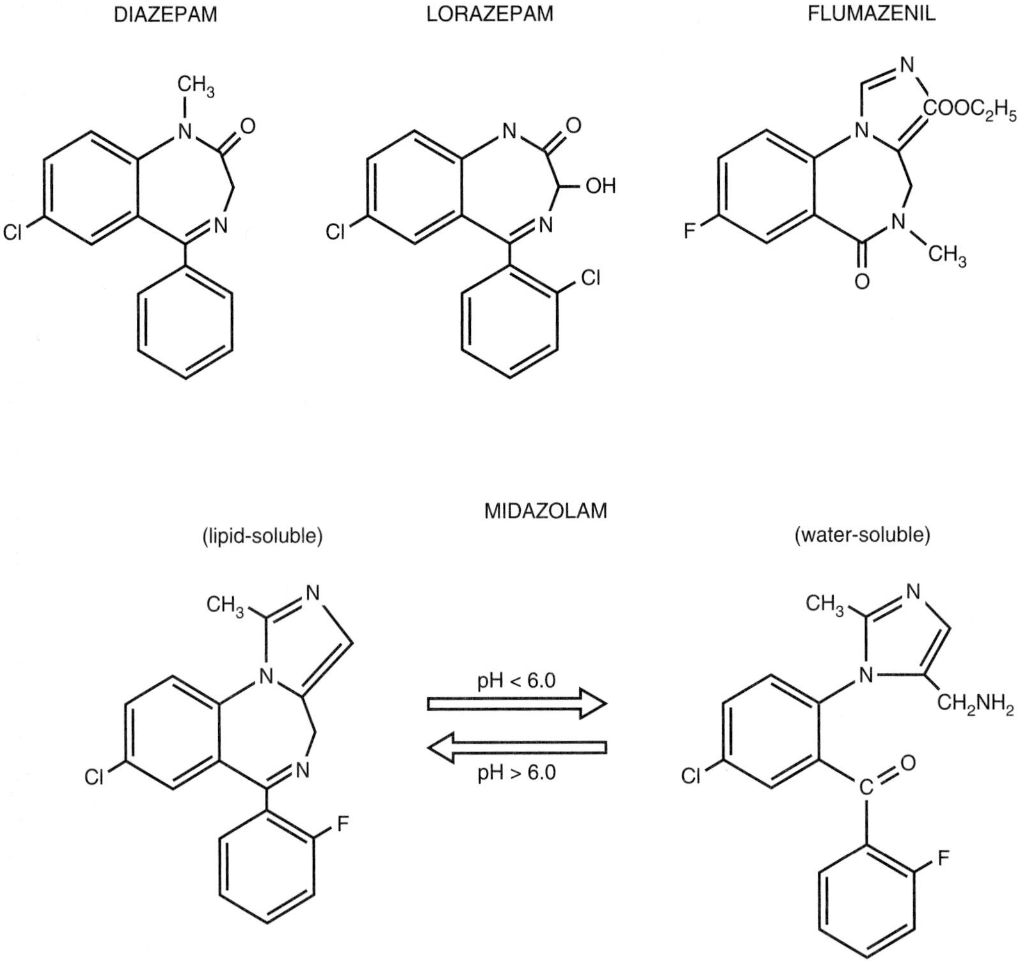

Figure 8–5. The structures of commonly used benzodiazepines and their antagonist, flumazenil, share a seven-member diazepine ring. (Modified and reproduced, with permission, from White PF: Pharmacologic and clinical aspects of preoperative medication. Anesth Analg 1986;65:963. With permission from the International Anesthesia Research Society.)

Pharmacokinetics

A. ABSORPTION:

Benzodiazepines are commonly administered orally, intramuscularly, and intravenously to provide sedation or induction of general anesthesia (Table 8–3). Diazepam and lorazepam are well absorbed from the gastrointestinal tract, with peak plasma levels usually achieved in 1 and 2 hours, respectively. Although oral midazolam has not been approved by the US Food and Drug Administration, this route of administration has been popular for pediatric premedication. Likewise, intranasal (0.2–0.3 mg/kg), buccal (0.07 mg/kg), and sublingual (0.1 mg/kg) midazolam have been demonstrated to provide effective preoperative sedation.

Intramuscular injection of diazepam is painful and unreliable. In contrast, midazolam and lorazepam are well absorbed after intramuscular injection, with peak levels achieved in 30 and 90 minutes, respectively. Induction of general anesthesia relies upon intravenous administration.

B. DISTRIBUTION:

Diazepam is quite lipid-soluble and rapidly penetrates the blood-brain barrier. Although midazolam is water-soluble at low pH, its imidazole ring closes at physiologic pH, causing an increase in its lipid solubility (Figure 8–5). The moderate lipid solubility of lorazepam accounts for its slower brain uptake and onset of action. Redistribution is fairly rapid for the benzodiazepines (initial distribution half-life is 3–10 minutes) and, like the barbiturates, is responsible for awakening. Although midazolam is frequently used as an induction agent, none of the benzodiazepines can match thiopental's

rapid onset and short duration of action. All three benzodiazepines are highly protein-bound (90–98%).

C. BIOTRANSFORMATION:

The benzodiazepines rely on the liver for biotransformation into water-soluble glucuronide end products. The phase I metabolites of diazepam are pharmacologically active.

Slow hepatic extraction and a large V_d result in a long elimination half-life for diazepam (30 hours). Although lorazepam also has a low hepatic extraction ratio, its lower lipid solubility limits its V_d, resulting in a shorter elimination half-life (15 hours). Nonetheless, the clinical duration of lorazepam is often quite prolonged owing to a very high receptor affinity. In contrast, midazolam shares diazepam's V_d, but its elimination half-life (2 hours) is the shortest of the group because of its high hepatic extraction ratio.

D. EXCRETION:

The metabolites of benzodiazepine biotransformation are excreted chiefly in the urine. Enterohepatic circulation produces a secondary peak in diazepam plasma concentration 6–12 hours following administration. Renal failure may lead to prolonged sedation in patients receiving midazolam due to the accumulation of a conjugated metabolite (alpha-hydroxymidazolam).

Effects on Organ Systems

A. CARDIOVASCULAR:

The benzodiazepines display minimal cardiovascular depressant effects even at induction doses. Arterial blood pressure, cardiac output, and peripheral vascular resistance usually decline slightly, while heart rate sometimes rises. Midazolam tends to reduce blood pressure and peripheral vascular resistance more than does diazepam. Heart rate variability changes during midazolam sedation suggest decreased vagal tone (ie, drug-induced vagolysis).

B. RESPIRATORY:

Benzodiazepines depress the ventilatory response to CO_2. This depression is usually insignificant unless the drugs are administered intravenously or in association with other respiratory depressants. Although apnea may be less common after benzodiazepine induction than after barbiturate induction, even small intravenous doses of diazepam and midazolam have resulted in respiratory arrest. The steep dose-response curve, slightly prolonged onset (compared with thiopental or diazepam), and high potency of midazolam necessitate careful titration to avoid overdosage and apnea. Ventilation must be monitored in all patients receiving intravenous benzodiazepines,

Table 8–3. Uses and doses of commonly used benzodiazepines.

Agent	Use	Route	Dose
Diazepam	Premedication	Oral	0.2–0.5 mg/kg[1]
	Sedation	IV	0.04–0.2 mg/kg
	Induction	IV	0.3–0.6 mg/kg
Midazolam	Premedication	IM	0.07–0.15 mg/kg
	Sedation	IV	0.01–0.1 mg/kg
	Induction	IV	0.1–0.4 mg/kg
Lorazepam	Premedication	Oral	0.05 mg/kg[2]
		IM	0.03–0.05 mg/kg[2]
	Sedation	IV	0.03–0.04 mg/kg[2]

IV = intravenous; IM = intramuscular.
[1]Maximum dose 15 mg.
[2]Not recommended for children.

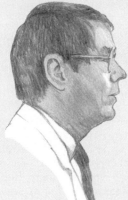

J.G. Reves, MD

RATIONAL ADMINISTRATION OF INTRAVENOUS ANESTHESIA

General anesthesia requires that adequate levels of anesthetic drugs be rapidly attained in the brain, and that they be maintained during the time required for surgery. This is a concept that applies equally to general anesthesia achieved by inhalational anesthetics and intravenous drugs. However, the routine clinical practice of anesthesia by many clinicians seems to approach the attainment and maintenance of therapeutic levels of anesthesia differently depending on whether inhalational or intravenous anesthetics are being used. This mystifies me. Why do clinicians administer inhalational drugs continuously, using a vaporizer, but administer intravenous drugs intermittently by bolus injection with hand-held syringes? With inhalational drugs administered continuously, a relatively constant brain level is achieved and maintained. With the intermittent intravenous bolus technique, however, markedly high and low levels of drug are attained in the blood and brain—usually an overdose (defined as far more than required) with the initial bolus and then as time passes redistribution occurs until an underdose (defined as less than required) is present. It has always seemed irrational to me that intravenous drugs are not routinely administered by continuous infusion.

Why is it more rational to administer intravenous drugs continuously rather than intermittently? The reason becomes obvious in considering a second question, "Why are inhalational drugs given continuously?" Of course the answer to both questions is that a relatively constant level of drug is maintained when it is administered continuously. Figure 1 shows the contrast between continuous infusion and intermittent bolus administration. Problems with a bolus

technique are obvious; there are great variations in the blood levels, which cause anesthesia to be too deep, right after the bolus and then too light before the next bolus. Repeated bolus administrations also tend to promote drug accumulation in patients, making it more difficult to arouse patients at the conclusion of surgery.

Why in the past has it not been routine to administer intravenous drugs continuously? There were two principal reasons; 1) most anesthetic drugs were not suited for continuous infusions, and 2) infusion pumps were not simple and easy to operate. These reasons are no longer valid. Drugs such as midazolam, propofol, alfentanil and remifentanil are ideally suited to continuous infusion. Also, infusion technology has advanced to the point that sophisticated pumps with preset programs that make it easy to set a precise, individualized infusion rate are readily available.

Another important advance in infusion anesthesia has been the use of a computer to administer anesthetics continuously using pharmacokinetic principles.[1,2] This technology may be termed "computer-assisted continuous infusion" (CACI), or "target controlled infusion" (TCI). The pharmacokinetics of the anesthetic drug to be used is in a chip within the computer-controlled syringe pump. The clinician sets a desired therapeutic blood or brain level of anesthetic, and the computer infuses the drug, first by bolus to attain a therapeutic level, and then by continuous infusion at an exponentially declining

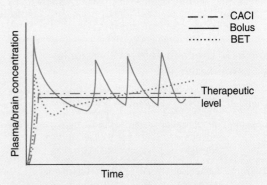

Figure 1. The object of anesthesia is to maintain a safe, constant therapeutic level of drug throughout the surgical period. Using intravenous drugs, this can be done in one of three ways: bolus injection (solid line), bolus injection followed by constant infusion (BET, dotted line), or by computer-assisted continuous infusion (CACI, hatched line). CACI provides the most constant plasma and brain concentrations.

rate to keep the drug level constant in the patient. This technology has been described for propofol,[3] and has been described in detail elsewhere.[4]

Is there an advantage to CACI over other continuous infusion methods? I am aware of only one study that has examined this question.[5] Although there were some advantages to CACI administration, the differences between CACI and continuous manual infusion were not great. Perhaps this is because with years of experience clinicians have determined how to attain and maintain stable, adequate levels of anesthesia without knowing the brain or plasma drug concentration. I am not aware of any study that compares intermittent bolus administration with either CACI or manual continuous infusion. I would predict that there would be less hemodynamic variability and less awareness with the continuous infusion technique.

In the future, intravenous anesthetic drugs will be delivered by intelligent infusion pumps that are able to individualize the administration based on the pharmacokinetics of the drug in that patient, and maintain a desired brain concentration. The intelligent pump would be able to titrate brain levels up or down to suit the individual patient's needs. Some patients may require even more sophisticated automation. Even more sophisticated would be a closed-loop intravenous and inhalational anesthesia system (Figure 2). The clinician would activate the system by choosing a desired drug level utilizing the processed electroencephalographic (EEG) reading. Processed EEG signaling similar to the existing bispectral system (BIS) now available will undoubtedly be used to close the loop.[6] Such an automated system will be able, for example, to administer anesthetic drugs in such a manner as to maintain the patient at the desired level of anesthesia. The depth of anesthesia and sedation will be maintained automatically, akin to speed control of an automobile. This technology will also have applications in intensive care units, emergency departments, and in a host of other sedation settings. Anesthesiologists will need to teach others the science behind the seemingly simple patient care applications of these new drug delivery technologies. This roboticlike approach to anesthesia and sedation cannot be viewed as a threat to the practice of anesthesia, but must be embraced as another step in the progress of the field of anesthesiology. It will allow anesthesiologists to improve patient care in multiple settings even when not personally present.

1. Schuttler J, Schwilden H, Stockel H: Pharmacokinetics as applied to total intravenous anesthesia: practical implications. Anaesthesia 1983;38:53.

2. Alvis JM, Reves JG, Govier AV, et al: Computer-assisted continuous infusions of fentanyl during cardiac anesthesia: comparison with a manual method. Anesthesiology 1985;63:41.

3. White M, Kenny GNC: Intravenous propofol using a computerized infusion system. Anaesthesia 1990;45:204.

4. Glass PSA, Shafer SL, Jacobs, JR, Reves JR: Intravenous drug delivery systems. In Miller RD (editor), *Anesthesia*, 4th ed. Churchill Livingstone, 1994.

5. Theil DR, Stanley TE, White WD, Goodman DK, Glass PSA, Reves JG: Midazolam and fentanyl continuous intravenous anesthesia for cardiac surgery: a comparison of two infusion systems. J Cardiothorac Vasc Anesth 1993;7:300.

6. Reves JG, Greene MN: Anesthesiology and the academic medical center: place and promise at the start of the new millennium. Internat Anesthesiol Clin, Lippincott, Williams & Wilkins 2000.

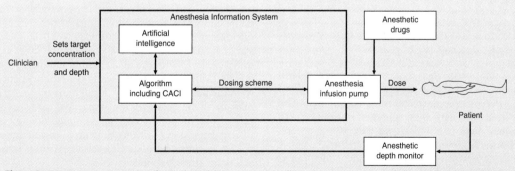

Figure 2. Future intravenous anesthesia drug delivery systems will involve automation and closed-loop drug administration. The clinician will set the appropriate drug concentration, and the desired level of unconsciousness (anesthesia) using an automated EEG monitor. The anesthetic dose and depth for that patient will then be maintained at the prescribed level by closed-loop technology. (CACI, computer-assisted continuous infusion) (Reproduced, with permission, from Reves JG, Greene MN: Anesthesiology and the academic medical center: place and promise at the start of the new millennium. Internat Anesthesiol Clin, Lippincott, Williams & Wilkins 2000.)

and resuscitation equipment must be immediately available.

C. CEREBRAL:

Benzodiazepines reduce cerebral oxygen consumption, cerebral blood flow, and intracranial pressure but not to the extent the barbiturates do. They are very effective in preventing and controlling grand mal seizures. Oral sedative doses often produce antegrade amnesia, a useful premedication property. The mild muscle-relaxant property of these drugs is mediated at the spinal cord level, not at the neuromuscular junction. The antianxiety, amnesic, and sedative effects seen at low doses progress to stupor and unconsciousness at induction doses. Compared with thiopental, induction with benzodiazepines is associated with a slower loss of consciousness and a longer recovery. Benzodiazepines have no direct analgesic properties.

Drug Interactions

Cimetidine binds to cytochrome P-450 and reduces the metabolism of diazepam. Erythromycin inhibits midazolam metabolism and causes a 2- to 3-fold prolongation and intensification of its effects. Heparin displaces diazepam from protein-binding sites and increases the free drug concentration (200% increase after 1000 units of heparin).

The combination of opioids and diazepam markedly reduces arterial blood pressure and peripheral vascular resistance. This synergistic interaction is especially pronounced in patients with ischemic or valvular heart disease.

Benzodiazepines reduce the minimum alveolar concentration of volatile anesthetics as much as 30%.

Ethanol, barbiturates, and other central nervous system depressants potentiate the sedative effects of the benzodiazepines.

OPIOIDS

Mechanisms of Action

Opioids bind to specific receptors located throughout the central nervous system and other tissues. Four major types of opioid receptor have been identified (Table 8–4): **mu** (**μ**, with subtypes **μ-1** and **μ-2**), **kappa** (**κ**), **delta** (**δ**), and **sigma** (**σ**). While opioids provide some degree of sedation, they are most effective at producing analgesia. The pharmacodynamic properties of specific opioids depend on which receptor is bound, the binding affinity, and whether the receptor is activated. Although both opioid agonists and antagonists bind to opioid receptors, only agonists are capable of receptor activation. Agonist-antagonists (eg, nalbuphine, nalorphine, butorphanol, and pentazocine)

Table 8–4. Classification of opioid receptors.

Receptor	Clinical Effect	Agonists
Mu	Supraspinal analgesia (μ-1) Respiratory depression (μ-2) Physical dependence Muscle rigidity	Morphine Met-enkephalin* Beta-endorphin* Fentanyl
Kappa	Sedation Spinal analgesia	Morphine Nalbuphine Butorphanol Dynorphin* Oxycodone
Delta	Analgesia Behavioral Epileptogenic	Leu-enkephalin* Beta-endorphin*
Sigma	Dysphoria Hallucinations Respiratory stimulation	Pentazocine Nalorphine Ketamine?

Note: The relationships between receptor, clinical effect, and agonist are more complex than indicated in this table. For example, pentazocine is an antagonist at mu receptors, a partial agonist at kappa receptors, and an agonist at sigma receptors.
*Endogenous opioid.

are drugs that have opposite actions at different receptor types. The pure opioid antagonist naloxone is discussed in Chapter 15.

Endorphins, enkephalins, and **dynorphins** are endogenous peptides that bind to opioid receptors. These three families of opioid peptides differ in their protein precursors, anatomic distributions, and receptor affinities.

Opioid-receptor activation inhibits the presynaptic release and postsynaptic response to excitatory neurotransmitters (eg, acetylcholine, substance P) from nociceptive neurons. The cellular mechanism for this neuromodulation may involve alterations in potassium and calcium ion conductance. Transmission of pain impulses can be interrupted at the level of the dorsal horn of the spinal cord with intrathecal or epidural administration of opioids. Modulation of a descending inhibitory pathway from the periaqueductal gray through the nucleus raphe magnus to the dorsal horn of the spinal cord may also play a role in opioid analgesia. Although opioids exert their greatest effect within the central nervous system, opioid receptors have also been isolated from somatic and sympathetic peripheral nerves.

Structure-Activity Relationships

Opioid-receptor interaction is shared by a chemically diverse group of compounds. Nonetheless, there are common structural characteristics, which are shown in

Figure 8–6. Small molecular changes can convert an agonist into an antagonist. Note that the levorotatory isomers are generally more potent than the dextrorotatory isomers.

Pharmacokinetics

A. ABSORPTION:

Rapid and complete absorption follows the intramuscular injection of morphine and meperidine, with peak plasma levels usually reached after 20–60 minutes. Oral transmucosal fentanyl citrate absorption (fentanyl "lollipop") is an effective method of producing analgesia and sedation and provides rapid onset (10 minutes) of analgesia and sedation in children (15–20 μg/kg) and adults (200 to 800 μg).

Fentanyl's low molecular weight and high lipid solubility also allow transdermal absorption (the fentanyl patch). The amount of fentanyl released depends primarily on the surface area of the patch but can vary with local skin conditions (eg, blood flow). Establishing a reservoir of drug in the upper dermis delays systemic absorption for the first few hours. Serum concentrations of fentanyl reach a plateau within 14–24 hours of application (peak levels occur later in elderly patients than in young adult patients) and remain constant for up to 72 hours. Continued absorption from the dermal reservoir accounts for a prolonged fall in serum levels after patch removal. A high incidence of nausea and variable blood levels have limited the acceptance of fentanyl patches for postoperative pain relief.

Experimental studies have explored the possibility of an inhalational delivery of liposome-encapsulated fentanyl by the lungs.

B. DISTRIBUTION:

Table 8–5 summarizes the physical characteristics that determine distribution and uptake of opioid anesthetics. The distribution half-lives of all of the narcotics are fairly rapid (5–20 minutes). The low fat solubility of morphine slows passage across the blood-brain barrier, however, so that its onset of action is slow and its duration of action prolonged. This contrasts with the high lipid solubility of fentanyl and sufentanil, which allows a rapid onset and short duration of action. Interestingly, alfentanil has a more rapid onset of action and shorter duration of action than fentanyl following a bolus injection, even though it is less lipid-soluble than fentanyl. The high nonionized fraction of alfentanil at physiologic pH and its small V_d increase the amount of drug available for binding in the brain. Significant amounts of lipid-soluble opioids can be retained by the lungs (first-pass uptake) and later diffuse back into the systemic circulation. The amount of pulmonary uptake depends on prior accumulation of another drug (de-

creases), a history of tobacco use (increases), and coincident inhalational anesthetic administration (decreases). Redistribution terminates the action of small doses of all of these drugs, while larger doses must depend on biotransformation to adequately lower plasma levels.

C. BIOTRANSFORMATION:

Most opioids depend primarily on the liver for biotransformation. Their high hepatic extraction ratio causes their clearance to be dependent on liver blood flow. The small V_d of alfentanil is responsible for a short elimination half-life (1½ hours). Morphine undergoes conjugation with glucuronic acid to form morphine 3-glucuronide and morphine 6-glucuronide. Meperidine is N-demethylated to normeperidine, an active metabolite associated with seizure activity. The end products of fentanyl, sufentanil, and alfentanil are inactive.

The unique ester structure of remifentanil, an ultra-short-acting opioid with a terminal elimination half-life of less than 10 minutes, makes it susceptible to rapid ester hydrolysis by nonspecific esterases in blood (red cells) and tissue (see Figure 8–6) in a manner similar to esmolol (see Chapter 12). Biotransformation is so rapid and so complete that the duration of a remifentanil infusion has little effect on wake-up time (Figure 8–7). Its **context-sensitive half-time** (the time required for the plasma drug concentration to decline by 50% after termination of an infusion) is approximately 3 minutes regardless of the duration of infusion. This lack of drug accumulation following repeated boluses or prolonged infusions differs from other currently available opioids. Extrahepatic hydrolysis also implies the absence of metabolite toxicity in patients with hepatic dysfunction. Patients with pseudocholinesterase deficiency have a normal response to remifentanil.

D. EXCRETION:

The end products of morphine and meperidine biotransformation are eliminated by the kidneys, with less than 10% undergoing biliary excretion. Because 5–10% of morphine is excreted unchanged in the urine, renal failure prolongs its duration of action. The accumulation of morphine metabolites (morphine 3-glucuronide and morphine 6-glucuronide) in patients with renal failure has been associated with narcosis and ventilatory depression lasting several days. In fact, morphine-6-glucuronide is a more potent and longer-lasting opioid agonist than is morphine. Similarly, renal dysfunction increases the chance of toxic effects from normeperidine accumulation. Normeperidine has an excitatory effect on the central nervous system, leading to myoclonic activity and seizures that are not reversed by naloxone. A late secondary peak in fentanyl plasma lev-

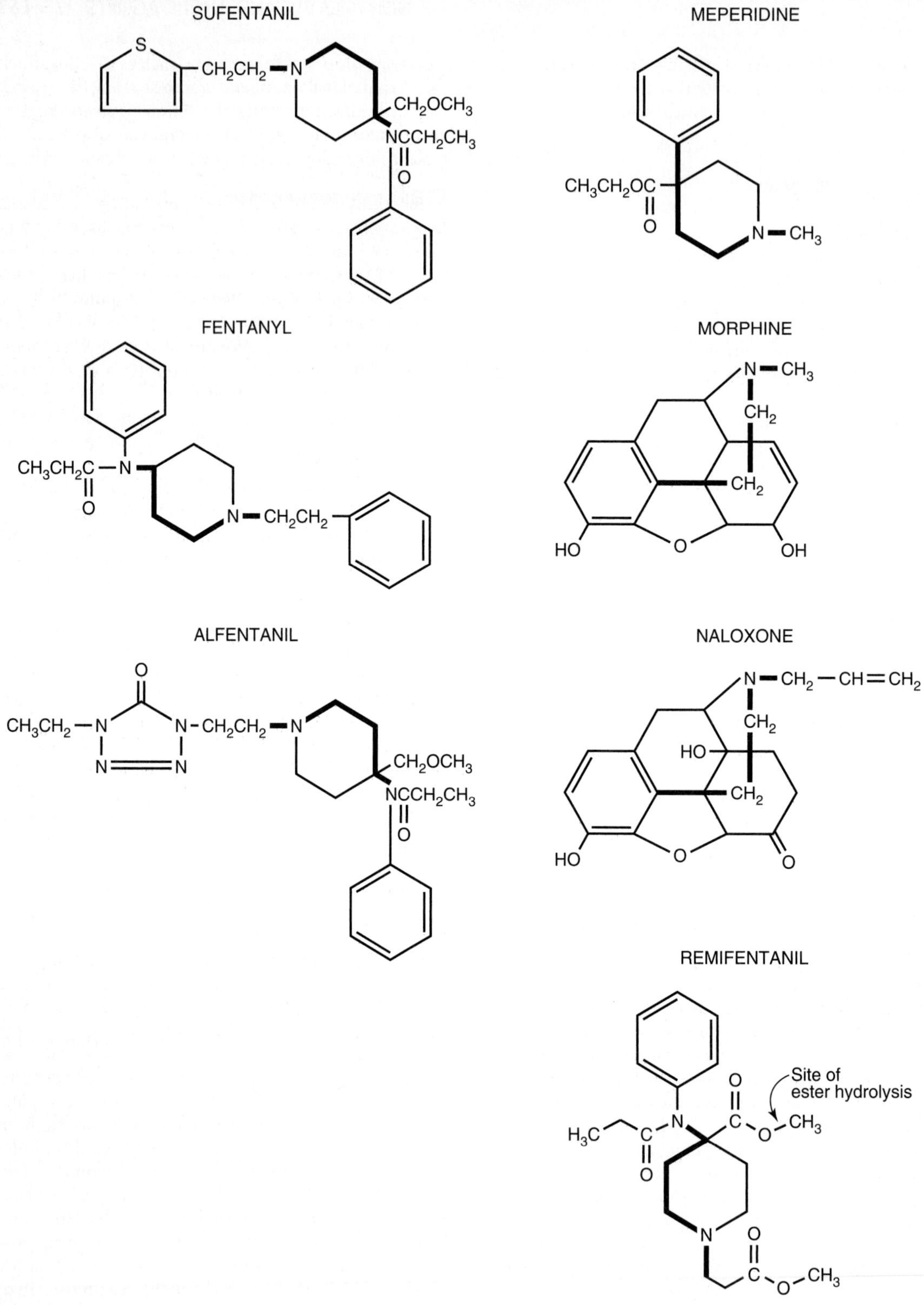

Figure 8-6. Opioid agonists and antagonists share part of their chemical structure, which is outlined in bold.

Table 8–5. Physical characteristics of opioids that determine distribution.

Agent	Nonionized Fraction	Protein Binding	Lipid Solubility
Morphine	++	++	+
Meperidine	+	+++	++
Fentanyl	+	+++	++++
Sufentanil	++	++++	++++
Alfentanil	++++	++++	+++
Remifentanil	+++	+++	++

+ = very low.
++ = low.
+++ = high.
++++ = very high.

els occurs up to 4 hours after the last intravenous dose and may be explained by enterohepatic recirculation or mobilization of sequestered drug. Metabolites of sufentanil are excreted in urine and bile. The main metabolite of remifentanil is eliminated renally but is several thousand times less potent than its parent compound, and thus is unlikely to produce any noticeable opioid effects. Even severe liver disease does not affect the pharmacokinetics or pharmacodynamics of remifentanil.

Effects on Organ Systems

A. CARDIOVASCULAR:

In general, opioids do not seriously impair cardiovascular function. Meperidine tends to increase heart rate (it is structurally similar to atropine), while high doses of morphine, fentanyl, sufentanil, remifentanil, and alfentanil are associated with a vagus-mediated bradycardia. With the exception of meperidine, the opioids do not depress cardiac contractility. Nonetheless, arterial blood pressure often falls as a result of bradycardia, venodilation, and decreased sympathetic reflexes, sometimes requiring vasopressor (eg, ephedrine) support. Furthermore, meperidine and morphine evoke histamine release in some individuals that can lead to profound drops in arterial blood pressure and systemic vascular resistance. The effects of histamine release can be minimized in susceptible patients by slow opioid infusion, adequate intravascular volume, or pretreatment with H_1 and H_2 histamine antagonists (see Chapter 15).

Intraoperative hypertension during opioid anesthesia, particularly morphine and meperidine, is not uncommon. It is often attributable to inadequate anesthetic depth and can be controlled with the addition of

vasodilators or volatile anesthetic agents. The combination of opioids with other anesthetic drugs (eg, nitrous oxide, benzodiazepines, barbiturates, volatile agents) can result in significant myocardial depression.

B. RESPIRATORY:

Opioids depress ventilation, particularly respiratory rate. Resting $PaCO_2$ increases and the response to a CO_2 challenge is blunted, resulting in a shift of the CO_2 response curve downward and to the right (Figure 8–8). These effects are mediated through the respiratory centers in the brainstem. The **apneic threshold**—the highest $PaCO_2$ at which a patient remains apneic—is elevated, and **hypoxic drive** is decreased. Gender differences may exist in these effects, with women demonstrating more respiratory depression. Morphine and meperidine can cause histamine-induced bron-

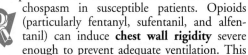 chospasm in susceptible patients. Opioids (particularly fentanyl, sufentanil, and alfentanil) can induce **chest wall rigidity** severe enough to prevent adequate ventilation. This centrally mediated muscle contraction is most frequent after large drug boluses and is effectively treated with muscle relaxants. Opioids can effectively blunt the bronchoconstrictive response to airway stimulation such as that occurring during intubation.

C. CEREBRAL:

The effects of opioids on cerebral perfusion and intracranial pressure appear to be variable. In general, opioids reduce cerebral oxygen consumption, cerebral

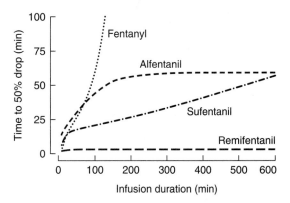

Figure 8–7. In contrast to other opioids, the time necessary to achieve a 50% decrease in remifentanil plasma concentration (its **context-sensitive half-time**) is very short and not influenced by the duration of the infusion. (Reproduced, with permission, from Egan TD: The pharmacokinetics of the new short-acting opioid remifentanil [GI87084B] in healthy adult male volunteers. Anesthesiology 1993;79:881.)

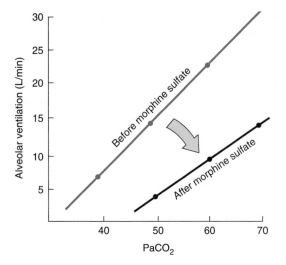

Figure 8–8. Opioids depress ventilation. This is graphically displayed by a shift of the CO_2 curve downward and to the right.

blood flow, and intracranial pressure, but to a much lesser extent than do barbiturates or benzodiazepines. These effects presume a maintenance of normocarbia by artificial ventilation; however, there are some reports of mild—and usually transient—increases in cerebral artery blood flow velocity and intracranial pressure following opioid boluses in patients with brain tumors or head trauma. Because opioids also tend to produce a mild decrease in mean arterial pressure, the resulting fall in CPP may be significant in some patients with abnormal intracranial compliance. Any small rise in intracranial pressure that opioids may cause must be compared with the potentially large increases in intracranial pressure during intubation in an inadequately anesthetized patient. The effect of most opioids on the EEG is minimal, although high doses are associated with slow delta-wave activity. High doses of fentanyl may rarely cause seizure activity; however, some cases may actually be severe opioid-induced muscle rigidity. EEG activation has been attributed to meperidine.

Stimulation of the medullary chemoreceptor trigger zone is responsible for a high incidence of nausea and vomiting. Physical dependence is a significant problem associated with repeated opioid administration. Unlike the barbiturates or benzodiazepines, relatively large doses of opioids are required to render patients unconscious (Table 8–6). Regardless of the dose, however, opioids do not reliably produce amnesia. Intravenous opioids have been the mainstay of pain control for more than a century. The relatively recent use of opi-

oids in epidural and subdural spaces has revolutionized pain management (see Chapter 18).

Unique among opioids, meperidine and structurally similar sameridine have local anesthetic qualities when administered into the subarachnoid space. Meperidine's clinical use has been limited by classic opioid side effects (nausea, sedation, and pruritus), which may not be as pronounced with sameridine. Intravenous meperidine (25 mg) has been found to be the

Table 8–6. Uses and doses of common opioids.

Agent	Use	Route	Dose*
Morphine	Premedication	IM	0.05–0.2 mg/kg
	Intraoperative anesthesia	IV	0.1–1 mg/kg
	Postoperative analgesia	IM	0.05–0.2 mg/kg
		IV	0.03–0.15 mg/kg
Meperidine	Premedication	IM	0.5–1 mg/kg
	Intraoperative anesthesia	IV	2.5–5 mg/kg
	Postoperative analgesia	IM	0.5–1 mg/kg
		IV	0.2–0.5 mg/kg
Fentanyl	Intraoperative anesthesia	IV	2–150 μg/kg
	Postoperative analgesia	IV	0.5–1.5 μg/kg
Sufentanil	Intraoperative anesthesia	IV	0.25–30 μg/kg
Alfentanil	Intraoperative anesthesia		
	Loading dose	IV	8–100 μg/kg
	Maintenance infusion	IV	0.5–3 μg/kg/min
Remifentanil	Intraoperative anesthesia		
	Loading dose	IV	1.0 μg/kg
	Maintenance infusion	IV	0.5–20 μg/kg/min
	Postoperative analgesia/ sedation	IV	0.05–0.3 μg/kg/min

IM = intramuscular; IV = intravenous.
***Note:** The wide range of opioid doses reflects a large therapeutic index and depends upon which other anesthetics are simultaneously administered. For obese patients, dose should be based on ideal body weight or lean body mass, not total body weight. Tolerance can develop rapidly (ie, within 2 hours) during IV infusion of opioids, necessitating higher infusion rates. Dose correlates with other variables besides body weight that need to be considered (eg, age). The relative potencies of fentanyl, sufentanil, and alfentanil are estimated to be 1:9:1/7.

most effective opioid for decreasing shivering (see Chapter 6).

D. GASTROINTESTINAL:

Opioids slow gastric emptying time by reducing peristalsis. Biliary colic may result from opioid-induced contraction of the sphincter of Oddi. Biliary spasm, which can mimic a common bile-duct stone on cholangiography, is effectively reversed with the pure opioid antagonist naloxone. Patients receiving long-term opioid therapy (for cancer pain, for example) usually become tolerant to most of the side effects, except constipation because of the decreased gastrointestinal motility.

E. ENDOCRINE:

The stress response to surgical stimulation is measured in terms of the secretion of specific hormones, including catecholamines, antidiuretic hormone, and cortisol. Opioids block the release of these hormones more completely than do volatile anesthetics. This is particularly true of the more potent opioids such as fentanyl, sufentanil, alfentanil, and remifentanil. Patients with ischemic heart disease may especially benefit from attenuation of the stress response.

Drug Interactions

The combination of opioids—particularly meperidine—and monoamine oxidase inhibitors may result in respiratory arrest, hypertension or hypotension, coma, and hyperpyrexia. The cause of this dramatic interaction is not understood.

Barbiturates, benzodiazepines, and other central nervous system depressants can have synergistic cardiovascular, respiratory, and sedative effects with opioids.

The biotransformation of alfentanil, but not sufentanil, may be impaired following a 7-day course of erythromycin, leading to prolonged sedation and respiratory depression.

KETAMINE

Mechanisms of Action

Ketamine has multiple effects throughout the central nervous system, including blocking polysynaptic reflexes in the spinal cord and inhibiting excitatory neurotransmitter effects in selected areas of the brain. In contrast to the depression of the reticular activating system induced by the barbiturates, ketamine functionally "dissociates" the thalamus (which relays sensory impulses from the reticular activating system to the cerebral cortex) from the limbic cortex (which is involved with the awareness of sensation). While some brain neurons are inhibited, others are tonically excited. Clinically, this state of **dissociative anesthesia** causes the

patient to appear conscious (eg, eye opening, swallowing, muscle contracture) but unable to process or respond to sensory input. Ketamine has been demonstrated to be an N-methyl-D-aspartate receptor (a subtype of the glutamate receptor) antagonist. The existence of specific ketamine receptors and interactions with opioid receptors has been postulated.

Structure-Activity Relationships

Ketamine (Figure 8–9) is a structural analogue of phencyclidine. It is one-tenth as potent, yet retains many of phencyclidine's psychotomimetic effects. Even subtherapeutic doses of ketamine can cause hallucinogenic effects. The increased anesthetic potency and decreased psychotomimetic side effects of one isomer (S+ versus R–) implies the existence of stereospecific receptors.

Pharmacokinetics

A. ABSORPTION:

Ketamine is administered intravenously or intramuscularly (Table 8–7). Peak plasma levels are usually achieved within 10–15 minutes after intramuscular injection.

B. DISTRIBUTION:

Ketamine is more lipid-soluble and less protein-bound than thiopental; it is equally ionized at physiologic pH. These characteristics, along with a ketamine-induced increase in cerebral blood flow and cardiac output, lead

Table 8–7. Uses and doses of ketamine, etomidate, propofol, and droperidol.

Agent	Use	Route	Dose
Ketamine	Induction	IV	1–2 mg/kg
		IM	3–5 mg/kg
Etomidate	Induction	IV	0.2–0.5 mg/kg
Propofol	Induction	IV	1–2.5 mg/kg
	Maintenance infusion	IV	50–200 µg/kg/min
	Sedation infusion	IV	25–100 µg/kg/min
Droperidol	Premedication	IM	0.04–0.07 mg/kg
	Sedation	IV	0.02–0.07 mg/kg
	Antiemetic	IV	0.05 mg/kg*

IV = intravenous; IM = intramuscular.
*Maximum adult dose without prolonging emergence is 1.25–2.5 mg.

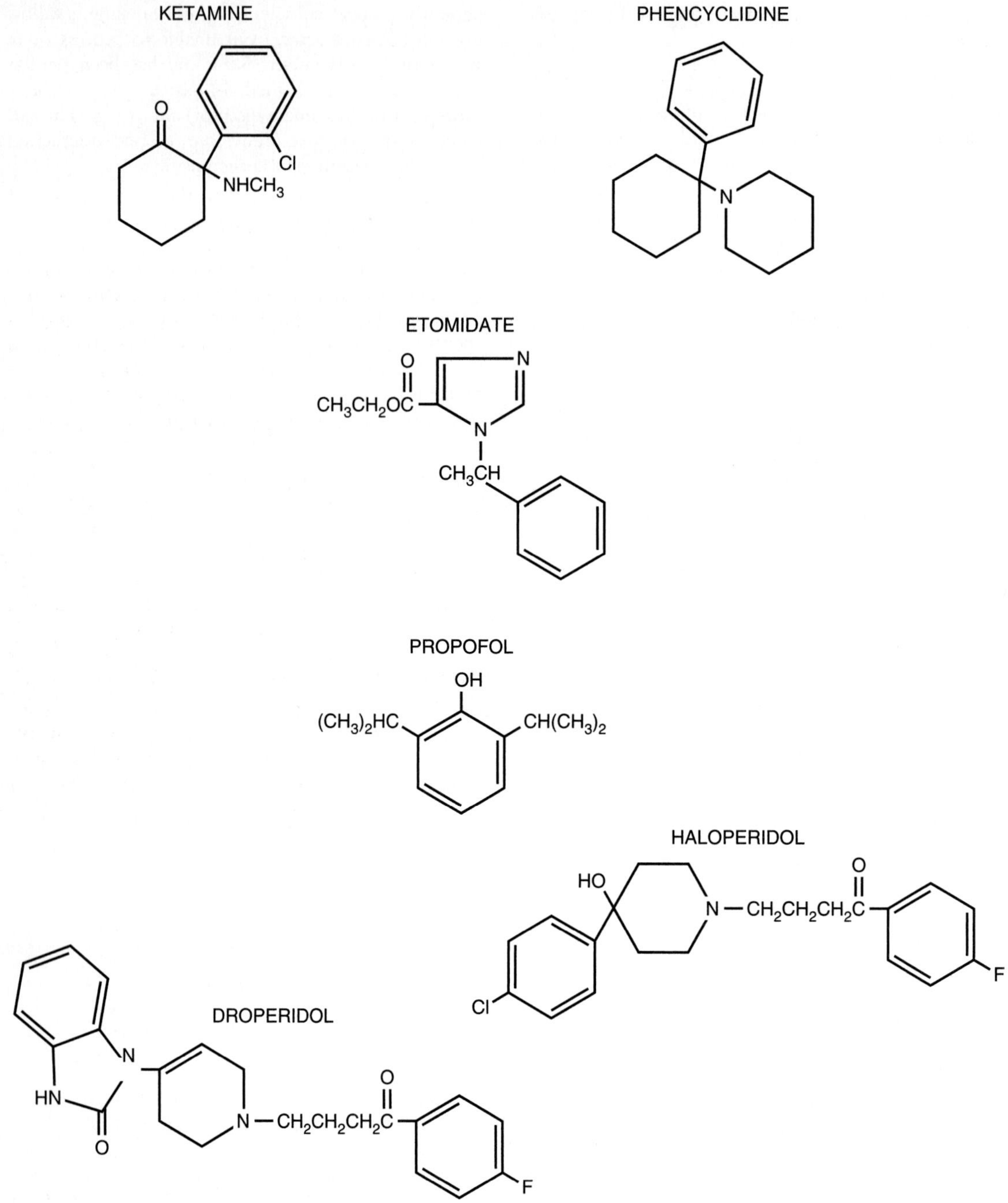

Figure 8–9. The structures of ketamine, etomidate, propofol, and droperidol. Note the similarities between ketamine and phencyclidine and between droperidol and haloperidol.

to rapid brain uptake and subsequent redistribution (distribution half-life is 10–15 minutes). Once again, awakening is due to redistribution to peripheral compartments.

C. BIOTRANSFORMATION:

Ketamine is biotransformed in the liver to several metabolites, some of which (eg, norketamine) retain anesthetic activity. Induction of hepatic enzymes may partially explain the development of tolerance in patients who receive multiple doses of ketamine. Extensive hepatic uptake (hepatic extraction ratio of 0.9) explains ketamine's relatively short elimination half-life (2 hours).

D. EXCRETION:

End products of biotransformation are excreted renally.

Effects on Organ Systems

A. CARDIOVASCULAR:

 In sharp contrast to other anesthetic agents, ketamine increases arterial blood pressure, heart rate, and cardiac output (Table 8–8). These indirect cardiovascular effects are due to central stimulation of the sympathetic nervous system and inhibition of the reuptake of norepinephrine. Accompanying these changes are increases in pulmonary artery pressure and myocardial work. For these reasons, ketamine should be avoided in patients with coronary artery disease, uncontrolled hypertension, congestive heart failure, and arterial aneurysms. The direct myocardial depressant effects of large doses of ketamine, probably due to inhibition of calcium transients, are unmasked by sympathetic blockade (eg, spinal cord

Table 8–8. Summary of nonvolatile anesthetic effects on organ systems.

Agent	Cardiovascular		Respiratory		Cerebral		
	HR	MAP	Vent	B'dil	CBF	CMRO$_2$	ICP
Barbiturates							
Thiopental	↑↑	↓↓	↓↓↓	↓	↓↓↓	↓↓↓	↓↓↓
Thiamylal	↑↑	↓↓	↓↓↓	↓	↓↓↓	↓↓↓	↓↓↓
Methohexital	↑↑	↓↓	↓↓↓	0	↓↓↓	↓↓↓	↓↓↓
Benzodiazepines							
Diazepam	0/↑	↓	↓↓	0	↓↓	↓↓	↓↓
Lorazepam	0/↑	↓	↓↓	0	↓↓	↓↓	↓↓
Midazolam	↑	↓↓	↓↓	0	↓↓	↓↓	↓↓
Opioids							
Meperidine*	↑	*	↓↓↓	*	↓	↓	↓
Morphine*	↓	*	↓↓↓	*	↓	↓	↓
Fentanyl	↓↓	↓	↓↓↓	0	↓	↓	↓
Sufentanil	↓↓	↓	↓↓↓	0	↓	↓	↓
Alfentanil	↓↓	↓↓	↓↓↓	0	↓	↓	↓
Remifentanil	↓↓	↓↓	↓↓↓	0	↓	↓	↓
Ketamine	↑↑	↑↑	↓	↑↑↑	↑↑↑	↑	↑↑↑
Etomidate	0	↓	↓	0	↓↓↓	↓↓↓	↓↓↓
Propofol	0	↓↓↓	↓↓↓	0	↓↓↓	↓↓↓	↓↓↓
Droperidol	↑	↓↓	0	0	↓	0	↓

*The effects of meperidine and morphine on MAP and bronchodilation depend upon the extent of histamine release.
HR = heart rate; MAP = mean arterial pressure; Vent = ventilatory drive; B'dil = bronchodilation; CBF = cerebral blood flow; CMRO$_2$ = cerebral oxygen consumption; ICP = intracranial pressure.
0 = no effect.
0/↑ = no change or mild increase.
↓ = decrease (mild, moderate, marked).
↑ = increase (mild, moderate, marked).

transection) or exhaustion of catecholamine stores (eg, severe end-stage shock). On the other hand, ketamine's indirect stimulatory effects are often beneficial to patients with acute hypovolemic shock.

B. RESPIRATORY:

Ventilatory drive is minimally affected by the customary induction doses of ketamine, although rapid intravenous bolus administration or pretreatment with opioids occasionally produces apnea. Ketamine is a potent bronchodilator, making it a good induction agent for asthmatic patients. Although upper airway reflexes remain largely intact, patients at increased risk for aspiration pneumonia should be intubated (see Case Discussion, Chapter 15). The increased salivation associated with ketamine can be attenuated by premedication with an anticholinergic agent.

C. CEREBRAL:

Consistent with its cardiovascular effects, ketamine increases cerebral oxygen consumption, cerebral blood flow, and intracranial pressure. These effects preclude its use in patients with space-occupying intracranial lesions. Myoclonic activity is associated with increased subcortical electrical activity, which is not apparent on surface EEG. Undesirable psychotomimetic side effects (eg, illusions, disturbing dreams, and delirium) during emergence and recovery are less common in children and in patients premedicated with benzodiazepines. Of the nonvolatile agents, ketamine may be the closest to being a "complete" anesthetic since it induces analgesia, amnesia, and unconsciousness.

Drug Interactions

Nondepolarizing muscle relaxants are potentiated by ketamine (see Chapter 9). The combination of theophylline and ketamine may predispose patients to seizures. Diazepam attenuates ketamine's cardiostimulatory effects and prolongs its elimination half-life. Propranolol, phenoxybenzamine, and other sympathetic antagonists unmask the direct myocardial depressant effects of ketamine. Ketamine produces myocardial depression when given to patients anesthetized with halothane or, to a lesser extent, other volatile anesthetics. Lithium may prolong the duration of action of ketamine.

ETOMIDATE

Mechanisms of Action

Etomidate depresses the reticular activating system and mimics the inhibitory effects of GABA. Specifically, etomidate (particularly the R(+) isomer) appears to bind to a subunit of the GABA type A receptor, increasing its affinity for GABA. Unlike barbiturates, it may have disinhibitory effects on the parts of the nervous system that control extrapyramidal motor activity. This disinhibition is responsible for a 30–60% incidence of myoclonus.

Structure-Activity Relationships

Etomidate, which contains a carboxylated imidazole, is structurally unrelated to other anesthetic agents (see Figure 8–9). The imidazole ring provides water solubility in acidic solutions and lipid solubility at physiologic pH. Etomidate is dissolved in propylene glycol. This solution often causes pain on injection that can be lessened by a prior injection of lidocaine.

Pharmacokinetics

A. ABSORPTION:

Etomidate is available only for intravenous administration and is used chiefly for induction of general anesthesia (see Table 8–7).

B. DISTRIBUTION:

Despite being highly protein-bound, etomidate is characterized by a very rapid onset of action owing to its high lipid solubility and large nonionized fraction at physiologic pH. Redistribution is responsible for decreasing the plasma concentration to awakening levels.

C. BIOTRANSFORMATION:

Hepatic microsomal enzymes and plasma esterases rapidly hydrolyze etomidate to an inactive metabolite. The rate of biotransformation is five times greater for etomidate than for thiopental.

D. EXCRETION:

The end product of hydrolysis is primarily excreted in the urine.

Effects on Organ Systems

A. CARDIOVASCULAR:

Etomidate has minimal effects on the cardiovascular system. A mild reduction in peripheral vascular resistance is responsible for a slight decline in arterial blood pressure. Myocardial contractility and cardiac output are usually unchanged. Etomidate does not release histamine.

B. RESPIRATORY:

Ventilation is affected less with etomidate than with barbiturates or benzodiazepines. Even induction doses usually do not result in apnea unless opioids have also been administered.

C. CEREBRAL:

Etomidate decreases the cerebral metabolic rate, cerebral blood flow, and intracranial pressure to the same extent as does thiopental. Because of minimal cardiovascular effects, CPP is well maintained. Although changes on EEG resemble those associated with barbiturates, etomidate enhances somatosensory evoked potentials. Postoperative nausea and vomiting are more common than following barbiturate induction, but can be minimized by antiemetic medications. Etomidate is a sedative-hypnotic but lacks analgesic properties.

D. ENDOCRINE:

 Induction doses of etomidate transiently inhibit enzymes involved in cortisol and aldosterone synthesis. Long-term infusions lead to **adrenocortical suppression** that may be associated with an increased mortality rate in critically ill patients.

Drug Interactions

Fentanyl increases the plasma level and prolongs the elimination half-life of etomidate.

Opioids decrease the myoclonus characteristic of an etomidate induction.

PROPOFOL

Mechanisms of Action

The mechanism by which propofol induces a state of general anesthesia may involve facilitation of inhibitory neurotransmission mediated by GABA.

Structure-Activity Relationships

Propofol (2,6-diisopropylphenol) consists of a phenol ring with two isopropyl groups attached (Figure 8–9). Altering the side-chain length of this alkylphenol influences potency, induction, and recovery characteristics. Propofol is not water-soluble, but a 1% aqueous solution (10 mg/mL) is available for intravenous administration as an oil-in-water emulsion containing soybean oil, glycerol, and egg lecithin. A history of egg allergy does not necessarily contraindicate the use of propofol because most egg allergies involve a reaction to egg white (egg albumin), while egg lecithin is extracted from egg yolk. This formulation can cause pain during injection (less common in elderly patients) that can be lessened by prior injection of lidocaine or mixing the lidocaine with propofol prior to injection (2 mL of 1% lidocaine in 18 mL propofol). Other formulations of propofol (eg, 1% propofol in 16% polyoxyethylated castor oil) may lessen injection discomfort. More im-

 portant, since propofol formulations can support the growth of bacteria, good sterile technique must be observed in preparation and handling, including cleaning the rubber stopper or ampule neck surface with an alcohol swab prior to opening it. Administration should be completed within 6 hours of opening the ampule. Sepsis and death have been linked to contaminated propofol preparations. Current formulations of propofol contain 0.005% disodium edetate or 0.025% sodium metabisulfite to help retard the rate of growth of microorganisms; however, these are still not antimicrobially preserved products under United States Pharmacopeia standards.

Pharmacokinetics

A. ABSORPTION:

Propofol is available only for intravenous administration for the induction of general anesthesia (see Table 8–7).

B. DISTRIBUTION:

The high lipid solubility of propofol results in an onset of action that is almost as rapid as that of thiopental (one-arm-to-brain circulation time). Awakening from a single bolus dose is also rapid owing to a very short initial distribution half-life (2–8 minutes). Most investigators feel that recovery from propofol is more rapid and accompanied by less hangover than recovery from methohexital, thiopental, or etomidate. This makes it a good agent for outpatient anesthesia. A lower induction dose is recommended in elderly patients because of their smaller V_d. Women may require a higher dose of propofol than men and appear to awaken faster.

C. BIOTRANSFORMATION:

The clearance of propofol exceeds hepatic blood flow, implicating the existence of extrahepatic metabolism. This exceptionally high clearance rate (10 times that of thiopental) probably contributes to relatively rapid recovery after a continuous infusion. Conjugation in the liver results in inactive metabolites that are eliminated by renal clearance. The pharmacokinetics of propofol do not appear to be affected by moderate cirrhosis. Use of propofol infusion for long-term sedation of children undergoing intensive care has been associated with cases of lipemia, metabolic acidosis, and death.

D. EXCRETION:

Although metabolites of propofol are primarily excreted in the urine, chronic renal failure does not affect clearance of the parent drug.

Effects on Organ Systems

A. CARDIOVASCULAR:

The major cardiovascular effect of propofol is a decrease in arterial blood pressure owing to a drop in systemic vascular resistance (inhibition of sympathetic vasoconstrictor activity), cardiac contractility, and preload. Hypotension is more pronounced than with thiopental but is usually reversed by the stimulation accompanying laryngoscopy and intubation. Factors exacerbating the hypotension include large doses, rapid injection, and old age. Propofol markedly impairs the normal arterial baroreflex response to hypotension particularly in conditions of normocarbia or hypocarbia. Rarely, a marked drop in preload may lead to a vagally mediated reflex bradycardia. Changes in heart rate and cardiac output are usually transient and insignificant in healthy patients but may be severe enough to lead to asystole, particularly in patients at the extremes of age, on negative chronotropic medications, or undergoing surgical procedures associated with the oculocardiac reflex (see Chapter 38). Patients with impaired ventricular function may experience a significant drop in cardiac output as a result of decreases in ventricular filling pressures and contractility. Although myocardial oxygen consumption and coronary blood flow decrease to a similar extent, coronary sinus lactate production increases in some patients. This indicates a regional mismatch between myocardial oxygen supply and demand.

B. RESPIRATORY:

Like the barbiturates, propofol is a profound respiratory depressant that usually causes apnea following an induction dose. Even when used for conscious sedation in subanesthetic doses, propofol infusion inhibits hypoxic ventilatory drive and depresses the normal response to hypercarbia. This underscores the necessity that only properly trained personnel use this technique. Propofol-induced depression of upper airway reflexes exceeds that of thiopental and can prove helpful during intubation or laryngeal mask placement in the absence of paralysis. Although propofol can cause histamine release, induction with propofol is accompanied with a lower incidence of wheezing in asthmatic and nonasthmatic patients compared with barbiturates or etomidate and is not contraindicated in asthmatic patients.

C. CEREBRAL:

Propofol decreases cerebral blood flow and intracranial pressure. In patients with elevated intracranial pressure, propofol can cause a critical reduction in CPP (< 50 mm Hg) unless steps are taken to support mean arterial blood pressure. Propofol and thiopental probably provide a similar degree of cerebral protection during focal ischemia. A unique characteristic of propofol is its antipruritic properties. Its antiemetic effects (requiring a blood propofol concentration of 200 ng/mL) make it a preferred drug for outpatient anesthesia. Induction is occasionally accompanied by excitatory phenomena such as muscle twitching, spontaneous movement, opisthotonus, or hiccupping possibly due to subcortical glycine antagonism. Although these reactions may occasionally mimic tonic-clonic seizures, propofol appears to have predominately anticonvulsant properties (ie, burst suppression), has been successfully used to terminate status epilepticus, and may be safely administered to epileptic patients. Propofol decreases intraocular pressure. Tolerance does not develop after long-term propofol infusions.

Drug Interactions

Nondepolarizing muscle relaxants may be potentiated by previous formulations of propofol, which contained Cremophor. Newer formulations do not share this interaction.

Fentanyl and alfentanil concentrations may be increased by concomitant administration of propofol. Some clinicians administer a small amount of midazolam (eg, 30 μg/kg) prior to induction with propofol; they believe the combination produces synergistic effects (eg, faster onset and lower total dose requirements). However, this technique of "coinduction" has questionable efficacy.

DROPERIDOL

Mechanisms of Action

Droperidol antagonizes the activation of dopamine receptors. For example, in the central nervous system, the caudate nucleus and the medullary chemoreceptor trigger zone are affected. Droperidol also interferes with transmission mediated by serotonin, norepinephrine, and GABA. These central actions account for droperidol's tranquilizer and antiemetic properties. Peripheral actions include α-adrenergic blockade (see Chapter 12).

Structure-Activity Relationships

Droperidol, a butyrophenone, is structurally related to haloperidol (see Figure 8–9). Structural differences between the two drugs explain the neuroleptic characteristics of the former and the antipsychotic activity of the latter.

Pharmacokinetics

A. ABSORPTION:

Although droperidol is occasionally administered intramuscularly as part of a premedication regimen, it is usually given intravenously (see Table 8–7).

B. DISTRIBUTION:

Despite a rapid distribution phase ($t_{1/2}$ = 10 minutes), the sedative effects of droperidol are delayed by a relatively high molecular weight and extensive protein binding, which hinder penetration of the blood-brain barrier. A prolonged duration of action (3–24 hours) may be explained by tenacious receptor binding.

C. BIOTRANSFORMATION:

Droperidol is extensively metabolized in the liver, as evidenced by a hepatic clearance as rapid as that of ketamine and etomidate.

D. EXCRETION:

The end products of biotransformation are excreted primarily in the urine.

Effects on Organ Systems

A. CARDIOVASCULAR:

Droperidol's mild α-adrenergic blocking effects decrease arterial blood pressure by peripheral vasodilation. Hypovolemic patients can experience exaggerated blood pressure declines. The α-adrenergic blocking actions may be responsible for an antidysrhythmic effect. Patients with pheochromocytoma should not receive droperidol because it can induce catecholamine release from the adrenal medulla, resulting in severe hypertension.

B. RESPIRATORY:

Droperidol, administered alone and in usual doses, does not significantly depress respiration and may actually stimulate hypoxic ventilatory drive.

C. CEREBRAL:

Droperidol decreases cerebral blood flow and intracranial pressure by inducing cerebral vasoconstriction. However, droperidol does not reduce cerebral oxygen consumption—unlike the barbiturates, benzodiazepines, and etomidate. The EEG is not markedly changed. Droperidol is a potent antiemetic; however, delayed awakening limits its intraoperative use to low doses (0.05 mg/kg, to a maximum of 2.5 mg). The antidopaminergic activity of droperidol rarely precipitates extrapyramidal reactions (eg, oculogyric crises, torticollis, agitation), which can be treated with diphenhydramine. Nonethe-

less, droperidol should be avoided in patients with Parkinson's disease.

Although patients premedicated with droperidol appear placid and sedated, they are often extremely apprehensive and fearful. For this reason, droperidol has fallen into disfavor as a sole premedication. The addition of an opioid decreases the incidence of dysphoria. Droperidol is a tranquilizer, and it does not produce analgesia, amnesia, or unconsciousness at usual doses. The combination of fentanyl and droperidol (Innovar) produces a state characterized by analgesia, immobility, and variable amnesia (classically referred to as **neuroleptanalgesia**). The addition of nitrous oxide or a hypnotic agent leads to unconsciousness and general anesthesia (**neuroleptanesthesia**) similar to the dissociative state induced by ketamine.

Drug Interactions

Droperidol antagonizes the effects of levodopa and may precipitate parkinsonian symptoms. The renal effects of dopamine are countered by droperidol.

Theoretically, droperidol could antagonize the central α-adrenergic action of clonidine and precipitate rebound hypertension.

Droperidol attenuates the cardiovascular effects of ketamine.

CASE DISCUSSION: PREMEDICATION OF THE SURGICAL PATIENT

An extremely anxious 17-year-old woman presents for uterine dilatation and curettage. She demands to be asleep before going to the operating room and does not want to remember anything.

What are the goals of administering preoperative medication?

Anxiety is a normal emotional response to impending surgery. Minimizing anxiety is usually the major goal of preoperative medication. For many patients, the preoperative interview with the anesthesiologist allays fears more effectively than do sedative drugs. Other psychological objectives of preoperative medication include preoperative pain relief and perioperative amnesia.

There may also be specific medical indications for preoperative medication: prophylaxis against aspiration pneumonia (eg, antacids), prevention of allergic reactions (eg, antihistamines), or decreasing upper airway secretions (eg, anticholinergics). The goals of preoperative medication de-

pend on many factors, including the health and emotional status of the patient, the proposed surgical procedure, and the anesthetic plan. For this reason, the choice of anesthetic premedication is not routine and must follow a thorough preoperative evaluation.

What is the difference between sedation and anxiety relief?

This distinction is well illustrated by the paradoxic effects of droperidol. Patients may appear to an observer to be adequately sedated but on questioning may be quite anxious. Anxiety relief can be measured only by the patient.

Do all patients require preoperative medication?

No—customary levels of preoperative anxiety do not harm most patients. Some patients dread intramuscular injections, and others find altered states of consciousness more unpleasant than nervousness. If the surgical procedure is brief, the effects of some sedatives may extend into the postoperative period and prolong recovery time. This is especially troublesome for patients undergoing ambulatory surgery. Specific contraindications for sedative premedication include severe lung disease, hypovolemia, impending airway obstruction, increased intracranial pressure, and depressed baseline mental status. Premedication with sedative drugs should never be given before informed consent has been obtained.

Which patients are most likely to benefit from preoperative medication?

Some patients are quite anxious despite the preoperative interview. Separation of young children from their parents is often a traumatic ordeal, especially if they have endured multiple prior surgeries. Chronic drug abusers may benefit from premedication to lessen the risk of withdrawal reactions. Medical conditions such as coronary artery disease or hypertension may be aggravated by psychological stress.

How does preoperative medication influence the induction of general anesthesia?

Some preoperative medications (eg, opioids) lessen anesthetic requirements and can smooth induction. Intravenous administration of these medications just prior to induction is a more reliable method of achieving the same benefits, however.

What governs the choice between the preoperative medications commonly administered?

After the goals of premedication have been determined, the clinical effects of the agents dictate choice. For instance, in a patient experiencing preoperative pain from a femoral fracture, the analgesic effects of an opioid (eg, morphine, meperidine) will lessen the discomfort associated with transportation to the operating room and positioning on the operating room table. Respiratory depression (drops in oxygen saturation), orthostatic hypotension, and nausea and vomiting make opioid premedication less desirable.

Barbiturates are effective sedatives but lack analgesic properties and can produce respiratory depression. Benzodiazepines relieve anxiety, often provide amnesia, and are relatively free of side effects. Like barbiturates, however, they are not analgesics. Diazepam and lorazepam are available orally. Intramuscular midazolam has a rapid onset (30 minutes) and short duration (90 minutes). Dysphoria, prolonged sedation, and α-adrenergic blockade limit the clinical usefulness of droperidol. Other preoperative medications are discussed in subsequent chapters: anticholinergics in Chapter 11; antihistamines, antiemetics, and antacids in Chapter 15.

Which factors must be considered in selecting the anesthetic premedication for this patient?

First, it must be made clear to the patient that, for safety reasons, anesthesia is not induced outside the operating room. Long-acting agents such as morphine or droperidol would not be a good choice for an outpatient procedure. Lorazepam and diazepam can also affect mental function for several hours. One alternative is to establish an intravenous line in the preoperative holding area and titrate small doses of midazolam, with or without fentanyl, using slurred speech as an end point. At that time, the patient can be taken to the operating room. Vital signs—particularly respiratory rate—must be continuously monitored.

SUGGESTED READING

Bissonnette B, Swan H, Ravussin P, Un V: Neuroleptanesthesia: Current status. Can J Anesth 1999;46:154. This article discusses several intravenous drugs used for conscious sedation.

Cammarano WB, Pittet J, Weitz S: Acute withdrawal syndrome related to the administration of analgesic and sedative medications in adult intensive care unit patients. Crit Care Med 1998;26:676. Symptoms of acute withdrawal are not uncommon in ICU patients receiving prolonged continuous infusions of opioids and benzodiazepines.

Feldman SA, Paton W, Scurr C (editors): *Mechanisms of Drugs in Anaesthesia,* 2nd ed. Oxford University Press, 1993.

Fragen RJ (editor): *Drug Infusions in Anesthesiology* 2nd ed. Lippincott Williams & Wilkins, 1996. The pharmacokinetic and hardware information necessary to fully utilize intravenous drug delivery systems.

Gan TJ, Glass PS, Sigl J: Women emerge from general anesthesia with propofol/alfentanil/nitrous oxide faster than men. Anesthesiology 1999;90:1283. Faster recovery may a higher incidence of intraoperative recall in women.

Miller RD (editor): Lessons learned from a phase IV study of propofol: Analysis of data of over 25,000 patients. Anesth Analg 1993;77(4S):S1. This supplement to Anesthesia and Analgesia provides a glimpse into what kind of research effort is involved in bringing a new drug to market and the subsequent safety follow-up and monitoring.

O'Hare R, McAtamney D, Mirakhur RK, Hughes D, Carabine U: Bolus dose remifentanil for control of haemodynamic response to tracheal intubation during rapid sequence induction of anaesthesia. Br J Anaesth 1999;82:283. This article found that a dose of 1 μg/kg effectively blunted the cardiovascular response to intubation 1 minute later.

Quinlan JJ, Homanics GE, Firestone LL: Anesthesia sensitivity in mice that lack the beta-3 subunit of the gamma aminobutyric acid type A receptor. Anesthesiology 1998;88:775. Mice that lack this subunit appear resistant to the obtunding effects of midazolam and etomidate but not pentobarbital, enflurane, or halothane.

Reich DL, Silvay G: Ketamine: An update on the first twenty-five years of clinical experience. Can J Anaesth 1989;36:186. Evolution of the multiple uses of ketamine.

Smith I, White PF, Nathanson M, Gouldson R: Propofol: An update on its use. Anesthesiology 1994;81:1005.

Stein C: Peripheral mechanisms of opioid analgesia. Anesth Analg 1993;76:182.

Stoelting RK: *Pharmacology and Physiology in Anesthetic Practice,* 3rd ed. Lippincott, 1999.

Neuromuscular Blocking Agents

KEY CONCEPTS

 It is important to realize that muscle relaxation does not ensure unconsciousness, amnesia, or analgesia.

 Depolarizing muscle relaxants act as acetylcholine (ACh) receptor agonists, while nondepolarizing muscle relaxants function as competitive antagonists.

 Because depolarizing muscle relaxants are not metabolized by acetylcholinesterase, they diffuse away from the neuromuscular junction and are hydrolyzed in the plasma and liver by another enzyme, pseudocholinesterase (nonspecific cholinesterase, plasma cholinesterase).

 With the exception of mivacurium, nondepolarizing agents are not significantly metabolized by either acetylcholinesterase or pseudocholinesterase. Reversal of their blockade depends on redistribution, gradual metabolism and excretion of the relaxant by the body, or administration of specific reversal agents (eg, cholinesterase inhibitors) that inhibit acetylcholinesterase enzyme activity.

 Muscle relaxants owe their paralytic properties to mimicry of ACh. For example, succinylcholine consists of two joined ACh molecules.

 Compared with patients with low enzyme levels or heterozygous atypical enzyme in whom blockade duration is doubled or tripled, patients with homozygous atypical enzyme will have a very long blockade (eg, 6–8 hours) following succinylcholine administration.

 Succinylcholine is considered contraindicated in the routine management of children and adolescents because of the risk of rhabdomyolysis, hyperkalemia, and cardiac arrest in children with undiagnosed myopathies.

 Normal muscle releases enough potassium during succinylcholine-induced depolarization to raise serum potassium by 0.5 mEq/L. While this is usually insignificant in patients with normal baseline potassium levels, a life-threatening potassium elevation is possible in patients with burn injury, massive trauma, neurologic disorders, and several other conditions.

 Tubocurarine, doxacurium, pancuronium, vecuronium, and pipecuronium are partially excreted by the kidneys, and their action is prolonged in patients with renal failure. Renal failure decreases clearance of rapacuronium, but does not affect its duration of action.

 Rapacuronium would clearly be the best choice of nondepolarizing muscle relaxant for rapid-sequence inductions because of its rapid onset of action, minimal cardiovascular side effects even at large doses, and short duration of action. However, at the time of publication, it was no longer available, having been withdrawn by the manufacturer.

 Cirrhotic liver disease and chronic renal failure often result in an increased volume of distribution and a lower plasma concentration for a given dose of water-soluble drugs, such as muscle relaxants. On the other hand, drugs dependent on hepatic or renal excretion may demonstrate prolonged clearance. Thus, depending on the drug, a greater initial dose—but smaller maintenance doses—might be required in these diseases.

(continued)

(continued)

 Atracurium and cisatracurium undergo degradation in plasma at physiologic pH and temperature by organ independent Hofmann elimination. The resulting metabolites (a monoquaternary acrylate and laudanosine) have no intrinsic neuromuscular blocking effects.

 Mivacurium, like succinylcholine, is metabolized by pseudocholinesterase. It is only minimally metabolized by true cholinesterase.

 Hypertension and tachycardia may occur in patients given pancuronium. These cardiovascular effects are caused by the combination of vagal blockade and catecholamine release from adrenergic nerve endings.

 Long-term administration of vecuronium to patients in intensive care units has resulted in pro- *longed neuromuscular blockade (up to several days), possibly from accumulation of its 3-hydroxy metabolite, changing drug clearance, or the development of a polyneuropathy.*

 Rocuronium (0.9–1.2 mg/kg) has an onset of action similar to but slightly longer than succinylcholine (60–90 seconds), making it suitable for rapid-sequence inductions, but at the cost of a much longer duration of action.

 Rapacuronium appears to be the least potent nondepolarizing muscle relaxant, supporting the apparent inverse relationship between potency and onset of action (less potent drugs require a higher dose, resulting in increased drug delivery to the neuromuscular junction and shorter onset time).

Skeletal muscle relaxation can be produced by deep inhalational anesthesia, regional nerve block, or neuromuscular junction blocking agents (commonly called *muscle relaxants*). In 1942, Harold Griffith published the results of a study using a refined extract of curare (a South American arrow poison) during anesthesia. Muscle relaxants rapidly became a routine part of the anesthesiologist's drug arsenal. As Griffith noted, it is important to realize that neuromuscular junction blocking agents produce paralysis, not anesthesia. In other words, muscle relaxation does not ensure unconsciousness, amnesia, or analgesia. This chapter reviews the principles of neuromuscular transmission and presents the mechanisms of action, physical structures, routes of elimination, recommended dosages, and side effects of several muscle relaxants.

■ NEUROMUSCULAR TRANSMISSION

The region of approximation between a motor neuron and a muscle cell is the **neuromuscular junction** (Figure 9–1). The cell membranes of the neuron and muscle fiber are separated by a narrow (20-nm) gap, the **synaptic cleft.** As a nerve's action potential depolarizes its terminal, an influx of calcium ions into the nerve cytoplasm allows **storage vesicles** to fuse with the **terminal membrane** and release their contents of acetylcholine (ACh). The ACh molecules diffuse across the synaptic cleft to bind with **nicotinic cholinergic receptors** on a specialized portion of the muscle membrane, the **motor end-plate.**

Each ACh receptor consists of five protein subunits, two of which (α subunits) are identical and capable of binding ACh molecules. If both binding sites are occupied by ACh, a conformational change in the subunits briefly (1 msec) opens an ion channel in the core of the receptor (Figure 9–2).

Cations flow through the open channel (sodium and calcium in; potassium out), generating an **end-plate potential.** The contents of a single vesicle, a quantum of ACh (10^4 molecules per quantum), produce a **miniature end-plate potential.** If enough receptors are occupied by ACh, the end-plate potential will be sufficiently strong to depolarize the perijunctional membrane. Sodium channels within this portion of the muscle membrane open when a voltage is developed across them, as opposed to end-plate receptors that open when ACh is applied. The resulting **action potential** propagates along the muscle membrane and T-tubule system, opening sodium channels and releasing calcium from the sarcoplasmic reticulum. This intracellular calcium allows the contractile proteins actin and myosin to interact, bringing about muscle contraction. The amount of ACh usually released and the number of re-

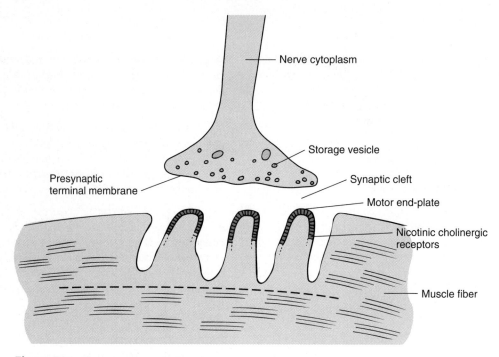

Figure 9-1. The neuromuscular junction.

ceptors subsequently activated far exceed the minimum required for the initiation of an action potential. This normal margin of safety is overwhelmed in Eaton-Lambert myasthenic syndrome (decreased release of ACh) and myasthenia gravis (decreased number of receptors).

ACh is rapidly hydrolyzed into acetate and choline by the substrate-specific enzyme acetylcholinesterase. This enzyme (also called **specific cholinesterase** or **true cholinesterase**) is embedded into the motor endplate membrane immediately adjacent to the ACh re-

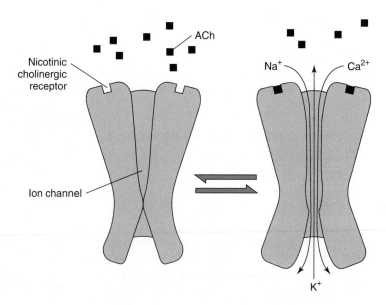

Figure 9-2. Binding of ACh to receptors on muscle end-plate causes channel opening and ion flux.

ceptors. Eventually, the receptors' ion channels close, causing the end-plate to repolarize. When action potential generation ceases, the sodium channels in the muscle membrane also close. Calcium is resequestered in the sarcoplasmic reticulum, and the muscle cell relaxes.

■ DISTINCTIONS BETWEEN DEPOLARIZING & NONDEPOLARIZING BLOCKADE

Neuromuscular blocking agents are divided into two classes: depolarizing and nondepolarizing (Table 9–1). This division reflects distinct differences in the mechanism of action, response to peripheral nerve stimulation, and reversal of block.

MECHANISM OF ACTION

Depolarizing muscle relaxants physically resemble ACh and therefore bind to ACh receptors, generating a muscle action potential. Unlike ACh, however, these drugs are *not* metabolized by acetylcholinesterase, and their concentration in the synaptic cleft does not fall as rapidly, resulting in a prolonged depolarization of the muscle end-plate.

Continuous end-plate depolarization causes muscle relaxation in the following way. As has been explained, an end-plate potential of sufficient strength will result in generation of an action potential in the neighboring perijunctional muscle membrane. The subsequent opening of perijunctional sodium channels is time-limited, however. After initial excitation and opening, these channels close. Furthermore, these sodium channels cannot reopen until the end-plate repolarizes, which is not possible as long as a depolarizer continues to bind to ACh receptors. Once the perijunctional channels close, the action potential disappears and the membrane downstream returns to its resting state, resulting in muscle relaxation. This is a **phase I block.**

Nondepolarizing muscle relaxants also bind to ACh receptors but are incapable of inducing the conformational change necessary for ion channel opening. Since ACh is prevented from binding to its receptors, no end-plate potential develops.

Thus, depolarizing muscle relaxants act as ACh receptor agonists, while nondepolarizing muscle relaxants function as competitive antagonists. This basic difference in mechanism of action explains their varying effects in certain disease states. For example, conditions associated with a chronic decrease in ACh release (eg, muscle denervation injuries) stimulate a compensatory increase in the number of ACh receptors within muscle membranes. This **up-regulation** causes an exaggerated response to depolarizing muscle relaxants (with more receptors being depolarized), but a resistance to nondepolarizing relaxants (more receptors that must be blocked). In contrast, conditions associated with fewer ACh receptors (eg, **down-regulation** in myasthenia gravis) demonstrate a resistance to depolarizing relaxants and an increased sensitivity to nondepolarizing relaxants.

RESPONSE TO PERIPHERAL NERVE STIMULATION

The use of peripheral nerve stimulators to monitor neuromuscular function is discussed in Chapter 6. Four patterns of electrical stimulation with supramaximal square-wave pulses are considered:

Tetany: A sustained stimulus of 50–100 Hz, usually lasting 5 seconds.

Twitch: A single pulse 0.2 msec in duration.

Train-of-four: A series of four twitches in 2 seconds (2-Hz frequency), each 0.2 msec long.

Double-burst stimulation: Three short (0.2 msec) high-frequency stimulations separated by a 20-msec interval (50 Hz) and followed 750 msec later by two ($DBS_{3,2}$) or three ($DBS_{3,3}$) additional impulses (see Figure 6–35).

The occurrence of **fade,** a gradual diminution of evoked response during prolonged or repeated nerve stimulation, is indicative of a nondepolarizing block (Table 9–2). Fade may be due to a prejunctional effect

Table 9–1. Depolarizing and nondepolarizing muscle relaxants.

Depolarizing	Nondepolarizing
Short-acting	Long-acting
Succinylcholine	Tubocurarine
Decamethonium	Metocurine
	Doxacurium
	Pancuronium
	Pipecuronium
	Gallamine
	Intermediate-acting
	Atracurium
	Cisatracurium
	Vecuronium
	Rocuronium
	Short-acting
	Mivacurium
	Rapacuronium

Table 9–2. Evoked responses during depolarizing (phase I and phase II) and nondepolarizing block.

Evoked Stimulus	Depolarizing Block		Nondepolarizing block
	Phase I	Phase II	
Train-of-four	Constant but diminished	Fade	Fade
Tetany	Constant but diminished	Fade	Fade
Double-burst stimulation (DBS$_{3,2}$)	Constant but diminished	Fade	Fade
Posttetanic potentiation	Absent	Present	Present

of nondepolarizing relaxants that reduces the amount of ACh in the nerve terminal available for release during stimulation (blockade of ACh mobilization). Adequate clinical recovery correlates well with the absence of fade. Because fade is more obvious during sustained tetanic stimulation or double-burst stimulation than following a train-of-four pattern or repeated twitches, the first two patterns are the preferred methods for determining adequacy of recovery from a nondepolarizing block.

The ability of tetanic stimulation during a partial nondepolarizing block to increase the evoked response to a subsequent twitch is termed **posttetanic potentiation.** This phenomenon may relate to a compensatory increase in ACh mobilization following tetanic stimulation.

In contrast, a phase I depolarization block does not exhibit fade during tetanus or train-of-four; neither does it demonstrate posttetanic potentiation. If enough depolarizer is administered, however, the quality of the block changes to resemble a nondepolarizing block.

This so-called **phase II block** appears to be caused by ionic and conformational changes that accompany prolonged muscle membrane depolarization.

REVERSAL OF BLOCK

Because depolarizing muscle relaxants are not metabolized by acetylcholinesterase, they diffuse away from the neuromuscular junction and are hydrolyzed in the plasma and liver by another enzyme, **pseudocholinesterase** (nonspecific cholinesterase, plasma cholinesterase). Fortunately, this is a fairly rapid process, since no specific agent to reverse a depolarizing blockade is available.

With the exception of mivacurium, nondepolarizing agents are not significantly metabolized by either acetylcholinesterase or pseudocholinesterase. Reversal of their blockade depends on redistribution, gradual metabolism and excretion of the relaxant by the body, or administration of specific reversal agents (eg, cholinesterase inhibitors) that inhibit acetylcholinesterase enzyme activity (see Chapter 10). Because this inhibition increases the amount of ACh available at the neuromuscular junction to compete with the nondepolarizing agents, clearly, the reversal agents are of no benefit in reversing a depolarizing block. In fact, by increasing neuromuscular junction ACh concentration and inhibiting pseudocholinesterase, *cholinesterase inhibitors prolong depolarization blockade.*

■ DEPOLARIZING MUSCLE RELAXANTS

SUCCINYLCHOLINE

The only depolarizing muscle relaxant in general use today is **succinylcholine.**

Physical Structure

Muscle relaxants owe their paralytic properties to mimicry of ACh. For example, all are quaternary ammonium compounds. In fact, succinylcholine—also called suxamethonium and diacetylcholine—consists of two joined ACh molecules (Figure 9–3). This copycat structure is responsible for succinylcholine's mechanism of action, side effects, and metabolism.

Metabolism & Excretion

The continued popularity of succinylcholine is due to its rapid onset of action (30–60 seconds) and short duration of action (typically less than 10 minutes). Its rapid onset of action is largely due to its low lipid solubility (all muscle relaxants are highly charged and water-soluble) and the relative overdose that is usually administered.

As succinylcholine enters the circulation, most of it is rapidly metabolized by pseudocholinesterase into succinylmonocholine. This process is so efficient that only a fraction of the injected dose ever reaches the neuromuscular junction. As drug serum levels fall, succinylcholine molecules diffuse away from the neuromuscular junction, limiting the duration of action.

The duration of action is prolonged by high doses or by abnormal metabolism. The latter may result from hypothermia, low enzyme levels, or a genetically aberrant enzyme. Hypothermia decreases the rate of hydrolysis. Low levels of pseudocholinesterase (measured as units per liter) accompany pregnancy, liver disease, renal failure, and certain drug therapies (Table 9–3).

One in 50 patients has one normal and one abnormal gene, resulting in a slightly prolonged block (20–30 minutes). Even fewer (1 in 3000) patients have two abnormal genes (homozygous atypical) that produce an enzyme with 1/100 the normal affinity for suc-

cinylcholine. In contrast to the doubling or tripling of blockade duration seen in patients with low enzyme levels or heterozygous atypical enzyme, patients with homozygous atypical enzyme will have a *very* long blockade (eg, 6–8 hours) following succinylcholine administration. Of the recognized abnormal genes, the dibucaine variant is the most common.

Dibucaine, a local anesthetic, inhibits normal pseudocholinesterase activity by 80% but inhibits the homozygous atypical enzyme by only 20%. The heterozygous enzyme is characterized by an intermediate 40–60% inhibition. The percentage of inhibition of pseudocholinesterase activity is termed the **dibucaine number.** The dibucaine number is proportional to pseudocholinesterase function and independent of the amount of enzyme. Therefore, adequacy of pseudocholinesterase can be determined in the laboratory quantitatively in units per liter (a minor factor) and qualitatively by dibucaine number (the major factor). Prolonged paralysis from succinylcholine caused by **abnormal pseudocholinesterase (atypical cholinesterase)** should be treated with continued mechanical ventilation until muscle function returns to normal. A heat-treated preparation of human plasma cholinesterase is available in some countries—but not the United States. Although fresh plasma could be used, its infectious risks clearly outweigh its potential benefit.

Drug Interactions

The effects of muscle relaxants can be modified by concurrent drug therapy (Table 9–4). Succinylcholine is involved in two interactions deserving special comment.

A. CHOLINESTERASE INHIBITORS:

Although cholinesterase inhibitors reverse nondepolarizing paralysis, they markedly prolong a depolarizing phase I block by two mechanisms: By inhibiting acetylcholinesterase, they lead to a higher ACh concentration at the nerve terminal, which intensifies depolarization. They also reduce the hydrolysis of succinylcholine by inhibiting pseudocholinesterase. Organophosphate pesticides, for example, cause an irreversible inhibition of acetylcholinesterase and can prolong the action of succinylcholine by 20–30 minutes.

B. NONDEPOLARIZING RELAXANTS:

In general, small doses of nondepolarizing relaxants antagonize a depolarizing phase I block. Because the drugs

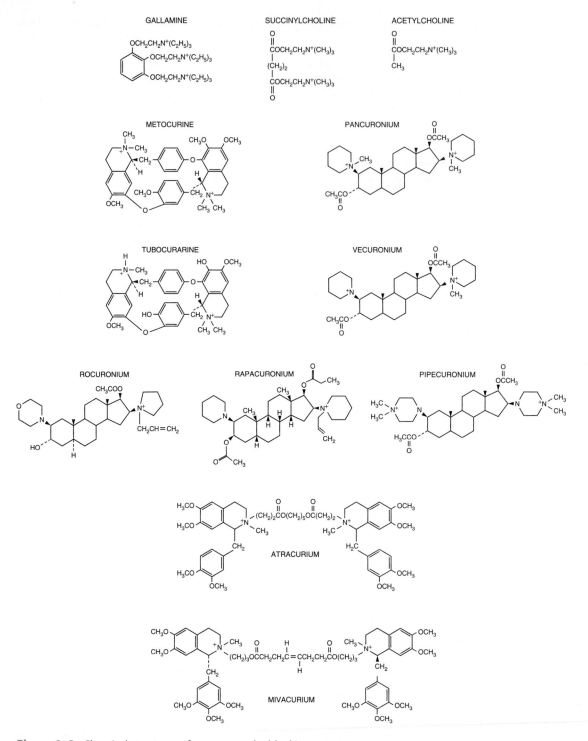

Figure 9–3. Chemical structures of neuromuscular blocking agents.

Table 9–3. Drugs causing quantitative decreases in pseudocholinesterases.

Drug	Description
Echothiophate	Irreversible cholinesterase inhibitor used for treatment of glaucoma
Neostigmine, pyridostigmine	Reversible cholinesterase inhibitors
Hexafluorenium	A seldom used nondepolarizer
Phenelzine	A monoamine oxidase inhibitor
Cyclophosphamide, mechlorethamine	Antineoplastic agents
Trimethaphan	An antihypertensive

occupy some ACh receptors, depolarization by succinylcholine is partially prevented. An exception to this interaction is pancuronium, which augments succinylcholine blockade by inhibiting pseudocholinesterase. If enough depolarizing agent is administered to

develop a phase II block, a nondepolarizer will potentiate paralysis. Similarly, an intubating dose of succinylcholine reduces nondepolarizer requirements for at least 30 minutes.

Dosage

Because of its rapid onset, short duration, and low cost, many clinicians feel that succinylcholine is still a good choice for routine intubation in adults, particularly since the withdrawal of rapacuronium. The adult dose of succinylcholine for intubation is usually 1–1.5 mg/kg intravenously. Repeated small boluses (10 mg) or a succinylcholine drip (1 g in 500 or 1000 mL, titrated to effect) are used during some surgical procedures that require brief but intense paralysis (eg, otolaryngologic endoscopies). Methylene blue indicator dye is often added to succinylcholine drips to prevent confusion with other intravenous fluids. In addition, neuromuscular function should be constantly monitored with a nerve stimulator to prevent overdosing and the development of phase II block. The availability of short-acting nondepolarizing muscle relaxants (eg, mi-

Table 9–4. Potentiation (+) and resistance (–) of neuromuscular blocking agents by other drugs.

Drug	Effect on Depolarizing Blockade	Effect on Nondepolarizing Blockade	Comments
Antibiotics	+	+	Streptomycins, colistin, polymyxin, tetracycline, lincomycin, clindamycin, bacitracin
Anticonvulsants	?	–	Phenytoin, carbamazepine, primidone, sodium valproate
Antidysrhythmics	+	+	Quinidine, lidocaine, calcium channel blockers, procainamide
Antihypertensives	+	+	Trimethaphan, nitroglycerin (only affects pancuronium)
Cholinesterase inhibitors	+	–	Neostigmine, pyridostigmine, edrophonium
Dantrolene	?	+	Used in treatment of malignant hyperthermia (has quaternary ammonium group)
Furosemide <10 μg/kg 1–4 mg/kg	 + –	 + –	Biphasic effect depending on dose
Inhalational anesthetics	+	+	See text
Ketamine	?	+	
Local anesthetics	+	+	
Lithium carbonate	+	?	Prolongs onset and duration of succinylcholine; one case reported of prolonged block with nondepolarizer
Magnesium sulfate	+	+	Used to treat preeclampsia and eclampsia of pregnancy

vacurium and perhaps rapacuronium) has reduced the popularity of this technique.

Since succinylcholine is not lipid-soluble, its distribution is limited to the extracellular space. Per kilogram, infants and neonates have a larger extracellular space than do adults. Therefore, pediatric dosage requirements are often greater than for adults. If succinylcholine is administered *intramuscularly* to children, a dose as high as 4–5 mg/kg does not always produce complete paralysis.

Side Effects & Clinical Considerations

Succinylcholine is a relatively safe drug—assuming that its many potential complications are understood and avoided. Because of the risk of rhabdomyolysis, hyperkalemia, and cardiac arrest in children with undiagnosed myopathies, however, succinylcholine is considered contraindicated in the routine management of children and adolescent patients.

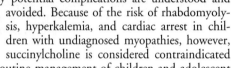

A. CARDIOVASCULAR:

Because of the resemblance of muscle relaxants to ACh, it is not surprising that they affect cholinergic receptors in addition to those at the neuromuscular junction. The entire parasympathetic nervous system and parts of the sympathetic nervous system (sympathetic ganglions, adrenal medulla, and sweat glands) depend on ACh as a neurotransmitter.

Succinylcholine not only stimulates nicotinic cholinergic receptors at the neuromuscular junction, it stimulates all ACh receptors. Stimulation of nicotinic receptors in parasympathetic and sympathetic ganglia and muscarinic receptors in the sinoatrial node of the heart can increase or decrease blood pressure and heart rate.

A succinylcholine metabolite, succinylmonocholine, excites cholinergic receptors in the sinoatrial node, resulting in bradycardia. Although children are particularly susceptible, bradycardia is commonly seen in adults if a second dose of succinylcholine is administered. Intravenous atropine (0.02 mg/kg in children, 0.4 mg in adults) is often given prophylactically in children and *always* before a second dose of succinylcholine. Other arrhythmias such as nodal bradycardia and ventricular ectopy have been reported.

B. FASCICULATIONS:

The onset of paralysis by succinylcholine is usually signaled by visible motor unit contractions called **fasciculations.** These can be prevented by pretreatment with a small dose of nondepolarizing relaxant. Since this pretreatment usually antagonizes a depolarizing block, a higher dose of succinylcholine is subsequently required (1.5 mg/kg).

C. HYPERKALEMIA:

Normal muscle releases enough potassium during succinylcholine-induced depolarization to raise serum potassium by 0.5 mEq/L. While this is usually insignificant in patients with normal baseline potassium levels, a life-threatening potassium elevation is possible in patients with burn injury, massive trauma, neurologic disorders, and several other conditions (Table 9–5). Subsequent cardiac arrest can prove to be quite refractory to routine cardiopulmonary resuscitation, requiring calcium, insulin, glucose, bicarbonate, cation-exchange resin, dantrolene, and even cardiopulmonary bypass to reduce metabolic acidosis and serum potassium levels. In denervation injuries, ACh receptors develop outside the neuromuscular junction (up-regulation). These extrajunctional receptors allow succinylcholine to effect widespread depolarization and extensive potassium release. Life-threatening potassium release is *not* reliably prevented by pretreatment with a nondepolarizer. The risk of hyperkalemia usually appears to peak in 7–10 days following the injury, but the exact time of onset and the duration of the risk period vary.

D. MUSCLE PAINS:

Patients who have received succinylcholine have an increased incidence of postoperative myalgia. This complaint is most common in healthy female outpatients. Pregnancy and extremes of age seem to be protective. The efficacy of nondepolarizing pretreatment is controversial.

E. INTRAGASTRIC PRESSURE ELEVATION:

Abdominal wall muscle fasciculations increase intragastric pressure, which is offset by an increase in lower

Table 9–5. Conditions causing susceptibility to succinylcholine-induced hyperkalemia.

Burn injury
Massive trauma
Severe intra-abdominal infection
Spinal cord injury
Encephalitis
Stroke
Guillain-Barré syndrome
Severe Parkinson's disease
Tetanus
Prolonged total body immobilization
Ruptured cerebral aneurysm
Polyneuropathy
Closed head injury
Near drowning
Hemorrhagic shock with metabolic acidosis
Myopathies (eg, Duchenne's dystrophy)

esophageal sphincter tone. Therefore, the risk of gastric reflux or pulmonary aspiration is probably not increased by succinylcholine. Although pretreatment with nondepolarizers abolishes the rise in gastric pressure, it also prevents the increase in lower esophageal sphincter tone.

F. INTRAOCULAR PRESSURE ELEVATION:

Extraocular muscle differs from other striated muscle in that it has multiple motor end-plates on each cell. Prolonged membrane depolarization and contraction of extraocular muscles following succinylcholine administration raises intraocular pressure and could compromise an injured eye (see Case Discussion, Chapter 38). The intraocular pressure elevation is not always prevented by nondepolarizer pretreatment.

G. MALIGNANT HYPERTHERMIA:

Succinylcholine is a potent triggering agent in patients susceptible to malignant hyperthermia, a hypermetabolic disorder of skeletal muscle. Paradoxic contraction of jaw musculature following succinylcholine administration is often a premonitory sign of malignant hyperthermia and has been associated with a mutation of the adult skeletal muscle sodium channel alpha-subunit gene (see Case Discussion, Chapter 44). Although the signs and symptoms of neuroleptic malignant syndrome (NMS) resemble those of malignant hyperthermia, the pathogenesis completely differs and there is no need to avoid succinylcholine in patients with NMS.

H. GENERALIZED CONTRACTIONS:

Patients afflicted with myotonia may develop myoclonus after succinylcholine administration.

I. PROLONGED PARALYSIS:

As discussed above, patients with low levels of normal pseudocholinesterase may have a longer than normal duration of action, while patients with atypical pseudocholinesterase will experience markedly prolonged paralysis. This is a dangerous complication if ventilation is not adequately maintained.

J. INTRACRANIAL PRESSURE:

Succinylcholine may lead to an activation of the electroencephalogram and slight increases in cerebral blood flow and intracranial pressure in some patients. Muscle fasciculations stimulate muscle stretch receptors, which subsequently increase cerebral activity. The increase in intracranial pressure can be attenuated by maintaining good airway control and instituting hyperventilation. It can be prevented by pretreating with a nondepolarizing muscle relaxant and administering intravenous lidocaine (1.5–2.0 mg/kg) 2–3 minutes prior to intubation.

The effects of intubation on intracranial pressure far outweigh any increase caused by succinylcholine.

■ NONDEPOLARIZING MUSCLE RELAXANTS

Unique Pharmacologic Characteristics

In contrast to depolarizing muscle relaxants, there is a wide selection of nondepolarizers (Table 9–6). Choice of a particular drug depends on its unique characteristics, which are often related to its structure. For example, steroidal compounds tend to be vagolytic, while benzyl isoquinolines tend to release histamine. Because of structural similarities, an allergic history to one muscle relaxant highly suggests the possibility of allergic reactions to other muscle relaxants.

A. AUTONOMIC SIDE EFFECTS:

In clinical doses, the nondepolarizers significantly differ in their effects on nicotinic and muscarinic cholinergic receptors. Tubocurarine and, to a lesser extent, metocurine block autonomic ganglia. This compromises the sympathetic nervous system's ability to increase heart contractility and rate in response to hypotension and other intraoperative stresses. In contrast, pancuronium and gallamine block vagal muscarinic receptors in the sinoatrial node, resulting in tachycardia. Gallamine's potent vagolytic effect has severely limited its clinical usefulness. Atracurium, cisatracurium, mivacurium, doxacurium, vecuronium, pipecuronium, and rapacuronium are devoid of significant autonomic effects in their recommended dosage ranges.

B. HISTAMINE RELEASE:

Histamine release from mast cells can result in bronchospasm, skin flushing, and hypotension from peripheral vasodilation. Nondepolarizers capable of triggering histamine release are tubocurarine > metocurine > atracurium and mivacurium. Slow injection rates and H_1 and H_2 antihistamine pretreatment ameliorate these side effects.

C. HEPATIC CLEARANCE:

Only pancuronium, vecuronium, and rapacuronium are metabolized to any significant degree by the liver. Vecuronium and rocuronium depend heavily on biliary excretion. Clinically, liver failure prolongs pancuronium and rocuronium blockade, with less effect on vecuronium, and no effect on pipecuronium or rapacuronium. Atracurium and mivacurium, while extensively metabolized, depend on extrahepatic mechanisms. Nonetheless, although severe liver disease does not sig-

Table 9–6. A summary of the pharmacology of nondepolarizing muscle relaxants.

Relaxant	Metabolism	Primary Excretion	Onset	Duration	Histamine Release	Vagal Blockade	Relative Potency[1]	Relative Cost[2]
Tubocurarine	Insignificant	Renal	++	+++	+++	0	1	Low
Metocurine	Insignificant	Renal	++	+++	++	0	2	Moderate
Atracurium	+++	Insignificant	++	++	+	0	1	High
Cisatracurium	+++	Insignificant	++	++	0	0	5	High
Mivacurium	+++	Insignificant	++	+	+	0	2.5	Moderate
Doxacurium	Insignificant	Renal	+	+++	0	0	12	High
Pancuronium	+	Renal	++	+++	0	++	5	Low
Pipecuronium	+	Renal	++	+++	0	0	6	High
Vecuronium	+	Biliary	++	++	0	0	5	High
Rocuronium	Insignificant	Biliary	+++	++	0	+	1	High
Rapacuronium	+	Renal	+++	+	+	0	0.3	High

[1]For example, pancuronium and vecuronium are five times more potent than tubocurarine or atracurium.
[2]Based on average wholesale price per 10 mL; does not necessarily reflect duration and potency.
[3]Rapacuronium not available at time of publication (see text).
Onset: + = slow; ++ = moderately rapid; +++ = rapid.
Duration: + = short; ++ = intermediate; +++ = long.
Histamine release: 0 = no effect; + = slight effect; ++ = moderate effect; +++ marked effect.
Vagal blockade: 0 = no effect; + = slight effect; ++ = moderate effect.

nificantly affect atracurium clearance, an associated decrease in pseudocholinesterase levels may slow mivacurium metabolism.

D. RENAL EXCRETION:

Metocurine and gallamine are almost entirely dependent on renal excretion, and their use in renal failure is therefore ill-advised. Since these agents are ionized, however, they can be removed by dialysis. Tubocurarine, doxacurium, pancuronium, vecuronium, and pipecuronium are partially excreted by the kidneys, and their action is prolonged in patients with renal failure. Renal failure decreases clearance of rapacuronium, but does not affect its duration of action. The elimination of atracurium, mivacurium, and rocuronium is independent of kidney function.

E. SUITABILITY FOR INTUBATION:

Only rapacuronium can equal succinylcholine's rapid onset of action; however, the onset of nondepolarizing relaxants can be quickened by using either a larger dose or a priming dose. Although a larger intubating dose speeds onset, it exacerbates side effects and prolongs blockade. For example, a dose of 0.15 mg/kg of pancuronium may produce intubating conditions in 90 seconds, but at the cost of more pronounced hypertension and tachycardia—and a block that may be irreversible for more than 45 minutes. The consequence of a long duration of action is the ensuing difficulty to completely reverse the blockade and a subsequent in-

creased incidence of postoperative pulmonary complications, especially in elderly patients and those undergoing abdominal surgery. The introduction of short- and intermediate-acting agents has resulted in the greater use of **priming doses.** Theoretically, giving 10–15% of the usual intubating dose 5 minutes before induction will occupy enough receptors so that paralysis will quickly follow when the balance of relaxant is administered. A priming dose does not usually lead to clinically significant paralysis because that requires that 75–80% of the receptors be blocked (a neuromuscular **margin of safety**). In some patients, however, the priming dose occupies enough receptors to produce dyspnea or dysphagia. In the former situation, the patient should be reassured and induction of anesthesia should proceed without delay. Priming can cause significant decreases in respiratory function (eg, forced vital capacity) and may lead to oxygen desaturation in patients with marginal pulmonary reserve. These negative side effects are more common in elderly patients. Use of a priming dose, however, has produced conditions suitable for intubation within 60 seconds following rocuronium or 90 seconds following other intermediate-acting nondepolarizers. Rapacuronium would clearly be the best choice of nondepolarizing muscle relaxant for rapid-sequence inductions because of its rapid onset of action, minimal cardiovascular side effects even at large doses, and short duration of action. However, at the time of publication, it was no longer available after being withdrawn by the manufacturer (see below).

It is important to keep in mind that muscle groups vary in their sensitivity to muscle relaxants (see Chapter 6 and Muscle Groups below). For example, the laryngeal muscles—whose relaxation is important during intubation—are quicker to recover from blockade than the adductor pollicis, which is commonly monitored by the peripheral nerve stimulator.

F. SUITABILITY FOR PREVENTING FASCICULATIONS:

To prevent fasciculation, 10–15% of a nondepolarizer intubating dose can be administered 5 minutes before succinylcholine. While most nondepolarizers have been successfully used for this purpose, tubocurarine and rocuronium appear to be particularly efficacious (**precurarization**). Because of the antagonism between most nondepolarizers and a phase I block, the subsequent dose of succinylcholine should be raised to 1.5 mg/kg.

G. POTENTIATION BY INHALATIONAL ANESTHETICS:

Volatile agents decrease nondepolarizer dosage requirements by at least 15%. The actual degree of this postsynaptic augmentation depends on both the inhalational anesthetic (desflurane > sevoflurane > isoflurane and enflurane > halothane > N_2O/O_2/narcotic) and the muscle relaxant employed (tubocurarine and pancuronium > vecuronium and atracurium).

H. POTENTIATION BY OTHER NONDEPOLARIZERS:

Some combinations of nondepolarizers (eg, tubocurarine and pancuronium; mivacurium and pancuronium) produce a greater than additive neuromuscular blockade. Some of these combinations have the added advantage of offsetting side effects, such as the attenuation of tubocurarine's hypotensive effect by pancuronium. The lack of augmentation by closely related compounds (eg, vecuronium and pancuronium) lends credence to the theory that potentiation results from slightly differing mechanisms of action.

General Pharmacologic Characteristics

Some variables affect all nondepolarizing muscle relaxants.

A. TEMPERATURE:

Hypothermia prolongs blockade by decreasing metabolism (eg, mivacurium, atracurium) and delaying excretion (eg, tubocurarine, metocurine, pancuronium).

B. ACID-BASE BALANCE:

Respiratory acidosis potentiates the blockade of most nondepolarizing relaxants and antagonizes its reversal. This could prevent complete neuromuscular recovery in a hypoventilating postoperative patient. Conflicting findings regarding the neuromuscular effects of other acid-base changes may be due to coexisting alterations

in extracellular pH, intracellular pH, electrolyte concentrations, or structural differences between drugs (eg, monoquaternary versus bisquaternary; steroidal versus isoquinolinium).

C. ELECTROLYTE ABNORMALITIES:

Hypokalemia and hypocalcemia augment a nondepolarizing block. The response of a patient with hypercalcemia is unpredictable. Hypermagnesemia, as may be seen in preeclamptic patients being managed with magnesium sulfate, potentiates a nondepolarizing blockade by competing with calcium at the motor end-plate.

D. AGE:

Neonates have an increased sensitivity to nondepolarizing relaxants because of their immature neuromuscular junctions. This sensitivity does not necessarily decrease dosage requirements, since the neonate's greater extracellular space provides a larger volume of distribution.

E. DRUG INTERACTIONS:

As noted earlier, many drugs augment nondepolarizing blockade (see Table 9–4). They have multiple sites of interaction: prejunctional structures, postjunctional cholinergic receptors, and muscle membranes.

F. CONCURRENT DISEASE:

The presence of neurologic or muscular disease can have profound effects on an individual's response to muscle relaxants (Table 9–7). Cirrhotic liver disease and chronic renal failure often result in an increased volume of distribution and a lower plasma concentration for a given dose of water-soluble drugs, such as muscle relaxants. On the other hand, drugs dependent on hepatic or renal excretion may demonstrate prolonged clearance. Thus, depending on the drug chosen, a greater initial (loading) dose—but smaller maintenance doses—might be required in these diseases.

G. MUSCLE GROUPS:

The onset and intensity of blockade vary among muscle groups. This may be due to differences in blood flow, distance from the central circulation, or different fiber types. Furthermore, the relative sensitivity of a muscle group may depend on the choice of muscle relaxant. In general, the diaphragm, laryngeal muscles, and orbicularis oculi respond to and recover from muscle relaxation sooner than the thumb. While they are a fortuitous safety feature, persistent diaphragmatic contractions can be disconcerting in the face of complete adductor pollicis paralysis. Glottic musculature is also quite resistant to blockade, as is often confirmed during laryngoscopy.

Considering the multitude of factors influencing the duration and magnitude of muscle relaxation, it be-

Table 9–7. Diseases with altered responses to muscle relaxants.

Disease	Response to Depolarizers	Response to Nondepolarizers
Amyotrophic lateral sclerosis	Contracture	Hypersensitivity
Autoimmune disorders (systemic lupus erythematosus, polymyositis, dermatomyositis)	Hypersensitivity	Hypersensitivity
Burn injury	Hyperkalemia	Resistance
Cerebral palsy	Slight hypersensitivity	Resistance
Familial periodic paralysis (hyperkalemic)	Myotonia and hyperkalemia	Hypersensitivity?
Guillain-Barré syndrome	Hyperkalemia	Hypersensitivity
Hemiplegia	Hyperkalemia	Resistance on affected side
Muscular denervation (peripheral nerve injury)	Hyperkalemia and contracture	Normal response or resistance
Muscular dystrophy (Duchenne type)	Hyperkalemia and malignant hyperthemia	Hypersensitivity
Myasthenia gravis	Resistance and proneness to phase II block	Hypersensitivity
Myasthenic syndrome	Hypersensitivity	Hypersensitivity
Myotonia (dystrophica, congenita, paramyotonia)	Generalized muscular contractions	Normal or hypersensitivity
Severe chronic infection (tetanus, botulism)	Hyperkalemia	Resistance

comes clear that an individual's response to neuromuscular blocking agents should be monitored. Dosage recommendations, including those in this chapter, should be considered guidelines that require modification for individual patients.

TUBOCURARINE

Physical Structure

Tubocurarine (*d*-tubocurarine) is a monoquaternary compound with a tertiary amine group (Figure 9–3). The quaternary ammonium group mimics ACh and is responsible for receptor binding, while the cumbersome ring structure prevents receptor activation.

Metabolism & Excretion

Tubocurarine is not metabolized to a significant extent. Elimination is primarily renal (50% of the injected dose in the first 24 hours) and secondarily biliary (10%). Renal failure prolongs its duration of action.

Dosage

For intubation, 0.5–0.6 mg/kg of tubocurarine is administered slowly over 3 minutes. Intraoperative relaxation is achieved with a dose of 0.15 mg/kg initially, followed by incremental doses of 0.05 mg/kg. The average 70-kg patient usually receives a 9-mg loading dose followed by 3-mg increments every 20–30 minutes.

Initial dosage requirements are not usually less in children, although subsequent doses may be less frequently required. Neonates can display a marked variation in response.

Tubocurarine is packaged as 3 mg/mL and does not require refrigeration.

Side Effects & Clinical Considerations

A. Hypotension and Tachycardia:

These cardiovascular effects are primarily related to histamine release. Tubocurarine's ability to block autonomic ganglia is of secondary importance.

B. BRONCHOSPASM:

This also is related to increased histamine levels, and tubocurarine is best avoided in asthmatics.

METOCURINE

Physical Structure

Metocurine is a bisquaternary derivative of tubocurarine and is also known as dimethyl tubocurarine. Tubocurarine and metocurine share many pharmacologic properties and side effects because their structures are so closely related.

Metabolism & Excretion

Like tubocurarine, metocurine is not metabolized and is primarily excreted by the kidneys (50% in the first 24 hours). The duration of action of metocurine is prolonged in patients with renal failure because of decreased clearance. Biliary excretion plays a minor role (< 5%).

Dosage

Conditions suitable for intubation are achieved by administering 0.3 mg/kg over 1–2 minutes to minimize side effects. Intraoperative relaxation is provided by 0.08 mg/kg initially, followed by incremental doses of 0.03 mg/kg.

Dosage considerations are similar to those described for tubocurarine in pediatric patients. Regardless of age, metocurine is twice as potent as tubocurarine.

Metocurine is packaged in 20-mL vials containing 2 mg/mL and does not require refrigeration.

Side Effects & Clinical Considerations

In equipotent doses, metocurine releases half as much histamine as does tubocurarine. Nonetheless, if large doses are administered, side effects include hypotension and tachycardia, bronchospasm, and allergic reactions. Patients allergic to iodine (eg, those with fish allergies) may be hypersensitive to metocurine preparations since they too contain iodide.

ATRACURIUM

Physical Structure

Like all muscle relaxants, atracurium has a quaternary group; however, a benzyl isoquinoline structure is responsible for its unique method of degradation.

Metabolism & Excretion

Atracurium is so extensively metabolized that its pharmacokinetics are independent of renal and hepatic function, and less than 10% is excreted unchanged by renal and biliary routes. Two separate processes are responsible for metabolism.

A. ESTER HYDROLYSIS:

This action is catalyzed by nonspecific esterases, not by acetylcholinesterase or pseudocholinesterase.

B. HOFMANN ELIMINATION:

A spontaneous nonenzymatic chemical breakdown occurs at physiologic pH and temperature.

Dosage

A dose of 0.5 mg/kg is administered intravenously over 30–60 seconds for intubation. Intraoperative relaxation is achieved with 0.25 mg/kg initially, then in incremental doses of 0.1 mg/kg every 10–20 minutes. An infusion of 5–10 μg/kg/min can effectively replace intermittent boluses.

Although dosage requirements do not significantly vary with age, atracurium may be shorter-acting in children and infants than in adults.

Atracurium is available as a solution of 10 mg/mL. It must be stored at 2–8 °C, since it loses 5–10% of its potency for each month it is exposed to room temperature.

Side Effects & Clinical Considerations

Atracurium triggers the release of histamine to a lesser extent than does either tubocurarine or metocurine.

A. HYPOTENSION AND TACHYCARDIA:

Cardiovascular side effects are unusual unless doses in excess of 0.5 mg/kg are administered. Atracurium may also cause a transient drop in systemic vascular resistance and an increase in cardiac index independent of any histamine release. A slow rate of injection minimizes these effects.

B. BRONCHOSPASM:

Atracurium should be avoided in asthmatic patients. Nonetheless, severe bronchospasm is possible even in patients without a history of asthma.

C. LAUDANOSINE TOXICITY:

Laudanosine is a breakdown product of atracurium's Hofmann elimination and has been associated with central nervous system excitation, resulting in elevation of the minimum alveolar concentration and even precipitation of seizures. These are probably irrelevant considerations unless a patient has received an extremely high total dose or has hepatic failure (laudanosine is metabolized by the liver).

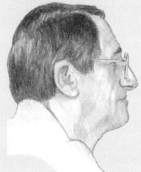

John J. Savarese, MD

A CURRENT PRACTICE OF RELAXATION

Amid much recent debate about the high cost of medical care, there has been a modest amount of discussion concerning economy in the practice of anesthesia. Some of these ideas, which focus on the cost of relaxation, have advocated a return to practice patterns of 25 years ago, when the standard relaxant drugs were succinylcholine and pancuronium, now the least expensive relaxants on the market. It is unfortunate that some practitioners have gone back to this pattern in a misguided attempt to save a few dollars. In fact, when the cost of relaxation is viewed carefully and completely, this modification of practice actually involves added expense and a great deal of added risk , as well as revealing ignorance of current advances in technology and thinking.

In case anyone still believes strongly in practicing with succinycholine and pancuronium, I say emphatically: "Give it up!" The new relaxants, in the long run, save money and decrease risk, as well as increase patient satisfaction. Economy of practice involves all of the above, not simply the bean counting of adding up drug acquisition cost and dosage over time. Here are a few relatively recent comparisons that provide hard data strongly suggesting that any apparent acquisition cost savings accrued by the succinylcholine/pancuronium practice pattern are largely overbalanced by various added and easily identified expenses related to the use of older long-acting relaxants.

Ballantyne compared recovery room costs in a carefully balanced study of patients who had received either pancuronium or an intermediate-duration relaxant (atracurium or vecuronium).[1] Because the intermediate-duration drugs were associated with 30 minutes less postanesthesia care unit (PACU) time, their cost per patient was about $15 less than that of pancuronium.

Berg et al conducted a study of the incidence and severity of postoperative pulmonary complications, such as bronchitis, aspiration, and pneumonia, in patients throughout Denmark.[2] In a well-matched comparison, patients undergoing abdominal surgery had a three times greater incidence of pulmonary complications postoperatively with the use of pancuronium for neuromuscular blockade than with an agent of in-

D. TEMPERATURE AND pH SENSITIVITY:

Because of its unique metabolism, atracurium's duration of action can be markedly prolonged in hypothermic or acidotic patients.

E. CHEMICAL INCOMPATIBILITY:

Atracurium will precipitate as a free acid if it is introduced into an intravenous line containing an alkaline solution such as thiopental.

CISATRACURIUM

Physical Structure

Cisatracurium is one of ten stereoisomers that constitute atracurium.

Metabolism & Excretion

Like atracurium, cisatracurium undergoes degradation in plasma at physiologic pH and temperature by organ independent Hofmann elimination. The resulting metabolites (a monoquaternary acrylate and laudanosine) have no intrinsic neuromuscular blocking effects. Nonspecific esterases do not appear to be involved in the metabolism of cisatracurium. Metabolism and elimination appear to be independent of renal or liver failure. Minor variations in pharmacokinetic patterns due to age do not tend to result in clinically significant changes in duration of action.

Dosage

Cisatracurium produces good intubating conditions following a dose of 0.1–0.15 mg/kg within 2 minutes

*termediate duration. This clearly increased risk trans-
lates into significantly added cost for increased hospitalization time, treatment, medical consultation, etc.
The issue of cost of complications is probably the
most significant comparison in the general debate
over relaxant expense. Without getting into any detail, the additional spending per patient, per complication is probably at least $10,000.*

*The major risk issue involved in everyday practice
with relaxants is residual paralysis. It is easy to show
that the risk of residual paralysis in the PACU is directly related to the half-life (speed of recovery) of
the relaxant.[3,4] This greater risk translates into added
costs, such as PACU/ventilator time and treatment
of aspiration. As the half-life of relaxants decreases,
the above risk-cost issue decreases, most likely to
zero in the case of the ultra-short-acting relaxants
with very rapid recoveries.*

*A final consideration is that several authors have
shown that neuromuscular function of the upper airway, jaw, and pharynx does not recover to control
levels until the train-of-four (TOF) value is 90% or
more.[5,6] This implies that there is a longer period of
risk involved in the use of longer-acting relaxants
than we have hitherto understood. In fact, practice
with longer-acting relaxants would most likely result
in more than 50% of patients being returned to the
PACU with inadequate (as defined by TOF < 0.90)
function. Again, this added risk must translate into
cost.[7]*

*So, the rationale of modern anesthesiologists for
practicing with new drugs and techniques and
employing new technologies is, in fact, that these*

*methods are safer and cheaper. Your patients, your
surgeons, your lawyers, and your hospital adminis-
trators will appreciate that. Therefore, for the greatest economy and safety, practice with shorter-acting
drugs given by infusion and by pump, and do not
underestimate the multifaceted value of new discov-
eries.*

1. Ballantyne JC, Chang YC: The impact of choice of relaxant on postoperative recovery time: A retrospective study. Anesth Analg 1997;85:476.

2. Berg H, Viby-Morgensen J, Chraemmer Jorgensen B, et al: Residual neuromuscular block is a risk factor for postoperative pulmonary complications. A prospective, randomized, and blinded study of postoperative pulmonary complications after atracurium, vecuronium, and pancuronium. Acta Anaesthesiol Scand 1997;41:1095.

3. Bevan DR, Bevan JC, Donati F: Postoperative neuromuscular blockade: a comparison between atracurium, vecuronium and pancuronium. Anesthesiology 1988;69: 272.

4. Kopman AF: Recovery times following edrophonium and neostigmine reversal of pancuronium, atracurium, and vecuronium steady-state infusions. Anesthesiology 1986;65:572.

5. Erikson LI, Sundman E, Olsson R et al: Functional assessment of the pharynx at rest and during swallowing in partially paralyzed humans. Anesthesiology 1997;87: 1035.

6. Kopman AF, Yee PS, and Neuman GG: Relationship of train-of-four fade to clinical signs and symptoms of residual paralysis in awake volunteers. Anesthesiology 1997;86:765.

7. Caldwell JE: The problem with long-acting muscle relaxants? They cost more! [Editorial] Anesth Analg 1997;85: 473.

and results in muscle blockade of intermediate duration. The average infusion rate ranges from 1.0–2.0 µg/kg/min. Thus, it is equipotent with vecuronium and more potent than atracurium.

Cisatracurium should be stored under refrigeration (2–8 °C), and should be used within 21 days after removal from refrigeration and exposure to room temperature.

Side Effects & Clinical Considerations

Cisatracurium differs from atracurium in that with the former there is no consistent, dose-dependent increase in plasma histamine levels following its administration. Cisatracurium does not affect heart rate or blood pressure, nor does it produce autonomic effects, even at doses as high as 8 times ED$_{95}$.

Cisatracurium shares with atracurium the considerations discussed above with regard to laudanosine toxicity (although levels appear to be lower due to its greater potency), pH and temperature sensitivity, and chemical incompatibility.

MIVACURIUM

Physical Structure

Mivacurium is a benzyl isoquinoline derivative.

Metabolism & Excretion

 Mivacurium, like succinylcholine, is metabolized by pseudocholinesterase. It is only minimally metabolized by true cholinesterase. This introduces the possibility of prolonged action in patients with low pseudocholinesterase levels (see Table 9–3) or variants of the pseudocholinesterase gene. In fact, patients who are heterozygous for the atypical gene will experience a block approximately twice the normal duration, while atypical homozygous patients will remain paralyzed for hours. Because atypical homozygotes cannot metabolize mivacurium, the block resembles that caused by a long-acting, unmetabolized drug. In contrast to succinylcholine-induced paralysis in these patients, pharmacologic antagonism with cholinesterase inhibitors will quicken reversal of mivacurium blockade once some response to nerve stimulation becomes apparent. Edrophonium more effectively reverses mivacurium blockade than does neostigmine because the latter has a greater inhibition of plasma cholinesterase activity (see Chapter 10), but edrophonium increases mivacurium plasma concentrations. Although mivacurium metabolism and excretion do not directly depend on the kidneys or liver, duration of action can be prolonged in patients with renal or hepatic failure or in patients who are pregnant or postpartum as a result of decreased plasma cholinesterase levels.

Dosage

The usual intubating dose of mivacurium is 0.15–0.2 mg/kg. Steady-state infusion rates for intraoperative relaxation vary with pseudocholinesterase levels but can be initiated at 4–10 µg/kg/min. Children require higher dosages than adults if dosage is calculated in terms of body weight, but not if based on surface area.

Side Effects & Clinical Considerations

Mivacurium releases histamine to about the same degree as does atracurium. The consequent cardiovascular side effects can be minimized by slow injection over 1 minute. Nonetheless, patients with cardiac disease may rarely experience a significant drop in arterial blood pressure after doses larger than 0.15 mg/kg, despite a slow injection rate. Mivacurium's onset time is similar to that of atracurium (2–3 minutes). Its principal advantage is its brief duration of action (20–30 minutes), which is still two to three times longer than a phase I block from succinylcholine—but half the duration of atracurium, vecuronium, or rocuronium. The short duration of mivacurium's action can be markedly prolonged by prior administration of pancuronium. Children tend to exhibit a faster onset and shorter duration of action than adults. Despite relatively rapid recovery after mivacurium, neuromuscular function must be monitored in all patients to determine whether or not pharmacological reversal is necessary. Mivacurium has a shelf-life of 18 months when stored at room temperature.

DOXACURIUM

Physical Structure

Doxacurium is a benzyl isoquinoline compound closely related to mivacurium and atracurium.

Metabolism & Excretion

This potent, long-acting relaxant undergoes a minor degree of slow hydrolysis by plasma cholinesterase. Like other long-acting muscle relaxants, however, its primary route of elimination is renal excretion. Predictably, the duration of action of doxacurium is prolonged and more variable in patients with renal disease. Hepatobiliary excretion appears to play a minor role in doxacurium clearance.

Dosage

Adequate conditions for tracheal intubation within 5 minutes require 0.05 mg/kg. Intraoperative relaxation is achieved with an initial dose of 0.02 mg/kg followed by doses of 0.005 mg/kg. Doxacurium may be given in similar weight-adjusted dosages to young and elderly patients, although the latter demonstrate a prolonged duration of action.

Side Effects & Clinical Considerations

Doxacurium is essentially devoid of cardiovascular and histamine-releasing side effects. Owing to its greater potency (more potent drugs require a lower dose, resulting in decreased drug delivery to the neuromuscular junction and longer onset time), doxacurium has an onset of action slightly slower than that of other long-acting nondepolarizing relaxants (4–6 minutes). Its duration of action is similar to that of pancuronium (60–90 minutes).

PANCURONIUM

Physical Structure

Pancuronium consists of a steroid ring on which two modified ACh molecules are positioned (a bisquaternary relaxant). To an ACh receptor, pancuronium resembles ACh enough to bind—but not enough to open the lock.

Metabolism & Excretion

Unlike tubocurarine or metocurine, pancuronium is metabolized (deacetylated) by the liver, but to a limited degree. Its metabolic products have some neuromuscular blocking activity. Excretion is primarily renal (40%), although some of the drug is cleared by the bile (10%). Not surprisingly, pancuronium elimination is slowed and neuromuscular blockade is prolonged by renal failure. Patients with cirrhosis may require a higher initial dose due to an increased volume of distribution but have lower maintenance requirements because of a decreased rate of plasma clearance.

Dosage

Pancuronium is approximately half as potent as doxacurium. A dose of 0.08–0.12 mg/kg of pancuronium provides adequate relaxation for intubation in 2–3 minutes. Intraoperative relaxation is achieved by administering 0.04 mg/kg initially followed every 20–40 minutes by 0.01 mg/kg.

Children may require moderately higher doses of pancuronium.

Pancuronium is available as a solution of 1 or 2 mg/mL and is stored at 2–8 °C.

Side Effects & Clinical Considerations

A. HYPERTENSION AND TACHYCARDIA:

These cardiovascular effects are caused by the combination of vagal blockade and catecholamine release from adrenergic nerve endings. Pancuronium should be given with caution to patients in whom an increased heart rate would be particularly detrimental (eg, coronary artery disease, idiopathic hypertrophic subaortic stenosis).

B. DYSRHYTHMIAS:

Increased atrioventricular conduction and catecholamine release increase the likelihood of ventricular dysrhythmias in predisposed individuals. The combination of pancuronium, tricyclic antidepressants, and halothane has been reported to be particularly dysrhythmogenic.

C. ALLERGIC REACTIONS:

Patients who are hypersensitive to bromides may exhibit allergic reactions to pancuronium (pancuronium bromide).

VECURONIUM

Physical Structure

Vecuronium is pancuronium minus a quaternary methyl group (a monoquaternary relaxant). This minor structural change beneficially alters side effects without affecting potency.

Metabolism & Excretion

Vecuronium is metabolized to a small extent by the liver. Vecuronium depends primarily on biliary excretion and secondarily (25%) on renal excretion. While it is a satisfactory drug for renal failure patients, its duration of action is somewhat prolonged. Vecuronium's brief duration of action is explained by its shorter elimination

half-life and more rapid clearance compared with pancuronium. Long-term administration of vecuronium to patients in intensive care units has resulted in prolonged neuromuscular blockade (up to several days), possibly from accumulation of its 3-hydroxy metabolite, changing drug clearance, or the development of a polyneuropathy. Risk factors appear to include female gender, renal failure, long-term or high-dose corticosteroid therapy, and sepsis. Thus, these patients must be closely monitored and the dose of vecuronium carefully titrated. Long-term relaxant administration and the subsequent prolonged lack of ACh binding at the postsynaptic nicotinic ACh receptors may mimic a chronic denervation state and cause lasting receptor dysfunction and paralysis. The neuromuscular effects of vecuronium may be prolonged in patients with AIDS. Tolerance to nondepolarizing muscle relaxants can also develop after long-term use.

Dosage

Vecuronium is equipotent with pancuronium, and the intubating dose is 0.08–0.12 mg/kg. A dose of 0.04 mg/kg initially followed by increments of 0.01 mg/kg every 15–20 minutes provides intraoperative relaxation. Alternatively, an infusion of 1–2 μg/kg/min produces good maintenance of relaxation.

Age does not affect initial dose requirements, although subsequent doses are required less frequently in neonates and infants. Women appear to be approximately 30% more sensitive than men to vecuronium as evidenced by a greater degree of blockade and longer duration of action (this has also been seen with pancuronium and rocuronium). The cause for this sensitivity may be related to gender-related differences in fat and muscle mass, protein binding, volume of distribution, or metabolic activity. The duration of action of vecuronium may be further prolonged in postpartum patients owing to alterations in hepatic blood flow or liver uptake.

Vecuronium is packaged as 10 mg of powder, which is reconstituted with 5 or 10 mL of preservative-free water immediately before use. Unused portions are discarded after 24 hours. Vecuronium and thiopental can form a precipitate that can obstruct flow through an intravenous line and lead to pulmonary embolization.

Side Effects & Clinical Considerations

A. CARDIOVASCULAR:

Even at doses of 0.28 mg/kg, vecuronium is devoid of significant cardiovascular effects.

B. LIVER FAILURE:

Although it is dependent on biliary excretion, vecuronium's duration of action is usually not significantly prolonged in patients with cirrhosis unless doses greater than 0.15 mg/kg are given. Vecuronium requirements are reduced during the anhepatic phase of liver transplantation.

PIPECURONIUM

Physical Structure

Pipecuronium has a bisquaternary steroidal structure very similar to that of pancuronium.

Metabolism & Excretion

Like other long-acting nondepolarizers, metabolism of pipecuronium plays a minor role. Elimination depends on excretion, which is primarily renal (70%) and secondarily biliary (20%). The duration of action is increased in patients with renal failure, but not in those with hepatic insufficiency.

Dosage

Pipecuronium is slightly more potent than pancuronium, and the usual intubating dose ranges from 0.06 to 0.1 mg/kg. Likewise, maintenance relaxation doses can be reduced by approximately 20% compared with pancuronium. Infants require less pipecuronium on a per kilogram basis than children or adults. Pipecuronium's pharmacologic profile is relatively unchanged in elderly patients.

Side Effects & Clinical Considerations

The principal advantage of pipecuronium over pancuronium is its lack of cardiovascular side effects due to a decreased binding to cardiac muscarinic receptors. Pipecuronium is not associated with histamine release. The onset of action and duration of action are similar for both drugs.

ROCURONIUM

Physical Structure

This monoquaternary steroid analogue of vecuronium was designed to provide a rapid onset of action.

Metabolism & Excretion

Rocuronium undergoes no metabolism and is eliminated primarily by the liver and slightly by the kidneys. Its duration of action is not significantly affected by renal disease, but it is modestly prolonged by severe hepatic failure and pregnancy. Because rocuronium does not have active metabolites, it may be a better choice than vecuronium for prolonged infusions (eg, the intensive care unit

setting). Elderly patients may experience a prolonged duration of action due to decreased liver mass.

Dosage

Rocuronium is less potent than most other steroidal muscle relaxants (potency appears to be inversely related to speed of onset). It requires 0.45–0.9 mg/kg intravenously for intubation and 0.15 mg/kg boluses for maintenance. Intramuscular rocuronium (1 mg/kg for infants; 2 mg/kg for children) provides adequate vocal cord and diaphragmatic paralysis for intubation, but not until after 3 to 6 minutes (deltoid injection has a faster onset than quadriceps), and can be reversed after about 1 hour. The infusion requirements for rocuronium range from 5 to 12 μg/kg/min. Rocuronium can produce a prolonged duration of action in elderly patients. Initial dosage requirements are modestly increased in patients with advanced liver disease, presumably due to a larger volume of distribution.

Side Effects & Clinical Considerations

 Rocuronium (at a dose of 0.9–1.2 mg/kg) has an onset of action similar to but slightly longer than succinylcholine (60–90 seconds), making it suitable for rapid-sequence inductions, but at the cost of a much longer duration of action. This intermediate duration of action is comparable to vecuronium or atracurium.

Some clinicians compensate for rocuronium's longer onset of action (compared with that of succinylcholine) by administering it 20 seconds before thiopental (the "timing principle"). Disadvantages to this technique include the possibility of delayed administration of induction agent (eg, due to intravenous line precipitate) resulting in a conscious but paralyzed patient.

Rocuronium (0.1 mg/kg) has been shown to be a rapid (90 seconds) and effective agent (decreased fasciculations and postoperative myalgias) for precurarization prior to succinylcholine administration. Rocuronium has slightly greater vagolytic tendencies than does vecuronium.

RAPACURONIUM

Physical Structure

Rapacuronium bromide, a new short-acting nondepolarizing muscle relaxant, has an aminosteroid structure very similar to vecuronium. The rapid onset and offset of this drug have been explained by a very rapid equilibrium between plasma concentration and effect site, and weaker binding to ACh receptors. Furthermore, rapacuronium appears to be the least potent nondepolarizing muscle relaxant, supporting the apparent inverse relationship between potency and onset of action (less potent drugs require a higher dose, resulting in increased drug delivery to the neuromuscular junction and shorter onset time). Unfortunately, several reports of serious bronchospasm, including a few unexplained fatalities, prompted the manufacturer of rapacuronium to voluntarily withdraw the product in March 2001. At the time of publication this association was under investigation and the drug's future still unknown.

Metabolism & Excretion

Rapacuronium undergoes hepatic metabolism (hydrolysis) to a 3-desacetyl metabolite that possesses neuromuscular blocking properties. However, hepatic cirrhosis does not affect onset time, plasma clearance, elimination half-life, or duration of action of a single dose of rapacuronium.

Both rapacuronium and its chief metabolite are excreted by renal clearance. Although drug clearance decreases, patients with renal failure experience unchanged onset and duration of action of a single dose.

Dosage

Rapacuronium (1.5 mg/kg) has a more rapid onset of action than rocuronium or mivacurium with good to excellent tracheal intubating conditions within 1 minute in 85% of adult patients, and a duration of action of approximately 10–20 minutes. Rapacuronium's clinical efficacy rivals that of succinylcholine, but with slightly slower onset and longer duration. Onset of action is faster at the vocal cords than the adductor pollicis or laryngeal muscles. Somewhat higher dosages have been recommended for children aged 1 to 12 years (2 mg/kg) and patients undergoing cesarean section (2.5 mg/kg), while infants younger than 12 months require lower dosages (0.3–0.9 mg/kg). Intramuscular rapacuronium (3 mg/kg in infants, 5 mg/kg in children) allows good intubating conditions within 3 minutes.

Side Effects & Clinical Considerations

Rapacuronium tends to lower blood pressure by vasodilatation and raise heart rate, however these effects are mild and transient. As mentioned above, severe bronchospasm has been reported following rapacuronium administration. However, plasma histamine levels in earlier clinical trials appeared to be elevated only following higher dosages (2–3 mg/kg).

Administering neostigmine (40–50 μg/kg) 2 minutes after rapacuronium decreases the time to recovery by almost half, approaching the recovery speed of succinylcholine. Patients receiving phenytoin may demonstrate resistance to rapacuronium blockade.

CASE DISCUSSION: DELAYED RECOVERY FROM GENERAL ANESTHESIA

A 72-year-old man has undergone general anesthesia for transurethral resection of the prostate. Twenty minutes after conclusion of the procedure, he is still intubated and shows no evidence of spontaneous respiration or consciousness.

What is your general approach to this diagnostic dilemma?

Clues to the solution of complex clinical problems are usually found in a pertinent review of the medical and surgical history, the history of drug ingestions, the physical examination, and laboratory results. In this case, the perioperative anesthetic management should also be considered.

What medical illnesses predispose a patient to delayed awakening or prolonged paralysis?

Chronic hypertension alters cerebral blood flow autoregulation and decreases the brain's tolerance to episodes of hypotension. Liver disease reduces hepatic drug metabolism and biliary excretion, resulting in prolonged drug action. Reduced serum albumin levels increase free drug (active drug) availability. Hepatic encephalopathy can alter consciousness. Kidney disease lessens the renal excretion of many drugs. Uremia can also affect consciousness. Diabetic patients are prone to hypoglycemia and hyperosmotic, hyperglycemic, and nonketotic coma. A prior stroke or symptomatic carotid bruit increases the risk of intraoperative cerebral vascular accident. Right-to-left heart shunts, especially in children with congenital heart disease, allow air emboli to pass directly from the venous circulation to the systemic (possibly cerebral) arterial circulation. A paradoxic air embolism can result in permanent brain damage. Severe hypothyroidism is associated with impaired drug metabolism and, rarely, myxedema coma.

Does an uneventful history of general anesthesia narrow the differential?

Hereditary atypical pseudocholinesterase is ruled out by uneventful prior general anesthesia, assuming succinylcholine was administered. Decreased levels of normal enzyme would not result in postoperative apnea unless the surgery was of very short duration. Malignant hyperthermia does not typically present as delayed awakening, although prolonged somnolence is not unusual. Un-

eventful prior anesthetics do not, however, rule out malignant hyperthermia. Persons unusually sensitive to anesthetic agents (eg, geriatric patients) may have a history of delayed emergence.

How do drugs that a patient takes at home affect awakening from general anesthesia?

Drugs that decrease minimum alveolar concentration, such as reserpine or methyldopa, predispose patients to anesthetic overdose. Acute ethanol intoxication decreases barbiturate metabolism and acts independently as a sedative. Drugs that decrease liver blood flow, such as cimetidine, will limit hepatic drug metabolism. Antiparkinsonian drugs and tricyclic antidepressants have anticholinergic side effects that augment the sedation produced by scopolamine. Long-acting sedatives, such as the benzodiazepines, can delay awakening.

Does anesthetic technique alter awakening?

Preoperative medications can affect awakening. In particular, anticholinergics (with the exception of glycopyrrolate, which does not cross the blood-brain barrier), narcotics, and sedatives can interfere with postoperative recovery. Patients with low cardiac output may have delayed absorption of intramuscular injections.

Anesthetic maintenance techniques influence the recovery rate. Specifically, nitrous-narcotic (eg, N_2O/fentanyl) techniques tend to be associated with rapid return of early signs of awakening, such as eye opening or response to verbal commands. Nitrous-narcotic and volatile anesthetics do not significantly differ in the time required for complete recovery, however.

Intraoperative hyperventilation is a common cause of postoperative apnea. Since volatile agents raise the apneic threshold, the $PaCO_2$ level at which spontaneous ventilation ceases, moderate postoperative hypoventilation may be required to stimulate the respiratory centers. Severe intraoperative hypotension or hypertension may lead to cerebral hypoxia and edema.

Hypothermia decreases minimum alveolar concentration, antagonizes muscle relaxation reversal, and limits drug metabolism. Arterial hypoxia or severe hypercapnia ($PaCO_2 > 70$ mm Hg) can alter consciousness.

Certain surgical procedures, such as carotid endarterectomy, cardiopulmonary bypass, and intracranial procedures, are associated with an increased incidence of postoperative neurologic deficits. Transurethral resection of the prostate is associated with hyponatremia from the dilutional effects of absorbed irrigating solution.

What clues does a physical examination provide?

Pupil size is not always a reliable indicator of central nervous system integrity. Fixed and dilated pupils in the absence of anticholinergic medication or ganglionic blockade (eg, trimethaphan), however, may be an ominous sign. Response to physical stimulation, such as a forceful jaw thrust, may differentiate somnolence from paralysis. Peripheral nerve stimulation also differentiates paralysis from coma.

What specific laboratory findings would you order?

Arterial blood gases and serum electrolytes, particularly sodium, may be helpful. Computed tomographic scanning may be recommended by a neurologic consultant.

What therapeutic interventions should be considered?

Supportive mechanical ventilation should be continued in the unresponsive patient. Naloxone, flumazenil, physostigmine, doxapram, or aminophylline may be indicated, depending on the probable cause of the delayed emergence.

SUGGESTED READING

Feldman S: *Neuromuscular blockade.* Butterworth-Heinemann, 1996. Excellent chapters on neuromuscular transmission, acetylcholine pharmacology, and mechanisms of muscle relaxant actions.

Haywood PT, Divekar N, Karalliedde LD: Concurrent medication and the neuromuscular junction. Eur J Anaesthesiol 1999;16:77. This review article examines the interaction between drugs (eg, antibiotics, anticonvulsants, and diuretics) and muscle relaxants.

Kopman AF, Klewicka MM, Koman DJ: Molar potency is predictive of the speed of onset of neuromuscular block for agents of intermediate, short, and ultrashort duration. Anesthesiology 1999;90:425. Fast onset and short duration correlate inversely with potency.

Martyn JAJ, White DA, Gronert GA, Jaffe RS, Ward JM: Up-and-down regulation of skeletal muscle acetylcholine receptors. Anesthesiology 1992;76:822. A definitive look at the effects of disease states on the number of acetylcholine receptors and the clinical response to muscle relaxants.

Onrust SV, Foster RH: Rapacuronium bromide, a review of its use in anaesthetic practice. Drugs 1999;58:887.

Wright PMC, Brown R, Lau M, Fisher DM: A pharmacodynamic explanation for the rapid onset/offset of rapacuronium bromide. Anesthesiology 1999;90:16.

Cholinesterase Inhibitors

10

KEY CONCEPTS

 The primary clinical use of cholinesterase inhibitors, also called anticholinesterases, is to reverse nondepolarizing muscle blockade.

 Acetylcholine is the neurotransmitter for the entire parasympathetic nervous system (parasympathetic ganglions and effector cells), parts of the sympathetic nervous system (sympathetic ganglions, adrenal medulla, and sweat glands), some neurons in the central nervous system, and somatic nerves innervating skeletal muscle.

 Neuromuscular transmission is blocked when nondepolarizing muscle relaxants compete with acetylcholine to bind to nicotinic cholinergic receptors. The cholinesterase inhibitors indirectly increase the amount of acetylcholine available to compete with the nondepolarizing agent, thereby reestablishing neuromuscular transmission.

 In excessive doses, acetylcholinesterase inhibitors can paradoxically potentiate a nondepolarizing neuromuscular blockade. In addition, these drugs prolong the depolarization blockade of succinylcholine.

 Any prolongation of action of a nondepolarizing muscle relaxant from renal or hepatic insufficiency will probably be accompanied by a corresponding increase in the duration of action of a cholinesterase inhibitor.

 The time required to fully reverse a nondepolarizing block depends on several factors, including the choice and dose of cholinesterase inhibitor administered, the muscle relaxant being antagonized, and the extent of the blockade before reversal.

 A reversal agent should be routinely given to patients who have received nondepolarizing muscle relaxants unless full reversal can be demonstrated or the postoperative plan includes continued intubation and ventilation.

 In monitoring a patient's recovery from neuromuscular blockade, the suggested end points are sustained tetanus for 5 seconds in response to a 100-Hz stimulus in anesthetized patients or sustained head lift in awake patients. If neither of these end points is achieved, the patient should remain intubated and ventilation should continue.

 The primary clinical use of cholinesterase inhibitors, also called **anticholinesterases,** is to reverse nondepolarizing muscle blockade. However, this drug group has effects on cholinergic receptors beyond the neuromuscular end plate. This chapter reviews cholinergic pharmacology, explores the mechanisms of acetylcholinesterase inhibition, and presents the clinical pharmacology of commonly used cholinesterase inhibitors (neostigmine, edrophonium, pyridostigmine, and physostigmine).

■ CHOLINERGIC PHARMACOLOGY

The term **cholinergic** refers to the effects of the neurotransmitter acetyl*choline,* as opposed to the **adrenergic** effects of nor*adrenaline* (norepinephrine). Acetylcholine is synthesized in the nerve terminal by the enzyme

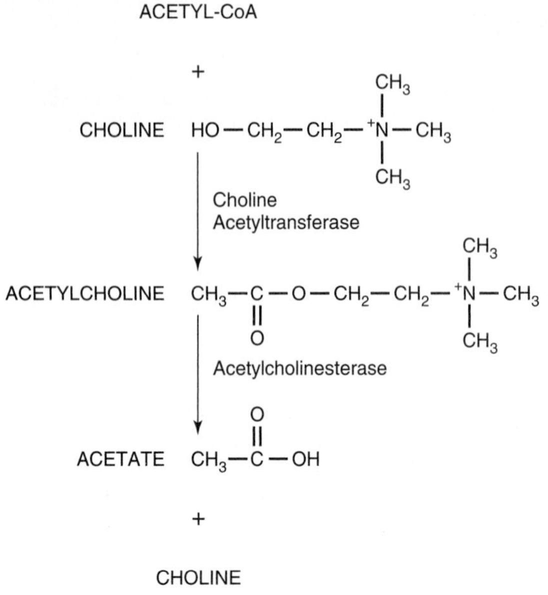

ACETYL-CoA

+

CHOLINE $HO-CH_2-CH_2-{}^+N-CH_3$
with CH_3 groups above and below

Choline
Acetyltransferase

ACETYLCHOLINE $CH_3-C-O-CH_2-CH_2-{}^+N-CH_3$
with O below the carbonyl and CH_3 groups above and below the nitrogen

Acetylcholinesterase

ACETATE CH_3-C-OH
with O above

+

CHOLINE

Figure 10–1. The synthesis and hydrolysis of acetylcholine.

choline acetyltransferase, which catalyzes the reaction between acetylcoenzyme A and choline (Figure 10–1). After its release, acetylcholine is rapidly hydrolyzed by acetylcholinesterase (true cholinesterase) into acetate and choline.

Acetylcholine is the neurotransmitter for the entire parasympathetic nervous system (parasympathetic ganglions and effector cells), parts of the sympathetic nervous system (sympathetic ganglions, adrenal medulla, and sweat glands), some neurons in the central nervous system, and somatic nerves innervating skeletal muscle (Figure 10–2).

Cholinergic receptors have been subdivided into two major groups depending on their reaction to the alkaloids **muscarine** and **nicotine** (Figure 10–3). Nicotine stimulates the autonomic ganglia and skeletal muscle receptors (**nicotinic receptors**), while muscarine activates end-organ effector cells in bronchial smooth muscle, salivary glands, and the sinoatrial node (**muscarinic receptors**). Nicotinic receptors are blocked by nondepolarizing muscle relaxants (see Chapter 9), and muscarinic receptors are blocked by anticholinergic drugs such as atropine (see Chapter 11). Although nicotinic and muscarinic receptors differ in their response to some agonists (eg, nicotine, muscarine) and some antagonists (eg, pancuronium, atropine), they both respond to acetylcholine (Table 10–1). The primary goal of muscle relaxant reversal is to maximize nicotinic transmission while minimizing muscarinic side effects.

MECHANISM OF ACTION

Neuromuscular transmission depends on acetylcholine binding to nicotinic cholinergic receptors on the motor end plate. Nondepolarizing muscle relaxants act by competing with acetylcholine for these binding sites, thereby blocking neuromuscular transmission. Reversal of blockade depends on gradual diffusion, redistribution, metabolism, and excretion from the body of the nondepolarizing relaxant (spontaneous reversal) or on the administration of specific reversal agents (pharmacologic reversal). The cholinesterase inhibitors *indirectly* increase the amount of acetylcholine available to compete with the nondepolarizing agent, thereby reestablishing neuromuscular transmission.

Cholinesterase inhibitors inactivate acetylcholinesterase by reversibly binding to the enzyme. The stability of the bond influences the duration of action: The electrostatic attraction and hydrogen bonding of **edrophonium** are short-lived; the covalent bonds of **neostigmine** and **pyridostigmine** are longer lasting. The clinical duration of the cholinesterase inhibitor effect, however, is probably most influenced by the rate of drug disappearance from the plasma. Differences in duration of action can be overcome by dosage adjustments. Reversible cholinesterase inhibitors are also used in the diagnosis and treatment of myasthenia gravis.

Table 10–1. Characteristics of cholinergic receptors.

	Nicotinic	Muscarinic
Location	Autonomic ganglia Sympathetic ganglia Parasympathetic ganglia Skeletal muscle	Glands Lacrimal Salivary Gastric Smooth muscle Bronchial Gastrointestinal Bladder Blood vessels Heart Sinoatrial node Atrioventricular node
Agonists	Acetylcholine Nicotine	Acetylcholine Muscarine
Antagonists	Nondepolarizing relaxants	Antimuscarinics Atropine Scopolamine Glycopyrrolate

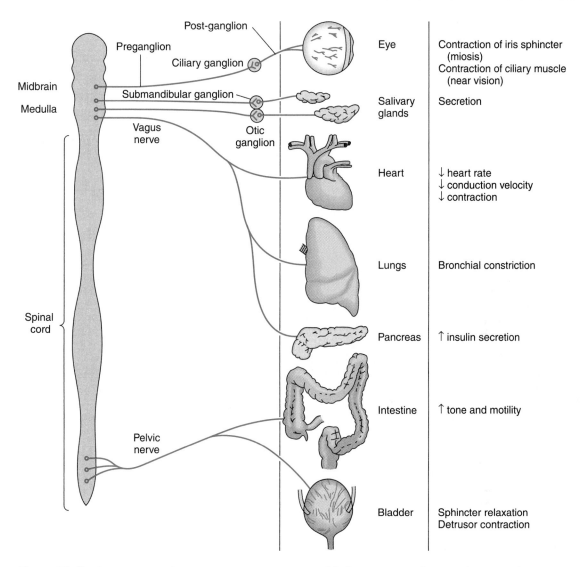

Figure 10-2. The parasympathetic nervous system uses acetylcholine as preganglionic and postganglionic neurotransmitter.

The **organophosphates,** another class of cholinesterase inhibitors, form very stable irreversible bonds to the enzyme. The use of organophosphates, such as echothiophate, to treat glaucoma can result in a significant prolongation of blockade from succinylcholine, because these drugs also inhibit pseudocholinesterase (plasma cholinesterase; see Chapter 38).

Mechanisms of action other than acetylcholinesterase inactivation may contribute to the restoration of neuromuscular function. For example, neostigmine has a direct (but weak) agonist effect on nicotinic recep-

tors. Furthermore, acetylcholine mobilization and release by the nerve may be enhanced (a presynaptic mechanism).

In excessive doses, acetylcholinesterase inhibitors can paradoxically potentiate a nondepolarizing neuromuscular blockade. In addition, these drugs prolong the depolarization blockade of succinylcholine. Two mechanisms may explain this latter effect: an increase in acetylcholine (which increases motor end plate depolarization) and inhibition of pseudocholinesterase activity. Neostig-

NICOTINE

MUSCARINE

Figure 10–3. The molecular structures of nicotine and muscarine. Compare these alkaloids with acetylcholine (Figure 10–1).

Table 10–2. Muscarinic side effects of cholinesterase inhibitors.

Organ System	Muscarinic Side Effects
Cardiovascular	Decreased heart rate, dysrhythmias
Pulmonary	Bronchospasm, bronchial secretions
Cerebral	Diffuse excitation*
Gastrointestinal	Intestinal spasm, increased salivation
Genitourinary	Increased bladder tone
Ophthalmologic	Pupillary constriction

*Applies only to physostigmine.

mine is stronger than edrophonium as an inhibitor of pseudocholinesterase, yet its inhibition of acetylcholinesterase still predominates. Thus, although neostigmine could slightly slow mivacurium metabolism, its net effect is to speed the reversal of mivacurium blockade. In large doses, neostigmine can itself cause a weak depolarizing neuromuscular blockade.

CLINICAL PHARMACOLOGY

General Pharmacologic Characteristics

The increase in acetylcholine caused by cholinesterase inhibitors affects more than the nicotinic receptors of skeletal muscle (Table 10–2). Cholinesterase inhibitors can act at cholinergic receptors of several other organ systems, including the following:

Cardiovascular receptors–The predominant muscarinic effect on the heart is a vagal-like bradycardia that can progress to sinus arrest. This effect has even been reported in the newly transplanted (denervated) heart but is more likely in a heart transplanted more than 6 months earlier (reinnervated).

Pulmonary receptors–Muscarinic stimulation can result in bronchospasm (smooth muscle contraction) and increased respiratory tract secretions.

Cerebral receptors–Physostigmine is a cholinesterase inhibitor that crosses the blood-brain barrier and can cause diffuse activation of the electroencephalogram by stimulating muscarinic and nicotinic receptors within the central nervous system (CNS). Inactivation of nicotinic acetylcholine receptors in the CNS may play a role in the action of general anesthetics (see Chapter 7).

Gastrointestinal receptors–Muscarinic stimulation increases peristaltic activity (esophageal, gastric, and intestinal) and glandular secretions (eg, salivary, parietal). Perioperative bowel anastomotic leakage, nausea and vomiting, and fecal incontinence have been attributed to the use of cholinesterase inhibitors.

Unwanted muscarinic side effects are minimized by prior or concomitant administration of anticholinergic medications such as atropine sulfate or glycopyrrolate (see Chapter 11).

The duration of action is similar among the cholinesterase inhibitors. Clearance is due to both hepatic metabolism (25–50%) and renal excretion 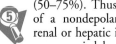 (50–75%). Thus, any prolongation of action of a nondepolarizing muscle relaxant from renal or hepatic insufficiency will probably be accompanied by a corresponding increase in the duration of action of a cholinesterase inhibitor.

Dosage requirements of cholinesterase inhibitors depend on the degree of neuromuscular block that is being reversed. This is usually estimated by the response to peripheral nerve stimulation. As a rule, no amount of cholinesterase inhibitor can immediately reverse a block so intense that there is no response to tetanic peripheral nerve stimulation. Excessive doses of cholinesterase inhibitors may actually prolong recovery.

The time required to fully reverse a nondepolarizing block depends on several factors, including the choice and dose of cholinesterase inhibitor administered, the muscle relaxant being antagonized, and the extent of the blockade before reversal. For example, edrophonium reversal is usually faster than neostigmine; large doses of neostigmine lead to faster reversal than do small doses; intermediate-acting relaxants reverse sooner than long-acting relaxants; and a shallow block is easier to reverse than a deep block (ie, twitch height < 10%). Short- and intermediate-acting muscle relaxants therefore require a lower dose of reversal agent (for the same degree of blockade) than long-acting agents do, and concurrent excretion or metabolism provides a proportionally faster reversal of the short- and intermediate-acting agents. These advantages can be lost in conditions associated with severe end-organ disease (eg, the use of vecuronium in a patient with liver failure) or enzyme deficiencies (eg, mivacurium in a patient with homozygous atypical pseudocholinesterase). Depending on the dose of muscle relaxant that has been given, spontaneous recovery to a level adequate for pharmacologic reversal may take more than an hour with long-acting muscle relaxants because of their insignificant metabolism and slow excretion. Factors associated with faster reversal are associated with a lower incidence of residual paralysis in the recovery room and a lower risk of postoperative respiratory complications.

Although the time to recovery of neuromuscular function does not significantly depend on when reversal is attempted, some clinicians recommend waiting until at least some evidence of spontaneous recovery appears (ie, 10% twitch height). A reversal agent should be routinely given to patients who have received nondepolarizing muscle relaxants unless *full* reversal can be demonstrated or the postoperative plan includes continued intubation and ventilation. In the latter situation, adequate sedation must also be provided.

The use of a peripheral nerve stimulator to monitor recovery from neuromuscular blockade is discussed in Chapters 6 and 9. In general, the higher the frequency of stimulation, the greater the sensitivity of the test (100 Hz tetany > 50 Hz or train-of-four > single-twitch

height). Since peripheral nerve stimulation is uncomfortable, alternative tests of neuromuscular function must be used in awake patients. These also vary in sensitivity (sustained head lift > inspiratory force > vital capacity > tidal volume). Therefore, the suggested end points of recovery are sustained tetanus for 5 seconds in response to a 100-Hz stimulus in anesthetized patients or sustained head lift in awake patients. If neither of these end points is achieved, the patient should remain intubated and ventilation should continue.

■ SPECIFIC ANTICHOLINERGIC AGENTS

NEOSTIGMINE

Physical Structure

Neostigmine consists of a carbamate moiety and a quaternary ammonium group (Figure 10–4). The former provides covalent bonding to acetylcholinesterase. The latter renders the molecule lipid-insoluble, so that it cannot pass through the blood-brain barrier.

Dosage & Packaging

The maximum recommended dose of neostigmine is 0.08 mg/kg (up to 5 mg in adults), but smaller amounts often suffice (Table 10–3). Neostigmine is

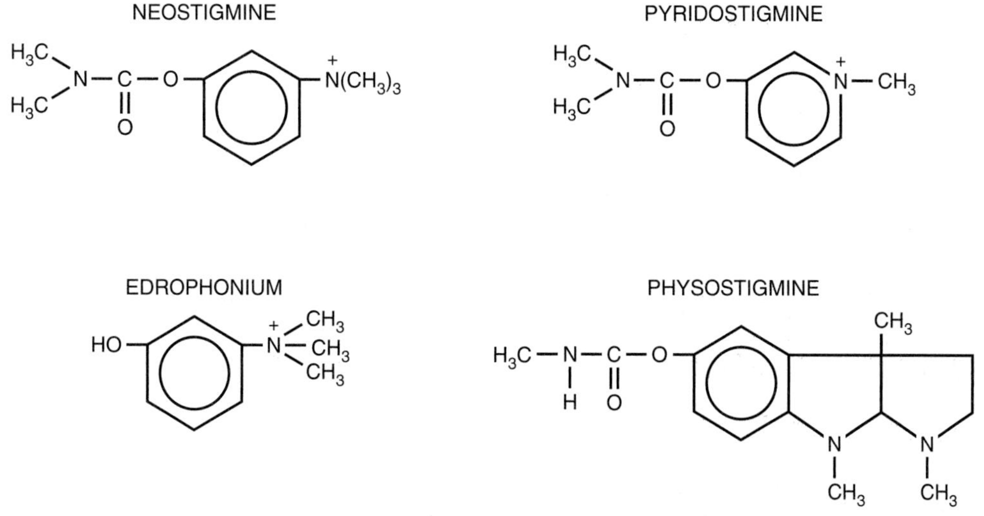

NEOSTIGMINE

PYRIDOSTIGMINE

EDROPHONIUM

PHYSOSTIGMINE

Figure 10–4. Molecular structures of neostigmine, pyridostigmine, edrophonium, and physostigmine.

Table 10–3. The choice and dose of cholinesterase inhibitor determine the choice and dose of anticholinergic.

Cholinesterase Inhibitor	Usual Dose of Cholinesterase Inhibitor	Recommended Anticholinergic	Usual Dose of Anticholinergic per mg of Cholinesterase Inhibitor	Cost* of Reversal
Neostigmine	0.04–0.08 mg/kg	Glycopyrrolate	0.2 mg	L
Pyridostigmine	0.1–0.4 mg/kg	Glycopyrrolate	0.05 mg	L
Edrophonium	0.5–1 mg/kg	Atropine	0.014 mg	M
Physostigmine	0.01–0.03 mg/kg	Usually not necessary	NA	NA

*Based on average wholesale price; L = low; M = moderate; NA = not applicable.

most commonly packaged as 10 mL of a 1 mg/mL solution, although 0.5 mg/mL and 0.25 mg/mL concentrations are also available.

Clinical Considerations

The effects of neostigmine (0.04 mg/kg) are usually apparent in 5–10 minutes and last more than an hour. Pediatric and elderly patients appear to be more sensitive to its effects, experiencing a more rapid onset and requiring a smaller dose. The duration of action is prolonged in geriatric patients. Muscarinic side effects are minimized by prior or concomitant administration of an anticholinergic agent. The onset of action of glycopyrrolate (0.2 mg glycopyrrolate per 1 mg of neostigmine) is similar to that of neostigmine and is associated with less tachycardia than is experienced with atropine (0.4 mg of atropine per 1 mg of neostigmine). Neostigmine has been reported to cross the placenta resulting in fetal bradycardia. Thus, atropine may be a better choice of an anticholinergic agent than glycopyrrolate in pregnant patients receiving neostigmine. Neostigmine is also used to treat myasthenia gravis, urinary bladder atony, and paralytic ileus. Neostigmine (50–100 μg) has been used as an adjunct to intrathecal anesthesia causing a prolongation of sensory and motor blockade, presumably by inhibiting the breakdown of spinal cord acetylcholine. However, side effects include nausea, vomiting, fecal incontinence, delayed recovery room discharge, and atropine-resistant bradycardia at higher doses (200 μg).

PYRIDOSTIGMINE

Physical Structure

Pyridostigmine is structurally similar to neostigmine except that the quaternary ammonium is incorporated into the phenol ring. Pyridostigmine shares neostigmine's covalent binding to acetylcholinesterase and its lipid insolubility.

Dosage & Packaging

Pyridostigmine is one-fifth as potent as neostigmine and may be administered in doses up to 0.4 mg/kg (a total of 20 mg in adults). It is available as a solution of 5 mg/mL.

Clinical Considerations

The onset of action of pyridostigmine is slower (10–15 minutes) than that of neostigmine, and its duration is slightly longer (> 2 hours). Equivalent doses of anticholinergic medications are required to prevent bradycardia. Again, glycopyrrolate (0.05 mg per 1 mg of pyridostigmine) is preferred because its onset of action is slower than that of atropine (0.1 mg per 1 mg of pyridostigmine).

EDROPHONIUM

Physical Structure

Because it lacks a carbamate group, edrophonium must rely on noncovalent bonding to the acetylcholinesterase enzyme. The quaternary ammonium group limits lipid solubility.

Dosage & Packaging

Edrophonium is less than one-tenth as potent as neostigmine. The recommended dosage is 0.5–1 mg/kg. Edrophonium is available as a solution containing 10 mg/mL; it is available with atropine as a combination drug (Enlon-Plus; 10 mg edrophonium and 0.14 mg atropine per milliliter).

Clinical Considerations

Edrophonium has the most rapid onset of action (1–2 minutes) and the shortest duration of effect of any of the cholinesterase inhibitors. Low doses should not be used, because longer-acting muscle relaxants may outlast edrophonium's effects. Higher doses prolong the duration of action to more than an hour. Patients at the extremes of age are not more sensitive to edrophonium reversal (unlike the case with neostigmine). Edrophonium may not be as effective as neostigmine at reversing intense neuromuscular blockade, but it may be more effective in reversing a mivacurium blockade. In equipotent doses, edrophonium's muscarinic effects are less pronounced than those of neostigmine or pyridostigmine, requiring only half the amount of anticholinergic agent. Edrophonium's rapid onset is well matched to that of atropine (0.014 mg of atropine per 1 mg of edrophonium). Although glycopyrrolate (0.007 mg per 1 mg of edrophonium) can also be used, it should be given several minutes prior to edrophonium to avoid the possibility of bradycardia.

PHYSOSTIGMINE

Physical Structure

Physostigmine, a tertiary amine, has a carbamate group but no quaternary ammonium. Therefore, it is lipid-soluble and is the only cholinesterase inhibitor available for clinical use that freely passes the blood-brain barrier.

Dosage & Packaging

The dose of physostigmine is 0.01–0.03 mg/kg. It is packaged as a solution containing 1 mg/mL.

Clinical Considerations

Physostigmine's lipid solubility and CNS penetration limit its usefulness as a reversal agent for nondepolarizing blockade. For the same reasons, it is effective in the treatment of central anticholinergic toxicity caused by overdoses of atropine or scopolamine (see Chapter 11). In addition, physostigmine reverses some of the CNS depression and delirium associated with benzodiazepines and volatile anesthetics. Physostigmine (0.04 mg/kg) has been shown to be effective in preventing postoperative shivering. Physostigmine reportedly antagonizes morphine-induced respiratory depression, presumably because morphine reduces acetylcholine release in the brain. These effects are transient, and repeated doses may be required. Bradycardia is infrequent in the recommended dosage range, but atropine or glycopyrrolate should be immediately available. Because glycopyrrolate does not cross the blood-brain barrier, it will not reverse the CNS effects of physostigmine (see Chapter 11). Other possible muscarinic side effects include excessive salivation, vomiting, and convulsions. In contrast to other cholinesterase inhibitors, physostigmine is almost completely metabolized by plasma esterases, so that renal excretion is not important.

CASE DISCUSSION: RESPIRATORY FAILURE IN THE RECOVERY ROOM

A 66-year-old woman weighing 85 kg is brought to the recovery room following cholecystectomy. She had received an anesthetic technique that included isoflurane and pancuronium for muscle relaxation. At the conclusion of the procedure, the anesthesiologist administered 6 mg of morphine sulfate for postoperative pain control and 3 mg of neostigmine with 0.6 mg of glycopyrrolate to reverse any residual neuromuscular blockade. The dose of cholinesterase inhibitor was empirically based on clinical judgment. Although she was apparently breathing normally on arrival in the recovery room, the patient's tidal volume progressively diminished. Arterial blood gas measurements revealed a $PaCO_2$ of 62 mm Hg, a PaO_2 of 110 mm Hg, and a pH of 7.26 on an FiO_2 (fraction of inspired oxygen) of 40%.

Which drugs administered to this patient could explain her hypoventilation?

Isoflurane, morphine sulfate, and pancuronium all interfere with a patient's ability to maintain a normal ventilatory response to an elevated $PaCO_2$.

Why would the patient's breathing worsen in the recovery room?

Possibilities include the delayed onset of action of morphine sulfate, a lack of sensory stimulation in the recovery area, fatigue of respiratory muscles, and splinting as a result of upper abdominal pain.

Could the patient still have residual neuromuscular blockade?

If the dose of neostigmine was not determined by the response to a peripheral nerve stimulator, or if the recovery of muscle function was inadequately tested after the reversal drugs were given, persistent neuromuscular blockade is possible. Assume, for example, that the patient had minimal or no response to initial tetanic stimulation at 100 Hz. Even the maximal dose of neostigmine (5 mg) might not yet have adequately reversed the paralysis. Because of enormous patient variability, the response to peripheral nerve stimulation must always be monitored when intermediate or long-acting muscle relaxants are administered. Even if partial reversal is achieved, paralysis may worsen if the patient hypoventilates. Other factors (besides respiratory *acidosis) that impair the reversal of nondepolarizing muscle relaxants include intense neuromuscular paralysis, electrolyte disturbances (hypermagnesemia, hypokalemia, and hypocalcemia), hypothermia (temperature < 32 °C), drug interactions (see Table 9–4), metabolic alkalosis (from accompanying hypokalemia and hypocalcemia), and coexisting diseases (see Table 9–7).*

How could the extent of reversal be tested?

Tetanic stimulation is a sensitive but uncomfortable test of neuromuscular transmission in an awake patient. Because of its shorter duration, double-burst stimulation is better tolerated than tetany by conscious patients. Many other tests of neuromuscular transmission, such as vital capacity and tidal volume, are insensitive since they may still appear normal when 70–80% of receptors are still blocked. In fact, 70% of receptors may remain blocked despite an apparently normal response to train-of-four stimulation. The ability to sustain a head lift for 5 seconds, however, indicates that fewer than 33% of receptors are occupied by muscle relaxant.

What treatment would you suggest?

Ventilation should be assisted to reduce the respiratory acidosis. Even if diaphragmatic function appears to be adequate, residual blockade can lead to airway obstruction and poor airway protection. More neostigmine (with an anticholinergic) could be administered up to a maximum recommended dose of 5 mg. If this does not adequately reverse paralysis, mechanical ventilation and airway protection should be instituted and continued until neuromuscular function is fully restored.

SUGGESTED READING

Bevan DR, Donati F, Kopman AF: Reversal of neuromuscular blockade. Anesthesiology 1992;77:785. This article covers methods of determining adequacy of reversal, anticholinesterase pharmacology, and clinical conditions affecting reversal.

Bevan JC, Collins L, Fowler C, et al: Early and late reversal of rocuronium and vecuronium with neostigmine in adults and children. Anesth Analg 1999;89:333-339. One study demonstrating no advantage to delaying reversal of blockade until some degree of spontaneous reversal.

Fuchs-Buder T, Ziegenfub T, Lysakowski K, Tassonyi E: Antagonism of vecuronium-induced neuromuscular block in patients pretreated with magnesium sulphate: dose-effect relationship of neostigmine. Br J Anaesth 1999;82:61-65. Magnesium sulfate treatment prolongs neuromuscular blockade by slowing spontaneous reversal but does not appear to affect reversal of blockade by neostigmine.

Joshi GP, Garg SA, Hailey A, Yu SY: The effects of antagonizing residual neuromuscular blockade by neostigmine and glycopyrrolate on nausea and vomiting after ambulatory surgery. Anesth Analg 1999;89:628-631. Reversal with neostigmine did not increase the incidence of nausea and vomiting or the need for antiemetic therapy in outpatient surgery.

Klamt JG, Garcia LV, Prado WA: Analgesic and adverse effects of a low dose of intrathecally administered hyperbaric neostigmine alone or combined with morphine in patients submitted to spinal anesthesia: Pilot studies. Anaesthesia 1999; 54:27-31. Multiple side effects of intrathecal neostigmine, even at relatively low doses, are described.

Stoelting RK: *Pharmacology and Physiology in Anesthetic Practice,* 3rd ed. Lippincott William & Wilkins, 1999. An up-to-date presentation of cholinesterase inhibitors.

Taylor P: Anticholinesterase agents. Chapter 8 in: *Goodman and Gilman's Pharmacological Basis of Therapeutics,* 9th ed. Hardman JG (editor). McGraw-Hill, 1996. An excellent overview of this drug class.

Anticholinergic Drugs

11

KEY CONCEPTS

Ester linkage is essential for effective binding of the anticholinergics to the acetylcholine receptors. This competitively blocks binding by acetylcholine and prevents receptor activation. The cellular effects of acetylcholine, which are mediated through second messengers such as cyclic guanosine monophosphate (cGMP), are prevented.

Anticholinergic effect on the respiratory system is relaxation of bronchial smooth musculature, which reduces airway resistance and increases anatomic dead space.

Overall, the anticholinergic drugs are not especially advantageous in the prevention of aspiration pneumonia.

Atropine has particularly potent effects on the heart and bronchial smooth muscle and is the most efficacious anticholinergic for treating bradyarrhythmias.

Ipratropium solution (0.5 mg in 2.5 mL) appears especially effective in the treatment of acute chronic obstructive pulmonary disease when combined with a β-agonist drug (eg, albuterol).

Scopolamine is a more potent antisialagogue than atropine and causes greater central nervous system effects.

Because of a quaternary structure, glycopyrrolate cannot cross the blood-brain barrier and is almost always devoid of central nervous system and ophthalmic activity.

One group of cholinergic antagonists has already been discussed: the nondepolarizing neuromuscular blocking agents (see Chapter 9). These drugs act chiefly at the **nicotinic receptors** in skeletal muscle. This chapter presents the pharmacology of drugs that block **muscarinic receptors**. Although the classification *anticholinergic* usually refers to this latter group, a more precise term would be *antimuscarinic*.

In this chapter, the mechanism of action and clinical pharmacology are introduced for three common anticholinergics: atropine, scopolamine, and glycopyrrolate. The clinical uses of these drugs in anesthesia relate to their effect on the cardiovascular, respiratory, cerebral, gastrointestinal, and other organ systems (Table 11–1).

MECHANISMS OF ACTION

Anticholinergics are esters of an aromatic acid combined with an organic base (Figure 11–1). The ester linkage is essential for effective binding of the anticholinergics to the acetylcholine receptors. This competitively blocks binding by acetylcholine and prevents receptor activation. The cellular effects of acetylcholine, which are mediated through second messengers such as cyclic guanosine monophosphate (cGMP), are prevented. The tissue receptors vary in their sensitivity to blockade. In fact, muscarinic receptors are not homogeneous, and receptor subgroups have been identified: neuronal (M_1), cardiac (M_2) and glandular (M_3) receptors.

CLINICAL PHARMACOLOGY

General Pharmacologic Characteristics

In clinical doses, only muscarinic receptors are blocked by the anticholinergic drugs discussed in this chapter. The extent of the anticholinergic effect depends on the

Table 11–1. Pharmacologic characteristics of anticholinergic drugs.

	Atropine	Scopolamine	Glycopyrrolate
Tachycardia	+++	+	++
Bronchodilatation	++	+	++
Sedation	+	+++	0
Antisialagogue effect	++	+++	+++

0 = no effect.
+ = minimal effect.
++ = moderate effect.
+++ = marked effect.

degree of baseline vagal tone. Several organ systems are affected:

A. CARDIOVASCULAR:

Blockade of muscarinic receptors in the sinoatrial node results in tachycardia. This effect is especially useful in reversing bradycardia due to vagal reflexes (eg, baroreceptor reflex, peritoneal stimulation, or oculocardiac reflex). A transient slowing of heart rate in response to low doses of anticholinergics has been reported. The mechanism of this paradoxic response may be a weak peripheral agonist effect, suggesting that these drugs are not pure antagonists. Facilitation of conduction through the atrioventricular node shortens the P–R interval on the electrocardiogram and often decreases heart block caused by vagal activity. Atrial dysrhythmias and nodal rhythms occasionally occur. Anticholinergics have little effect on ventricular function or pe-

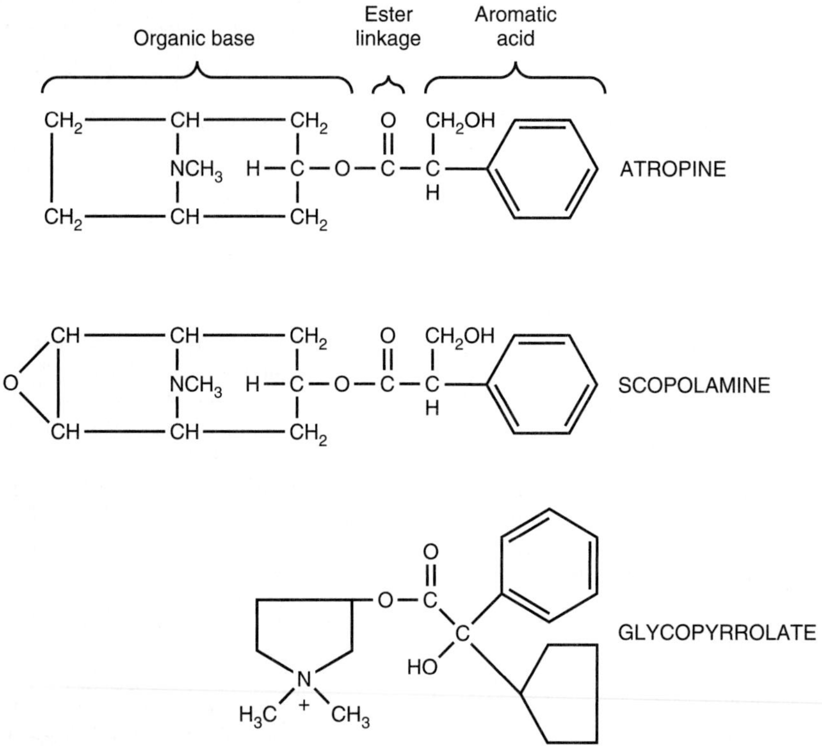

Figure 11–1. Physical structures of anticholinergic drugs.

ripheral vasculature because of the paucity of direct cholinergic innervation of these areas despite the presence of cholinergic receptors. Large doses of anticholinergic agents can result in dilatation of cutaneous blood vessels (**atropine flush**).

B. RESPIRATORY:

The anticholinergics inhibit the secretions of the respiratory tract mucosa, from the nose to the bronchi. This drying effect was more important before the advent of 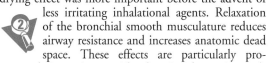 less irritating inhalational agents. Relaxation of the bronchial smooth musculature reduces airway resistance and increases anatomic dead space. These effects are particularly pronounced in patients with chronic obstructive pulmonary disease or asthma.

C. CEREBRAL:

Anticholinergic medications can cause a spectrum of central nervous system effects ranging from stimulation to depression, depending on drug choice and dosage. Stimulation may present as excitation, restlessness, or hallucinations. Depression can cause sedation and amnesia. Physostigmine, a cholinesterase inhibitor that crosses the blood-brain barrier, promptly reverses these actions (see Chapter 10).

D. GASTROINTESTINAL:

Salivary secretions are markedly reduced by anticholinergic drugs. Gastric secretions are also decreased, but larger doses are necessary. Decreased intestinal motility and peristalsis prolong gastric emptying time. Lower 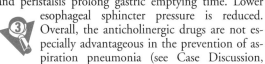 esophageal sphincter pressure is reduced. Overall, the anticholinergic drugs are not especially advantageous in the prevention of aspiration pneumonia (see Case Discussion, Chapter 15).

E. OPHTHALMIC:

Anticholinergics cause mydriasis (pupillary dilation) and cycloplegia (an inability to accommodate to near vision); acute angle-closure glaucoma is unlikely following systemic administration of most anticholinergic drugs.

F. GENITOURINARY:

Anticholinergics may decrease ureter and bladder tone as a result of smooth muscle relaxation and lead to urinary retention, particularly in elderly men with prostatic hypertrophy.

G. THERMOREGULATION:

Inhibition of sweat glands may lead to a rise in body temperature (**atropine fever**).

H. IMMUNE-MEDIATED HYPERSENSITIVITY:

Decreasing intracellular cGMP would theoretically be useful in the treatment of hypersensitivity reactions. Clinically, anticholinergics appear to have little efficacy in these situations.

■ SPECIFIC ANTICHOLINERGIC DRUGS

ATROPINE

Physical Structure

Atropine is a tertiary amine consisting of tropic acid (an aromatic acid) and tropine (an organic base). The naturally occurring levorotatory form is active, but the commercial mixture is racemic (Figure 11–1).

Dosage & Packaging

As a premedication, atropine is administered intravenously or intramuscularly in a range of 0.01–0.02 mg/kg up to the usual adult dose of 0.4–0.6 mg. Larger intravenous doses up to 2 mg may be required to completely block the cardiac vagal nerves in treating severe bradycardia. The appropriate dose for minimizing the side effects of cholinesterase inhibitors during reversal of nondepolarizing blockade is shown in Table 10–3. Atropine sulfate is available in a multitude of concentrations.

Clinical Considerations

 Atropine has particularly potent effects on the heart and bronchial smooth muscle and is the most efficacious anticholinergic for treating bradyarrhythmias. Patients with coronary artery disease may not tolerate the increased myocardial oxygen demand and decreased oxygen supply associated with the tachycardia caused by atropine. A derivative of atropine (ipratropium bromide) is available in a metered-dose inhaler for the treatment of bronchospasm. Ipratropium solution (0.5 mg to 2.5 mL) appears especially effective in the treatment of acute chronic obstructive pulmonary disease when combined with a β-agonist drug (eg, albuterol). The central nervous system effects of atropine are minimal after the usual doses, even though this tertiary amine can rapidly cross the blood-brain barrier. Atropine has been associated with mild postoperative memory deficits, and toxic doses are usually associated with excitatory reactions. An intramuscular dose of 0.01–0.02 mg/kg reliably provides an antisialagogue effect. Atropine should be used cautiously in patients with narrow-angle glaucoma, prostatic hypertrophy, or bladder-neck obstruction.

SCOPOLAMINE

Physical Structure

Scopolamine differs from atropine by incorporating an oxygen bridge into the organic base to form scopine.

Dosage & Packaging

The premedication dose of scopolamine is the same as that of atropine, and it is usually given intramuscularly. Scopolamine hydrobromide is available as solutions containing 0.3, 0.4, and 1 mg/mL.

Clinical Considerations

 Scopolamine is a more potent antisialagogue than atropine and causes greater central nervous system effects. Clinical dosages usually result in drowsiness and amnesia, although restlessness and delirium are possible. The sedative effects may be desirable for premedication but can interfere with awakening following short procedures. Scopolamine has the added virtue of preventing motion sickness. The lipid solubility allows transdermal absorption. Because of its pronounced ocular effects, scopolamine is best avoided in patients with closed-angle glaucoma.

GLYCOPYRROLATE

Physical Structure

Glycopyrrolate is a synthetic quaternary ammonium containing mandelic acid in the place of tropic acid.

Dosage & Packaging

The usual dose of glycopyrrolate is one-half that of atropine. For instance, the premedication dose is 0.005–0.01 mg/kg up to 0.2–0.3 mg in adults. Glycopyrrolate for injection is packaged as a solution of 0.2 mg/mL.

Clinical Considerations

Because of a quaternary structure, glycopyrrolate cannot cross the blood-brain barrier and is almost always devoid of central nervous system and ophthalmic activity. Potent inhibition of salivary gland and respiratory tract secretions is the primary rationale for using glycopyrrolate as a premedication. Heart rate usually increases after intravenous—but not intramuscular—administration. Glycopyrrolate

has a longer duration of action than atropine (2–4 hours versus 30 minutes after intravenous administration).

CASE DISCUSSION:
CENTRAL ANTICHOLINERGIC SYNDROME

An elderly patient is scheduled for enucleation of a blind, painful eye. Scopolamine, 0.4 mg intramuscularly, is administered as premedication. In the preoperative holding area, the patient becomes agitated and disoriented. The only other medication the patient has received is 1% atropine eye drops.

How many milligrams of atropine are in 1 drop of a 1% solution?

A 1% solution contains 1 g dissolved in 100 mL, or 10 mg/mL. Eyedroppers vary in the number of drops formed per milliliter of solution but average 20 drops/mL. Therefore, 1 drop usually contains 0.5 mg of atropine.

How are ophthalmic drops systemically absorbed?

Absorption by vessels in the conjunctival sac is similar to subcutaneous injection. More rapid absorption is possible by the nasolacrimal duct mucosa.

What are the signs and symptoms of anticholinergic poisoning?

*Reactions from an overdose of anticholinergic medication involve several organ systems. The **central anticholinergic syndrome** refers to central nervous system changes that range from unconsciousness to hallucinations. Agitation and delirium are not unusual in elderly patients. Other systemic manifestations include dry mouth, tachycardia, atropine flush, atropine fever, and impaired vision.*

What other drugs possess anticholinergic activity that could predispose patients to the central anticholinergic syndrome?

Tricyclic antidepressants, antihistamines, and antipsychotics have antimuscarinic properties that could potentiate the side effects of anticholinergic drugs.

What drug is an effective antidote to anticholinergic overdosage?

Cholinesterase inhibitors indirectly increase the amount of acetylcholine available to compete with anticholinergic drugs at the muscarinic receptor. Neostigmine, pyridostigmine, and edrophonium possess a quaternary ammonium group that prevents penetration of the blood-brain barrier. Physostigmine, a tertiary amine, is lipid-soluble and effectively reverses central anticholinergic toxicity. An initial dose of 0.01–0.03 mg/kg may have to be repeated after 15–30 minutes.

Should this case be canceled or allowed to proceed?

Enucleation to relieve a painful eye is clearly an elective procedure. The most important question that must be addressed for elective cases is whether the patient is optimally medically managed. In other words, would canceling surgery allow further fine-tuning of any medical problems? For example, if this anticholinergic overdose were accompanied by tachycardia, it would probably be prudent to postpone surgery in this elderly patient. On the other hand, if the patient's mental status responds to physostigmine and there appear to be no other significant anticholinergic side effects, surgery could proceed.

SUGGESTED READING

Brown JH, Taylor P: Muscarinic receptor agonists and antagonists. Chapter 7 in: *Goodman and Gilman's The Pharmacological Basis of Therapeutics,* 9th ed. Hardman JG (editor): McGraw-Hill, 1996. Mechanisms of action, structure-activity relationships, and therapeutic uses.

Katzung BG (editor): Cholinoceptor-blocking drugs. Chapter 8 in: *Basic and Clinical Pharmacology,* 8th ed. McGraw-Hill, 2001.

Naguib M, Yaksh TL: Characterization of muscarinic receptor subtypes that mediate antinociception in the rat spinal cord. Anesth Analg 1997;85:847-853. A discussion of the function of muscarinic receptor subtypes.

Adrenergic Agonists & Antagonists 12

KEY CONCEPTS

 1 Direct agonists bind to the receptor, while indirect agonists increase endogenous neurotransmitter activity. Mechanisms of indirect action include increased release or decreased reuptake of norepinephrine.

 2 The primary effect of phenylephrine is peripheral vasoconstriction with a concomitant rise in systemic vascular resistance and arterial blood pressure.

 3 Clonidine appears to decrease anesthetic and analgesic requirements and to provide sedation and anxiolysis.

 4 Ephedrine is commonly used as a vasopressor during anesthesia. As such, its administration should be viewed as a temporizing measure while the cause of hypotension is determined and remedied.

 5 Small doses (≤ 2 μg/kg/min) of dopamine have minimal adrenergic effects but activate dopaminergic receptors. Stimulation of these non-

adrenergic receptors (specifically, DA_1 receptors) vasodilates the renal vasculature and promotes diuresis.

 6 Favorable effects on myocardial oxygen balance make dobutamine a good choice for patients with the combination of congestive heart failure and coronary artery disease, particularly if peripheral vascular resistance and heart rate are already elevated.

 7 Because labetalol has combined α- and β-effects, it lowers blood pressure without reflex tachycardia.

 8 Esmolol is an ultra-short-acting selective $β_1$-antagonist that reduces heart rate and, to a lesser extent, blood pressure.

 9 Discontinuation of β-blocker therapy for 24–48 hours may trigger a withdrawal syndrome characterized by hypertension, tachycardia, and angina pectoris.

The three previous chapters presented the pharmacology of drugs that affect cholinergic activity. This chapter introduces an analogous group of agents that interact at adrenergic receptors—**adrenoceptors.** The clinical effects of these drugs can be deduced from an understanding of adrenoceptor physiology and a knowledge of which receptors each drug activates or blocks.

ADRENOCEPTOR PHYSIOLOGY

The term **adrenergic** originally referred to the effects of epinephrine (*adren*aline), as opposed to the **cholinergic** effects of acetyl*choline*. It is now known that norepi-

nephrine (noradrenaline) is the neurotransmitter responsible for most of the adrenergic activity of the sympathetic nervous system. With the exception of eccrine sweat glands and some blood vessels, norepinephrine is released by postganglionic sympathetic fibers at end-organ tissues (Figure 12–1). In contrast, as was explained in Chapter 10, acetylcholine is released by preganglionic sympathetic fibers and all parasympathetic fibers.

Norepinephrine is synthesized in the cytoplasm and packaged into vesicles of sympathetic postganglionic fibers (Figure 12–2). After release by a process of exocytosis, the action of norepinephrine is termi-

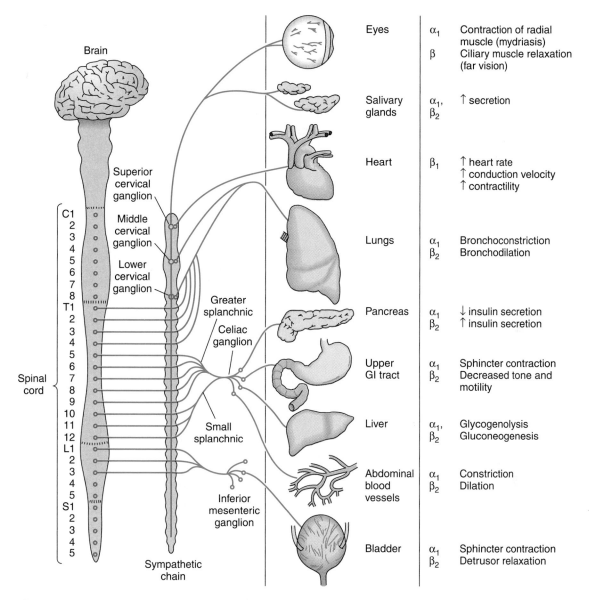

Organ	Receptor	Response
Eyes	α_1	Contraction of radial muscle (mydriasis)
	β	Ciliary muscle relaxation (far vision)
Salivary glands	α_1, β_2	↑ secretion
Heart	β_1	↑ heart rate ↑ conduction velocity ↑ contractility
Lungs	α_1	Bronchoconstriction
	β_2	Bronchodilation
Pancreas	α_1	↓ insulin secretion
	β_2	↑ insulin secretion
Upper GI tract	α_1	Sphincter contraction
	β_2	Decreased tone and motility
Liver	α_1, β_2	Glycogenolysis Gluconeogenesis
Abdominal blood vessels	α_1	Constriction
	β_2	Dilation
Bladder	α_1	Sphincter contraction
	β_2	Detrusor relaxation

Figure 12–1. The sympathetic nervous system. Organ innervation, receptor type, and response to stimulation. The origin of the sympathetic chain is the thoracoabdominal (T1–L3) spinal cord, in contrast to the craniosacral distribution of the parasympathetic nervous system. Another anatomic difference is the greater distance from the sympathetic ganglion to the visceral structures.

nated by reuptake into the postganglionic nerve ending (inhibited by tricyclic antidepressants), diffusion from receptor sites, or metabolism by monoamine oxidase (inhibited by monoamine oxidase inhibitors) and catechol-O-methyltransferase (Figure 12–3). Pro-

longed adrenergic activation leads to desensitization and hyporesponsiveness to further stimulation.

Adrenergic receptors are divided into two general categories: α and β. Each of these has been further subdivided into at least two subtypes: α_1 and α_2, and β_1 and β_2.

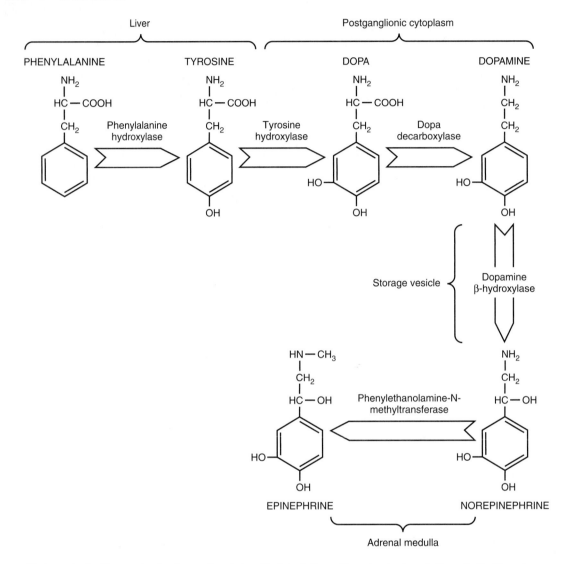

Figure 12–2. The synthesis of norepinephrine. Hydroxylation of tyrosine to dopa is the rate-limiting step. Dopamine is actively transported into storage vesicles. Norepinephrine can be converted to epinephrine in the adrenal medulla.

α_1-Receptors

α_1-Receptors are postsynaptic adrenoceptors located in smooth muscle throughout the body, in the eye, lung, blood vessels, uterus, gut, and genitourinary system. Activation of these receptors increases intracellular calcium ion concentration, which leads to muscle contraction. Thus, α_1-agonists are associated with mydriasis (pupillary dilation due to contraction of the radial eye muscles), bronchoconstriction, vaso-constriction, uterine contracture, and contraction of sphincters in the gastrointestinal and genitourinary tracts. α_1-Stimulation also inhibits insulin secretion and lipolysis. The myocardium may possess α_1-receptors that have slightly positive inotropic and negative chronotropic effects. Nonetheless, the most important cardiovascular effect of α_1-stimulation is vasoconstriction, which increases peripheral vascular resistance, left ventricular afterload, and arterial blood pressure.

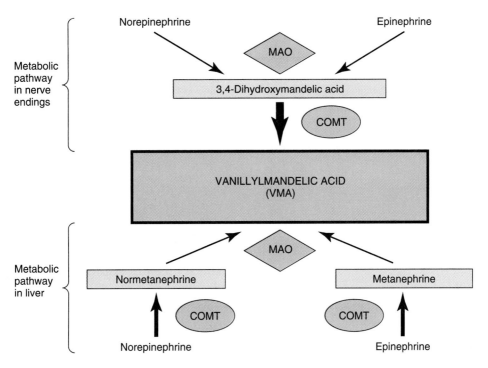

Figure 12–3. Sequential metabolism of norepinephrine and epinephrine. Monoamine oxidase (MAO) and catechol-O-methyltrasnferase (COMT) produce a common end product, vanillylmandelic acid (VMA).

α₂-Receptors

In contrast to α₁-receptors, α₂-receptors are located chiefly on the presynaptic nerve terminals. Activation of these adrenoceptors inhibits adenylate cyclase activity. This decreases the entry of calcium ions into the neuronal terminal, which limits subsequent exocytosis of storage vesicles containing norepinephrine. Thus, α₂-receptors create a negative feedback loop that inhibits further norepinephrine release from the neuron. In addition, vascular smooth muscle contains postsynaptic α₂-receptors that produce vasoconstriction. More important, stimulation of postsynaptic α₂-receptors in the central nervous system causes sedation and reduces sympathetic outflow, which leads to peripheral vasodilation and lower blood pressure.

β₁-Receptors

The most important β₁-receptors are located on postsynaptic membranes in the heart. Stimulation of these receptors activates adenylate cyclase, which converts adenosine triphosphate to cyclic adenosine monophosphate and initiates a kinase phosphorylation cascade. Initiation of the cascade has positive **chronotropic** (in-creased heart rate), **dromotropic** (increased conduction), and **inotropic** (increased contractilty) effects.

β₂-Receptors

β₂-Receptors are chiefly postsynaptic adrenoceptors located in smooth muscle and gland cells. They share a common mechanism of action with β₁-receptors: adenylate cyclase activation. Despite this commonality, β₂-stimulation relaxes smooth muscle, resulting in bronchodilation, vasodilation, and relaxation of the uterus (tocolysis), bladder, and gut. Glycogenolysis, lipolysis, gluconeogenesis, and insulin release are stimulated by β₂-receptor activation. β₂-Agonists also activate the sodium-potassium pump, which drives potassium intracellularly and can induce hypokalemia and dysrhythmias.

■ ADRENERGIC AGONISTS

Adrenergic agonists interact with varying specificity (selectivity) at α- and β-adrenoceptors (Table 12–1). Overlapping of activity complicates the prediction of

Table 12–1. Receptor selectivity of adrenergic agonists.

Drug	α_1	α_2	β_1	β_2	DA$_1$	DA$_2$
Phenylephrine	+++	+	+	0	0	0
Methyldopa	+	+++	0	0	0	0
Clonidine	+	+++	0	0	0	0
Epinephrine[1]	++	++	+++	++	0	0
Ephedrine[2]	++	?	++	+	0	0
Fenoldopam	0	0	0	0	+++	0
Norepinephrine[1]	++	++	++	0	0	0
Dopamine[1]	++	++	++	+	+++	+++
Dopexamine	0	0	+	+++	++	+++
Dobutamine	0/+	0	+++	+	0	0
Terbutaline	0	0	+	+++	0	0

[1]The α_1 effects of epinephrine, norepinephrine, and dopamine become more prominent at high doses.
[2]The primary mode of action of ephedrine is indirect stimulation.
  0 = no effect.
  + = agonist effect (mild, moderate, marked).
  ? = unknown effect.
DA$_1$ and DA$_2$ = dopaminergic receptors.

clinical effects. For example, epinephrine stimulates α_1-, α_2-, β_1-, and β_2-adrenoceptors. Its net effect on arterial blood pressure depends on the balance between α_1-vasoconstriction, α_2- and β_2-vasodilation, and β_1-inotropic influences. Moreover, this balance changes at different doses.

Adrenergic agonists can also be categorized as direct or indirect. **Direct agonists** bind to the receptor, while **indirect agonists** increase endogenous neurotransmitter activity. Mechanisms of indirect action include increased release or decreased reuptake of norepinephrine. The differentiation between direct and indirect mechanisms of action is particularly important in patients who have abnormal endogenous norepinephrine stores, as may occur with use of some antihypertensive medications or monoamine oxidase inhibitors. Intraoperative hypotension in these patients should be treated with direct agonists, since their response to indirect agonists will be altered.

Another feature distinguishing adrenergic agonists from each other is their chemical structure. Adrenergic agonists that have a 3,4-dihydroxybenzene structure (Figure 12–4) are known as catecholamines. These drugs are typically short-acting because of their metabolism by monoamine oxidase and catechol-O-methyltransferase. Patients taking monoamine oxidase in-

hibitors or tricyclic antidepressants may therefore demonstrate an exaggerated response to catecholamines. The naturally occurring catecholamines are epinephrine, norepinephrine, and dopamine (DA). Changing the side-chain structure (R_1, R_2, R_3) of naturally occurring catecholamines has led to the development of synthetic catecholamines (eg, isoproterenol and dobutamine), which tend to be more receptor-specific.

Adrenergic agonists commonly used in anesthesiology are discussed individually below. Note that the recommended doses for continuous infusion are expressed as μg/kg/min for some agents and μg/min for others. In either case, these recommendations should be regarded only as guidelines, since individual responses are quite variable.

PHENYLEPHRINE

Clinical Considerations

Phenylephrine is a noncatecholamine with predominantly direct α_1-agonist activity; (high doses may stimulate α_2- and β-receptors). Its primary effect is peripheral vasoconstriction with a concomitant rise in systemic vascular resistance and arterial blood pressure. Reflex bradycardia can reduce cardiac output. Coronary blood flow increases because any direct vasoconstrictive effect of phenylephrine on the coronary arteries is overridden by vasodilation induced by the release of metabolic factors (Table 12–2).

Dosage & Packaging

Small intravenous boluses of 50–100 μg (0.5–1 μg/kg) of phenylephrine rapidly reverse blood pressure reductions caused by peripheral vasodilation (eg, spinal anesthesia). A continuous infusion (100 μg/mL at a rate of 0.25–1 μg/kg/min) will maintain arterial blood pressure but at the expense of renal blood flow. Tachyphylaxis occurs with phenylephrine infusions requiring up-

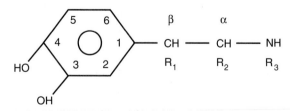

Figure 12–4. Adrenergic agonists that have a 3,4-dihydroxybenzene structure are known as catecholamines. Substitutions at the R_1, R_2, and R_3 sites affect activity and selectivity.

Table 12–2. Effects of adrenergic agonists on organ systems.

Drug	Heart Rate	Mean Arterial Pressure	Cardiac Output	Peripheral Vascular Resistance	Bronchodilation	Renal Blood Flow
Phenylephrine	↓	↑↑↑	↓	↑↑↑	0	↓↓↓
Epinephrine	↑↑	↑	↑↑	↑/↓	↑↑	↓↓
Ephedrine	↑↑	↑↑	↑↑	↑	↑↑	↓↓
Fenoldopam	↑↑	↓/↓↓	↓/↑	↓↓	0	↑↑↑
Norepinephrine	↓	↑↑↑	↓/↑	↑↑↑	0	↓↓↓
Dopamine	↑/↑↑	↑	↑↑↑	↑	0	↑↑↑
Dopexamine	↑/↑↑	↓/↑	↑↑	↑	0	↑
Isoproterenol	↑↑↑	↓	↑↑↑	↓↓	↑↑↑	↓/↑
Dobutamine	↑	↑	↑↑↑	↓	0	↑

0 = no effect.
↑ = increase (mild, moderate, marked).
↓ = decrease (mild, moderate, marked).
↓/↑ = variable effect.
↑/↑↑ = mild-to-moderate increase.

ward titration of the infusion. Phenylephrine must be diluted from a 1% solution (10 mg/1 mL ampule), usually to a 100 µg/mL solution.

α_2-AGONISTS

Clinical Considerations

Methyldopa, a prototypical drug, is an analogue of levodopa. Methyldopa enters the norepinephrine-synthesis pathway and is converted to α-methylnorepinephrine and α-methylepinephrine. These false transmitters activate α-adrenoceptors, particularly central α_2-receptors. As a result, norepinephrine release and sympathetic tone are diminished. A fall in peripheral vascular resistance is responsible for a drop in arterial blood pressure (peak effect within 4 hours). Renal blood flow is maintained or increased. Because methyldopa relies on metabolites to be effective, it is being replaced by drugs with direct α_2-activity, although it is still recommended for treating high blood pressure in pregnancy.

Clonidine is an α_2-agonist that is now commonly used for its antihypertensive (decreased systemic vascular resistance) and negative chronotropic effects. More recently, it and other α_2-agonists have been found to have sedative properties. Investigational studies have examined the anesthetic effects of oral (3–5 µg/kg), intramuscular (2 µg/kg), intravenous (1–3 µg/kg), transdermal (0.1–0.3 mg released per day), intrathecal (75–150 µg), and epidural (1–2 µg/kg) clonidine administra-

tion. In general, clonidine appears to decrease anesthetic and analgesic requirements and to provide sedation and anxiolysis. During general anesthesia, clonidine reportedly enhances intraoperative circulatory stability by reducing catecholamine levels. During regional anesthesia, including peripheral nerve block, clonidine prolongs the duration of the block. Direct effects on the spinal cord may be mediated by α_2-postsynaptic receptors within the dorsal horn. Other possible benefits include decreased postoperative shivering, inhibition of opioid-induced muscle rigidity, attenuation of opioid withdrawal symptoms, and the treatment of some chronic pain syndromes. Side effects include bradycardia, hypotension, sedation, respiratory depression, and dry mouth.

Dexmedetomidine is a novel lipophylic α-methylol derivative with a higher affinity for α_2-receptors than clonidine. It has sedative, analgesic, and sympatholytic effects that blunt many of the cardiovascular responses (hypertension, tachycardia) seen during the perioperative period. When used intraoperatively, it reduces intravenous and volatile anesthetic requirements; when used postoperatively, it reduces concurrent analgesic and sedative requirements. Patients remain sedated when undisturbed but arouse readily with stimulation. Similar to methyldopa and clonidine, dexmedetomidine is a **sympatholytic** because sympathetic outflow is reduced. It may be a useful agent for decreasing intraoperative anesthetic requirements and for sedating ventilated patients postoperatively in the postanesthesia care unit and in the intensive care unit because of its anxiolytic and analgesic effects. It does so without significant ventilatory depression. Rapid administration may elevate blood pressure, but hypotension and bradycardia may occur during ongoing therapy.

Although methyldopa and clonidine are adrenergic agonists, they are also considered to be **sympatholytic** because sympathetic outflow is reduced.

Dosage & Packaging

Clonidine is available as an oral, transdermal, or parenteral preparation (see Clinical Considerations in the α_2-Agonists section for dosages). The latter is approved only for epidural or intrathecal use as an adjunct to regional analgesia/anesthesia. However, it is widely used in Europe at an intravenous bolus dose of 50 μg for blood pressure or heart rate control. It has a slow onset of action.

EPINEPHRINE

Clinical Considerations

Direct stimulation of β_1-receptors by epinephrine raises cardiac output and myocardial oxygen demand by increasing contractility and heart rate (increased rate of spontaneous phase IV depolarization). α_1-Stimulation decreases splanchnic and renal blood flow but increases coronary and cerebral perfusion pressure. Systolic blood pressure rises, although β_2-mediated vasodilation in skeletal muscle may lower diastolic pressure. β_2-Stimulation also relaxes bronchial smooth muscle.

Epinephrine administration is the principal pharmacologic treatment for anaphylaxis and can be used to treat ventricular fibrillation (see Chapters 47 and 48). Complications of epinephrine administration include cerebral hemorrhage, coronary ischemia, and ventricular dysrhythmias. Volatile anesthetics, particularly halothane, potentiate the dysrhythmic effects of epinephrine.

Dosage & Packaging

In emergency situations (eg, shock and allergic reactions), epinephrine is administered as an intravenous bolus of 0.05–1 mg depending on the severity of cardiovascular compromise. To improve myocardial contractility or heart rate, a continuous infusion is prepared (1 mg in 250 mL D_5W [4 μg/mL]) and run at a rate of 2–20 μg/min. Some local anesthetic solutions containing epinephrine at a concentration of 1:200,000 (5 μg/mL) or 1:100,000 (10 μg/mL) are characterized by less systemic absorption and a longer duration of action. Epinephrine is available in vials at a concentration of 1:1000 (1 mg/mL) and prefilled syringes at a concentration of 1:10,000 (0.1 mg/mL [100 μg/mL]). A 1:100,000 (10 μg/mL) concentration is available for pediatric use.

EPHEDRINE

Clinical Considerations

The cardiovascular effects of ephedrine are similar to those of epinephrine: increase in blood pressure, heart rate, contractility, and cardiac output. Likewise, ephedrine is also a bronchodilator. There are important differences, however: ephedrine has a longer duration of action because it is a noncatecholamine, is much less potent, has indirect and direct actions, and stimulates the central nervous system (it raises minimum alveolar concentration). The indirect agonist properties of ephedrine may be due to central stimulation, peripheral postsynaptic norepinephrine release, or inhibition of norepinephrine reuptake.

 Ephedrine is commonly used as a vasopressor during anesthesia. As such, its administration should be viewed as a temporizing measure while the cause of hypotension is determined and remedied. Unlike direct-acting α_1-agonists, ephedrine does not decrease uterine blood flow. This makes it the preferred vasopressor for most obstetric uses. Ephedrine has also been reported to possess antiemetic properties, particularly in association with hypotension following spinal anesthesia. Clonidine premedication augments the effects of ephedrine.

Dosage & Packaging

In adults, ephedrine is administered as a bolus of 2.5–10 mg; in children it is given as a bolus of 0.1 mg/kg. Subsequent doses are increased to offset the development of tachyphylaxis, which is probably due to depletion of norepinephrine stores. Ephedrine is available in 1-mL ampules containing 25 or 50 mg of the agent.

NOREPINEPHRINE

Clinical Considerations

Direct α_1-stimulation in the absence of β_2-activity induces intense vasoconstriction of arterial and venous vessels. Increased myocardial contractility from β_1-effects may contribute to a rise in arterial blood pressure, but increased afterload and reflex bradycardia prevent any elevation in cardiac output. Decreased renal blood flow and increased myocardial oxygen requirements limit the usefulness of norepinephrine to the treatment of refractory shock, which requires potent vasoconstriction to maintain tissue perfusion pressure.

Norepinephrine has been used with an α-blocker (eg, phentolamine) in an attempt to take advantage of its β-activity without the profound vasoconstriction caused by its α-stimulation. Extravasation of norepinephrine at the site of intravenous administration can cause tissue necrosis.

Dosage & Packaging

Norepinephrine is administered as a bolus (0.1 µg/kg) or as a continuous infusion (4 mg of drug to 500 mL D$_5$W [8 µg/mL]) at a rate of 2–20 µg/min. Ampules contain 4 mg of norepinephrine in 4 mL of solution.

DOPAMINE

Clinical Considerations

The clinical effects of DA, a nonselective direct and indirect adrenergic agonist, vary markedly with the dose. Small doses (≤ 2 µg/kg/min) have minimal adrenergic effects but activate dopaminergic receptors. Stimulation of these nonadrenergic receptors (specifically, DA$_1$ receptors) vasodilates the renal vasculature and promotes diuresis. At moderate doses (2–10 µg/kg/min), β$_1$-stimulation increases myocardial contractility, heart rate, and cardiac output. Myocardial oxygen demand typically increases more than supply. α$_1$-Effects become prominent at higher doses (10–20 µg/kg/min), causing an increase in peripheral vascular resistance and a fall in renal blood flow. The indirect effects of DA are due to release of norepinephrine, which it resembles at doses above 20 µg/kg/min.

DA is commonly used in the treatment of shock to improve cardiac output, support blood pressure, and maintain renal function. It is often used in combination with a vasodilator (eg, nitroglycerin or nitroprusside), which reduces afterload and further improves cardiac output (see Chapter 13). The chronotropic and dysrhythmogenic effects of DA limit its usefulness in some patients.

Dosage & Packaging

DA is administered as a continuous infusion (400 mg in 1000 mL D$_5$W; 400 µg/mL) at a rate of 1–20 µg/kg/min. It is most commonly supplied in 5-mL ampules containing 200 or 400 mg of DA.

ISOPROTERENOL

Isoproterenol is of interest because it is a pure β-agonist. β$_1$-Effects increase heart rate, contractility, and cardiac output. β$_2$-Stimulation decreases peripheral vascular resistance and diastolic blood pressure. Myocardial oxygen demand increases while oxygen supply falls,

making isoproterenol or any pure β-agonist a poor inotropic choice in most situations. Isoproterenol's availability is decreasing in the United States.

DOBUTAMINE

Clinical Considerations

Dobutamine is a relatively selective β$_1$-agonist. Its primary cardiovascular effect is a rise in cardiac output as a result of increased myocardial contractility. A slight decline in peripheral vascular resistance caused by β$_2$-activation usually prevents much of a rise in arterial blood pressure. Left ventricular filling pressure decreases, while coronary blood flow increases. Heart rate increases are less marked than with other β-agonists.

 These favorable effects on myocardial oxygen balance make dobutamine a good choice for patients with the combination of congestive heart failure and coronary artery disease, particularly if peripheral vascular resistance and heart rate are already elevated.

Dosage & Packaging

Dobutamine is administered as an infusion (1 g in 250 mL [4 mg/mL]) at a rate of 2–20 µg/kg/min. It is supplied in 20-mL vials containing 250 mg.

DOPEXAMINE

Clinical Considerations

Dopexamine is structural analogue of DA that has potential advantages over dopamine because it has less β$_1$-adrenergic (arrhythmogenic) and α-adrenergic effects. Because of the lesser β-adrenergic effects and its specific effect on renal perfusion, it may have advantages over dobutamine. The drug has been clinically available since 1990 but has not gained widespread acceptance in practice.

Dosage & Packaging

Dopexamine comes in a concentration of 50 mg/mL and should be diluted in D$_5$W. The infusion should be started at a rate of 0.5 µg/kg/min, increasing to 1 µg/kg/min at intervals of 10 to 15 minutes to a maximum infusion rate of 6 µg/kg/min.

FENOLDOPAM

Clinical Considerations

Fenoldopam is a selective DA$_1$-receptor agonist that has many of the benefits of DA but with little or no α- or β-adrenoceptor or DA$_2$-receptor agonist activity. Fenoldopam has been shown to exert hypotensive effects characterized by a decrease in peripheral vascular resistance, along with an increase in renal blood flow, diuresis, and natriuresis. It is indicated for patients undergoing cardiac surgery and aortic aneurysm repair, because of its antihypertensive and renal sparing properties. It is also indicated for patients who have severe hypertension, particularly those with renal impairment.

Dosage & Packaging

Fenoldopam is supplied in 1-, 2-, and 5-mL ampules, 10 mg/mL. It is started as a continuous infusion of 0.1 μg/kg/min, increased by increments of 0.1 μg/kg/min at 15- to 20-minute intervals until target blood pressure is achieved. Lower doses have been associated with less reflex tachycardia.

■ ADRENERGIC ANTAGONISTS

Adrenergic antagonists bind but do not activate adrenoceptors. They act by preventing adrenergic agonist activity. Like the agonists, the antagonists differ in their spectrum of receptor interaction (Table 12–3).

α-BLOCKERS—PHENTOLAMINE

Clinical Considerations

Phentolamine produces a competitive (reversible) blockade of α-receptors. α_1-Antagonism and direct smooth muscle relaxation are responsible for peripheral vasodilation and a decline in arterial blood pressure. The drop in blood pressure provokes reflex tachycardia. This tachycardia is augmented by antagonism of α_2-receptors in the heart because α_2-blockade promotes norepinephrine release by eliminating negative feedback. These cardiovascular effects are usually apparent within 2 minutes and last up to 15 minutes. As with all of the adrenergic antagonists, the extent of the response to receptor blockade depends on the degree of existing sympathetic tone. Reflex tachycardia and postural hypotension limit the usefulness of phentolamine to the treatment of hypertension caused by excessive α-stimulation (eg, pheochromocytoma, clonidine withdrawal).

Dosage & Packaging

Phentolamine is administered intravenously as intermittent boluses (1–5 mg in adults) or as a continuous infusion (10 mg in 100 mL D_5W [100 μg/mL]). To prevent tissue necrosis following extravasation of intra-

Table 12–3. Receptor selectivity of adrenergic antagonists.

Drug	α_1	α_1	β_1	β_2
Prazosin	–	0	0	0
Phenoxybenzamine	–	–	0	0
Phentolamine	–	–	0	0
Labetalol*	–	0	–	–
Metoprolol	0	0	–	–
Esmolol	0	0	–	–
Propranolol	0	0	–	–

*Labetalol may also have some β_2-agonist activity.
0 = no effect.
– = antagonist effect (mild, moderate, marked).

venous fluids containing an α-agonist (eg, norepinephrine), 5–10 mg of phentolamine in 10 mL of normal saline can be locally infiltrated. Phentolamine is packaged as a lyophilized powder (5 mg).

MIXED ANTAGONISTS—LABETALOL

Clinical Considerations

Labetalol blocks α_1-, β_1-, and β_2-receptors. The ratio of α-blockade to β-blockade has been estimated to be approximately 1:7 following intravenous administration. This mixed blockade reduces peripheral vascular resistance and arterial blood pressure. Heart rate and cardiac output are usually slightly depressed or unchanged. Thus, labetalol lowers blood pressure without reflex tachycardia because of its combination of α- and β- effects. Peak effect usually occurs within 5 minutes after an intravenous dose. Left ventricular failure, paradoxic hypertension, and bronchospasm have been reported.

Dosage & Packaging

The initial recommended dose of labetalol is 0.1–0.25 mg/kg administered intravenously over 2 minutes. Twice this amount may be given at 10-minute intervals until the desired blood pressure response is obtained. Labetalol can also be administered as a slow continuous infusion (200 mg in 250 mL D_5W) at a rate of 2 mg/min. However, owing to its long elimination half-life (> 5 hours), prolonged infusions are not recommended. Labetalol (5 mg/mL) is available in 20- and 40-mL multidose containers, and in 4- and 8-mL single-dose prefilled syringes.

β-BLOCKERS

β-Receptor blockers have variable degrees of selectivity for the β_1-receptors. Those that are more β_1-selective have less influence on bronchopulmonary and vascular β_2-receptors (Table 12–4). Theoretically, a selective β_1-blocker would have less of an inhibitory effect on β_2-receptors and, therefore, might be preferred in patients with chronic obstructive lung disease or peripheral vascular disease. Patients with peripheral vascular disease could potentially have a decrease in blood flow if β_2-receptors, which are dilating the arterioles, are blocked.

β-Blockers are also classified by the amount of intrinsic sympathomimetic activity (ISA) they have. Many of the β-blockers have some slight agonist activity; although they would not produce effects similar to full agonists, such as epinephrine, β-blockers with ISA may not be as beneficial as β-blockers without ISA in treating patients with cardiovascular disease.

β-Blockers can be further classified by those that are eliminated by hepatic metabolism (such as atenolol or metoprolol), those that are excreted by the kidneys unchanged (such as atenolol), or those that are hydrolyzed in the blood (such as esmolol).

ESMOLOL

Clinical Considerations

Esmolol is an ultra-short-acting selective β_1-antagonist that reduces heart rate and, to a lesser extent, blood pressure. It has been successfully used to prevent tachycardia and hypertension in response to perioperative stimuli, such as intubation, surgical stimulation, and emergence. For example, esmolol (1 mg/kg) attenuates the rise in blood pressure and heart rate that usually accompanies electroconvulsive therapy, without affecting seizure duration. Esmolol is as effective as propranolol in controlling the ventricular rate of patients with atrial fibrillation or flutter. Although esmolol is considered to be cardioselective, at higher doses it inhibits β_2-receptors in bronchial and vascular smooth muscle.

Its short duration of action is due to rapid redistribution (distribution half-life is 2 minutes) and hydrolysis by red blood cell esterase (elimination half-life is 9 minutes). Side effects can be reversed within minutes by discontinuing its infusion. As with all β_1-antagonists, esmolol should be avoided in patients with sinus bradycardia, heart block greater than first-degree, cardiogenic shock, or overt heart failure.

Dosage & Packaging

Esmolol is administered as a bolus (0.2–0.5 mg/kg) for short-term therapy, such as attenuating the cardiovascular response to laryngoscopy and intubation. Long-term treatment is typically initiated with a loading dose of 0.5 mg/kg administered over 1 minute, followed by a continuous infusion of 50 μg/kg/min to maintain the therapeutic effect. If this fails to produce a sufficient response within 5 minutes, the loading dose may be repeated and the infusion increased by increments of 50 μg/kg/min every 5 minutes to a maximum of 200 μg/kg/min.

Esmolol is supplied as multidose vials for bolus administration containing 10 mL of drug (10 mg/mL). Ampules for continuous infusion (2.5 g in 10 mL) are also available but must be diluted prior to administration to a concentration of 10 mg/mL.

PROPRANOLOL

Clinical Considerations

Propranolol nonselectively blocks β_1- and β_2-receptors. Arterial blood pressure is lowered by several mechanisms, including decreased myocardial contractility, lowered heart rate, and diminished renin release. Car-

Table 12–4. Pharmacology of β-blockers.

	Selectivity for β_1-Receptors	ISA	α_2 Blockade	Hepatic Metabolism	$T^{1/2}$
Atenolol	+	0	0	0	6–7
Esmolol	+	0	0	0	$-\frac{1}{4}$
Labetalol	0	0	+	+	4
Metoprolol	+	0	0	+	3–4
Propranolol	0	0	0	+	4–6

ISA = intrinsic sympathomimetic activity.
+ = mild effect.
0 = no effect.

diac output and myocardial oxygen demand are reduced. Propranolol is particularly useful during myocardial ischemia related to increased blood pressure and heart rate. Impedance of ventricular ejection is beneficial in patients with obstructive cardiomyopathy and aortic aneurysm. Propranolol slows atrioventricular conduction and stabilizes myocardial membranes, although the latter effect may not be significant at clinical doses. Propranolol is particularly effective in slowing the ventricular response to supraventricular tachycardia, and it occasionally controls recurrent ventricular tachycardia or fibrillation caused by myocardial ischemia. Propranolol blocks the β-adrenergic effects of thyrotoxicosis and pheochromocytoma.

Side effects include bronchospasm (β$_2$-antagonism), congestive heart failure, bradycardia, and atrioventricular heart block (β$_1$-antagonism). Propranolol may worsen the myocardial depression of volatile anesthetics (eg, enflurane) or unmask the negative inotropic characteristics of indirect cardiac stimulants (eg, isoflurane). Concomitant administration of propranolol and verapamil (a calcium channel blocker) can synergistically depress heart rate, contractility, and atrioventricular node conduction. Discontinuation of propranolol therapy for 24–48 hours may trigger a withdrawal syndrome characterized by hypertension, tachycardia, and angina pectoris. This effect appears to be caused by an increase in the number of β-adrenergic receptors (**up-regulation**). Propranolol is extensively protein-bound and is cleared by hepatic metabolism. Its elimination half-life of 100 minutes is quite long compared with that of esmolol.

Dosage & Packaging

Individual dosage requirements of propranolol depend on baseline sympathetic tone. Generally, propranolol is titrated to the desired effect, beginning with 0.5 mg and progressing by 0.5 mg increments every 3–5 minutes. Total doses rarely exceed 0.15 mg/kg. Propranolol is supplied in 1-mL ampules containing 1 mg.

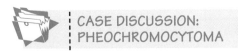

CASE DISCUSSION: PHEOCHROMOCYTOMA

A 45-year-old man with a history of paroxysmal attacks of headache, hypertension, sweating, and palpitations is scheduled for resection of an abdominal pheochromocytoma.

What is a pheochromocytoma?

A pheochromocytoma is a vascular tumor of chromaffin tissue (most commonly the adrenal medulla) that produces and secretes norepineph-

rine and epinephrine. The diagnosis and management of pheochromocytoma are based on the effects of abnormally high circulating levels of these endogenous adrenergic agonists.

How is the diagnosis of pheochromocytoma made in the laboratory?

Urinary excretion of vanillylmandelic acid (an end product of catecholamine metabolism), norepinephrine, and epinephrine are often markedly increased. Elevated levels of urinary normetanephrines and metanephrines (Figure 12–3) provide a highly accurate diagnosis. The total plasma concentration of catecholamines may also be elevated. The location of the tumor can be determined by magnetic resonance imaging, computed tomographic scan, ultrasound, or scintigraphy.

What pathophysiology is associated with chronic elevations of norepinephrine and epinephrine?

α$_1$-Stimulation increases peripheral vascular resistance and arterial blood pressure. Hypertension can lead to intravascular volume depletion (increasing hematocrit), renal failure, and cerebral hemorrhage. Elevated peripheral vascular resistance also increases myocardial work, which predisposes patients to myocardial ischemia, ventricular hypertrophy, and congestive heart failure. Prolonged exposure to epinephrine and norepinephrine may lead to a catecholamine-induced cardiomyopathy. Hyperglycemia results from decreased insulin secretion in the face of increased glycogenolysis and gluconeogenesis. β$_1$-Stimulation increases automaticity and ventricular ectopy.

Which adrenergic antagonists might be helpful in controlling the effects of norepinephrine and epinephrine hypersecretion?

***Phenoxybenzamine,** an α$_1$-antagonist (see Table 12–3), effectively reverses the vasoconstriction, resulting in a drop in arterial blood pressure and an increase in intravascular volume (hematocrit drops). Glucose intolerance is often corrected. Phenoxybenzamine can be administered orally and is longer-acting than phentolamine, another α$_1$-antagonist. For these reasons, phenoxybenzamine is often administered preoperatively to control symptoms.*

Intravenous phentolamine is often used intraoperatively to control hypertensive episodes. Compared with some other hypotensive agents (see Chapter 13), however, phentolamine has a slow onset and long duration of action; furthermore, tachyphylaxis often develops.

β_1-Blockade with an agent such as labetalol is recommended for patients with tachycardia or ventricular dysrhythmias.

Why should α_1-receptors be blocked with phenoxybenzamine before administration of a β-antagonist?

If β-receptors are blocked first, norepinephrine and epinephrine will produce unopposed α-stimulation. β_2-Mediated vasodilation will not be able to offset α_1-vasoconstriction, and peripheral vascular resistance would increase. This may explain the paradoxic hypertension that has been reported in a few patients with pheochromocytoma treated only with labetalol. Finally, the myocardium might not be able to handle its already elevated workload without the inotropic effects of β_1-stimulation.

Which anesthetic agents should be specifically avoided?

Succinylcholine-induced fasciculations of the abdominal musculature will increase intra-abdominal pressure, which might cause release of catecholamines from the tumor. Ketamine is a sympathomimetic and would exacerbate the effects of adrenergic agonists. Halothane sensitizes the myocardium to the dysrhythmogenic effects of epinephrine. Vagolytic drugs (eg, anticholinergics and pancuronium) will worsen the imbalance of autonomic tone. Since histamine provokes catecholamine secretion by the tumor, drugs associated with histamine release (eg, tubocurarine, atracurium, morphine sulfate, and meperidine) are best avoided. Vecuronium, rocuronium, and pipecuronium are probably the muscle relaxants of choice. Although droperidol is an α-antagonist, it has been associated with hypertensive crises in some patients with pheochromocytoma.

Would an epidural or spinal technique effectively block sympathetic hyperactivity?

A major regional block—such as an epidural or spinal anesthetic—could block sensory (afferent) nerves and sympathetic (efferent) discharge in the area of the surgical field. The catecholamines released from a pheochromocytoma during surgical manipulation would still be able to bind and activate adrenergic receptors throughout the body, however. Therefore, these regional techniques cannot block the sympathetic hyperactivity associated with pheochromocytoma, which is further discussed in Chapter 36.

SUGGESTED READING

Bonet S, Agusti A, Arnau JM, et al: β-Adrenergic blocking agents in heart failure: Benefits of vasodilating and nonvasodilating agents according to patients' characteristics: A meta-analysis of clinical trials. Arch Intern Med 2000;160:621.

Chernow B: *Critical Care Pharmacotherapy,* Williams & Wilkins, 1995.

Ebert TJ: Is gaining control of the autonomic nervous system important to our specialty? Anesthesiology 1999;90:651.

Kamibayashi T, Harasawa K, Maze T: Alpha-2 adrenergic agonists. Can J Anaesth 1997;44:R13.

Moss J, Renz C: The autonomic nervous system. Chapter 14 in: *Anesthesia,* 5th ed. Miller RD (editor). Churchill Livingstone, 2000. Excellent discussion of the autonomic nervous system and drugs with adrenergic activity.

Piper SN, Boldt J, Schmidt CC, et al: Influence of dopexamine on hemodynamics, intramucosal pH, and regulators of the macrocirculation and microcirculation in patients undergoing abdominal aortic surgery. J Cardiothorac Vasc Anesth 2000;14:281.

Schwinn DA: Cardiac pharmacology. Chapter 2 in: *Cardiac Anesthesia: Principles and Clinical Practice.* Estafanous FG, Barash PG, Reves JG (editors). JB Lippincott, 1994. A succinct discussion of adrenergic receptors, cardiac medications, and their use in the acute and chronic setting.

Stoelting RK: *Pharmacology and Physiology in Anesthetic Practice,* 3rd ed. Lippincott-Raven, 1999. Chapter 12 contains an excellent review and discussion of sympathomimetic drugs. Chapter 14 contains an excellent summary of the α- and β-adrenergic receptor antagonists and blockers. Chapter 42 reviews the physiology of the autonomic nervous system.

Hypotensive Agents

13

A multitude of drugs are capable of lowering blood pressure, including volatile anesthetics (see Chapter 7) and sympathetic antagonists (see Chapter 12). This chapter examines six additional agents that may be useful to the anesthesiologist for intraoperative control of arterial blood pressure: sodium nitroprusside, nitroglycerin, hydralazine, trimethaphan, adenosine, and fenoldopam (Figure 13–1 and Table 13–1). Although all these drugs lower blood pressure by dilating peripheral vessels, they are not identical in their mechanisms

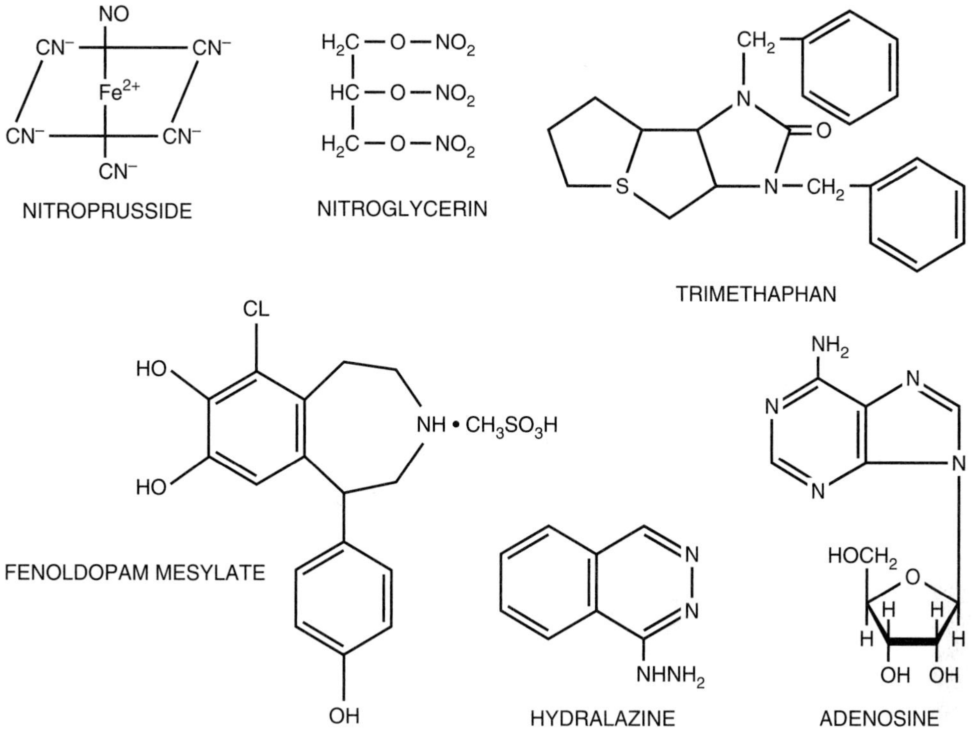

Figure 13–1. Structures of hypotensive agents.

of action, clinical uses, routes of metabolism, effects on organ systems, or drug interactions.

SODIUM NITROPRUSSIDE

Mechanism of Action

Sodium nitroprusside relaxes both arteriolar and venous smooth muscle. Its primary mechanism of action is shared with other nitrates (eg, hydralazine and nitroglycerin). These drugs form **nitric oxide,** which activates guanylyl cyclase. This enzyme is responsible for the synthesis of guanosine 3′,5′-monophosphate (cGMP), which controls the phosphorylation of several proteins, including some involved in control of free intracellular calcium and smooth muscle contraction.

Nitric oxide, a naturally occurring potent vasodilator released by endothelial cells (endothelium-derived relaxing factor), plays an important role in regulating vascular tone throughout the body. Its ultrashort half-life (< 5 sec) provides sensitive endogenous control of regional blood flow. Clinical trials have shown *inhaled* nitric oxide to be a selective pulmonary vasodilator that may be bene-

ficial in the treatment of reversible pulmonary hypertension. By improving perfusion only in ventilated areas of the lung, inhaled nitric oxide may improve oxygenation in patients with acute respiratory distress syndrome or during one-lung ventilation (see Chapter 24). Nitric oxide may also have anti-inflammatory effects that could promote lung healing.

Clinical Uses

Sodium nitroprusside is a potent and reliable antihypertensive. It is usually diluted to a concentration of 100 μg/mL and administered as a continuous intravenous infusion (0.5–10 μg/kg/min). Its extremely rapid onset of action (1–2 minutes) and fleeting duration of action allow precise titration of arterial blood pressure. A bolus of 1–2 μg/kg minimizes blood pressure elevation during laryngoscopy but can cause transient hypotension in some patients. The potency of this drug requires frequent blood pressure measurements—or, preferably, intra-arterial monitoring—and the use of mechanical infusion pumps. Solutions of sodium nitroprusside must be protected from light because of photodegradation.

Table 13–1. Comparative pharmacology of hypotensive agents.

	Nitroprusside	Nitroglycerin	Hydralazine	Trimethaphan	Adenosine	Fenoldopam
Organ effects						
Heart rate	↑↑	↑	↑↑↑	↑	↑	↑↑
Preload	↓↓	↓↓↓	0	↓↓	0	?
Afterload	↓↓↓	↓↓	↓↓↓	↓↓	↓↓	↓↓
Cerebral blood flow, intracranial pressure	↑↑	↑↑	↑↑	0	↑↑	?
Kinetics						
Onset	1 min	1 min	5–10 min	3 min	< 1 min	< 15 min
Duration	5 min	5 min	2–4 hours	10 min	1 min	1 hour
Metabolism	Blood, kidney	Blood, liver	Liver	Blood?	Blood	Liver
Dose						
Bolus	50–100 μg	50–100 μg	5–20 mg	NA	6–12 mg	NA
Infusion (μg/kg/min)	0.5–10	0.5–10	0.25–1.5	10–100	60–120	0.01–1.6
Relative cost*	Low	Low	Low	Moderate	High	Very high

0 = no change.
↑ = increase (slight, moderate, marked).
↓ = decrease (slight, moderate, marked).
? = Incomplete data or variable results reported.
NA = not applicable.
*Based on cost of 1-hour infusion.

Metabolism

After parenteral injection, sodium nitroprusside enters red blood cells, where it receives an electron from the iron of oxyhemoglobin (Fe^{2+}). This nonenzymatic electron transfer results in an unstable nitroprusside radical and methemoglobin (Fe^{3+}). The former moiety spontaneously decomposes into five cyanide ions and the active nitroso (N=O) group.

The cyanide ions can be involved in one of three possible reactions: binding to methemoglobin to form cyanmethemoglobin; undergoing a reaction in the liver and kidney catalyzed by the enzyme rhodanase (thiosulfate + cyanide → thiocyanate); or binding to tissue cytochrome oxidase, which interferes with normal oxygen utilization (Figure 13–2).

The last of these reactions is responsible for the development of acute cyanide toxicity, which is characterized by metabolic acidosis, cardiac dysrhythmias, and increased venous oxygen content (as a result of the inability to metabolize oxygen). Another early sign of cyanide toxicity is the acute resistance to the hypotensive effects of increasing doses of sodium nitroprusside (**tachyphylaxis**). It should be noted that tachyphylaxis implies acute tolerance to the drug following multiple rapid injections, as opposed to **tolerance,** which is caused by more chronic exposure. Cyanide toxicity can usually be avoided if the cumulative dose of sodium nitroprusside is less than 0.5 mg/kg/hour. Patients with cyanide toxicity should be mechanically ventilated with 100% oxygen to maximize oxygen availability. The pharmacologic treatment of cyanide toxicity depends on increasing the kinetics of the two reactions by administering sodium thiosulfate (150 mg/kg over 15 minutes) or 3% sodium nitrate (5 mg/kg over 5 minutes), which oxidizes hemoglobin to methemoglobin. Hydroxocobalamin, an experimental drug, combines with cyanide to form cyanocobalamin (vitamin B_{12}).

SNP + Oxyhemoglobin ⟶ $(SNP)^-$ + Methemoglobin
$(SNP)^-$ ⟶ $5CN^-$

CN^- + Methemoglobin ⟶ Cyanmethemoglobin

or

CN^- + Thiosulfate ⟶ (Rhodanase, vitamin B_{12}) Thiocyanate

or

CN^- + Cytochrome oxidase ⟶ Cyanide toxicity

Figure 13–2. The metabolism of sodium nitroprusside.

Thiocyanate is slowly cleared by the kidney. Accumulation of large amounts of thiocyanate (eg, in patients with renal failure) may result in a milder toxic reaction that includes thyroid dysfunction, muscle weakness, nausea, hypoxia, and an acute toxic psychosis. The risk of cyanide toxicity is not increased by renal failure, however. Methemoglobinemia from excessive doses of sodium nitroprusside or sodium nitrate can be treated with methylene blue (1–2 mg/kg of a 1% solution over 5 minutes), which reduces methemoglobin to hemoglobin.

Effects on Organ Systems

A. Cardiovascular:

The combined dilatation of venous and arteriolar vascular beds by sodium nitroprusside results in reductions of preload and afterload. Arterial blood pressure falls owing to the decrease in peripheral vascular resistance. Although cardiac output is usually unchanged in normal patients, the reduction in afterload may increase cardiac output in patients with congestive heart failure, mitral regurgitation, or aortic regurgitation. In contrast to the pure afterload reduction produced by hydralazine, sodium nitroprusside primarily reduces preload, which decreases myocardial work and the likelihood of ischemia. In opposition to any favorable changes in myocardial oxygen requirements are reflex-mediated responses to the fall in arterial blood pressure. These include tachycardia (less pronounced than with hydralazine) and increased myocardial contractility. In addition, dilatation of coronary arterioles by sodium nitroprusside may result in an intracoronary steal of blood flow away from ischemic areas that are already maximally dilated.

B. Cerebral:

Sodium nitroprusside dilates cerebral vessels and abolishes cerebral autoregulation. Cerebral blood flow is maintained or increases unless arterial blood pressure is markedly reduced. The resulting increase in cerebral blood volume tends to increase intracranial pressure, especially in patients with reduced intracranial compliance (eg, brain tumors). This intracranial hypertension can be minimized by slow administration of sodium nitroprusside and institution of hypocapnia.

C. Respiratory:

The pulmonary vasculature also dilates in response to sodium nitroprusside infusion. Reductions in pulmonary artery pressure may decrease the perfusion of some normally ventilated alveoli, increasing physiologic dead space. By dilating pulmonary vessels, sodium nitroprusside may prevent the normal vasoconstrictive response of the pulmonary vasculature to hypoxia (**hypoxic pulmonary vasoconstriction**). Both these effects tend to mismatch pulmonary ventilation to perfusion and decrease arterial oxygenation.

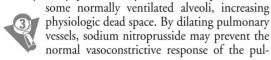

D. Renal:

In response to decreased arterial blood pressure, renin and catecholamines are released during nitroprusside administration. This hormonal response, which can lead to a pressure rebound after discontinuation of the drug, is blocked by propranolol or a high epidural block (T1 level). Renal function is fairly well maintained during sodium nitroprusside infusion despite moderate drops in arterial blood pressure and renal perfusion.

Drug Interactions

Sodium nitroprusside does not directly interact with muscle relaxants. Nonetheless, a decrease in muscle blood flow caused by arterial hypotension could indirectly delay the onset and prolong the duration of neuromuscular blockade. By inhibiting phosphodiesterase, aminophylline increases cGMP and potentiates the hypotensive effects of these agents.

NITROGLYCERIN

Mechanism of Action

Nitroglycerin relaxes vascular smooth muscle, with venous dilatation predominating over arterial dilatation. Its mechanism of action is presumably similar to sodium nitroprusside: metabolism to nitric oxide which activates guanylyl cyclase, leading to increased cGMP, decreased intracellular calcium, and vascular smooth muscle relaxation.

Clinical Uses

Nitroglycerin relieves myocardial ischemia, hypertension, and ventricular failure. Like sodium nitroprusside, nitroglycerin is commonly diluted to a concentration of 100 μg/mL and administered as a continuous intravenous infusion (0.5–10 μg/kg/min). Glass containers and special intravenous tubing are recommended because of the adsorption of nitroglycerin to polyvinylchloride. Nitroglycerin can also be administered by a sublingual (peak effect in 4 minutes) or transdermal (sustained release for 24 hours) route. Some patients appear to require higher than expected doses of nitroglycerin to achieve a given drop in blood pressure, particularly after chronic administration (tolerance). Tolerance may be due to depletion of reactants necessary for nitric oxide formation, compensatory secretion of vasoconstrictive substances, or volume expansion. Dosing regimens that provide for intermittent periods of low or no drug exposure may minimize the development of tolerance.

Metabolism

Nitroglycerin undergoes rapid reductive hydrolysis in the liver and blood by glutathione-organic nitrate reductase. One metabolic product is nitrite, which can covert hemoglobin (Fe^{2+}) to methemoglobin (Fe^{3+}). Significant methemoglobinemia is rare and can be treated with intravenous methylene blue (1–2 mg/kg over 5 minutes).

Effects on Organ Systems

A. CARDIOVASCULAR:

Nitroglycerin reduces myocardial oxygen demand and increases myocardial oxygen supply by several mechanisms:

- The pooling of blood in the large-capacitance vessels reduces venous return and preload. The accompanying decrease in ventricular end-diastolic pressure reduces myocardial oxygen demand and increases endocardial perfusion.
- Any afterload reduction from arteriolar dilatation will decrease both end-systolic pressure and oxygen demand. Of course, a fall in diastolic pressure may lower coronary perfusion pressure and actually decrease myocardial oxygen supply.
- Nitroglycerin redistributes coronary blood flow to ischemic areas of the subendocardium.
- Coronary artery spasm may be relieved.
- Nitroglycerin decreases platelet aggregation and may improve patency of coronary vessels.

 The beneficial effect of nitroglycerin in patients with coronary artery disease contrasts with the coronary steal phenomenon seen with sodium nitroprusside. A drop in preload decreases cardiac output in the absence of congestive heart failure. Preload reduction makes nitroglycerin an excellent drug for the relief of cardiogenic pulmonary edema. Heart rate is unchanged or minimally increased. Rebound hypertension is less likely after discontinuation of nitroglycerin than following discontinuation of sodium nitroprusside. The prophylactic administration of low-dose nitroglycerin (0.5–2.0 μg/kg/min) during anesthesia of patients at high risk for perioperative myocardial ischemia remains controversial.

B. CEREBRAL:

The effects of nitroglycerin on cerebral blood flow and intracranial pressure are similar to those of sodium ni-

troprusside. Headache from dilatation of cerebral vessels is a common side effect of nitroglycerin.

C. RESPIRATORY:

In addition to the dilating effects on the pulmonary vasculature (previously described for sodium nitroprusside), nitroglycerin relaxes bronchial smooth muscle.

D. OTHER:

Nitroglycerin (50–100 μg boluses) has been demonstrated to be an effective but transient uterine relaxant that can be beneficial during certain obstetrical procedures if the placenta is still present in the uterus (eg, retained placenta, uterine inversion, uterine tetany, breech extraction, and external version of the second twin). Nitroglycerin therapy has been shown to diminish platelet aggregation, an effect enhanced by administration of N-acetylcysteine.

Drug Interactions

Nitroglycerin has been reported to potentiate the neuromuscular blockade produced by pancuronium.

HYDRALAZINE

Mechanism of Action

 Hydralazine relaxes arteriolar smooth muscle, causing dilatation of precapillary resistance vessels. The mechanism of this effect may be interference with calcium utilization or activation of guanylyl cyclase.

Clinical Uses

Intraoperative hypertension is usually controlled with an intravenous dose of 5–20 mg of hydralazine. The onset of action is within 15 minutes, and the antihypertensive effect usually lasts 2–4 hours. Continuous infusions (0.25–1.5 μg/kg/min) are less frequently used owing to their rather slow onset and long duration of action. Hydralazine is frequently used to control pregnancy-induced hypertension (see Chapter 43).

Metabolism

Hydralazine undergoes acetylation and hydroxylation in the liver.

Effects on Organ Systems

A. CARDIOVASCULAR:

The lowering of peripheral vascular resistance causes a drop in arterial blood pressure. The body reacts to the fall in blood pressure by increasing heart rate, myocardial contractility, and cardiac output. These compensatory responses can be detrimental to patients with coronary artery disease and are minimized by the concurrent administration of a β–adrenergic antagonist. Conversely, the decline in afterload often proves beneficial to patients in congestive heart failure.

B. CEREBRAL:

Hydralazine is a potent cerebral vasodilator and inhibitor of cerebral blood flow autoregulation. Unless blood pressure is markedly reduced, cerebral blood flow and intracranial pressure will rise.

C. RENAL:

Because renal blood flow is usually maintained or increased by hydralazine, it is often selected for patients with renal disease. Renin secretion by juxtaglomerular cells is stimulated.

Drug Interactions

Hydralazine may induce enflurane defluorination, increasing its potential for nephrotoxicity.

TRIMETHAPHAN

Mechanism of Action

Trimethaphan produces peripheral vasodilatation by direct smooth muscle relaxation and by blockade of acetylcholine receptors in autonomic ganglia. Two other groups of cholinergic antagonists have been described in previous chapters: the antinicotinic nondepolarizing neuromuscular blocking agents (see Chapter 9) and the antimuscarinic drugs (see Chapter 11). Like the nondepolarizing agents, trimethaphan competitively blocks nicotinic receptors; however, these nicotinic receptors are located in autonomic ganglia instead of skeletal muscle. Because both sympathetic and parasympathetic ganglia are cholinergic, trimethaphan results in a mixed autonomic blockade.

Clinical Uses

Trimethaphan is used to control arterial blood pressure and to manage **autonomic hyperreflexia** (a syndrome of massive sympathetic discharge seen in patients with upper spinal cord injuries). A continuous intravenous infusion of 0.1% trimethaphan (1 mg/mL) is titrated to the desired blood pressure response (usually 10–100 μg/kg/min). Trimethaphan acts rapidly, but its duration of action is longer than that of sodium nitroprusside. Tachyphylaxis is common after prolonged administration.

Metabolism

Trimethaphan does not depend on the kidney or liver for termination of its action. Because trimethaphan interferes with plasma cholinesterase activity, it has been postulated that this enzyme may play a role in its metabolism.

Effects on Organ Systems

A. CARDIOVASCULAR:

Trimethaphan decreases arterial blood pressure by arteriolar and venous dilatation. The latter decreases venous return to the heart and lowers cardiac output. This characteristic is valuable when increases in cardiac output are best avoided (eg, during dissecting aortic aneurysm repair). Heart rate often increases, not from sympathetic reflexes but because of parasympathetic ganglionic blockade. Patients are particularly susceptible to postural hypotension (eg, reverse Trendelenburg). In the event of sudden hypotension caused by acute blood loss, trimethaphan's sympathetic ganglion blocking action will prevent restoration of cardiac output by abolishing the arterial baroreflex response. This may provide a lower margin of safety than nitroprusside or nitroglycerin in some clinical situations.

B. CEREBRAL:

Trimethaphan is a highly ionized quaternary ammonium and does not easily pass the blood-brain barrier. Unlike the other peripheral vasodilators discussed in this chapter, trimethaphan is not associated with cerebral vasodilation or increases in cerebral spinal fluid pressure. Nonetheless, cerebral blood flow is usually adequately maintained at mean arterial pressures above 60 mm Hg. These factors lead to preservation of spinal cord perfusion pressure and may result in improved neurologic outcome following thoracic aortic cross-clamping, compared with sodium nitroprusside. Pupillary dilation accompanying ganglionic blockade can interfere with the interpretation of neurologic examinations.

C. RENAL AND GASTROINTESTINAL:

Trimethaphan's parasympathetic effects can result in urinary retention and paralytic ileus following prolonged infusions.

D. ENDOCRINE:

Unlike sodium nitroprusside, trimethaphan-induced hypotension does not activate catecholamine and renin release, but trimethaphan can cause histamine release.

Drug Interactions

Trimethaphan inhibits plasma cholinesterase and can double the duration of action of succinylcholine. Since both autonomic ganglia and skeletal neuromuscular junctions contain nicotinic cholinergic receptors, it is not surprising that trimethaphan also potentiates non-depolarizing muscle blockade.

ADENOSINE

Mechanism of Action

Adenosine, a purine endogenous to all cells of the body, acts on specific adenosine receptors located in several vascular beds and on the atrioventricular (AV) node. Its mechanism of action may involve activation of adenylate cyclase and depression of action potentials. Specifically, adenosine is thought to open potassium channels, hyperpolarizing nodal tissue and making it less likely to fire. This leads to an atrioventricular block and a slowing of the sinus rate in patients with supraventricular tachycardia. Adenosine has little effect on atrial or ventricular muscle tissue.

Clinical Uses

Adenosine is a potent vasodilator that can be used to reduce arterial blood pressure during anesthesia. It selectively affects arteriolar resistance vessels (afterload), with little effect on venous capacitance (preload). Because of a very short half-life (< 10 seconds), a continuous infusion (60–120 µg/kg/min) is required for controlled hypotension.

Currently, the only indication approved by the Food and Drug Administration for adenosine is conversion to sinus rhythm of paroxysmal supraventricular tachycardia, including that associated with Wolff-Parkinson-White syndrome, by an intravenous bolus injection of 6 mg over 1–2 seconds (6 mg/2 mL). If this proves ineffective, a 12-mg bolus should be administered and may be repeated once. Its ultrashort duration of action prevents cumulative effects after repeat doses. Intravenous bolus of adenosine for paroxysmal supraventricular tachycardia can induce the onset of atrial fibrillation and thus should only be administered in an appropriate setting (eg, cardioversion capability). Wide complex tachycardias arising in the ventricle, as opposed to the AV node, will not be affected by adenosine. Similarly, atrial dysrhythmias (eg, atrial fibrillation, atrial flutter, multifocal atrial tachycardia) will only demonstrate a transient slowing of ventricular rate. Intrathecal adenosine (0.5–1.0 mg) has undergone successful preliminary study for the treatment of chronic neuropathic pain.

Metabolism

Erythrocytes and vascular endothelial cells rapidly take up adenosine from the circulation and metabolize it to inosine and adenosine monophosphate.

Effects on Organ Systems

A. CARDIOVASCULAR:

Adenosine decreases arterial blood pressure by lowering systemic vascular resistance. Cardiac index, heart rate, and stroke volume increase. Myocardial blood flow increases as a result of coronary vasodilatation without an increase in oxygen consumption or work. Unfavorable changes in distribution of regional coronary blood flow (intracoronary steal) have led to myocardial ischemia in patients with coronary artery disease, however—which may greatly limit its usefulness during anesthesia.

Adenosine also slows AV conduction (increases P–R interval) and can interrupt reentrant dysrhythmias that involve the AV node. Large doses of adenosine depress sinus node and ventricular automaticity, leading to brief periods of sinus pause that resolve spontaneously. Although it is best avoided in patients with second- or third-degree heart block or sick sinus syndrome, adverse reactions are rare and of brief duration. Hypotension has not been reported to be a significant side effect of bolus administration of the dose recommended for treatment of paroxysmal supraventricular tachycardia.

B. PULMONARY:

Adenosine decreases pulmonary vascular resistance, increases intrapulmonary shunt, and can lead to a drop in arterial oxygen saturation as a result of the inhibition of pulmonary hypoxic vasoconstriction. Adenosine may rarely cause bronchospasm in predisposed individuals.

C. RENAL:

Surprisingly, adenosine causes renal vasoconstriction with a resulting drop in renal blood flow, glomerular filtration rate, filtration fraction, and urinary output.

Drug Interactions

Methylxanthines (eg, aminophylline) competitively antagonize adenosine, while blockers of nucleoside transport (eg, dipyridamole) potentiate its actions.

FENOLDOPAM

Mechanism of Action

Fenoldopam mesylate causes rapid vasodilatation by selectively activating D1-dopamine receptors. It has also demonstrated moderate affinity for α_2-adrenoceptors.

The R-isomer is responsible for the racemic mixture's biologic activity due to its much greater receptor affinity, compared with the S-isomer.

Clinical Uses

 Fenoldopam mesylate (infusion rates studied in clinical trials range from 0.01–1.6 µg/kg/min) reduces systolic and diastolic blood pressure in patients with malignant hypertension to an extent comparable to nitroprusside. Side effects include headache, flushing, nausea, tachycardia, hypokalemia, and hypotension. The onset of the hypotensive effect occurs within 15 minutes and discontinuation of an infusion quickly reverses this effect without rebound hypertension. There may be some degree of tolerance that develops after 48 hours of infusion. As with most new drugs, fenoldopam's clinical profile has yet to be fully determined. However, its eventual place in anesthetic practice may be greatly influenced by its very high cost.

Metabolism

Fenoldopam undergoes conjugation without participation of the cytochrome P-450 enzymes, and its metabolites are inactive. Clearance of fenoldopam remains unaltered despite the presence of renal or hepatic failure, and no dosage adjustments are necessary for these patients.

Effects on Organ Systems

A. CARDIOVASCULAR:

Fenoldopam decreases systolic and diastolic blood pressure. Heart rate typically increases. Low initial doses (0.03–0.1 µg/kg/min) titrated slowly have been associated with less reflex tachycardia than higher doses (> 0.3 µg/kg/min). Tachycardia lessens over time but remains substantial at higher doses.

B. OPHTHALMIC:

Fenoldopam can lead to rises in intraocular pressure and should be administered with caution or avoided in patients with a history of glaucoma or intraocular hypertension.

C. RENAL:

As would be expected from a D1-dopamine receptor agonist, fenoldopam markedly increases renal blood flow. Despite a drop in arterial blood pressure, glomerular filtration rate is well maintained. Fenoldopam increases urinary flow rate, urinary sodium extraction, and creatinine clearance compared with sodium nitroprusside. Fenoldopam was found to vasodilate renal efferent and afferent arterioles in animal studies.

Warnings

The preservative sodium metabisulfite may cause allergic reactions and even anaphylactic reactions. Patients with asthma and those with a history of sulfite sensitivity appear to be at higher risk.

Drug Interactions

To date, there have been no formal interaction studies; however, fenoldopam has been safely administered with digitalis and sublingual nitroglycerin.

CASE DISCUSSION: CONTROLLED HYPOTENSION

A 59-year-old man is scheduled for total hip arthroplasty under general anesthesia. The surgeon requests a controlled hypotensive technique.

What is controlled hypotension, and what are its advantages?

Controlled hypotension is the elective lowering of arterial blood pressure. The primary advantages of this technique are minimization of surgical blood loss and better wound visualization.

How is controlled hypotension achieved?

The primary methods of electively lowering blood pressure are proper positioning, positive pressure ventilation, and the administration of hypotensive drugs. Positioning involves elevation of the surgical site so that the blood pressure at the wound is selectively reduced. The increase in intrathoracic pressure that accompanies positive pressure ventilation lowers venous return, cardiac output, and mean arterial pressure. Numerous pharmacologic agents effectively lower blood pressure: volatile anesthetics, sympathetic antagonists, calcium channel blockers, and the peripheral vasodilators discussed in this chapter. Owing to their rapid onset and short duration of action, sodium nitroprusside, nitroglycerin, trimethaphan, and adenosine have the advantage of precise control. An additional method of producing hypotension is creation of a high sympathetic block with an epidural or spinal anesthetic.

What surgical procedures might benefit most from a controlled hypotensive technique?

Controlled hypotension has been successfully used during cerebral aneurysm repair, brain tumor resection, total hip arthroplasty, radical neck dis-

section, radical cystectomy, and other operations associated with significant blood loss. Controlled hypotension may allow safer surgery of patients whose religious beliefs prohibit blood transfusions (eg, Jehovah's Witnesses; see Case Discussion, Chapter 40). Decreasing extravasation of blood may improve the result of some plastic surgery procedures.

What are some relative contraindications to controlled hypotension?

Some patients have predisposing illnesses that lessen the margin of safety for adequate organ perfusion: severe anemia, hypovolemia, atherosclerotic vascular disease, renal or hepatic insufficiency, cerebrovascular disease, or uncontrolled glaucoma.

What are the possible complications of controlled hypotension?

As the above list of contraindications suggests, the risks of low arterial blood pressure include cerebral thrombosis, hemiplegia (due to decreased spinal cord perfusion), acute tubular necrosis, massive hepatic necrosis, myocardial infarction, cardiac arrest, and blindness (from retinal artery thrombosis or ischemic optic neuropathy). These complications are more likely in patients with coexisting anemia.

What is a safe level of hypotension?

This depends on the patient. Healthy young individuals tolerate mean arterial pressures as low as 50–60 mm Hg without complications. On the other hand, chronically hypertensive patients have altered autoregulation of cerebral blood flow and may tolerate a mean arterial pressure no more than 25% lower than baseline. Patients with a history of transient ischemic attacks may not tolerate any decline in cerebral perfusion.

What special monitoring is indicated during controlled hypotension?

Intra-arterial blood pressure monitoring and electrocardiography with ST-segment analysis are strongly recommended. Central venous monitoring and measurement of urinary output by an indwelling catheter are indicated if extensive surgery is anticipated. Monitors of neurologic function (eg, electroencephalography) have not gained widespread acceptance.

SUGGESTED READING

Oates JA: Antihypertensive agents and the drug therapy of hypertension. Chapter 33 in: *Goodman and Gilman's The Pharmaceutical Basis of Therapeutics,* 9th ed. Gilman AG et al (editors). McGraw-Hill, 1996.

Lauretti GR, de Oliveira R, Reis MP: Transdermal nitroglycerine enhances spinal sufentanil postoperative analgesia following orthopedic surgery. Anesthesiology 1999;90:734. Nitroglycerin possesses analgesic properties.

Marshman LAG, Morice AH, Thompson JS: Increased efficacy of sodium nitroprusside in middle cerebral arteries following acute subarachnoid hemorrhage: Indications for its use after rupture. J Neurosurg Anesthesiol 1998;10:171.

Van Aken H, Miller ED: Deliberate hypotension. Chapter 41, in: *Anesthesia,* 5th ed. Miller RD (editor). Churchill Livingstone, 2000.

Parker JD, Parker JO: Nitrate therapy for stable angina pectoris. N Engl J Med 1998;338:520. A comprehensive review of organic nitrates including nitroglycerin and isosorbide dinitrate.

Rinde-Hoffman D, Glasser SP, Arnett DK: Update on nitrate therapy. J Clin Pharmacol 1991;31:697.

Tobias JD: Fenoldopam: applications in anesthesiology, perioperative medicine, and critical care medicine. Am J Anesthesiol 2000;27:395.

Williams-Russo P, Sharrock NE, Mattis S: Randomized trial of hypotensive epidural anesthesia in older adults. Anesthesiology 1999;91:926. Cognitive outcome following hip arthroplasty did not differ between a low blood pressure group (MAP 45–55 mm Hg) and higher blood pressure group (MAP 55–70 mm Hg).

Local Anesthetics

14

KEY CONCEPTS

 There are multiple measurements of local anesthetic potency that are analogous to the minimum alveolar concentration (MAC) of inhalational anesthetics. Cm is the minimum concentration of local anesthetic that will block nerve impulse conduction. This measure of relative potency is affected by several factors, including fiber size, type, and myelination; pH (acidic pH antagonizes block); frequency of nerve stimulation (access of local anesthetic to the sodium receptor is enhanced by repeatedly opening the sodium channel); and electrolyte concentrations (hypokalemia and hypercalcemia antagonize blockade).

 The pH at which the amount of ionized and nonionized drug is equal is the pK_a of the drug.

 Local anesthetics with a pK_a closer to physiologic pH will have a higher concentration of nonionized base that can pass through the nerve cell membrane, and onset will be more rapid.

 The rate of systemic absorption is proportionate to the vascularity of the site of injection: intravenous > tracheal > intercostal > caudal > paracervical > epidural > brachial plexus > sciatic > subcutaneous.

 The metabolism of local anesthetics differs depending on their structure. Ester local anesthetics are predominantly metabolized by pseudocholinesterase (plasma cholinesterase). Amide local anesthetics are metabolized by microsomal enzymes in the liver.

 Cardiac dysrhythmia or circulatory collapse is often the presenting sign of local anesthetic overdose during general anesthesia.

 Unintentional intravascular injection of bupivacaine during regional anesthesia has produced severe cardiotoxic reactions, including hypotension, atrioventricular heart block, and dysrhythmias such as ventricular fibrillation.

 Cocaine inhibits the reuptake of norepinephrine, thereby potentiating the effects of adrenergic stimulation.

 The central nervous system (CNS) is the site of premonitory signs of local anesthetic overdose in awake patients. Early symptoms are circumoral numbness, tongue paresthesia, and dizziness. Sensory complaints may include tinnitus and blurred vision. Excitatory signs (eg, restlessness, agitation, nervousness, paranoia) often precede CNS depression (eg, slurred speech, drowsiness, unconsciousness).

Regional anesthetic techniques depend on a group of drugs—local anesthetics—that produce transient loss of sensory, motor, and autonomic function in a discrete portion of the body. This chapter presents the mechanism of action, structure-activity relationships, and clinical pharmacology of local anesthetic drugs. Commonly used nerve blocks are presented in Section III (see Chapters 16 and 17).

THEORIES OF LOCAL ANESTHETIC ACTION

Nerve cells maintain a **resting membrane potential** by active transport and passive diffusion of ions. The sodium-potassium pump transports sodium out of the cell and potassium into the cell. This creates a concentration gradient that favors the extracellular diffusion of potassium and the intracellular diffusion of sodium. The cell membrane is much more permeable to potassium than to sodium, however, so a relative excess of negatively charged ions (**anions**) accumulates intracellularly. This accounts for the **negative resting potential** difference (−70 mV polarization).

After chemical, mechanical, or electrical excitation, an impulse is conducted along a nerve axon. The impulse propagation is usually accompanied by depolarization of the nerve membrane. If the depolarization exceeds the **threshold level** (a membrane potential of −55 mV), sodium channels in the membrane are activated, allowing a sudden and spontaneous influx of sodium ions. This increase in sodium permeability causes a relative excess of positively charged ions (cations) intracellularly, resulting in a membrane potential of +35 mV. A consequent drop in sodium permeability (caused by inactivation of the sodium channels) and an increase in potassium conductance (allowing more potassium to exit the cell) return the membrane to its resting potential. Baseline concentration gradients are eventually reestablished by the sodium-potassium pump. These changes in axon membrane potential are collectively called the **action potential.**

Most local anesthetics bind to sodium channels in the inactivated state, preventing subsequent channel activation and the large transient sodium influx associated with membrane depolarization. This does not alter the resting membrane potential or the threshold level, but it slows the rate of depolarization. The action potential is not propagated because the threshold level is never attained. Specific receptors in the interior of the sodium channels are probably the exact site of local anesthetic action.

Some local anesthetics may penetrate the membrane, causing membrane expansion and channel distortion analogous to the **critical volume hypothesis** of general anesthetics (see Chapter 7). Alternatively, the **surface charge theory** postulates that partial penetra-

tion by local anesthetics of the axonal membrane could increase the transmembrane potential and inhibit depolarization.

STRUCTURE-ACTIVITY RELATIONSHIPS

Local anesthetics consist of a **lipophilic group**—usually a benzene ring—separated from a **hydrophilic group**—usually a tertiary amine—by an intermediate chain that includes an **ester** or **amide linkage.** Local anesthetics are weak bases that usually carry a positive charge at the tertiary amine group at physiologic pH. The nature of the intermediate chain is the basis of the classification of local anesthetics as esters or amides (Table 14–1). Physicochemical properties of local anesthetics depend on the substitutions in the aromatic ring, the type of linkage in the intermediate chain, and the alkyl groups attached to the amine nitrogen.

Potency correlates with lipid solubility; that is, potency depends on the ability of the local anesthetic to penetrate a hydrophobic environment. In general, potency and hydrophobicity increase with an increase in the total number of carbon atoms in the molecule. More specifically, potency is increased by adding a halide to the aromatic ring (2-chloroprocaine as opposed to procaine), an ester linkage (procaine versus procainamide), and large alkyl groups on the tertiary amide nitrogen (etidocaine versus lidocaine). There are multiple measurements of local anesthetic potency that are analogous to the minimum alveolar concentration (MAC) of inhalational anesthetics. **Cm** is the minimum concentration of local anesthetic that will block nerve impulse conduction. This measure of relative potency is affected by several factors, including fiber size, type, and myelination; pH (acidic pH antagonizes block); frequency of nerve stimulation (access of local anesthetic to the sodium receptor is enhanced by repeatedly opening the sodium channel); and electrolyte concentrations (hypokalemia and hypercalcemia antagonize blockade). Minimum local analgesic concentration (**MLAC**), another measure of relative potency of local anesthetic agents, has been defined as the median effective local analgesia concentration in a 20 mL volume for epidural analgesia in the first stage of labor. Minimum effective anesthetic concentration (**MEAC**) is defined as the concentration at which a spinal anesthetic agent produces surgical anesthesia within 20 minutes of administration in 50% of patients.

Onset of action depends on many factors, including the relative concentration of the nonionized lipid-soluble form (B) and the ionized water-soluble form (BH$^+$). The pH at which the amount of ionized and nonionized drug is equal is the **pK$_a$** of the drug. For instance, the pK$_a$ of lido-

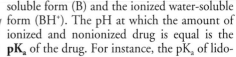

caine is 7.8. When lidocaine is exposed to a higher hydrogen ion concentration (eg, a pH of 7.4), more than half of it will exist as the charged cation form (BH⁺).

Although both forms of local anesthetic are involved in blockade, only the lipid-soluble form diffuses across the neural sheath (epineurium) and nerve membrane. Local anesthetics with a pK_a closer to physiologic pH will have a higher concentration of nonionized base that can pass through the nerve cell membrane, and onset will be more rapid. Once inside the cell, the nonionized base will reach an equilibrium with its ionized form. Only the charged cation actually binds to the receptor within the sodium channel. Not all local anesthetics exist in a charged form (eg, benzocaine), however. These anesthetics probably act by an alternative mechanism (eg, expanding the lipid membrane).

The importance of the ionized and nonionized forms has many clinical implications. Local anesthetic solutions are prepared commercially as water-soluble hydrochloride salt (pH 6–7). Because epinephrine is unstable in alkaline environments, local anesthetic solutions containing it are made even more acidic (pH 4–5). Because of the lower concentration of free base, these commercial preparations have a slower onset than when epinephrine is added at the time of use. Similarly, the extracellular base-to-cation ratio is decreased and onset is delayed when local anesthetics are injected into acidic (eg, infected) tissues. **Tachyphylaxis**—the decreased efficacy of repeated doses—is explained by the eventual consumption of local extracellular buffering capacity by the acidic local anesthetic solution. Conversely, if carbonated solutions of local anesthetic rather than the hydrochloride salts are used, onset of action may be shortened. This appears to be due to improved intracellular distribution of the ionized form. Although controversial, some researchers have reported that alkalinization of an anesthetic solution (particularly commercially prepared solutions containing epinephrine that tend to be quite acidic) by the addition of sodium bicarbonate (eg, 1 mL 8.4% sodium bicarbonate per 10 mL 1% lidocaine) speeds onset, improves quality of block, and prolongs blockade by increasing the amount of free base available. It is interesting to note that this combination also decreases pain during subcutaneous infiltration.

Onset of action of local anesthetics in *isolated* nerve fiber preparations directly correlates with pK_a. However, *clinical* onset of action is not necessarily identical for local anesthetics with the same pK_a. Other factors, such as ease of diffusion through connective tissue, can affect the onset of action in vivo.

Duration of action is associated with plasma protein binding (α_1-acid glycoprotein), presumably because the local anesthetic receptor is also a protein. The pharmacokinetic factors that determine absorption also affect duration of action. Liposomal encapsulation systems for delivery of local anesthetics may significantly prolong their duration of action.

CLINICAL PHARMACOLOGY

Pharmacokinetics

A. ABSORPTION:

Traditionally, local anesthetics have been applied to mucous membranes (eg, ocular conjunctiva) or injected into a variety of tissues and compartments. Most mucous membranes provide a weak barrier to local anesthetic penetration, leading to a rapid onset of action. Intact skin, on the other hand, requires a high water concentration for its penetration and a high concentration of lipid soluble local anesthetic base to ensure analgesia. **EMLA cream** (eutectic [easily melted] mixture of local anesthetic) consists of a 1:1 mixture of 5% lidocaine and 5% prilocaine in an oil-in-water emulsion. Dermal analgesia sufficient for beginning an intravenous line requires a contact time of at least 1 hour under an occlusive dressing. Depth of penetration (usually 3–5 mm), duration of action (usually 1–2 hours), and amount of drug absorbed depends on application time, dermal blood flow, keratin thickness, and total dose administered. Typically, 1–2 g of cream are applied per 10 cm^2 area of skin, with a maximum application area of 2000 cm^2 in an adult (100 cm^2 in children weighing less than 10 kg). Split-thickness skin-graft harvesting, laser removal of port-wine stains, lithotripsy, and circumcision have been successfully performed with EMLA cream. Side effects include skin blanching, erythema, and edema. EMLA cream should not be used on mucous membranes, broken skin, infants less than 1 month old, or patients with a predisposition to methemoglobinemia (see Metabolism, below).

Systemic absorption of injected local anesthetics depends on blood flow, which is determined by the following factors:

 1. Site of injection—The rate of systemic absorption is proportionate to the vascularity of the site of injection: intravenous > tracheal > intercostal > caudal > paracervical > epidural > brachial plexus > sciatic > subcutaneous.

2. Presence of vasoconstrictors—The addition of epinephrine—or, less commonly, phenylephrine or norepinephrine—causes vasoconstriction at the site of administration. The consequent decreased absorption increases neuronal uptake, enhances the quality of analgesia, prolongs duration of action, and limits toxic side effects. The effects of vasoconstrictors are more pronounced with shorter-acting agents. For example, the

Table 14–1. Physicochemical properties of local anesthetics.

Generic (Proprietary)	Ring	Structure Chain	Amine	Potency and Lipid Solubility	pKa	Duration and Protein Binding	Uses	Maximum Dose (mg/kg)
Amides								
Bupivacaine (Marcaine)	2,6-dimethylphenyl	NHCO	piperidine with C$_4$H$_9$, N	+++	8.1	++++	Epidural, caudal, spinal; infiltration; peripheral nerve block	3
Dibucaine (Nupercaine)	quinoline, OC$_4$H$_9$	CONHCH$_2$	N with C$_2$H$_5$, C$_2$H$_5$	+++	8.8	++++	Spinal; topical	1
Etidocaine (Duranest)	2,6-dimethylphenyl	NHCOCH–C$_2$H$_5$	N with C$_2$H$_5$, C$_3$H$_7$	+++	7.7	++++	Epidural, caudal infiltration; peripheral nerve block	4
Lidocaine (Xylocaine)	2,6-dimethylphenyl	NHCOCH$_2$	N with C$_2$H$_5$, C$_2$H$_5$	++	7.8	++	Epidural, caudal, spinal; infiltration; peripheral nerve block; topical	4.5[1] 7[2]
Mepivacaine (Carbocaine)	2,6-dimethylphenyl	NHCO	piperidine with CH$_3$, N	++	7.6	++	Epidural, caudal; infiltration; peripheral nerve block	4.5[1] 7[2]

Prilocaine (Citanest) — 7.8 — ++ — ++ — Epidural, caudal; infiltration; peripheral nerve block — 8

Ropivacaine — 8.1 — +++ — ++ — Epidural, caudal, spinal; infiltration; peripheral nerve block — 3

Esters

Chloroprocaine (Nesacaine)[3] — 9.0 — + — + — Epidural, caudal; infiltration; peripheral nerve block — 12

Cocaine — 8.7 — ++ — ++ — Topical — 3

Procaine — 8.9 — + — + — Spinal; infiltration; peripheral nerve block — 12

Tetracaine (Pontocaine) — 8.2 — +++ — +++ — Spinal; topical — 3

[1] Maximum dose without epinephrine.
[2] Maximum dose with epinephrine.
[3] Chloroprocaine is metabolized too rapidly to measure lipid solubility or protein binding. It has a rapid onset of action despite a high pK_a.

addition of epinephrine to lidocaine usually extends the duration of anesthesia by at least 50%, but epinephrine has no significant effect when added to bupivacaine, whose long duration of action is due to a high degree of protein binding.

3. Local anesthetic agent—Local anesthetics that are highly tissue-bound are more slowly absorbed (eg, etidocaine). The agents also vary in their intrinsic vasodilator properties.

B. Distribution:

Distribution depends on organ uptake, which is determined by the following factors:

1. Tissue perfusion—The highly perfused organs (brain, lung, liver, kidney, and heart) are responsible for initial rapid uptake (alpha phase), which is followed by a slower redistribution (beta phase) to moderately perfused tissues (muscle and gut). In particular, the lung extracts significant amounts of local anesthetic.

2. Tissue/blood partition coefficient—Strong plasma protein binding tends to retain anesthetic in the blood, while high lipid solubility facilitates tissue uptake.

3. Tissue mass—Muscle provides the greatest reservoir for local anesthetic agents because of its large mass.

C. Metabolism and Excretion:

The metabolism and excretion of local anesthetics differ depending on their structure.

1. Esters—Ester local anesthetics are predominantly metabolized by **pseudocholinesterase (plasma cholinesterase)**. Ester hydrolysis is very rapid, and the water-soluble metabolites are excreted in the urine. One metabolite, p-aminobenzoic acid, has been associated with allergic reactions. Patients with genetically abnormal pseudocholinesterase are at increased risk for toxic side effects, since metabolism is slower. Cerebrospinal fluid lacks esterase enzymes, so the termination of action of intrathecally injected ester local anesthetics depends on their absorption into the bloodstream. In contrast to other ester anesthetics, cocaine is partially metabolized in the liver and partially excreted unchanged in the urine.

2. Amides—Amide local anesthetics are metabolized by microsomal enzymes in the liver. The rate of metabolism depends on the specific agent (prilocaine is faster than lidocaine, which is faster than bupivacaine) but is much slower than ester hydrolysis. Decreases in hepatic function (eg, cirrhosis of the liver) or liver blood flow (eg, congestive heart failure) will reduce the metabolic rate and predispose patients to systemic toxicity. Very little drug is excreted unchanged by the kid-

neys, although the metabolites are dependent on renal clearance.

Metabolites of prilocaine (o-toluidine derivatives), which accumulate after large doses of drug (> 10 mg/kg), convert hemoglobin to **methemoglobin.** Neonates of mothers who have received prilocaine epidural anesthesia during labor and patients with limited cardiopulmonary reserve are particularly susceptible to the alteration in oxygen transport. Benzocaine, a common ingredient in local anesthetic sprays, also can cause methemoglobinemia. Treatment of significant methemoglobinemia includes intravenous administration of methylene blue (1–2 mg/kg of 1% solution over 5 minutes). Methylene blue reduces methemoglobin (Fe^{3+}) to hemoglobin (Fe^{2+}).

Effects on Organ Systems

Since blockade of sodium channels affects action potential propagation throughout the body, it is not surprising that local anesthetics have the capability for systemic toxicity. While organ system effects are discussed for these drugs as a group, it must be recognized that individual drugs differ in their pharmacology.

Toxicity is often directly proportionate to potency. Maximum safe doses are listed in Table 14–1. Mixtures of local anesthetics should be considered to have roughly additive toxic effects: A solution containing 50% of the toxic dose of lidocaine and 50% of the toxic dose of bupivacaine will have roughly 100% of the toxic effects of either drug.

A. Cardiovascular:

In general, local anesthetics depress myocardial automaticity (spontaneous phase IV depolarization) and reduce the duration of the refractory period. Myocardial contractility and conduction velocity are depressed at higher concentrations. These effects result from direct cardiac muscle membrane changes (ie, cardiac sodium channel blockade) and inhibition of the autonomic nervous system. Smooth muscle relaxation causes some degree of arteriolar dilatation. The ensuing combination of bradycardia, heart block, and hypotension may cul-

minate in cardiac arrest. Cardiac dysrhythmia or circulatory collapse is often the presenting sign of local anesthetic overdose during general anesthesia.

Lower concentrations of lidocaine provide effective treatment for some types of ventricular dysrhythmias. Myocardial contractility and arterial blood pressure are generally unaffected by the usual intravenous doses. The hypertension associated with laryngoscopy and intubation is attenuated in some patients by intravenous administration of lidocaine (1.5 mg/kg) 1–3 minutes prior to instrumentation.

Unintentional intravascular injection of bupivacaine during regional anesthesia has produced severe cardiotoxic reactions, including hypotension, atrioventricular heart block, and dysrhythmias such as ventricular fibrillation. Pregnancy, hypoxemia, and respiratory acidosis are predisposing risk factors. Electrophysiologic studies have demonstrated that bupivacaine is associated with more pronounced depolarization changes than is lidocaine. Bupivacaine blocks cardiac sodium channels and alters mitochondrial function; its high degree of protein binding makes resuscitation prolonged and difficult.

Ropivacaine, a relatively new amide local anesthetic, shares many physicochemical properties with bupivacaine, except that it is half as lipid-soluble. Potency, onset time, and duration of action are similar (ropivacaine provides less motor block, which may be due to an overall lower potency demonstrated by some studies). However, ropivacaine has a larger therapeutic index because it is 70% less likely to cause severe cardiac dysrhythmias than is bupivacaine, and ropivacaine has been associated with greater central nervous system tolerance. This improved safety profile may be due to its lower lipid solubility or its availability as a pure S(−) isomer, as opposed to bupivacaine's racemic mixture. The S(−) isomer of bupivacaine (levobupivacaine) has been reported to have fewer cardiovascular and cerebral side effects than the racemic mixture. Otherwise, levobupivacaine and bupivacaine appear to exhibit similar anesthetic effects.

Cocaine's cardiovascular reactions are unlike those of any other local anesthetic. Adrenergic nerve terminals normally reabsorb norepinephrine after its release. Cocaine inhibits this reuptake, thereby potentiating the effects of adrenergic stimulation. Cardiovascular responses to cocaine include hypertension and ventricular ectopy. The latter contraindicates its use in patients anesthetized with halothane. Cocaine-induced dysrhythmias have been successfully treated with adrenergic and calcium channel antagonists. Cocaine produces vasoconstriction when applied topically.

B. Respiratory:

Lidocaine depresses **hypoxic drive** (the ventilatory response to low PaO$_2$). Apnea can result from phrenic and intercostal nerve paralysis or depression of the medullary respiratory center following direct exposure to local anesthetic agents (eg, postretrobulbar apnea syndrome; see Chapter 38). Local anesthetics relax bronchial smooth muscle. Intravenous lidocaine (1.5 mg/kg) may be effective in blocking the reflex bronchoconstriction sometimes associated with intubation. Lidocaine administered as an aerosol can lead to

bronchospasm in some patients with reactive airway disease.

C. Neurological:

The central nervous system is especially vulnerable to local anesthetic toxicity and is the site of premonitory signs of overdose in awake patients. Early symptoms are circumoral numbness, tongue paresthesia, and dizziness. Sensory complaints may include tinnitus and blurred vision. Excitatory signs (eg, restlessness, agitation, nervousness, paranoia) often precede central nervous system depression (eg, slurred speech, drowsiness, unconsciousness). Muscle twitching heralds the onset of tonic-clonic seizures. Respiratory arrest often follows. The excitatory reactions are a result of selective blockade of inhibitory pathways. By decreasing cerebral blood flow and drug exposure, benzodiazepines and hyperventilation raise the threshold of local anesthetic-induced seizures. Thiopental (1–2 mg/kg) quickly and reliably terminates seizure activity. Adequate ventilation and oxygenation must be maintained.

Intravenous lidocaine (1.5 mg/kg) decreases cerebral blood flow and attenuates the rise in intracranial pressure that accompanies intubation in patients with decreased intracranial compliance. Infusions of lidocaine and procaine have been used to supplement general anesthetic techniques, since they are capable of reducing the MAC of volatile anesthetics by up to 40%.

Cocaine stimulates the central nervous system and usually causes a sense of euphoria. An overdose is heralded by restlessness, emesis, tremors, convulsions, and respiratory failure.

Local anesthetics only temporarily block neuronal function. Nonetheless, large volumes of chloroprocaine unintentionally injected into the subarachnoid instead of the epidural space have caused prolonged neurologic deficit. The cause of this neural toxicity may be the low pH of the combination of chloroprocaine and a preservative, sodium bisulfate, which has been replaced with an antioxidant, a derivative of disodium ethylenediaminetetraacetic acid (EDTA). Chloroprocaine has also been associated with severe back pain following epidural administration. Possible etiologies include large volumes (> 40 mL) of, or local infiltration with, chloroprocaine; low pH; and the EDTA preservative. Chloroprocaine has more recently become available in a preservative-free formulation, which should be used for epidural blockade.

Repeated doses of 5% lidocaine and 0.5% tetracaine may be responsible for neurotoxicity (**cauda equina syndrome**) following infusion through small-bore catheters used in continuous spinal anesthesia. This may be due to pooling of drug around the cauda equina, resulting in high concentrations and permanent neuronal damage.

Transient neurologic symptoms, which consist of dysesthesia, burning pain, and aching in the lower extremities and buttocks have been reported following spinal anesthesia with a variety of local anesthetic agents. The etiology for these symptoms has been attributed to radicular irritation, and the symptoms typically resolve within 1 week. Risk factors include lidocaine (versus mepivacaine, bupivacaine, or tetracaine), lithotomy position, obesity, and outpatient status.

D. IMMUNOLOGIC:

True hypersensitivity reactions to local anesthetic agents—as distinct from systemic toxicity caused by excessive plasma concentration—are quite uncommon. Esters are more likely to induce an allergic reaction because they are derivatives of *p*-aminobenzoic acid, a known allergen. Commercial multidose preparations of amides often contain **methylparaben,** which has a chemical structure similar to that of *p*-aminobenzoic acid. This preservative may be responsible for most of the rare allergic responses to amide agents. The signs and treatment of allergic drug reactions are discussed in Chapter 47. Local anesthetics may inhibit neutrophil function and theoretically retard wound healing.

E. MUSCULOSKELETAL:

When directly injected into skeletal muscle (eg, trigger-point injection), local anesthetics are myotoxic (bupivacaine > lidocaine > procaine). Histologically, myofibril hypercontraction progresses to lytic degeneration, edema, and necrosis. Regeneration usually occurs after 3–4 weeks. Concomitant steroid or epinephrine injection worsens the myonecrosis.

F. HEMATOLOGIC:

Lidocaine has been demonstrated to decrease coagulation (prevention of thrombosis and decrease platelet aggregation) and enhance fibrinolysis of whole blood as measured by thromboelastography. These effects may relate to the reduced efficacy of epidural autologous blood patch shortly following local anesthetic administration and the lower incidence of embolic events in patients receiving epidural anesthetics.

Drug Interactions

Nondepolarizing muscle relaxant blockade is potentiated by local anesthetics.

Succinylcholine and ester local anesthetics depend on pseudocholinesterase for metabolism. Concurrent administration may potentiate the effects of both drugs.

Dibucaine, an amide local anesthetic, inhibits pseudocholinesterase and is used to detect genetically abnormal enzyme (see Chapter 9).

Pseudocholinesterase inhibitors can lead to decreased metabolism of ester local anesthetics (see Table 9–3).

Cimetidine and propranolol decrease hepatic blood flow and lidocaine clearance. Higher lidocaine blood levels increase the potential for systemic toxicity.

Opioids (eg, fentanyl, morphine) and α_2-adrenergic agonists (eg, epinephrine, clonidine) potentiate local anesthetic pain relief. Epidural chloroprocaine may interfere with the analgesic actions of intraspinal morphine, however, as may bupivacaine with fentanyl.

CASE DISCUSSION: LOCAL ANESTHETIC OVERDOSE

An 18-year-old woman in the active stage of labor requests an epidural anesthetic for delivery. Immediately following the epidural injection of 12 mL of 2% lidocaine, the patient complains of lip numbness and becomes very apprehensive.

What is your presumptive diagnosis?

The temporal relationship of the numbness and apprehension to the administration of local anesthetic suggests an unintentional intravascular injection. These prodromal signs do not always precede a seizure.

What prophylactic measures should be immediately taken?

Because hypocapnia increases the seizure threshold of local anesthetics, the patient should be instructed to hyperventilate. Simultaneously, a very small dose of thiopental sodium (50 mg) could be administered intravenously. Unconsciousness should be strictly avoided, because pregnant patients are considered to have a full stomach. The patient should already be receiving supplemental oxygen.

If symptoms progress to a generalized convulsion, what treatment should be initiated?

The laboring patient is always considered to be at risk for aspiration (see Chapter 43). Therefore, protecting the airway is of utmost importance. Immediate administration of succinylcholine should be followed by a rapid-sequence intubation (see Case Discussion, Chapter 15). While the succinylcholine will eliminate tonic-clonic activity, it will not address the underlying cerebral excitability. An anticonvulsant such as diazepam (2.5–10 mg) or thiopental sodium (50–75 mg) should be administered. It is clear from this sequence of events that whenever large doses of local anesthetic are administered, the same drugs and equipment must be available as for a general anesthetic.

What could have been expected if a large dose of bupivacaine—instead of lidocaine—had been given intravascularly?

Bupivacaine is more cardiotoxic than lidocaine, especially in the presence of acute respiratory acidosis. Ventricular dysrhythmias and conduction disturbances may lead to cardiac arrest and death. Bupivacaine is considered a more potent cardiac sodium channel blocker because the channels recover more slowly than after lidocaine blockade. Bretylium should be considered as the preferred alternative to lidocaine in the treatment of local anesthetic-induced ventricular tachyarrhythmias. Isoproterenol may effectively reverse some of the electrophysiologic abnormalities characteristic of bupivacaine toxicity. The reason for the higher incidence of cardiotoxicity during pregnancy is unclear. Although total dose rather than concentration determines toxicity, the Food and Drug Administration no longer recommends 0.75% bupivacaine for anesthesia during labor.

What could have prevented the toxic reaction described?

The risk of intravascular injection of toxic doses of local anesthetic during epidural anesthesia is minimized by using an adequate test dose (see Chapter 16), fractionation of the therapeutic dose into safe aliquots, and administering the minimum total dose of local anesthetic possible.

SUGGESTED READING

Bowdle TA: *Pharmacologic Basis of Anesthesiology: Basic Science and Practical Applications.* WB Saunders and Company, 1994. The second section of this book consists of three well-written chapters on local anesthetic pharmacology.

Butterworth JF, Strichartz GR: Molecular mechanisms of local anesthetics: A review. Anesthesiology 1990;72:711. Recent advances in electrophysiologic techniques have contributed to understanding of local anesthetic action.

Catterall WA, Mackie K: Local anesthetics. Chapter 15 in: *Goodman and Gilman's The Pharmacological Basis of Therapeutics,* 9th ed. Hardman JG (editor). McGraw-Hill, 1996.

Covino BG, Wildsmith JAW: Clinical pharmacology of local anesthetic agents. In: *Neural Blockade in Clinical Anesthesia and Management of Pain,* 3rd ed. Cousins MJ (editor). Lippincott Williams & Wilkins, 1998.

Freedman JM: Transient neurologic symptoms after spinal anesthesia: An epidemiologic study of 1,863 patients. Anesthesiology 1998;89:633. Conclusions of the Spinal Anesthesia Study Group that include the increased incidence of neurologic symptoms following spinal anesthesia with lidocaine compared with bupivacaine or tetracaine.

Gajraj NM, Pennant JH, Watcha MF: Eutectic mixture of local anesthetics (EMLA) cream. Anesth Analg 1994;78:574. A review of the pharmacology and clinical applications of EMLA cream.

Graf BM, Martin E, Bosnjak ZJ: Stereospecific effect of bupivacaine isomers on atrioventricular conduction in the isolated perfused guinea pig heart. Anesthesiology 1997;86:410. The R(+) isomer had a greater effect on AV conduction than the racemic mixture or the S(–) isomer (levobupivacaine), which had the least effect.

Tetzlaff JE: *Clinical Pharmacology of Local Anesthetics.* Butterworth-Heinemann, 2000.

Adjuncts to Anesthesia

15

KEY CONCEPTS

 H_2-blockers reduce the perioperative risk of aspiration pneumonia by decreasing gastric fluid volume and raising the pH of gastric contents.

 Metoclopramide increases lower esophageal sphincter tone, speeds gastric emptying, and lowers gastric fluid volume by enhancing the stimulatory effects of acetylcholine on intestinal smooth muscle.

 Ketorolac is a parenterally administered nonsteroidal anti-inflammatory drug that provides analgesia by inhibiting prostaglandin synthesis.

 Long-term administration of ketorolac may lead to renal toxicity (eg, papillary necrosis) or GI tract ulceration with bleeding and perforation. Because ketorolac depends on elimination by the kidneys, it should not be given to patients in renal failure.

 Selective activation of carotid chemoreceptors by low doses of doxapram stimulates hypoxic drive, producing an increase in tidal volume and a slight increase in respiratory rate. However, doxapram is not a specific reversal agent and should not replace standard supportive therapy (ie, mechanical ventilation).

 Naloxone reverses the agonist activity associated with endogenous or exogenous opioid compounds.

 Flumazenil has proved useful in the reversal of benzodiazepine sedation and treatment of benzodiazepine overdose.

 Aspiration does not necessarily result in aspiration pneumonia. The seriousness of the lung damage depends on the volume and composition of the aspirate. Patients are at risk if their gastric volume is greater than 25 mL (0.4 mL/kg) and their gastric pH is less than 2.5.

This final pharmacology chapter describes several drugs of particular interest to the anesthesiologist. Because some of these are histamine-receptor antagonists, the physiology of histamine is briefly reviewed. Diphenhydramine represents the classic antihistaminic drug. Cimetidine, ranitidine, and famotidine are helpful in the preoperative preparation of patients at risk for aspiration pneumonia. The chapter reviews other drugs (eg, metoclopramide, antacids, and proton pump inhibitors) that may be used to lessen the risk of aspiration as well as serotonin antagonists, which have proved to be potent antiemetics. The chapter concludes with a discussion of a respiratory stimulant (doxapram), an opiate antagonist (naloxone), and a benzodiazepine antagonist (flumazenil).

HISTAMINE-RECEPTOR ANTAGONISTS

Histamine Physiology

Histamine is found in central nervous system (histaminergic neurons), the gastric mucosa, and in other peripheral tissues. It is synthesized by decarboxylation of the amino acid **histidine.** The highest concentrations of histamine are found in the storage granules of mast cells and basophils. Histamine release (degranulation) can be triggered by chemical, mechanical, or immunologic stimulation. Two receptors, H_1 and H_2, mediate histamine's effects. The H_1-receptor activates phospholipase C, while the H_2-receptor increases intracellular cyclic adenosine monophosphate (cAMP). An H_3-receptor is primarily located on histamine-secreting cells and mediates negative feedback, inhibiting the synthesis and release of additional histamine. Histamine-N-methyltransferase metabolizes histamine to inactive metabolites that are excreted in the urine. This enzymatic reaction is inhibited by droperidol.

A. CARDIOVASCULAR:

Histamine reduces arterial blood pressure but increases heart rate and myocardial contractility. H_1-receptor stimulation increases capillary permeability and enhances ventricular irritability, while H_2-receptor stimulation increases heart rate and increases contractility. Both types of receptors mediate peripheral arteriolar dilation and some coronary vasodilation.

B. RESPIRATORY:

Histamine constricts bronchiolar smooth muscle via the H_1-receptor. H_2-receptor stimulation may produce mild bronchodilation. Histamine has variable effects on the pulmonary vasculature; the H_1-receptor appears to mediate pulmonary vasodilation while the H_2-receptor may be responsible for histamine-mediated pulmonary vasoconstriction.

C. GASTROINTESTINAL:

Activation of H_2-receptors in parietal cells increases gastric acid secretion. Stimulation of H_1-receptors leads to contraction of intestinal smooth muscle.

D. DERMAL:

The classic wheal-and-flare response of the skin to histamine results from increased capillary permeability and vasodilation and is primarily via H_1-receptor activation.

E. IMMUNOLOGIC:

Histamine is a major mediator of type 1 hypersensitivity reactions (see Chapter 47). H_1-receptor stimulation attracts leukocytes and induces prostaglandin synthesis. In contrast, the H_2-receptor appears to activate suppressor T lymphocytes.

1. H_1-Receptor Antagonists

Mechanism of Action

Diphenhydramine (an ethanolamine) is an example of a diverse group of drugs that competitively block H_1-receptors (Table 15–1). Many drugs with H_1-receptor antagonist properties have considerable antimuscarinic, or atropine-like, activity (eg, dry mouth), and some also have antiserontinergic activity (antiemetic).

Clinical Uses

Like other H_1-receptor antagonists, diphenhydramine has a multitude of therapeutic uses: suppression of allergic symptoms (eg, urticaria, rhinitis, conjunctivitis); vertigo, nausea and vomiting (eg, motion sickness, Ménière's disease); sedation; suppression of cough; and dyskinesia (eg, parkinsonism, drug-induced extrapyramidal side effects). Some of these actions are predictable from the understanding of histamine physiology, while others are due to the drugs' antimuscarinic and antiserotoninergic effects. Although H_1-blockers prevent the bronchoconstrictive response to histamine, they are ineffective in treating bronchial asthma, which is primarily due to other mediators (see Chapters 23 and 47). Like-

Table 15–1. Properties of commonly used H_1-receptor antagonists.

Drug	Route	Dose	Duration	Sedation	Antiemesis
Diphenhydramine (Benadryl)	PO, IM, IV	25–100 mg	3–6 hours	+++	++
Dimenhydrinate (Dramamine)	PO, IM, IV	50–100 mg	3–6 hours	+++	++
Chlorpheniramine (Chlor-Trimeton)	PO IM, IV	2–12 mg 5–20 mg	4–8 hours	++	0
Hydroxyzine (Atarax, Vistaril)	PO, IM	25–100 mg	4–12 hours	+++	++
Promethazine (Phenergan)	PO, IM, IV	12.5–50 mg	4–12 hours	+++	+++

0 = no effect.
++ = moderate activity.
+++ = marked activity.

wise, H_1-blockers will not completely prevent the hypotensive effect of histamine unless an H_2-blocker is administered concomitantly. Thus, the usefulness of H_1-blockers during an acute anaphylactic reaction is quite limited. The antiemetic and mild hypnotic effects of antihistaminic drugs (particularly diphenhydramine, promethazine, and hydroxyzine) have led to their use for premedication. Although H_1-blockers cause significant sedation, ventilatory drive is usually unaffected or augmented in the absence of other sedative medications.

Dosage

The usual adult dose of diphenhydramine is 25–50 mg (0.5–1.5 mg/kg) orally, intramuscularly, or intravenously every 4–6 hours. The doses of other H_1-receptor antagonists are listed in Table 15–1.

Drug Interactions

The sedative effects of H_1-receptor antagonists can potentiate other central nervous system depressants such as barbiturates and opioids.

2. H_2-Receptor Antagonists

Mechanism of Action

H_2-receptor antagonists include cimetidine, famotidine, nizatidine, and ranitidine (Table 15–2). These agents competitively inhibit histamine binding to H_2-receptors, thereby reducing gastric acid output and raising gastric pH. Nizatidine is only available in an oral formulation.

Clinical Uses

All H_2-receptor antagonists are equally effective in the treatment of peptic duodenal and gastric ulcers, hypersecretory states (Zollinger-Ellison syndrome), and gastroesophageal reflux disease (GERD). Intravenous preparations are also used to prevent stress ulceration in critically ill patients (see Chapter 50). Duodenal and gastric ulcers are usually associated with *Helicobacter pylori* infection, which is also treated with combinations of bismuth, tetracycline, and metronidazole. Ranitidine bismuth citrate with clarithromycin may also be used for peptic ulcers associated with *H pylori* infection. By decreasing gastric fluid volume and hydrogen ion content, H_2-blockers reduce the perioperative risk of aspiration pneumonia. These drugs affect the pH of only those gastric secretions occurring after their administration.

The combination of H_1- and H_2-receptor antagonists provides some protection against drug-induced allergic reactions (eg, intravenous radiocontrast, chymopapain injection for lumbar disk disease, protamine). Although pretreatment with these agents does not reduce histamine release, it does lessen subsequent hypotension.

Table 15–2. Pharmacology of aspiration pneumonia prophylaxis.

Drug	Route	Dose	Onset	Duration	Acidity	Volume	LES Tone
Cimetidine (Tagamet)	PO	300–800 mg	1–2 h	4–8 h	——	—	0
	IV	300 mg					
Ranitidine (Zantac)	PO	150–300 mg	1–2 h	10–12 h	——	—	0
	IV	50 mg					
Famotidine (Pepcid)	PO	20–40 mg	1–2 h	10–12 h	——	—	0
	IV	20 mg					
Nizatidine (Axid)	PO	150–300 mg	0.5–1 h	10–12 h	——	—	0
Nonparticulate antacids (Bicitra, Polycitra)	PO	15–30 mL	5–10 min	30–60 min	——	+	0
Metoclopramide (Reglan)	IV	10 mg	1–3 min	1–2 h	0	—	++
	PO	10–15 mg		30–60 min*			

*Oral metoclopramide has a quite variable onset of action and duration of action.
0 = no effect.
— = moderate decrease.
—— = marked decrease.
+ = slight increase.
++ = moderate increase.
LES = lower esophageal sphincter.

Side Effects

Rapid intravenous injection of cimetidine and raniti-dine has been rarely associated with hypotension, bradycardia, arrhythmias, and cardiac arrest. These adverse cardiovascular effects are more frequent following the administration of cimetidine to critically ill patients. In contrast, famotidine can be safely injected intravenously over a 2-minute period. H_2-receptor antagonists change the gastric flora by virtue of their pH effects. The clinical significance of this alteration has yet to be determined. Complications of long-term cimetidine therapy include hepatotoxicity (elevated serum transaminases), interstitial nephritis (elevated serum creatinine), granulocytopenia, and thrombocytopenia. Cimetidine also binds to androgen receptors, occasionally causing gynecomastia and impotence. Finally, cimetidine has been associated with mental status changes ranging from lethargy and hallucinations to seizures, particularly in elderly patients. In contrast, ranitidine, nizatidine, and famotidine do not affect androgen receptors and penetrate the blood-brain barrier poorly.

Dosage

As a premedication to reduce the risk of aspiration pneumonia, H_2-receptor antagonists should be administered at bedtime and again at least 2 hours before surgery (Table 15–2). Because all four drugs are eliminated primarily by the kidneys, the dose should be reduced in patients with significant renal dysfunction.

Drug Interactions

Cimetidine reduces hepatic blood flow and binds to the cytochrome P-450 mixed-function oxidases. These effects slow the metabolism of a multitude of drugs, including lidocaine, propranolol, diazepam, theophylline, phenobarbital, warfarin, and phenytoin. Ranitidine also decreases hepatic blood flow, but it is a weak inhibitor of the cytochrome P-450 system, and no significant drug interactions have been demonstrated. Famotidine and nizatidine do not appear to affect the cytochrome P-450 system.

ANTACIDS

Mechanism of Action

Antacids neutralize the acidity of gastric fluid by providing a base (usually hydroxide, carbonate, bicarbonate, citrate, or trisilicate) that reacts with hydrogen ions to form water.

Clinical Uses

Common uses of antacids include the treatment of gastric and duodenal ulcers, GERD, and Zollinger-Ellison syndrome. In anesthesiology, antacids provide protection against the harmful effects of aspiration pneumonia by raising the pH of gastric contents. Unlike H_2-receptor antagonists, antacids have an immediate effect. Unfortunately, they increase intragastric volume. Aspiration of particulate antacids (aluminum or magnesium hydroxide) produces abnormalities in lung function comparable to those that occur following acid aspiration. Nonparticulate antacids (sodium citrate or sodium bicarbonate) are much less damaging to lung alveoli if aspirated. Furthermore, nonparticulate antacids mix with gastric contents better than particulate solutions. Timing is critical, since nonparticulate antacids lose their effectiveness within 30–60 minutes after ingestion.

Dosage

The usual adult dose of a 0.3-M solution of sodium citrate—Bicitra (sodium citrate and citric acid) or Polycitra (sodium citrate, potassium citrate, and citric acid)—is 15–30 mL orally, 15–30 minutes prior to induction.

Drug Interactions

Because antacids alter gastric and urinary pH, they change the absorption and elimination of many drugs. The rate of absorption of digoxin, cimetidine, and ranitidine is slowed, while the rate of phenobarbital elimination is quickened.

METOCLOPRAMIDE

Mechanism of Action

Metoclopramide acts peripherally as a cholinomimetic (ie, facilitates acetylcholine transmission at selective muscarinic receptors) and centrally as a dopamine antagonist. Its action as a prokinetic agent in the upper gastrointestinal (GI) tract is not dependent on vagal innervation but is abolished by anticholinergic agents. It does not stimulate secretions.

Clinical Uses

 By enhancing the stimulatory effects of acetylcholine on intestinal smooth muscle, metoclopramide increases lower esophageal sphincter tone, speeds gastric emptying, and lowers gastric fluid volume. These properties account for its efficacy in the treatment of patients with diabetic gastroparesis or GERD as well as those at risk for aspiration pneumonia. Metoclopramide does not affect the secretion of gastric acid or the pH of gastric fluid.

Metoclopramide produces an antiemetic effect by blocking dopamine receptors in the chemoreceptor trigger zone of the central nervous system. Its usefulness as an antiemetic during cancer chemotherapy is better documented than is its usefulness following general anesthesia.

Metoclopramide provides some degree of analgesia in conditions associated with smooth muscle spasm (eg, renal or biliary colic, uterine cramping), presumably because of its cholinergic and dopaminergic effects. It has also reduced the analgesic requirements in patients undergoing prostaglandin-induced termination of pregnancy.

Side Effects

Rapid intravenous injection may cause abdominal cramping, and metoclopramide is contraindicated in patients with intestinal obstruction or pheochromocytoma. Sedation, nervousness, and extrapyramidal signs from dopamine antagonism (eg, akathisia) are rare and reversible. Nonetheless, metoclopramide is best avoided in patients with Parkinson's disease. Metoclopramide-induced increases in aldosterone and prolactin secretion are probably inconsequential during short-term therapy. Metoclopramide may rarely result in hypotension and dysrhythmias.

Dosage

An adult dose of 10–20 mg of metoclopramide (0.25 mg/kg) is effective orally, intramuscularly, or intravenously (injected over 5 minutes). Higher doses (1–2 mg/kg) have been used to prevent emesis during chemotherapy. Onset of action is much more rapid following parenteral (3–5 minutes) than oral (30–60 minutes) administration. Because metoclopramide is excreted in the urine, its dose should be decreased in patients with renal dysfunction.

Drug Interactions

Antimuscarinic drugs (eg, atropine, glycopyrrolate) block the GI effects of metoclopramide. Metoclopramide decreases the absorption of orally administered cimetidine. Concurrent use of phenothiazines or butyrophenones (droperidol) increases the likelihood of extrapyramidal side effects. Metoclopramide decreases dosage requirements for thiopental induction of anesthesia. It does not reverse the effects of low-dose dopamine infusion on the renal vasculature.

PROTON PUMP INHIBITORS

Mechanism of Action

These agents, including omeprazole, lansoprazole, rabeprazole, and pantoprazole, bind to the proton pump of parietal cells in the gastric mucosa and inhibit secretion of hydrogen ions.

Clinical Uses

Proton pump inhibitors are indicated for the treatment of duodenal ulcer, GERD, and Zollinger-Ellison syndrome. They may heal peptic ulcers and erosive GERD faster than H_2-receptor blockers. The use of proton pump inhibitors in aspiration prophylaxis prior to general anesthesia is limited. Some studies have shown that compared with omeprazole, H_2-receptor blockers are more reliable in consistently raising gastric pH and reducing gastric volume; lansoprazole may be as effective as H_2-receptor blockers. Two doses of lansoprazole (the evening before surgery and the morning of surgery) appear to be more effective than a single dose prophylaxis. Data on the use of newer intravenous agents (pantoprazole) for aspiration prophylaxis is limited.

Side Effects

Proton pump inhibitors are generally well tolerated causing few side effects. Adverse side effects are primarily GI (nausea, abdominal pain, constipation, and diarrhea). On rare occasions, they have been associated with myalgias, anaphylaxis, angioedema, and severe dermatologic reactions. Long-term treatment has also been associated with gastric enterochromaffin-like cell hyperplasia.

Dosage

Recommended oral doses for adults are omeprazole 20 mg, lansoprazole 15 mg, rabeprazole 20 mg, and pantoprazole 40 mg. Only pantoprazole is available for intravenous use in the United States. Because these drugs are primarily eliminated by the liver, repeat doses should be decreased in patients with severe liver impairment.

Drug Interactions

Omeprazole interferes with hepatic P-450 enzymes and decreases the clearance of diazepam, warfarin, and phenytoin. Other agents do not appear to have significant drug interactions.

5-HT₃ RECEPTOR ANTAGONISTS

Serotonin Physiology

Serotonin, 5-hydroxytryptamine (5HT), is present in platelets, the GI tract, and the central nervous system. It is formed by hydroxylation and decarboxylation of tryptophan. Monoamine oxidase inactivates serotonin into 5-hydroxyindolacetic acid. Serotonin physiology is complex because there are at least seven receptor types, some with multiple subtypes. The 5-HT_3 receptor is related to vomiting and found in the GI tract and the brain (area postrema). The 5-HT_2 receptors are responsible for smooth muscle contraction and platelet aggregation; 5-HT_4 receptors in the GI tract mediate secretion and peristalsis; and 5-HT_7 receptors, which are located primarily in the limbic system, may play a role in depression.

Mechanism of Action

Ondansetron, granisetron, dolasetron, and tropisetron selectively block serotonin 5-HT_3 receptors, with little or no effect on dopamine receptors (Figure 15–1). 5-HT_3 receptors, which are located peripherally (abdominal vagal afferents) and centrally (chemoreceptor trigger zone of the area postrema and the nucleus tractus solitarius), appear to play an important role in the initiation of the vomiting reflex. Unlike metoclopramide,

ONDANSETRON

5-HYDROXYTRYPTAMINE (serotonin)

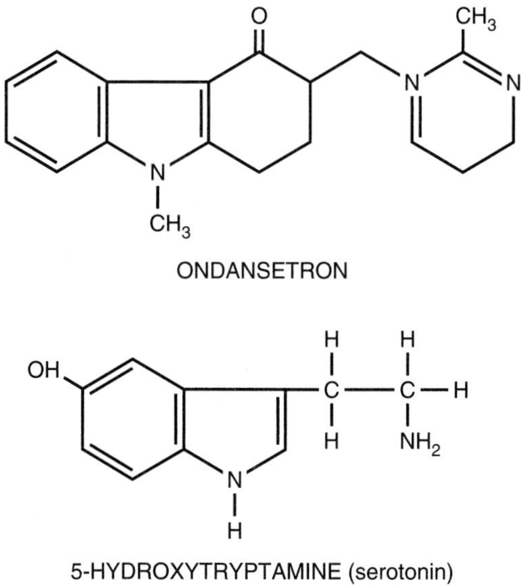

Figure 15–1. Ondansetron is structurally related to serotonin.

these agents do not affect GI motility or lower esophageal sphincter tone.

Clinical Uses

All these agents have proved to be effective antiemetics in the postoperative period. In some studies, 5-HT_3 receptor antagonists, as single agents, provided superior antiemetic prophylaxis compared with metoclopramide or droperidol alone. Other studies suggest that metoclopramide and droperidol together can provide equivalent prophylaxis to ondansetron alone. Because of their expense, some clinicians feel that 5-HT_3 receptor antagonists should not be used for routine prophylaxis but rather for symptomatic treatment of nausea or vomiting. Indeed, studies suggest no differences in outcome when antiemetics are given for symptomatic treatment and when they are administered prophylactically. Prophylaxis should, however, be seriously considered in patients with a prior history of postoperative nausea; those who are undergoing procedures at high risk for nausea (eg, laparoscopy); those in whom nausea and vomiting must be avoided (eg, neurosurgery); and those experiencing nausea and vomiting, to prevent further episodes. At this time, only ondansetron and dolasetron are approved by the Food and Drug Administration (FDA) for postoperative nausea and vomiting; granisetron is approved only for prevention of chemotherapy-induced nausea and vomiting.

Side Effects

5-HT_3 receptor antagonists are essentially devoid of serious side effects, even in amounts several times the recommended dose. They do not appear to cause sedation, extrapyramidal signs, or respiratory depression. The most common reported side effect is headache. Dolasetron can prolong the QT interval and should be used cautiously in patients taking antiarrhythmic drugs or those with a prolonged QT interval.

Dosage

The recommended adult intravenous dose of ondansetron for prevention of perioperative nausea and vomiting is 4 mg either prior to the induction of anesthesia or at the end of surgery. Postoperative nausea and vomiting can also be treated with a 4-mg dose, repeated as needed every 4–8 hours. Ondansetron undergoes extensive metabolism in the liver via hydroxylation and conjugation by cytochrome P-450 enzymes. Liver failure impairs clearance several-fold, and the dose should be reduced accordingly. The recommended intravenous dose for dolasetron is 12.5 mg. In clinical studies examining postoperative nausea, doses of 3 mg and 5 mg have been used for granisetron and tropisetron, respectively.

Drug Interactions

No significant drug interactions with 5-HT$_3$ receptor antagonists have been reported.

KETOROLAC

Mechanism of Action

 Ketorolac is a parenterally administered nonsteroidal anti-inflammatory drug (NSAID) that provides analgesia by inhibiting prostaglandin synthesis.

Clinical Uses

Ketorolac is indicated for the short-term (less than 5 days) management of pain, and appears to be particularly useful in the immediate postoperative period. A standard dose of ketorolac provides analgesia equivalent to 6–12 mg of morphine administered by the same route. Its time to onset is also similar to morphine, but ketorolac has a longer duration of action (6–8 hours).

Ketorolac, a peripherally acting drug, has become a popular alternative to opioids for postoperative analgesia because of its minimal central nervous system side effects. Specifically, ketorolac does not cause respiratory depression, sedation, or nausea and vomiting. In fact, ketorolac does not cross the blood-brain barrier to any significant degree. However, this does not mean that nausea, vomiting, or respiratory depression cannot occur postoperatively in patients treated with this drug; rather, it implies that ketorolac is not a likely cause. Because of the cost associated with its use, ketorolac may be most beneficial in patients at increased risk for postoperative respiratory depression or emesis. The analgesic effects of ketorolac may be more pronounced following orthopedic procedures than following intraabdominal surgery.

Side Effects

As with other NSAIDs, ketorolac inhibits platelet aggregation and prolongs bleeding time. It should therefore be used with caution, if at all, in patients at risk for postoperative hemorrhage. Long-term administration may lead to renal toxicity (eg, papillary necrosis) or GI tract ulceration with bleeding and perforation. Because ketorolac depends on elimination by the kidneys, it should not be given to patients in renal failure. Ketorolac is contraindicated in patients allergic to aspirin or NSAIDs. Asthmatic patients have an increased incidence of aspirin sensitivity (approximately 10%), particularly if they also have a history of nasal polyps (approximately 20%).

Dosage

Ketorolac has been approved for intramuscular administration (a loading dose of 30–60 mg; a maintenance dose of 15–30 mg every 6 hours) and intravenous administration (a loading dose of 15–30 mg; a maintenance dose of 15 mg every 6 hours). Elderly patients clear ketorolac more slowly and should receive reduced doses.

Drug Interactions

Aspirin decreases the protein binding of ketorolac, increasing the amount of active unbound drug. Ketorolac does not affect minimum alveolar concentration of inhalational anesthetic agents, and its administration does not alter the hemodynamics of anesthetized patients. It decreases the postoperative requirement for opioid analgesics.

DOXAPRAM

Mechanism of Action

Doxapram is a peripheral and central nervous system stimulant. Selective activation of carotid chemoreceptors by low doses of doxapram stimulates hypoxic drive, producing an increase in tidal volume and a slight increase in respiratory rate. At higher doses, the central respiratory centers in the medulla are stimulated.

Clinical Uses

Because doxapram mimics a low PaO$_2$, it may be useful in patients with chronic obstructive pulmonary disease who are dependent on hypoxic drive yet require supplemental oxygen. Drug-induced respiratory and central nervous system depression, including that seen immediately postoperatively, can be *temporarily* overcome. Doxapram is not a specific reversal agent, however, and should not replace standard supportive therapy (mechanical ventilation). For example, doxapram will not reverse paralysis caused by muscle relaxants, although it may transiently mask respiratory failure. The most common cause of postoperative hypoventilation—airway obstruction—will not be alleviated by doxapram. For these reasons, many anesthesiologists believe that doxapram has very limited usefulness.

Side Effects

Stimulation of the central nervous system leads to a variety of possible side effects: mental status changes (confusion, dizziness, seizures), cardiac abnormalities (tachycardia, dysrhythmias, hypertension), and pulmonary dysfunction (wheezing, tachypnea). Vomiting and laryngospasm are of particular concern to the anesthesiologist in the postoperative period. Doxapram should be avoided in patients with a history of epilepsy, cerebrovascular disease, acute head injury, coronary artery disease, hypertension, or bronchial asthma.

Dosage

Bolus intravenous administration (0.5–1 mg/kg) results in transient increases in minute ventilation (onset of action 1 minute; duration of action 5–12 minutes). Continuous intravenous infusions (1–3 mg/min) provide longer-lasting effects (maximum dose 4 mg/kg).

Drug Interactions

The sympathetic stimulation produced by doxapram may exaggerate the cardiovascular effects of monoamine oxidase inhibitors or adrenergic agents. Doxapram should be avoided in patients awakening from halothane anesthesia, since the latter sensitizes the myocardium to catecholamines.

NALOXONE

Mechanism of Action

Naloxone is a competitive antagonist at opioid receptors. Its affinity for μ receptors appears to be much greater than for κ or δ receptors (see Chapter 8). Naloxone has no significant agonist activity.

Clinical Uses

Naloxone reverses the agonist activity associated with endogenous (enkephalins, endorphins) or exogenous opioid compounds. A dramatic example is the reversal of unconsciousness that occurs in a patient with opioid overdose who has received naloxone. Perioperative respiratory depression caused by overzealous opioid administration is rapidly antagonized (1–2 minutes). Some degree of opioid analgesia can often be spared if the dose of naloxone is limited to the minimum required to maintain adequate ventilation. Low doses of intravenous naloxone reverse the side effects of epidurally administered opioids (see Chapter 18) without necessarily reversing the analgesia.

Side Effects

Abrupt reversal of opioid analgesia can result in sympathetic stimulation (tachycardia, ventricular irritability, hypertension, pulmonary edema) caused by pain perception, an acute withdrawal syndrome in patients who are opioid-dependent, or vomiting. The extent of these side effects is proportional to the amount of opioid being reversed and the speed of the reversal.

Dosage

In postoperative patients experiencing respiratory depression from excessive opioid administration, intravenous naloxone (0.4 mg/mL vial diluted to 0.04 mg/mL) can be titrated in increments of 0.5–1 μg/kg every 3–5 minutes until adequate ventilation and alertness are achieved. Intravenous doses in excess of 0.2 mg are rarely indicated. The brief duration of action of intravenous naloxone (30–45 minutes) is due to rapid redistribution from the central nervous system. A more prolonged effect is almost always necessary to prevent the recurrence of respiratory depression from longer-acting opioids. Therefore, intramuscular naloxone (twice the required intravenous dose) or a continuous infusion (4–5 μg/kg/hour) is recommended. Neonatal respiratory depression resulting from maternal opioid administration is treated with 10 μg/kg, repeated in 2 minutes if necessary. Neonates of opioid-dependent mothers will exhibit withdrawal symptoms if given naloxone. The primary treatment of respiratory depression is always airway establishment and artificial ventilation.

Drug Interactions

The effect of naloxone on nonopiate anesthetic agents such as nitrous oxide is controversial and probably insignificant. Naloxone may antagonize the antihypertensive effect of clonidine.

Similar Agents

Naltrexone and nalmefene are also pure opioid antagonists with a high affinity for the μ receptor. Both have significantly longer half-lives than naloxone. Naltrexone is used orally for maintenance treatment of opioid addicts. Nalmefene is currently not available in the United States.

FLUMAZENIL

Mechanism of Action

Flumazenil, an imidazobenzodiazepine, is a specific and competitive antagonist of benzodiazepines at benzodiazepine receptors (see Figure 8–5).

Clinical Uses

Flumazenil has proved useful in the reversal of benzodiazepine sedation and treatment of benzodiazepine overdose. Although it promptly (onset < 1 minute) reverses the hypnotic effects of benzodiazepines, amnesia has proved to be less reliably prevented. Some evidence of respiratory depression may linger despite an alert and awake appearance. Specifically, tidal volume and minute ventilation return to normal, but the slope of the carbon dioxide response curve remains depressed (see Figure 8–8). Elderly patients appear to be particularly difficult to reverse fully and are more prone to resedation.

Side Effects & Drug Interactions

Rapid administration of flumazenil may cause anxiety reactions in previously sedated patients and symptoms of withdrawal in those on long-term benzodiazepine therapy. Flumazenil reversal has been associated with increases in intracranial pressure in patients with head injuries and abnormal intracranial compliance. Flumazenil may induce seizure activity if benzodiazepines have been given as anticonvulsants or in conjunction with an overdose of tricyclic antidepressants. Flumazenil reversal following a midazolam-ketamine anesthetic technique may increase the incidence of emergence dysphoria and hallucinations. Nausea and vomiting are not uncommon following flumazenil administration.

The reversal effect of flumazenil is based on its strong affinity for benzodiazepine receptors, a *pharmacodynamic* (not pharmacokinetic) effect. Flumazenil does not affect the minimum alveolar concentration of inhalational anesthetics.

Dosage

Gradual titration of flumazenil is usually accomplished by intravenous administration of 0.2 mg every minute until reaching the desired degree of reversal. The usual total dose is 0.6–1.0 mg. Because of flumazenil's rapid hepatic clearance, repeat doses may be required after 1–2 hours to avoid resedation and premature recovery room or outpatient discharge. A continuous infusion (0.5 mg/hour) may be helpful in the case of an overdose of a longer-acting benzodiazepine. Liver failure prolongs the clearance of flumazenil and benzodiazepines.

CASE DISCUSSION: MANAGEMENT OF PATIENTS AT RISK FOR ASPIRATION PNEUMONIA

A 58-year-old man is scheduled for elective inguinal hernia repair. His past history reveals a persistent problem with heartburn and passive regurgitation of gastric contents into the pharynx. He has been told by his internist that these symptoms are due to a hiatal hernia.

Why would a history of hiatal hernia concern the anesthesiologist?

*Perioperative aspiration of gastric contents (**Mendelson's syndrome**) is a potentially fatal complication of anesthesia. Hiatal hernia is commonly associated with symptomatic gastroesophageal reflux disease (GERD), which is considered a predisposing factor for aspiration. Mild or occasional heartburn may not significantly increase the risk of aspiration. In contrast, symptoms related to passive reflux of gastric fluid, such as acid taste or sensation of refluxing liquid into the mouth, should alert the clinician to a high risk of pulmonary aspiration. Paroxysms of coughing and/or wheezing, especially at night or when the patient is flat, may be indicative of chronic aspiration. Aspiration can occur on induction, during maintenance or upon emergence from anesthesia.*

Which patients are predisposed to aspiration?

Patients with altered airway reflexes (eg, drug intoxication, general anesthesia, encephalopathy, neuromuscular disease) or abnormal pharyngeal or esophageal anatomy (eg, hiatal hernia, scleroderma, pregnancy, obesity) are prone to pulmonary aspiration.

Does aspiration consistently result in aspiration pneumonia?

Not necessarily. The seriousness of the lung damage depends on the volume and composition of the aspirate. Patients are considered to be at risk if their gastric volume is greater than 25 mL (0.4 mL/kg) and their gastric pH is less than 2.5. Some investigators believe that controlling acidity is more important than volume and that the criteria should be revised to a pH less than 3.5 with a volume greater than 50 mL.

Patients who have eaten immediately prior to emergency surgery are obviously at risk. Traditionally, "NPO after midnight" implied a preoperative fast of at least 6 hours. Current opinion allows clear liquids until 2–4 hours before induction of anesthesia, although solids are still taboo for 6 hours in adult patients. Some patients who have fasted for 8 hours or more before elective surgery also meet the at-risk criteria, however. Certain patient populations are especially likely to have large volumes of acidic gastric fluid: patients with an acute abdomen or peptic ulcer disease, children, the elderly, diabetic patients, pregnant women, and obese patients. Furthermore, pain, anxiety, or opioid-agonists may delay gastric emptying. Note that pregnancy and obesity place patients in double jeopardy by increasing the chance of aspiration (increased intra-abdominal pressure and distortion of the lower esophageal sphincter) and the risk of aspiration pneumonia (increased acidity and volume of gastric contents). Aspiration is more common in patients undergoing esophageal, upper abdominal, or emergency laparoscopic surgery.

Which drugs lower the risk of aspiration pneumonia?

H_2-receptor antagonists decrease gastric acid secretion. Although they will not affect gastric contents already in the stomach, they will inhibit further acid production. Both gastric pH and volume are affected. In addition, the long duration of action of ranitidine and famotidine may provide protection in the recovery room.

Metoclopramide shortens gastric emptying time, increases lower esophageal sphincter tone, and is an antiemetic. It does not affect gastric pH, and it cannot clear large volumes of food in a few hours. Nonetheless, the combination of metoclopramide with ranitidine is a good combination for most at-risk patients.

Antacids usually raise gastric fluid pH, but at the same time, they increase gastric volume. While antacid administration technically removes a patient from the at-risk category, aspiration of a substantial volume of particulate matter will lead to serious physiologic damage. For this reason, clear antacids (eg, sodium citrate) are strongly preferred. In contrast to H_2 antagonists, antacids are immediately effective and alter the acidity of existing gastric contents. Thus, they are useful in emergency situations and in patients who have recently eaten.

Anticholinergic drugs (see Chapter 11), particularly glycopyrrolate, decrease gastric secretions if large doses are administered; however, lower esophageal sphincter tone is reduced. Overall, anticholinergic drugs do not reliably reduce the risk of aspiration pneumonia.

The role of proton pump inhibitors is not clear and is discussed in the preceding section on proton pump inhibitors.

What anesthetic techniques are used in full-stomach patients?

If the full stomach is due to recent food intake and the surgical procedure is elective, the operation should be postponed. If the risk factor is not reversible (eg, hiatal hernia) or the case is emergent, proper anesthetic technique can minimize the risk of aspiration pneumonia. Regional anesthesia with minimal sedation should be considered in all patients at increased risk for aspiration pneumonia. If local anesthetic techniques are impractical, the patient's airway must be protected. Delivering anesthesia by mask or laryngeal mask airway is definitely contraindicated. As in every anesthetic case, the availability of suction must be confirmed before induction. If there are signs suggesting a difficult airway, intubation should precede induction (see Case Discussion, Chapter 5). Otherwise, a rapid-sequence induction is indicated.

How does a rapid-sequence induction differ from a routine induction?

- The patient is always preoxygenated prior to induction. Four maximal breaths of oxygen are sufficient to denitrogenate normal lungs. Patients with lung disease require 3–5 minutes of preoxygenation.

- Prior curarization with a nondepolarizing muscle relaxant may prevent the increase in intra-abdominal pressure that accompanies the fasciculations caused by succinylcholine. This step is often omitted, however, since it can decrease lower esophageal sphincter tone. If rocuronium has been selected for relaxation, a small priming dose (0.1 mg/kg) given 2–3 minutes prior to induction may speed its onset of action.

- A wide assortment of blades and endotracheal tubes are prepared in advance. It is prudent to begin with a stylet and an endotracheal tube one-half size smaller than usual to maximize the chances of an easy intubation.

- An assistant applies firm pressure over the cricoid cartilage prior to induction (**Sellick's maneuver**). Because the cricoid cartilage forms an uninterrupted and incompressible ring, pressure over it is transmitted to underlying tissue. The esophagus is collapsed, and passively regurgitated gastric fluid cannot reach the hypopharynx. Excessive cricoid pressure (beyond that which can be tolerated by a conscious person) applied during active regurgitation has been associated with rupture of the posterior wall of the esophagus.

- No test dose of thiopental is given. The induction dose is given as a bolus. Obviously, this dose must be modified if there is any indication that the patient's cardiovascular system is unstable. Other rapid-acting induction agents can be substituted for thiopental (eg, propofol, etomidate, ketamine).

- Succinylcholine (1.5 mg/kg) or rocuronium (0.9–1.2 mg/kg) is administered immediately following the thiopental, even if the patient has not yet lost consciousness.

- The patient is not artificially ventilated, to avoid filling the stomach with gas and thereby increasing the risk of emesis. Once spontaneous efforts have ceased or muscle response to nerve stimulation has disappeared, the patient is rapidly intubated. Cricoid pressure is maintained until the endotracheal tube cuff is inflated and tube position is confirmed. A modification of the classic rapid sequence induction allows gentle ventilation as long as cricoid pressure is maintained.

- If the intubation proves difficult, cricoid pressure is maintained and the patient is gently ventilated with oxygen until another intubation attempt can be performed. If intubation is still unsuccessful, spontaneous ventilation should be allowed to return and an awake intubation performed (see Figure 5–21).

- After surgery, the patient should remain intubated until airway reflexes have returned and consciousness has been regained.

What are the relative contraindications to rapid-sequence inductions?

Rapid-sequence inductions are usually associated with increases in intracranial pressure, arterial blood pressure, and heart rate. This technique shares the contraindications of thiopental (eg, hypovolemic shock) and succinylcholine (eg, thermal burns).

Describe the pathophysiology and clinical findings associated with aspiration pneumonia.

The pathophysiologic changes depend on the composition of the aspirate. Acid solutions cause atelectasis, alveolar edema, and loss of surfactant. Particulate aspirate will also result in small-airway obstruction and alveolar necrosis. Granulomas may form around food or antacid particles. The earliest physiologic change following aspiration is intrapulmonary shunting, resulting in hypoxia.

Other changes may include pulmonary edema, pulmonary hypertension, and hypercapnia.

Wheezing, tachycardia, and tachypnea are common physical findings. Hypotension signals significant fluid shifts into the alveoli and is associated with massive lung injury. Chest roentgenography may not demonstrate diffuse bilateral infiltrates for several hours after the event. Arterial blood gases reveal hypoxemia, hypercapnia, and respiratory acidosis.

What is the treatment of aspiration pneumonia?

As soon as regurgitation is suspected, the patient should be placed in a head-down position so that gastric contents drain out of the mouth instead of into the trachea. The pharynx and, if possible, the trachea should be thoroughly suctioned. The mainstay of therapy in patients who subsequently become hypoxic is positive pressure ventilation. Intubation and the institution of positive end-expiratory pressure or continuous positive airway pressure are often required. Bronchoscopy, pulmonary lavage, broad-spectrum antibiotics, and corticosteroids are controversial treatments and are rarely indicated.

SUGGESTED READING

Birmacombe JR, Berry AM: Cricoid pressure. Can J Anaesth 1997;44:414.

Bovill JG, Howie MB: *Clinical Pharmacology for Anaesthetists.* WB Saunders and Company, 1999.

Ferrari LR, Rooney FM, Rockoff MA: Preoperative fasting practices in pediatrics. Anesthesiology 1999;90:978.

Kovac AL: Prevention and treatment of postoperative nausea and vomiting. Drugs 2000;59:213.

Practice Guidelines for preoperative fasting and the use of pharmacologic agents to reduce the risk of pulmonary aspiration: Application to healthy patients undergoing elective procedures. A report by the American Society of Anesthesiologists Task Force on Preoperative Fasting. Anesthesiology 1999;90:896.

Schreiner MS: Gastric fluid volume: Is it really a risk factor for pulmonary aspiration? Anesth Analg 1998;86:754.

Warner MA, Warner ME, Warner DO, et al: Clinical significance of pulmonary aspiration during the perioperative period. Anesthesiology 1993;78:56.

Whitwam JG, Amrein R: Pharmacology of flumazenil. Acta Anaesthesiol Scand Suppl 1995;108:3.

SECTION III

Regional Anesthesia & Pain Management

Spinal, Epidural, & Caudal Blocks* | 16

*Wayne Kleinman, MD***

KEY CONCEPTS

 1 Performing a lumbar (subarachnoid) puncture below L1 in an adult (L3 in a child) avoids needle trauma to the cord; damage to the cauda equina is unlikely because these nerve roots float in the dural sac below L1 and tend to be pushed away (rather than pierced) by an advancing needle.

 2 The principal site of action for neuraxial blockade is the nerve root. Local anesthetic is injected into CSF (spinal anesthesia) or the epidural space (epidural and caudal anesthesia) and bathes the nerve root in the subarachnoid space or epidural space, respectively.

 3 Differential blockade typically results in sympathetic blockade (judged by temperature sensitivity) that may be two segments higher than the sensory block (pain, light touch), which in turn is two segments higher than motor blockade.

 4 Neuraxial blockade of sympathetic nerves causes vasodilation of the venous capacitance vessels, pooling of blood, and decreased venous return to the heart; in some instances, arterial vasodilation may also decrease systemic vascular resistance.

 5 Deleterious cardiovascular effects should be anticipated and steps undertaken to minimize the degree of hypotension. Volume loading with 10–20 mL/kg of intravenous fluid for a healthy patient will partially compensate for the venous pooling. Excessive or symptomatic bradycardia should be treated with atropine, and hypotension should be treated with vasopressors. If profound hypotension and/or bradycardia persist despite these interventions, epinephrine should be administered promptly.

(continued)

---

* This chapter has been revised and updated from an original chapter written by John E. Tetzlaff, MD, Section Head, Acute Perioperative Care, Department of General Anesthesiology, The Cleveland Clinic Foundation, Cleveland, Ohio.
** Director of Obstetric Anesthesia, Encino-Tarzana Regional Medical Center in Los Angeles, California.

(continued)

 Major contraindications to neuraxial anesthesia are patient refusal, bleeding diathesis, severe hypovolemia, elevated intracranial pressure, infection at the site of injection, and severe stenotic valvular heart disease.

 A line drawn between both iliac crests usually crosses either the body of L4 or the L4–L5 interspace. The anatomic midline is often easier to palpate when the patient is sitting than when the patient is in the lateral position. This is especially true with very obese patients.

 For epidural anesthesia, a sudden loss of resistance is encountered as the needle penetrates the ligamentum flavum and enters the epidural space. For spinal anesthesia, the needle is advanced further and penetrates the dura-subarachnoid membranes as signaled by free flowing CSF.

 In a lateral position, a hyperbaric spinal will have a greater effect on the dependent (down) side, while a hypobaric solution will achieve a higher level on the nondependent (up) side. An isobaric solution tends to remain at the level of injection.

 Epidural anesthesia is slower in onset (10–20 minutes) and usually not as dense as spinal anesthesia. This can be manifested as a more pronounced differential block or a segmental block.

Spinal, caudal, and epidural blocks were first used for surgical procedures at the turn of the last century (see Chapter 1). These central blocks were widely used prior to the 1940s until increasing reports of permanent neurologic injury appeared. Publication of a large-scale epidemiological study in the 1950s showed that complications were rare when these blocks were performed skillfully with attention to asepsis and newer, safer local anesthetics were used. Resurgence in the use of central blocks ensued, and today, they are once again widely used in clinical practice.

Spinal, epidural, and caudal blocks are also known as neuraxial anesthesia. Each of these blocks can be performed as a single injection or with a catheter to allow intermittent boluses or continuous infusions. Neuraxial anesthesia greatly expands the anesthesiologists' armamentarium to allow alternatives to general anesthesia when appropriate. They may also be used simultaneously with general anesthesia or afterwards for postoperative analgesia and in the management of acute and chronic pain disorders (see Chapter 18).

Some clinical studies suggest that postoperative morbidity—and possibly mortality—may be reduced when neuraxial blockade is used either alone or in combination with general anesthesia in some settings. Neuraxial blocks may reduce the incidence of venous thrombosis and pulmonary embolism, cardiac complications in high-risk patients, bleeding and transfusion requirements, vascular graft occlusion, and pneumonia and respiratory depression following upper abdominal or thoracic surgery in patients with chronic lung disease. Neuraxial blocks may also allow earlier return of gastrointestinal function following surgery. Proposed beneficial effects include amelioration of the hypercoagulable state associated with surgery, sympathectomy-mediated increases in blood flow, improved oxygenation from decreased splinting, and suppression of the neuroendocrine stress response to surgery. For patients with coronary artery disease, a decreased stress response may translate into less perioperative ischemia and reduced morbidity and mortality. Reduction of parenteral opiate requirements may decrease the incidence of aspiration pneumonia and hypoventilation. Postoperative epidural analgesia may significantly reduce the time until extubation and need for mechanical ventilation after major abdominal or thoracic surgery.

Perhaps neuraxial anesthesia has had its greatest impact in obstetric anesthesia (see Chapter 43). Currently, epidural anesthesia is widely used for analgesia in women in labor as well as during vaginal delivery of the neonate. Cesarean section is most commonly performed under epidural or spinal anesthesia. Both blocks allow a mother to remain awake and experience the birth of her child. Large population studies in Great Britain and in the United States have shown that regional anesthesia is associated with less maternal morbidity and mortality than is general anesthesia, which may be largely due to reducing the incidence of pulmonary aspiration and failed intubation.

Neuraxial techniques have proved to be extremely safe when managed well; however, there is still a risk for complications. Adverse reactions and complications range from self-limited back soreness to debilitating permanent neurologic deficits and even death. The practitioner must therefore have a good understanding of the anatomy involved, be thoroughly familiar with the pharmacology and toxic dosages of the agents employed, diligently employ sterile technique, and anticipate and quickly treat physiologic derangement.

ANATOMY

THE VERTEBRAL COLUMN

The spinal cord and its nerve roots lie within the central bony canal of the vertebral column, which provides them with structural support and protection. The vertebral column is made up of 7 cervical, 12 thoracic, 5 lumbar, 5 sacral, and 4 coccygeal vertebrae. With some notable exceptions, most vertebrae have similar features: a vertebral body, two pedicles, and two laminae. The spinal canal is bounded anteriorly by the vertebral bodies, laterally by the pedicles, and posteriorly by lamina (Figure 16–1). Each has a midline spinous process that arises between the laminae and two transverse processes that arise laterally at the junction of the lamina and pedicle. These processes serve as attachments for ligaments and muscles. Each vertebra also has four articular processes: two that project upward and two that project downward (Figure 16–1). Articular processes serve as synovial joints between vertebra. The joint formed between the articular processes of adjacent vertebra is commonly referred to as the facet joint. Adjacent vertebral bodies are attached via fibrocartilaginous intervertebral disks (Figure 16–2). Pedicles have large notches on their inferior surface and smaller notches on their superior surface. Notches from adjacent vertebrae form intervertebral foramina, through which nerve roots exit the spinal column (Figure 16–2).

The first cervical vertebra, the atlas, lacks a body and has unique articulations with the base of the skull and the second vertebra. The latter, also called the axis, consequently has atypical articulating surfaces. All 12 thoracic vertebrae articulate with their corresponding rib. Sacral vertebrae normally fuse into one large bone, the sacrum, but each one retains discrete anterior and posterior intervertebral foramina. Moreover, the lamina of S5 and all or part of that of S4 normally do not fuse, leaving a caudal opening to the spinal canal, the sacral hiatus. Coccygeal vertebrae are small rudimentary structures that also fused.

The spinal column normally forms a double C, being convex anteriorly in the cervical and lumbar regions (Figure 16–3). Ligamentous elements provide structural support and together with supporting muscles help maintain the unique shape. Ventrally, the vertebral bodies and intervertebral disks are connected and supported by the anterior and posterior longitudinal ligaments (Figure 16–1). Dorsally, the ligamentum

flavum, interspinous ligament, and supraspinous ligament provide additional stability.

THE SPINAL CORD

The spinal canal contains the spinal cord with its coverings (the meninges), fatty tissue, and a venous plexus (Figure 16–4). The meninges are composed of three layers: the pia mater, arachnoid mater, and the dura mater; all are contiguous with their cranial counterparts. The pia mater is closely adherent to the spinal cord, while the arachnoid mater is usually closely adherent to the thicker and denser dura mater. Cerebrospinal fluid (CSF) is contained between the pia and arachnoid maters in the subarachnoid space (see Chapter 25). The spinal subdural space is generally a poorly demarcated, potential space that exists between the dura and arachnoid membranes. The epidural space is a better defined potential space within the spinal canal that is bounded by the dura and the ligamentum flavum (Figure 16–5). The anatomy of the spinal cord is further discussed in Chapter 18.

The spinal cord normally extends from the foramen magnum to the level of L1 in adults (Figure 16–3). In children, the spinal cord ends at L3 but moves up as they grow older. The anterior and posterior nerve roots at each spinal level join one another and exit the intervertebral foramina forming spinal nerves from C1 to S5 (Figure 16–3). At the cervical level, the nerves arise above their respective vertebra, but starting at T1 they exist below their vertebra. As a result, there are eight cervical nerve roots but only seven cervical vertebra. Moreover, at the cervical and upper thoracic levels, the roots emerge from the spinal cord and exit the vertebral foramina nearly at the same level (Figure 16–3). But because the spinal cord normally ends at L1, lower nerve roots must travel an increasing distance (within the lumbar and sacral subarachnoid and epidural spaces) from the spinal cord to the intervertebral foramina. These lower spinal nerves form the cauda equina ("horse's tail"; Figure 16–3). Therefore, performing a lumbar (subarachnoid) puncture below L1 in an adult (L3 in a child) avoids needle trauma to the cord; damage to the cauda equina is unlikely as these nerve roots float in the dural sac below L1 and tend to be pushed away (rather than pierced) by an advancing needle.

A dural sheath invests most nerve roots for a small distance even after they exit the spinal canal. Nerve blocks close to the intervertebral foramen therefore carry a risk of subdural or subarachnoid injection (see Chapter 17). The dural sac and the subarachnoid and subdural spaces usually extend to S2 in adults and often S3 in children. Therefore, caudal anesthesia in children carries a greater risk of subarachnoid injection than in

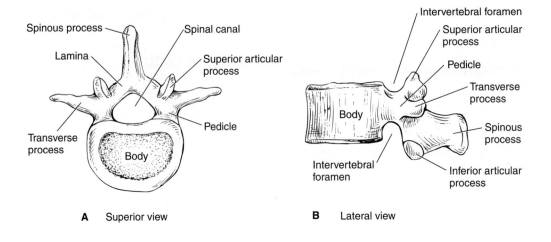

A Superior view

B Lateral view

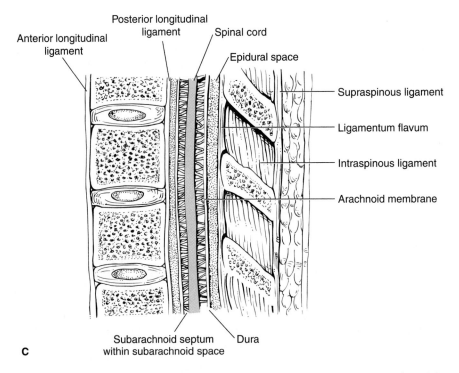

C

Figure 16–1. Common features of vertebrae (**A, B**). Saggital section through lumbar vertabrae (**C**).

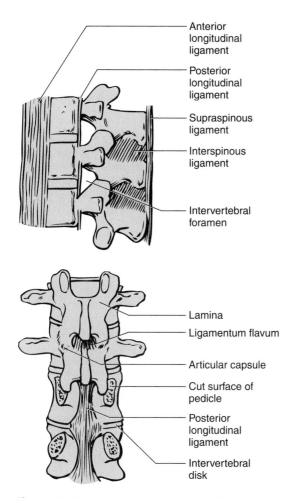

Anterior longitudinal ligament

Posterior longitudinal ligament

Supraspinous ligament

Interspinous ligament

Intervertebral foramen

Lamina

Ligamentum flavum

Articular capsule

Cut surface of pedicle

Posterior longitudinal ligament

Intervertebral disk

Figure 16–2. Ligaments of the spinal column.

adults. An extension of the pia mater, the filum terminale, penetrates the dura and attaches the terminal end of the spinal cord (conus medullaris) to the periostium of the coccyx.

The blood supply to the spinal cord and nerve roots is derived from a single anterior spinal artery and paired posterior spinal arteries (Figure 16–6A). The anterior spinal artery is formed from the vertebral artery at the base of the skull and courses down along the anterior surface of the cord. The anterior spinal artery supplies the anterior two-thirds of the cord, whereas the two posterior spinal arteries supply the posterior one-third. The posterior spinal arteries arise from the posterior inferior cerebellar arteries and course down along the dorsal surface of the cord medial to the dorsal nerve roots (see Chapter 25). The anterior and posterior spinal arteries receive additional blood flow from the intercostal arteries in the thorax and the lumbar arteries in the ab-

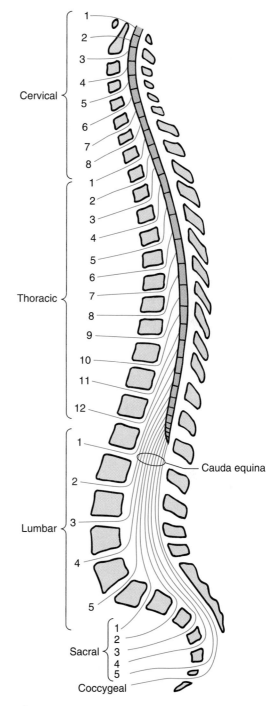

Cervical

Thoracic

Lumbar

Sacral

Coccygeal

Cauda equina

Figure 16–3. The vertebral column. (Adapted, with permission, from Waxman SG: *Correlative Neuroanatomy,* 24th ed. McGraw-Hill, 2000.)

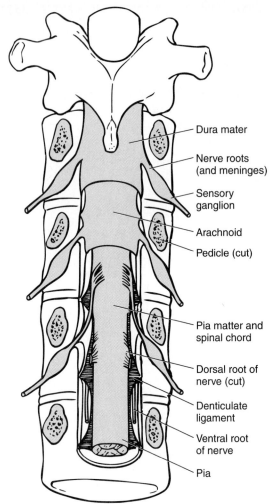

Figure 16–4. The spinal cord.

and bathes the nerve root in the subarachnoid space or epidural space, respectively. In the case of spinal anesthesia, the CSF concentration of local anesthetic is thought to have minimal effect on the spinal cord itself. Direct injection of local anesthetic into CSF, however, allows a relatively small quantity and volume of local anesthetic to achieve high levels of sensory and motor blockade. In contrast, the same local anesthetic concentration is achieved at nerve roots only with much higher volumes and quantities of local anesthetic with epidural and caudal anesthesia. Moreover, the injection site for epidural anesthesia must generally be close to the nerve roots that must be blocked. Blockade of neural transmission in the posterior nerve root fibers interrupts somatic and visceral sensation while blockade of anterior nerve root fibers prevents efferent motor and autonomic outflow (see Chapter 18).

SOMATIC BLOCKADE

By interrupting the transmission of painful stimuli and abolishing skeletal muscle tone, neuraxial blocks can provide excellent operating conditions. Sensory blockade interrupts both somatic and visceral painful stimuli while motor blockade produces skeletal muscle relaxation. The mechanism of action for local anesthetic agents is discussed in Chapter 14. The effect of local anesthetics on nerve fibers varies according to the size of the nerve fiber, whether or not it is myelinated, and the concentration achieved and the duration of contact. Table 16–1 contains the most commonly used classification systems for nerve fibers. Spinal nerve roots contain varying mixtures of these fiber types. Although

domen. One of these radicular arteries is typically large, the artery of Adamkiewicz, or arteria radicularis magna, arising from the aorta (Figures 16–6B and 16–6C). It is typically unilateral and nearly almost arises on the left side, providing the major blood supply to the anterior, lower two-thirds of the spinal cord. Injury to this artery can result in the anterior spinal artery syndrome (see Chapters 21 and 33).

■ PHYSIOLOGY

 The principal site of action for neuraxial blockade is the nerve root. Local anesthetic is injected into CSF (spinal anesthesia) or the epidural space (epidural and caudal anesthesia)

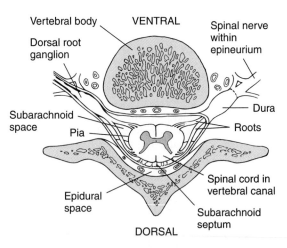

Figure 16–5. Exit of the spinal nerves. (Adapted, with permission, from Waxman SG: *Correlative Neuroanatomy,* 24th ed. McGraw-Hill, 2000.)

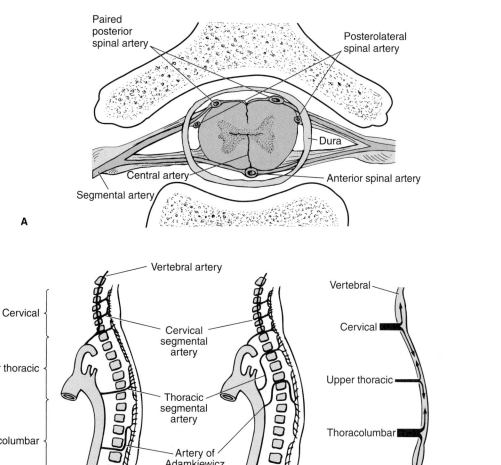

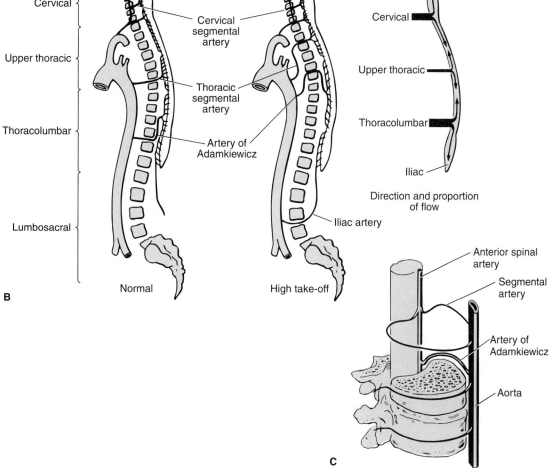

Figure 16–6. Arterial supply to the spinal cord (**A**). Segmental arterial blood supply to the vertebral cord (**B**) showing segmental distribution (**C**).

Table 16–1. Nerve fiber classification.*

Fiber Type	Sensory Classification	Modality Served	Diameter (mm)	Conduction (m/sec)
Aα		Motor	12–20	70–120
Aα	Type Ia	Proprioception	12–20	70–120
Aα	Type Ib	Proprioception	12–30	70–120
Aβ	Type II	Touch pressure Proprioception	5–12	30–70
Aγ		Motor (muscle spindle)	3–6	15–30
Aδ	Type III	Pain Cold temperature Touch	2–5	12–30
B		Preganglionic autonomic fibers	<3	3–14
C Dorsal root	Type IV	Pain Warm and cold temperature Touch	0.4–1.2	0.5–2
C Sympathetic		Postganglionic sympathetic fibers	0.3–1.3	0.7–2.3

*Peripheral nerve fibers and their respective neurons are classified from A–C according to axonal diameter, covering (myelinated or unmyelinated), and conduction velocity. Sensory fibers also are categorized as I–IV. Type C (sensory type IV) are unmyelinated fibers, while type Aδ fibers are lightly myelinated.

smaller and myelinated fibers are generally said to be more easily blocked than larger and unmyelinated ones, the phenomena of **differential blockade** appears to be more complex, especially for neuraxial anesthesia. In general, the concentration of local anesthetic decreases with increasing distance from the level of injection as does the concentration gradients. Differential blockade typically results in sympathetic blockade (judged by temperature sensitivity) that may be two segments higher than the sensory block (pain, light touch), which in turn is two segments higher than motor blockade.

AUTONOMIC BLOCKADE

Interruption of efferent autonomic transmission at the spinal nerve roots can produce sympathetic and some parasympathetic blockade (see Chapters 11 and 12). Sympathetic outflow from the spinal cord may be described as thoracolumbar, while parasympathetic outflow is craniosacral. Sympathetic preganglionic nerve fibers exit the spinal cord with the spinal nerves from T1 to the L2 level and may course many levels up or down the sympathetic chain before synapsing with a postganglionic cell in a sympathetic ganglia. In con-trast, parasympathetic preganglionic fibers exit the spinal cord with the cranial and sacral nerves. Neuraxial anesthesia does not block the vagal nerve. Neuraxial blocks therefore primarily result in varying degrees of sympathetic blockade and physiologic responses, resulting from decreased sympathetic tone and/or unopposed parasympathetic tone.

Cardiovascular Manifestations

Neuraxial blocks typically produce variable decreases in blood pressure that may be accompanied by a decrease in heart rate and cardiac contractility. These effects are generally proportional to the degree (level) of the sympathectomy. Vasomotor tone is primarily determined by sympathetic fibers arising from T5 to L1, innervating arterial and venous smooth muscle. Blocking these nerves causes vasodilation of the venous capacitance vessels, pooling of blood, and decreased venous return to the heart; in some instances, arterial vasodilation may also decrease systemic vascular resistance. The effects of arterial vasodilation may be minimized by compensatory vasoconstriction above the level of the block. A high sympathetic block not only prevents compensatory vasoconstriction but also blocks the sympathetic cardiac accelerator fibers that arise at T1–T4 (see Chapter 12). It should also be noted that blockade of cardiac sympathetic innervation with dilute local anesthetic (postoperatively via a thoracic epidural catheter) can reduce myocardial ischemia in patients with coronary artery disease. Profound hypotension may result from vasodilation combined with bradycardia and decreased contractility. These effects are exaggerated if venous return is further compromised by a head-up position or from the weight of a gravid uterus. Unopposed vagal tone in some persons may explain cardiac arrest with spinal anesthesia (see Chapter 47).

Deleterious cardiovascular effects should be anticipated and steps undertaken to minimize the degree of hypotension. Volume loading with 10–20 mL/kg of intravenous fluid for a healthy patient will partially compensate for the venous pooling. Left uterine displacement in the third trimester of pregnancy helps minimize the obstruction to venous return (see Chapter 42). Despite these efforts, hypotension may still occur and should be treated promptly. Fluid administration can be increased, and autotransfusion may be accomplished by placing the patient in the head-down position. Excessive or symptomatic bradycardia should be treated with atropine, and hypotension should be treated with vasopressors. Direct α-adrenergic agonists (such as phenylephrine) increase venous tone and produce arteriolar constriction, increasing both venous return and systemic vascular resistance. Ephedrine has direct β-adrenergic effects that increase heart rate and contractility and indirect effects that also produce some vasoconstriction. If profound hypotension and/or bradycardia persist despite these interventions, epinephrine should be administered promptly.

Pulmonary Manifestations

Clinically significant alterations in pulmonary physiology are usually minimal with neuraxial blocks. Even with high thoracic levels, tidal volume is unchanged; there is but a small decrease in vital capacity, which results from a loss of the abdominal muscles' contribution to forced expiration. Phrenic nerve (C3–C5) block may not occur even with total spinal anesthesia as apnea often resolves with hemodynamic resuscitation, suggesting that brainstem hypoperfusion is responsible rather than phrenic nerve block. The concentration of local anesthetic, even with a cervical sensory level, is reported to be below that required to block the large Aα fibers of the phrenic nerve.

Patients with severe chronic lung disease may rely upon accessory muscles of respiration (intercostal and abdominal muscles) to actively inspire or exhale. These muscles will be impaired below the level of the block. Similarly, effective coughing and clearing of secretions requires these muscles for expiration. For these reasons, neuraxial blocks should be used with caution in patients with limited respiratory reserve. These deleterious effects need to be weighed against the advantages of avoiding airway instrumentation and positive pressure ventilation. For surgical procedures above the umbilicus, a pure regional technique may not be the best choice for patients with severe lung disease. On the other hand, these patients may benefit from the effects of thoracic epidural analgesia in the postoperative period. Thoracic or upper abdominal surgery is associated with decreased diaphragmatic function postoperatively (from decreased phrenic nerve activity) and decreased functional residual capacity (FRC), which can lead to atelectasis and hypoxia via ventilation/perfusion ($\dot{V}/\dot{Q}$) mismatch. Some evidence suggests that postoperative thoracic epidural analgesia in high-risk patients can improve pulmonary outcome by decreasing the incidence of pneumonia and respiratory failure, improving oxygenation, and decreasing the duration of mechanical ventilatory support.

Gastrointestinal Manifestations

Sympathetic outflow originates at the T5–L1 level. It serves to decrease peristalsis, maintain sphincter tone, and oppose vagal tone. Neuraxial-block induced sympathectomy allows vagal tone dominance and results in a small, contracted gut with active peristalsis that can provide excellent operative conditions for some operations. Postoperative epidural analgesia has been shown to hasten return of gastrointestinal function.

Hepatic blood flow will decrease with reductions in mean arterial pressure from any anesthetic technique. For intra-abdominal surgery, the decrease in hepatic perfusion is more related to surgical manipulation than anesthetic technique (see Chapter 34).

Urinary Tract Manifestations

Renal blood flow is maintained through autoregulation, and there is little clinical effect upon renal function from neuraxial block. Neuraxial anesthesia at the lumbar and sacral levels blocks both sympathetic and parasympathetic control of bladder function. Loss of autonomic bladder control results in urinary retention until the block wears off. If no urinary catheter is anticipated perioperatively, it is prudent to use the shortest acting and least amount of drug necessary for the surgical procedure and limit the amount of intravenous fluid administration (if possible).

Metabolic & Endocrine Manifestations

Surgical trauma produces a neuroendocrine response via a localized inflammatory response and activation of somatic and visceral afferent nerve fibers. This response includes increases in adrenocorticotropic hormone, cortisol, epinephrine, norepinephrine, and vasopressin levels as well as activation of the renin-angiotensin-aldosterone system. Clinical manifestations include intraoperative and postoperative hypertension, tachycardia, hyperglycemia, protein catabolism, suppressed immune responses, and altered renal function. Neuraxial blockade can partially suppress (during major invasive surgery) or totally block (during lower extremity surgery) this stress response. A T11 block can block adrenal pathways and blunt hyperglycemia. By reducing catecholamine release, neuraxial blocks may decrease perioperative arrhythmias and possibly reduce the incidence ischemia. To maximize this blunting of the neuroendocrine stress response, neuraxial block should precede incision and extend into the postoperative period.

■ CLINICAL CONSIDERATIONS COMMON TO SPINAL & EPIDURAL BLOCKS

Indications

Neuraxial blocks may be used alone or in conjunction with general anesthesia for nearly any procedure below the neck. Indeed in some European centers, cardiac surgery has been routinely performed under thoracic epidural anesthesia (typically with light general anesthesia). As a primary anesthetic, neuraxial blocks have proved most useful for lower abdominal, inguinal, urogenital, rectal, and lower extremity surgery. Lumbar spinal surgery may also be performed under spinal anesthesia. Upper abdominal procedures (eg, cholecystectomy) can be performed with spinal or epidural anesthesia, but it can be difficult to achieve a sensory level adequate for patient comfort yet avoid the complications of a high block. Spinal anesthesia has been used for neonatal surgery.

If a neuraxial anesthetic is being considered, the risks and benefits need to be discussed with the patient, and an informed consent should be obtained. It is important to ascertain that the patient is mentally prepared for neuraxial anesthesia, that the choice of anesthesia is appropriate for the type of surgery, and that there are no contraindications. Patients should understand that they will have little or no motor function until the block resolves. Procedures that involve major

blood loss, maneuvers that might compromise respiratory function, or unusually prolonged surgery should generally be performed under general anesthesia with or without neuraxial bloackade.

Contraindications

 Major contraindications to neuraxial anesthesia are patient refusal, bleeding diathesis, severe hypovolemia, elevated intracranial pressure, infection at the site of injection, and severe stenotic valvular heart disease. Left ventricular outflow obstruction (valvular aortic or hypertrophic subaortic stenosis) and mitral stenosis limit compensatory increases in cardiac output in response to hypotension; regional anesthesia-induced sympathectomy can result in severe refractory hypotension with these cardiac lesions.

Relative and controversial contraindications are also listed in (Table 16–2). Physical examination of the back can reveal important information, such as the presence of surgical scars, scoliosis, skin lesions, and whether or not the spinous processes are palpable. Although no preoperative screening tests are required for healthy patients undergoing neuraxial blockade, coagulation studies and platelet count should be checked when the clinical history suggests the possibility of a bleeding diathesis. Neur-

Table 16–2. Contraindications to neuraxial blockade.

Absolute
Infection at the site of injection
Patient refusal
Coagulopathy or other bleeding diathesis
Severe hypovolemia
Increased intracranial pressure
Severe aortic stenosis
Severe mitral stenosis
Relative
Sepsis
Uncooperative patient*
Preexisting neurologic deficits
Demyelinating lesions
Stenotic valvular heart lesions
Severe spinal deformity
Controversial
Prior back surgery at the site of injection
Inability to communicate with patient*
Complicated surgery*
Prolonged operation
Major blood loss
Maneuvers that compromise respiration

*May be performed in conjunction with general anesthesia.

axial anesthesia in the presence of sepsis or bacteremia may predispose patients to hematogenous spread of the infectious agents into the epidural or subarachnoid space, but this is controversial.

Patients with preexisting neurologic deficits or demyelinating diseases may report worsening symptoms following a block. It may be impossible to discern effects or complications of the block from preexisting deficits or unrelated exacerbation of preexisting disease. For these reasons, many practitioners argue against neuraxial anesthesia in such patients.

Regional anesthesia requires at least some degree of patient cooperation. This may be difficult or impossible for patients with dementia, psychosis, or emotional instability. The decision needs to be individualized. Young children may similarly not be suitable for pure regional techniques.

Awake or Asleep?

If a regional anesthetic is to be used in conjunction with general anesthesia, should it be performed before or after induction of general anesthesia? This is a very controversial topic. The major arguments for having the patient asleep are that most patients, if given a choice, would prefer to be asleep and the possibility of sudden patient movement causing injury is markedly diminished. It may, however, be difficult to achieve ideal spinal flexion in some patients under general anesthesia. The major argument for neuraxial blockade while the patient is still awake is that the patient can alert the clinician to paresthesias and pain on injection, both of which have been associated with postoperative neurologic deficits. A few anecdotal reports of needle injections into the spinal cord itself during neuraxial blocks and interscalene nerve blocks in anesthetized patients have strengthened the latter argument, but studies showing an increased incidence of neurologic complications in anesthetized patients are lacking. Experts continue to argue both sides. Pediatric neuraxial blocks, especially caudal blocks, are nearly always performed under general anesthesia.

Technical Considerations

Neuraxial blocks should only be performed in a facility where all the equipment and drugs needed for intubation and resuscitation are immediately available. Regional anesthesia is greatly facilitated with adequate patient premedication. Nonpharmacologic patient preparation is also very helpful. The patient should be told what to expect so any surprises are eliminated and anxiety is minimized. This is especially important in those situations when premedication is not used, as is typically the case in obstetric anesthesia. Supplemental

oxygen via a face mask or nasal cannula helps avoid hypoxemia, especially if sedation is used. Minimum monitoring requirements include blood pressure and pulse oximetry for labor analgesia and pain management applications. Monitoring for surgical anesthesia is the same as for a general anesthetic.

Surface Anatomy

Spinous processes are generally palpable and help define the midline of the back. The spinous processes of the cervical and lumbar spine are nearly horizontal whereas those in the thoracic spine slant in a caudal direction and can overlap significantly. Therefore, when performing a lumbar or cervical epidural block (with maximum spinal flexion), the needle is directed nearly horizontally with a slight cephalad angle, whereas for a thoracic block the needle must be angled significantly more cephalad to enter the thoracic epidural space. In the cervical area, the first palpable spinous process is that of C2, but the most prominent one is that of C7 (vertebra prominens). With the arms at the side, the spinous process of T7 is usually at the same level as the inferior angle of the scapulae. A line drawn between both iliac crests usually crosses either the body of L4 or the L4–L5 interspace. Counting spinous processes up or down from these reference points identifies other spinal levels. A parallel line drawn connecting the posterior superior iliac spines crosses the S2 posterior foramina. In slender persons, the sacrum is easily palpable, and the sacral hiatus is felt as a depression just above or between the gluteal clefts and above the coccyx.

Patient Positioning

SITTING POSITION:

The anatomic midline is often easier to palpate when the patient is sitting than when the patient is in the lateral position. This is especially true with very obese patients. The patient sits on the edge of the operating table or bed with their feet either on the floor or preferably on a stool. They are asked to lean forward with elbows resting on their thighs or a bedside table, or with the arms crossed. The back should be maximally flexed (arched "like a mad cat"). Spinal flexion maximizes the opening between the interspaces and stretches the skin against deeper structures.

LATERAL DECUBITUS:

Many clinicians prefer the lateral position for central blocks (Figure 16–7). The patient lies on their side on edge of the table or bed and close to the anesthesiologist. The hips and knees are maximally flexed, and the chest and neck are flexed toward the knees. It may help

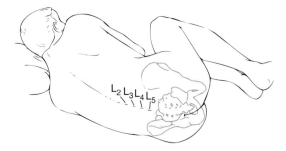

Figure 16–7. Identification of lumbar interspaces.

to ask the patient to assume the "fetal position" or "hug the knees like the cannonball position." The lateral decubitus position is useful for patients with hip or leg fracture who cannot sit up. It can also be useful for those who cannot fully cooperate, since an assistant can hold the hips and shoulders to optimally flex the spine. For unilateral surgical procedures, a hyperbaric spinal is usually administered to the patient in the lateral decubitus position with the surgical site down. In contrast, with a hypobaric technique, the patient is placed in lateral decubitus position where the surgical site is nondependent (up). Some practitioners prefer to always have the patient in the same (left or right) position to minimize variability and maximize their success rate.

PRONE POSITION:

This position may be used with spinal anesthesia for anorectal procedures. The patient is placed in the jackknife position, and lumbar puncture is performed. The advantage is that the patient does not have to be moved or turned, and with a hypobaric spinal solution, the uphill drift will provide the necessary sacral anesthesia. The main disadvantage is difficulty in verifying correct lumbar puncture because CSF often does not drip (against gravity) from the needle when the subarachnoid space is entered but has to be aspirated.

Anatomic Approach

Anatomic landmarks for the desired level of the block are first identified (see Surface Anatomy). A sterile field is established with a povidone-iodine or similar solution that is applied with three abrasive sponges. The solution is applied starting at the anticipated injection site and proceeding outward in a widening circle. A fenestrated sterile drape is applied. After the preparation solution has dried, it should be wiped away with sterile gauze to avoid introduction of this solution into the

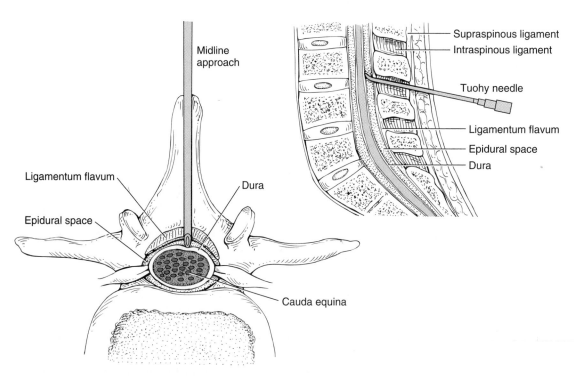

Figure 16–8. Lumbar epidural anesthesia; midline approach.

subarachnoid space, resulting in a chemical meningitis. A skin wheal is raised at the level of the chosen interspace with local anesthetic using a small gauge (25 g) needle. A longer (22-gauge) needle can then be used for deeper local anesthetic infiltration.

MIDLINE APPROACH:

(Figure 16–8) The spine is palpated and the patient's body position is examined to ensure that the plane of the back is perpendicular to that of the floor. This ensures that a needle passed parallel to the floor will stay midline as it courses deeper. The depression between the spinous processes of the vertebra above and below the level to be used is palpated; this will be the needle entry site. After prepping and anesthetizing the skin as above, the procedure needle is introduced in the midline. Remembering that the spinous processes course downward from the spine toward the skin, the needle will be directed slightly cephalad. The subcutaneous tissues offer little feeling of resistance to the needle. As the needle courses deeper, it will enter the supraspinous and interspinous ligaments, felt as an increase in tissue

density. The needle also feels more firmly implanted in the back. If bone is contacted superficially, the needle is likely hitting the lower spinous process. Contact with bone at a deeper depth usually indicates the needle is in the midline and hitting the upper spinous process or it is lateral to the midline and hitting a lamina. In either case the needle must be redirected. As the needle penetrates the ligamentum flavum an obvious increase in resistance is usually encountered. At this point, the procedure for spinal and epidural anesthesia differ (see Spinal Anesthesia and Epidural Anesthesia). For epidural anesthesia, a sudden loss of resistance is encountered as the needle penetrates the ligamentum flavum and enters the epidural space. For spinal anesthesia, the needle is advanced further and penetrates the dura-subarachnoid membranes as signaled by free flowing CSF.

PARAMEDIAN APPROACH:

(Figure 16–9) The paramedian technique may be selected if epidural or subarachnoid block is difficult, particularly in patients who cannot be positioned easily

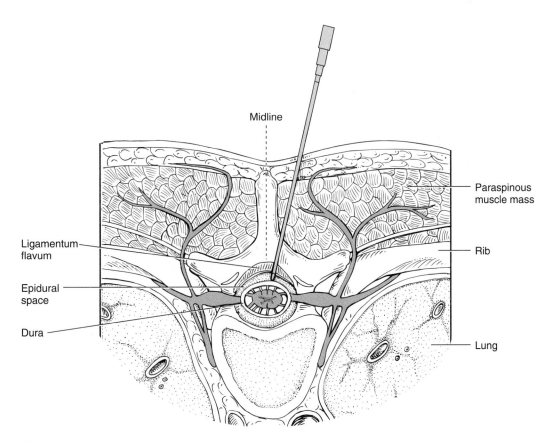

Figure 16–9. Lumbar spinal anesthesia; paramedian approach.

and those with severe arthritis, kyphoscoliosis, or prior lumbar spine surgery. As can readily be appreciated from a model of the spine the paramedian approach offers a much larger opening into the spinal canal than the midline approach. The skin wheal for a paramedian approach is raised 2-cm lateral to the superior spinous process of the desired level. Because this approach is lateral to most of the interspinous ligaments and penetrates the paraspinous muscles, the needle may encounter little resistance initially and may not feel to be in firm tissue. It is directed and advanced at a 10–25 degree angle toward the midline. Identification of the ligamentum flavum and entry into the epidural space with loss of resistance is often more subtle than with the midline approach.

ASSESSING LEVEL OF BLOCKADE:

The sensory level achieved by a block can be assessed with pinprick, whereas the level of sympathectomy is assessed by measuring skin temperature. The Bromage scale can be used to evaluate motor blockade: "no block" (the ability to flex the knees and feet), "partial block" (ability to flex the knees and resist gravity with full movement of the feet), "almost complete block" (inability to flex the knees but retained ability to flex the feet), and "complete block" (inability to move the legs or feet).

■ SPINAL ANESTHESIA

Spinal anesthesia blocks nerve roots as they course through the subarachnoid space. The spinal subarachnoid space extends from the foramen magnum to the S2 in adults and S3 in children. Injection of local anesthetic below L1 in adults and L3 in children helps avoid direct trauma to the spinal cord. Spinal anesthesia is also referred to a subarachnoid block or intrathecal injection.

Spinal Needles

These needles are precisely made, without any surface irregularities, and have a tightly fitting removable stylet that completely occludes the lumen to avoid tracking epithelial cells into the subarachnoid space. They are commercially available in an array of sizes (16 to 30 gauge), lengths, and bevel and tip designs (Figure 16–10). Broadly, they can be divided into either sharp (cutting) tipped or blunt tipped needles. The **Quincke** needle is a cutting needle with end-injection. The **Whitacre** and other pencil-point needles have rounded points and side-injection. The **Sprotte** is a side-injection needle with a long opening. It has the advantage of more vigorous CSF

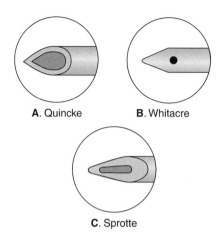

A. Quincke   **B.** Whitacre

C. Sprotte

Figure 16–10. Spinal needles.

flow compared with similar gauge needles. However, this can lead to a failed block if the distal part of the opening is subarachnoid (with free flow CSF) while the proximal part is not past the dura and the full dose of medication is not delivered. Blunt tipped needles are associated with less incidence of dural puncture headache; in general, the smaller the needle, the lower the incidence of post-puncture headache.

Spinal Catheters

Very small subarachnoid catheters are currently no longer approved by the US Food and Drug Administration (FDA). The withdrawal of these catheters was prompted by their association with cauda equina syndrome. Larger catheters designed for epidural use are associated with relatively high complication rates when placed subarachnoid. They may be used for spinal anesthesia after inadvertent dural puncture ("wet tap").

Specific Technique for Spinal Anesthesia

The midline, paramedian, or prone approach can be used for spinal anesthesia. As previously discussed, the needle is advanced from skin through the deeper structures until two "pops" are felt. The first is penetration of the ligamentum flavum and the second is penetration of the dura-arachnoid membrane. Successful dural puncture is confirmed by withdrawing the stylet to verify free flow of CSF. With small gauge needles (< 25 g), especially in the presence of low CSF pressure (eg, a dehydrated patient), aspiration may be necessary to detect CSF. The needle may be rotated 360 degrees to verify free flow in each quadrant, and the syringe is then connected, CSF aspirated, and the medication injected. If free flow does not occur in all quadrants, the needle tip may be near the dural sleeve. Injecting here may result in an incomplete block, and may cause damage to the spinal nerve by hydrostatic compression. If CSF cannot be aspirated after attaching the syringe, the needle may have moved. Persistent paresthesia or pain upon injection should alert the clinician to withdraw and redirect the needle.

Factors Influencing Level of Block

Table 16–3 lists factors that have been shown to affect level of neural blockade following spinal anesthesia. The most important determinants are baricity, position of the patient during and immediately after injection, and drug dosage. In general, the higher the dosage or site of injection, the higher the level of anesthesia obtained. Moreover, migration of the local anesthetic cephalad in CSF depends on its specific gravity relative to CSF (baricity). CSF has a specific gravity of 1.003–1.008 at 37 °C. Table 16–4 lists the specific gravity of the commonly used local anesthetic solutions. A **hyperbaric solution** of local anesthetic is denser (heavier) than CSF while a **hypobaric solution** is less dense (lighter) than CSF. The local anesthetic solutions can be made hyperbaric by the addition of glucose and hypobaric by the addition of sterile water. Thus, with a head-down position, a hyperbaric solution spreads cephalad and a hypobaric anesthetic solution moves caudad. Head-up position causes a hyperbaric solution to settle caudad and the hypobaric solution ascends cephalad. Similarly, in a lateral position, a hyperbaric spinal will have a greater effect on the dependent (down) side, while a hypobaric solution will achieve a higher level on the nondepen-

Table 16–3. Factors affecting the level of spinal anesthesia.

Most important factors
Baricity of anesthetic solution
Position of the patient
During injection
Immediately after injection
Drug dosage
Site of injection
Other factors
Age
Cerebrospinal fluid
Curvature of the spine
Drug volume
Intra-abdominal pressure
Needle direction
Patient height
Pregnancy

Table 16–4. Specific gravities of some spinal anesthetic agents.

Agent	Specific Gravity
Procaine	
1.5% in water	1.0052
2.5% in D₅W	1.0203
Lidocaine	
2% plain	1.0004–1.0066
5% in 7.5% dextrose	1.0262–1.0333
Tetracaine, 0.5% in D₅W	1.0133–1.0203
Tetracaine, 0.5% in water	0.9977–0.9997
Bupivacaine	
0.5% in 8.25% dextrose	1.0227–1.0278
0.5% plain	0.9990–1.0058

dent (up) side. An **isobaric solution** tends to remain at the level of injection. Anesthetic agents are mixed with CSF (at least 1:1) to make their solutions isobaric. Other factors affecting the level of neural blockade include the level of injection and the patient's height and vertebral column anatomy. The direction of the needle bevel or injection port may also play a role; if the injection is directed cephalad higher levels of anesthesia are achieved than if point of injection is oriented laterally or caudad.

Hyperbaric solutions tend move to the most dependent area of the spine (normally T4–T8 in the supine position). With normal spinal anatomy, the apex of the thoracolumbar curvature is T4. In the supine position, this should limit a hyperbaric solution to produce a level of anesthesia at or below T4. Abnormal curvatures of the spine, such as scoliosis and kyphoscoliosis, have multiple effects on spinal anesthesia; Placing the block becomes more difficult because of the rotation and angulation of the vertebral bodies and spinous processes. Finding the midline and the interlaminar space may be difficult. The paramedian approach to lumbar puncture may be preferable in patients with severe scoliosis and kyphoscoliosis, especially if there is associated degenerative joint disease. Reviewing radiographs of the spine before attempting the block may be useful. Spinal curvature affects the ultimate level by changing the contour of the subarachnoid space. Previous spinal surgery can similarly present technical difficulties in placing a block. Correctly identifying the interspinous and interlaminar spaces may be difficult at the levels of previous laminectomy or spinal fusion. The paramedian approach may be easier, or a level above the surgical site can be chosen. The block may be incomplete, or the level different than anticipated, due to postsurgical anatomic changes.

CSF volume inversely correlates with level of anesthesia. Increased intra-abdominal pressure or conditions that cause engorgement of the epidural veins, thus decreasing CSF volume, are associated with higher blocks. This would include conditions such as pregnancy, ascites, and large abdominal tumors. In these clinical situations, higher levels of anesthesia are achieved with a given dose of local anesthetic than would otherwise be expected. For spinal anesthesia on a term parturient, the dosage of anesthetic can be reduced by one-third compared with a nonpregnant patient (see Chapters 42 and 43). Age-related decreases in CSF volume are likely responsible for the higher anesthetic levels achieved in the elderly for a given dosage of spinal anesthetic. Severe kyphosis or kyphoscoliosis can be associated with a decreased volume of CSF and often results in a higher than expected level, especially with a hypobaric technique or rapid injection. Conflicting opinion exists as to whether increased CSF pressure caused by coughing or straining, or turbulence on injection has any effect on the spread of local anesthetic in the CSF.

Spinal Anesthetic Agents

Many local anesthetics have been used for spinal anesthesia in the past, but only a few are currently in use (Table 16-5). There is renewed interest in some older medications because of reports documenting an increased incidence of transient neurologic symptoms with 5% lidocaine (see Complications of Neuraxial Anesthesia). Only preservative-free local anesthetic solutions are used. Addition of vasoconstrictors (α-adrenergic agonists) and opioids greatly enhances the quality and prolongs the duration of spinal anesthesia (see Chapter 18). Vasoconstrictors include epinephrine (0.1–0.2 mg) and phenylephrine (1–2 mg). Both agents

appear to decrease the uptake and clearance of local anesthetics from CSF and may have weak spinal analgesic properties. Clonidine and neostigmine also have spinal analgesic properties, but experience with them as additives for spinal anesthesia is limited.

Hyperbaric bupivacaine and tetracaine are the most commonly used agents for spinal anesthesia. Both are relatively slow in onset (5–10 minutes) and have a prolonged duration (90–120 minutes). Although both agents produce similar sensory levels, spinal tetracaine generally produces more motor blockade than the equivalent dose of bupivacaine. Addition of epinephrine to spinal bupivacaine only modestly prolongs its duration. In contrast, epinephrine can prolong the duration of tetracaine anesthesia by more than 50%. Phenylephrine also prolongs tetracaine anesthesia but has no effect on bupivacaine spinal blocks. Ropivacaine has also been used for spinal anesthesia, but experience with it is more limited. A 12-mg intrathecal dose of ropivacaine is roughly equivalent to 8 mg of bupivacaine, but it appears to have no particular advantages for spinal anesthesia. Lidocaine and procaine have a rapid onset (3–5 minutes) and short duration of action (60–90 minutes). There are conflicting data as whether or not their duration is prolonged by vasoconstrictors; any effect appears to be modest. Some clinicians no longer use 5% lidocaine for spinal anesthesia.

Hyperbaric spinal anesthesia is more commonly used than the hypobaric or isobaric techniques. The level of anesthesia then is dependent on the patient's position during and immediately following the injection. In the sitting position, "saddle block" can be achieved by keeping the patient sitting for 3–5 minutes following injection so that only the lower lumbar nerves and sacral nerves are blocked. If the patient is placed from the sitting position to the supine position immediately after injection, the agent will move more cephalad to the dependent region defined by the thoracolumbar curve, as full protein binding has not yet oc-

Table 16–5. Dosages and actions of commonly used spinal anesthetic agents.

| Drug | Preparation | Doses | | | Duration | |
		Perineum, Lower Limbs	Lower Abdomen	Upper Abdomen	Plain (min)	Epinephrine (min)
Procaine	10% solution	75 mg	125 mg	200 mg	45	60
Bupivacaine	0.75% in 8.25% dextrose	4–10 mg	12–14 mg	12–18 mg	90–120	100–150
Tetracaine	1% solution in 10% glucose	4–8 mg	10–12 mg	10–16 mg	90–120	120–240
Lidocaine	5% in 7.5% glucose	25–50 mg	50–75 mg	75–100 mg	60–75	60–90
Ropivacaine	0.2–1% solution	8–12 mg	12–16 mg	16–18 mg	90–120	90–120

curred. Hyperbaric anesthetics injected intrathecally with the patient in the lateral decubitus position are useful for unilateral lower extremity procedures. The patient is placed laterally with the extremity to be operated on in a dependent position. If the patient is kept in this position for 5 minutes or so following injection, the block will tend to be denser and achieve a higher level on the operative dependent side.

■ EPIDURAL ANESTHESIA

Epidural anesthesia is a neuraxial technique offering a wider range of applications than the typical all-or-nothing spinal anesthetic. An epidural block can be performed at the lumbar, thoracic, or cervical levels. Sacral epidural anesthesia is referred to as a caudal block and is described at the end of the chapter. Epidural techniques are widely used for operative anesthesia, obstetric analgesia, postoperative pain control, and chronic pain management. It can be used as a single shot technique or with a catheter that allows intermittent boluses and/or continuous infusion. The motor block can range from none to complete. All these variables are controlled by the choice of drug, concentration, dosage, and level of injection.

The epidural space surrounds the dura mater posteriorly, laterally, and anteriorly. Nerve roots travel in this space as they exit laterally through the foramen and course outward. Other contents include fatty connective tissue, lymphatics, and a rich venous (Batson's) plexus. Recent fluoroscopic studies have suggested the presence of septa or connective tissue bands. Advancing age is associated with a decrease in epidural adipose tissue.

 Epidural anesthesia is slower in onset (10–20 minutes) and usually not as dense as spinal anesthesia. This can be manifested as a more pronounced differential block or a segmental block, a feature that can be useful clinically. For example, by using relatively dilute concentrations of local anesthetic combined with an opiate, an epidural can block the smaller sympathetic and sensory fibers while sparing the larger motor fibers, providing analgesia without motor block. This is commonly employed for labor analgesia and postoperative analgesia. Moreover, a segmental block is possible because the anesthetic is not spread readily by CSF and can be confined close to the level where it was injected. A segmental block is characterized by a well-defined band of anesthesia at certain nerve roots, while those above *and* below are not blocked. This can be seen with a thoracic epidural that provides upper abdominal anesthesia while sparing cervical and lumbar nerve roots.

Lumbar epidural is the most common anatomic insertion site for epidural anesthesia and analgesia. The midline or paramedian approach can be used. Lumbar epidural anesthesia can be used for any procedure below the diaphragm. Because the spinal cord typically terminates at the L1 level, there is an extra measure of safety in performing the block in the lower lumbar interspaces, especially if an inadvertent dural puncture occurs (see Complications).

Thoracic epidural blocks are technically more difficult to accomplish than lumbar blocks and the risk of spinal cord injury, though small with good technique, is greater than that at the lumbar level. They can be accomplished with the midline or paramedian approach. Some clinicians feel that the paramedian approach is easier because of the extreme oblique course of the thoracic spinous processes. Rarely used as a primary anesthetic, the thoracic epidural technique is most commonly used for intra- and postoperative analgesia. Single shot or catheter techniques are used for chronic pain management. Infusions via an epidural catheter are very useful for providing analgesia and may obviate or shorten postoperative ventilation for patients with underlying lung disease and following chest surgery.

Cervical blocks are usually performed with the patient sitting, the neck flexed, and using the midline approach. Clinically, they are used primarily for pain management (see Chapter 18).

Epidural Needles

The standard epidural needle is typically 17–18-gauge, 3 or 3.5 inches long, and has a blunt bevel with a gentle curve of 15–30 degrees at the tip. The Tuohy needle is most commonly used (Figure 16–11). The blunt, curved tip helps push away the dura after passing through the ligamentum flavum instead of penetrating it. Straight needles without a curved tip (Crawford needles) may have a higher incidence of dural puncture but facilitated passage of an epidural catheter. Needle modifications include winged tips and introducer devices set into the hub designed for guiding catheter placement.

Epidural Catheters

Placing a catheter into the epidural space allows for continuous infusion or intermittent bolus techniques. Besides extending the duration of the block, it may allow a lower total dose of anesthetic to be used, and therefore, lessen the hemodynamic insults if incremental initial dosing is used.

Epidural catheters are useful for intraoperative epidural anesthesia and/or postoperative analgesia. Typically, a 19- or 20-gauge catheter is introduced through a 17- or 18-gauge epidural needle. When using

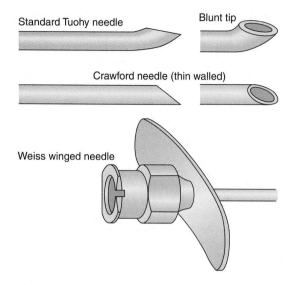

Figure 16–11. Epidural needles.

a curved tipped needle, the bevel opening is directed either cephalad or caudad, and the catheter is advanced 2–6 cm into the epidural space. The shorter the distance the catheter is advanced, the more likely it is to become dislodged. Conversely, the further the catheter is advanced, the higher the chance of a unilateral block that may be due to the catheter tip either exiting the epidural space via an intervertebral foramen or coursing into the anterolateral recesses of the epidural space. After advancing the catheter the desired depth, the needle is removed leaving the catheter in place. The catheter can be taped or otherwise secured along the back. Catheters either have a single port at the distal end or multiple side ports close to a closed tip. Some have a stylet for easier insertion. Spiral wire reinforced catheters are very resistant to kinking. The spiral or spring tip is associated with fewer, less intense paresthesias and may be associated with a lower incidence of inadvertent intravascular insertion.

Specific Technique for Epidural Anesthesia

Using the midline or paramedian approaches detailed previously, the epidural needle courses from the skin just through the ligamentum flavum. Epidural anesthesia requires that the needle stop short of piercing the dura. Two techniques exist for recognizing when the tip of the needle has entered the potential (epidural) space: the "loss of resistance" and "hanging drop" techniques.

The **loss of resistance technique** is preferred by most clinicians. The needle is advanced through the subcutaneous tissues with the stylet in place until the interspinous ligament is entered as noted by an increase in tissue resistance. The stylet or introducer is removed and a glass syringe filled with approximately 2 mL of fluid or air is attached to the hub of the needle. If the tip of the needle is within the ligament, gentle attempts at injection are met with resistance and injection is not possible. The needle is then slowly advanced, millimeter by millimeter, with either continuous or rapidly repeating attempts at injection. As the tip of the needle just enters the epidural space there is a sudden loss of resistance and injection is easy.

Once into the interspinous ligament and the stylet is removed, the **hanging drop technique** requires that the hub of the needle be filled with solution so that a drop hangs from its outside opening. The needle is then slowly advanced deeper. As long as the tip of the needle remains within the ligamentous structures, the drop remains "hanging." However, as the tip of the needle enters the epidural space it creates negative pressure and the drop of fluid is sucked into the needle. If the needle becomes plugged the drop will not be drawn into the hub of the needle and inadvertent dural puncture may occur. Some clinicians prefer to use this technique for the paramedian approach and for cervical epidurals.

Activating an Epidural

The quantity (volume and concentration) of local anesthetic needed for epidural anesthesia is relatively large compared with spinal anesthesia. Significant toxicity can occur if this amount is injected intrathecally or intravascularly. Safeguards against this include the epidural test dose and incremental dosing. This is true whether the injection is through the needle or through an epidural catheter.

A **test dose** is designed to detect both subarachnoid injection and intravascular injection. The classic test dose combines local anesthetic and epinephrine typically 3 mL of 1.5% lidocaine with 1:200,000 epinephrine (0.005 mg/mL). The 45 mg of lidocaine, if injected intrathecally, will produce spinal anesthesia that should be rapidly apparent. The 15 µg of epinephrine, if injected intravascularly, should produce a noticeable increase in heart rate (20% or more). Some have suggested lower doses of local anesthetic should be used, as unintended injection of 45 mg of intrathecal lidocaine can be difficult to manage in some areas such as labor rooms. Similarly, epinephrine as a marker of intravenous injection is not ideal. False-positives can occur (a uterine contraction causing pain and increase heart rate coincidental to test dosing) as well as false-negatives (patients taking β-blockers). Fentanyl has been advocated as an intravenous injection test dose, as have larger doses of local anesthetic without epinephrine. Some suggest that simply aspirating prior to injection is sufficient to avoid inadvertent intravenous injection. However, most experienced practitioners have encountered false-negative aspirations through a needle and with a catheter.

Incremental dosing is a very effective method of avoiding serious complications. If aspiration is negative, a fraction of the total intended local anesthetic dose is injected, typically 5 mL. This dose should be large enough that mild symptoms of intravascular injection occur but small enough to avoid seizure or cardiovascular compromise. This is especially important in the scenario of the labor epidural that is to be used for cesarean section. If the initial labor epidural bolus was delivered through the needle and then the catheter was inserted, it may be erroneously assumed that the catheter is well positioned because the patient is still comfortable from the initial bolus. If the catheter was inserted intravascularly, or has since migrated intravascularly, systemic toxicity will likely result if the full anesthetic dose is injected. Catheters can migrate intrathecally or intravascularly from an initial correct epidural position anytime after initial placement. Some cases of "catheter migration" may represent delayed recognition.

If one uses an initial test dose, is diligent about aspirating prior to each injection, and always uses incremental dosing, significant systemic toxicity and inadvertent intrathecal injections are rare.

Factors Affecting Level of Block

Factors affecting the level of epidural anesthesia may not be as predictable as with spinal anesthesia. In adults, 1–2 mL of local anesthetic per segment to be blocked is a generally accepted guideline. For example, to achieve a T4 sensory level from an L4–L5 injection would require about 12–24 mL. For segmental or analgesic blocks, less volume is needed.

The dose required to achieve the same level of anesthesia decreases with age. This is probably a result of age-related decreases in the size or compliance of the epidural space. Because escape of the local anesthetic solution through intervertebral foramina tends to limit cephalad spread of local anesthetic, age-related narrowing of intervertebral foramina was previously thought to be responsible, but this has been disputed. While there is little correlation between body weight and epidural dosage requirements, patient height affects the extent of cephalad spread. Thus, shorter patients may require only 1 mL of local anesthetic per segment to be blocked, while taller patients generally require 2 mL per segment. Although less dramatic than with spinal anesthesia, spread of epidural local anesthetics tends to be partially affected by gravity. The lateral decubitus, Trendelenburg, and reverse Trendelenburg positions can be used to help achieve blockade in the desired dermatomes. Injection in the sitting position appears to deliver more local anesthetic to the larger L5–S1 and S2 nerve roots; patchy anesthesia or sparing of those dermatomes is sometimes encountered with lumbar epidural anesthesia.

Additives to the local anesthetic, especially opioids, tend to have a greater effect on the quality of epidural anesthesia more than the duration of the block. Epinephrine in concentrations of 0.005 mg/mL prolongs the effect of epidural lidocaine, mepivacaine, and chloroprocaine more than that of bupivacaine, etidocaine, and ropivacaine. In addition to prolonging the duration and improving the quality of block, epinephrine decreases vascular absorption and peak systemic blood levels of epidurally administered local anesthetics. Phenylephrine generally is less effective than epinephrine as a vasoconstrictor for epidural anesthesia.

Epidural Anesthetic Agents

The epidural agent is chosen based on the desired clinical effect, whether it is to be used as a primary anesthetic, for supplementation of general anesthesia, or for analgesia. The anticipated duration of the procedure may call for a short- or long-acting single shot anesthetic or the insertion of a catheter (Table 16–6). Commonly used short- to intermediate-acting agents for surgical anesthesia include 1.5–2% lidocaine, 3% chloroprocaine, and 2% mepivacaine. Long-acting agents include 0.5–0.75% bupivacaine, 0.5–1% ropivacaine, and etidocaine. Experience with levobupivacaine, the less toxic S-enantiomer of bupivacaine, is limited. Only preservative-free local anesthetic solutions or those specifically labeled for epidural or caudal use are employed.

Following the initial 1–2 mL per segment bolus (in fractionated doses), repeat doses delivered through an epidural catheter are either done on a fixed time interval, based on the practitioners experience with the agent, or when the block demonstrates some degree of regression. The "time to two-segment regression" is a characteristic feature of each local anesthetic and is defined as the time it takes for a sensory level to decrease by two dermatome levels (Table 16–7). When a two-segment regression has occurred, one can generally safely reinject one-third to half the initial activation dose.

It should be noted that chloroprocaine, an ester with rapid onset, short duration, and extremely low toxicity, may interfere with the analgesic effects of epidural opiates. Previous chloroprocaine formulations with preservatives, specifically bisulfite and EDTA (ethylenediaminetetraacetic acid) proved to be problematic. Bisulfite preparations caused neurotoxicity when inadvertently injected in large volume intrathecally, while

Table 16–6. Agents for epidural anesthesia.

Agent	Concentration	Onset	Sensory Block	Motor Block
Chloroprocaine	2%	Fast	Analgesic	Mild to moderate
	3%	Fast	Dense	Dense
Lidocaine	≤ 1%	Intermediate	Analgesic	Minimal
	1.5%	Intermediate	Dense	Mild to moderate
	2%	Intermediate	Dense	Dense
Mepivacaine	1%	Intermediate	Analgesic	Minimal
	2%	Intermediate	Dense	Dense
Prilocaine	2%	Fast	Dense	Minimal
	3%	Fast	Dense	Dense
Bupivacaine	≤ 0.25%	Slow	Analgesic	Minimal
	0.375–0.5%	Slow	Dense	Mild to moderate
	0.75%	Slow	Dense	Moderate to dense
Ropivacaine	≤ 0.2%	Slow	Analgesic	Minimal
	0.3–0.5%	Slow	Dense	Mild to moderate
	0.6–1.0%	Slow	Dense	Moderate to dense

EDTA formulations were associated with severe back pain (presumably due to localized hypocalcemia). Current chloroprocaine preparations are preservative-free and without these complications.

Bupivacaine, an amide local anesthetic with a slow onset and long duration of action, has a high potential for systemic toxicity (see Chapter 14). Surgical anesthesia is obtained with the 0.5% or 0.75% formulation. The 0.75% concentration is not recommended for obstetric anesthesia. Its use in the past for cesarean section was associated with several reports of cardiac arrest resulting from inadvertent intravenous injection. The difficulty in resuscitation and resultant high mortality rate results from the high protein binding and lipid solubility of bupivacaine, which causes the agent to accumulate in the cardiac conduction system leading to refractory re-entrant arrhythmias. Very dilute concentrations of bupivacaine (eg, 0.0625%) are commonly combined with fentanyl and used for analgesia for labor and post-operative pain (see Chapters 18 and 43). The S-enantiomer of bupivacaine, levobupivacaine, appears to be primarily responsible for the local anesthetic action on nerve conduction but not the systemic toxic effects. Ropivacaine, a mepivacaine analogue introduced and marketed as a less toxic alternative to bupivacaine, is roughly equivalent to bupivacaine in potency, onset, duration, and quality of block. It is purported to have less motor block at lower concentrations while maintaining a good sensory block.

LOCAL ANESTHETIC pH ADJUSTMENT:

Local anesthetic solutions have a pH between 3.5 and 5.5 for chemical stability and bacteriostasis. Because they are weak bases, they exist chiefly in the ionic form in commercial preparations. Unfortunately, the onset of neural block depends on penetration of the lipid nerve cell membranes by the nonionic form of the local anesthetic. Increasing the pH of the solutions increases the concentration of the nonionic form of the local anesthetic. Addition of sodium bicarbonate (1 mEq per 10 mL of local anesthetic) immediately before injection may therefore accelerate the onset of the neural blockade. This approach is most useful for agents that can be adjusted to physiologic pH, such as lidocaine, mepivacaine, and chloroprocaine. Bupivacaine precipitates above a pH of 6.8.

Failed Epidural Blocks

Unlike spinal anesthesia, where the end point is usually very clear (free flowing CSF) and the technique is asso-

Table 16–7. Time to two-segment regression.

Agent	Time Range (min)
Chloroprocaine	50–70
Prilocaine	90–130
Lidocaine	90–150
Mepivacaine	120–160
Bupivacaine	200–260

ciated with a very high success rate, epidural anesthesia is critically dependent on detection of a more subjective loss of resistance (or hanging drop). Also, the more variable anatomy of the epidural space and less predictable spread of local anesthetic in it make epidural anesthesia inherently less predictable.

Misplaced injections of local anesthetic can occur in a number of situations. In some young adults, the spinal ligaments are soft and either good resistance is never appreciated or a false loss of resistance is encountered. Similarly, entry into the paraspinous muscles during an off-center midline approach may cause a false loss of resistance. Other causes of failed epidural anesthesia (such as intrathecal, subdural, and intravenous injection) are discussed in the complications section of this chapter.

Even if an adequate concentration and volume of an anesthetic was delivered into the epidural space, and sufficient time was allowed for the block to take effect, some epidural blocks are not successful. A **unilateral block** can occur if the medication is delivered through a catheter that has either exited the epidural space or coursed laterally. The chance of this occurring increases as the distance the catheter is threaded into the epidural space increases. When unilateral block occurs, the problem may be overcome by withdrawing the catheter 1–2 cm and reinjecting it with the patient turned with the unblocked side down. **Segmental sparing,** which may be due to septations within the epidural space, may also be corrected by injecting additional local anesthetic with the unblocked segment down. The large size of the L5, S1, and S2 nerve roots may prevent adequate penetration of local anesthetic and is thought to be responsible for **sacral sparing.** The latter is especially a problem for surgery on the lower leg; in such cases, elevating the head of the bed and reinjecting the catheter can sometimes achieve a more intense block of these large nerve roots. Patients may complain of **visceral pain** despite a seemingly good epidural block. In some cases (traction on the inguinal ligament and spermatic cord), a high thoracic sensory level may alleviate the pain, while in others (traction on the peritoneum), intravenous supplementation with opiates or other agents may be necessary. Visceral afferent fibers that travel with the vagus nerve may be responsible.

■ CAUDAL ANESTHESIA

Caudal epidural anesthesia is one of the most commonly regional techniques used in pediatric patients. It may also be used in adults. The caudal space is the sacral portion of the epidural space, as described previously it may be accessed a needle or catheter that is inserted through the **sacral hiatus.** The hiatus is covered by the sacrococcygeal ligament and may be felt as a groove or notch above the coccyx and between two bony prominences, the sacral cornuae (Figure 16–12). Its anatomy is more easily appreciated in infants and children. Calcification of the sacrococcygeal ligament may make caudal anesthesia difficult or impossible in older adults. Within the sacral canal, the dural sac extends to the first sacral vertebra in adults and to about the third sacral vertebra in infants, making inadvertent intrathecal injection more common in infants.

In children, caudal anesthesia is typically combined with general anesthesia for intraoperative supplementation and postoperative analgesia. It is commonly used for procedures below the diaphragm, including urogenital, rectal, inguinal, and lower extremity surgery. Pediatric caudal blocks are most commonly performed after the induction of general anesthesia. The patient is placed in the lateral or prone position with one or both hips flexed, and the sacral hiatus is palpated. After sterile skin preparation, a needle or intravenous catheter (18–23 gauge) is advanced at a 45 degree angle cephalad until a pop is felt as the needle pierces the sacrococcygeal ligament. The angle of the needle is then flattened and advanced (Figure 16–13). Aspiration for blood and CSF is performed, and if negative, injection can proceed. Some clinicians recommend test dosing as with other epidural techniques, although many simply rely on incremental dosing with frequent aspiration. Clinical data have shown that the complication rate for "kiddie caudals" is very low. Complications include total spinal and intravenous injection causing seizure or cardiac arrest. Intraosseous injection has also been reported to cause systemic toxicity.

A dosage of 0.5–1.0 mL/kg of 0.125% to 0.25% bupivacaine (or ropivacaine) with or without epinephrine can be used. Opioids may also be added (eg, 50–70 µg of morphine), although they are not recommended for outpatients because of the risk of delayed respiratory depression. The analgesic effects of the block extend for hours into the postoperative period. Pediatric outpatients can safely be discharged home even with mild residual motor block and without urinating, as most children will urinate within 8 hours.

Repeated injections can be accomplished in two ways. If the initial block is done with an intravenous catheter, the catheter can be left in place and covered with an occlusive dressing after being connected to extension tubing. Second, epidural catheters can be threaded cephalad into the lumbar or even thoracic epidural space from the caudal approach in infants and children. Smaller catheters are technically difficult to pass due to kinking. Catheters advanced into the thoracic epidural space have been used to achieve T2–T4

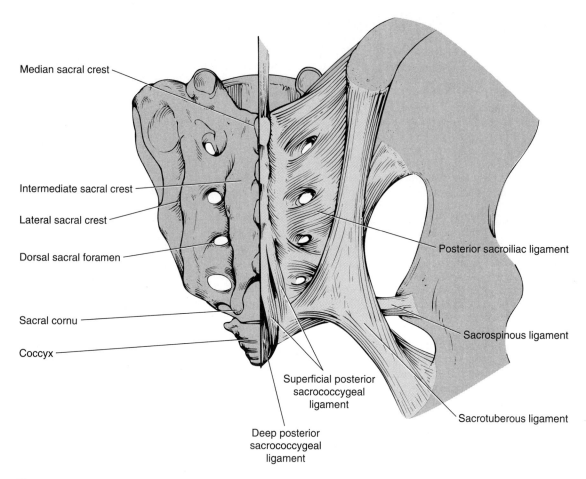

Median sacral crest

Intermediate sacral crest

Lateral sacral crest

Dorsal sacral foramen

Sacral cornu

Coccyx

Superficial posterior
sacrococcygeal
ligament

Deep posterior
sacrococcygeal
ligament

Posterior sacroiliac ligament

Sacrospinous ligament

Sacrotuberous ligament

Figure 16–12. Dorsal surface of the sacrum.

blocks for ex-premature infants undergoing inguinal hernia repair. This is achieved using chloroprocaine 1 mL/kg as an initial bolus and incremental doses of 0.3 mL/kg until the desired level is achieved.

For adults undergoing anorectal procedures, caudal anesthesia can provide dense sacral sensory blockade with limited cephalad spread. Furthermore, the injection can be given with the patient in the prone, jack-knifed position, which is used for surgery. A dose of 15–20 mL of 1.5% lidocaine with or without epinephrine is usually effective. Fentanyl 50–100 μg may also be added. This technique should be avoided in patients with pilonidal cysts because the needle may pass through the cyst track and can potentially introduce bacteria into the caudal epidural space. Although no longer commonly used for obstetric analgesia, a caudal block can be useful for the second stage of labor in situations where the epidural is not reaching the sacral

nerves, or when repeated attempts at epidural blockade have been unsuccessful.

■ COMPLICATIONS OF NEURAXIAL BLOCKS

The complications of epidural, spinal, or caudal anesthetics range from the bothersome to the crippling and life-threatening. Broadly, the complications can be thought of as those resulting from the medication introduced or the needle used to perform the procedure. Backache, headache, nerve injury, vascular injury, and infection can result from the procedure needle. Medications can result in excessively high blockade, systemic toxicity, local toxicity (nerve injury), or in-

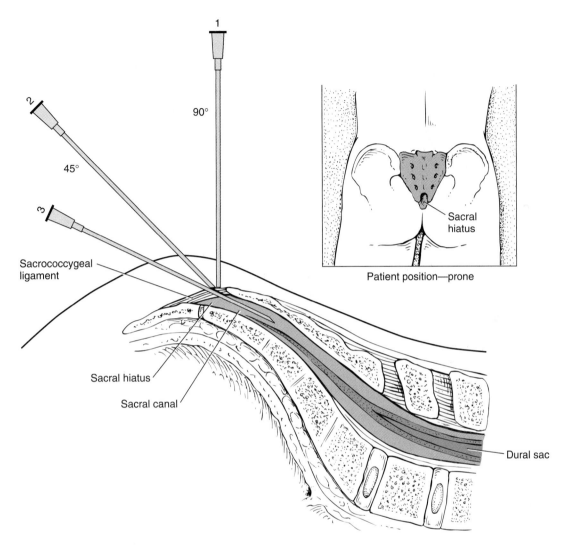

Figure 16–13. Caudal block.

fection. Ischemic injury may result from a combination of factors. Cardiac arrest can occur with spinal anesthesia. A very large survey from France of regional anesthesia gives one an idea of the incidence of serious complications from spinal and epidural anesthesia (Table 16–8).

Backache

A needle that passes through skin, subcutaneous tissues, muscle, and ligaments can result in a backache. A localized inflammatory response with or without reflex muscle spasm may be responsible. It should be noted that up to 25–30% of patients receiving only general anesthesia also complain of backache postoperatively. The soreness or ache is usually mild and self-limited, although it may last for a number of weeks. If treatment is sought, acetaminophen, nonsteroidal anti-inflammatory medication, and warm or cold compresses should suffice. Although backache is usually benign, remember that it may also be an important clinical sign of the much more serious complications, such as epidural hematoma and abscess (see below).

Headache

Any breach of the dura may result in a **post-dural puncture headache** (PDPH). This may follow a diagnostic lumbar puncture, a myelogram, a spinal anesthetic, or an epidural "wet tap" in which the epidural

Table 16–8. Incidence of serious complications from spinal and epidural anesthesia

Technique	Cardiac Arrest	Death	Seizure	Cauda Equina Syndrome	Paraplegia	Radiculopathy
Spinal (n = 40,640)	26	6	0	5	0	19
Epidural (n = 30,413)	3	0	4	0	1	5

Data from Auroy Y, et al: Serious complications related to regional anesthesia, results of a prospective survey in France. Anesthesiology 1997; 87:479.

needle passed through the epidural space and entered the subarachnoid space. Similarly, an epidural catheter might puncture the dura and result in PDPH. An epidural wet tap is usually immediately recognized as CSF drips from the needle. However, PDPH can follow a seemingly uncomplicated epidural anesthetic and may be the result of just the tip of the needle scratching through the dura. Typically, the headache is bilateral, frontal or retro-orbital, occipital and extending into the neck. It may be throbbing or constant and associated with photophobia and nausea. The hallmark of PDPH is its association with body position. The pain is aggravated by sitting or standing and relieved or lessened by lying down flat. The onset of headache is usually 12–72 hours following the procedure; however, it may be seen sooner. Untreated, the pain may last weeks, and in rare instances has required surgical repair.

PDPH is believed to result from decreased intracranial pressure as CSF leaks from the dural defect at a greater rate than it is being produced. The incidence is related to needle size, needle type, and patient population. The larger the needle, the greater the incidence of PDPH. Cutting point needles are associated with a higher incidence of PDPH than pencil point needles of the same gauge. A cutting needle introduced with the bevel parallel to the longitudinal fibers of the dura is said to separate these fibers rather than transecting them, therefore reducing the chance of PDPH. Factors that increase the risk of PDPH include young age, female sex, and pregnancy. The highest incidence, then, would be expected following an inadvertent wet tap with a large epidural needle in an obstetric patient (perhaps as high as 20–50%). The lowest incidence would be expected with an elderly male using a 27 g pencil point needle (< 1%). Studies of obstetric patients undergoing spinal anesthesia for cesarean section with small gauge pencil point needles have shown rates as low as 3% or 4%.

Conservative treatment involves recumbent positioning, analgesics, intravenous or oral fluid administration, and caffeine. Keeping the patient supine will lessen the hydrostatic pressure driving fluid out of the dural hole while minimizing the headache. Analgesic medication may range from acetaminophen to nonsteroidal anti-inflammatory drugs. Hydration and caffeine work to stimulate production of CSF. Caffeine further helps by vasoconstricting intracranial vessels. Stool softeners and soft diet are used to minimize Valsalva straining. Headache may persist for days despite conservative therapy.

Epidural blood patch is a very effective treatment for PDPH. It involves injecting 15–20 mL of autologous blood into the epidural space at, or one interspace below, the level of the dural puncture. It is believed to stop further leakage of CSF by either mass effect or coagulation. The effects may be immediate or may take some hours as CSF production slowly builds intracranial pressure. Approximately 90% of patients will respond to a single blood patch, and 90% of initial nonresponders will get relief from a second injection. Prophylactic blood patching has been advocated by injecting blood through an epidural catheter that was placed after a wet tap. However, not all patients will develop PDPH, and the tip of the catheter may be many levels away from the dural defect. Similarly, a saline bolus has been injected through the epidural catheter but does not appear to be as effective as blood patching. Most practitioners either offer the epidural blood patch when PDPH becomes apparent, or allow conservative therapy a trial of 12–24 hours.

Urinary Retention

Local anesthetic block of S2–S4 root fibers decreases urinary bladder tone and inhibits the voiding reflex. Epidural opioids can also interfere with normal voiding. These effects are most pronounced in male patients. Urinary bladder catheterization should be used for all but the shortest acting blocks. If a catheter is not present postoperatively, close observation for voiding is necessary. Persistent bladder dysfunction can also be a manifestation of serious neural injury as discussed below.

Maternal Fever

Epidural analgesia for labor is associated with a higher incidence of temperature elevation in parturients compared with those delivering without the benefit of epidural analgesia. Maternal fever is often interpreted as chorioamnionitis and may trigger an invasive neonatal sepsis evaluation. There is no evidence, however, that neonatal sepsis is actually increased with epidural analgesia. This temperature elevation may result from epidural-induced shivering or inhibition of sweating and hyperventilation. A selection bias may also exist, with nulliparous women with prolonged labors being more likely to receive epidural analgesia.

Transient Neurologic Symptoms

First described in 1993, transient neurologic symptoms (TNS) is characterized by back pain radiating to the legs without sensory or motor deficits, occurring after the resolution of spinal block and resolving spontaneously within several days. It is most commonly associated with hyperbaric lidocaine (incidence up to 11.9%) but has also been reported with tetracaine (1.6%), bupivacaine (1.3%), mepivacaine, prilocaine, procaine, and subarachnoid ropivacaine. There are also case reports of TNS following epidural anesthesia. The incidence of this syndrome is highest among outpatients (early ambulation) after surgery in the lithotomy position and lowest among inpatients in positions other than lithotomy. There is a paucity of reports of TNS following spinal lidocaine for cesarean section. The pathogenesis of TNS is unclear and controversy exists as to whether it represents neurotoxicity (a mild form of the cauda equina syndrome), or myofascial pain resulting from musculoskeletal strain.

High or Total Spinal Anesthesia

Spinal anesthesia ascending into the cervical levels causes severe hypotension, bradycardia, and respiratory insufficiency. Unconsciousness, apnea, and hypotension resulting from high levels of spinal anesthesia are referred to as a "high spinal" or "total spinal." It can also occur following attempted epidural/caudal anesthesia if there is inadvertent intrathecal injection. Onset is usually rapid, especially with inadvertent injections of large amounts of anesthetic intended for the epidural space. Severe sustained hypotension with lower sensory blocks can also lead to apnea through medullary hypoperfusion.

Treatment of high spinal anesthesia consists of support of the airway, maintaining adequate ventilation, and supporting the circulation. When respiratory insufficiency becomes evident, supplemental oxygen is mandatory. Assisted ventilation, intubation, and mechanical ventilation may be necessary. Hypotension can be treated with rapid administration of intravenous fluids, a head-down position, and aggressive use of vasopressors. Epinephrine should be used early if ephedrine, phenylephrine or metaraminol are insufficient. Dopamine infusion may be helpful. Bradycardia should be treated with atropine. Ephedrine or epinephrine will also increase heart rate.

If respiratory and hemodynamic control can be achieved and maintained after high or total spinal anesthesia, surgery may proceed. Apnea is often transient, and unconsciousness leaves the patient amnestic without adverse recall.

Subdural Injection

A subdural injection may occur during attempted epidural anesthesia. It has a similar clinical presentation to the high spinal, with the exception that the onset may be delayed in onset for 15–30 minutes. The spinal subdural space is a potential space between the dura and the arachnoid containing a small amount of serous fluid. Unlike the epidural space, the subdural space extends intracranially, so that anesthetic injected into the spinal subdural space can ascend to higher levels than epidural medications. As with the high spinal, treatment is supportive and may require intubation, mechanical ventilation, and cardiovascular support. The effects generally last from 1 to several hours.

Cardiac Arrest During Spinal Anesthesia

Examination of data from the American Society of Anesthesiologists (ASA) Closed Claim Project identified several cases of cardiac arrest during spinal anesthesia. Since most of these cases predated the routine use of pulse oximetry, many physicians believed oversedation and unrecognized hypoventilation and hypoxia was the cause. However, in the years since, large prospective studies continue to report a relatively high incidence of cardiac arrest in patients having received a spinal anesthetic, perhaps as high as 1:1500. Many of the arrests were preceded by bradycardia and occurred in young healthy patients. The mortality rate has been reported to be high. A recent examination of this problem has identified vagal responses to a decreased preload to be a key factor and suggests that patients with high vagal tone are particularly at risk (see Chapter 47). Prophylactic volume expansion is recommended, as is early vagolytic (atropine) treatment of bradycardia followed by ephedrine and epinephrine if necessary.

Systemic Toxicity

Extremely high levels of local anesthetics affect the central nervous system (seizure and unconsciousness) and the cardiovascular system (hypotension, arrhythmia, and cardiovascular collapse). Absorption of excessive amounts or inadvertent intravascular injection of local anesthetics can produce very high serum levels. Because the dosage of medication for spinal anesthesia is relatively small, this complication is seen primarily with epidural and caudal blocks. Excessive absorption from epidural or caudal blocks is rare if the maximum safe dosage of local anesthetic is not exceeded. (This is in contrast to other regional techniques with greater surrounding blood supply.) Injection of local anesthetic directly into a vessel either directly through a needle or through a catheter is an occasional complication of both epidural and caudal anesthesia. The incidence can be minimized by carefully aspirating the needle or catheter before injection, by using a test dose, and by injecting incremental doses and observing for early signs of intravascular injection (tinnitus, lingual sensations).

The local anesthetics vary in their toxicity (see Chapter 14). Chloroprocaine is the least toxic; lidocaine, mepivacaine, and ropivacaine are intermediate; and bupivacaine is the most toxic. As previously discussed, the use of epidural 0.75% bupivacaine for cesarean section resulted in many reports of death from intravascular injection.

Cauda Equina Syndrome & Other Neurologic Deficits

Perhaps no complication is more perplexing or distressing than persistent neurologic deficits following an apparently routine neuraxial block in which epidural hematoma or abscess is ruled out. Most peripheral neuropathies resolve spontaneously, but some are permanent. Some of these deficits have been associated with paresthesia from the needle or catheter or pain during injection. Some studies have suggested that multiple attempts during a technically difficult block are also a risk factor. These cases may represent direct physical trauma to the nerve roots. Any sustained paresthesia should alert the clinician to redirect the needle. Injections should be immediately stopped and the needle withdrawn if they are associated with pain. Direct injection into the spinal cord can cause paraplegia. Damage to the conus medullaris may cause isolated sacral dysfunction, including paralysis of the biceps femoris muscles, anesthesia in the posterior thigh, saddle area, or great toes, and loss of bowel or bladder functions. Some animal studies suggest catheters can cause inflammation or even demyelination in nerve tissue. Neurotoxicity of local anesthetics is another cause of persistent neurologic deficits, sometimes being a presumptive explanation of exclusion.

It must be remembered that not all neurologic deficits that occur after a regional anesthetic are a result of the block. Surveys of complications have reported many instances of postoperative neurologic deficits that were attributed to regional anesthesia when in fact only general anesthesia was used. Postpartum deficits including lateral femoral cutaneous neuropathy, foot drop, and paraplegia were recognized before the modern era of anesthesia and still occur in the absence of anesthetics. Less clear are the postanesthetic cases complicated by concurrent conditions such as atherosclerosis, diabetes mellitus, intervertebral disk disease, and spinal disorders.

Cauda equina syndrome (CES) is characterized by bowel and bladder dysfunction together with evidence of multiple nerve root injury. There is lower motor neuron type injury with paresis of the legs. Sensory deficits may be patchy, typically occurring in a peripheral nerve pattern. There may be pain characteristic of nerve root compromise. A cluster of cases of CES with the use of microcatheters used for repeated dose or continuous infusion of subarachnoid local anesthetic led the FDA to withdraw these catheters from the US market. It appears that pooling (maldistribution) of hyperbaric solutions of lidocaine can lead to neurotoxicity of the nerve roots of the cauda equina. However, there are reports of CES occurring after uneventful single shot lidocaine spinals. CES has also been reported following epidural anesthesia.

Meningitis & Arachnoiditis

Infection of the subarachnoid space can follow neuraxial blocks as the result of contamination of the equipment or injected solutions, or as a result of organisms tracked in from the skin. Indwelling catheters may become colonized with organisms that then track deep, causing infection. Fortunately, these are rare occurrences. Arachnoiditis, another reported rare complication of neuraxial anesthesia, may be infectious or noninfectious. Clinically, it is marked by pain and other neurologic symptoms and on radiographic imaging is seen as a clumping of the nerve roots. Cases of arachnoiditis have been traced to detergent in a spinal procaine preparation. Lumbar arachnoiditis has been reported from subarachnoid steroid injection but is more commonly seen following spinal surgery. Prior to the use of disposable spinal needles, caustic cleaning solutions caused cases of chemical meningitis resulting in severe neurologic dysfunction.

Epidural Abscess

Spinal epidural abscess (EA) is a rare but potentially devastating complication of neuraxial anesthesia. The reported incidence varies widely from 1:6500 to 1:500,000 epidurals. Most cases in the literature are isolated case reports. Several prospective studies, including over 140,000 blocks, have failed to report one EA. EA can occur in patients who did not receive regional anesthesia; risk factors in such cases include back trauma, injecting drug use, and neurosurgical procedures. Most reported anesthesia-related cases involve epidural catheters. In one reported series, there was a mean of 5 days from catheter insertion to the development of symptoms, although presentation can be delayed for weeks.

There are four classic clinical stages of EA, although progression and time course can vary. Initially, symptoms include back or vertebral pain that is intensified by percussion over the spine. Second, nerve root or radicular pain develops. The third stage is marked by motor and/or sensory deficits or sphincter dysfunction. Paraplegia or paralysis marks the fourth stage. Ideally, the diagnosis is made in the early stages. Prognosis has consistently been shown to correlate to the degree of neurologic dysfunction at the time the diagnosis is made. Back pain and fever after epidural anesthesia should alert the clinician to consider EA. Radicular pain or neurologic deficit heightens the urgency to investigate. Once EA is suspected, the catheter should be removed (if still present) and the tip cultured. The injection site is examined for evidence of infection, if pus is expressed it is sent for culture. Blood cultures should be obtained. If suspicion is high and cultures have been obtained, anti-staphylococcus coverage can be instituted, as the most common organisms causing EA are *Staphylococcus aureus* and *Staphylococcus epidermidis.* Magnetic resonance imaging (MRI) or computed tomographic (CT) scanning should be performed to confirm or rule out the diagnosis. Early neurosurgical consultation is advisable.

In addition to antibiotics, treatment of EA usually involves decompression (laminectomy) although percutaneous drainage with fluoroscopic or CT guidance has been reported. There are a few reports of patients with no neurologic signs being treated with antibiotic alone.

Suggested strategies for guarding against the occurrence of EA include (1) minimizing catheter manipulations and maintaining a closed system when possible, (2) using a micropore (0.22 micron) bacterial filter, and (3) removing an epidural catheter after 96 hours or at least changing the catheter, filter, and solution every 96 hours. Although these interventions seem logical, they remain unproved. Sometimes the system can become disconnected and the clinician needs to decide whether to remove the catheter or try to reconnect using aseptic technique. No universal guidelines for performing an epidural exist; some practitioners use a cap and mask, and thoroughly wash hands prior to gloving as a minimum in addition to sterile skin preparation and maintaining a sterile field.

Spinal or Epidural Hematoma

Needle or catheter trauma to epidural veins often causes minor bleeding in the spinal canal although this is usually benign and self-limiting. A clinically significant spinal hematoma can occur following spinal or epidural anesthesia, especially in the presence of abnormal coagulation or bleeding disorder. The incidence of such hematomas has been estimated to be about 1:150,000 for epidural blocks and 1:220,000 for spinal anesthetics. The vast majority of reported cases have occurred in patients with abnormal coagulation either secondary to disease or pharmacologic therapies. Some have emphasized the association with a technically difficult or bloody block. It should be noted that many hematomas have occurred immediately after the removal of an epidural catheter. Thus, insertion and removal of an epidural catheter is a risk factor.

The pathologic insult to the spinal cord and nerves is analogous to epidural abscess where a mass effect compresses neural tissue causing direct pressure injury and ischemia. As with epidural abscess, the need for rapid diagnosis and intervention is paramount if permanent neurologic sequelae are to be avoided. The onset of symptoms is typically more sudden compared with epidural abscess. Symptoms include sharp back and leg pain with a progression to numbness and motor weakness and/or sphincter dysfunction. When hemotoma is suspected, neurologic imaging (MRI, CT, or myelography) must be obtained immediately and neurosurgical consultation should be requested. Most cases of good neurologic recovery have occurred in patients who have undergone surgical decompression within 8–12 hours.

Neuraxial anesthesia is best avoided in patients with coagulopathy, significant thrombocytopenia, platelet dysfunction, or those who have received fibrinolytic/thrombolytic therapy.

Neuraxial Blockade in the Setting of Anticoagulants & Antiplatelet Agents

The issue of performing a block in the setting of anticoagulants and antiplatelet agents can be problematic. A 1998 statement of a consensus conference of the American Society of Regional Anesthesia can be summarized as follows:

ORAL ANTICOAGULANTS:

If neuraxial anesthesia is to be used in patients on long-term warfarin therapy, it must be stopped and a normal prothrombin time (PT) and international normalized ratio (INR) should be documented prior to the block. For perioperative thromboembolic prophylaxis, if the initial dose was given more than 24 hours prior to the block, or if more than one dose was given, the PT and INR need to be checked. If only one dose was given within 24 hours, it should be safe to proceed. Removing an epidural catheter on patients receiving low-dose warfarin (5 mg/d) has been reported to be safe.

ANTIPLATELET DRUGS:

By themselves, antiplatelet drugs do not appear to increase the risk of spinal hematoma from neuraxial anesthesia or epidural catheter removal. This assumes a normal patient with a normal coagulation profile and not receiving other medications that might affect clotting mechanisms. (It should be noted that specific data for newer agents such as clopidogrel and abciximab is not available.)

Standard (Unfractionated) Heparin: Minidose subcutaneous prophylaxis is not a contraindication to neuraxial anesthesia. For patients who are to receive heparin intraoperatively, blocks may be performed 1 hour or more before heparin administration. A bloody epidural or spinal does not necessarily require cancellation of surgery but discussion of the risks with the surgeon and careful postoperative monitoring is needed. Removal of an epidural catheter should occur 1 hour prior to, or 4 hours following, subsequent heparin dosing. The risk of spinal hematoma is undetermined in the setting of full anticoagulation for cardiac surgery. Neuraxial anesthesia should be avoided in patients on therapeutic doses of heparin and increased partial thromboplastin time (PTT). If the patient is started on heparin after the placement of an epidural catheter, its removal should only occur after discontinuation or interruption of heparin infusion and evaluation of the coagulation status.

LOW MOLECULAR WEIGHT HEPARIN (LMWH):

Many cases of spinal hematoma associated with neuraxial anesthesia followed the introduction of LMWH in the United States in 1993. Many of these cases involved intraoperative or early postoperative LMWH use, and several patients were receiving concomitant antiplatelet medication. It is recommended that if bloody needle or catheter placement occurs, LMWH should be delayed until 24 hours postoperatively, because this trauma may significantly increase the risk of spinal hematoma. If postoperative LMWH thromboprophylaxis will be utilized, epidural catheters should be removed 2 hours prior to the first LMWH dose. If already present, the catheter should be removed at least 10 hours after a dose of LMWH and subsequent dosing should not occur for 2 more hours.

FIBRINOLYTIC OR THROMBOLYTIC THERAPY:

Neuraxial anesthesia is best avoided if a patient has received fibrinolytic or thrombolytic therapy.

CASE DISCUSSION: NEURAXIAL ANESTHESIA FOR LITHOTRIPSY

A 56-year-old male presents for extracorporeal shock wave lithotripsy (ESWL) of a large kidney stone. The procedure involves immersing the patient in a water bath through which high-energy waves are focused onto the stone (see Chapter 33). The patient has a long history of spinal problems and has undergone fusion of the cervical spine (C3–C6) and laminectomy with fusion of the lower lumbar spine (L3–L5). On examination, he has no neck flexion or extension and has a Mallampati class IV airway (see Chapter 5).

What types of anesthesia are appropriate for this patient?

High-energy lithotripsy usually requires general or neuraxial anesthesia. A significant advantage of general anesthesia is that diaphragmatic excursion and secondary movement of the stone can be controlled by adjusting tidal volume and respiratory rate. Selection of the type of anesthesia as always should be based on patient preference after informed consent. This patient presents potential difficulties for both general and regional anesthesia. The limited excursion of the cervical spine together with the anatomy of a class IV airway makes difficulty in intubation and possibly ventilation almost certain. Induction of general anesthesia would be safest after the airway is secured with an awake fiberoptic intubation.

Regional anesthesia also presents a problem in that the patient has had previous back surgery in the lumbar area where neuraxial anesthesia is most commonly performed. Some clinicians consider prior back surgery to be a relative contraindication to neuraxial anesthesia. Postoperative distortion of the anatomy makes the block technically challenging and may increase the likelihood of a failure, inadvertent dural puncture during epidural anesthesia, paresthesias, and an unpredictable spread of the local anesthetics. Many clinicians believe that the neuraxial blockade can be safely done above or below the level of surgery. Indeed, lumbar laminectomy can facilitate spinal anesthesia at the level of the surgery.

If the patient chooses to have neuraxial anesthesia, would spinal or epidural anesthesia be more appropriate?

Many clinicians feel that epidural anesthesia is more appropriated for ESWL in a tub. Use of an epidural catheter may allow better control of the sensory level and duration of anesthesia. The associated sympathectomy and subsequent drop in blood pressure are more gradual than that following spinal anesthesia. Because the patient will be placed in a chair for the procedure, spinal anesthesia may be associated with a more marked degree of hypotension until the patient is placed in the tub (see Chapter 33). With either type of anesthesia, significant hypotension should be treated aggressively with intravenous fluids, vasoconstrictors; bradycardia should be treated with atropine. Placing the patient in a sitting position immediately after spinal anesthesia also increases the risk of a post-dural puncture headache (PDPH). If spinal anesthesia is elected, use of a small gauge needle (25 gauge or less pencil point needle) may help minimize the risk of PDPH.

After an explanation of the options, the patient appears to understand the risks of both types of anesthesia and desires epidural anesthesia. Placement of an epidural catheter is attempted at the L1–L2 interspace but inadvertent dural puncture occurs.

What options are now available?

Options include inject a spinal dose of local anesthetic through the epidural needle to induce spinal anesthesia; attempt epidural anesthesia at another level; attempt spinal anesthesia at a lower level; abandon regional anesthesia and proceed with an awake fiberoptic intubation. If a spinal dose of local anesthetic is to be injected, the syringe and needle should be kept in place for a few moments to prevent significant back leakage of anesthetic through the large dural hole. Threading an epidural catheter through the needle into the subarachnoid space allows subsequent redosing, but above L1 it carries some risk of injury to the spinal cord (conus medullaris). Without radiographic confirmation, even experienced clinicians can misjudge the actual level of needle insertion by one to two spinal levels; thus the dural puncture site could be as high as the T11–T12 interspace. Even when a catheter is advanced in the subarachnoid space well below L2 it should not be advanced more than 2–3 cm to avoid injury to the cauda equina.

How might a dural puncture affect subsequent epidural or spinal anesthesia?

A potential hazard of epidural anesthesia at a level adjacent to a large dural puncture is the possibility that some local anesthetic might pass through the dural puncture into the subarachnoid space. This could result in a higher than expected level of sensory and motor blockade. Careful incremental injection of local anesthetic may help avoid this problem.

Conversely, a large dural puncture can theoretically diminish the effect of subsequent spinal anesthesia at an adjacent level. Because only a small amount is used, leakage of local anesthetic with CSF through dural puncture can theoretically limit the cephalad spread of the solution.

What can be done to prevent the occurrence of a spinal headache?

Studies suggest that successfully placing an epidural catheter after a wet tap at a different level decreases the incidence of PDPH by as much as 50%. Unfortunately, the same difficult anatomy that might have led to the dural puncture may increase the likelihood of a second inadvertent puncture. Observation is generally recommended. The management of PDPH was discussed earlier in this chapter.

SUGGESTED READING

Aouad MT, Siddik SS, Jalbout MI, Baraka AS: Does pregnancy protect against intrathecal lidocaine-induced transient neurologic symptoms? Anesth Analg 2001;92:401.

Auroy Y, Narchi P, Messiah A, et al: Serious complications related to regional anesthesia: Results of a prospective survey in France. Anesthesiology 1997;87:479.

Ben-David B, Frankel R, Arzumonov T, Marchevsky Y, Volpin G: Minidose bupivacaine-fentanyl spinal anesthesia for surgical repair of hip fracture in the aged. Anesthesiology 2000;92:6.

Broadman LM, Hannallah RS, Norden JM, McGill WA: "Kiddie caudals": Experience with 1154 consecutive cases without complications. Anesth Analg 1987;66:S18.

Brookman CA, Rutledge ML: Epidural abscess: Case report and literature review. Reg Anesth Pain Med 2000;25:428.

Brown DL: *Atlas of Regional Anesthesia,* 2nd ed. WB Saunders and Company, 1999.

Burrow GN, Ferris TF: *Medical Complications During Pregnancy,* 2nd ed. WB Saunders and Company, 1982 p 466.

Cousins MJ: *Neural Blockade in Clinical Anesthesia and Pain Management,* 3rd ed. Lippincott Williams & Wilkins, 1998.

Crews JC: New developments in epidural anesthesia and analgesia. Anesth Clin North Am 2000;18:251.

Dahlgren N, Tornebrandt K: Neurological complications after anaesthesia. A follow-up of 18,000 spinal and epidural anaesthetics performed over three years. Acta Anaesthesiol Scand 1995;39:872.

Finucane BT: *Complications of Regional Anesthesia.* Churchill Livingstone, 1999.

Gautier PE, De Kock M, Van Steenberge A, et al: Intrathecal ropivacaine for ambulatory surgery. Anesthesiology 1999; 91:1239.

Grass JA: The role of epidural anesthesia and analgesia in postoperative outcome. Anesth Clin North Am 2000;18:407.

Greene NM: *Physiology of Spinal Anesthesia,* 4th ed. Williams & Wilkins, 1993.

Hodgson PS, Liu SS: New developments in spinal anesthesia. Anesth Clin North Am 2000;18:235.

Horlocker TT: Complications of spinal and epidural anesthesia. Anesth Clin North Am 2000;18:461.

Khalil S, Campos C, Farag AM, et al: Caudal block in children. Anesthesiology 1999;91:1279.

Kindler C, Seeberger M, Siegemund M, Schneider M: Extradural abscess complicating lumbar extradural anaesthesia and analgesia in an obstetric patient. Acta Anaesthesiol Scand 1996;40:858.

Liu SS, McDonald SB: Current issues in spinal anesthesia. Anesthesiology 2001;94:888.

Pollard JB: Cardiac arrest during spinal anesthesia: Common mechanisms and strategies for prevention. Anesth Analg 2001;92:252.

Richardson MG: Regional anesthesia for obstetrics. Anesth Clin North Am 2000;18:383.

Rodgers A, Walker N, Schug S, et al: Reduction of postoperative mortality and morbidity with epidural or spinal anaesthesia: Results from overview of randomised trials. BMJ 2000; 321:1493.

Sarubbi FA, Vasquez JE: Spinal epidural abscess associated with the use of temporary epidural catheters: Report of two cases and review. Clin Infect Dis 1997;25:1155.

Strong WE: Epidural abscess associated with epidural catheterization: A rare event? Anesthesiology 1991;74:944.

Tetzlaff JE: The pharmacology of local anesthetics. Anesth Clin North Am 2000;18:217.

Viscomi CM, Manullang T: Maternal fever, neonatal sepsis evaluation, and epidural labor analgesia. Reg Anesth Pain Med 2000;25:549.

Wang LP, Hauerberg J, Schmidt JF: Incidence of spinal epidural abscess after epidural analgesia: A national 1-year survey. Anesthesiology 1999;91:1928.

Peripheral Nerve Blocks*

KEY CONCEPTS

 The greatest immediate risk of nerve blocks is systemic toxicity from inadvertent intravascular injection. Delayed toxicity can follow the initial injection when rapid or excessive amounts of local anesthetics are absorbed systemically.

 Good surgical anesthesia is obtained only when local anesthetic is injected in close proximity to the nerve or nerves that are to be blocked. Injection techniques include use of a field block, reliance on fixed anatomic relationships, elicitation of paresthesias, and use of a nerve stimulator.

 A perineural injection may produce a brief accentuation of the paresthesia, whereas an intraneural injection produces an intense, searing pain that serves as a warning to immediately terminate the injection and reposition the needle.

 Surgical anesthesia of the upper extremity and shoulder can be obtained following neural blockade of the brachial plexus (C5–T1) or its terminal branches at several sites.

 A fascial sleeve that is derived from the prevertebral and scalene fascia encloses the brachial plexus. This sheath extends from the intervertebral foramina to the upper arm and serves as the anatomic basis for brachial plexus blocks. Injection into this sheath at any point allows local anesthetic to spread and block the C5–T1 nerve roots.

 The interscalene approach is most optimal for procedures on the shoulder, arm, and forearm. Injection at the interscalene level tends to produce a block that is most intense at the C5–C7 dermatomes and least intense in the C8–T1 dermatomes.

 The axillary approach to the brachial plexus is most optimal for procedures from the elbow to the hand. This approach tends to produce the most intense block in the distribution of C7–T1 (ulnar nerve).

 Intravenous regional anesthesia, also called a Bier block, can provide intense surgical anesthesia for short surgical procedures (< 45–60 minutes) on the forearm and hand.

 A femoral nerve block can used to provide anesthesia for the anterior thigh, knee, and a small part of the medial foot. Twenty to 40 mL of local anesthetic can be injected to produced a "three-in-one" block of the femoral, obturator, and lateral femoral cutaneous nerves.

 A sciatic nerve block may be used for all procedures on the lower extremity that do not require a pneumatic tourniquet on the thigh. The sciatic nerve provides sensation to the knee and lower leg. When combined with a "three-in-one" block, it can anesthetize the entire lower extremity.

 Ankle block is commonly performed for surgery of the foot in frail patients who may not tolerate the hemodynamic effects associated with neuraxial or general anesthesia. Epinephrine is usually not added for ankle block to reduce the risk of ischemic injury to the foot.

 Epinephrine or other vasoconstrictors should be avoided in a penile block to prevent end artery spasm and ischemic injury.

---

*This chapter has been revised and updated from an original chapter written by John E. Tetzlaff, MD, Section Head, Acute Perioperative Care, Department of General Anesthesiology, The Cleveland Clinic Foundation, Cleveland, Ohio.

Shortly after the purification of cocaine in 1860, the famous surgeon William Halsted demonstrated how this naturally occurring substance with local anesthetic properties could be used for surgical anesthesia. Using his expertise in anatomy, he could produce regional anesthesia by blocking specific peripheral nerves or nerve groups (facial nerves, brachial plexus, and the pudendal and posterior tibial nerves). The first synthetic local anesthetic, procaine (Novocaine) was discovered in 1904 and within a year found clinical use as a local anesthetic by Heinrich Braun, who subsequently also demonstrated that addition of epinephrine could prolong the action of local anesthetics. August Bier shortly afterwards described the technique of intravenous regional anesthesia (Bier block). Unfortunately, enthusiasm for regional anesthesia was eventually overshadowed by major developments and improvements in general anesthetic agents and techniques (see Chapter 1). It was not until the discovery of newer and safer local anesthetic agents, refinements in equipment and techniques and, most importantly, better training in anesthesiology residency programs served as an impetus for renewed interest in peripheral nerve blocks in the last few decades. The recent emergence of pain management as a formal subspeciality and the increasing importance of outpatient (ambulatory) surgery in anesthetic practices have further bolstered interest in peripheral nerve blocks.

Peripheral nerve blocks may be used for surgical anesthesia alone or in conjunction with general anesthesia, for postoperative pain control, and for acute and chronic pain management. This chapter considers peripheral nerve blocks that are used for anesthesia of the arms, legs, and trunk. Chapter 18 discusses nerve blocks that are primarily for pain management. The term regional anesthesia is broad and often used to refer to peripheral nerve blocks and neuraxial anesthesia (see Chapter 16). Plexus anesthesia (eg, brachial plexus block) is often used to describe a peripheral nerve block that simultaneously blocks multiple nerves as they travel together in a discrete fascial compartment.

INDICATIONS

The choice of anesthesia is determined by the patient (or guardian) based on an informed consent that includes understanding all available options and their risks and benefits. Important considerations in discussing anesthetic choices include the suitability of the technique for the type of surgery, the surgeon's preference, the experience of the anesthetist, and the physiologic and mental state of the patient.

Peripheral nerve blocks may be used as the sole anesthetic for surgery (with or without sedation), in conjunction with general anesthesia, or for postoperative analgesia. Peripheral nerve blocks may be used for procedures on the arm, shoulder, trunk, or legs. Regional anesthesia may be especially useful in certain clinical settings, such as emergency surgery in a patient with a full stomach and closed reductions of fractures. Major *potential* benefits of peripheral nerve block techniques may include postoperative analgesia, less physiologic derangements, more rapid postoperative recovery, avoidance of airway instrumentation, and a reduced incidence of potential complications associated with general anesthesia (nausea/vomiting, aspiration, inability to ventilate/intubate, and malignant hyperthermia). Although controversial, some clinical studies suggest that when compared with general anesthesia regional anesthesia may reduce postoperative complications (see Chapter 16), and produce a preemptive analgesic effect (see Chapter 18).

The principal disadvantages of regional anesthesia are that it may require patient cooperation and there is a risk of systemic toxicity from local anesthetics. Moreover, most techniques are performed in a blind fashion, relying on indirect signs that the needle placement and injection are in close proximity to the nerves to be blocked. All techniques therefore have a small but finite failure rate that is generally directly related to clinical experience. Even if a nerve block is initially successful, early resolution or an unanticipated prolongation of the surgery may make it inadequate and necessitate general anesthesia. Many if not most clinicians alert patients to this possibility preoperatively and therefore have the patient consent for the use of general anesthesia as well.

CONTRAINDICATIONS

With some exceptions, major contraindications to peripheral nerve blocks are generally similar to those for neuraxial anesthesia (see Table 16–2). One major difference is that peripheral nerve blocks are not associated with a sympathectomy and do not affect intracranial pressure. These blocks are therefore generally not contraindicated in patients with stenotic valvular heart disease or elevated intracranial pressure. Coagulation studies, platelet count, and a bleeding time should be checked when the clinical history suggests the possibility of a bleeding diathesis. Hematogenous spread of an infection to the block site is not as great a concern as with neuraxial blocks in the presence of sepsis or bacteremia. Preexisting neurologic deficits in the area to be blocked are only a relative contraindication because to discern effects or complications of the block from preexisting deficits or unrelated exacerbation of preexisting disease may be impossible.

Regional anesthesia requires at least some degree of patient cooperation. Some techniques (eg, elicitation of paresthesia) rely on the patient's feedback to determine correct needle placement. Some clinicians also believe it is important for the patient to be able to communicate pain on injection, which may be indicative of an undesirable intraneural injection. Such injections can lead to ischemic nerve injury. This type of feedback may not be possible in very young patients; those who are unable to communicate; or in patients with dementia, psychosis, or emotional instability. As with neuraxial blockade, the issue of performing peripheral nerve blocks in anesthetized or heavily sedated patients is controversial. In such cases, elicitation of paresthesia cannot be used; alternate techniques such as relying on nerve stimulation must be used. Studies showing an increased incidence of neurologic complications following blocks in anesthetized patients are lacking. Pediatric blocks are typically performed under general anesthesia.

TECHNICAL CONSIDERATIONS

Peripheral nerve blocks may be performed in the operating room, preoperative holding area, or in a procedure room ("block room"). Regardless of the location, in addition to nerve block supplies and equipment, adequate monitoring capabilities, oxygen, and resuscitation drugs and equipment should be immediately available. Minimum monitoring for performing a peripheral nerve block include pulse oximetry and blood pressure; an electrocardiogram is also desirable. Other monitoring requirements are dictated by any surgical procedure and patient's physical status.

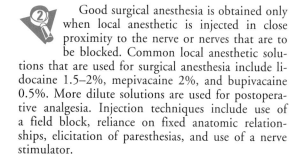 The greatest immediate risk of nerve blocks is systemic toxicity from inadvertent intravascular injection (see Chapters 14 and 16). Delayed toxicity can follow the initial injection when rapid or excessive amounts of local anesthetics are absorbed systemically. Peak blood levels occur at various times after the block. A high index of suspicion is required to detect early signs of systemic toxicity. In addition to aspiration of the syringe, many clinicians always use a 3 mL test dose of local anesthetic with 1:200,000 epinephrine (15 μg/mL) to detect intravascular placement of a needle or catheter. An abrupt increase in heart rate greater than 20% over baseline is generally indicative of an intravascular injection. Incremental dosing (5 mL injections at a time; see Chapter 16) with frequent intermittent aspiration helps avoid systemic toxicity. The "immobile needle" technique is often used to prevent needle movement during injection: intravenous tubing is attached between the needle and syringe such that the needle can be easily stabilized in the correct position and is not readily displaced by injection. An assistant usually aspirates and injects on the syringe so that the operator can use one hand for palpation and the other to control the needle.

Good surgical anesthesia is obtained only when local anesthetic is injected in close proximity to the nerve or nerves that are to be blocked. Common local anesthetic solutions that are used for surgical anesthesia include lidocaine 1.5–2%, mepivacaine 2%, and bupivacaine 0.5%. More dilute solutions are used for postoperative analgesia. Injection techniques include use of a field block, reliance on fixed anatomic relationships, elicitation of paresthesias, and use of a nerve stimulator.

Premedication

Premedication with small doses of a benzodiazepine and/or opioid helps reduce anxiety and raise the pain threshold. The degree of sedation varies according to practitioner, but in general only light sedation is desirable when the elicitation of paresthesias is to be used for nerve localization. Use of a nerve stimulator allows heavier degrees of sedation. Supplemental oxygen should generally be administered to all patients via nasal cannula or face mask to reduce the incidence of hypoxemia following sedation.

Field Block

A single or multiple injections of a relatively large volume of local anesthetic in the general location of cutaneous nerves produces a field block. The superficial cervical plexus block is an example of a field block. Field blocks are also commonly used to supplement axillary brachial plexus and ankle blocks. Surgeons often use field blocks for minor, superficial operations. The technique may also be used to supplement patchy peripheral nerve blocks or when the level of neuraxial begins to recede. When a large volume of local anesthetic is to be injected, use of dilute concentration and addition of epinephrine (1:200,000 or 5 μg/mL) help reduce systemic absorption and the likelihood of systemic toxicity.

Fixed Anatomic Relationships

Some nerve block techniques rely on a constant anatomic relationship to locate correct needle position. High in the axilla, the brachial plexus is always in close association with the axillary artery in the axillary sheath. As described later, in the transarterial technique of a brachial plexus block, the artery is located and local anesthetic is injected just above and below it. Similarly, the musculocutaneous nerve can be blocked as it travels in the body of the coracobrachialis muscle; injection of coracobrachialis muscle can therefore be used to supplement axillary or interscalene brachial plexus anesthesia. Intercostal nerves travel in a neurovascular bundle on the undersurface of the inferior border of each rib. The nerve maintains an inferior position in the bundle; from superior to inferior the order is vein, artery, and nerve (VAN). Each intercostal nerve can therefore be blocked by an injection at the inferior border of the corresponding rib. Similarly, the femoral nerve has a constant position in a neurovascular bundle as it travels in the femoral canal. The femoral nerve is always lateral to the artery; from lateral to medial the order is nerve, artery, vein, (empty space), and lymphatics (NAVEL).

ELICITATION OF PARESTHESIAS

When a needle makes direct contact with a sensory nerve, a paresthesia is elicited in its area of sensory distribution. With this technique, it is important to ascertain that the needle is making contact with the nerve rather than within it, and that the injection is in proximity to the nerve (perineural) rather than within its substance (intraneural). The high pressures generated by a direct intraneural injection can cause hydrostatic (ischemic) injury to nerve fibers. A perineural injection may produce a brief accentuation of the paresthesia, whereas an intraneural injection produces an intense, searing pain that serves as a warning to immediately terminate the injection and reposition the needle. Pain intensity and duration help differentiate between accentuation and intraneural injection. Use of blunt bevel (B-bevel) needles appears to reduce the small incidence of nerve trauma associated with peripheral nerve blocks. Blunt-bevel (B-bevel) needles have a less blunt tip and smaller cutting edge than regular needles. This design helps push nerves aside upon contact, instead of piercing them. Many clinicians also believe that the blunt tip gives better feedback of allowing better appreciation of tissue planes and penetration of fascial compartments.

Nerve Stimulation

Low level electrical current applied from the tip of a needle can elicit specific muscle contractions when the needle is in close proximity to a motor nerve. One lead of a low-output nerve stimulator is attached to needle and the other lead is grounded elsewhere on the patient. Lower current is required when the negative lead is attached to the exploring needle. The special needles that are used are insulated and permit current flow only at the tip for precise localization of nerves, while the nerve stimulators used deliver a linear, constant current output of 0.1–6.0 mA. Muscle contractions occur and increase in intensity as the needle approaches the nerve and diminish when the needle moves away. Moreover, the evoked contractions require much less current as the needle approaches the nerve. Optimal positioning produces evoked contractions with 0.5 mA or less, but

successful blocks can often be obtained with needle positions that produce contractions with as much as 1 mA. Characteristically, the evoked response rapidly diminishes after injection of 1–2 mL of local anesthetic. Transient augmentation may be observed before extinction of the motor response because the ionic anesthetic solutions transiently facilitate conduction of the current.

SOMATIC BLOCKADE OF THE UPPER EXTREMITY

Surgical anesthesia of the upper extremity and shoulder can be obtained following neural blockade of the brachial plexus (C5–T1) or its terminal branches at several sites (Figure 17–1). It may also be necessary to block additional nerves independently for shoulder surgery and for procedures in which use of a pneumatic upper arm tourniquet is planned. Some areas of the anterior shoulder are innervated by the superficial cervical plexus (C1–4). These nerve roots converge lateral to their respective transverse processes, and pass through the platysma at the posterior border of the sternocleidomastoid muscle where a field block can be used to supplement a brachial plexus block (Figure 17–2). The medial brachial cutaneous (C8–T1) and intercostobrachial (T2) nerves must also be blocked separately to reliably prevent pain from an arm tourniquet. They innervate the skin of the medial and posterior proximal upper arm (Figure 17–3). The medial brachial cutaneous nerve often leaves the sheath just below the clavicle and may therefore be missed with the axillary approach to the brachial plexus, while the intercostobrachial nerve does not travel in the sheath at all.

ANATOMY OF THE BRACHIAL PLEXUS

The brachial plexus is formed by the union of the anterior primary divisions (ventral rami) of the fifth through the eighth cervical nerves and the first thoracic nerves (see Figure 17–1). Contributions from C4 and T2 are often minor or absent. As the nerve roots leave the intervertebral foramina, they converge, forming trunks, divisions, cords, and then finally terminal nerves. Three distinct trunks are formed between the anterior and middle scalene muscles. Because they are vertically arranged, they are named superior, middle, and inferior. The superior trunk is predominantly derived from C5–6, the middle trunk is derived from C7, and the inferior trunk originates from C8–T1. As the trunks pass over the lateral border of the first rib and

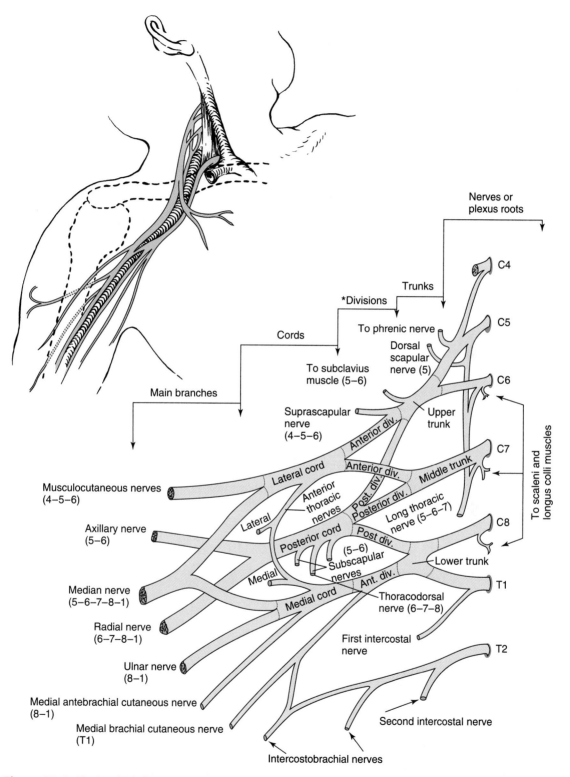

Figure 17–1. The brachial plexus. (Reproduced, with permission, from Waxman SG: *Correlative Neuroanatomy*, 24th ed. McGraw-Hill, 2000.)

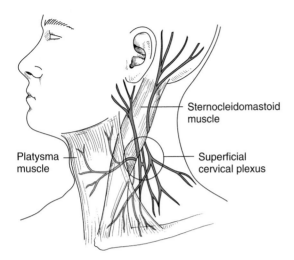

Figure 17–2. Superficial cervical plexus.

under the clavicle, each trunk divides into anterior and posterior divisions. As the brachial plexus emerges below the clavicle, the fibers combine again to form three cords that are named according to their relationship to the axillary artery: lateral, medial, and posterior. The lateral cord is the union of the anterior divisions of the superior and middle trunks; the medial cord is the continuation of anterior division of the inferior trunk; while the posterior cord is formed by the posterior division of the all three trunks. At the lateral border of the pectoralis minor muscle, each cord gives off a large branch before terminating as a major terminal nerve. The lateral cord gives off the lateral branch of the median nerve and terminates as the musculocutaneous nerve; the medial cord gives off the medial branch of the median nerve and terminates as the ulnar nerve; and the posterior cord gives off the axillary nerve and terminates as the radial nerve.

TECHNIQUES FOR BRACHIAL PLEXUS BLOCK

A fascial sleeve that is derived from the prevertebral and scalene fascia encloses the brachial plexus. This sheath extends from the intervertebral foramina to the upper arm and serves as the anatomic basis for brachial plexus blocks. Injection into this sheath at any point allows local anesthetic to spread and block the C5–T1 nerve roots. The degree of neural blockade, however, may vary somewhat depending on the level of injection.

The interscalene approach is most optimal for procedures on the shoulder, arm, and forearm. It may be especially useful when the arm

cannot be positioned for the axillary approach. Injection at the interscalene level tends to produce a block that is most intense at the C5–C7 dermatomes and least intense in the C8–T1 dermatomes. The interscalene approach may therefore not provide optimal surgical anesthesia for procedures in the ulnar nerve distribution. In contrast, the axillary approach to the brachial plexus is most optimal for procedures from the elbow to the hand.

This approach tends to produce the most intense block in the distribution of C7–T1 (ulnar nerve) but is usually inadequate for procedures on the shoulder and upper arm (C5–C6). The supraclavicular and infraclavicular approaches to the brachial plexus result in a more even distribution of local anesthetic and can be used for procedures on the arm, forearm, and hand.

Interscalene Brachial Plexus Block

A. ANATOMY:

The cervical spinal nerves blend into trunks between the anterior and middle scalene muscles. This interscalene groove lies at the level of the cricoid cartilage and is a relatively easy place to enter the brachial plexus sheath to elicit a paresthesia or obtain an evoked motor response with a nerve stimulator.

B. TECHNIQUE:

(Figure 17–4) Palpation of the interscalene groove is usually accomplished with the patient supine and the head rotated 30 degrees to the contralateral side. The external jugular vein often crosses the interscalene groove at the level of the cricoid cartilage. The intersca-

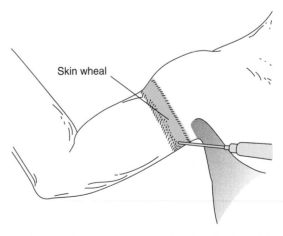

Figure 17–3. Intercostobrachial and medial brachial cutaneous nerve blocks.

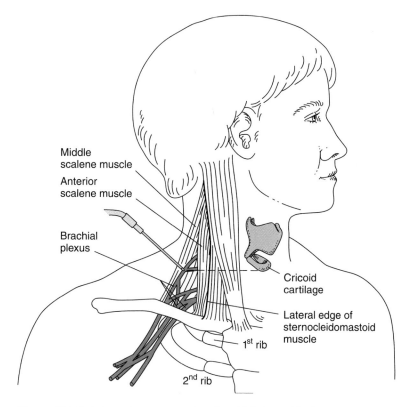

Figure 17–4. Interscalene approach to brachial plexus block.

lene groove should not be confused with the groove between the sternocleidomastoid and the anterior scalene muscle, which lies more anteriorly. Having the patient lift and turn the head against resistance often helps delineate the anatomy. After injection of a skin wheal with a 25-gauge needle at the level of the cricoid cartilage, a 22-gauge, 1.5-inch B-bevel needle is introduced nearly perpendicular to the skin and advanced in slightly medial and caudal directions until a paresthesia or evoked muscle contraction in the arm is elicited. Some clinicians apply proximal pressure on the sheath to favor distal spread of local anesthetic. A total of 30–40 mL of local anesthetic solution is used.

C. COMPLICATIONS:

The proximity of the stellate ganglion, the phrenic nerve, and the recurrent laryngeal nerve to this location explains their high rate of incidental blockade. Thus patients may display a Horner's syndrome (myosis, ptosis, and anhidrosis), dyspnea, and hoarseness, respectively. The proximity of the vertebral artery to the injection site increases the risk of an intra-arterial injection. Even a very small amount (1–3 mL) of local anesthetic injected into a vertebral artery can produce a seizure be-

cause the entire amount goes directly to the brain. Venous injection and rapid absorption can result in a slower onset of central nervous system toxicity. Inadvertent epidural, subarachnoid, or subdural injection can occur because of the close proximity of the cervical neural foramina and the presence of dural sleeves on nerve roots (see Chapter 16). Advancing the needle too far, especially in lateral direction, can result in puncture of the pleura and a pneumothorax.

Supraclavicular (Subclavian) Brachial Plexus Block

A. ANATOMY:

At the lateral border of the anterior scalene muscle, the brachial plexus passes down between the first rib and clavicle to enter the axilla. The trunks are tightly oriented vertically on top of the first just posterior to the subclavian artery.

B. TECHNIQUE:

(Figure 17–5.) The patient is positioned supine with the head turned about 30 degrees to the contralateral

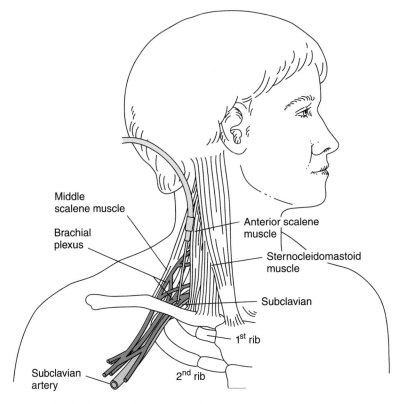

Middle
scalene muscle

Brachial
plexus

Anterior scalene
muscle

Sternocleidomastoid
muscle

Subclavian

1st rib

Subclavian
artery

2nd rib

Figure 17–5. Supraclavicular approach to brachial plexus block.

side. The interscalene groove is palpated at its most in-ferior point, which is just posterior to the subclavian artery pulse; the latter can be felt in a plane just medial to the midpoint of the clavicle. After a skin wheal, a 22-gauge, 1.5-inch B-bevel needle is directed just above and posterior to the subclavian pulse and di-rected caudally at a very flat angle against the skin. The needle is advanced until a paresthesia is encountered where 25–40 mL of local anesthetic is injected. If the rib is encountered without a paresthesia or if blood is encountered, the needle is withdrawn and the landmarks as well as the plane of the needle are reeval-uated.

C. COMPLICATIONS:

Although this is an excellent technique in experienced hands, a relatively high incidence of pneumothorax (1–6%) causes many clinicians to avoid this approach. Hemothorax has also been reported. As with the inter-scalene approach, Horner's syndrome and phrenic nerve block often occur.

Infraclavicular Brachial Plexus Block

A. ANATOMY:

The brachial plexus lies underneath the midpoint of the clavicle, anterior to the coracoid process, and posterior and lateral to the subclavian artery.

B. TECHNIQUE:

(Figure 17–6.) With the patient supine, a skin wheal is raised 1 inch beneath the midpoint of the clavicle. A 3.5-inch, 22-gauge spinal needle is then directed laterally from this site at a 45 degree angle *away* from the chest wall and toward the humeral head or coracoid process. Once a paresthesia or evoked con-traction is elicited, 20–25 mL of local anesthetic is in-jected.

C. COMPLICATIONS:

Pneumothorax, hemothorax, and chylothorax (with a left-sided block) are possible and occur at a higher rate than with the supraclavicular approach.

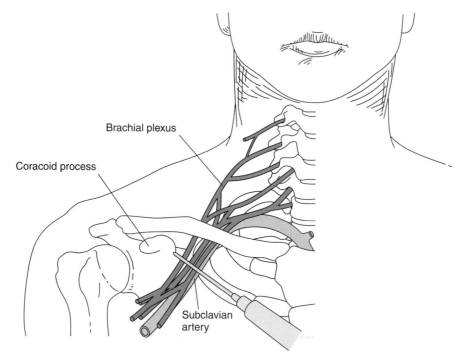

Figure 17–6. Infraclavicular block.

Axillary Brachial Plexus Block

A. ANATOMY:

The subclavian artery becomes the axillary artery beneath the clavicle, where the trunks of the brachial plexus split into anterior and posterior divisions. At the lateral border of the pectoralis minor muscle, the cords form large terminal branches. It should be noted that in the axilla, the musculocutaneous nerve has already left the sheath and lies within the coracobrachialis muscle. Moreover, imaging studies suggest that the fascial sheath is multicompartmental and that fascial septa may be responsible for the "patchy" anesthesia observed in some patients. Fascial septa may result in incomplete spread of local anesthetic within the plexus sheath.

B. TECHNIQUE:

(Figure 17–7) Axillary block is most commonly performed by one of three techniques that use axillary arterial pulse as a starting point. The patient is positioned supine with the arm abducted and the elbow flexed at 90 degrees. After a skin wheal is raised over the pulse, a 22-gauge, 1.5-inch B-bevel needle is introduced. As the needle is advanced, a distinct "pop" is often felt when the needle enters the brachial plexus sheath. Regardless of the subsequent technique, it should be noted that the medial brachial cutaneous nerve leaves the sheath just below the clavicle and will be missed with the axillary approach. A field block must therefore be performed in the subcutaneous tissue over the artery, to anesthetize this nerve as well as the intercostobrachial nerve; this supplementation allows the use of a pneumatic arm tourniquet. Injection of the coracobrachialis muscle may also be necessary to block the musculocutaneous nerve.

1. Transarterial technique—The pulse of the axillary artery is identified as high (proximal) in the axilla as possible. Using an "immobile needle" technique, a 22-gauge, 1.5-inch B-bevel needle is inserted until bright red blood is aspirated. The needle is then moved slightly forward or withdrawn until blood aspiration ceases. Injection can be performed either posteriorly, anteriorly, or in both locations in relation to the artery. A total of 40 mL of local anesthetic is usually injected; distal pressure on the sheath during the injection may promote better cephalad spread of the solution within the sheath. Some clinicians inject the entire quantity either anterior or posterior to the artery, while those who worry about septa in the sheath inject 20 mL anterior and 20 mL posterior to the artery.

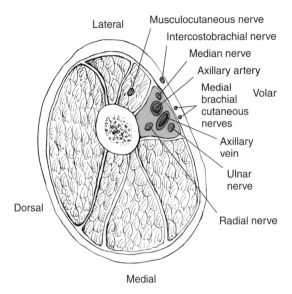

Lateral

Musculocutaneous nerve

Intercostobrachial nerve

Median nerve

Axillary artery

Medial brachial cutaneous nerves **Volar**

Axillary vein

Ulnar nerve

Dorsal

Radial nerve

Medial

Figure 17–7. Axillary block, showing relationships of the nerves to the artery.

2. Elicitation of paresthesia technique—With this technique, the needle is directed toward the axillary artery to elicit a single, specific or multiple paresthesias. If the artery is entered, the needle is redirected until a paresthesia is obtained. Many practitioners try to elicit any parestheisa in the brachial plexus distribution, while others always try to specifically elicit paresthesias in the nerve distribution of the operative area before injection. Yet, other clinicians who are concerned about septations in the plexus sheath, try to elicit paresthesias in the ulnar, median, and radial nerve distributions, injecting some local anesthetic at each site. Regardless of whether one or multiple paresthesias are elicited, a total of 40 mL of local anesthetic is usually injected.

3. Nerve stimulator technique—As with the elicitation of paresthesia technique, the nerve stimulator technique may be used to evoked contraction in any muscle innervated by the brachial plexus, a contraction specific to the innervation of the operative area, or contractions in the ulnar, median, and radial nerve distributions.

C. COMPLICATIONS:

The axillary approach to the brachial plexus is associated with a very low complication rate, providing intravascular injection is avoided. Although controversial, repeated elicitation of paresthesia at multiple sites may increase the incidence of postoperative neuropathies. Hematoma and infection are very rare.

Midhumeral Brachial Plexus Block

All four major nerves of the arm can be blocked separately at the level of the midhumerus. This relatively new technique uses a nerve stimulator to locate each nerve as it passes in the humeral canal. The success rate of this approach appears to be similar to the classic axillary block but the onset of the blockade is slower.

PERIPHERAL NERVE BLOCKS

Intercostobrachial & Medial Brachial Cutaneous Nerves

The intercostobrachial and the medial brachial nerves originate in the lower neck and upper thorax and become cutaneous on the medial upper arm. Both must be blocked proximal to the axilla for shoulder surgery or for any upper extremity procedure that involves use of a pneumatic tourniquet. The intercostobrachial nerve derives from the T2 somatic intercostal nerve, while the medial brachial cutaneous nerve derives from C8 and T1. Both become superficial and cutaneous at the pectoral ridge over the humeral head. They are easily blocked, with the arm abducted, by means of a linear injection (field block) from the deltoid prominence superiorly to the most inferior aspect of the medial upper arm (see Figure 17–3). A total of 5 mL of local anesthesia is used.

Musculocutaneous Nerve

The musculocutaneous nerve is the most proximal of the major nerves of the brachial plexus. Because of its early take-off proximal to the insertion of the pectoralis minor muscle, axillary brachial plexus blocks often fail to block the musculocutaneous nerve, and supplemental blockade is necessary for complete motor block of the arm or sensory block in the musculocutaneous distribution of the forearm and wrist.

The nerve enters the arm by piercing the coracobrachialis and then travels ventral to the humerus between the biceps and the brachialis muscles, which it innervates. The terminal sensory limit is cutaneous on the lateral aspect of the forearm and is called the lateral cutaneous nerve of the forearm.

Using a 22-gauge, 1.5-inch needle, one of two techniques may be used to block the musculocutaneous nerve. The first is a field block of 5–8 mL of local anesthetic into the belly of the coracobrachialis muscle (Figure 17–8). The second blocks it behind the brachial artery near the biceps muscle.

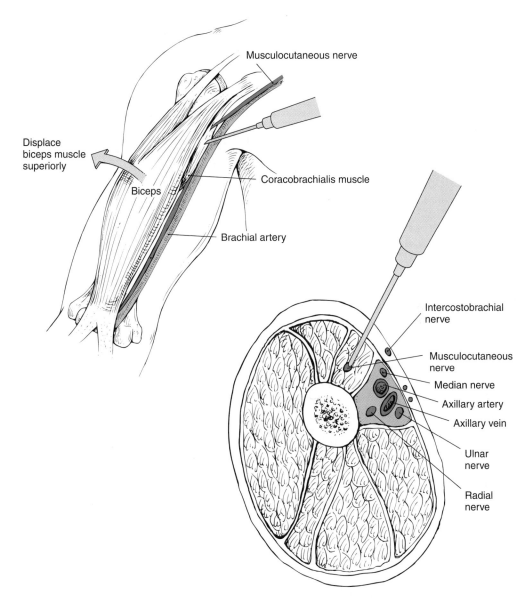

Figure 17–8. Musculocutaneous block, showing injection into coracobrachialis.

Radial Nerve

An isolated radial nerve block is typically used to supplement an incomplete brachial plexus block that spares the radial distribution.

A. ANATOMY:

The radial nerve—the terminal branch of the posterior cord of the brachial plexus—courses posterior to the humerus, innervating the triceps muscle, and enters the musculospiral groove of the humerus before it moves laterally at the elbow. Terminal sensory branches include the lateral cutaneous nerve of the arm and the posterior cutaneous nerve of the forearm. After exiting the musculospiral groove as it approaches the lateral epicondyle, it branches into superficial and deep branches. The deep branch remains close to periosteum and innervates the postaxial extensor group of the forearm. The superficial branch comes close to the dermis and follows the radial artery to innervate the radial aspects of the dorsal wrist and the dorsal aspect of the lateral 3½ digits.

B. TECHNIQUES:

1. At the upper arm—(Figure 17–9) The radial nerve exits the musculospiral groove between the two heads of the triceps. Palpation of a line between this site and the lateral epicondyle often reveals a palpable nerve. Three to 4 cm proximal to the epicondyle, a 22-gauge, B-bevel needle is inserted toward the nerve or the periosteum and withdrawn 0.5 cm, and 5 mL of local anesthetic is injected. Mild paresthesia is acceptable, but the intense paresthesia of intraneural injection must be avoided. At this level, localization with a nerve stim-

ulator is possible with motor-evoked response of wrist extensors (wrist extension).

2. At the elbow—(Figure 17–10) From the antecubital space, the lateral aspect of the biceps tendon is identified at the flexion crease. A 22-gauge, 1.5-inch B-bevel needle is inserted almost parallel to the forearm. It is directed just superficial to the radial head toward the lateral epicondyle until paresthesia is elicited or periosteum is encountered. With paresthesia, the needle is withdrawn slightly and injection then proceeds as long as intense paresthesia is not encountered. At the periosteum, the needle is withdrawn 1 cm, and 5 mL of local anesthetic is injected.

3. At the distal forearm—(Figure 17–11) At the level of the ulnar styloid, sensory branches to the lateral side of the thumb lie between the radial artery and the

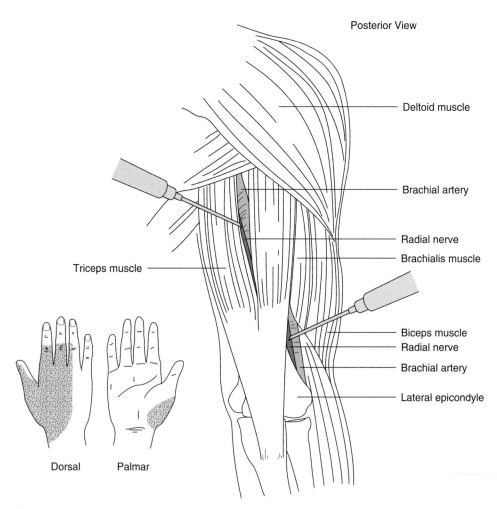

Figure 17–9. Radial nerve block, showing injection under biceps muscle.

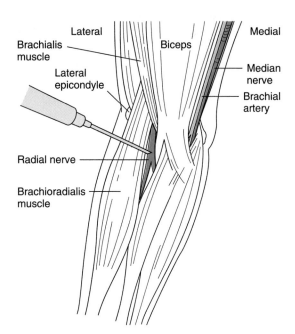

Figure 17–10. Radial nerve block in the antecubital space.

flexor carpi radialis tendon. One to 2 mL of local anesthetic deposited in this interval, deep to flexor carpi radialis tendon, will block this sensation. More proximally, dorsal branches are given off. In some persons, this is palpable as the nerve moves from volar to dorsal. If palpable, 2–3 mL of local anesthetic as a directed field block can be performed. If not palpable, a linear field block at the level of the ulnar styloid from the volar lateral edge of the radius to the mid forearm will anesthetize the dorsal aspect of the lateral 3½ fingers.

C. COMPLICATIONS:

Radial artery injection and intraneural injection may occur.

Median Nerve

Isolated median nerve block is performed usually used as a supplement to a brachial plexus.

A. ANATOMY:

The median nerve is derived from the lateral and medial cords of the brachial plexus. It enters the arm and runs just medial to the brachial artery. As it enters the antecubital space, it lies medial to the brachial artery near the insertion of the biceps tendon. Just distal to this, it gives off numerous motor branches to the wrist

and finger flexors and follows the interosseous membrane to the wrist. At the level of the proximal wrist flexion crease, it lies directly behind palmaris longus tendon in the carpal tunnel.

B. TECHNIQUES:

1. At the elbow—(Figure 17–12) The brachial artery can be identified in the antecubital crease just medial to the biceps insertion. A 22-gauge, 1.5-inch B-bevel needle is inserted just medial to the artery and directed toward the medial epicondyle until a paresthesia, motor-evoked response (wrist flexion), or periosteum is encountered. If periosteum is encountered, the needle is withdrawn 0.5–1 cm. Three to 5 mL of anesthetic is injected.

2. At the wrist—(Figure 17–13) Asking the patient to flex the wrist against resistance can identify the palmaris longus tendon. It is marked at the proximal flexion crease. A 22–25 gauge, B-bevel needle is inserted just medial and deep to the palmaris longus, and 3–5 mL of anesthetic is injected.

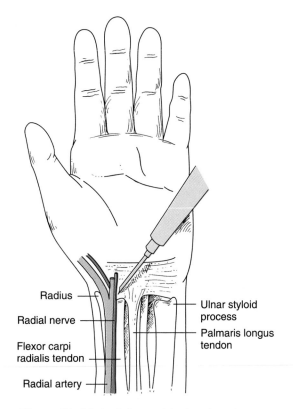

Figure 17–11. Radial nerve block at the wrist.

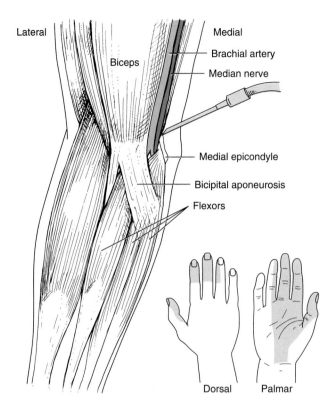

Figure 17–12. Median nerve block in the antecubital space.

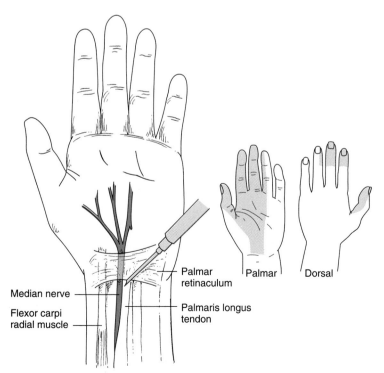

Figure 17–13. Median nerve block at the wrist.

C. Complications:

Brachial artery injection or intraneural injection may occur.

Ulnar Nerve

An ulnar nerve block can also be used to supplement a patchy axillary or interscalene block or for minor surgical procedures in the distribution of the ulnar nerve.

A. Anatomy:

The ulnar nerve is the continuation of the medial cord of the brachial plexus and maintains a medial position to the axillary and brachial arteries in the upper arm. At the distal third of the humerus, the nerve moves more medially and passes under the arcuate ligament of the medial epicondyle. The nerve is frequently palpable just proximal to the medial epicondyle. In the mid forearm, the nerve lies between the flexor digitorum profundus and the flexor carpi ulnaris. At the wrist, it is lateral to the flexor carpi ulnaris tendon and medial to the ulnar artery.

B. Techniques:

1. At the elbow—(Figure 17–14) A 22-gauge, B-bevel needle is inserted approximately one finger breadth proximal to the arcuate ligament and advanced until paresthesia or motor-evoked response is elicited (finger movement). Three to 5 mL of anesthetic is injected.

2. At the wrist—(Figure 17–15) A 22-gauge, B-bevel needle is directed just medial to the ulnar artery pulse, or immediately lateral to the flexor carpi ulnaris if no pulse is palpable. A total of 3–5 mL of anesthetic is injected.

C. Complications:

Intraneural injection may occur at the elbow and intraneural or intra-arterial injection at the wrist.

Digital Nerves

These nerve blocks are used for minor operations on the fingers and to supplement brachial plexus blocks.

A. Anatomy:

Sensory innervation of each finger is provided by four small digital nerves that enter each digit at its base in each of the four corners.

B. Technique:

(Figure 17–16) A 23–25 gauge needle inserted at the medial and lateral aspects of the base of the selected digit. Two to 3 mL of local anesthetic without epinephrine is injected on each side near the periosteum. Addition of a vasoconstrictor (epinephrine) can seriously compromise blood flow to the digit.

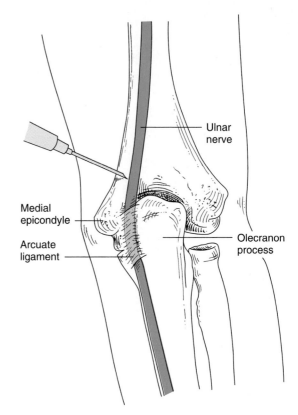

Figure 17–14. Ulnar nerve block at the elbow.

C. Complications:

Nerve injury is the chief risk of a digital block.

INTRAVENOUS REGIONAL ANESTHESIA OF THE ARM

 Intravenous regional anesthesia, also called a Bier block, can provide intense surgical anesthesia for short surgical procedures (< 45–60 minutes) on the forearm and hand. It is most commonly used for a carpal tunnel release. An intravenous catheter is usually on the dorsum of the hand and a double pneumatic tourniquet is placed on the arm (Figure 17–17). The extremity is elevated and exsanguinated by tightly wrapping an Eschmark elastic bandage from a distal to proximal direction. The upper (proximal) tourniquet inflated, Eschmark is removed, and 40–50 mL of 0.5% lidocaine is injected over 2–3 minutes through the catheter, which is removed at the end of the injection. Anesthesia is usually well established after 5–10 minutes. Patients often complain of tourniquet pain after 20–30 minutes. When this occurs, the lower (distal) tourniquet is inflated and only then the

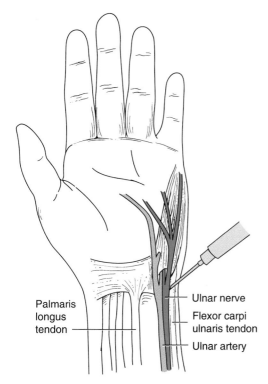

Figure 17–15. Ulnar nerve block at the wrist.

Palmaris longus tendon — Ulnar nerve
Flexor carpi ulnaris tendon
Ulnar artery

proximal is deflated. Patients usually tolerate the lower tourniquet for another 15–20 minutes because it is inflated over an anesthetized area. With very short procedures, the tourniquet must be left inflated for a total of at least 15–20 minutes to avoid a rapid intravenous systemic bolus of local anesthetic that can cause a seizure. Slow deflation my also provide a safety margin.

■ SOMATIC BLOCKADE OF THE LOWER EXTREMITY

Spinal and epidural anesthesia (see Chapter 16) are most often employed for regional anesthesia of the lower extremities. Peripheral nerve blocks in the lower extremity can also provide excellent surgical anesthesia for some procedures but require multiple injections and may be technically more challenging in some cases. Ankle block is the easiest and most commonly used lower extremity block; it is typically used for foot surgery.

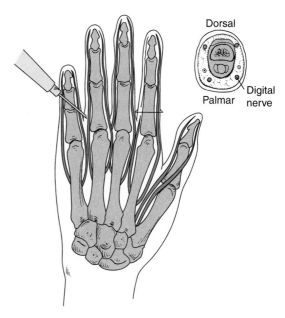

Dorsal
Palmar
Digital nerve

Figure 17–16. Digital block of the hand.

Four major nerves innervate the lower extremities: the femoral (L2–L4), obturator (L2–L4), lateral femoral (L1–L3), and sciatic nerves (L4–S3). The first three nerves are part of the lumbar plexus; they lie within the substance of the psoas muscle and emerge within a common fascial sheath that extends into the proximal thigh. The common peroneal and tibial nerves are continuations of the sciatic nerve in the lower leg.

Femoral Nerve and "Three-in One" Block

 A femoral nerve block can used to provide anesthesia for the anterior thigh, knee, and a small part of the medial foot. It is typically

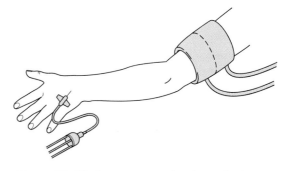

Figure 17–17. Intravenous regional anesthesia.

used in conjunction with other lower extremity blocks. It may also be for postoperative pain relief following knee surgery.

A. ANATOMY:

After passing through the psoas compartment, the femoral nerve enters the thigh lateral to the femoral artery just below the inguinal ligament. Distal to this point, motor branches to the quadriceps, sartorius, and pectineus muscles arise as well as numerous sensory branches to the medial and anterior thigh. The nerve is encased in a sheath that extends from the psoas muscle to just below the inguinal ligament.

B. TECHNIQUE:

(Figure 17–18) With the patient supine, the femoral pulse is identified and a 22-gauge, 1.5-inch B-bevel needle is directed just lateral to the artery. A distinct "pop" is often felt as the surrounding sheath is entered and a paresthesia or a motor-evoked response (quadriceps muscle) can usually be elicited. Twenty to 40 mL of local anesthetic can be injected to produce a "three-in-one" block of the femoral, obturator, and lateral femoral cutaneous nerves. Distal pressure during injection may help direct the anesthetic solution proximally into the psoas sheath.

C. COMPLICATIONS:

Careful aspiration and incremental dosing help avoid intravascular injection and systemic local anesthetic toxicity.

Obturator Nerve Block

An obturator nerve block provides anesthesia to the medial thigh and muscle relaxation of the adductor muscles of the hip. It may be used for an adductor release procedure.

A. ANATOMY:

The obturator nerve exits the pelvis and enters the medial thigh through the obturator foramen, which lies beneath the superior pubic ramus. It supplies sensation to the medial thigh and the hip joint and motor innervation to the adductor muscles of the thigh.

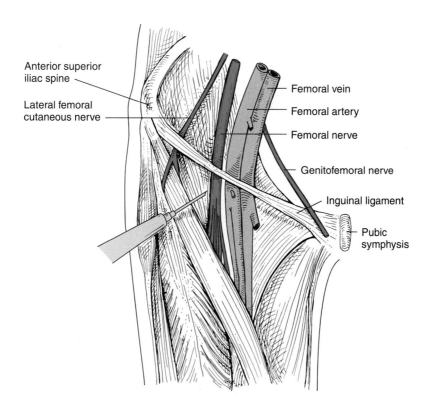

Figure 17–18. Femoral nerve block.

B. Technique:

(Figure 17–19) A 3.5-inch, 22-gauge needle is inserted through a skin wheal 2 cm lateral and 2 cm inferior to the pubic tubercle. As the needle is advanced medially toward the superior pubic ramus, small amounts of local anesthetic are injected to decrease patient discomfort. The needle is then "walked off" the superior ramus and advanced 3–4 cm until it enters the obturator foramen. Fifteen to 20 mL of local anesthetic is injected. The obturator nerve may also be blocked by the "three-in-one" block technique.

C. Complications:

Careful aspiration and incremental dosing help avoid intravascular injection and systemic local anesthetic toxicity.

Lateral Femoral Cutaneous Nerve Block

The lateral femoral cutaneous nerve block may be used for procedures on lateral thigh, such as muscle biopsy.

A. Anatomy:

The lateral femoral cutaneous exits the psoas muscle and courses ventrally and laterally, becoming superficial near the anterior superior iliac spine at the level of the inguinal ligament. It provides sensation to the lateral thigh sometimes as far as the knee.

B. Technique:

(Figure 17–20) With the patient supine, the anterior superior iliac spine is identified. A skin wheal is raised 2 cm medial and 2 cm caudal to the anterior superior iliac spine and a 22-gauge, 1.5-inch needle is inserted and advanced through the fascia lata. A distinct "pop" is often appreciated as the needle penetrates the fascia; 10–15 mL of local anesthetic is injected in a fanlike manner. The lateral femoral' cutaneous nerve may also be blocked by the "three-in-one" block technique.

C. Complications:

Persistent paresthesias from intraneural injection can occur.

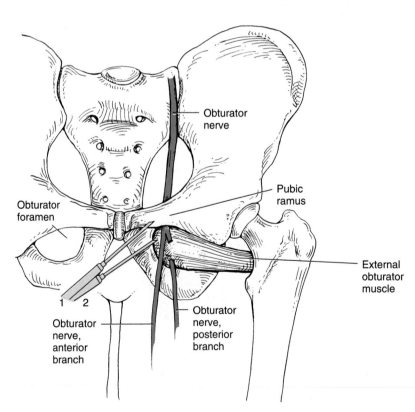

Figure 17–19. Obturator nerve block.

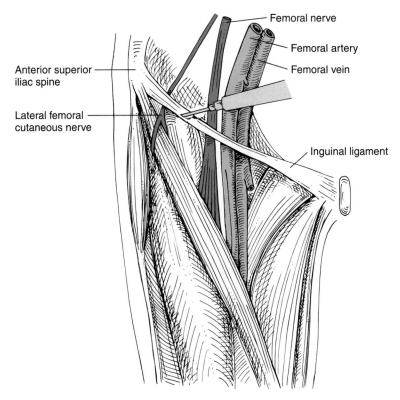

Figure 17–20. Lateral femoral cutaneous nerve block.

Sciatic Nerve Block

A sciatic nerve block may be used for all procedures on the lower extremity that do not require a pneumatic tourniquet on the thigh. The sciatic nerve provides sensation to the knee and lower leg. When combined with a "three-in-one" block, it can anesthetize the entire lower extremity.

A. Anatomy:

The sciatic nerve leaves the pelvis below the piriformis muscle in the sciatic notch. It passes distally just dorsal to the lesser trochanter of the femur. In a lateral position (with the hip flexed), the nerve courses midway between the greater trochanter and posterior-superior iliac spine. It divides into the tibial and common peroneal nerves.

B. Techniques:

1. Anterior approach—(Figure 17–21) This technique, which is more painful than the posterior approach, may be used for patients who are unable to flex the hip. With the patient supine and the legs in slight external rotation, a skin wheal is raised 2 cm medial to the femoral artery. A 22-gauge, 3.5-inch spinal needle is then directed dorsally until the periosteum of the lesser trochanter is encountered (4–6 cm depth) and "walked-off" superiorly and advanced until a paresthesia or a motor-evoked response (dorsiflexion or plantar flexion of the foot) is elicited. Twenty milliliters of local anesthetic is injected.

2. Posterior approach—(Figure 17–22) The patient is placed in the lateral decubitus position; the ipsilateral hip and knee are flexed, and a line is drawn connecting the prominence of the greater trochanter with the posterior superior iliac spine. At the midpoint, a 4-cm perpendicular line is drawn caudally. These lines are referred to as Labatt's lines and identify a constant position of the sciatic nerve, in the sciatic notch, proximal to its branching. Through a skin wheal, a 22-gauge, 3⅓-inch spinal needle is inserted perpendicular to the skin, and at 4–6 cm from the surface—depending on patient's weight and muscle mass—the nerve can be felt. Confirmatory paresthesia or motor-evoked response (dorsiflexion or plantar flexion of the foot) is desirable. Twenty milliliters of local anesthetic is in-

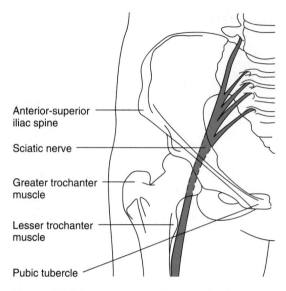

Figure 17–21. Sciatic nerve block, anterior approach.

jected. Searing pain suggests intraneural injection and requires needle redirection.

3. Lithotomy approach—With the patient supine, the ipsilateral leg is flexed 90 degrees at the knee and 90–120 degrees at the hip. A 22-gauge, 3.5- to 5-inch needle is advanced at a right angle to the skin through a skin wheal at the midpoint of a line connecting the greater trochanter and the ischial tuberosity. Twenty milliliters of local anesthetic is injected when paresthesia is encountered.

C. COMPLICATIONS:

Partial block due to injection distal to branching of the sciatic nerve and intraneural injection are the most frequent complications.

Popliteal Block

Nerve block in the popliteal fossa can be performed for procedures of the foot and ankle, when more proximal block (hip) is not feasible, when no tourniquet is used, or when a calf tourniquet is adequate. In combination with saphenous nerve block, popliteal nerve block provides complete anesthesia to the foot and ankle.

A. ANATOMY:

The sciatic nerve divides into the tibial and common peroneal nerves, high in the popliteal fossa. The upper popliteal fossa is bounded laterally by the biceps femoris tendon and medially by the semitendinosus and semimembranosus tendons. Cephalad to the flexion crease of the knee, the popliteal artery is immediately lateral to the semitendinosus tendon. The popliteal vein is lateral to the artery, and the tibial and common peroneal nerves (within a sheath) are just lateral to the vein and medial to the biceps tendon, 4–6 cm deep to the skin. The tibial nerve continues deep behind the gastrocnemius muscle, while the common peroneal nerve leaves the popliteal fossa by passing between the head and neck of the fibula to supply to the lower leg.

B. TECHNIQUE:

(Figure 17–23) The patient is positioned prone and the outline of the popliteal fossa is identified proximal to the flexion crease of the knee. If the popliteal artery can be identified, it serves as a landmark. If not, the midline is identified. Two inches proximal to the crease, a skin wheal is raised. A 22-gauge spinal needle is inserted 1 cm lateral to the pulse—or in the midline if the pulse cannot be felt—and advanced 2–4 cm until paresthesia or motor-evoked response (plantar flexion or dorsiflexion of foot) is elicited. Twenty to 30 mL of local anesthetic is injected. It may be necessary to block the com-

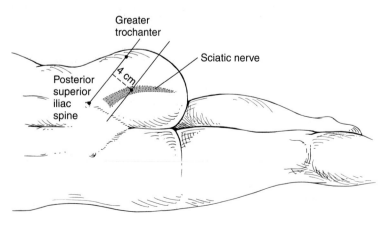

Figure 17–22. Sciatic nerve block, posterior approach.

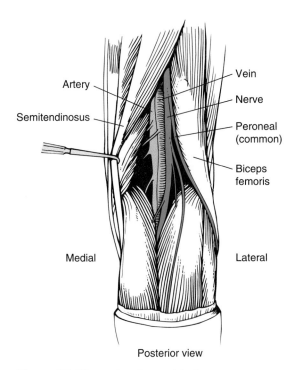

Artery

Vein

Nerve

Semitendinosus

Peroneal
(common)

Biceps
femoris

Medial

Lateral

Posterior view

Figure 17–23. Popliteal nerve block.

mon peroneal nerve separately, should it branch above the popliteal fossa. The nerve can often be felt subcutaneously at the junction of the head and neck of the fibula just below the knee, where it can be blocked by 5 mL of local anesthetic. The saphenous nerve can be blocked with 5–10 mL of local anesthetic injected just below the medial surface of the tibial condyle.

C. COMPLICATIONS:

Intravascular or intraneural injections are possible.

Ankle Block

 Ankle block is commonly performed for surgery of the foot in frail patients who may not tolerate the hemodynamic effects associated with neuraxial or general anesthesia.

A. ANATOMY:

Five nerves supply sensation to the foot. The saphenous nerve is a terminal branch of the femoral nerve and the only innervation of the foot not a part of the sciatic system. It supplies superficial sensation to the anteromedial foot and is most constantly located just anterior to the medial malleolus. The deep peroneal nerve runs in the anterior leg as a continuation of the common peroneal nerve; innervates toe extensors; enters the ankle

between the flexor hallucis longus and the extensor digitorum longus tendons; and provides sensation to the medial half of the dorsal foot, especially the first and second digits. The deep peroneal nerve has a constant location just lateral to the flexor hallucis longus at the level of the medial malleolus; the anterior tibial artery (which becomes the dorsalis pedis artery) lies between the nerve and this tendon. The superficial peroneal nerve, also a branch of the common peroneal nerve, descends toward the ankle in the lateral compartment, entering the ankle just lateral to the extensor digitorum longus and providing cutaneous sensation to the dorsum of the foot as well as all five toes. It is most constantly located lateral to the extensor digitorum longus at the level of the lateral malleolus superficially. The posterior tibial nerve is a direct continuation of the tibial nerve and enters the foot posterior to the medial malleolus, branching into lateral and medial plantar nerves. It is constantly located behind the posterior tibial artery at the level of the medial malleolus, and is sensory to the heel, the medial sole, and part of the lateral sole of the foot. The sural nerve is the continuation of the tibial nerve and enters the foot between the Achilles tendon and the lateral malleolus to provide sensation to the lateral foot.

B. TECHNIQUE:

The superficial peroneal and saphenous nerves are blocked with subcutaneous infiltration on the dorsal foot from the medial malleolus to the extensor digitorum longus tendon with 3–5 mL of local anesthetic (Figure 17–24). Through the numb area from saphenous infiltration, a 22-gauge, 1.5-inch needle is inserted at the intermalleolar line between the extensor digitorum longus and extensor hallucis longus tendons to periosteum or elicitation of paresthesia and 5 mL is injected to block the deep peroneal nerve (Figure 17–25). The posterior tibial nerve is blocked posterior to the medial malleolus (Figure 17–26). The posterior tibial artery is palpated and the needle directed just adjacent to the pulse until paresthesia or bone contact is encountered. If paresthesia is encountered, the needle is slightly withdrawn before 5 mL of local anesthetic is injected. The sural nerve is blocked laterally between the lateral malleolus and the Achilles tendon with a deep subcutaneous fan infiltration of 3–5 mL (Figure 17–27). Epinephrine is usually not added for ankle block to reduce the risk of ischemic injury to the foot.

C. COMPLICATIONS:

Aggressive injection, especially with excessively large volumes, may cause hydrostatic damage to small nerves, particularly those within closed ligamentous spaces, like the tibial nerve.

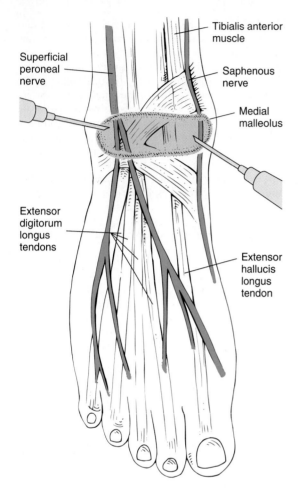

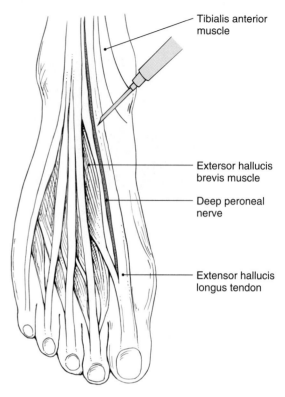

Figure 17–25. Ankle block, deep peroneal nerve.

Figure 17–24. Ankle block, saphenous and superficial peroneal nerves.

posterior to the sternocleidomastoid muscle. It supplies sensation to the jaw, neck, the occiput posteriorly, and areas of the chest and shoulder close to the clavicle.

■ SOMATIC BLOCKADE OF THE TRUNK

B. TECHNIQUE:

(see Figure 17–2) The patient is positioned supine with the neck slightly turned, and the posterior border of the sternocleidomastoid muscle is identified. A 22-gauge spinal needle is selected; the sternocleidomastoid is di-

Superficial Cervical Plexus Block

The superficial cervical plexus block is performed for unilateral procedures on the neck, such as carotid endarterectomy. This block is also done as an adjunct to interscalene block for shoulder surgery, especially with very anterior incisions. Blockade of the deep cervical plexus is discussed in Chapter 18.

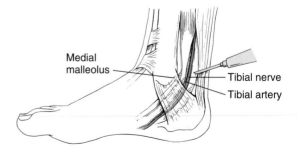

Figure 17–26. Ankle block, tibial nerve.

A. ANATOMY:

The cervical plexus is formed from the anterior rami of C1–4, which emerge from the platysma muscle

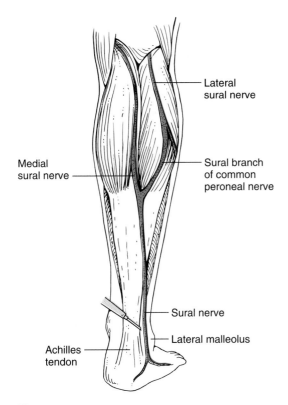

Figure 17–27. Ankle block, sural nerve.

vided into thirds, and at the junction of the upper and middle thirds, a skin wheal is raised. The spinal needle is directed cephalad toward the mastoid along the posterior border of the sternocleidomastoid in a subcutaneous plane and injected with 2–3 mL as the needle is withdrawn. Care is taken to avoid entering the external jugular vein. As the needle reaches the wheal, it is rotated 180 degrees and directed subcutaneously caudad toward the clavicle along the posterior border of the sternocleidomastoid. A similar amount is injected as the needle is withdrawn.

C. COMPLICATIONS:

Rapid systemic absorption and intravascular injection of local anesthetic are the most common complications.

Intercostal Block

Intercostal blocks are rarely employed as the sole anesthetic technique for surgery. They are more commonly used as supplements to general anesthesia, for postoperative analgesia following thoracic and upper abdominal surgery, and for relief of pain associated with rib fractures, herpes zoster, and cancer.

A. ANATOMY:

The intercostal nerves arise from the dorsal and ventral rami of the thoracic spinal nerves. They exit from the spine at the intervertebral foramen and enter a groove on the underside of the corresponding rib, running with the intercostal artery and vein; the nerve is generally the most inferior structure in the neurovascular bundle. Branches are given off for sensation in the correct dermatome from the midline dorsally all the way to across the midline ventrally.

B. TECHNIQUE:

(Figure 17–28) With the patient in the lateral decubitus or supine position, the level of each rib is palpated and marked in the mid and posterior axillary line. A skin wheal is raised over the inferior border at the selected ribs, and a 22- to 25-gauge needle is inserted down to the inferior edge of the rib and "walked-off" until it steps off the rib inferiorly. The needle is advanced 0.5 cm underneath the rib, and following a negative aspiration (for blood or air), 3–5 mL of local anesthetic is injected at each level.

C. COMPLICATIONS:

Intercostal blocks result in the highest blood levels of local anesthetic per volume injected of any block in the body. Care must be taken to avoid toxic levels of local anesthetic. Careful aspiration may help prevent intravascular injection. The risk of pneumothorax is obvious, and any indication of entering the chest should be investigated with a chest film.

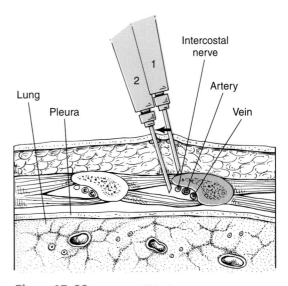

Figure 17–28. Intercostal block.

Thoracic Paravertebral Block

Thoracic paravertebral blocks may be useful at the upper thoracic segments where the scapula and shoulder block access to the intercostal nerves. Thoracic paravertebral blocks can also be used for analgesia in patients in whom a thoracic epidural block may be difficult or contraindicated.

A. ANATOMY:

Intercostal nerves originate just inferior to the transverse process of the spinal segment whose intervertebral foramen it has just exited.

B. TECHNIQUE:

(Figure 17–29) The patient is positioned prone, and a 22-gauge spinal needle is selected. The spinous process superior to the level to be blocked identifies the level of the transverse process; a skin wheal is raised 4 cm lateral to this, and the needle is inserted until the transverse process is contacted. The depth of the insertion is noted and marked. The needle is withdrawn to subcutaneous tissue and redirected to walk off the inferior edge of the transverse process and advanced no more than 2 cm beyond the depth of the transverse process; paresthesias should be encountered. At the point where paresthesia occurs (or 2 cm of penetration), 5 mL is injected. Under no circumstances should the needle be advanced

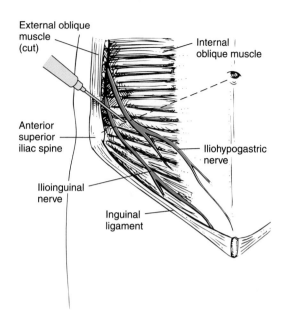

Figure 17–30. Ilioinguinal-iliohypogastric nerve block.

farther or repetitively moved in and out (seeking to elicit paresthesia), since the risk of pneumothorax is greatly increased by these maneuvers.

C. COMPLICATIONS:

The most common complication of paravertebral block is pneumothorax, which related to the number of levels and the experience of the operator. If air is aspirated, chest film is mandatory. Intravascular injection and failed block are other possible problems.

Inguinal Nerve Block

Ilioinguinal and iliohypogastric blocks can be used for inguinal or genital operations, such as inguinal herniorrhaphy or orchiopexy, or for postoperative pain relief. Supplementation with genitofemoral nerve block may be necessary.

A. ANATOMY:

The ilioinguinal and iliohypogastric nerves arise primarily from L1 but may derive fibers from T12. The iliohypogastric splits into two branches prior to becoming cutaneous. The lateral branch is sensory to the lateral aspect of the buttock and hip. The anterior branch becomes superficial just medial to the anterior superior iliac spine, where it sends off a network of branches that innervate the lower abdomen. The ilioinguinal nerve follows the same course and exits peritoneum to enter the inguinal canal, where it provides

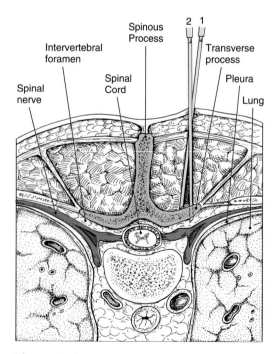

Figure 17–29. Paravertebral block.

sensation to the scrotum, penis, and medial thigh in the male, or equivalent area of the labia and mons pubis in the female. Both nerves pierce the transversalis abdominis and internal oblique muscles approximately 2 cm medial to the anterior superior iliac spine. The genitofemoral nerve is derived from L1 and L2. Its femoral branch travels with the femoral artery to provide cutaneous sensation just below the inguinal ligament, while its genital branch travels in the inguinal canal to supply the scrotum in men and the labium majus in women.

B. TECHNIQUE:

(Figure 17–30) A skin wheal is raised 2 cm medial to the upper aspect of the anterior superior iliac spine, and a 22-gauge, 3.5-inch spinal needle is inserted perpendicular to the skin until it is just under the fascia, and 8–10 mL of anesthetic is injected fanwise to block both the ilioinguinal and iliohypogastric nerves. The genital branch of the genitofemoral nerve is blocked with 2–3 mL of local anesthetic injected just lateral to the pubic tubercle; the femoral branch can be anesthetized with 3–5 mL injected subcutaneously just below the inguinal ligament.

C. COMPLICATIONS:

Patient discomfort and persistent paresthesia from intraneural injection are potential sequelae.

Penile Block

Penile block is performed for penile surgery or postoperative pain relief afterward.

A. ANATOMY:

Innervation of the penis is derived from the pudendal nerve, which gives off the dorsal nerve of the penis bilaterally. It enters the penis deep to Buck's fascia and divides into dorsal and ventral branches. The genitofemoral and ilioinguinal nerves may additionally provide sensation to the base of the penis via subcutaneous branches.

B. TECHNIQUE:

(Figure 17–31) A fan-shaped (triangular) field block with 10–15 mL of local anesthetic injected at the base of the penis and 2–4 cm lateral to the base on both sides of the penis, can block the sensory nerves without risk of vascular injury. If more profound block is necessary, or if extensive surgery is planned, the dorsal nerve is blocked just lateral to the base of the penis bilaterally with a 25-gauge, ¾- to 1-inch needle just penetrating Buck's fascia at the 10:30 and 1:30 o'clock positions; 1 mL of local anesthetic is injected on each side, with care taken to avoid pressure. Epinephrine or other vasoconstrictors should be avoided to prevent end artery spasm and ischemic injury.

C. COMPLICATIONS:

 Careful aspiration is necessary to avoid intravascular injection. Injecting large volumes of local anesthetic or epinephrine-containing solutions may compromise blood flow to the penis.

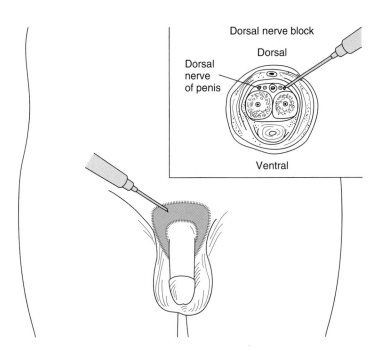

Figure 17–31. Penile field block.

CASE DISCUSSION: DYSPNEA FOLLOWING INTERSCALENE BLOCK

An anxious 54-year-old woman with a humeral fracture desires regional anesthesia for open reduction and internal fixation. An interscalene block with 25 mL of 2% lidocaine with epinephrine (1:200,000) is administered using an "immobile needle" with incremental injection and careful aspiration. After 5 minutes, the patient notes numbness of the operative arm but starts to complain of increasing dyspnea.

What would be appropriate management?

Dyspnea following an interscalene block may be due to multiple causes that are often not immediately apparent. Familiarity with the complication of the block, a high index of suspicion, careful monitoring, and preparations for managing these complications can help avoid an adverse outcome. Immediate management should emphasize maintenance of adequate oxygenation and ventilation and maintaining hemodynamic stability. If not already present, full monitoring should be instituted (electrocardiogram, blood pressure readings every 2–3 minutes, and pulse oximetry), and supplemental oxygen should be given regardless of pulse oximetry readings to provide additional reserves should apnea suddenly develop. Preparations should be made for induction of general anesthesia, endotracheal intubation, controlled ventilation, and administration of vasopressors and atropine. Mental status and ventilatory exchange should be also followed carefully. Small amounts of midazolam (0.5 mg) may help alleviate anxiety but excessive sedation should be avoided until the cause of the dyspnea is determined.

What are the most likely causes?

Possible causes include anxiety, ipsilateral phrenic nerve block, pneumothorax, cervical epidural anesthesia, and a dural sleeve injection resulting in spinal anesthesia. Anxiety-related dyspnea is a diagnosis of exclusion. An immediate onset of dyspnea is suggestive of inadvertent spinal anesthesia. Other causes are typically more delayed in onset and become apparent only with time. Mental obtundation, apnea, hypotension, and bradycardia are characteristic of high spinal and inadvertent cervical epidural anesthesia. Pneumothorax and phrenic nerve block are usually asymptomatic but can decrease arterial oxygen saturation. A chest radiograph can help confirm the diagnosis.

Clinical studies suggest that phrenic nerve block is an unavoidable complication of interscalene blocks; patients who are unusually anxious and those with preexisting pulmonary compromise are more likely to complain of dyspnea.

Why does inadvertent epidural or spinal injection cause apnea?

The relatively large volume of local anesthetic used for interscalene blocks can produce very high neuraxial anesthesia. Intrathecal injection at the cervical level results in total spinal anesthesia, while epidural injection results in bilateral blockade of the C3–5 nerve roots that innervate the diaphragm. A subdural injection at this level also has similar effects. Moreover, the sudden and profound sympathectomy associated with neuraxial anesthesia at this level can produce apnea from hypoperfusion of the brainstem.

How should an inadvertent epidural or spinal injection be managed?

Immediate ventilation with 100% oxygen should be instituted. Atropine 1–3 mg should be given to reverse bradycardia. Ephedrine 10–25 mg is administered for hypotension. If either the bradycardia or hypotension does not resolve immediately, 10–100 μg of epinephrine is administered. Rapid intubation of the trachea and controlled ventilation is usually necessary until spontaneous ventilation returns. Intravenous fluid administration also partially offsets the decreased venous return from the sympathectomy. Repeat administration or a continuous infusion of vasopressor may be necessary. The surgery should generally be postponed until the patient recovers and the neurologic function can be assessed.

SUGGESTED READING

Aeschbach A, Mekhail NA: Common nerve blocks in chronic pain management. Anesth Clin North Am 2000;18:429.

Brown DL: *Atlas of Regional Anesthesia,* 2nd ed. WB Saunders and Company, 1999.

Chelly JE: *Peripheral Nerve Blocks; A Color Atlas.* Lippincott Williams & Wilkins, 1999.

Cousins MJ: *Neural Blockade in Clinical Anesthesia and Pain Management,* 3rd ed. Lippincott Williams & Wilkins, 1998.

Finucane BT: *Complications of Regional Anesthesia,* Churchill Livingstone, 1999.

Jankovic D, Wells C: *Regional Nerve Blocks.* Blackwell Science, 2000.

Richardson J, Lönnqvist PA: Thoracic paravertebral block. Br J Anaesth 1998;81:230.

Pain Management

18

KEY CONCEPTS

 1 Pain can be classified according to pathophysiology (eg, nociceptive or neuropathic pain), etiology (eg, postoperative or cancer pain), or the affected area (eg, headache or low back pain).

 2 Nociceptive pain is due to activation or sensitization of peripheral nociceptors, specialized receptors that transduce noxious stimuli. Neuropathic pain is the result of injury or acquired abnormalities of peripheral or central neural structures.

 3 Acute pain can be defined as that which is caused by noxious stimulation due to injury, a disease process, or abnormal function of muscle or viscera. It is nearly always nociceptive.

 4 Chronic pain is defined as that which persists beyond the usual course of an acute disease or after a reasonable time for healing to occur; this period varies between 1 to 6 months in most definitions. Chronic pain may be nociceptive, neuropathic, or a combination of both.

 5 Modulation of pain occurs peripherally at the nociceptor, in the spinal cord, or in supraspinal structures. This modulation can either inhibit (suppress) or facilitate (aggravate) pain.

 6 Moderate to severe acute pain, regardless of site, can affect nearly every organ function and may adversely influence postoperative morbidity and mortality.

 7 Neural blockade with local anesthetics can be useful in delineating pain mechanisms, but more importantly, it plays a major role in the management of patients with acute or chronic pain. The role of the sympathetic system and its pathways can be evaluated.

 8 Antidepressants are generally most useful in patients with neuropathic pain, eg, from postherpetic neuralgia and diabetic neuropathy. These agents demonstrate an analgesic effect that occurs at a lower dose than their antidepressant action.

 9 Anticonvulsants have been found to be extremely useful in patients with neuropathic pain, especially trigeminal neuralgia and diabetic neuropathy.

 10 Spinal cord stimulation is most effective for neuropathic pain. Proposed mechanisms include activation of descending modulating systems and inhibition of sympathetic outflow. Accepted indications include sympathetically mediated pain, spinal cord lesions with localized segmental pain, phantom limb pain, ischemic lower extremity pain due to peripheral vascular disease, and adhesive arachnoiditis.

 11 Studies show patient-controlled analgesia (PCA) to be a cost-effective technique that produces superior analgesia with very high patient satisfaction. Total drug consumption is less, compared with intramuscular injections. The routine use of a basal ("background") infusion is controversial.

(continued)

(continued)

12 *The administration of local anesthetics, opioids, or a combination neuraxially (subarachnoid or epidural) is an excellent technique for managing postoperative pain following abdominal, pelvic, thoracic, or orthopedic procedures on the lower extremities. Patients often have better preservation of pulmonary function, are able to ambulate early, and benefit from early physical therapy. Patients may be at lower risk for postoperative venous thrombosis.*

13 *The most serious side effect of epidural or intrathecal opioids is dose-dependent, delayed respiratory depression. Most cases of serious respiratory depression occur in patients receiving concomitant parenteral opioids or sedatives. Elderly patients*

and those with sleep apnea appear to be especially vulnerable and require reduced dosing.

14 *Physical dependence occurs in all patients on large doses of opioids for extended periods. A withdrawal phenomenon can be precipitated by the administration of opioid antagonists.*

15 *Multiple triggers can induce sympathetically maintained pain, which is often overlooked or misdiagnosed. Patients often dramatically respond to sympathetic blocks. The likelihood of a cure is high (over 90%) if treatment is initiated within 1 month of symptoms and appears to decrease with time.*

Pain—the most common symptom that brings patients to see a physician—nearly always manifests a pathologic process. Any treatment plan must be directed at the underlying process as well as at controlling pain. Patients are generally referred for pain management by primary care practitioners or specialists once a diagnosis has been made and treatment of any underlying process has been initiated. Notable exceptions are patients with chronic pain in which the cause remains obscure after preliminary investigations; serious and life-threatening illnesses should, however, have been excluded.

The term "pain management" in a general sense applies to the entire discipline of anesthesiology, but its modern usage is restricted to management of pain outside the operating room. This type of practice may be broadly divided into acute and chronic pain management. The former primarily deals with patients recovering from surgery or with acute medical conditions in a hospital setting, while the latter includes diverse groups of patients in the outpatient setting. Unfortunately, this distinction is artificial because considerable overlap exists; a good example is the cancer patient who frequently requires short- and long-term pain management, both in and out of the hospital.

The practice of pain management is not just limited to anesthesiologists but other practitioners that include physicians (such as internists, oncologists, and neurologists) and nonphysicians (psychologists, chiropractors, acupuncturists, and hypnotists). Clearly, the most effective approach is multidisciplinary, where the patient is evaluated by one physician (the case manager) who conducts the initial evaluation and formulates a treatment plan, and where the services and resources of

other specialists are readily available. Moreover, the case manager and the various consultants meet regularly in formal case conferences to discuss patients. Single specialty pain clinics tend to be either syndrome- or modality-oriented. The former specialize in chronic back pain, headache, and temporomandibular joint dysfunction, while the latter offer nerve block, acupuncture, hypnosis, and biofeedback.

Anesthesiologists trained in pain management are in a unique position to coordinate multidisciplinary pain management centers because of broad training in dealing with a wide diversity of patients from surgical, obstetric, pediatric, and medical subspecialties, as well as expertise in clinical pharmacology and applied neuroanatomy, including the use of peripheral and central nerve blocks (see Chapters 16 and 17).

DEFINITIONS & CLASSIFICATION OF PAIN

Like other conscious sensations, normal pain perception depends on specialized neurons that function as receptors, detecting the stimulus, and then transducing and conducting it into the central nervous system. Sensation is often described as either **protopathic** (noxious) or **epicritic** (non-noxious). Epicritic sensation (light touch, pressure, proprioception, and temperature discrimination) is characterized by low-threshold receptors and generally conducted by large myelinated nerve fibers (see Table 16–1). In contrast, protopathic sensation (pain) is subserved by high-threshold receptors and conducted by smaller, lightly myelinated (Aδ) and unmyelinated (C) nerve fibers.

What Is Pain?

Pain is not just a sensory modality but an experience. The International Association for the Study of Pain defines pain as "an unpleasant sensory and emotional experience associated with actual or potential tissue damage, or described in terms of such damage." This definition recognizes the interplay between the objective, physiologic sensory aspects of pain and its subjective, emotional, and psychological components. The response to pain can be highly variable between persons as well as in the same person at different times.

The term "nociception," which is derived from *noci* (Latin for harm or injury), is used only to describe the neural response to traumatic or noxious stimuli. All nociception produces pain, but not all pain results from nociception. Many patients experience pain in the absence of noxious stimuli. It is therefore clinically useful to divide pain into one of two categories: (1) acute pain, which is primarily due to nociception, and (2) chronic pain, which may be due to nociception but in which psychological and behavioral factors often play a major role. Table 18–1 lists terms frequently used in describing pain.

Pain can also be classified according to pathophysiology (eg, nociceptive or neuropathic pain), etiology (eg, postoperative or cancer pain), or the affected area (eg, headache or low back pain). Such classifications are useful in the selection of treatment modalities and drug therapy. **Nociceptive pain** is due to activation or sensitization of peripheral nociceptors, specialized receptors that transduce noxious stimuli. **Neuropathic pain** is the result of injury or acquired abnormalities of peripheral or central neural structures.

A. ACUTE PAIN:

Acute pain can be defined as that which is caused by noxious stimulation due to injury, a disease process, or abnormal function of muscle or viscera. It is nearly always nociceptive. Nociceptive pain serves to detect, localize, and limit tissue damage. Four physiologic processes are involved: transduction, transmission, modulation, and perception. This type of pain is typically associated with a neuroendocrine stress that is proportional to intensity. Its most common forms include posttraumatic, postoperative, and obstetric pain as well as that associated with acute medical illnesses, such as myocardial infarction, pancreatitis, and renal calculi. Most forms of acute pain are self-limited or resolve with treatment in a few days or weeks. When the pain fails to resolve because of either abnormal healing or inadequate treatment, the pain becomes chronic (below). Two types of acute (nociceptive) pain—somatic and visceral—are differentiated based on origin and features.

Table 18–1. Terms used in pain management.

Term	Description
Allodynia	Perception of an ordinarily nonnoxious stimulus as pain
Analgesia	Absence of pain perception
Anesthesia	Absence of all sensation
Anesthesia dolorosa	Pain in an area that lacks sensation
Dysesthesia	Unpleasant or abnormal sensation with or without a stimulus
Hypalgesia (Hypoalgesia)	Diminished response to noxious stimulation (eg, pin prick)
Hyperalgesia	Increased response to noxious stimulation
Hyperesthesia	Increased response to mild stimulation
Hyperpathia	Presence of hyperesthesia, allodynia, and hyperalgesia usually associated with overreaction, and persistence of the sensation after the stimulus
Hypesthesia (Hypoesthesia)	Reduced cutaneous sensation (eg, light touch, pressure, or temperature)
Neuralgia	Pain in the distribution of a nerve or a group of nerves
Paresthesia	Abnormal sensation perceived without an apparent stimulus
Radiculopathy	Functional abnormality of one or more nerve roots

1. Somatic pain—Somatic pain can be further classified as superficial or deep. Superficial somatic pain is due to nociceptive input arising from skin, subcutaneous tissues, and mucous membranes. It is characteristically well-localized and described as a sharp, pricking, throbbing, or burning sensation.

Deep somatic pain arises from muscles, tendons, joints, or bones. In contrast to superficial somatic pain, it usually has a dull, aching quality and is less well-localized. An additional feature is that both the intensity and duration of the stimulus affect the degree of localization. For example, pain following brief minor trauma to the elbow joint is localized to the elbow, but severe or sustained trauma often causes pain in the whole arm.

2. Visceral pain—This form of acute pain is due to a disease process or abnormal function of an internal organ or its covering (eg, parietal pleura, pericardium, or peritoneum). Four subtypes are described: (1) true localized visceral pain, (2) localized parietal pain, (3) referred visceral pain, and (4) referred parietal pain. True visceral pain is dull, diffuse, and usually midline. It is frequently associated with either abnormal sympathetic or parasympathetic activity causing nausea, vomiting, sweating, and changes in blood pressure and heart rate. Parietal pain is typically sharp and often described as a stabbing sensation that is either localized to the area around the organ or referred to a distant site (Table 18–2). The phenomenon of visceral or parietal pain referred to cutaneous areas results from patterns of embryologic development and migration of tissues, and the convergence of visceral and somatic afferent input into the central nervous system. Thus, pain associated with disease processes involving the peritoneum or pleura over the central diaphragm is frequently referred to the neck and shoulder, whereas disease affecting the parietal surfaces of the peripheral diaphragm is referred to the chest or upper abdominal wall.

B. CHRONIC PAIN:

Chronic pain is defined as that which persists beyond the usual course of an acute disease or after a reasonable time for healing to occur; this period varies between 1 to 6 months in most definitions. Chronic pain may be nociceptive,

Table 18–2. Patterns of referred pain.

Location	Cutaneous Dermatome
Central diaphragm	C4
Lungs	T2–T6
Heart	T1–T4
Aorta	T1–L2
Esophagus	T3–T8
Pancreas and spleen	T5–T10
Stomach, liver, and gallbladder	T6–T9
Adrenals	T8–L1
Small intestine	T9–T11
Colon	T10–L1
Kidney, ovaries, and testes	T10–L1
Ureters	T10–T12
Uterus	T11–L2
Bladder and prostate	S2–S4
Urethra and rectum	S2–S4

neuropathic, or a combination of both. A distinguishing feature is that psychological mechanisms or environmental factors frequently play a major role. Patients with chronic pain often have an attenuated or absent neuroendocrine stress response, and have prominent sleep and affective (mood) disturbances. Neuropathic pain is classically spontaneous, has a burning quality, and is associated with hyperpathia. When it is also associated with loss of sensory input (eg, amputation) into the central nervous system, it is termed "**deafferentation pain.**" When the sympathetic system plays a major role, it is often termed "**sympathetically maintained pain.**"

The most common forms of chronic pain include those associated with musculoskeletal disorders, chronic visceral disorders, lesions of peripheral nerves, nerve roots, or dorsal root ganglia (including causalgia, phantom limb pain, and postherpetic neuralgia), lesions of the central nervous system (stroke, spinal cord injury, and multiple sclerosis), and cancers invading the nervous system. Some clinicians use the term "chronic benign pain" when pain does not result from cancer. This is to be discouraged, because pain is never benign from the patient's point of view, regardless of its cause.

■ ANATOMY & PHYSIOLOGY OF NOCICEPTION

PAIN PATHWAYS

To simplify for the sake of illustration, pain is conducted along three-neuron pathways that transmit noxious stimuli from the periphery to the cerebral cortex (Figure 18–1). Primary afferent neurons are located in the dorsal root ganglia, which lie in the vertebral foramina at each spinal cord level. Each neuron has a single axon that bifurcates, sending one end to the peripheral tissues it innervates and the other into the dorsal horn of the spinal cord. In the dorsal horn, the primary afferent neuron synapses with a second-order neuron whose axons cross the midline and ascend in the contralateral spinothalamic tract to reach the thalamus. Second-order neurons synapse in thalamic nuclei with third-order neurons, which in turn send projections through the internal capsule and corona radiata to the postcentral gyrus of the cerebral cortex.

First-Order Neurons

The majority of first-order neurons send the proximal end of their axons into the spinal cord via the dorsal (sensory) spinal root at each cervical, thoracic, lumbar, and sacral level. Some unmyelinated afferent (C) fibers

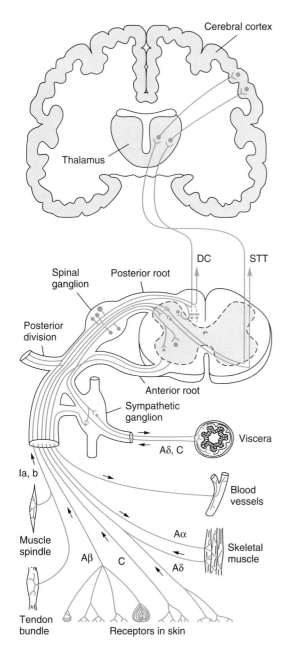

Figure 18–1. Pain pathways.

have been shown to enter the spinal cord via the ventral nerve (motor) root, accounting for observations that some patients continue to feel pain even after transection of the dorsal nerve root (rhizotomy) and report pain following ventral root stimulation. Once in the dorsal horn, in addition to synapsing with second-order neurons, the axons of first-order neurons may synapse

with interneurons, sympathetic neurons, and ventral horn motor neurons.

Pain fibers originating from the head are carried by the trigeminal (V), facial (VII), glossopharyngeal (IX), and vagal (X) nerves. The gasserian ganglion contains the cell bodies of sensory fibers in the ophthalmic, maxillary, and mandibular divisions of the trigeminal nerve. Cell bodies of first-order afferent neurons of the facial nerve are located in the geniculate ganglion; those of the glossopharyngeal nerve lie in its superior and petrosal ganglia; and those of the vagal nerve are located in the jugular ganglion (somatic) and the ganglion nodosum (visceral). The proximal axonal processes of the first-order neurons in these ganglia reach the brainstem nuclei via their respective cranial nerves, where they synapse with second-order neurons in brainstem nuclei.

Second-Order Neurons

As afferent fibers enter the spinal cord, they segregate according to size, with large, myelinated fibers becoming medial, and small, unmyelinated fibers becoming lateral. Pain fibers may ascend or descend one to three spinal cord segments in Lissauer's tract before synapsing with second-order neurons in the gray matter of the ipsilateral dorsal horn. In many instances they communicate with second-order neurons through interneurons.

Spinal cord gray matter was divided by Rexed into 10 lamina (Figure 18–2 and Table 18–3). The first six lamina, which make up the dorsal horn, receive all afferent neural activity, and represent the principal site of modulation of pain by ascending and descending neural pathways. Second-order neurons are either nociceptive-specific or wide dynamic range (WDR) neurons. Nociceptive-specific neurons serve only noxious stimuli, but WDR neurons also receive non-noxious afferent input from Aβ, Aδ, and C fibers. Nociceptive-specific neurons are arranged somatotopically in lamina I and have discrete, somatic receptive fields; they are normally silent and respond only to high-threshold noxious stimulation, poorly encoding stimulus intensity. WDR neurons are the most prevalent cell type in the dorsal horn. Although they are found throughout the dorsal horn, WDR neurons are most abundant in lamina V. During repeated stimulation, WDR neurons characteristically increase their firing rate exponentially in a graded fashion ("wind-up"), even with the same stimulus intensity. They also have large receptive fields compared with nociceptive-specific neurons.

Most nociceptive C fibers send collaterals to, or terminate on, second-order neurons in laminas I, II, and to a lesser extent lamina V. In contrast, nociceptive Aδ fibers synapse mainly in laminas I, V, and to a lesser degree lamina X. Lamina I responds primarily to noxious (nociceptive) stimuli from cutaneous and deep somatic

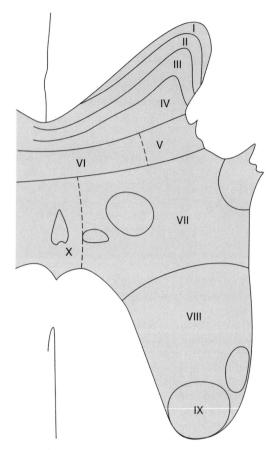

Figure 18–2. Rexed's spinal cord laminae.

tissues. Lamina II, also called the substantia gelatinosa, contains many interneurons and is believed to play a major role in processing and modulating nociceptive input from cutaneous nociceptors. It is also of special interest because it is believed to a major site of action for opioids. Laminas III and IV receive primarily non-nociceptive sensory input. Laminas VIII and IX make up the anterior (motor) horn. Lamina VII is called the intermediolateral column and contains the cell bodies of preganglionic sympathetic neurons.

Visceral afferents terminate primarily in lamina V, and to a lesser extent lamina I. These two lamina represent points of central convergence between somatic and visceral inputs. Lamina V responds to both noxious and non-noxious sensory input and receives both visceral and somatic pain afferents. The phenomenon of convergence between visceral and somatic sensory input is manifested clinically as referred pain (Table 18–3). Compared with somatic fibers, visceral nociceptive fibers are fewer in number, more widely distributed,

proportionately activate a larger number of spinal neurons, and are not organized somatotopically.

A. THE SPINOTHALAMIC TRACT:

The axons of most second-order neurons cross the midline close to their level of origin (at the anterior commissure) to the contralateral side of the spinal cord before they form the spinothalamic tract and send their fibers to the thalamus, the reticular formation, the nucleus raphe magnus, and the periaqueductal gray. The spinothalamic tract, which is classically considered the major pain pathway, lies anterolaterally in the white matter of the spinal cord. This ascending tract can be divided as lateral and medial. The lateral spinothalamic (neospinothalamic) tract projects mainly to the ventral posterolateral nucleus of the thalamus and carries discriminative aspects of pain, such as location, intensity, and duration. The medial spinothalamic (paleospinothalamic) tract projects to the medial thalamus and is responsible for mediating the autonomic and unpleasant emotional perceptions of pain. Some spinothalamic fibers also project to the periaqueductal gray and thus may be an important link between the ascending and descending pathways. Collateral fibers also project to the reticular activating system and the hypothalamus; these are likely responsible for the arousal response to pain.

B. ALTERNATE PAIN PATHWAYS:

As with epicritic sensation, pain fibers ascend diffusely, ipsilaterally, and contralaterally; hence, some patients continue to perceive pain following ablation of the contralateral spinothalamic tract. Thus, other ascending pain pathways are also important. The spinoreticular tract is thought to mediate arousal and autonomic responses to pain. The spinomesencephalic tract may be important in activating anti-nociceptive, descending pathways, because it has some projections to periaqueductal gray. The spinohypothalamic and spinotelencephalic tracts activate the hypothalamus and evoke emotional behavior. The spinocervical tract ascends uncrossed to the lateral cervical nucleus, which relays the fibers to the contralateral thalamus; this tract is likely a major alternative pain pathway. Lastly, some fibers in the dorsal columns (which mainly carry light touch and proprioception) are responsive to pain; they ascend medially and ipsilaterally.

C. INTEGRATION WITH THE SYMPATHETIC AND MOTOR SYSTEMS:

Somatic and visceral afferents are fully integrated with the skeletal motor and sympathetic systems in the spinal cord, brainstem, and higher centers. Afferent dorsal horn neurons synapse both directly and indirectly with anterior horn motor neurons. These synapses are responsible for reflex muscle activity—whether normal or abnor-

Table 18–3. Spinal cord lamina.

Lamina	Predominant Function	Input	Name
I	Somatic nociception thermoreception	Aδ, C	Marginal layer
II	Somatic nociception thermoreception	C, Aδ	Sustantia gelatinosa
III	Somatic mechanoreception	Aβ, Aδ	Nucleus proprius
IV	Mechanoreception	Aβ, Aδ	Nucleus proprius
V	Visceral and somatic nociception and mechanoreception	Aβ, Aδ, (C)	Nucleus proprius WDR neurons
VI	Mechanoreception	Aβ	Nucleus proprius
VII	Sympathetic		Intermediolateral column
VIII		Aβ	Motor horn
IX	Motor	Aβ	Motor horn
X		Aβ	Central canal

mal—that is associated with pain. In a similar fashion, synapses between afferent nociceptive neurons and sympathetic neurons in the intermediolateral column result in reflex sympathetically mediated vasoconstriction, smooth muscle spasm, and the release of catecholamines, both locally and from the adrenal medulla.

Third-Order Neurons

Third-order neurons are located in the thalamus and send fibers to somatosensory areas I and II in the postcentral gyrus of the parietal cortex and the superior wall of the sylvian fissure, respectively. Perception and discrete localization of pain take place in these cortical areas. While most neurons from the lateral thalamic nuclei project to the primary somatosensory cortex, those from the intralaminar and medial nuclei project to the anterior cingulate gyrus and likely mediate the suffering and emotional components of pain.

PHYSIOLOGY OF NOCICEPTION

1. Nociceptors

Nociceptors are characterized by a high threshold for activation and encode the intensity of stimulation by increasing their discharge rates in a graded fashion. Following repeated stimulation, they characteristically display delayed adaptation, sensitization, and afterdischarges.

Noxious sensations can often be broken down into two components: a fast, sharp, and well-localized sensation ("first pain") which is conducted with a short latency (0.1 s) by Aδ fibers (tested by pinprick); and a duller, slower onset, and often poorly localized sensation ("second pain") which is conducted by C fibers. In contrast to epicritic sensation, which is transduced by specialized end-organs on the afferent neuron, protopathic sensation is transduced mainly by free nerve endings.

Most nociceptors are free nerve endings that sense heat, mechanical, and chemical tissue damage. Several types are described: (1) mechanonociceptors, which respond to pinch and pinprick, (2) silent nociceptors, which respond only in the presence of inflammation, and (3) polymodal mechanoheat nociceptors. The last are most prevalent and respond to excessive pressure, extremes of temperature (> 42 °C and < 18 °C), and alogens (pain-producing substances). Alogens include bradykinin, histamine, serotonin (5-hydroxytryptamine or 5-HT), H^+, K^+, some prostaglandins, and possibly adenosine triphosphate. Polymodal nociceptors are slow to adapt to strong pressure and display heat sensitization. Specialized heat, cold, and chemical nociceptors have been described but appear to be rare.

Cutaneous Nociceptors

Nociceptors are present in both somatic and visceral tissues. Primary afferent neurons reach tissues by traveling along spinal somatic, sympathetic, or parasympathetic nerves. Somatic nociceptors include those in skin (cutaneous) and deep tissues (muscle, tendons, fascia, and bone), while visceral nociceptors include those in internal organs. The cornea and tooth pulp are unique in that they are almost exclusively innervated by nociceptive Aδ and C fibers.

Deep Nociceptors

Deep somatic nociceptors are less sensitive to noxious stimuli than cutaneous nociceptors, but are easily sensitized by inflammation. The pain arising from them is characteristically dull and poorly localized. Specific nociceptors may exist in muscles and joint capsules; they respond to mechanical, thermal, and chemical stimuli.

Visceral Nociceptors

Visceral organs are generally insensitive tissues that mostly contain silent nociceptors. Some organs appear to have specific nociceptors, such as the heart, lung, testis, and bile ducts. Most other organs, such as the intestines, are innervated by polymodal nociceptors that respond to smooth muscle spasm, ischemia, and inflammation (alogens). These receptors generally do not respond to the cutting, burning, or crushing that occurs during surgery. A few organs, such as the brain, lack nociceptors altogether; however, the brain's meningeal coverings do contain nociceptors.

Like somatic nociceptors, those in the viscera are the free nerve endings of primary afferent neurons whose cell bodies lie in the dorsal horn. These afferent nerve fibers, however, frequently travel with efferent sympathetic nerve fibers to reach the viscera. Afferent activity from these neurons enters the spinal cord between T1 and L2. Nociceptive C fibers from the esophagus, larynx, and trachea travel with the vagus nerve to enter the nucleus solitarius in the brainstem. Afferent pain fibers from the bladder, prostate, rectum, cervix and urethra, and genitalia are transmitted into the spinal cord via parasympathetic nerves at the level of the S2 to S4 nerve roots.

2. Chemical Mediators or Pain

Several neuropeptides and excitatory amino acids function as neurotransmitters for afferent neurons subserving pain (Table 18–4). Many if not most neurons contain more than one neurotransmitter which is simultaneously coreleased. The most important of these peptides are substance P (sP) and calcitonin gene-related peptide (CGRP). Glutamate is the most important excitatory amino acid.

Substance P is an 11 amino acid peptide that is synthesized and released by first-order neurons both peripherally and in the dorsal horn; sP facilitates transmis-

Table 18–4. Major neurotransmitters mediating or modulating pain.

Neurotransmitter	Receptor	Effect on Nociception
Substance P	NK–1	Excitatory
Calcitonin gene-related peptide		Excitatory
Glutamate	NMDA, AMPA, kainite, quisqualate	Excitatory
Aspartate	NMDA, AMPA, kainite, quisqualate	Excitatory
Adenosine triphosphate (ATP)	P_1, P_2	Excitatory
Somatostatin		Inhibitory
Acetylcholine	Muscarinic	Inhibitory
Enkephalins	μ, δ, κ	Inhibitory
β-Endorphin	μ, δ, κ	Inhibitory
Norepinephrine	α_2	Inhibitory
Adenosine	A_1	Inhibitory
Serotonin	5-HT_1, (5-HT_3)	Inhibitory
γ-Aminobutyric acid (GABA)	A, B	Inhibitory
Glycine		Inhibitory

sion in pain pathways via NK-1 receptor activation. In the periphery, sP neurons send collaterals that are closely associated with blood vessels, sweat glands, hair follicles, and mast cells in the dermis. Substance P sensitizes nociceptors, degranulates histamine from mast cells and serotonin (5-HT) from platelets, and is a potent vasodilator and chemoattractant for leukocytes. Substance P-releasing neurons also innervate the viscera and send collateral fibers to paravertebral sympathetic ganglia; intense stimulation of viscera, therefore, can cause direct postganglionic sympathetic discharge.

Both opioid and α_2-adrenergic receptors have been described on or near the terminals of unmyelinated peripheral nerves. Although their physiologic role is not clear, the latter may explain the observed analgesia of peripherally applied opioids, especially in the presence of inflammation.

3. Modulation of Pain

 Modulation of pain occurs peripherally at the nociceptor, in the spinal cord, or in supraspinal structures. This modulation can either inhibit (suppress) or facilitate (aggravate) pain.

Peripheral Modulation

Nociceptors and their neurons display sensitization following repeated stimulation. Sensitization may be manifested as an enhanced response to noxious stimulation or a newly acquired responsiveness to a wider range of stimuli, including non-noxious stimuli.

A. PRIMARY HYPERALGESIA:

Sensitization of nociceptors results in a decrease in threshold, an increase in the frequency response to the same stimulus intensity, a decrease in response latency, and spontaneous firing even after cessation of the stimulus (afterdischarges). Such sensitization commonly occurs with injury and following application of heat. Primary hyperalgesia is mediated by the release of alogens from damaged tissues. Histamine is released from mast cells, basophils, and platelets, while serotonin is released from mast cells and platelets. Bradykinin is released from tissues following activation of factor XII. Bradykinin activates free nerve endings via specific receptors (B1 and B2).

Prostaglandins are produced following tissue damage by the action of phospholipase A_2 on phospholipids released from cell membranes to form arachidonic acid (Figure 18–3). The cyclooxygenase (COX) pathway then converts the latter into endoperoxides, which in turn are transformed into prostacyclin and prostaglandin E_2 (PGE$_2$). PGE$_2$ directly activates free nerve endings, while prostacyclin potentiates the edema from bradykinin. The lipoxygenase pathway converts arachidonic acid into hydroperoxy compounds, which are subsequently converted into leukotrienes. The role of the latter is not well-defined, but they also appear to potentiate certain types of pain. Pharmacologic agents

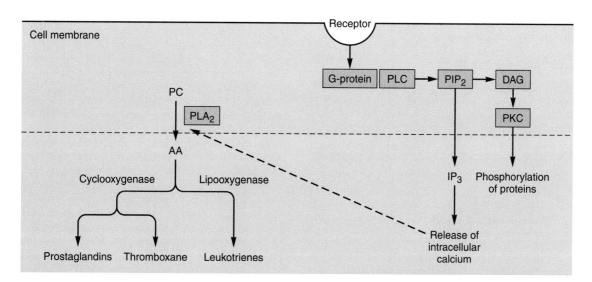

Figure 18–3. Phospholipase C (PLC) catalyses the hydrolysis of phosphatidylinositol 4,5-bisphosphate (PIP$_2$) to produce inositol triphosphate (IP$_3$) and diacyclglycerol (DAG). Protein kinase C (PKC) is also important. Phospholipase A_2 (PLA$_2$) catalyses the conversion of phosphatidylcholine (PC) to arachadonic acid (AA).

such as acetylsalicylic acid (ASA, or aspirin), acetaminophen, and nonsteroidal anti-inflammatory drugs (NSAIDs) produce analgesia by inhibition of COX. The analgesic effect of corticosteroids is likely the result of inhibition of prostaglandin production through blockade of phospholipase A_2 activation.

B. Secondary Hyperalgesia:

Neurogenic inflammation, also called secondary hyperalgesia, also plays an important role in peripheral sensitization following injury. It is manifested by the "triple response" of a red flush around the site of injury (flare), local tissue edema, and sensitization to noxious stimuli. Secondary hyperalgesia is primarily due to antidromic release of sP (and probably CGRP) from collateral axons of the primary afferent neuron. Substance P degranulates histamine and 5-HT, vasodilates blood vessels, causes tissue edema, and induces the formation of leukotrienes. The neural origin of this response is emphasized by the following: (1) it can be produced by antidromic stimulation of a sensory nerve, (2) it is not observed in denervated skin, and (3) it is diminished by injection of local anesthetic such as lidocaine. The compound capsaicin, which is derived from the Hungarian red pepper, degranulates and depletes sP. When applied topically, capsaicin diminishes neurogenic inflammation, and appears to be useful for some patients with postherpetic neuralgia.

Central Modulation

A. Facilitation:

At least three mechanisms are responsible for central sensitization in the spinal cord:

(1) Wind-up and sensitization of second-order neurons. WDR neurons increase their frequency of discharge with the same repetitive stimuli, and exhibit prolonged discharge, even after afferent C fiber input has stopped.

(2) Receptor field expansion. Dorsal horn neurons increase their receptive fields such that adjacent neurons become responsive to stimuli (whether noxious or not) to which they were previously unresponsive.

(3) Hyperexcitability of flexion reflexes. Enhancement of flexion reflexes is observed both ipsilaterally and contralaterally.

Neurochemical mediators of central sensitization include sP, CGRP, VIP, cholecystokinin (CCK), angiotensin, and galanin, as well as the excitatory amino acids L-glutamate and L-aspartate. These substances trigger changes in membrane excitability by interacting with G protein-coupled membrane receptors on neurons, activating intracellular second messengers, which in turn phosphorylate substrate proteins. A common pathway is an increase in intracellular calcium concentration (Figure 18–3).

Glutamate and aspartate play an important role in wind-up, via activation of N-methyl-D-aspartate (NMDA) and non-NMDA receptor mechanisms. These amino acids are believed to be largely responsible for the induction and maintenance of central sensitization. Activation of NMDA receptors increases intracellular calcium concentration in spinal neurons and activates phospholipase C (PLC). Increased intracellular calcium concentration activates phospholipase A_2 (PLA_2), catalyzes the conversion of phosphatidylcholine (PC) to arachidonic acid (AA), and induces the formation of prostaglandins. Phospholipase C catalyzes the hydrolysis of phosphatidylinositol 4,5-bisphosphate (PIP_2) to produce inositol triphosphate (IP_3) and diacylglycerol (DAG), which functions as a second messenger; DAG, in turn, activates protein kinase C (PKC).

Activation of NMDA receptors also induces nitric oxide synthetase, resulting in the formation of nitric oxide. Both prostaglandins and nitric oxide facilitate the release of excitatory amino acids in the spinal cord. Thus, COX inhibitors such as ASA and NSAIDs also appear to have important analgesic actions in the spinal cord.

B. Inhibition:

Transmission of nociceptive input in the spinal cord can be inhibited by segmental activity in the cord itself, as well as descending neural activity from supraspinal centers.

1. Segmental inhibition—Activation of large afferent fibers subserving epicritic sensation inhibits WDR neuron and spinothalamic tract activity. Moreover, activation of noxious stimuli in noncontiguous parts of the body inhibits WDR neurons at other levels; ie, pain in one part of the body inhibits pain in other parts. These two observations support a "gate" theory for pain processing in the spinal cord.

Glycine and γ-aminobutyric acid (GABA) are amino acids that function as inhibitory neurotransmitters. They likely play an important role in segmental inhibition of pain in the spinal cord. Antagonism of glycine and GABA results in powerful facilitation of WDR neurons and produces allodynia and hyperesthesia. There are two subtypes of GABA receptors: $GABA_A$, of which muscimol is an agonist, and $GABA_B$, of which baclofen is an agonist. Segmental inhibition appears to be mediated by $GABA_B$ receptor activity, which increases K^+ conductance across the cell membrane. The $GABA_A$ receptor functions as a Cl^- channel, which increases Cl^- conductance across the cell membrane. Benzodiazepines potentiate this action. Activation of glycine receptors also increases Cl⁻ conductance across neuronal cell membranes. Strychnine and tetanus toxoid are glycine receptor antagonists. The action of glycine is more complex than GABA, because the former also has a facilitatory (excitatory) effect on the NMDA receptor.

Adenosine also modulates nociceptive activity in the dorsal horn. At least two receptors are known: A_1, which inhibits adenylcyclase, and A_2, which stimulates adenylcyclase. The A_1 receptor mediates adenosine's antinociceptive action. Methylxanthines can reverse this effect through phosphodiesterase inhibition.

2. Supraspinal inhibition—Several supraspinal structures send fibers down the spinal cord to inhibit pain in the dorsal horn. Important sites of origin for these descending pathways include the periaqueductal gray, reticular formation, and nucleus raphe magnus (NRM). Stimulation of the periaqueductal gray area in midbrain produces widespread analgesia in humans. Axons from these tracts act presynaptically on primary afferent neurons and postsynaptically on second-order neurons (or interneurons). These pathways mediate their antinociceptive action via α_2-adrenergic, serotonergic, and opiate (μ, δ, and κ) receptor mechanisms. The role of monoamines in pain inhibition explains the analgesic action of antidepressants that block reuptake of catecholamines and serotonin. Activity at these receptors (which are also coupled to G proteins) activates secondary intracellular messenger, opening K^+ channels and inhibiting increases in intracellular calcium concentration.

Inhibitory adrenergic pathways originate primarily from the periaqueductal gray area and the reticular formation. Norepinephrine mediates this action via activation of presynaptic or postsynaptic α_2 receptors. At least part of the descending inhibition from the periaqueductal gray is relayed first to the NRM and medullary reticular formation; serotonergic fibers from the NRM then relay the inhibition to dorsal horn neurons via the dorsolateral funiculus.

The endogenous opiate system (primarily the NRM and reticular formation) act via methionine enkephalin, leucine enkephalin, and β-endorphin, which are antagonized by naloxone. These opioids act presynaptically to hyperpolarize primary afferent neurons and inhibit the release of substance P; they also appear to cause some postsynaptic inhibition. In contrast, exogenous opioids may preferentially act postsynaptically on the second-order neurons or interneurons in the substantia gelatinosa.

4. Preemptive Analgesia

The importance of peripheral and central modulation in nociception has fostered the concept of "preemptive analgesia" in patients undergoing surgery. This type of management pharmacologically induces an effective analgesic state *prior* to the surgical trauma. This may involve infiltration of the wound with local anesthetic, central neural blockade, or the administration of effective doses of opioids, NSAIDs, or ketamine. Experimental evidence suggests that preemptive analgesia can effectively attenuate peripheral and central sensitization to pain. Although some studies have failed to demonstrate preemptive analgesia in humans, other studies have reported significant reductions in postoperative analgesic requirements in patients receiving preemptive analgesia.

PATHOPHYSIOLOGY OF CHRONIC PAIN

Chronic pain may be caused by a combination of peripheral, central, or psychological mechanisms. Sensitization of nociceptors plays a major role in the origin of pain associated with peripheral mechanisms, such as chronic musculoskeletal and visceral disorders.

Peripheral-central and central mechanisms are complex and generally associated with partial or complete lesions of peripheral nerves, dorsal root ganglia, nerve roots, or more central structures (Table 18–5). Systemic administration of local anesthetics and anticonvulsants have been shown to suppress the spontaneous firing of sensitized or traumatized neurons. This observation is supported by the efficacy of agents such as lidocaine, mexiletine, and carbamazepine in many patients with neuropathic pain.

The sympathetic nervous system appears to play a major role in some patients with peripheral-central and

Table 18–5. Peripheral-central and central mechanisms of chronic pain.

(1) Spontaneous self-sustaining neuronal activity in the primary afferent neuron (such as a neuroma).

(2) Marked mechanosensitivity associated with chronic nerve compression.

(3) Short-circuits between pain fibers and other types of fibers following demyelination, resulting in activation of nociceptive fibers by nonnoxious stimuli at the site of injury (ephaptic transmission).

(4) Functional reorganization of receptive fields in dorsal horn neurons such that sensory input from surrounding intact nerves emphasizes or aggravates any input from the area of injury.

(5) Spontaneous electrical activity in dorsal horn cells or thalamic nuclei.

(6) Release of segmental inhibition in the spinal cord.

(7) Loss of descending inhibitory influences that are dependent on normal sensory input.

(8) Lesions of the thalamus or other supraspinal structures.

Table 18–6. Psychological mechanisms
or environmental factors associated
with chronic pain.

---

(1) Psychophysiologic mechanisms in which emotional factors act as the initiating cause for somatic or visceral dysfunction (eg, tension headaches).
(2) Learned or operant behavior in which chronic behavior patterns are rewarded (eg, by attention of a spouse) following an often minor injury.
(3) Psychopathology due to psychiatric disorders such as major affective disorders (depression), schizophrenia, and somatization disorders (conversion hysteria) in which the patient has an abnormal preoccupation with bodily functions.
(4) Pure psychogenic mechanisms (somatoform pain disorder), in which real suffering is experienced despite the absence of any nociceptive input.

---

central mechanisms. The efficacy of sympathetic nerve blocks in some patients supports the concept of sympathetically maintained pain. Painful disorders that often respond to sympathetic blocks include reflex sympathetic dystrophy, deafferentation syndromes due to nerve avulsion or amputations, and postherpetic neuralgia (shingles). The simplistic theory of heightened sympathetic activity resulting in vasoconstriction, edema, and hyperalgesia fails to account for the warm and erythematous phase observed in some patients. Similarly, clinical and experimental observations do not satisfactorily support the theory of ephaptic transmission between pain fibers and demyelinated sympathetic fibers.

Psychological mechanisms or environmental factors are rarely sole mechanisms for chronic pain, but are commonly associated with other mechanisms (Table 18–6). Patients with psychogenic pain typically experienced pain that was associated with great anxiety, fear of bodily harm, and loss of love early in life; later in life, anxiety is perceived as pain.

SYSTEMIC RESPONSES TO PAIN

Acute Pain

Acute pain is typically associated with a neuroendocrine stress response that is proportional to pain intensity. The pain pathways mediating the afferent limb of this response are discussed above. The efferent limb is mediated by the sympathetic nervous and endocrine systems. Sympathetic activation increases efferent sympathetic tone to all viscera and releases catecholamines from the adrenal medulla. The hormonal response results from increased sympathetic tone and hypothalamically mediated reflexes.

Minor or superficial operations are associated with little or no stress, whereas major upper abdominal and thoracic procedures produce major stress. Pain following abdominal and thoracic operations or trauma additionally has direct effects on respiratory function. Immobilization or bed rest due to pain in peripheral sites can also indirectly affect respiratory as well as hematologic function. Moderate to severe acute pain, regardless of site, can affect nearly every organ function and may adversely influence postoperative morbidity and mortality. The latter suggests that effective postoperative pain management is not only humane but a very important aspect of postoperative care.

A. Cardiovascular Effects:

Cardiovascular effects are often prominent and include hypertension, tachycardia, enhanced myocardial irritability, and increased systemic vascular resistance. Cardiac output increases in most normal persons but may decrease in patients with compromised ventricular function. Because of the increase in myocardial oxygen demand, pain can aggravate or precipitate myocardial ischemia.

B. Respiratory Effects:

An increase in total body oxygen consumption and carbon dioxide production necessitates a concomitant increase in minute ventilation. The latter increases the work of breathing, especially in patients with underlying lung disease. Pain due to abdominal or thoracic incisions further compromises pulmonary function because of guarding (splinting). Decreased movement of the chest wall reduces tidal volume and functional residual capacity; this promotes atelectasis, intrapulmonary shunting, hypoxemia, and, less commonly, hypoventilation. Reductions in vital capacity impair coughing and the clearing of secretions. Regardless of the pain's location, prolonged bed rest or immobilization can produce similar changes in pulmonary function.

C. Gastrointestinal & Urinary Effects:

Enhanced sympathetic tone increases sphincter tone and decreases intestinal and urinary motility, promoting ileus and urinary retention, respectively. Hypersecretion of gastric acid can promote stress ulceration, and together with reduced motility, potentially predisposes patients to severe aspiration pneumonitis. Nausea, vomiting, and constipation are common. Abdominal distention further aggravates loss of lung volume and pulmonary dysfunction.

D. Endocrine Effects:

The hormonal response to stress increases catabolic hormones (catecholamines, cortisol, and glucagon) and decreases anabolic hormones (insulin and testosterone).

Patients develop a negative nitrogen balance, carbohydrate intolerance, and increased lipolysis. The increase in cortisol, together with increases in renin, aldosterone, angiotensin, and antidiuretic hormone results in sodium retention, water retention, and secondary expansion of the extracellular space.

E. HEMATOLOGIC EFFECTS:

Stress-mediated increases in platelet adhesiveness, reduced fibrinolysis, and hypercoagulability have been reported.

F. IMMUNE EFFECTS:

The stress response produces leukocytosis with lymphopenia and has been reported to depress the reticuloendothelial system. The latter predisposes patients to infection.

G. GENERAL SENSE OF WELL-BEING:

The most common reaction to acute pain is anxiety. Sleep disturbances are also typical. When the duration of the pain becomes prolonged, depression is not unusual. Some patients react with anger that is frequently directed at the medical staff.

Chronic Pain

The neuroendocrine stress response is absent or attenuated in most patients with chronic pain. The stress response is generally observed only in patients with severe recurring pain due to peripheral (nociceptive) mechanisms and in patients with prominent central mechanisms such as pain associated with paraplegia. Sleep and affective disturbances, especially depression, are often prominent. Many patients also experience significant changes in appetite (increase or decrease) and stresses on social relationships.

■ EVALUATING THE PATIENT WITH PAIN

The physician must first distinguish between acute and chronic pain. The management of acute pain is primarily therapeutic, whereas that of chronic pain additionally involves investigative measures. Thus, the patient with postoperative pain requires significantly less evaluation than the patient with a 10-year history of chronic low back pain who has sought multiple medical opinions and treatments. The former requires only a pertinent history and examination, including quantitative evaluation of pain severity, while the latter requires a careful history and physical examination, a review of

prior medical evaluations and treatments, and thorough psychological and sociological evaluations.

The first evaluation is very important from both the physician and patient points of view. In addition to its diagnostic utility, this evaluation helps the physician demonstrate a sympathetic attitude to the patient. A written questionnaire can elicit valuable information about the nature of the pain, its onset and duration, and previous medication and treatments. Diagrams can be useful in defining patterns of radiation. The written questionnaire can help define the effect of the patient's pain on bodily functions, daily activities, and social interactions, and can offer insight about pain relief. The physical examination should emphasize the musculoskeletal and neurologic systems. Imaging studies are often necessary and may include plain radiographs, computed tomography (CT), magnetic resonance imaging (MRI), or bone scans. These studies can often detect unsuspected trauma, tumors, or metabolic bone disease. MRI is especially useful for soft tissue analysis and can show nerve compression.

PAIN MEASUREMENT

Reliable quantitation of pain severity helps determine therapeutic interventions and evaluate the efficacy of treatments. This is a challenge, however, because pain is a subjective experience that is influenced by psychological, cultural, and other variables. Clear definitions are necessary, because pain may be described in terms of tissue destruction, or bodily or emotional reaction. Descriptive scales such as mild, moderate, and severe pain or verbal numerical scales are noncontinuous and generally unsatisfactory.

The visual analog scale (VAS) and the McGill Pain Questionnaire (MPQ) are most commonly used clinically. The VAS is a 10-cm horizontal line labeled "no pain" at one end and "worst pain imaginable" on the other end. The patient is asked to mark on this line where the intensity of the pain lies. The distance from "no pain" to the patient's mark numerically quantitates the pain. The VAS is a simple, efficient, and minimally intrusive method that correlates well with other reliable methods. Unfortunately, VAS assumes pain is unidimensional; it describes intensity but not quality.

The MPQ is a checklist of words describing symptoms. The MPQ attempts to define the pain in three major dimensions: (1) sensory-discriminative (nociceptive pathways), (2) motivational-affective (reticular and limbic structures), and (3) cognitive-evaluative (cerebral cortex). It contains 20 sets of descriptive words that are divided into four major groups: (1) 10 sensory, (2) 5 affective, (3) 1 evaluative, and (4) 4 miscellaneous. The patient selects the sets that apply to his or her pain, and circles the words in each set that best describe the pain. The words in each class are given rank according to severity of pain. A pain rating index is derived based on the words chosen; scores may also be analyzed in each dimension (sensory, affective, evaluative, and miscellaneous). The MPQ is reliable and can be completed in 5–15 minutes. More importantly, the choice of descriptive words that characterize the pain correlates with pain syndromes and thus can be useful diagnostically. Unfortunately, high levels of anxiety and psychological disturbance can obscure the MPQ's discriminative capacity.

PSYCHOLOGICAL EVALUATION

Psychological evaluation is most useful whenever medical evaluation fails to reveal an apparent cause for pain, or when pain intensity is disproportionate to disease or injury. These types of evaluations help define the role of psychological or behavioral factors. The most commonly used tests are the Minnesota Multiphasic Personality Inventory (MMPI) and Beck Depression Inventory.

The MMPI consists of a 566-item true-false questionnaire that attempts to define the patient's personality on 10 clinical scales. Three validity scales serve to identify patients deliberately trying to hide traits or alter the results. It must be noted that cultural differences can affect scores. Moreover, the test is lengthy and some patients find its questions insulting. The MMPI is used primarily to confirm clinical impressions about the role of psychological factors; it cannot reliably distinguish between "organic" and "functional" pain.

Depression is very common in patients with chronic pain. It is often difficult to determine depression's contribution to the suffering associated with pain. The Beck Depression Inventory is a useful test for identifying patients with major depression.

ELECTROMYOGRAPHY AND NERVE CONDUCTION STUDIES

These two studies, which complement one another, are useful for confirming the diagnosis of entrapment syndromes, radicular syndromes, neural trauma, and polyneuropathies. They can often distinguish between neurogenic and myogenic disorders. Patterns of abnormalities can localize a lesion to the spinal cord, nerve root, limb plexus, or peripheral nerve. In addition, they may also be useful in excluding "organic" disorders when psychogenic pain or a "functional" syndrome is suspected.

Electromyography employs needle electrodes to record potentials in individual muscles. Muscle potentials are recorded first while the muscle is at rest and then as the patient is asked to move the muscle. Abnormal findings suggestive of denervation include persistent insertion potentials, the presence of positive sharp

waves, fibrillary activity, or fasciculation potentials. A triphasic motor unit action potential is normally seen as the patient voluntarily moves the muscle. Abnormalities in muscles produce changes in amplitude and duration, and polyphasic action potentials.

Peripheral nerve conduction studies employ supramaximal stimulations of motor or mixed sensory-motor nerve while muscle potentials are recorded over the appropriate muscle. The time between the onset of the stimulation and the onset of the muscle potential (latency) is a measurement of the fastest conducting motor fibers in the nerve. The amplitude of the recorded potential indicates the number of functional motor units, while its duration reflects the range of conduction velocities in the nerve. Conduction velocity can be obtained by stimulating the nerve from two points and comparing the latencies. When a pure sensory nerve is evaluated, the nerve is stimulated while action potentials are recorded either proximally or distally (antidromic conduction).

Nerve conduction studies distinguish between mononeuropathies (due to trauma, compression, or entrapment) and polyneuropathies. The latter include systemic disorders which may produce abnormalities that are widespread and symmetrical, or random (mononeuropathy multiplex). Moreover, the polyneuropathy may be due to axonal loss, demyelination, or both. Demyelination neuropathies slow nerve conduction, disperse action potentials, and prolong latencies. In contrast, axonal neuropathies decrease the amplitude of action potentials with preservation of nerve conduction velocities. Toxic, inherited, traumatic, and ischemic diseases typically cause axonal loss, while some inherited and most autoimmune diseases cause demyelination. Diabetic neuropathy frequently presents with mixed findings of both axonal loss and demyelination.

THERMOGRAPHY

This technique relies on the heat emitted in the form of infrared energy from body surfaces; this emission is normally symmetrical in homologous areas. Differences between each side should generally be no more than 0.5 °C. Neurogenic pathophysiologic changes in the skin frequently result in asymmetry. Telethermography measures infrared energy and displays images where differences in emission are represented by colors or shades of gray (sensitivity 0.5–1.0 °C). Contact thermography is a less expensive technique in which only one part of the body is pressed against elastometric sheets; cholesterol derivatives in the sheets respond to the heat emitted by producing different color bands.

Neuropathic conditions involving somatic or autonomic nerves produce asymmetric segmental abnormalities of hyperemission or hypoemission. Hyperemission is more common in acute stages while hypoemission is more typical of chronicity. The thermography is useful in diagnosing patients with early reflex dystrophy. Myofascial syndromes and ligamentous disorders often produce multifocal hyperemissions that correspond to trigger points or areas of muscle spasm. Bone and joint disorders cause hyperemissions in areas of increased blood flow, while peripheral vascular disease produces hypoemission in the affected extremity.

■ DIAGNOSTIC & THERAPEUTIC NEURAL BLOCKADE

Neural blockade with local anesthetics can be useful in delineating pain mechanisms, but more importantly, it plays a major role in the management of patients with acute or chronic pain. The role of the sympathetic system and its pathways can be evaluated. Pain relief following diagnostic neural blockade often carries favorable prognostic implications for a therapeutic series of blocks. Although the utility of **differential neural blockade** in differentiating between somatic and sympathetic mechanisms may be questionable, this technique can identify patients displaying a placebo response and those with psychogenic mechanisms. In selected patients, "permanent" neural blockade may be appropriate.

The efficacy of neural blockade is presumably due to interruption of afferent nociceptive activity. This is in addition to, or in combination with, blockade of afferent and efferent limbs of abnormal reflex activity (sympathetic and skeletal muscle). The pain relief frequently outlasts the known pharmacologic duration of the agent employed by hours (or sometimes weeks). Selection of the type of block depends on the location of pain, its presumed mechanism, and the skills of the treating physician. Local anesthetic may be applied locally (infiltration), or at a peripheral nerve, somatic plexus, sympathetic ganglia, or nerve root. It can be applied centrally in the neuraxis. Spinal and epidural anesthesias are described in Chapters 16; somatic nerve blocks, which are commonly used for surgery, are described in Chapter 17.

SOMATIC BLOCKS

Trigeminal Nerve Blocks

A. INDICATIONS:

The two principal indications are **trigeminal neuralgia** and intractable cancer pain in the face. Depending on the site of pain, these blocks may be performed on the

gasserian ganglion itself, one of the major divisions (ophthalmic, maxillary, or mandibular), or one of their smaller branches.

B. ANATOMY:

The rootlets of cranial nerve V arise from the brainstem and join one another to form a crescent-shaped sensory (gasserian) ganglion in Meckel's cave. Most of the ganglion is invested with a dural sleeve. The three subdivisions of the trigeminal nerve arise from the ganglia and exit the cranium separately. The ophthalmic division enters the orbit through the superior orbital fissure. The maxillary division exits the cranium via the foramen rotundum to enter the pterygopalatine fossa, where it divides into its various branches. The mandibular nerve exits through the foramen ovale, after which it divides into an anterior trunk, which is mainly motor to the muscles of mastication, and a posterior trunk, which further divides into the various sensory branches (Figure 18–4A).

C. TECHNIQUE:

1. Gasserian ganglion block—To undertake this procedure (Figure 18–4B), radiographic guidance is mandatory. An anterolateral approach is most commonly employed. An 8- to 10-cm 22-gauge needle is inserted approximately 3 cm lateral to the angle of the mouth at the level of the upper second molar; it is advanced posteromedially and angled superiorly such that the needle is aligned with the pupil in the anterior plane and with the mid zygomatic arch in the lateral plane. Without entering the mouth, the needle should pass between the mandibular ramus and the maxilla, and lateral to the pterygoid process to enter the cranium through the foramen ovale. After a negative aspiration for cerebrospinal fluid and blood, 2 mL of anesthetic is injected.

2. Blockade of the ophthalmic nerve and its branches—In this procedure, to avoid keratitis, the ophthalmic division itself is not blocked, so only the supraoptic branch is blocked in most cases (Figure 18–4C). The nerve is easily located and blocked with 2 mL of local anesthetic at the supraoptic notch, which is located on the supraoptic ridge above the pupil. The supratrochlear branch can also be blocked with 1 mL at the superior medial corner of the orbital ridge.

3. Blockade of the maxillary nerve and its branches—With the patient's mouth slightly opened, an 8- to 10-cm 22-gauge needle is inserted between the zygomatic arch and the notch of the mandible (Figure 18–4D). After contact with the lateral pterygoid plate (at about 4 cm depth), the needle is partially withdrawn and angled slightly superiorly and anteriorly to pass into the pterygopalatine fossa. Four to 6 mL of anes-

A. Blocks of the trigeminal nerve

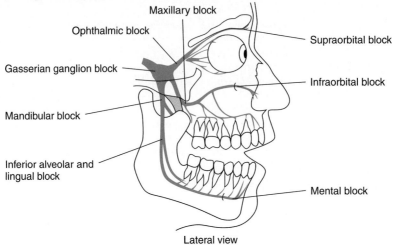

Maxillary block
Ophthalmic block
Supraorbital block
Gasserian ganglion block
Infraorbital block
Mandibular block
Inferior alveolar and lingual block
Mental block

Lateral view

B. Gasserian ganglion block

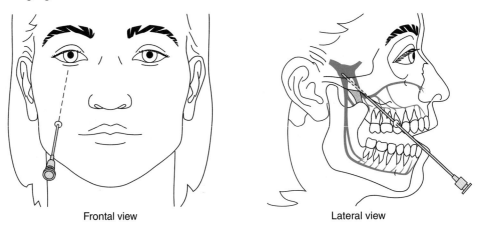

Frontal view

Lateral view

C. Supraorbital nerve block

Supraorbital nerve, medial branch

Supraorbital nerve, lateral branch

Supraorbital notch

Frontal view

Figure 18–4. Trigeminal nerve blocks.

D. Maxillary nerve block

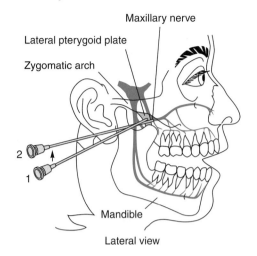

Lateral view

E. Mandibular nerve block

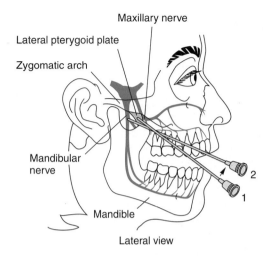

Lateral view

F. Lingual and inferior alveolar nerve block

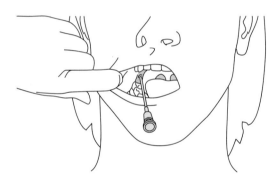

Frontal view

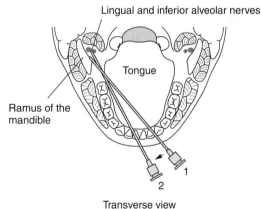

Transverse view

Figure 18–4. (Continued).

thetic is injected once paresthesias are elicited. Both the maxillary nerve and the pterygopalatine ganglia are anesthetized by this technique. The pterygopalatine (sphenopalatine) ganglion (and anterior ethmoid nerves) can be anesthetized transmucosally with topical anesthetic applied through the nose; several cotton applicators soaked with local anesthetic (cocaine or lidocaine) are inserted along the medial wall of the nasal cavity into the area of the sphenopalatine recess.

The infraorbital branch passes through the infraorbital foramen, where it can be blocked with 2 mL of anesthetic. This foramen is approximately 1 cm below the orbit and is usually located with a needle inserted about 2 cm lateral to the nasal ala and directed superiorly, posteriorly, and slightly laterally.

4. Blockade of the mandibular nerve and its branches—This procedure is undertaken with the patient's mouth slightly opened (Figure 18–4E). An 8- to 10-cm 22-gauge needle is inserted between the zygomatic arch and the mandibular notch. After contact with the lateral pterygoid plate, the needle is partially withdrawn and angled slightly superiorly and posteriorly towards the ear. Four to 6 mL of anesthetic is injected once paresthesias are elicited.

The lingual and inferior mandibular branches of the mandibular nerve may be blocked intraorally utilizing a 10-cm 22-gauge needle (Figure 18–4F). The patient is asked to open the mouth maximally and the coronoid notch is palpated with the index finger of the nonoperative hand. The needle is then introduced at the same level (approximately 1 cm above the surface of the last molar), medial to the finger but lateral to the pterygomandibular plicae (fold). It is advanced posteriorly 1.5–2 cm along the medial side of the mandibular ramus, making contact with the bone. Both nerves are usually blocked following injection of 2–3 mL of local anesthetic.

The terminal portion of the inferior alveolar nerve may be blocked as it emerges from the mental foramen at the mid-mandible just beneath the corner of the mouth. Two milliliters of local anesthetic is injected once paresthesias are elicited or the needle is felt to enter the foramen.

D. Complications:

Complications of a gasserian ganglion block include accidental intravascular injection, subarachnoid injection, Horner's syndrome, and motor block of the muscles of mastication. The potential for serious hemorrhage is greatest for blockade for the maxillary nerve. The facial nerve may be unintentionally blocked during blockade of the mandibular division.

Facial Nerve Block

A. Indications:

Blockade of the facial nerve is occasionally indicated to relieve spastic contraction of the facial muscles and to treat herpes zoster affecting this nerve. This procedure is also used during certain eye surgery (see Chapter 38).

B. Anatomy:

The facial nerve exits the cranium through the stylomastoid foramen, where it can be blocked. A small sensory component supplies special sensation (taste) to the anterior two-thirds of the tongue and general sensation to the tympanic membrane, the external auditory meatus, soft palate, and part of the pharynx.

C. Technique:

The injection point is just anterior to the mastoid process, beneath the external auditory meatus, and at the midpoint of the mandibular ramus (see Chapter 38). The nerve is approximately 1–2 cm deep and is blocked with 2–3 mL of local anesthetic, just below the stylomastoid process.

D. Complications:

If the needle is inserted too deeply past the level of the styloid bone, the glossopharyngeal and vagal nerves may also be blocked. Careful aspiration is necessary because of the facial nerve's proximity to the carotid artery and the internal jugular vein.

Glossopharyngeal Block

A. Indications:

Glossopharyngeal nerve block may be used for patients with pain due to with malignant growths at the base of the tongue, the epiglottis, and palatine tonsils. It can also be used to distinguish glossopharyngeal neuralgia from trigeminal and geniculate neuralgia.

B. Anatomy:

The nerve exits from the cranium via the jugular foramen medial to the styloid process and courses anteromedially to supply the posterior third of the tongue, pharyngeal muscles, and mucosa. The vagus and spinal accessory nerves also exit the cranium via the jugular foramen and descend alongside the glossopharyngeal nerve; the carotid artery and internal jugular vein are closely associated structures.

C. Technique:

The block is performed with 2 mL using a 5-cm 22-gauge needle inserted just posterior to the angle of the mandible (Figure 18–5). The nerve is approximately 3–4 cm deep; use of a nerve stimulator facilitates correct placement of the needle. An alternative approach is from a point midway between the mastoid process and the angle of the mandible and over the styloid process; the nerve is located just anterior to the styloid process.

D. Complications:

Complications include dysphagia and vagal blockade resulting in ipsilateral vocal cord paralysis and tachycardia. Block of the accessory nerve and hypoglossal nerves causes ipsilateral paralysis of the trapezius muscle and the tongue, respectively. Careful aspiration is necessary to prevent intravascular injection.

Occipital Nerve Block

A. Indications:

Occipital nerve block is useful diagnostically and therapeutically in patients with occipital headaches and neuralgias.

B. Anatomy:

The greater occipital nerve is derived from the dorsal primary rami of the C2 and C3 spinal nerves, whereas the lesser occipital nerve arises from the ventral rami of the same roots.

C. Technique:

The greater occipital nerve is blocked with 5 mL of anesthetic approximately 3 cm lateral to the occipital prominence at the level of the superior nuchal line (Figure 18–6); the nerve is just medial to the occipital

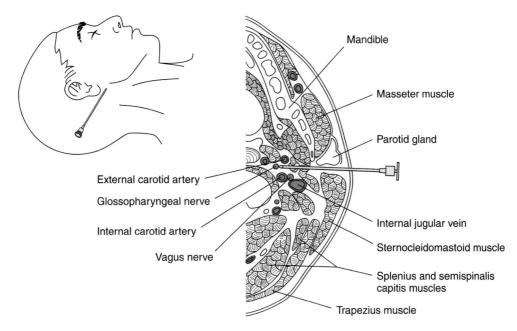

Figure 18–5. Glossopharyngeal nerve block.

artery, which is often palpable. The lesser occipital is blocked with another 2–3 mL injected 2–3 cm more laterally along the nuchal ridge.

D. COMPLICATIONS:

Rarely, intravascular injections may occur.

Phrenic Nerve Block

A. INDICATIONS:

Blockade of the phrenic nerve may occasionally provide relief for pain arising from the central portion of the diaphragm. It can also be useful in patients with refractory hiccups (singultation).

B. ANATOMY:

The phrenic nerve arises from the C3–C5 nerve roots at the lateral border of the anterior scalenus muscle.

C. TECHNIQUE:

The nerve is blocked at a point 3 cm above the clavicle, just lateral to the posterior border of the sternocleidomastoid, and above the anterior scalene muscles. Five to 10 mL of anesthetic solution is injected.

D. COMPLICATIONS:

In addition to serious intravascular injection, pulmonary compromise may occur in patients with preexisting lung disease or injury. Simultaneous bilateral phrenic nerve block should never be performed.

Suprascapular Nerve Block

A. INDICATIONS:

This block is useful for painful conditions arising from the shoulder (most commonly arthritis and bursitis).

B. ANATOMY:

The suprascapular nerve is the major sensory nerve of the shoulder joint. It arises from the brachial plexus (C4–C6) and passes over the upper border of the scapula in the suprascapular notch to enter the suprascapular fossa.

C. TECHNIQUE:

The nerve is blocked with 5 mL of anesthetic solution at the supraspinal notch, which is located at the junction of the lateral and middle thirds of the superior scapular border (Figure 18–7). Correct placement of the needle is determined by paresthesia, or the use of a nerve stimulator.

D. COMPLICATIONS:

Pneumothorax is possible if the needle is advanced too far anteriorly. Paralysis of the supraspinatus and infraspinatus muscles can be troublesome.

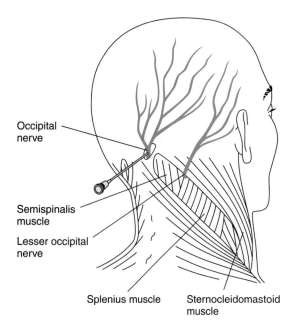

Figure 18–6. Occipital nerve blocks.

Cervical Paravertebral Nerve Block

A. INDICATIONS:

Selective paravertebral blockade at the cervical level can be useful diagnostically and therapeutically for cancer patients with pain originating from the cervical spine or the shoulder.

B. ANATOMY:

The cervical spinal nerves lie in the sulcus of the transverse process of their respective vertebral levels. The transverse processes can be palpated in most persons. Note that in contrast to thoracic and lumbar spinal nerves, cervical spinal nerves exit above their respective vertebral levels (see Chapter 16).

C. TECHNIQUE:

The lateral approach is most commonly used to block C2–C7 (Figure 18–8). The patient is asked to turn his head to the opposite side while in the sitting position. A line is then drawn between the mastoid process and the Chassaignac's tubercle (the tubercle of the C6 transverse process). A series of 2-mL injections are made with a 5-cm 22-gauge needle along a second parallel line 0.5 cm posterior to the first line. Because the transverse process of C2 is usually difficult to palpate, the injection for this level is placed 1.5 cm beneath the mastoid process. The other transverse processes are usually interspaced 1.5 cm apart and are 2.5–3 cm deep. Fluo-

roscopy is useful in identifying vertebral levels during diagnostic blocks.

D. COMPLICATIONS:

Unintentional intrathecal, subdural, or epidural anesthesia at this level rapidly causes respiratory paralysis and hypotension. Injection of even small volumes of local anesthetic into the vertebral artery causes unconsciousness and seizures. Other complications include Horner's syndrome, as well as blockade of the recurrent laryngeal and phrenic nerves.

Thoracic Paravertebral Nerve Block

A. INDICATIONS:

Unlike an intercostal nerve block, a thoracic paravertebral nerve block anesthetizes both the dorsal and ventral rami of spinal nerves (see Chapter 17). It is therefore useful in patients with pain originating from the thoracic spine, thoracic cage, or abdominal wall, including compression fractures, proximal rib fractures, and acute herpes zoster. This technique must be used for blockade of upper thoracic segments, because the scapula interferes with the intercostal technique at these levels.

B. ANATOMY:

Each thoracic nerve root exits from the spinal canal just inferior to the transverse process of its corresponding spinal segment.

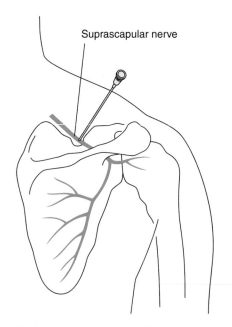

Figure 18–7. Suprascapular nerve block.

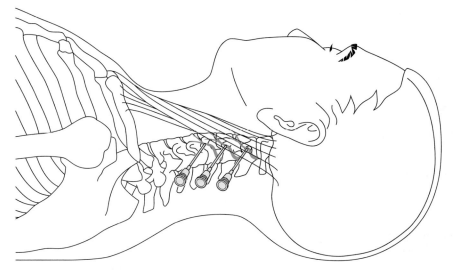

Figure 18–8. Cervical paravertebral nerve block.

C. TECHNIQUE:

This block may be performed with the patient prone or in the lateral position. A 5- to 8-cm 22-gauge spinal needle with an adjustable marker (bead or rubber stopper) is used. With the classic technique, the needle is inserted 4–5 cm lateral to the midline at the spinous process of the level above. The needle is directed anteriorly and medially using a 45-degree angle with the midsagittal plane, and advanced until it contacts the transverse process of the desired level. The needle is then partially withdrawn, and redirected to pass just under the transverse process. The adjustable marker on the needle is used to mark the depth of the spinous process; when the needle is subsequently withdrawn and redirected, it should not be advanced more than 2 cm beyond this mark. Normally, 5 mL of local anesthetic are injected at each level.

An alternative technique that may decrease the risk of pneumothorax uses a more medial insertion point and a loss of resistance technique much similar to epidural anesthesia (see Chapter 17). The needle is inserted in a sagittal plane 1.5 cm lateral to the midline at the level of the spinous process above, and it is advanced until it contacts the lateral edge of the lamina of the level to be blocked. It is then withdrawn to subcutaneous position and reinserted 0.5 cm more laterally but still in a sagittal plane; as the needle is advanced, it engages the superior costotransverse ligament, just lateral to the lamina and inferior to the transverse process. The correct position may be identified by loss of resistance to injection of saline when the needle penetrates the costotransverse ligament.

D. COMPLICATIONS:

The most common complication of paravertebral block is pneumothorax; others include accidental subarachnoid, subdural, epidural, and intravascular injections. Sympathetic blockade and hypotension may be obtained if multiple segments are blocked or a large volume is injected at one level. A chest radiograph is mandatory afterward to rule out a pneumothorax.

Lumbar Paravertebral Somatic Nerve Block

A. INDICATIONS:

Paravertebral block at this level is useful in evaluating pain due to disorders involving the lumbar spine or spinal nerves.

B. ANATOMY:

The lumbar spinal nerves enter the psoas compartment as soon as they exit through the intervertebral foramina beneath the transverse processes. This compartment is formed by the psoas fascia anteriorly, the quadratus lumborum fascia posteriorly, and the vertebral bodies medially.

C. TECHNIQUE:

The approach to lumbar spinal nerves is essentially the same as that for thoracic paravertebral blockade (Figure 18–9). An 8-cm 22-gauge needle is usually used. Radiographic confirmation of the correct level is helpful. For diagnostic blocks, only 2 mL of local anesthetic is injected at any one level, because larger volumes block

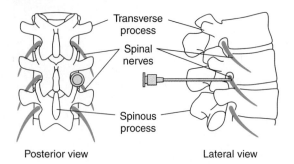

Transverse process

Spinal nerves

Spinous process

Posterior view   Lateral view

Figure 18–9. Lumbar paravertebral nerve blocks.

more than level. Five milliliters of local anesthetic is used for therapeutic blocks, and yet even larger volumes (25 mL) at the level of L3 can produce complete somatic and sympathetic blockade of the lumbar nerves.

D. COMPLICATIONS:

Complications are primarily those of unintentional subarachnoid, subdural, or epidural anesthesia.

Lumbar Medial Branch & Facet Blocks

A. INDICATIONS:

These blocks may establish the contribution of lumbar facet (zygapophyseal) joint disease in back pain. Corticosteroids are commonly injected with the local anesthetic when the intra-articular technique is chosen.

B. ANATOMY:

Each facet joint is innervated by the medial branches of the posterior primary division of the spinal nerves above and below the joint. Thus, every joint is supplied by two or more adjacent spinal nerves. Each medial branch crosses the upper border of the lower transverse process running in a groove between the root of the transverse process and the superior articular process.

C. TECHNIQUE:

These blocks should be performed under fluoroscopic guidance with the patient in prone position (Figure 18–10). A 6- to 8-cm 22-gauge needle is inserted 5–6 cm lateral to the spinous process of the desired level and directed medially toward the upper border of the root of the transverse process; 1–1.5 mL of local anesthetic is injected to block the medial branch of the posterior division of the spinal nerve.

Alternatively, local anesthetic with or without corticosteroid may be directly injected into the joint itself. Positioning the patient prone with slight obliquity (by placing a pillow beneath the anterior iliac crest on the affected side) facilitates identification of the joint space

during fluoroscopy. Correct placement of the needle should be confirmed by injecting 0.5 mL of radiocontrast prior to injection of local anesthetic.

D. COMPLICATIONS:

Injection into a dural sleeve results in a subarachnoid block, while injection near the spinal nerve root results in sensory and motor blockade at that level.

Trans-Sacral Nerve Block

A. INDICATIONS:

This technique is useful in the diagnosis and treatment of pelvic and perineal pain. Blockade of the S1 spinal root can help define its role in back pain.

B. ANATOMY:

The five paired sacral spinal nerves and one pair of coccygeal nerves descend in the sacral canal, forming the cauda equina. Each nerve then travels through its respective intervertebral foramen. The S5 and coccygeal nerves exit through the sacral hiatus.

C. TECHNIQUE:

While the patient is prone, the sacral foramina are identified with a needle along a line drawn 1.5 cm medial to the posterior superior iliac spine and 1.5 cm lateral to the ipsilateral sacral cornu (Figure 18–11). Correct positioning requires entry of the needle into the posterior sacral foramen and usually produces paresthesias. The S1 nerve root is usually 1.5 cm above the level of the posterior superior iliac spine along this imaginary line. Two milliliters of local anesthetic is injected for diagnostic blocks while 5 mL is used for therapeutic blocks. Blockade of the S5 and coccygeal nerves can be

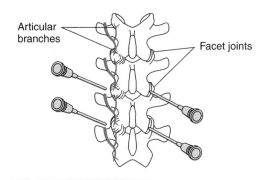

Articular branches

Facet joints

Posterior view

Figure 18–10. Lumbar medical branch nerve and facet blocks.

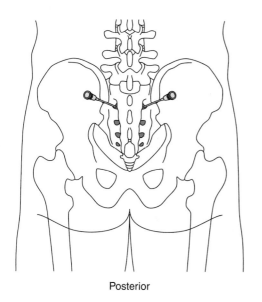

Posterior

Figure 18–11. Transsacral nerve block.

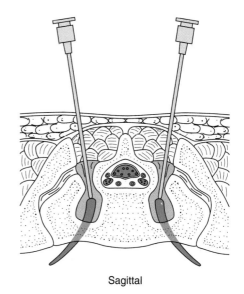

Sagittal

accomplished by injection at the sacral hiatus (see Chapter 17).

D. COMPLICATIONS:

Complications are rare but include nerve damage and intravascular injection.

Pudendal Nerve Block

A. INDICATIONS:

Pudendal nerve block is useful in evaluating patients with perineal pain.

B. ANATOMY:

The pudendal nerve arises from S2–S4 and courses between the sacrospinous and the sacrotuberous ligaments to reach the perineum.

C. TECHNIQUE:

This block is usually performed transperineally in the lithotomy position (Figure 18–12). Injection of 5–10 mL of anesthetic is carried out percutaneously just posterior to the ischial spine at the attachment of the sacrospinous ligament. The ischial spine can be palpated transrectally or transvaginally. A special guide is typically used for a transvaginal approach (see Chapter 43).

D. COMPLICATIONS:

Unintentional sciatic blockade and intravascular injection are common complications.

SYMPATHETIC BLOCKS

Sympathetic blockade can be accomplished by a variety of techniques including subarachnoid, epidural, as well as paravertebral blocks. Unfortunately, these approaches usually block both somatic and sympathetic

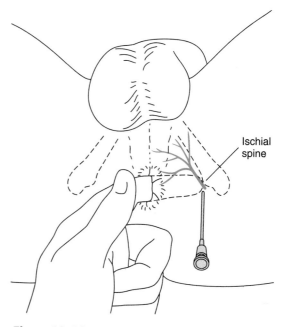

Ischial spine

Figure 18–12. Pudenal nerve block.

fibers. Problems with differential spinal and epidural techniques are discussed below. The following techniques specifically block sympathetic fibers and can be used to define the role of the sympathetic system in a patient's pain and possibly provide long-term pain relief. The most common indications include reflex sympathetic dystrophy, visceral pain, acute herpetic neuralgia, postherpetic pain, and peripheral vascular disease. Isolated sympathetic blockade to a region is characterized by unaltered somatic sensation but loss of sympathetic tone as evidenced by increased cutaneous blood flow and temperature. Other tests include loss of the skin conductance (sympathogalvanic) and sweat response (Ninhydrin, cobalt blue, or starch tests) following a painful stimulus.

Cervicothoracic (Stellate) Block

A. INDICATIONS:

This block is often used in patients with head, neck, arm, and upper chest pain. It is commonly referred to as a stellate block but in reality usually blocks the upper thoracic as well as all cervical ganglia. Injection of large volumes of anesthetic (> 10 mL) often blocks down to the T5 ganglia. Stellate blocks may also be used for vasospastic disorders of the upper extremity.

B. ANATOMY:

Sympathetic innervation of the head, neck, and most of the arm is derived from four cervical ganglia; the largest is the **stellate ganglion**. The latter usually represents a fusion of the lower cervical and first thoracic ganglia. Some sympathetic innervation of the arm (T1) as well as all innervation of the thoracic viscera are derived from the five upper thoracic ganglia. The sympathetic supply to the arm in some persons may also originate from T2–T3 via anatomically distinct nerves (Kuntz's nerves) that join the brachial plexus high in the axilla; these nerves may be missed by a stellate block but not an axillary block. The point of injection is at the level of the stellate, which lies posterior to the origin of the vertebral artery from the subclavian artery, anterior to the longus colli muscle and the first rib, anterolateral to the prevertebral fascia, and medial to the scalene muscles.

C. TECHNIQUE:

The paratracheal technique is most commonly used (Figure 18–13). With the patient's head extended, a 4- to 5-cm 22-gauge needle is inserted at the medial edge of the sternocleidomastoid muscle just below the level of the cricoid cartilage at the level of the transverse process of C6 (Chassaignac's tubercle) or C7 (3–5 cm above the clavicle). The nonoperative hand should be used to retract the muscle together with the carotid sheath prior to needle insertion. The needle is advanced to the transverse process and withdrawn 2–3 mm prior to injection. Aspiration must be carried out in two planes before a 1-mL test dose is used to exclude unintentional intravascular injection (into the vertebral or subclavian arteries) or subarachnoid injection into a dural sleeve. A total of 10–15 mL of local anesthetic may be injected.

Correct placement of the needle is usually promptly followed by an increase in the skin temperature of the ipsilateral arm and the onset of Horner's syndrome. The latter consists of ipsilateral ptosis, meiosis, enoph-

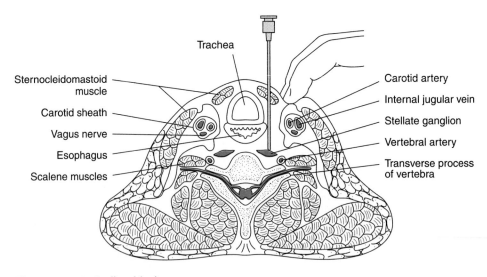

Figure 18–13. Stellate block.

thalmos, nasal congestion, and anhidrosis of the neck and face.

D. COMPLICATIONS:

In addition to intravascular and subarachnoid injection, other complications include hematoma, pneumothorax, epidural anesthesia, brachial plexus block, hoarseness due to blockade of the recurrent laryngeal nerve, and rarely, osteitis or mediastinitis following esophageal puncture.

Thoracic Sympathetic Chain Block

The thoracic sympathetic ganglia lie just lateral to the vertebral bodies and anterior to spinal nerve roots, but this block is generally not used because of a significant risk of pneumothorax.

Celiac Plexus Block

A. INDICATIONS:

Celiac block is indicated in patients with pain arising from the abdominal viscera, especially abdominal malignant growths. The technique usually also blocks the lumbar sympathetic chain.

B. ANATOMY:

The celiac ganglia vary in number (1–5), form, and position. They are generally clustered at the level of the body of L1, posterior to the vena cava on the right,

just lateral to aorta on left, and posterior to the pancreas.

C. TECHNIQUE:

The patient is placed prone and a 15-cm 22-gauge needle is used to inject 15–20 mL of local anesthetic from the left side or bilaterally (Figure 18–14). Fluoroscopic or CT guidance with injection of radiocontrast increases the success rate, reduces the volume required, and decreases the incidence of complications. Each needle is inserted 3–8 cm from the midline at the inferior edge of the spinous process of L1; it is advanced under radiographic guidance towards the midline, making approximately a 10–45-degree angle. The needle passes under the edge of the 12th rib and should be positioned anterior to the body of L1 in the lateral radiographic view and close to the midline overlying the same vertebral body on the anteroposterior view. When CT is used, the tip of the needle should come to lie anterolateral to the aorta at a level between the celiac and superior mesenteric arteries.

D. COMPLICATIONS:

The most common complication is postural hypotension, which is largely due to blockade of the lumbar sympathetic chain. Intravascular injection into the vena cava is more likely to produce a severe systematic reaction than accidental intra-aortic injection. Other less common complications include pneumothorax, retroperitoneal hemorrhage, injury to the kidneys or

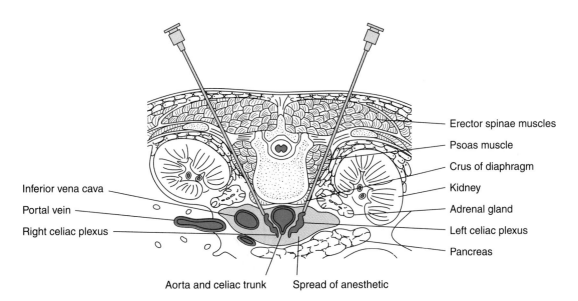

Inferior vena cava
Portal vein
Right celiac plexus

Erector spinae muscles
Psoas muscle
Crus of diaphragm
Kidney
Adrenal gland
Left celiac plexus
Pancreas

Aorta and celiac trunk   Spread of anesthetic

Figure 18–14. Celiac plexus block.

pancreas, sexual dysfunction, or rarely, paraplegia (due to injury of a lumbar artery of Adamkiewicz).

Splanchnic Nerve Block

Although similar to celiac plexus block, this technique is preferred by a few clinicians because it is less likely to block the lumbar sympathetic chain and requires less anesthetic volume. Three groups of splanchnic nerves (greater, lesser, and least) arise from the lower seven thoracic sympathetic ganglia on each side and descend alongside the vertebral bodies to communicate with the celiac ganglia. The needle is inserted 6–7 cm from the midline at the lower end of the T11 spinous process, and advanced under fluoroscopic guidance to anterolateral surface of T12. Ten milliliters of local anesthetic is injected on each side. The needle should maintain contact with the vertebral body at all times to avoid a pneumothorax. In addition to pneumothorax, possible complications include hypotension, and possible injuries to the azygous vein on the right, or the hemiazygos vein and the thoracic duct on the left.

Lumbar Sympathetic Block

A. INDICATIONS:

Lumbar sympathetic blockade may be indicated for painful conditions involving the pelvis or the lower extremities, and possibly in some patients with peripheral vascular disease.

B. ANATOMY:

The lumbar sympathetic chain contains three to five ganglia and is a continuation of the thoracic chain; it also supplies sympathetic fibers to the pelvic plexus and

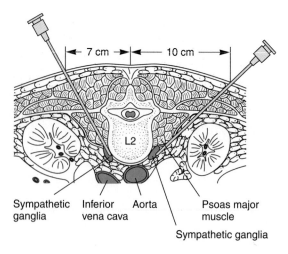

Figure 18–15. Lumbar sympathetic block.

ganglia. The lumbar sympathetic chain's ganglia lie in a more anteromedial position to the vertebral bodies than do the thoracic ganglia and are anterior to the psoas muscle and fascia. The lumbar chain is usually posterior to the vena cava on the right but is just lateral to the aorta on the left.

C. TECHNIQUE:

A two-needle technique at the L2 and L4 levels is most commonly employed with the patient either prone or in the lateral position (Figure 18–15). The needle is inserted at the upper edge of the spinous process and is directed above or just lateral to the transverse process of the vertebrae (depending on the distance from the midline). Fluoroscopic guidance with injection of radiocontrast solution increases the success rate and may reduce complications.

D. COMPLICATIONS:

Complications include intravascular injection (into the cava, aorta, or lumbar vessels), and somatic nerve block of the lumbar plexus.

Hypogastric Plexus Block

A. INDICATIONS:

This procedure is indicated for pain that originates from the pelvis, and that is unresponsive to lumbar or caudal epidural blocks. The hypogastric plexus contains visceral sensory fibers that bypass the lower spinal cord. This block is usually appropriate for patients with cancer of the cervix, uterus, bladder, prostate, or rectum. The block may also be effective in some women with chronic nonmalignant pelvic pain.

B. ANATOMY:

The hypogastric plexus not only contains postganglionic fibers derived from the lumbar sympathetic chain, but also visceral sensory fibers from cervix, uterus, bladder, prostate, and rectum. The superior hypogastric plexus usually lies just to the left of the midline at the L5 vertebral body and beneath the bifurcation of the aorta. The fibers of this plexus divide into left and right branches and descend to the pelvic organs via the right and left inferior hypogastric and pelvic plexuses. The inferior hypogastric plexus additionally receives preganglionic parasympathetic fibers from S2–S4 spinal nerve roots.

C. TECHNIQUE:

The patient is positioned prone, and a 15-cm needle is inserted approximately 7 cm lateral to the L4–L5 spinal interspace. The needle is directed medially and caudally at a 45-degree angle under fluoroscopic guidance so that it passes just over the transverse process of L5. In its final position, the needle should lie over the intervertebral disc between L5 and S1 and within 1 cm of the vertebral bodies in the anteroposterior view. Injection of radiocontrast dye confirms the correct position of the needle in the retroperitoneal space; 8–10 mL of local anesthetic is injected.

D. COMPLICATIONS:

Complications include intravascular injection and transient bowel and bladder dysfunction.

Ganglion Impar Block

A. INDICATIONS:

This block is effective in patients with visceral or sympathetically maintained pain in the perineal area.

B. ANATOMY:

The ganglion impar (ganglion of Walther) is the most caudal part of the sympathetic trunks. The two lowest pelvic sympathetic ganglia often fuse forming one ganglion in the midline just anterior to the coccyx.

C. TECHNIQUE:

The patient may be positioned in a lateral decubitus or lithotomy position. With the patient in the lateral decubitus position, a 22-gauge 8–10 cm curved needle is directed through the anococcygeal ligament upward into a position that is just anterior to the coccyx. Insertion of a finger in the rectum helps keep the needle in the midline and outside the rectal wall. An alternative approach utilizes a straight needle with the patient in lithotomy position; a straight needle can be used in this position because the curvature of the coccyx is reduced. After confirmation of correct position with radiocontrast dye, 4–6 mL of local anesthetic is injected.

D. COMPLICATIONS:

No complications have been reported, but intravascular injection and transient bowel or bladder dysfunction is possible.

Intravenous Regional Sympathetic Blockade

A Bier block (see Chapter 17) utilizing guanethidine (20–40 mg) can selectively interrupt sympathetic innervation to an extremity. Ten milliliters of lidocaine 0.5% can also be added to prevent burning. A tourniquet is placed proximally on the extremity and usually left inflated for at least 20 minutes. Guanethidine causes depletion of norepinephrine and inhibits its reuptake at the terminals of postganglionic neurons. The selective sympathetic blockade lasts 3–7 days. Premature release of the tourniquet can result in hypotension,

bradycardia, edema, diarrhea, and nausea. Reserpine (1–1.5 mg) and bretylium (5 mg/kg) can be used similarly. Intravenous regional sympathetic blockade is a safe alternative to standard sympathetic blocks in patients with hemostatic defects.

DIFFERENTIAL NEURAXIAL & BRACHIAL PLEXUS BLOCKS

Pharmacologic differential neural blockade has been advocated as a method of distinguishing somatic, sympathetic, and psychogenic pain mechanisms. This approach relies on the differential sensitivity of nerve fibers to local anesthetics (see Chapter 14). Preganglionic sympathetic (B) fibers are reported to be most sensitive, and closely followed by pain (C and Aδ), somatosensory (Aβ) fibers, and finally motor fibers (Aα). By using different concentrations of local anesthetic, it may be possible to selectively block certain types of fibers while preserving the function of others. Here the challenge is that the critical concentration to block sympathetic fibers can vary considerably between patients, and conduction block by local anesthetics is dependent not only on fiber size but the duration of contact and frequency of impulses conducted. Many clinicians have therefore abandoned the use of differential neural blocks; nonetheless, some continue to use this technique routinely in evaluating patients. Spinal or epidural blockade (see Chapter 16) is used for abdominal and lower extremity pain, while brachial plexus block (see Chapter 17) is used for arm pain.

Differential neuraxial blockade utilizes sequential injections of four different solutions with increasing anesthetic concentration (Table 18–7). After each injection, the patient is evaluated for pain relief, signs of sympathetic blockade (a decrease in blood pressure), sensation to pinprick and light touch, and motor function. If the pain disappears after the saline injection, the patient has either psychogenic pain (usually a profound long-lasting effect) or is displaying a placebo effect (usually short-lasting). If pain relief coincides with isolated signs

Table 18–7. Solutions for differential neuronal blockade.

Solution	Spinal	Epidural[1]
Placebo	Saline	Saline
Sympatholytic	0.25% procaine	0.5% lidocaine
Somatic	0.5% procaine	1% lidocaine
All fibers	1% procaine	2% lidocaine

[1]Chloroprocaine may be used instead.

of sympathetic blockade, then it is likely mediated by sympathetic fibers. If the pain relief only follows somatosensory blockade, then it is likely mediated by somatic fibers. Lastly, if the pain persists even after signs of motor blockade, then the pain is either central (supraspinal) or psychogenic.

A serious disadvantage of the standard differential technique, especially epidural blockade, is that it is very time-consuming. Most clinicians therefore use a modified two-injection technique: placebo injection followed by a maximally concentrated solution (5% hyperbaric procaine intrathecally, or 2% chloroprocaine or 2% lidocaine epidurally). The patient is still evaluated after each injection, but the pain is correlated with the recovery of motor, sensory, and sympathetic function.

RADIOFREQUENCY ABLATION & CRYONEUROLYSIS

Percutaneous radiofrequency ablation relies on the heat produced by current flow from an active electrode that is incorporated at the tip of a special needle. The needle is positioned under fluoroscopy. Electrical stimulation (2 Hz for motor responses and 50 Hz for sensory responses) via the electrode and impedance measurement prior to ablation also helps confirm correct positioning. Depending on the location of the block, the heating temperature generated at the electrode is precisely controlled (60–90 °C for 1–3 minutes) to ablate the nerve without causing excessive tissue damage. Radiofrequency ablation is commonly used for trigeminal rhizotomy, and medial branch (facet) rhizotomy. It has also been used for dorsal root rhizotomy and lumbar sympathectomy. Pain relief usually lasts 3–12 months.

Cryoanalgesia can produce temporary neurolysis for weeks to months by freezing and thawing tissue. The temperature at the tip of a cryoprobe rapidly drops as gas (carbon dioxide or nitrous oxide) at a high pressure is allowed to expand. The probe tip, which can achieve temperatures of −50 to −70 °C, is introduced via a 16–12 gauge catheter. Electrical stimulation (2–5 Hz for motor responses and 50–100 Hz for sensory responses) helps confirm correct positioning of the probe. Two or more 2-minute cycles of freezing and thawing are usually administered. Cryoanalgesia is most commonly used to achieve long-term blockade of peripheral nerve. It may be especially useful for postthoracotomy pain (see Chapter 24).

ALCOHOL & PHENOL NEUROLYTIC BLOCKS

Neurolytic blocks are indicated for patients with severe intractable cancer pain. They may occasionally be used in some patients with refractory neuralgia and rarely in patients with peripheral vascular disease. These blocks can be associated with considerable morbidity, so patients must be selected carefully. Moreover, the blocks are not permanent, because the original pain recurs or new (central) pain develops in a majority of patients within weeks to months. Temporary destruction of nerve fibers or ganglia can be accomplished by injection of alcohol or phenol. These agents are not selective, equally affecting visceral, sensory, and motor fibers. Ethyl alcohol (50–100%) causes extraction of membrane phospholipids and precipitation of lipoproteins in axons and Schwann cells, while phenol (6–12%) appears to coagulate proteins. Alcohol causes severe pain on injection. For peripheral nerve blocks, alcohol may be given undiluted, but for sympathetic blocks where large volumes are injected, it is given in a 1:1 mixture with bupivacaine. Phenol is painless when injected either as the aqueous solution (6–8%) or in glycerol; a 12% phenol solution can be prepared in radiocontrast dye.

At least one diagnostic block with a local anesthetic solution should be used before consideration of any neurolytic technique. This serves to confirm the pain pathways involved and determine the potential efficacy of neurolytic blockade. Local anesthetic should again be injected immediately prior to the neurolytic agent. Moreover, fluoroscopy (or CT) with radiocontrast should always be used whenever possible. Following injection of any neurolytic agent, the needle must be cleared with air or saline prior to withdrawal to prevent damage to superficial structures.

Neurolytic techniques are most commonly employed with celiac plexus, lumbar sympathetic chain, hypogastric plexus, and ganglion impar blocks in cancer patients but may be used for somatic or cranial nerves or even neural axial blocks. Many clinicians prefer alcohol for celiac plexus block but phenol for lumbar sympathetic blockade. With neurolytic subarachnoid techniques, very small amounts of the agent (0.1 mL) are injected, and the patient is carefully positioned such that the solution localizes to the appropriate level and is confined to the dorsal horn area. Alcohol is hypobaric, while phenol in glycerin is hyperbaric.

■ PHARMACOLOGIC INTERVENTIONS

Pharmacologic interventions in pain management include COX inhibitors, opioids, antidepressants, neuroleptic agents, anticonvulsants, corticosteroids, and systemic administration of local anesthetics. COX inhibitors are reviewed below in the discussion on postoperative pain management. Opioids, which are used primarily for acute moderate to severe pain and cancer pain, are discussed in Chapter 8 and below with cancer pain.

Antidepressants

These agents demonstrate an analgesic effect that occurs at a lower dose than their antidepressant action. Both actions are due to blockade of presynaptic reuptake of serotonin, norepinephrine, or both (see Chapter 27). Older tricyclic agents appear to be more effective analgesics than selective serotonin reuptake inhibitors (SSRIs). In contrast, SSRIs appear to be more effective antidepressants. Antidepressants are generally most useful in patients with neuropathic pain, eg, from postherpetic neuralgia and diabetic neuropathy. They potentiate the action of opioids and frequently normalize sleep patterns.

Available agents differ in side effects (Table 18–8), which include antimuscarinic effects, such as dry mouth (xerostomia), impaired visual accommodation, urinary retention and constipation; antihistaminic effects (H_1 and H_2), such as sedation and increased gastric pH; α-adrenergic blockade resulting in orthostatic hypotension; and a quinidine-like effect, especially with amitriptyline.

All agents undergo extensive first-pass hepatic metabolism and are highly protein bound. Most are highly lipophilic and have large volumes of distribution. Elimination half-lives vary between 1–4 days, and many have active metabolites.

Anticonvulsants

 Anticonvulsants have been found to be extremely useful in patients with neuropathic pain, especially trigeminal neuralgia and diabetic neuropathy. These agents can suppress the spontaneous neural discharges that play a major role in these disorders. The most commonly employed agents are phenytoin, carbamazepine, valproic acid, clonazepam, and gabapentin (Table 18–9; see also Chapter 27).

Table 18–8. Selected antidepressants.

Drug	Norepinephrine Blockade	Serotonin Blockade	Sedation	Anticholinergic Activity	Orthostatic Hypotension	Half-life (h)	Daily Dose (mg)
Desipramine (Norpramin)	++++	+++	Low	Low	Low	12–50	50–300
Nortriptyline (Pamelor)	++	+++	Moderate	Moderate	Low	15–90	40–150
Imipramine (Tofranil)	++	++++	Moderate	Moderate	High	6–20	75–400
Amitriptyline (Elavil)	++	++++	High	High	Moderate	30–40	25–300
Trazodone (Desyrel)	+	+++	Moderate	Low	Moderate	3–9	150–400
Doxepine (Sinequan)	+	++	High	Moderate	Moderate	8–24	75–400
Fluoxetine (Prozac)	+	++++	Low	Moderate	Low	160–200	20–80
Venlafaxine (Effexor)	+	++++	Low	Moderate	Low	5–11	75–100
Paroxeline (Paxil)	+	++++	Low	Moderate	Low	31	20–40
Sertraline (Zoloft)	+	++++	Low	Moderate	Low	26	50–200
Citalopram (Celexa)	+	++++	Low	Moderate	Low	35	20–40

Table 18–9. Anticonvulsants possibly useful in pain management.

Anticonvulsant	Half-life (h)	Daily Dose (mg)	Therapeutic level (μg/mL)
Phenytoin (Dilantin)	22	200–600	10–20
Carbamazepine (Tegratol)	10–20	200–1200	4–12
Clonazepam (Clonopin)	18–30	1–18	0.01–0.08
Gabapentin (Neurontin)	5–7	900–1800	Unknown
Valproic acid (Depakene)	6–16	750–1250	50–100

Lamotrigine and topiramate may also be effective. All are highly protein bound and have relatively long half-lives. Carbamazepine has slow and unpredictable absorption, which requires monitoring of blood levels for optimal efficacy. Side effects are discussed in Chapter 27.

Neuroleptics

Some clinicians find these agents useful in patients with refractory neuropathic pain. Neuroleptics may be most useful in patients with marked agitation or psychotic symptoms. The most commonly used agents are fluphenazine, haloperidol, chlorpromazine, and perphenazine. Their therapeutic action appears to be due to blockade of dopaminergic receptors in mesolimbic sites. Unfortunately, the same action in nigrostriatal pathways can produce undesirable extrapyramidal side effects, such as mask-like facies, a festinating gait, cogwheel rigidity, and bradykinesia. Some patients also can develop acute dystonic reactions such as oculogyric crisis and torticollis. Long-term side effects include akathisia (extreme restlessness) and tardive dyskinesia (involuntary choreoathetoid movements of the tongue, lipsmacking, truncal instability). Like antidepressants, many of these drugs also have antihistaminic, antimuscarinic, and α-adrenergic-blocking effects.

Corticosteroids

Glucocorticoids are used extensively in pain management for their anti-inflammatory and possibly analgesic actions. They may be given topically, orally, or parenterally (intravenously, subcutaneously, intrabursally, intrarticularly, epidurally). Table 18–10 lists the most commonly used agents, which differ in potency, relative glucocorticoid and mineralocorticoid activities, and duration. Large doses or prolonged administration results in significant side effects. Excess glucocorticoid activity can produce hypertension, hyperglycemia, increased susceptibility to infection, peptic ulcers, osteoporosis, aseptic necrosis of the femoral head, proximal myopa-

Table 18–10. Selected corticosteroids.

Drug	Routes Given	Glucocorticoid Activity	Mineralocorticoid Activity	Equivalent Dose (mg)	Half-life (h)
Hydrocortisone	O, I, T	1	1	20	8–12
Prednisone	O	4	0.8	5	12–36
Prednisolone	O, I	4	0.8	5	12–36
Methylprednisolone (Depo-Medrol, Solu-Medrol)	O, I, T	5	0.5	4	12–36
Triamcinolone (Aristocort)	O, I, T	5	0	4	12–36
Betamethasone (Celestone)	O, I, T	25	0	0.75	36–72
Dexamethasone (Decadron)	O, I, T	25	0	0.75	36–72

O = oral, I = injectable, T = topical.
*Adapted from Goodman and Gilman: The Pharmacologic Basis of Therapeutics, 8th ed., Pergamon, 1990.

thy, cataracts, and rarely, psychosis. Patients can also develop characteristic physical features of Cushing's syndrome (see Chapter 36). Excess mineralocorticoid activity causes sodium retention, hypokalemia, and can precipitate congestive heart failure.

Systemic Local Anesthetics

Local anesthetics (see Chapter 14) are occasionally used systemically in patients with neuropathic pain. They produce sedation and central analgesia; the analgesia frequently outlasts the pharmacokinetic profile of the local anesthetic and breaks the "pain cycle." Lidocaine, procaine, and chloroprocaine are the most commonly used agents. They are given either as slow bolus or by continuous infusion. Lidocaine is given by infusion over 5–30 minutes for a total of 1–5 mg/kg. Procaine 200–400 mg can be given intravenously over the course of 1–2 hours, while chloroprocaine (1% solution) is infused at a rate of 1 mg/kg/min for a total of 10–20 mg/kg. Monitoring should include the electrocardiogram (ECG), blood pressure, respirations, and mental status; full resuscitation equipment should also be immediately available. Signs of toxicity such as tinnitus, slurring, excessive sedation, or nystagmus necessitate slowing or discontinuing the infusion.

Patients who do not respond to anticonvulsants but respond to intravenous local anesthetics may benefit from chronic oral antiarrhythmic therapy. Mexiletine (150–300 mg every 6–8 hours) is the most commonly used agent and generally well tolerated.

■ THERAPEUTIC ADJUNCTS

PSYCHOLOGICAL INTERVENTIONS

These techniques are most effective when employed by psychologists or psychiatrists. They include cognitive therapy, behavioral therapy, biofeedback and relaxation techniques, and hypnosis. Cognitive interventions are based on the assumption that a patient's attitude toward pain can influence the perception of pain. Maladaptive attitudes contribute to suffering and disability. The patient is taught skills for coping with the pain either individually or in group therapy. The most common techniques include attention diversion and imagery. Behavioral (operant) therapy is based on the premise that behavior in patients with chronic pain is determined by the behavior's consequences. Positive reinforcers (such as attention from a spouse) tend to aggravate the pain, whereas negative reinforcers reduce pain behavior. The therapist identifies "unhealthy" pain behavior and tries to manipulate reinforcers; this type

of intervention requires the cooperation of family members and medical providers.

Relaxation techniques teach the patient to alter the arousal response and the increase in sympathetic tone associated with pain. The most commonly employed technique is a progressive muscle relaxation exercise. Biofeedback and hypnosis are closely related interventions. All forms of biofeedback are based on the principle that patients can be taught to control involuntary physiologic parameters. Once proficient in the technique, the patient may be able to control physiologic factors (eg, muscle tension) that aggravate pain, can induce a relaxation response, and can more effectively apply coping skills. The most commonly used physiologic parameters are muscle tension (electromyographic biofeedback) and temperature (thermal biofeedback). The effectiveness of hypnosis varies considerably between individuals. Hypnotic techniques teach patients to alter pain perception by having them focus on other sensations, localize the pain to another site, and dissociate themselves from a painful experience through imagery. Patients with chronic headaches and musculoskeletal disorders appear to benefit most from these relaxation techniques.

PHYSICAL THERAPY

Heat and cold can provide pain relief by alleviating muscle spasm. Heat additionally decreases joint stiffness and increases blood flow, while cold vasoconstricts and can reduce tissue edema. The analgesic action of heat and cold may also be at least partially explained by the gate theory of pain processing (above).

Superficial heating modalities include conductive (hot packs, paraffin baths, fluidotherapy), convective (hydrotherapy), and radiant (infrared) techniques. Techniques for application of deep heat include ultrasound, and shortwave and microwave diathermy; these modalities are more effective for pain involving deep joints and muscles. Cold is most effective for pain associated with acute injuries and edema. When applied selectively, cold can also relieve muscle spasm. Application may take the form of cold packs, ice massage, or vapocoolant sprays (ethyl-chloride or fluormethane).

Exercise should be part of any rehabilitation program for chronic pain. A graded exercise program prevents joint stiffness, muscle atrophy, and contractures, all of which can contribute to the patient's pain and functional disabilities.

ACUPUNCTURE

Acupuncture can be a useful adjunct for some patients with chronic pain, especially that associated with chronic musculoskeletal disorders and headaches. The technique involves insertion of needles into discrete anatomically defined points, called meridians. Stimulation of the needle after insertion takes the form of twirling or application of a mild electrical current. Insertion points appear to be unrelated to the conventional anatomy of the nervous system. Although the scientific literature concerning acupuncture's mechanism of action and role in pain management is conflicting, some studies suggest that acupuncture stimulates the release of endogenous opioids, because its effects can be antagonized by naloxone.

ELECTRICAL STIMULATION

Electrical stimulation of the nervous system can produce analgesia in patients with acute and chronic pain. Current may be applied transcutaneously, epidurally, or by electrodes implanted into the central nervous system.

Transcutaneous Stimulation

Transcutaneous electrical nerve stimulation (TENS) is thought to produce analgesia by stimulating large afferent fibers. It may have a role for patients with mild to moderate acute pain and those with chronic low back pain, arthritis, and neuropathic pain. The gate theory of pain processing suggests that the afferent input from large epicritic fibers competes with that from the smaller pain fibers. An alternative theory proposes that at high rates of stimulation, TENS causes conduction block in small afferent pain fibers. With conventional TENS, electrodes are applied to the same dermatome as the pain and are stimulated periodically by direct current from a generator (usually for 30 minutes several times a day). A current of 10–30 ma with a pulse width of 50–80 µs is applied at a frequency of 80–100 Hz. Some patients refractory to conventional TENS respond to low-frequency TENS (acupuncture-like TENS), which employs stimuli with a pulse width > 200 µs at frequencies < 10 Hz (for 5–15 minutes). Unlike conventional TENS, low-frequency stimulation is at least partly reversed by naloxone, suggesting a role for endogenous opioids.

Spinal Cord Stimulation

This technique is also called dorsal column stimulation because it was thought to produce analgesia by directly stimulating large Aβ fibers in the dorsal columns of the spinal cord. Proposed mechanisms include activation of descending modulating systems and inhibition of sympathetic outflow. Spinal cord stimulation is most effective for neuropathic pain. Accepted indications include sympathetically mediated pain, spinal cord lesions with localized segmental pain, phantom limb pain, ischemic lower extremity pain due to peripheral vascular disease, and adhesive arachnoiditis.

Temporary electrodes are initially placed epidurally and connected to an external generator to evaluate efficacy in a given patient. If a favorable response is obtained, a fully implantable system is placed; the permanent epidural electrodes are usually placed percutaneously, tunneled and connected to a subcutaneous generator. Unfortunately, the efficacy of the technique decreases with time in some patients.

Intracerebral Stimulation

Deep brain stimulation may be used for intractable cancer pain, and rarely for intractable neuropathic pain of nonmalignant origin. Electrodes are implanted stereotactically into the periaqueductal and periventricular gray areas for nociceptive pain (primarily cancer and chronic low back pain); for neuropathic pain, the electrodes are implanted into specific sensory thalamic nuclei. The most serious complications are intracranial hemorrhage and infection.

◼ POSTOPERATIVE PAIN

The concept of "preemptive" analgesia (above) suggests that the best postoperative pain management begins preoperatively. Some studies suggest that anesthetic technique can also influence the neuroendocrine stress response to surgery and pain. Studies suggest that regional anesthesia, especially epidural anesthesia (alone or combined with general anesthesia), can block the neuroendocrine response to surgery; the sensory level of the epidural anesthesia must be above L1 to have a significant effect on the cortisol response. Regional anesthetic techniques in which a catheter can be left in place also provide an excellent means for postoperative analgesia. Intercostal and epidural anesthesia can additionally improve respiratory function following thoracic and upper abdominal operations and encourage early ambulation. Epidural and possibly spinal anesthesia reduce the incidence of thromboembolism following hip surgery and attenuate the hypercoagulation state following vascular procedures.

Postoperative pain control is generally best managed by anesthesiologists, because they offer regional anesthetic techniques as well as pharmacologic expertise in analgesics. Concerns over increased cost may be unjustified because some studies have demonstrated lower mortality and morbidity, as well as reduced hospital costs with these techniques.

Postoperative analgesic modalities include oral or parenteral analgesics, peripheral nerve blocks, neuraxial blocks with local anesthetics, intraspinal opioids, as well as adjunctive techniques such as TENS and physical therapy. Selection of analgesic techniques is generally based on three factors: the patient, the procedure, and the setting (inpatient vs outpatient).

OUTPATIENTS

1. Oral Analgesics

Most patients who have mild to moderate pain following surgery can be managed with oral COX inhibitors, opioids, or a combination. Patients unable to resume an oral intake or with severe pain require inpatient admission regardless of the procedure.

Cyclooxygenase Inhibitors

Oral nonopioid analgesics include salicylates, acetaminophen, and NSAIDs (Table 18–11). These agents inhibit prostaglandin synthesis (COX) and have varying analgesic, antipyretic, and anti-inflammatory properties. Acetaminophen lacks significant anti-inflammatory activity. Analgesia is due to blockade of prostaglandin synthesis, which sensitizes and amplifies nociceptive input (above). Some types of pain, especially pain that follows orthopedic and gynecologic surgery, respond very well to these agents, suggesting an important role for prostaglandins. COX inhibitors likely have important peripheral and central nervous system actions. Their analgesic action is limited by side effects and toxicity at higher doses. At least two types COX are recognized. COX-1 is constitutive and widespread throughout the body, but COX-2 is expressed primarily with inflammation. Selective COX-2 inhibitors, such celecoxib and rofecoxib, appear to have lower toxicity, especially gastrointestinal side effects. Moreover, COX-2 inhibitors do not interfere with platelet aggregation.

All these agents are well-absorbed enterally. Food delays absorption but has no effect on bioavailability. Because most are highly protein-bound (> 80%), these agents can displace other highly bound drugs such as warfarin. All undergo hepatic metabolism and are renally excreted. Dosages should therefore be reduced in patients with hepatic or renal impairment.

Acetaminophen has the fewest side effects but is a hepatotoxin at very high doses. Isoniazid, zidovudine, and barbiturates can potentiate acetaminophen toxicity. Aspirin and NSAIDs most commonly produce

Table 18–11. Selected oral nonopioid analgesics.

Analgesic	Half-life (h)	Onset (h)	Dose (mg)	Dosing Interval (h)	Maximum Daily Dosage (mg)
Salicylates					
Acetylsalicylic acid (aspirin)	2–3	0.5–1.0	500–1000	4	3600–6000
Diflunisal (Dolobid)	8–12	1–2	500–1000	8–12	1500
Choline magnesium trisalicylate (Trilisate)	8–12	1–2	500–1000	12	2000–3000
p-Aminophenols					
Acetaminophen (Tylenol, others)	1–4	0.5	500–1000	4	1200–4000
Proprionic acids					
Ibuprofen (Motrin, others)	1.8–2.5	0.5	400	4–6	3200
Naproxen (Naprosyn)	12–15	1	250–500	12	1500
Naproxen sodium (Anaprox)	13	1–2	275–550	6–8	1375
Indoles					
Indomethacin (Indocin)	4	0.5	25–50	8–12	150–200
Ketorolac (Toradol)	4–6	0.5–1	10	4–6	40
COX-2 Inhibitors					
Celecoxib (Celebrex)	11	3	100–200	12	400
Rofecoxib (Vioxx)	17	2–3	12.5–50	24	50

stomach upset, heartburn, nausea, and dyspepsia; some patients develop ulceration of the gastric mucosa, which appears to be due to inhibition of prostaglandin-mediated mucus and bicarbonate secretion. Other side effects include dizziness, headache, and drowsiness. With the exception of acetaminophen and COX-2 inhibitors, all other COX inhibitors induce platelet dysfunction. Aspirin irreversibly acetylates platelets, inhibiting platelet adhesiveness for 1–2 weeks, while the antiplatelet effect of NSAIDs is reversible and lasts about five elimination half-lives (24–96 hours). This antiplatelet effect does not appear to appreciably increase the incidence of postoperative hemorrhage following most outpatient procedures. ASA and NSAIDs can exacerbate bronchospasm in patients with the triad of nasal polyps, rhinitis, and asthma. ASA should not be used in children with varicella or influenza infections because it may precipitate Reye's syndrome. Lastly, NSAIDs can cause acute renal insufficiency and renal papillary necrosis, especially in patients with underlying renal dysfunction (see Chapter 31).

Opioids

Moderate postoperative pain should be treated with oral opioids either on an as-needed basis (PRN) or on a fixed schedule (Table 18–12). They are commonly combined with oral COX inhibitors; combination therapy enhances analgesia and decreases side effects. The most commonly used agents are codeine, oxycodone, and hydrocodone. These agents are well-absorbed, but hepatic first-pass metabolism limits systemic delivery. Like other opioids (see Chapter 8), they undergo hepatic biotransformation and conjugation before renal elimination. Codeine is transformed by the liver into morphine. The side effects of orally administered opioids are similar to those of systemic opioids (see Chapter 8); when prescribed on a fixed schedule, stool softeners or laxatives may be indicated. Tramadol is a synthetic oral opioid that also blocks neuronal reuptake of norepinephrine and serotonin. It appears to have the same efficacy as the combination of codeine and acetaminophen but unlike others, it is associated with significantly less respiratory depression and has little effect on gastric emptying.

2. Infiltration of Local Anesthetic

Direct infiltration of an incision or a field block with local anesthetic is an easy and safe method of achieving good postoperative pain relief. Ilioinguinal and femoral nerve blocks can be used for hernia repairs and scrotal procedures, while a penile block can be utilized with circumcision (see Chapter 17). A local-acting anesthetic such as bupivacaine should be used (see Chapter 14). The analgesia often outlasts the pharmacokinetic duration of the local anesthetic. It is preferable to adminis-

Table 18–12. Oral opioids.

Opioid	Half-life (h)	Onset (h)	Duration (h)	Relative Potency	Initial Dose (mg)	Dosing Interval (h)
Codeine	3	0.25–1.0	3–4	20	30–60	4
Hydromorphone (Dilaudid)	2–3	0.3–0.5	2–3	0.6	2–4	4
Hydrocodone[1]	1–3	0.5–1.0	3–6	3	5–7.5	4–6
Oxycodone[2]	2–3	0.5	3–6	3	5–10	6
Levorphanol (Levo-Dromoran)	12–16	1–2	6–8	0.4	4	6–8
Methadone (Dolophine)	15–30	0.5–1.0	4–6	1	20	6–8
Propoxyphene (Darvon)[3]	6–12	1–2	3–6	30	100	6
Tramadol (Ultram)	6–7	1–2	3–6	30	50	4–6

[1]Preparations also contain acetaminophen (Vicodin, others).
[2]Preparations may contain acetaminphen (Percocet) or aspirin (Percodan).
[3]Some preparations contain acetaminophen (Darvocet).

ter the local anesthetic prior to the surgery to produce a preemptive analgesic effect (above).

Intra-articular injections of local anesthetics, opioids, or a combination thereof appear to be effective for many patients following arthroscopic procedures.

INPATIENTS

Most inpatients with moderate to severe postoperative pain require parenteral analgesics or neural blockade with local anesthetics during the first 1–6 days following surgery. Once the patient is able to resume an oral intake and pain intensity decreases, oral analgesics are initiated. Parenteral analgesics include NSAIDs (ketorolac), and opioids, and ketamine (see Chapter 8). Ketorolac may be given intramuscularly or intravenously, while opioids can be given subcutaneously, intramuscularly, intravenously, or intraspinally. Transdermal opioid preparations are not recommended for postoperative pain because of an increased risk of respiratory depression.

1. Opioids

Opioid analgesia is achieved at a specific blood level for each patient for a given pain intensity. Patients with severe pain typically continue to report pain until the analgesic blood level reaches a certain concentration above which the patient experiences analgesia and the severity of pain rapidly diminishes. That point is referred to as the **minimum effective analgesic concentration (MEAC)**. Small increases above this point produce a large increase in analgesia.

Subcutaneous and Intramuscular Injections

These two routes are least desirable because they are painful and produce unpredictable blood levels due to erratic absorption. Patient dissatisfaction is common

because of delays in drug administration and incorrect dosing. Cycles of sedation, analgesia, and inadequate analgesia are common.

Intravenous Administration

Intravenous administration solves problems with unpredictable absorption but not necessarily those of correct dosing. An optimal balance between adequate analgesia, sedation, and respiratory depression can be achieved by frequent, intermittent, small doses of opioid (eg, morphine 1–2 mg). Regardless of the drug selected, because of drug redistribution (see Chapter 8), a short duration of action is observed until several doses have been given; adequate blood levels can then be maintained by a continuous infusion. Unfortunately, this technique is very labor-intensive and requires close monitoring for respiratory depression. It must therefore be restricted to postanesthesia recovery, intensive care, and specialized oncology units.

Patient-Controlled Analgesia

Advances in computer technology have allowed the development of patient-controlled analgesia (PCA). By pushing a button, patients are able to self-administer precise doses of opioids intravenously (or intraspinally) on an as-needed basis. The physician programs the infusion pump to deliver a specific dose, the minimum interval between doses (lockout period) and the maximum amount of opioid that can be given in a given period (usually 1 or 4 hours); a basal infusion can also be simultaneously delivered (Table 18–13). When PCA is first initiated, a loading dose of the opioid must be given by the medical staff in attendance, or depending on the settings, the patient may be able to load him or herself in the first hour. When an intravenous morphine PCA is used following major surgery, most adult patients require 2–3 mg/hour in the first 24–48 hours and 1–2 mg/hour in the following 36–72 hours.

Table 18–13. General guidelines for patient-controlled analgesia (PCA) orders for the average adult.

Opioid	Bolus Dose	Lockout (min)	Infusion Rate[1]
Morphine	1–3 mg	10–20	0–1 mg/h
Meperidine (Demerol)	10–15 mg	5–15	0–20 mg/h
Fentanyl (Sublimaze)	15–25 μg	10–20	0–50 μg/h
Sufentanil (Sufenta)	2.5–5 μg	10–20	0–10 μg/h
Hydromorphone (Dilaudid)	0.2–0.5 mg	10–20	0–0.5 mg/h

[1]The authors do not recommend continuous infusion for most patients.

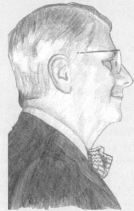

Carl C. Hug, Jr., MD, PhD

SHOULD PATIENTS SUFFER BECAUSE PHYSICIANS ARE AFRAID?

INAPPROPRIATE NONUSE OF OPIOID ANALGESICS

"For all the happiness that man can gain,

it is not in pleasure

but in rest from pain"

John Dryden, 17th Century writer

Morphine and it congeners are powerful analgesics able to assuage the suffering of painful conditions due to disease, trauma, and the interventions of physicians and surgeons. But they have to be used in sufficient doses. No single dose is adequate for all patients, even when administered on the basis of body weight. In fact, there is as much as a tenfold variation in dose requirements among similar patients. Furthermore, there are a number of misconceptions about the side effects and toxicities of morphine-type analgesics.

A prominent orthopedic surgeon and a past president of the Texas Medical Association underwent liver transplantation in 1986. He experienced excruciating abdominal pain both before and after transplantation, but was denied the benefits of morphine. Before transplantation the denial was based on the physicians' fear of overdose in the presence of liver failure. After transplantation it was the physicians' fear of a detrimental effect of morphine on his newly transplanted liver. Both of these concerns reflect a lack of knowledge about a basic tool of medicine. How would you evaluate a mechanic or plumber who does not know how to use a crescent wrench? How does one evaluate a physician who is reluctant, for whatever reason, to relieve pain, especially that which is acute during or after an intervention?

The following are some basic facts about morphine and other opioids acting on μ-type opioid receptors:

1. They relieve the suffering of pain by placing the patient in the frame of mind that the injury isn't bothersome. A typical statement is, "I'm still aware of the incision but I don't care about it."

2. As mentioned, the dose required for similar patients varies as much as tenfold. There is intrinsic (genetic) variation among healthy patients taking no other drugs. In addition, there are numerous factors that can affect the dose requirement within the same patient over time, most especially the presence of other drugs and a varying intensity of noxious stimulation.

3. Opioids depress spontaneous ventilation and the ventilatory responses to hypercarbia and hypoxemia. This depression occurs after analgesic doses and is antagonized by pain. Titrating the opioid dose to provide an adequate level of pain relief also produces respiratory depression of a moderate degree (eg, $PaCO_2$ between 45–55 mm Hg). Patients do not suffer ill effects from moderate hypercarbia, provided supplemental oxygen (eg, nasal prongs) is given to maintain adequate oxygenation of blood ($SpO_2 > 90\%$), respiratory rate is 12–18 breaths per minute (bpm), and lung function is normal. In fact, one way to access both the adequacy and safety of the opioid dose is to titrate it to a respiratory rate of 12–18 bpm.

4. Nonsteroidal anti-inflammatory drugs (NSAIDs) decrease the doses of opioids required for adequate analgesia by about one third. They also decrease the degree of ventilatory depression accordingly because the NSAIDs do not affect ventilation except by decreasing the tachypnea associated with pain. Intravenous doses of ketorolac in the range of 15–30 mg produce the maximum reduction of morphine used as patient-controlled analgesia (PCA) after major surgery. It is prudent to place limits on the total dose and duration of use of ketorolac to minimize the risks of its side effects on the stomach,

kidneys, and bone marrow. However, mild renal failure or a history of gastric ulcers are not absolute contraindications to using intravenous ketoralac for a short period of time in the postoperative patient (eg, to a total dose of 90 mg in an adult).

5. Natural sleep and the drugs producing sleep increase the ventilatory depressant effects of morphinelike analgesics in a synergistic manner. Sedative–hypnotic drugs other than antihistamines and major tranquilizers should be used very cautiously in spontaneously breathing patients receiving μ-type opioids. Falling asleep is a clear sign of patient comfort and adequate analgesia. It is irrational to arouse patients and ask if they are hurting. To administer additional doses of opioid in this situation is to risk serious respiratory depression when sleep recurs.

6. The most effective safe way to control pain using systemic opioids is by PCA. It is important to give a loading dose of the morphine-type analgesic to achieve adequate or near adequate analgesia. Then the patient can easily maintain the effect as pain waxes and wanes over time. It has been thoroughly documented in the scientific medical literature that a) more complete and satisfactory pain relief is achieved with lower doses than those typically administered by a nurse following a dose-time order by a physician; b) risky degrees of respiratory depression do not occur unless excessive doses of hypnotics are used; and c) patients being treated appropriately for pain do not become opioid addicts.

7. In addition to dose-related analgesic and respiratory depressant effects, morphinelike analgesics depress the cough reflex, including the reaction to the presence of an endotracheal tube. Morphine can and should be used according to the individual patient's need during weaning from mechanical ventilation. As long as the spontaneous respiratory rate remains above 15 bpm, the $PaCO_2$ or $ETCO_2$ is stable or declining from a moderately elevated level for that particular patient (ie, $PaCO_2 < 50$ or 55 mm Hg in a young healthy patient), and the other criteria for tracheal extubation are met, extubation can proceed without the fear that the patient will lapse into apnea.

8. Liver failure has to be nearly complete (> 80%) before accumulation of μ-type opioids becomes a problem. If their dose is titrated to adequate analgesia in the individual patient, there is no danger in their use. They do not damage the liver.

9. Opioid metabolites (eg, morphine-3-glucuronide, normeperidine and normeperidine acid) do accumulate over time in the presence of renal failure. Other μ-type opioids without active metabolites are available (eg, fentanyl).

10. Morphine effects are evident within 10–15 minutes but do not reach their peak levels after an intravenous dose until about 30 minutes. Once the peak effect is reached, the brain levels and the effects of morphine decline much more slowly than the blood levels. Hence, there is no accumulation of morphine with subsequent doses that are titrated to the individual patient's need. Its duration of action is not progressively prolonged. More lipid soluble μ-type opioids (eg, fentanyl) achieve their peak effect within 4–10 minutes after an intravenous dose, but they do accumulate in peripheral tissues with successive doses over time, and their duration of action lengthens progressively.

11. True antibody-mediated allergic reactions to opioids are extremely rare. Some opioids release histamine after injection, and in some patients this can lead to obvious and distressful flushing, itching, and even wheezing. Hypotension, related to both histamine release and decreased central sympathetic tone, can occur. It is especially evident in the hypovolemic patient and may be manifest as orthostatic hypotension. Nausea, retching, and vomiting are due to stimulation of the chemoreceptor trigger zone by the opioid and are exacerbated by movement (ie, vestibular stimulation). None of these side effects represents an allergic reaction.

The new regulations of the Joint Commission on Accreditation of Healthcare Organizations mandate the inclusion of pain intensity on a 10-point scale as a regular part of the recording of patient vital signs. Health care institutions will be evaluated on the timeliness and effectiveness of pain relief measures. It is my hope that this summary of the clinical pharmacology of morphine-type analgesics will lead to their more aggressive use in relieving real pain and suffering related to disease, trauma, and medical and surgical interventions. A competent, caring physician should be capable of using morphine-type analgesics effectively and safely.

Studies show PCA to be a cost-effective technique that produces superior analgesia with very high patient satisfaction. Moreover, total drug consumption is less, compared with intramuscular injections. Patients additionally like the control that is given to them; they are able to adjust the analgesia according to their pain severity, which varies with activity and the time of day. PCA therefore requires the understanding and cooperation of patient; this limits its use in very young or confused patients.

In addition to computerized drug-delivery safeguards, the inherent safety of PCA is based on the principle that if the patient becomes too sleepy, he or she will not be able to push the button that delivers opioid. Others (such as family members or nurses) should therefore not push the button for the patient. The routine use of a basal ("background") infusion is controversial. Clinicians that advocate a basal infusion suggest it prevents the analgesic level from appreciably decreasing when patients sleep; patients are presumably, then, less likely to awaken in severe pain. Other clinicians argue that because of highly variable pharmacokinetics between patients and the sometimes rapid decrease in analgesic requirements observed in postoperative patients, basal infusions are more likely to produce respiratory depression. Indeed factors associated with excessively respiratory depressions requiring naloxone administration during PCA include a basal infusion, advanced age, and hypovolemia. Patients that benefit most from a continuous basal infusion are those requiring large amounts of opioid. Thirty to fifty percent of the 24-hour consumption can be given as a basal infusion. Thus, a patient who is consuming 60 mg of morphine per day can safely be given a basal infusion of 1–1.5 mg/hour.

The most common side effects of opioids are nausea, vomiting, itching, and ileus (see Chapter 8). Nearly all opioid overdoses associated with PCA have been due to incorrect programming of parameters. Siphoning of a large amount of opioid into the patient's intravenous infusion (due to a crack in the delivery system) is a rare but potentially serious problem with older systems; in later systems, changes in mounting design and antisiphoning valves have virtually eliminated this problem. Mechanical malfunction of the PCA device is reported but appears to be very rare.

2. Peripheral Nerve Blocks

Intercostal, interpleural, brachial plexus, and femoral nerve blocks (see Chapter 17) can provide excellent postoperative analgesia. Catheter techniques allow intermittent or continuous infusions of local anesthetic (bupivacaine 0.125% or ropivacaine 0.125%) which can provide analgesia for 3–5 days postoperatively.

3. Central Neuraxial Blockade & Intraspinal Opioids

The administration of local anesthetics, opioids, or a combination neuraxially (subarachnoid or epidural) is an excellent technique for managing postoperative pain following abdominal, pelvic, thoracic, or orthopedic procedures on the lower extremities. Patients often have better preservation of pulmonary function, are able to ambulate early, and benefit from early physical therapy. Moreover, patients may be at lower risk for postoperative venous thrombosis.

Single-shot neuraxial injections (subarachnoid or epidural) of local anesthetic, opioid, or a combination thereof may be useful in providing preemptive analgesia and analgesia on the day of surgery. These techniques, however, are most effective when a catheter is left in place for intermittent or continuous infusions. Epidural catheters are most commonly used because of reports of the cauda equina syndrome with subarachnoid catheters (see Chapter 16).

Local Anesthetics Alone

Local anesthetic solutions alone can provide excellent analgesia but produce sympathetic and motor blockade. The former can cause hypotension while the latter limits ambulation. Dilute local anesthetic solutions can provide excellent analgesia with little motor blockade (see Chapter 14). The most commonly used agent is bupivacaine or ropivacaine 0.125–0.25%. The infusion rate must be individualized for each patient but generally depends on the level of the catheter tip relative to the dermatomes of the incision. With an optimally placed catheter, infusion rates of 5–10 mL/hour generally produce satisfactory analgesia.

Opioids Alone

The spinal analgesic action of opioids was discussed above. (See also Table 18–14.) Intrathecal morphine 0.2–0.4 mg can provide excellent analgesia for 4–24 hours. Epidural morphine 3–5 mg is similarly effective and is more commonly employed. Whether given epidurally or intrathecally, opiate penetration into the spinal cord is both time- and concentration-dependent. Epidurally administered hydrophilic agents (such as morphine) produce analgesia at much lower blood levels compared with lipophilic agents (such as fentanyl). The latter may produce segmental effects and thus should generally only be used when the catheter tip is close to the incisional dermatome. Systemic blood levels of fentanyl during epidural infusion are nearly equivalent to those during intravenous administration.

Table 18–14. Epidural opioids.

Opioid	Relative Lipid Solubility	Dose	Onset (min)	Peak (min)	Duration (h)	Infusion Rate
Morphine	1	2–5 mg	15–30	60–90	4–24	0.3–0.9 mg/h
Fentanyl	600	50–100 μg	5–10	10–20	1–3	25–50 μg/h
Meperidine	30	25–75 mg	5–10	15–30	4–6	5–20 mg/h
Sufentanil	1200	20–50 μg	5–15	20–30	2–6	10–25 μg/h
Methadone	80	1–5 mg	10–15	15–20	6–10	0.3–0.5 mg/h
Hydromorphone	1.5	0.75–1.5 mg	10–15	20–30	6–18	0.1–0.2 mg/h

The efficacy of epidurally administered alfentanil and possibly sufentanil appears to be almost entirely due to systemic absorption.

Hydrophilic agents spread rostrally with time; thus, low lumbar morphine injections can provide good (although delayed) analgesia for thoracic and upper abdominal procedures. Important factors that influence dose requirements include the location of the catheter tip relative to the incision and the age of the patient. The closer the catheter tip is to the incision dermatome, the less opiate is required. Older patients generally require less opiate. When epidural morphine is used as the sole analgesic by continuous infusion (0.1 mg/mL), a 3–5 mg bolus is given initially followed by 0.1–0.7 mg/hour infusion. An intermittent bolus technique can be used, but continuous infusions may lessen side effects such as urinary retention and itching.

Fentanyl is the most commonly used lipophilic agent and is administered as a 5–10 μg/mL solution at 5–10 mL/hour.

Local Anesthetic and Opiate Mixtures

Although intraspinal opioids alone can produce excellent analgesia, many patients experience significant dose-dependent side effects, especially with lipid soluble opioids. When dilute local anesthetic solutions are combined with opioids, significant synergy is observed. Bupivacaine 0.0625–0.125% (or ropivacaine 0.1–0.2%) combined with morphine 0.1 mg/mL (or fentanyl 5 μg/mL) provides excellent analgesia with lower drug requirements and fewer side effects.

Contraindications

Contraindications include patient refusal, coagulopathy, or platelet abnormalities, and the presence of infection or tumor at the site of puncture (see Chapter 16). The presence of a systemic infection is only a relative contraindication unless bacteremia is documented. Placement of intraspinal catheters in patients to undergo heparinization intraoperatively is controversial because of the possibility of epidural hematoma. Available evidence suggests that the risk is very small when the catheter is placed atraumatically prior to heparinization and removed only after coagulation normalizes.

Side Effects of Intraspinal Opioids

 The most serious side effect of epidural or intrathecal opioids is dose-dependent, delayed respiratory depression. Diffusion of the opiate into the cerebrospinal fluid and migration to the medullary respiratory center is thought to be responsible. Depression of the CO_2 response curve is typical (see Chapter 22); $PaCO_2$ values in the high 40s or low 50s are not unusual even in fully awake and alert patients. The incidence of respiratory depression is higher following intrathecal than after epidural administration. Early respiratory depression (within 1–2 hours) can also be observed with epidural opioids and is thought to be due to systemic uptake of opioids via spinal blood vessels. The incidence of serious respiratory depression requiring naloxone is low (0.1%) with epidural opioids.

Most cases of serious respiratory depression occur in patients receiving concomitant parenteral opioids or sedatives. Elderly patients and those with sleep apnea appear to be especially vulnerable and require reduced dosing. All patients require special monitoring, which are generally provided in intensive care or specially designated nursing units. Controversy exists concerning optimal monitoring. Pulse oximeters and apnea monitors may be used but are not adequate substitutes for close nursing observation. Changes in pulse oximetry readings may be late signs and apnea monitors produce high false-positive alarms. Excessive sedation appears to be a good clinical indicator of respiratory depression.

Decreases in respiratory rate may also be helpful but not entirely reliable because airway obstruction can be as lethal as apnea. Protocols should be established to allow the nursing staff to decrease or stop the opiate infusion, or even administer naloxone for severe respiratory depression. The amount of naloxone given should be according to the urgency of the clinical situation. Marked respiratory depression should be treated with large doses of naloxone (0.4 mg). A continuous naloxone infusion may be necessary because the half-life of naloxone is generally shorter than that of most opioids (see Chapter 8). Small doses of naloxone (0.04 mg increments) may reverse the respiratory depression but not the analgesia. Intravenous doxapram, 0.75–1 mg/ kg followed by 1–2 mg/min can also be used as a temporizing measure. The latter can reverse the respiratory depression without affecting analgesia.

Common side effects are itching, nausea, urinary retention, sedation, and ileus. Hydromorphone appears less likely than morphine to cause pruritus and nausea. The incidence of pruritus is up to 30%, while that of urinary retention is reported to be 40–100%. The same side effects are observed with parenteral opioids (see Chapter 8). The mechanism of the pruritus is poorly understood but is not related to histamine release. Small doses of naloxone (0.04 mg) have been reported to reverse pruritus without reversing the analgesia. Antihistamines such as diphenhydramine or hydroxyzine can also be used for itching but cause sedation. Nausea and vomiting may be treated with metoclopramide (5–10 mg), transdermal scopolamine, droperidol (0.625–1.25 mg), or ondansetron (4–6 mg). Urinary retention is generally not a problem, because many if not most patients have an indwelling urinary catheter for the first few days postoperatively.

Other Agents

Epidural butorphanol can also provide good analgesia (2–3 hours duration) with little pruritus, but excessive sedation may be a side effect. Epidural clonidine has been shown to be an effective analgesic, but it can be associated with hypotension and bradycardia. Newer, more selective α_2-adrenergic agonists, such as dexmedetomidine, may prove to have fewer side effects.

■ CANCER PAIN

Approximately 19 million people worldwide experience cancer pain every year. Forty to eighty percent of them suffer from moderate to severe pain. Their pain may be due to the cancerous lesion itself, metastatic disease, complications such as neural compression or infections,

treatment, or totally unrelated factors. The pain manager must therefore have a good understanding of the nature of the cancer, its stage, the presence of metastatic disease, and treatments.

Cancer pain can be managed with oral analgesics in most patients. The World Health Organization recommends a three-step approach: (1) nonopioid analgesics such as aspirin, acetaminophen, or NSAID for mild pain, (2) "weak" oral opioids (codeine and oxycodone) for moderate pain, and (3) stronger opioids (morphine and hydromorphone) for severe pain. Parenteral therapy is necessary for refractory pain and when the patient cannot take medication orally or has poor enteral absorption. Regardless of the agent selected, in most instances drug therapy should be on a fixed time schedule rather than PRN. COX inhibitors and the less potent oral opioids are discussed above. Adjuvant drug therapy, especially antidepressants, and other modalities should also be used liberally in cancer patients.

ORAL OPIATE THERAPY

Moderate to severe cancer pain is usually treated with an immediate-release morphine preparation (10–30 mg every 1–4 hours). These preparations have an effective half-life of 2–4 hours. Once the patient's daily requirements are determined, the same dose can be given in the form of a sustained-release preparation (MS Contin or Oramorph SR) which is dosed every 8–12 hours. The immediate-release preparation is then used only for breakthrough pain (PRN). Oral transmucosal fentanyl lozenges (Actif, 200–1600 µg) can also be used for breakthrough pain. Excessive sedation can be treated with dextroamphetamine or methylphenidate 5 mg in the morning and the early afternoon. Most patients require a stool softener such as docusate sodium, senna, cascara, magnesium citrate, milk of magnesia, or lactulose. Nausea may be treated with transdermal scopolamine, oral meclizine, or metoclopramide.

Hydromorphone (Dilaudid) is an excellent alternative to morphine, especially in elderly patients and those with impaired renal function. Methadone is reported to have a half-life of 15–30 hours, but clinical duration is shorter and quite variable (usually 6–8 hours). Patients who experience drug tolerance require escalating doses of opioid to maintain the same analgesic effect. Psychological tolerance, characterized by behavioral changes focusing on drug craving, is rare in cancer patients. Tolerance develops at different rates between persons and results in some desirable effects such as decreased sedation, nausea, and respiratory depression. Unfortunately, though, many patients continue to suffer from constipation. Physical dependence occurs in all patients on large doses of opioids for extended periods. A

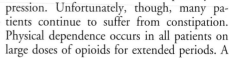

withdrawal phenomenon can be precipitated by the administration of opioid antagonists.

TRANSDERMAL OPIOIDS

Transdermal fentanyl is an excellent alternative to sustained-release morphine preparations, especially when oral medication is not possible. The currently available patches are constructed as a drug reservoir that is separated from the skin by a microporous rate-limiting membrane and an adhesive polymer. A very large quantity of fentanyl (10 mg) provides a large force for transdermal diffusion. The major obstacle to absorption is the stratum corneum. The transdermal route avoids hepatic first-pass metabolism. Transdermal fentanyl patches are available in 25, 50, 75, and 100 μg/hour sizes that provide drug for 2–3 days. The largest patch is equivalent to 60 mg/d of intravenous morphine.

The major disadvantage of this route is its slow onset and the inability to rapidly change dosage in response to changing opioid requirements. Blood fentanyl levels rise and reach a plateau in 12–18 hours, providing average concentrations of 1, 1.5, and 2 ng/mL for the 50, 75, and 100 patches respectively. Large interpatient variability results in actual delivery rates ranging from 50 to 200 μg/hour. The dermis acts as a secondary reservoir such that even after the patch is removed, fentanyl absorption continues for several hours.

PARENTERAL THERAPY

Severe uncontrolled cancer pain requires conversion from oral to parenteral or intraspinal opioids. When the character of the pain changes significantly, it is important to reevaluate the patient for disease progression. In many instances adjunctive treatments such as palliative surgery, radiation, or chemotherapy are helpful. Hormonal therapy should be used whenever possible. Surgery can debulk the tumor, alleviate compression, or fixate a fracture. Neurolytic techniques should also be considered whenever appropriate.

Parenteral opiate therapy is usually best accomplished by continuous intravenous infusion but can also be given subcutaneously through a butterfly needle. Modern portable infusion devices have PCA capability (above) allowing the patient to treat him or herself for breakthrough pain.

INTRASPINAL OPIOIDS

The use of intraspinal opioids is an excellent alternative for patients obtaining poor relief with other techniques or who experience excessive side effects. Epidural and subarachnoid opioids offer pain relief with substantially lower total doses of opiate and fewer side effects. Continuous infusion techniques reduce drug requirements (compared with intermittent boluses), minimize side effects, and decrease the likelihood of catheter occlusion.

Epidural or intrathecal catheters can be placed percutaneously or implanted to provide long-term effective pain relief. Tunneling the catheter reduces the risk of infection. Epidural catheters can be attached to lightweight external pumps which can be worn by ambulatory patients. A temporary catheter must be inserted first to assess the potential efficacy of the technique. Correct placement of the permanent catheter should be confirmed by fluoroscopy and radiocontrast. Completely implantable intrathecal catheters with externally programmable pumps can also be used for continuous infusion; their major disadvantage is cost. The reservoir of the implanted pump is periodically refilled percutaneously; an additional injection port allows injection into catheter directly. Implantable intrathecal systems are most appropriate for patients with a life expectancy of several months, while tunneled epidural catheters are appropriate for patients expected to live for only weeks.

The major problem with intraspinal opioids is tolerance. Generally a slow phenomenon, tolerance does develop rapidly in some patients. In such instances, adjuvant therapy must be used, including the intermittent use of local anesthetics or a mixture of opioids with local anesthetics (bupivacaine or ropivacaine 2–24 mg/d), epidural clonidine (48–800 μg/d), or the GABA agonist baclofen. Epidural clonidine is especially useful for neuropathic pain. In high doses, it is more likely to be associated with hypotension and bradycardia.

Complications include local skin infections and epidural abscess. Superficial infections can be reduced by the use of a silver-impregnated cuff close to the exit site. Other complications include hematoma, which may be immediate or delayed-onset (days). The use of invasive spinal techniques can be complicated by raised intracranial pressure (from mass lesions) and coagulopathy. The risk-benefit ratio must be weighed carefully in terminal patients.

NEUROLYTIC TECHNIQUES

Neurolytic celiac plexus block is very effective for intra-abdominal malignant growths, especially in pancreatic cancer. Lumbar sympathetic, hypogastric plexus, or ganglion impar neurolytic blocks can also be used for malignant tumors of the pelvis. Neurolytic intercostal blocks can be helpful for patients with rib metastases. In patients with refractory pelvic pain, a neurolytic saddle block can provide pain relief; however, bowel and bladder dysfunction should be expected. Because of the significant morbidity associated with neurolytic blocks (loss of motor and somatic sensory function) these techniques should be utilized after careful consideration of alternatives. Neurodestructive procedures, such as pituitary adenolysis and cordotomy, can be useful in terminal patients. Some centers additionally offer deep-brain stimulation.

■ SELECTED PAIN SYNDROMES

SYMPATHETICALLY MAINTAINED PAIN

 Multiple triggers can induce sympathetically maintained pain, which is often overlooked or misdiagnosed. The term "complex regional pain syndrome" (CRPS) has also been suggested to include these and related pain syndromes. The two most common syndromes are reflex sympathetic dystrophy (CRPS type I) and causalgia (CRPS type II).

Reflex Sympathetic Dystrophy (CRPS Type I)

This form of sympathetically maintained pain typically affects the extremities and follows relatively minor trauma. Common preceding events include trauma (contusion, crush, or laceration), surgery, sprain, fracture, or dislocation. It may follow carpal tunnel release, palmar fasciotomy, or arthroplasties. The trauma is sometimes occult. Similar syndromes may be associated with burns, postherpetic neuralgia, multiple sclerosis, diabetic neuropathy, myocardial infarction, stroke, cancer, herniated intervertebral discs, and degenerative joint disease. Three phases can often be identified (Table 18–15). A technetium bone scan shows increased uptake in small joints during the acute phase; thermography reveals asymmetric hyperemission. Although the pain can resolve spontaneously, most patients typically progress to severe functional disabilities.

Causalgia (CRPS Type II)

Causalgia means burning pain, and typically follows high velocity (eg, gunshot) injuries to large nerves. The pain frequently has an immediate onset and is associated with allodynia, hyperpathia, and vasomotor and sudomotor dysfunction. Anything that increases sympathetic tone, such as fear, anxiety, light, noise, or touch exacerbates the pain. The syndrome has a variable progression that can range from days to months. Causalgia most commonly affects the brachial plexus, especially the median nerve in the upper extremity, and the tibial division of sciatic nerve in the lower extremity. Early in the course of the disease patients obtain dramatic pain relief from sympathetic blockade.

Treatment

Patients often dramatically respond to sympathetic blocks, but treatment must be multidisciplinary to avoid long-term functional and psychological disability. Physical therapy plays a central role. Some patients recover spontaneously; but without treatment, most patients progress to severe functional and irreversible disability. Sympathetic blocks and intravenous regional sympatholytic blockade are equally effective. These blocks should be continued until the response plateaus or a cure is achieved. The sympathetic blocks facilitate physical therapy, which usually consists of active movement without weights. Most patients require three to seven blocks. The likelihood of a cure is high (over 90%) if treatment is initiated within 1 month of symptoms and appears to decrease with time. Some patients benefit from TENS. Dorsal column (spinal cord) stimulation may be effective in some patients with long-standing symptoms. Oral α-adrenergic blockers, such as phenoxybenzamine or prazosin, clonidine, anticonvulsants, and antidepressants may also be beneficial. Surgical sympathectomy

Table 18–15. Phases of reflex sympathetic dystrophy.

Characteristic	Phase		
	Acute	Dystrophic	Atrophic
Pain	Localized, severe, and burning	More diffuse, throbbing	Less severe; often involves other extremities
Extremity	Warm	Cold, cyanotic, and edematous; muscle wasting	Severe muscle atrophy; contractures
Skin	Dry and red	Sweaty	Glossy and atrophic
X-ray	Normal	Reveals osteoporosis	Reveals severe osteoporosis, and ankylosis of joints
Duration	1–3 months	3–6 months	Indefinite

for chronic cases is often disappointing because of only transient relief.

ENTRAPMENT SYNDROMES

Entrapment neuropathies are commonly overlooked entities that involve sensory, motor, or mixed nerves. Neural compression can occur wherever a nerve courses through an anatomically narrowed passage. Genetic factors and repetitive macrotrauma or microtrauma are likely involved; adjacent tenosynovitis is often responsible. Table 18–16 lists the most commonly recognized entrapment syndromes. When a sensory nerve is involved, patients complain of pain and numbness in its distribution distal to the site of entrapment; occasionally, a patient may complain of pain referred proximal to the site of entrapment. Entrapment of the sciatic nerve (the piriformis syndrome) can mimic a herniated intervertebral disease. Entrapment of a motor nerve produces weakness in the muscles it innervates. Even

entrapments of "pure" motor nerves can produce a vague pain that may be mediated by afferent fibers from muscles and joints. The diagnosis can usually be confirmed by electromyography and nerve conduction studies. Neural blockade of the nerve with local anesthetic, with or without corticosteroid, may be diagnostic and can provide temporary pain relief. Treatment is generally symptomatic with oral analgesics and temporary immobilization, whenever appropriate. Development of reflex sympathetic dystrophy requires sympathetic blockade. Refractory symptoms require surgical decompression.

MYOFASCIAL PAIN

Myofascial syndromes are common disorders characterized by aching muscle pain, muscle spasm, stiffness, weakness, and occasionally, autonomic dysfunction. Patients have discrete areas (trigger points) of marked tenderness in one or more muscles or the associated

Table 18–16. Entrapment neuropathies.

Nerve	Entrapment Site	Location of Pain
Cranial nerves VII, IX, and X	Styloid process or stylohyoid ligament	Ipsilateral tonsil, base of tongue, temporomandibular joint, and ear (Eagle's syndrome)
Brachial plexus	Scalenus anticus muscle or a cervical rib	Ulnar side of arm and forearm (scalenus anticus syndrome)
Suprascapular nerve	Suprascapular notch	Posterior and lateral shoulder
Median nerve	Pronator teres muscle	Proximal forearm and palmar surface of the first three digits (pronator syndrome)
Median nerve	Carpal tunnel	Palmar surface of the first three digits (carpal tunnel syndrome)
Ulnar nerve	Cubital fossa (elbow)	Fourth and fifth digits of the hand (cubital tunnel syndrome)
Ulnar nerve	Guyon's canal (wrist)	Fourth and fifth digits of the hand
Lateral femoral cutaneous nerve	Anterior iliac spine under the inguinal ligament	Anterolateral thigh (meralgia paresthetica)
Obturator nerve	Obturator canal	Upper medial thigh
Saphenous nerve	Subsartorial tunnel (adductor canal)	Medial calf
Sciatic nerve	Sciatic notch	Buttock and leg (piriformis syndrome)
Common peroneal nerve	Fibular neck	Lateral distal leg and foot
Deep peroneal nerve	Anterior tarsal tunnel	Big toe or foot
Superficial peroneal nerve	Deep fascia above the ankle	Anterior ankle and dorsum of foot
Posterior tibial nerve	Posterior tarsal tunnel	Undersurface of foot (tarsal tunnel syndrome)
Interdigital nerve	Deep transverse tarsal ligament	Between toes and foot (Morton's neuroma)

connective tissue. Palpation of the involved muscles may reveal tight, ropy bands over trigger points. Signs of autonomic dysfunction (vasoconstriction or piloerection) in the overlying muscles may be present. The pain characteristically radiates in a fixed pattern that does not follow dermatomes.

Gross trauma or repetitive microtrauma is thought to play a major role in initiating myofascial syndromes. Trigger points develop following acute injury; stimulation of these active trigger points produces pain, and the ensuing muscle spasm sustains the pain. When the acute episode subsides, the trigger points become latent (tender, but not pain-producing) only to be reactivated at a later time by subsequent stress. The pathophysiology is poorly understood, but the trigger points may represent areas of localized ischemia that develop as a result of muscle or vascular spasm.

The diagnosis of a myofascial syndrome is suggested by the character of the pain and palpation of discrete **trigger points** that reproduce it. Common syndromes produce trigger points in the levator scapulae, masseter, quadratus lumborum, and gluteus medius muscles. The latter two syndromes produce low back pain and should be considered in all patients with back pain; moreover, gluteal trigger points can mimic S1 radiculopathy.

Although myofascial pain can resolve spontaneously without sequelae, many patients continue to have latent trigger points. When trigger points are active, the treatment is directed at regaining muscle length and elasticity. Analgesia must be provided in the form of trigger point injections (1–3 mL) with local anesthetic. Topical cooling with vapocoolant, either an ethyl chloride or fluorocarbon (fluoromethane) spray, can also induce reflex muscle relaxation, and allows massage (stretch and spray) and ultrasound therapy. Ethyl chloride is preferable, because unlike fluorocarbons, it does not deplete the upper atmosphere's ozone layer. Physical therapy is important in maintaining a normal range of motion for affected muscles. Biofeedback may be helpful for some patients.

LOW BACK PAIN & RELATED SYNDROMES

Back pain is an extremely common complaint and a major cause of work disability worldwide. Lumbosacral strain, degenerative disk disease, and myofascial syndromes are the most common causes of low back pain. Many syndromes can also produce low back pain with or without associated leg pain. Causes can be congenital, traumatic, degenerative, inflammatory, infectious, metabolic, psychological, or cancerous. Moreover, back pain can be due to disease processes in the abdomen

and pelvis, especially those diseases affecting retroperitoneal structures (pancreas, kidneys, ureters, aorta, and tumors), the uterus and adnexa, prostate, and the rectosigmoid. Disorders of the hip can similarly mimic back disorders. A positive Patrick's sign helps identify pain due to hip disorder. This sign consists of pain in the hip while placing the ipsilateral heel on the contralateral knee and pressing the ipsilateral thigh. It is also called by the acronym FABERE (sign) because the movement of the leg involves *f*lexion, *ab*duction, *ex*ternal *r*otation, and *e*xtension.

1. Applied Anatomy of the Back

The back can be described as anterior or posterior. The anterior component consists of the cylindrical vertebral bodies that are interconnected by intervertebral disks and supported by anterior and posterior longitudinal ligaments. The posterior elements are bony arches that extend from each vertebral body, consisting of two pedicles, two transverse processes, two lamina, and a spinous process (see Chapter 16). The transverse and spinous processes provide points of attachment for the muscles that move and protect the spinal column. Adjacent vertebra also articulate posteriorly by two gliding facet joints, allowing some motion.

Spinal structures are innervated by the sinuvertebral branches and posterior rami of spinal nerves. The sinuvertebral nerve arises before each spinal nerve divides into anterior and posterior rami, and reenters the intervertebral foramen to innervate the posterior longitudinal ligament, the posterior annulus fibrosus, periosteum, dura, and epidural vessels. Paraspinal structures are supplied by the posterior primary ramus. Each facet joint is innervated by the medial branch of the posterior primary rami of the spinal nerves above and below the joint.

As lumbar spinal nerve roots exit from the dural sac, they travel down 1–2 cm laterally before exiting through their respective intervertebral foramina; thus, the L5 nerve root leaves the dural sac at the level of the L4–L5 disk (where it is more likely to be compressed) but leaves the spinal canal beneath the L5 pedicle opposite the L5–S1 disk.

2. Paravertebral Muscle & Lumbosacral Joint Sprain/Strain

Approximately 80–90% of low back pain is due to sprain or strain associated with lifting heavy objects, falls, or sudden abnormal movements of the spine. The term "sprain" is generally used when the pain is related to a well-defined acute injury, whereas strain is used when the pain is more chronic and likely related to repetitive minor injuries.

Injury to paravertebral muscles and ligaments results in reflex muscle spasm, which may or may not be associated with trigger points. The pain is usually dull and aching, and occasionally radiates down the buttocks or hips. Sprain is a self-limited benign process that resolves in 1–2 weeks. Symptomatic treatment consists of rest and oral analgesics.

The sacroiliac joint is especially vulnerable to rotational injuries. Acute or chronic injury can cause slippage or subluxation of the joint. Pain originating from this joint is characteristically located along the posterior ilium and radiates down the hips and posterior thigh to the knees. The diagnosis is suggested by tenderness on palpation and compression of the joints. Pain relief following injection of the joint with local anesthetic is diagnostic and may be therapeutic. The role of intra-articular steroid injection is not well established.

3. Intervertebral Disk Disease

Intervertebral disks bear at least one-third of the weight of the spinal column. Their central portion, which is called the nucleus pulposus, is composed of gelatinous material early in life. This material degenerates and becomes fibrotic with advancing age and following trauma. The nucleus pulposus is ringed by the annulus fibrosus which is thinnest posteriorly and bounded superiorly and inferiorly by cartilaginous plates. Disk pain may be due to one of two major mechanisms: (1) protrusion or extrusion of the nucleus pulposus posteriorly, or (2) loss of disk height, resulting in the reactive formation of bony spurs (osteophytes) from the rims of the vertebral bodies above and below the disk. Intervertebral disk disease most commonly affects the lumbar spine because it is subjected to the greatest motion and

the posterior longitudinal ligament is thinnest at L2–L5.

Herniated Disk

Weakness and degeneration of the annulus fibrosus and posterior longitudinal ligament can cause herniation of the nucleus pulposus posteriorly into the spinal canal. Ninety percent of disk herniations occur at L5–S1 or L4–L5. Symptoms usually develop following flexion injuries and may be associated with (1) bulging, (2) protrusion, or (3) extrusion of the disk. Disk herniation usually occurs posterolaterally and thus often compresses adjacent nerve roots, producing pain that radiates along that dermatome (radiculopathy). The term "sciatica" is sometimes used because compression of the lower lumbar nerve roots produces pain along the sciatic nerve. When disk material is extruded through the annulus fibrosus and posterior longitudinal ligament, free fragments can become wedged in the spinal canal or the intervertebral foramina; the pain may also be due to a chemical reaction to the glycoproteins released from the degenerating disk. Less commonly a large disk bulges or large fragments extrude posterocentrally, compressing the cauda equina in the dural sac; in these instances patients can experience bilateral pain, urinary retention, or less commonly, fecal incontinence.

The onset of disk pain is typically associated with heavy lifting. The pain is aggravated by bending, lifting, prolonged sitting or anything that increases intra-abdominal pressure, such as sneezing, coughing, or straining. It is usually relieved by lying down. Numbness or weakness is indicative of radiculopathy (Table 18–17). Bulging of the disk through the posterior longitudinal ligament can also produce low back pain that radiates to the hips or buttocks. Straight leg-raising tests may be used to assess nerve root compression. With the patient supine and the knee fully extended, the leg on

Table 18–17. Lumbar disk radiculopathies.

	Disk Level		
	L3–L4 (L4 Nerve)	**L4–L5 (L5 Nerve)**	**L5–S1 (S1 Nerve)**
Pain distribution	Anterolateral thigh, anteromedial calf to the ankle	Lateral thigh, anterolateral calf, medial dorsum of foot, especially between the first and second toes	Gluteal region, posterior thigh, posterolateral calf, lateral dorsum and undersurface of the foot, especially between fourth and fifth toes
Weakness	Quadriceps femoris	Dorsiflexion of the foot	Plantar flexion of foot
Reflex affected	Knee	None	Ankle

the affected side is raised and the angle at which the pain develops is noted; dorsiflexion of the ankle with the leg raised typically exacerbates the pain by further stretching the lumbosacral plexus. Pain while raising the contralateral leg is an even more reliable sign of nerve compression.

Plain radiographs of the lumbar spine are usually obtained in the anterior-posterior, lateral, and oblique views. Bone scans may be useful in older patients to exclude malignant growths. Although the most sensitive modality detecting disk herniation is MRI, this technology does not always accurately demonstrate bony detail like CT. Radiologic findings should be carefully correlated with symptoms, because up to 30–40% of asymptomatic persons have abnormalities on CT or MRI. CT employing myelography is the most sensitive test for evaluating subtle neural compression.

The natural history is generally benign and usually less than 2 months' duration. Over 75% of patients treated nonsurgically, even those with radiculopathy, have complete or near complete pain relief. The goals of treatment should therefore be to alleviate the pain, rehabilitate the patient to return to work, and improve fitness. Acute back pain due to a herniated disk should be treated with complete bed rest for 3 days and with analgesics. The bed rest allows the acute injury to subside. NSAIDs are especially useful. A short course of opioids may be indicated in patients with severe pain. After the acute symptoms subside, the patient should be sent to "back school" to improve back fitness. Physical therapy, including the application of cold or heat and massage, may also be helpful. Surgical decompression should be considered for patients with refractory pain, but a trial of epidural steroids should be considered first. For properly selected patients, laminectomy speeds recovery and reduces the incidence of recurrence.

When symptoms persist beyond 3 months, the pain may be considered chronic and to require a multidisciplinary approach. Physical therapy becomes a very important component of rehabilitation. NSAIDs and antidepressants are also helpful. Back supports should be discouraged because they may weaken paraspinal muscles.

Epidural Steroids

Epidural steroid injections are most effective for symptomatic relief of pain associated with nerve root compression (radiculopathy). Pathologic studies often demonstrate inflammation following disk herniation. Clinical improvement appears to correlate with the resolution of nerve root edema. Epidural steroid injections are clearly superior to local anesthetics alone. These injections are most effective when given within 2 weeks of

the onset of pain but appear to be of little benefit in the absence of neural compression or irritation. Long-term studies have failed to show any persistent benefit after 3 months.

The two most commonly used agents are methylprednisolone acetate (60–120 mg) and triamcinolone diacetate (50–75 mg). The steroid may be injected with diluent (saline) or local anesthetic in volumes of 6–10 mL or 10–20 mL for lumbar and caudal injections, respectively. Simultaneous injection of opioids offers no added benefit. The epidural needle should be cleared of the steroid prior to its withdrawal to prevent a formation of a fistula tract. Injection of local anesthetic along with the steroid can be helpful if the patient has significant muscle spasm, but it is associated with the risks of intrathecal, subdural, and intravascular complications (see Chapter 16). The local anesthetic provides immediate pain relief until the steroid's anti-inflammatory effects take place in 12–48 hours. The pain is often transiently intensified following injection. Epidural steroid injections may be most effective when injection is at the site of injury. Only a single injection is given if complete pain relief is achieved. If there is no initial response, a second injection may be given 1–4 weeks later. Most clinicians recommend only three injections because of the risk of adrenal suppression and systemic side effects.

Caudal injection may be preferable in patients with previous back surgery, because scarring and anatomic distortion often make lumbar epidural injections more difficult; unfortunately, the migration of the steroid to the site of injury may not be optimal. Subarachnoid steroid injections are not recommended because of the ethylene glycol preservative; this has been implicated in adhesive arachnoiditis following unintentional subarachnoid injections. Other reported complications include aseptic, cryptococcal, and tuberculous meningitis.

Spinal Stenosis

Degeneration of the nucleus pulposus reduces disk height and leads to osteophyte formation (spondylosis) at the rims of adjoining vertebral bodies and infolding of the spinal ligaments, leading to progressive narrowing of the intervertebral foramina and spinal canal. Neural compression can cause radiculopathy that mimics a herniated disk. Extensive osteophyte formation may compress multiple nerve roots and cause bilateral pain. When these growths encroach on the cauda equina, the term "spinal stenosis" is used.

Spinal stenosis is a disease of advancing age. The back pain usually radiates into both buttocks, thighs, and legs. It is characteristically worse with exercise and relieved by rest, especially sitting with the spine flexed. The term "pseudoclaudication" is occasionally used.

The diagnosis is suggested by the clinical presentation and confirmed by MRI, CT, or both of the spine, with myelography. Electromyography and somatosensory evoked potentials can be useful in evaluating neurologic compromise.

Conservative therapy and epidural steroids generally have a limited role. Patients with mild to moderate stenosis and radicular symptoms may benefit from epidural steroids. Severe symptoms are an indication for surgical decompression; the pseudoclaudication usually resolves but back pain may persist.

4. Facet Syndrome

Some patients complain of pain that is primarily related to degenerative changes in the facet (zygapophyseal) joints. The pain tends to be just off the midline and radiates down the back to the gluteal region, thigh, and knee; muscle spasm may also be present. Hyperextension and rotation of the spine usually exacerbates the pain. The diagnosis may be suggested by oblique radiographs or CT of the spine, and is confirmed by pain relief following intra-articular injection of local anesthetic into affected joints or blockade of the medial branch of the posterior division (ramus) of the spinal nerves that innervate them. Long-term studies suggest medial branch nerve blocks are more effective than facet joint injections. Medial branch rhizotomy can provide long-term analgesia for facet joint disease in the lumbar (and cervical) spine.

5. Congenital Abnormalities

Congenital abnormalities of the back are often asymptomatic and remain occult. Abnormal spinal mechanics may make the patient prone to back pain and in some instances progressive deformities. Common anomalies include sacralization of L5 (the vertebral body is fused to the sacrum), lumbarization of S1 (it functions as a sixth lumbar vertebra), spondylolysis (a bony defect develops between the pedicle and the lamina), and spondylolisthesis (the vertebral body, pedicles, and superior facet joints slide anteriorly leaving the posterior elements behind—most commonly at L5). The diagnosis is made radiographically. Spinal fusion may be necessary in patients with progressive symptoms and spinal instability.

6. Tumors

Spinal tumors in patients younger than 50 years old are generally benign, while those in older patients are usually malignant. Breast, lung, prostate, renal, gastrointestinal, and thyroid carcinomas, lymphomas, and multiple myelomas frequently metastasize to the lumbar spine. The pain is usually constant and may be associated with localized tenderness over involved vertebrae. Bony destruction, or neural or vascular compression produce the pain. Epidural or intradural tumors can present like a herniated disk and may rapidly progress to flaccid paralysis. The primary site may be asymptomatic or overlooked. The diagnosis is made radiographically or with a bone scan. Depending on the type of tumor, corticosteroids, radiation, or surgical decompression (with stabilization) may be indicated.

7. Infection

Bacterial infections of the spine usually affect the vertebral body, and can be due to pyogenic as well as tuberculous organisms. Patients, especially those with spinal tuberculosis, present with chronic back pain without fever or leukocytosis. In contrast, those with epidural abscesses present acutely with pain, fever, and leukocytosis; urgent surgical evacuation and antibiotic therapy are necessary to prevent progression to flaccid paralysis.

8. Arthritides

Ankylosing spondylitis is a familial disorder that is associated with histocompatibility antigen HLA-B27. It typically presents as low back pain associated with early morning stiffness in a young man. The pain has an insidious onset and may initially improve with activity. After a few months to years, the pain gradually intensifies and is associated with progressive restricted movement of the spine. Diagnosis can be difficult early in the disease, but radiographic evidence of sacroiliitis is usually present. As the disease progresses, the spine develops a characteristic "bamboo-like" radiographic appearance. Some patients develop arthritis of the hips and shoulders as well as extra-articular inflammatory manifestations. Treatment is primarily directed at maintaining functional preservation of posture. NSAIDs, especially indomethacin, are good analgesics and reduce the early morning stiffness.

Patients with Reiter's syndrome, psoriatic arthritis, or inflammatory bowel disease may also present with low back pain, but extraspinal manifestations are usually more prominent. Rheumatoid arthritis usually spares the spine except for the apophyseal joints of the cervical spine.

ACUTE HERPES ZOSTER & POSTHERPETIC NEURALGIA

Acute herpes zoster represents a reactivation of the varicella-zoster virus. During the initial childhood infection (chickenpox), the virus infects dorsal root ganglia, where it remains latent until reactivation. The disease presents as a vesicular, dermatomal rash that is usually associated with severe pain. Dermatomes T3–L3 are most commonly affected. The pain often precedes the rash by 48–72 hours; the rash usually lasts 1–2 weeks. Herpes zoster may occur at any age but is most common in elderly patients. It is typically a benign self-limited disorder in younger patients (< 50 years old). Treatment is primarily supportive consisting of oral analgesics and oral acyclovir or famciclovir. Antiviral therapy reduces the duration of the rash and speeds healing. Immunocompromised patients with disseminated infection require intravenous acyclovir therapy.

Older patients may continue to experience severe radicular pain, even after the rash resolves. The incidence of postherpetic neuralgia (PHN) is estimated to be 50% in patients older than 50 years of age. Moreover, PHN is often very difficult to treat. An oral course of corticosteroids during acute zoster may decrease the incidence of PHN but remains controversial. Corticosteroids may increase the likelihood of dissemination in immunocompromised patients. Sympathetic blockade during acute herpes zoster can produce excellent analgesia and is also reported to decrease the incidence of PHN. The latter suggests that PHN is sympathetically maintained. Studies suggest that when sympathetic blocks are initiated within 2 months of the rash, PHN resolves in up to 80% of patients. Once the neuralgia is well established, however, the sympathetic blocks (like other treatments) are generally ineffective. Antidepressants, anticonvulsants, opioids, and TENS may be useful in some patients. Application of a transdermal lidocaine patch 5% (Lidoderm, 700 mg) over the most painful area may help some patients.

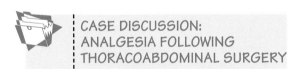

CASE DISCUSSION: ANALGESIA FOLLOWING THORACOABDOMINAL SURGERY

An obese 21-year-old male is admitted to the recovery room following a right thoracoabdominal lymph node dissection for a testicular malignant growth. The incision extends from the eighth rib to the pubis and a right thoracostomy (chest tube) is present. He had consented to an epidural catheter for managing his pain postoperatively. Unfortunately, placement of the catheter prior to surgery proved to be very difficult because of his obesity, and could not be accomplished. He is extubated and awakens from anesthesia in severe pain and is noted to have shallow breathing at a rate of 35/min ("splinting"). A total of 10 mg of morphine sulfate is given intravenously before he stops complaining of pain and becomes very drowsy again.

While the patient was receiving 50% oxygen by face mask, an arterial blood reading is as follows:

PaO_2, 58 mm Hg; $PaCO_2$, 53 mm Hg; pH, 7.25; and HCO_3^-, 21 mEq/L. The postoperative chest film reveals clear lung fields with diminished lung volumes.

Why is pain management very important in this patient?

The patient is at high risk for pulmonary complications because of his obesity and the extensive thoracoabdominal incision. He is unable to take deep breaths or cough effectively, and already has hypoxemia and respiratory acidosis. In fact, if his respiratory status cannot be improved promptly, endotracheal intubation and controlled mechanical should be considered. The chest film is very helpful in excluding residual right pneumothorax, significant hemothorax, or lobar atelectasis that could explain his marginal respiratory status. The most likely explanation of these findings is inadequate pain relief combined with opioid-induced respiratory depression. The hypoxemia is most likely due to microatelectasis and a low functional residual capacity (see Chapter 22), while the hypoventilation is due to splinting from incisional pain, residual effects of intraoperative anesthetics (including opioids), and postoperative morphine. Clearly, satisfactory opioid analgesia could not be obtained in this patient without significant respiratory depression and oversedation. Additional, more effective analgesic measures are indicated if postoperative mechanical ventilation is to be avoided.

What additional options are available to manage his pain more optimally?

Additional intravenous opioids would likely aggravate the respiratory depression and are to be avoided (unless the patient is reintubated). Intrathecal opioid administration may provide relatively rapid analgesia for the abdominal part of the incision but will require several hours for analgesia of its thoracic extension; the technique also predisposes to delayed respiratory depression. Moreover, performing a lumbar puncture in this setting is likely to be as difficult or more difficult than placing an epidural catheter preoperatively.

Intravenous ketorolac can offer additional analgesia without respiratory depression and can significantly reduce opioid requirements. The use of ketorolac immediately following such extensive surgical dissections, however, may be hazardous because of its antiplatelet effects and risk of postoperative hemorrhage.

Ketamine in low doses (10–20 mg/hour) is a very potent analgesic and is not a respiratory depressant. In higher doses, it is more likely to cause excessive sedation and psychotomimetic effects. Although a ketamine infusion may be a reasonable option, concerns about oversedating this patient are justified.

Multiple intercostal blocks (see Chapter 17) can provide excellent analgesia for thoracic incisions and are indicated in this patient. Splinting can be abolished, and vital capacity and arterial blood gases often improve. Four to five mL of 0.25% bupivacaine can be injected at the appropriate dermatomal levels where the rib can be palpated. Moreover, because the patient already has a chest tube, the risk of a significant pneumothorax is minimal. A similarly effective technique that may be easier to perform in this obese patient is interpleural analgesia.

What is interpleural analgesia?

The technique can provide analgesia over the chest wall and upper abdomen. It involves placement of a catheter into a tissue plane within the chest wall such that a single injection of local anesthetic spreads to several intercostal nerves. The terms "intrapleural" and "interpleural" have been used interchangeably, but the latter is generally preferred.

What is the anatomic basis of interpleural analgesia?

The intercostal space posteriorly has three layers: the external intercostal muscle, the posterior intercostal membrane (which is the aponeurosis of the internal intercostal muscle), and the intercostalis intimus muscle (part of the transversus thoracis group of muscles which are a continuation of the transversus abdominis). Intercostal nerves lie in between the posterior intercostal membrane and the intercostalis intimus muscle. While the posterior intercostal membrane forms a complete barrier beneath the external intercostal muscle, the intercostalis intimus muscle is incomplete and freely allows fluid to pass into the subpleural space. Thus, interpleural analgesia can be accomplished by placing a catheter either deep to the internal intercostal muscle but superficial to the parietal pleura, or between the parietal and visceral layers of the pleura. In either case, the local anesthetic injected will diffuse to adjacent intercostal nerves. The number of nerves affected depends on the level of the catheter, the volume of anesthetic injected, and the effects of gravity. In some instances the local anesthetic may reach the paravertebral space.

How is interpleural anesthesia performed?

A single epidural catheter is most commonly inserted through a Tuohy needle at a level between T6 and T8. The needle is inserted at a point anywhere between 8 cm lateral to the posterior midline and the posterior axillary line. It is then "walked off" the inferior edge of the rib (see intercostal nerve block, Chapter 17) and advanced to a position either just deep to the posterior intercostal membrane just beneath a rib, or between the parietal and visceral space. In the first instance, a "pop" may be encountered as the needle pierces the posterior intercostal membrane. In the second instance, a loss of resistance technique (similar to that for epidural anesthesia) can be used to identify entry into the pleural cavity. The catheter is then advanced 3–6 cm past the tip of the needle and fixed in position as the needle is withdrawn. Twenty to 25 mL of local anesthetic (usually 0.25% bupivacaine) is then injected. The mean duration of analgesia with bupivacaine is about 7 hours (range 2–18 hours). Peak plasma concentrations of the local anesthetic occur 15–20 minutes after injection. Adding epinephrine to the bupivacaine solution reduces and slightly delays the peak plasma concentration. Continuous infusions have also been employed at a rate of 0.125 mL/kg/hour.

What are other indications for interpleural analgesia?

Interpleural analgesia is most effective in providing analgesia to patients with multiple rib fractures and those who have undergone open cholecystectomy. Postoperative analgesia is inconsistent following thoracotomy when multiple chest tubes are in place and a significant amount of blood is likely to be present in the chest; a significant amount of the local anesthetic may be lost through the chest. The technique can also be used for chest wall pain due to cancer, acute herpes zoster, and postherpetic neuralgia.

What are the hazards of interpleural anesthesia?

Pneumothorax is a significant risk if a chest tube is not already in place. Unilateral sympathetic block may be observed and can result in a Horner's syndrome. Chest wall hematoma has been reported. Systemic absorption is significant; high plasma concentrations of local anesthetics can be observed with continuous infusions, espe-

cially after 2 days. Fortunately, clinical reports of systemic toxicity (seizures) are rare. Rarely, the local anesthetic can spread to the epidural space.

SUGGESTED READING

Abram SE, Hogan QH: Neural blockade for diagnosis and prognosis: a review. Anesthesiology 1997;86:216.

Abram SE: Treatment of lumbosacral radiculopathy with epidural steroids. Anesthesiology 1999;91:1937.

Aeschbach A, Mekhail NA: Common nerve blocks in chronic pain management. Anesth Clin North Am 2000;18:429.

Aronoff GM: *Evaluation & Treatment of Chronic Pain.* Lippincott Williams & Wilkins, 1999.

Brown DL: *Atlas of Regional Anesthesia,* 2nd ed. WB Saunders and Company, 1999.

Chelly JE: *Peripheral Nerve Blocks; A Color Atlas.* Lippincott Williams & Wilkins, 1999.

Collett B-J: Opioid tolerance: The clinical perspective. Br J Anaesth 1998;81:58.

Cousins MJ: *Neural Blockade in Clinical Anesthesia and Pain Management,* 3rd ed. Lippincott Williams & Wilkins, 1998.

Cousins MJ: Pain: The past, present and future of anesthesiology? Anesthesiology 1999;91:538.

Desborough JP: The stress response to trauma and surgery. Br J Anaesth 2000;85:109.

Dougherty PM, Staats PS: Intrathecal drug therapy for patients with chronic pain. Anesthesiology 1999;91:1891.

Duthie DJR: Remifentanil and tramadol. Br J Anaesth 1998;81:51.

Finucane BT: *Complications of Regional Anesthesia.* Churchill Livingstone, 1999.

Grubb BD: Peripheral and central mechanisms of pain. Br J Anaesth 1998;81:8.

Hollmann MW, Durieux ME: Local anesthetics and the inflammatory response. Anesthgesiology 2000;93:858.

Jacobson L, Mariano AJ, Chabal C, Chaney EF: Beyond the needle: Expanding the role of anesthesiologists in the management of chronic non-malignant pain. Anesthesiology 1997;87:1210.

Jankovic D, Wells C: *Regional Nerve Blocks.* Blackwell Science, 2000.

Jordan B, Devi LA: Molecular mechanisms of opioid receptor signal transduction. Br J Anaesth 1998;81:12.

Kamibayashi T, Maze M: Clinical uses of α_2-adrenergic agonists. Anesthesiology 2000;93:1345.

Kissin I: Preemptive analgesia. Anesthesiology 2000;93:1138.

Kohrs R, Durieux ME: Ketamine: teaching an old drug new tricks. Anesth Analg 1998;87:1186.

Loeser JD, Butler SH, Chapman CR: *Bonica's Management of Pain.* Lippincott Williams & Wilkins, 2001.

Macintyre PE, Ready LB: *Acute Pain Management: A Practical Guide,* 2nd edition. WB Saunders and Company, 2001.

Mayers I, Johnson D: The nonspecific inflammatory response to injury. Can J Anaesth 1998;45:871.

Morton NS: *Acute Paediatric Pain Management.* WB Saunders and Company, 1998

Park GR, Fulton B, Senthuran S: *Management of Acute Pain.* Oxford University Press, 2000.

Peng PWH, Sandler AN: A review of the use of fentanyl analgesia in the management of acute pain in adults. Anesthesiology 1999;90:576.

Perkins FM, Kehlet H: Chronic pain as an outcome of surgery. Anesthesiology 2000;93:1123.

Practice Guidelines for Chronic Pain Management: A Report by the American Society of Anesthesiologists Task Force on Pain Management, Chronic Pain Section. Anesthesiology 1997;86:995.

Raj PP: *Practical Management of Pain,* 3rd ed. Mosby, 2000.

Richardson J, Lönnqvist PA: Thoracic paravertebral block. Br J Anaesth 1998;81:230.

Rosenberg AD, Grande C, Bernstein RL: *Pain Management and Regional Anesthesia in Trauma.* WB Saunders and Company, 1999.

Sear JW: Recent advances and developments in the clinical use of i.v. opioids during the perioperative period. Br J Anaesth 1998;81:38.

Stanton-Hicks M, Baron R, Boas R, et al: Complex regional pain syndromes: Guidelines for therapy. Clin J Pain 1998;14:155.

Stein C: Opioid treatment of chronic nonmalignant pain. Anesth Analg 1997;84:912.

Steinbrook RA: Epidural anesthesia and gastrointestinal motility. Anesth Analg 1998;86:837.

Thomas S: *Image Guided Pain Management.* Lippincott Williams & Wilkins, 1997.

Waldman SD: *Atlas of Pain Management Injection Techniques.* WB Saunders and Company, 2000.

Waldman SD: *Interventional Pain Management,* 2nd ed. WB Saunders and Company, 2001.

Wall PD, Melzack OC: *Textbook of Pain,* 4th ed. Churchill Livingstone, 2000.

Warfield C: *Principles & Practice of Pain Management,* 2nd ed. McGraw-Hill, 2001.

SECTION IV

Physiology, Pathophysiology, & Anesthetic Management

Cardiovascular Physiology & Anesthesia

19

KEY CONCEPTS

 In contrast to action potentials in neurons, the spike in cardiac action potentials is followed by a plateau phase that lasts 0.2–0.3 seconds. While the action potential for skeletal muscle and nerves is due to abrupt opening of fast sodium channels in the cell membrane, that in cardiac muscle is due to the opening of both fast sodium channels (the spike) and slower calcium channels (the plateau).

 Halothane, enflurane, and isoflurane depress sinoatrial (SA) node automaticity. These agents appear to have only modest direct effects on the atrioventricular (AV) node, prolonging conduction time and increasing refractoriness. This combination of effects likely explains the frequent occurrence of junctional tachycardia when an anticholinergic is administered for sinus bradycardia during inhalational anesthesia; junctional pacemakers are accelerated more than those in the SA node.

 Studies suggest that all volatile anesthetics depress cardiac contractility by decreasing the entry of Ca^{2+} into cells during depolarization (affecting T- and L-type calcium channels), altering the kinetics of its release and uptake into the sarcoplasmic reticulum, and decreasing the sensitivity of contractile proteins to calcium.

 Because the normal cardiac index (CI) has a wide range, it is a relatively insensitive measurement of ventricular performance. Abnormalities in CI therefore usually reflect gross ventricular impairment.

 The mixed venous oxygen tension (or saturation) is the best measurement for determining the adequacy of cardiac output, in the absence of hypoxia or severe anemia.

 Because the atrial contribution to ventricular filling is important in maintaining low mean

(continued)

(continued)

ventricular diastolic pressures, patients with reduced ventricular compliance are most affected by loss of a normally timed atrial systole.

 Cardiac output in patients with marked right or left ventricular impairment is very sensitive to acute increases in afterload.

 Ventricular ejection fraction, the fraction of the end-diastolic ventricular volume ejected, is the most commonly used clinical measurement of systolic function.

 Left ventricular diastolic function can be assessed clinically by Doppler echocardiography on a transthoracic or transesophageal examination.

 Because the endocardium is subjected to the greatest intramural pressures during systole, it tends to be most vulnerable to ischemia during decreases in coronary perfusion pressure.

 The failing heart becomes increasingly dependent on circulating catecholamines. Abrupt withdrawal in sympathetic outflow or decreases in circulating catecholamine levels, such as can occur following induction of anesthesia, may lead to acute cardiac decompensation.

Anesthesiologists must have a thorough understanding of cardiovascular physiology both for its scientific significance in anesthesia and for its practical applications to modern patient management. This chapter reviews the physiology of the heart and the systemic circulation and the pathophysiology of heart failure. The pulmonary circulation and the physiology of blood and nutrient exchange are discussed in Chapters 22 and 28, respectively.

The circulatory system consists of the heart, the blood vessels, and the blood. Its function is to provide tissues with oxygen and nutrients and to carry away the by-products of metabolism. The heart propels blood through two vascular systems arranged in series. In the pulmonary circulation, blood flows past the alveolar-capillary membrane, takes up oxygen, and eliminates CO_2. In the systemic circulation, oxygenated blood is pumped to metabolizing tissues, and the by-products of metabolism are taken up for elimination by the lungs, kidneys, or liver.

■ THE HEART

Although anatomically one organ, the heart can be functionally divided into right and left pumps, each consisting of an atrium and a ventricle. The atria serve as both conduits and priming pumps, while the ventricles act as the major pumping chambers. The right ventricle receives systemic venous (deoxygenated) blood and pumps it into the pulmonary circulation, while the left ventricle receives pulmonary venous (oxygenated)

blood and pumps it into the systemic circulation. Four valves normally ensure unidirectional flow through each chamber. The normal pumping action of the heart is the result of a complex series of electrical and mechanical events.

The heart consists of specialized striated muscle in a connective tissue skeleton. Cardiac muscle can be divided into atrial, ventricular, and specialized pacemaker and conducting cells. The self-excitatory nature of cardiac muscle cells and their unique organization allow the heart to function as a highly efficient pump. Serial low-resistance connections (intercalated disks) between individual myocardial cells allow the rapid and orderly spread of electrical activity in each pumping chamber. Electrical activity readily spreads from one atrium to another and from one ventricle to another via specialized conduction pathways. The absence of direct connections between the atria and ventricles except through the atrioventricular (AV) node delays conduction and enables atrial contraction to prime the ventricle.

CARDIAC ACTION POTENTIALS

The myocardial cell membrane is normally permeable to K^+ but relatively impermeable to Na^+. A membrane-bound Na^+-K^+ adenosine triphosphatase (ATPase) concentrates K^+ intracellularly in exchange for extrusion of Na^+ out of cells (see Chapter 28). Intracellular sodium concentration is kept low, whereas intracellular potassium concentration is kept high relative to the extracellular space. Relative impermeability of the membrane to calcium also maintains a high extracellular to cytoplasmic calcium gradient. Movement of K^+ out of the cell and down its concentration gradient results in a net loss of positive charges from inside the cell. An electrical potential is established across the cell membrane, with the inside of the cell negative with respect to the extracellular environment, because anions do not accompany K^+. Thus, the resting membrane potential represents the balance between two opposing forces: the movement of K^+ down its concentration gradient and the electrical attraction of the negatively charged intracellular space for the positively charged potassium ions.

Normal ventricular cell resting membrane potential is -80 to -90 mV. As with other excitable tissues (nerve and skeletal muscle), when the cell membrane potential becomes less negative and reaches a threshold value, a characteristic action potential (depolarization) develops (Figure 19–1 and Table 19–1). The action potential transiently raises myocardial cell membrane potential to +20 mV. In contrast to action potentials in neurons (see Chapter 14), the spike in cardiac action potentials is followed by a plateau phase that lasts 0.2–0.3 seconds. While the action potential for skeletal muscle and nerves is due to abrupt opening of fast sodium channels in the cell membrane, that in cardiac muscle is due to the opening of both fast sodium channels (the spike) and slower calcium channels (the plateau). Depolarization is also accompanied by a transient decrease in potassium permeability. Subsequent restoration of normal potassium permeability and closure of sodium and calcium channels eventually restores membrane potential to normal.

Following depolarization, the cells are typically refractory to subsequent normal depolarizing stimuli until phase 4. The effective refractory period is the minimum interval between two depolarizing impulses that are propagated. In fast-conducting myocardial cells, this period is generally closely correlated with the duration of the action potential. In contrast, the effective refractory period in slowly conducting myocardial cells can outlast the duration of the action potential.

Table 19–2 lists the multiple types of ion channels in cardiac muscle membrane. Some are activated by a change in cell membrane voltage, while others open only when bound by ligands. The voltage-gated fast Na^+ channel has an outer (m) gate that opens at -60 to -70 mV and an inner (h) gate that then closes at -30 mV. T-type (transient) voltage-gated calcium channels play a role in phase 0 of depolarization. During the plateau phase (phase 2), calcium inflow occurs through slow L-type, voltage-gated calcium channels. Three major types of K^+ channels are responsible for repolarization. The first results in a transient outward potassium current (I_{T_o}), the second is responsible for a short rectifying current (I_{Kr}), and the third produces a slowly acting rectifying current (I_{Ks}) that restores cell membrane potential to normal.

INITIATION & CONDUCTION OF THE CARDIAC IMPULSE

The cardiac impulse normally originates in the **sinoatrial (SA) node,** a group of specialized pacemaker cells in the sulcus terminalis, posteriorly at the junction of the right atrium with the superior vena cava. These cells appear to have an outer membrane that leaks sodium (and possibly calcium). The slow influx of sodium results in a less negative, resting membrane potential (-50 to -60 mV) and has three important conse-

Table 19–1. Cardiac action potential.

Phase	Name	Event	Cellular Ion Movement
0	Upstroke	Activation (opening) of fast Na^+ channels	Na^+ in and decreased permeability to K^+
1	Early rapid repolarization	Inactivation of Na^+ channel and transient increase in K^+ permeability	K^+ out (I_{T_o})
2	Plateau	Activation of slow Ca^{2+} channels	Ca^{2+} in
3	Final repolarization	Inactivation of Ca^{2+} channels and increased permeability to K^+	K^+ out
4	Resting potential or Diastolic repolarization	Normal permeability restored (atrial and ventricular cells) Intrinsic slow leakage of sodium and possibly Ca^{2+} into cells that spontaneously depolarize	K^+ out Na^+ in ? Ca^{2+} in

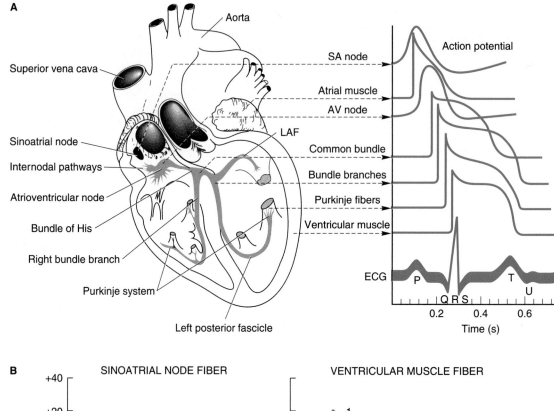

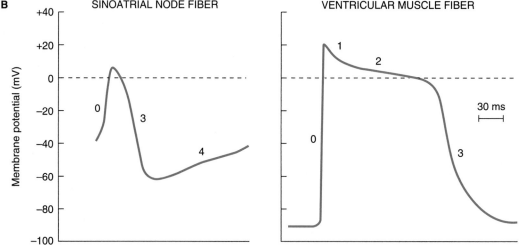

Figure 19–1. Cardiac action potentials. **A:** Note the characteristic action potentials of different parts of the heart. **B:** Pacemaker cells in the SA node lack the same distinct phases as atrial and ventricular muscle cells and display prominent spontaneous diastolic depolarization. See Table 19–1 for an explanation of the different phases of the action potential. (Modified and reproduced, with permission, from Ganong WF: *Review of Medical Physiology,* 20th ed. McGraw-Hill, 2001.)

Table 19–2. Cardiac ion channels.

Voltage-gated
Na^+
$T\ Ca^{2+}$
$L\ Ca^{2+}$
K^+
   Transient outward
   Inward rectifying
   Slow (delayed) rectifying
Ligand-gated K^+ channels
Ca^{2+}-activated
Na^+-activated
ATP-sensitive
Acetylcholine-activated
Arachadonic acid—activated

ATP = adenosine triphosphate.

quences: constant inactivation of fast sodium channels, an action potential with a threshold of −40 mV that is primarily due to ion movement across the slow calcium channels, and regular spontaneous depolarizations. During each cycle, intracellular leakage of sodium causes the cell membrane to become progressively less negative; when threshold potential is reached, calcium channels open, potassium permeability decreases, and an action potential develops. Restoration of normal potassium permeability returns the cells in the SA node to their normal resting membrane potential.

The impulse generated at the SA node is normally rapidly conducted across the atria and to the AV node. Specialized atrial fibers may speed up conduction to both the left atrium and the AV node. The **AV node,** which is located in the septal wall of the right atrium just anterior to the opening of the coronary sinus and above the insertion of the septal leaflet of the tricuspid valve, is actually made up of three distinct areas: an upper junctional (AN) region, a middle nodal (N) region, and a lower junctional (NH) region. Although the N region does not possess intrinsic spontaneous activity (automaticity), both junctional areas do. The normally slower rate of spontaneous depolarization in AV junctional areas (40–60 times/min) allows the faster SA node to control heart rate. Any factor that decreases the rate of SA node depolarization or increases the automaticity of AV junctional areas allows the junctional areas to function as the pacemaker for the heart.

Impulses from the SA node normally reach the AV node after about 0.04 seconds but leave after another 0.11 seconds. This delay is the result of the slowly conducting small myocardial fibers within the AV node, which depend on slow calcium channels for propagation of the action potential. In contrast, conduction of the impulse between adjoining cells in the atria and in the ventricles is due primarily to activation and inactivation of the fast sodium channels. The lower fibers of the AV node combine to form the **common bundle of His.** This specialized group of fibers passes into the interventricular septum before dividing into left and right branches to form the complex network of **Purkinje fibers** that depolarizes both ventricles. In sharp contrast to AV nodal tissue, His-Purkinje fibers have the fastest conduction velocities in the heart, resulting in nearly simultaneous depolarization of the entire endocardium of both ventricles (normally within 0.03 sec). Spread of the impulse from the endocardium to the epicardium through ventricular muscle requires an additional 0.03 seconds. Thus, an impulse arising from the SA node normally requires less than 0.2 seconds to depolarize the entire heart.

 Halothane, enflurane, and isoflurane depress SA node automaticity. These agents appear to have only modest direct effects on the AV node, prolonging conduction time and increasing refractoriness. This combination of effects likely explains the frequent occurrence of junctional tachycardia when an anticholinergic is administered for sinus bradycardia during inhalational anesthesia; junctional pacemakers are accelerated more than those in the SA node. The electrophysiologic effects of volatile agents on Purkinje fibers and ventricular muscle are complex due to autonomic interactions. Both antiarrhythmic and arrhythmogenic properties are described. The former may be due to direct depression of Ca^{2+} influxes, while the latter generally involves potentiation of catecholamines (see Chapter 7). The arrhythmogenic effect requires activation of both α_1- and β-adrenergic receptors. Intravenous induction agents have limited electrophysiologic effects in usual clinical doses. Opioids, especially fentanyl and sufentanil, can depress cardiac conduction, increasing AV node conduction and refractory period as well as prolonging Purkinje fiber action potential duration.

Local anesthetics have important electrophysiologic effects on the heart at blood concentrations that are generally associated with systemic toxicity. In the case of lidocaine, electrophysiologic effects at low blood concentrations can be therapeutic (see Chapter 48). At high blood concentrations, local anesthetics depress conduction by binding to fast sodium channels; at extremely high concentrations they also depress the SA node. The most potent local anesthetics—bupivacaine and, to lesser degrees, etidocaine and ropivacaine—appear to have the greatest effects on the heart, especially on Purkinje fibers and ventricular muscle. Bupivacaine binds inactivated fast sodium channels and dissociates from them slowly. It can cause profound sinus bradycardia and sinus node arrest as well as malignant ventricular arrhythmias.

Calcium channel blockers are organic compounds that block calcium influx through L-type but not T-type channels. Dihydropyridine blockers such as nifedipine simply plug the channel, whereas other agents such as verapamil and, to a lesser extent, diltiazem preferentially bind the channel in its depolarized inactivated state (use-dependent blockade).

MECHANISM OF CONTRACTION

Myocardial cells contract as a result of the interaction of two overlapping, rigid contractile proteins, **actin** and **myosin.** These proteins are fixed in position within each cell during both contraction and relaxation. Cell shortening occurs when the two proteins are allowed to fully interact and slide over one another (Figure 19–2). This interaction is normally prevented by two regulatory proteins, **troponin** and **tropomyosin;** troponin is made up of three subunits, troponin I, troponin C, and troponin T. Troponin is attached to actin at regular intervals, while tropomyosin lies within the center of the actin structure. An increase in intracellular calcium concentration (from about 10^{-7} to 10^{-5} mol/L) promotes contraction as calcium ions bind troponin C. The resulting conformational change in these regulatory proteins exposes the active sites on actin that allow interaction with myosin bridges (points of overlapping). The active site on myosin functions as a magnesium-dependent ATPase whose activity is enhanced by the increase in intracellular calcium concentration. A series of attachments and disengagements occur as each myosin bridge advances over successive active sites on actin. Adenosine triphosphate (ATP) is consumed during each attachment. Relaxation occurs as calcium is actively pumped back into the sarcoplasmic reticulum by a Ca^{2+}-Mg^{2+} ATPase; the resulting drop in intracellular calcium concentration allows the troponin-tropomyosin complex to again prevent the interaction between actin and myosin.

Excitation-Contraction Coupling

The quantity of calcium required to initiate contraction exceeds that entering the cell through slow channels during phase 2. The small amount that does enter through slow channels triggers the release of much larger amounts of calcium stored intracellularly (**calcium-dependent calcium release**) within cisterns in the sarcoplasmic reticulum.

The action potential of muscle cells depolarizes their T systems, tubular extensions of the cell membrane that transverse the cell in close approximation to the muscle fibrils, via dihydropyridine receptors (voltage-gated Ca^{2+} channels). This initial increase in intracellular Ca^{2+} triggers an even greater calcium inflow across ryanodine receptors, a nonvoltage-dependent calcium channel, in the sarcoplasmic reticulum. The force of contraction is directly dependent on the magnitude of the initial calcium influx. During relaxation, when the slow channels close, a membrane-bound ATPase actively transports calcium back into the sarcoplasmic reticulum. Calcium is also extruded extracellularly by an exchange of intracellular calcium for extracellular sodium by an ATPase in the cell membrane. Thus, relaxation of the heart also requires ATP.

The quantity of intracellular Ca^{2+} available, its rate of delivery, and its rate of removal determine, respectively, the maximum tension developed, the rate of contraction, and the rate of relaxation. Sympathetic stimulation increases the force of contraction by raising intracellular calcium concentration via a β_1-adrenergic receptor–mediated increase in intracellular cyclic adenosine monophosphate (cAMP) (see Chapter 12), through the action of a stimulatory G-protein (see Chapter 18). The increase in cAMP recruits additional open calcium channels. Moreover, adrenergic agonists enhance the rate of relaxation by enhancing calcium reuptake by the sarcoplasmic reticulum. Phosphodiesterase inhibitors, such as theophylline, amrinone, and milrinone produce similar effects by preventing the breakdown of intracellular cAMP. Digitalis increases intracellular calcium concentration through inhibition of the membrane-bound Na^+-K^+ ATPase; the resulting small increase in intracellular Na^+ allows for a greater influx of Ca^{2+} via the Na^+-Ca^{2+} exchange mechanism. Glucagon enhances contractility by increasing intracellular cAMP levels via activation of a specific nonadrenergic receptor. In contrast, release of acetylcholine following vagal stimulation depresses contractility through increased cyclic guanosine monophosphate (cGMP) levels and inhibition of adenylyl cyclase; these effects are mediated by an inhibitory G-protein. Acidosis blocks slow calcium channels and therefore also depresses cardiac contractility by unfavorably altering intracellular calcium kinetics.

Studies suggest that all volatile anesthetics depress cardiac contractility by decreasing the entry of Ca^{2+} into cells during depolarization (affecting T- and L-type calcium channels), altering the kinetics of its release and uptake into the sarcoplasmic reticulum, and decreasing the sensitivity of contractile proteins to calcium. Halothane and enflurane appear to depress contractility more than isoflurane, sevoflurane, and desflurane. Anesthetic-induced cardiac depression is potentiated by hypocalcemia, β-adrenergic blockade, and calcium channel blockers. Nitrous oxide also produces dose-dependent decreases in contractility by reducing intracellular Ca^{2+} availability during contraction. The mechanisms of direct cardiac depression from intravenous anesthetics are not well established but

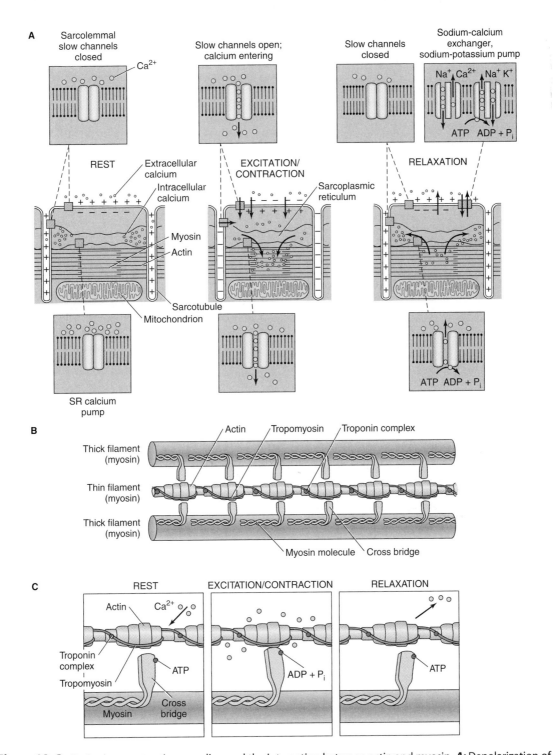

Figure 19–2. Excitation-contraction coupling and the interaction between actin and myosin. **A:** Depolarization of the muscle cell membrane allows entry of calcium into the cell and release of calcium stored in the sarcoplasmic reticulum. **B:** The structure of the actin-myosin complex. **C:** Calcium binds troponin, allowing the interaction between actin and myosin. (Modified and reproduced, with permission, from Katz AM, Smith VE: Hosp Pract 1985;19:69; and from Braunwald E: The Myocardium: *Failure and Infarction.* HP Publishing, 1974.)

presumably involve similar actions. Of all the major intravenous induction agents, ketamine appears to have the least direct depressant effect on contractility. Local anesthetic agents also depress cardiac contractility by reducing calcium influx and release in a dose-dependent fashion. Bupivacaine, tetracaine, and ropivacaine cause greater depression than lidocaine and chloroprocaine.

INNERVATION OF THE HEART

Parasympathetic fibers primarily innervate the atria and conducting tissues. Acetylcholine acts on specific cardiac muscarinic receptors (M_2) to produce negative chronotropic, dromotropic, and inotropic effects. In contrast, sympathetic fibers are more widely distributed throughout the heart. Cardiac sympathetic fibers originate in the thoracic spinal cord (T1–T4) and travel to the heart initially through the cervical ganglia (stellate), then as the cardiac nerves. Norepinephrine release causes positive chronotropic, dromotropic, and inotropic effects primarily through activation of β_1-adrenergic receptors. β_2-Adrenergic receptors are fewer in number and mainly found in the atria; activation increases heart rate and to a lesser extent contractility. α_1-Adrenergic receptors have a positive inotropic effect.

Cardiac autonomic innervation has an apparent *sidedness,* because the right sympathetic and right vagus nerves primarily affect the SA node while the left sympathetic and vagus nerves principally affect the AV node. Vagal effects frequently have a very rapid onset and resolution, while sympathetic influences generally have a more gradual onset and dissipation. Sinus arrhythmia is a cyclic variation in heart rate that correspond to respiration (increasing with inspiration and decreasing during expiration); it is due to cyclic changes in vagal tone.

THE CARDIAC CYCLE

The cardiac cycle can be defined by both electrical and mechanical events (Figure 19–3). *Systole* refers to contraction, while *diastole* refers to relaxation. Most diastolic ventricular filling occurs passively before atrial contraction. Contraction of the atria normally contributes 20–30% of ventricular filling. Three waves can generally be identified on atrial pressure tracings (Figure 19–3). The *a* **wave** is due to atrial systole. The *c* **wave** coincides with ventricular contraction and is said to be caused by bulging of the AV valve into the atrium. The *v* **wave** is due to the pressure buildup from venous return before the AV valve opens again. The *x* **descent** is the decline in pressure between the *c* and *v* waves and is thought to be due to a pulling down of the atrium by ventricular contraction. Incompetence of the AV valve on either side of the heart abolishes the *x* descent on that side, resulting in a prominent *cv* **wave.**

The *y* **descent** follows the *v* wave and represents the decline in atrial pressure as the AV valve opens. The notch in the aortic pressure tracing is referred to as the **incisura** and represents transient backflow of blood into the left ventricle just before aortic valve closure.

DETERMINANTS OF VENTRICULAR PERFORMANCE

Discussions of ventricular function usually refer to the left ventricle, but the same concepts apply to the right ventricle. Although the ventricles are often thought of as functioning separately, their interdependence has clearly been demonstrated. Moreover, factors affecting systolic and diastolic functions can be differentiated: Systolic function involves ventricular ejection, while diastolic function is related to ventricular filling.

Ventricular systolic function is most often equated with **cardiac output,** which can be defined as the volume of blood pumped by the heart per minute. Because the two ventricles function in series, their outputs are normally equal. Cardiac output (CO) is expressed by the following equation:

$$CO = SV \times HR$$

where SV is the stroke volume (the volume pumped per contraction) and HR is heart rate. To compensate for variations in body size, CO is often expressed in terms of total body surface area:

$$CI = \frac{CO}{BSA}$$

where CI is the **cardiac index** and BSA is total body surface area. BSA is usually obtained from nomograms based on height and weight. Normal CI is 2.5–4.2 L/min/m². Because the normal CI has a wide range, it is a relatively insensitive measurement of ventricular performance. Abnormalities in CI therefore usually reflect gross ventricular impairment. A more accurate assessment can be obtained if the response of the cardiac output to exercise is evaluated. Under these conditions, failure of the cardiac output to increase and keep up with oxygen consumption is reflected by a falling mixed venous oxygen saturation (see Chapter 22). A decrease in mixed venous oxygen saturation in response to increased demand usually reflects inadequate tissue perfusion. Thus, in the absence of hypoxia or severe anemia, the mixed venous oxygen tension (or saturation) is the best measurement for determining the adequacy of cardiac output.

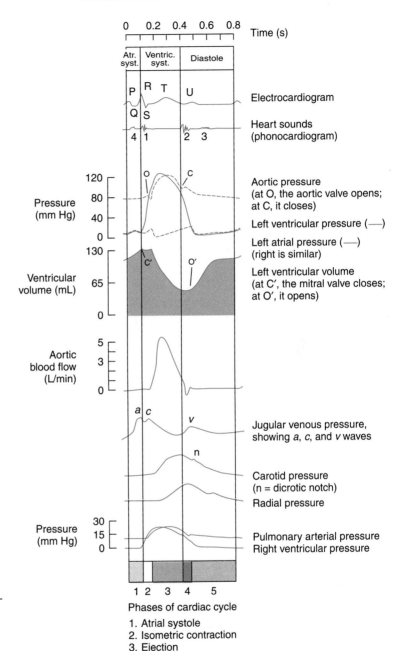

Figure 19–3. The normal cardiac cycle. Note the correspondence between electrical and mechanical events. (Modified and reproduced, with permission, from Ganong WF: *Review of Medical Physiology,* 20th ed. McGraw-Hill, 2001.)

1. Heart Rate

Cardiac output is generally directly proportional to heart rate (Figure 19–4). Heart rate is an intrinsic function of the SA node (spontaneous depolarization) but is modified by autonomic, humoral, and local factors. The normal intrinsic rate of the SA node in young adults is about 90–100 beats/min, but it decreases with age according to the following formula:

$$\text{Normal intrinsic heart rate} = 118 \text{ beats/min} - (0.57 \times \text{age})$$

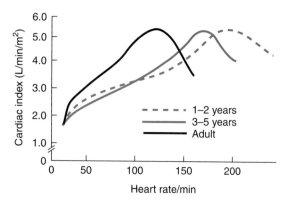

Figure 19–4. The relationship between heart rate and cardiac index. (Reproduced, with permission, from Wetsel RC: *Critical Care: State of the Art 1981.* Society of Critical Care Medicine, 1981.)

Enhanced vagal activity slows the heart rate via stimulation of M_2 cholinergic receptors, while enhanced sympathetic activity increases heart rate mainly through activation of β_1-adrenergic receptors and, to lesser extent, β_2-adrenergic receptors (see above).

2. Stroke Volume

Stroke volume is normally determined by three major factors: **preload, afterload,** and **contractility.** This analysis is analogous to laboratory observations on skeletal muscle preparations. Preload is muscle length prior to contraction, while afterload is the tension against which the muscle must contract. Contractility is an intrinsic property of the muscle that is related to the force of contraction but independent of both preload and afterload. Since the heart is a three-dimensional multichambered pump, both ventricular geometric form and valvular dysfunction can also affect stroke volume (Table 19–3).

Preload

Ventricular preload is end-diastolic volume, which is generally dependent on ventricular filling. The relationship between cardiac output and left ventricular end-diastolic volume is known as **Starling's law of the heart** (Figure 19–5). Note that when the heart rate is constant, cardiac output is directly proportional to preload, until excessive end-diastolic volumes are reached. At that point cardiac output does not appreciably change—or may even decrease. Overdistention of either ventricle can lead to excessive dilatation and incompetence of the AV valves.

Table 19–3. Major factors affecting cardiac stroke volume.

Preload
Afterload
Contractility
Wall motion abnormalities
Valvular dysfunction

A. DETERMINANTS OF VENTRICULAR FILLING:

Ventricular filling can be influenced by a variety of factors (Table 19–4), of which the most important is venous return. Because most of the other factors affecting venous return are usually fixed, venous tone is normally its major determinant. Increases in metabolic activity enhance venous tone, so that venous return to the heart increases as the volume of venous capacitance vessels decreases. Changes in blood volume and venous tone are important causes of intraoperative and postoperative changes in ventricular filling and cardiac output. Any factor that alters the normally small venous pressure gradient favoring blood return to the heart also affects cardiac filling. Such factors include changes in intrathoracic pressure (positive pressure ventilation or thoracotomy), posture (positioning during surgery), and pericardial pressure (pericardial disease).

The most important determinant of right ventricular preload is venous return. In the absence of significant pulmonary or right ventricular dysfunction, venous return is also the major determinant of left ventricular preload. Normally, the end-diastolic volumes of both ventricles are similar.

Both heart rate and rhythm can also affect ventricular preload. Increases in heart rate are associated with proportionately greater reductions in diastole than systole. Ventricular filling therefore progressively becomes impaired at high heart rates (> 120 beats/min in adults). Absent (atrial fibrillation), ineffective (atrial flutter), or altered timing of atrial contraction (low atrial or junctional rhythms) can also reduce ventricular fill- ing by 20–30%. Because the atrial contribution to ventricular filling is important in maintaining low mean ventricular diastolic pressures, patients with reduced ventricular compliance are most affected by loss of a normally timed atrial systole.

B. DIASTOLIC FUNCTION AND VENTRICULAR COMPLIANCE:

Ventricular end-diastolic volume is difficult to measure clinically. Even such imaging techniques as two-dimensional transesophageal echocardiography (TEE), radionuclide imaging, and contrast ventriculography pro-

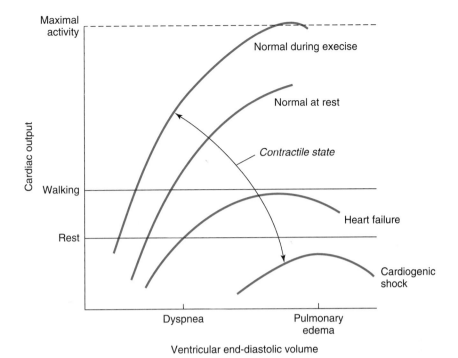

Figure 19–5. Starling's law of the heart.

vide only approximations of the volume. Left ventricular end-diastolic pressure (LVEDP) can be used as a measure of preload only if the relationship between ventricular volume and pressure (ventricular compliance) is constant. Unfortunately, ventricular compliance is normally nonlinear (Figure 19–6). Moreover, because altered diastolic functions reduces ventricular compliance, the same LVEDP represents a lesser preload. Many factors are known to influence ventricular diastolic function and compliance. Nonetheless, measurement of LVEDP or other pressures approximating LVEDP (such as pulmonary capillary wedge pressure) remains the most common means of estimating left

ventricular preload (see Chapter 6). Central venous pressure can be used as an index of right ventricular preload as well as left ventricular preload in most normal individuals.

Factors affecting ventricular compliance can be separated into those related to the rate of relaxation (early diastolic compliance) and passive stiffness of the ventricles (late diastolic compliance). Hypertrophy, ischemia, and asynchrony reduce early compliance, while hypertrophy and fibrosis reduce late compliance. Extrinsic factors (such as pericardial disease, overdistention of the contralateral ventricle, increased airway or pleural pressure, tumors, and surgical compression) can also reduce ventricular compliance. Because of its normally thinner wall, the right ventricle is more compliant than the left.

Table 19–4. Factors affecting ventricular preload.

Venous return
Blood volume
Distribution of blood volume
    Posture
    Intrathoracic pressure
    Pericardial pressure
    Venous tone
Rhythm (atrial contraction)
Heart rate

Afterload

Afterload for the intact heart is commonly equated with either ventricular wall tension during systole or arterial impedance to ejection. Wall tension may be thought of as the pressure the ventricle must overcome to reduce its cavity. If the ventricle is assumed to be spherical, ventricular wall tension can be expressed by Laplace's law:

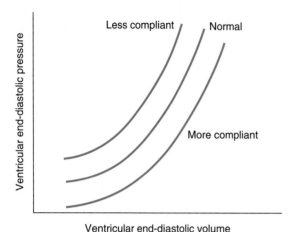

Figure 19–6. Normal and abnormal ventricular compliance.

$$\text{Circumferential stress} = \frac{P \times R}{2 \times H}$$

where P is intraventricular pressure, R is the ventricular radius, and H is wall thickness. Although the normal ventricle is usually ellipsoidal, this relationship is still useful. The larger the ventricular radius, the greater the wall tension required to develop the same ventricular pressure. Conversely, an increase in wall thickness reduces ventricular wall tension.

Systolic intraventricular pressure is dependent on the force of ventricular contraction; the viscoelastic properties of the aorta, its proximal branches, and blood (viscosity and density); and **systemic vascular resistance (SVR)**. Arteriolar tone is the chief determinant of SVR. Because viscoelastic properties are generally fixed in any given patient, left ventricular afterload is usually equated clinically with SVR, which is calculated by the following equation:

$$\text{SVR} = 80 \times \frac{\text{MAP} - \text{CVP}}{\text{CO}}$$

where MAP is mean arterial pressure in millimeters of mercury, CVP is central venous pressure in millimeters of mercury, and CO is cardiac output in liters per minute. Normal SVR is 900–1500 dynes·sec·cm^{-5}. Systolic blood pressure may also be used as an approximation of left ventricular afterload in the absence of chronic changes in the size, shape, or thickness of the ventricular wall or acute changes in systemic vascular

resistance. Some clinicians prefer to use CI instead of CO in calculating a systemic vascular resistance index (SVRI), so that SVRI = SVR × BSA.

Right ventricular afterload is mainly dependent on pulmonary vascular resistance and is expressed by the following equation:

$$\text{PVR} = 80 \times \frac{\text{PAP} - \text{LAP}}{\text{CO}}$$

where PAP is mean pulmonary artery pressure and LAP is left atrial pressure. In practice, PCWP is usually substituted as an approximation for LAP (see Chapter 6). Normal PVR is 50–150 dynes·sec·cm$^{-5.}$

Cardiac output is inversely related to afterload (Figure 19–7). The right ventricle is more sensitive to changes in afterload than is the left ventricle because of 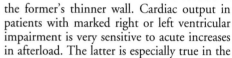 the former's thinner wall. Cardiac output in patients with marked right or left ventricular impairment is very sensitive to acute increases in afterload. The latter is especially true in the presence of myocardial depression (as often occurs during anesthesia).

Contractility

Cardiac contractility (**inotropism**) is the intrinsic ability of the myocardium to pump in the absence of changes in preload or afterload. Contractility is related to the rate of myocardial muscle shortening, which is in turn dependent on the intracellular calcium concentration during systole. Increases in heart rate can also enhance contractility under some conditions, perhaps because of the increased availability of intracellular calcium.

Contractility can be altered by neural, humoral, or pharmacologic influences. Sympathetic nervous system activity normally has the most important effect on contractility. Sympathetic fibers innervate atrial and ventricular muscle as well as nodal tissues. In addition to its positive chronotropic effect, norepinephrine release also enhances contractility via β_1-receptor activation. α-Adrenergic receptors are also present in the myocardium but appear to have only minor positive inotropic and chronotropic effects. Sympathomimetic drugs and epinephrine secretion from the adrenal glands similarly increase contractility via β_1-receptor activation.

Myocardial contractility is depressed by anoxia, acidosis, depletion of catecholamine stores within the heart, and loss of functioning muscle mass as a result of ischemia or infarction. Most anesthetics and antiarrhythmic agents are negative inotropes (ie, they decrease contractility).

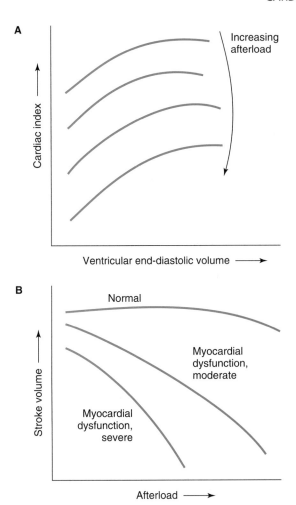

Figure 19–7. The relationship between cardiac output and afterload. *A:* The effect of increasing afterload on cardiac index. *B:* Note that patients with myocardial dysfunction become increasingly more sensitive to afterload.

Wall Motion Abnormalities

Regional wall motion abnormalities cause a breakdown of the analogy between the intact heart and skeletal muscle preparations. The abnormalities may be due to ischemia, scarring, hypertrophy, or altered conduction. When the ventricular cavity does not collapse symmetrically or fully, emptying becomes impaired. **Hypokinesis** (decreased contraction), **akinesis** (failure to contract), and **dyskinesis** (paradoxic bulging) during systole reflect increasing degrees of contraction abnormalities. Although contractility may be normal or even

enhanced in some areas, abnormalities in other areas of the ventricle can impair emptying and reduce stroke volume. The severity of the impairment depends on the size and number of abnormally contracting areas.

Valvular Dysfunction

Valvular dysfunction can involve any one of the four valves in the heart and can lead to stenosis, regurgitation (incompetence), or both. Stenosis of an AV (tricuspid or mitral) valve reduces stroke volume primarily by decreasing ventricular preload, while stenosis of a semilunar (pulmonary or aortic) valve reduces stroke volume chiefly by increasing ventricular afterload (see Chapter 20). In contrast, valvular regurgitation can reduce stroke volume without changes in preload, afterload, or contractility and without wall motion abnormalities. The effective stroke volume is reduced by the regurgitant volume with every contraction. When an AV valve is incompetent, a significant part of the ventricular end-diastolic volume can flow backward into the atrium during systole; the stroke volume is reduced by the regurgitant volume. Similarly, when a semilunar valve is incompetent, a fraction of end-diastolic volume returns backward into the ventricle during diastole.

ASSESSMENT OF VENTRICULAR FUNCTION

1. Ventricular Function Curves

Plotting cardiac output or stroke volume against preload is useful in evaluating pathologic states and understanding drug therapy. Normal right and left ventricular function curves are shown in Figure 19–8.

Ventricular pressure-volume diagrams are even more useful because they dissociate contractility from both preload and afterload. Two points are identified on such diagrams: the end-systolic point (ESP) and the end-diastolic point (EDP) (Figure 19–9). The former is reflective of systolic function while the latter is more reflective of diastolic function. For any given contractile state, all ESPs are on the same line—ie, the relationship between end-systolic volume and end-systolic pressure is fixed.

2. Assessment of Systolic Function

The change in ventricular pressure over time during systole (dP/dt) is defined by the first derivative of the ventricular pressure curve and is often used as a measure of contractility. Contractility is directly proportional to dP/dt, but accurate measurement of this value requires a high-fidelity ventricular catheter. Although

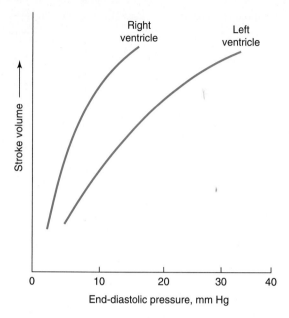

Figure 19–8. Function curves for the left and right ventricles.

arterial pressure tracings are distorted owing to properties of the vascular tree, the initial rate of rise in pressure (the slope) can serve as a rough approximation; the more proximal the catheter is in the arterial tree, the more accurate the extrapolation will be. The usefulness of dP/dt is also limited in that it may be affected by preload, afterload, and heart rate. Various correction factors have been used with only limited success.

Ejection Fraction

Ventricular ejection fraction (EF), the fraction of the end-diastolic ventricular volume ejected, is the most commonly used clinical measurement of systolic function. EF can be calculated by the following equation:

$$EF = \frac{EDV - ESV}{EDV}$$

where EDV is left ventricular diastolic volume and ESV is end-systolic volume. Normal EF is approximately 0.67 ± 0.08. Measurements can be made preoperatively from cardiac catheterization, radionucleotide studies, or transthoracic or TEE. Pulmonary artery catheters with fast-response thermistors allow measurement of the right ventricular EF. Unfortunately, when pulmonary vascular resistance increases, decreases in

right ventricular EF may reflect afterload rather than contractility.

3. Assessment of Diastolic Function

Left ventricular diastolic function can be assessed clinically by Doppler echocardiography on a transthoracic or transesophageal examination. Flow velocities are measured across the mitral valve during diastole. Three patterns of diastolic dysfunction are generally recognized based on isovolumetric relaxation time, the ratio of peak early diastolic flow (E) to peak atrial systolic flow (A), and the deceleration time of E (DT_E) (Figure 19–10).

■ SYSTEMIC CIRCULATION

The systemic vasculature can be divided functionally into arteries, arterioles, capillaries, and veins. Arteries are the high-pressure conduits that supply the various organs. Arterioles are the small vessels that directly feed and control blood flow through each capillary bed. Capillaries are thin-walled vessels that allow the exchange of nutrients between blood and tissues (see Chapter 28). Veins return blood from capillary beds to the heart.

The distribution of blood between the various components of the circulatory system is shown in Table 19–5. Note that most of the blood volume is in the systemic circulation—specifically, within systemic veins. Changes in systemic venous tone allow these vessels to function as a reservoir for blood. Following significant blood or fluid losses, a sympathetically mediated increase in venous tone reduces the caliber of these vessels and shifts blood into other parts of the vascular system. Conversely, venodilation allows these vessels to accommodate increases in blood volume. Sympathetic control of venous tone is an important determinant of venous return to the heart. Loss of this tone following induction of anesthesia frequently contributes to hypotension.

A multiplicity of factors influences blood flow in the vascular tree. These include local and metabolic control mechanisms, endothelium-derived factors, the autonomic nervous system, and circulating hormones.

AUTOREGULATION

Most tissue beds regulate their own blood flow (autoregulation). Arterioles generally dilate in response to reduced perfusion pressure or increased tissue demand. Conversely, arterioles constrict in response to increased pressure or reduced tissue demand. These phenomena are likely due to both an intrinsic response of vascular smooth muscle to stretch and the accumulation of va-

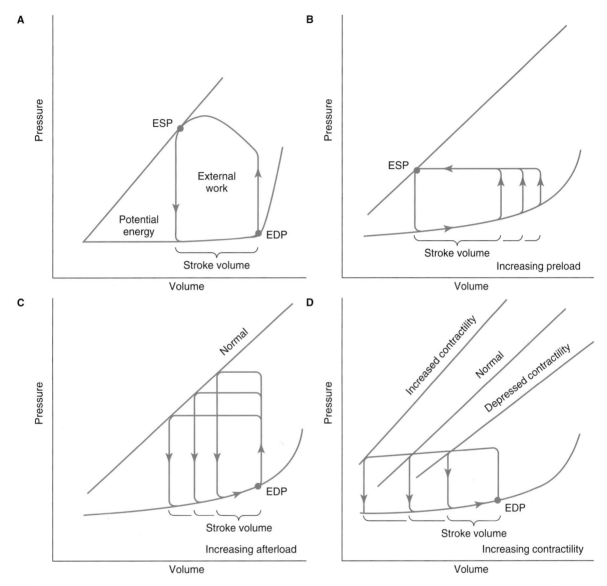

Figure 19–9. Ventricular pressure-volume diagrams. ***A:*** A single ventricular contraction. Note that stroke volume represents change in volume on the x axis (difference between end-systolic volume and end-diastolic volume). Note also that the circumscribed area represents external work performed by the ventricle. ***B:*** Increasing preload with constant contractility and afterload. ***C:*** Increasing afterload with constant preload and contractility. ***D:*** Increasing contractility with constant preload and afterload. ESP = end-systolic point; EDP = end-diastolic point.

sodilatory metabolic by-products. The latter may include K^+, H^+, CO_2, adenosine, and lactate.

ENDOTHELIUM-DERIVED FACTORS

The vascular endothelium is active metabolically in elaborating or modifying substances that directly or in-

directly play a major role in controlling blood pressure and flow. These include vasodilators (eg, nitric oxide, prostacyclin [PGI_2]), vasoconstrictors (endothelins, thromboxane A_2), anticoagulants (eg, thrombomodulin, protein C), fibrinolytics (tissue plasminogen activator), and factors that inhibit platelet aggregation (nitric oxide and PGI_2). Nitric oxide is synthesized from

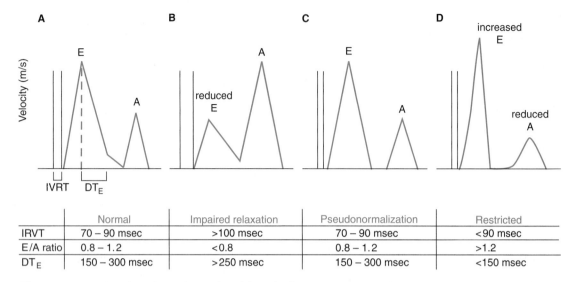

Figure 19–10. Doppler echocardiography of diastolic flow across the mitral valve. *A–D* (from left to right) represents increasing severity of diastolic dysfunction.

	Normal	Impaired relaxation	Pseudonormalization	Restricted
IRVT	70 – 90 msec	>100 msec	70 – 90 msec	<90 msec
E/A ratio	0.8 – 1.2	<0.8	0.8 – 1.2	>1.2
DT_E	150 – 300 msec	>250 msec	150 – 300 msec	<150 msec

arginine by nitric oxide synthetase. This substance has a number of functions (see Chapter 13). In the circulation, it is a potent vasodilator that may be tonically secreted. It binds guanylate cyclase, increasing cGMP levels and producing vasodilation. Endothelially derived vasoconstrictors, endothelins, are released in response to thrombin and epinephrine.

AUTONOMIC CONTROL OF THE SYSTEMIC VASCULATURE

Although both the sympathetic and parasympathetic systems can exert important influences on the circulation, autonomic control of the vasculature is primarily sympathetic. Sympathetic outflow to the circulation passes out of the spinal cord at all thoracic and the first two lumbar segments. These fibers reach blood vessels via specific autonomic nerves or by traveling along spinal nerves. Sympathetic fibers innervate all parts of

Table 19–5. Normal distribution of blood volume.

Heart	7%
Pulmonary circulation	9%
Systemic circulation	
Arterial	15%
Capillary	5%
Venous	64%

the vasculature except for capillaries. Their principal function is to regulate vascular tone. Variations of arterial vascular tone serve to regulate blood pressure and the distribution of blood flow to the various organs, while variations in venous tone alter venous return to the heart.

The vasculature has sympathetic vasoconstrictor and vasodilator fibers, but the former are more important physiologically in most tissue beds. Sympathetic-induced vasoconstriction (via α_1-adrenergic receptors) can be potent in skeletal muscle, kidneys, gut, and skin; it is least active in the brain and heart. The most important vasodilatory fibers are those to skeletal muscle, mediating an increase in blood flow (via β_2-adrenergic receptors) in response to exercise. **Vasodepressor (vasovagal) syncope,** which can occur following intense emotional strain associated with high sympathetic tone, results from reflex activation of both vagal and sympathetic vasodilator fibers.

Vascular tone and autonomic influences on the heart are controlled by vasomotor centers in the reticular formation of the medulla and lower pons. Distinct vasoconstrictor and vasodilator areas have been identified. Vasoconstriction is mediated by the anterolateral areas of the lower pons and upper medulla. The adrenergic cells in this area project to the intermediolateral columns (see Chapter 18). They are also responsible for the adrenal secretion of catecholamines as well as the enhancement of cardiac automaticity and contractility. Vasodilatory areas, which are located in the lower medulla, are also adrenergic but function by projecting inhibitory fibers upward to the vasoconstrictor areas. Vasomotor output is modified by inputs from throughout the central nervous system, including the hypothalamus, cerebral cortex, and the other areas in the brainstem. Areas in the posterolateral medulla receive input from both the vagal and the glossopharyngeal nerves and play an important role in mediating a variety of circulatory reflexes. The sympathetic system normally maintains some tonic vasoconstriction on the vascular tree. Loss of this tone following induction of anesthesia or sympathectomy frequently contributes to perioperative hypotension.

ARTERIAL BLOOD PRESSURE

Systemic blood flow is pulsatile in large arteries because of the heart's cyclic activity; by the time blood reaches the systemic capillaries, flow is continuous (laminar). The mean pressure in large arteries, which is normally about 95 mm Hg, falls nearly to zero in the large systemic veins that return blood to the heart. The largest pressure drop, nearly 50%, is across the arterioles, which account for the majority of SVR.

MAP is proportionate to the product of SVR × CO. This relationship is based on an analogy to Ohm's law as applied to the circulation:

$$MAP - CVP \approx SVR \times CO$$

Since CVP is normally very small compared with MAP, the former can usually be ignored. From this relationship, it is readily apparent that hypotension is the result of a decrease in SVR, CO, or both: In order to maintain arterial blood pressure, a decrease in one must be compensated by an increase in the other. MAP can be measured as the integrated mean of the arterial pressure waveform. Alternatively, MAP may be estimated by the following formula:

$$MAP = \text{Diastolic pressure} + \frac{\text{Pulse pressure}}{3}$$

where pulse pressure is the difference between systolic and diastolic blood pressure. Arterial pulse pressure is directly related to stroke volume but inversely proportional to the compliance of the arterial tree. Thus, decreases in pulse pressure may be due to a decrease in stroke volume, an increase in SVR, or both.

Transmission of the arterial wave from large arteries to smaller vessels in the periphery is faster than the actual velocity of blood; the wave travels at a rate 15 times the velocity of blood in the aorta. Moreover, reflections of the propagating waves off arterial walls widen pulse pressure before the pulse wave is completely dampened in very small arteries (see Chapter 6).

Control of Arterial Blood Pressure

Arterial blood pressure is regulated by a series of immediate, intermediate, and long-term adjustments that involve complex neural, humoral, and renal mechanisms.

A. IMMEDIATE CONTROL:

Minute-to-minute control of blood pressure is primarily the function of autonomic nervous system reflexes. Changes in blood pressure are sensed both centrally (in hypothalamic and brainstem areas) and peripherally by specialized sensors (baroreceptors). Decreases in arterial blood pressure enhance sympathetic tone, increase adrenal secretion of epinephrine, and suppress vagal activity. The resulting systemic vasoconstriction, elevation in heart rate, and enhanced cardiac contractility increase blood pressure. Conversely, hypertension decreases sympathetic outflow and enhances vagal tone.

Peripheral baroreceptors are located at the bifurcation of the common carotid arteries and the aortic arch. Elevations in blood pressure increase baroreceptor discharge, inhibiting systemic vasoconstriction and enhancing vagal tone (**baroreceptor reflex**). Reductions in blood pressure decrease baroreceptor discharge, allowing vasoconstriction and reduction of vagal tone. Carotid baroreceptors send afferent signals to circulatory brainstem centers via Hering's nerve (a branch of the glossopharyngeal nerve), while aortic baroreceptor afferent signals travel along the vagus nerve. Of the two peripheral sensors, the carotid baroreceptor is physiologically more important and is primarily responsible for minimizing blood pressure changes that are caused by acute events, such as a change in posture. Carotid baroreceptors sense MAP most effectively between pressures of 80 mm Hg and 160 mm Hg. Adaptation to acute blood pressure changes occurs over the course of 1–2 days, rendering this reflex ineffective for long-term blood pressure control. All volatile anesthetics depress the normal baroreceptor response, but isoflurane and desflurane appear to have the least effect. Cardiopulmonary stretch receptors located in the atria, left ventricle, and pulmonary circulation can cause a similar effect.

B. INTERMEDIATE CONTROL:

In the course of a few minutes, sustained decreases in arterial pressure together with enhanced sympathetic outflow activate the renin-angiotensin-aldosterone system (see Chapter 31), increase arginine vasopressin (AVP) secretion, and alter normal capillary fluid exchange (see Chapter 28). Both angiotensin II and AVP are potent arteriolar vasoconstrictors. Their immediate action is to increase SVR. In contrast to angiotensin II formation, however, moderate to marked hypotension is required for enough AVP secretion to produce vasoconstriction. Angiotensin constricts arterioles via AT_1 receptors. AVP mediates vasoconstriction via V_1 receptors and exerts its antidiuretic effect via V_2 receptors.

Sustained changes in arterial blood pressure can also alter fluid exchange in tissues by their secondary effects on capillary pressures. Hypertension increases interstitial movement of intravascular fluid, while hypotension increases reabsorption of interstitial fluid. Such compensatory changes in intravascular volume can serve to reduce fluctuations in blood pressure, especially in the absence of adequate renal function (see below).

C. Long-Term Control:

The effects of slower renal mechanisms become apparent within hours of sustained changes in arterial pressure. As a result, the kidneys alter total body sodium and water balance, in order to restore blood pressure to normal. Hypotension results in sodium (and water) retention, while hypertension generally increases sodium excretion in normal individuals (see Chapter 28).

ANATOMY & PHYSIOLOGY OF THE CORONARY CIRCULATION

1. Anatomy

Myocardial blood supply is derived entirely from the right and left coronary arteries (Figure 19–11). Blood flows from epicardial to endocardial vessels. After perfusing the myocardium, blood returns to the right atrium via the coronary sinus and the anterior cardiac veins. A small amount of blood returns directly into the chambers of the heart by way of the thebesian veins.

The right coronary artery (RCA) normally supplies the right atrium, most of the right ventricle and a variable portion of the left ventricle (inferior wall). In 85% of persons, the RCA gives rise to the posterior descending artery (PDA), which supplies the superior-posterior interventricular septum and inferior wall—a right dominant circulation; in the remaining 15% of persons, the PDA is branch of the left coronary artery—a left dominant circulation.

The left coronary artery normally supplies the left atrium and most of the interventricular septum and left ventricle (septal, anterior, and lateral walls). After a short course the left main coronary artery bifurcates into the left anterior descending artery (LAD) and the circumflex artery (CX); the former supplies the septum and anterior wall, while the CX supplies the lateral wall. In left a dominant circulation, the CX wraps around the AV groove and continues down as the PDA to also supply the most of the posterior septum and inferior wall.

The arterial supply to the SA node may be derived from either the RCA (60% of individuals) or the LAD (the remaining 40%). The AV node is usually supplied by the RCA (85–90%) or, less frequently, by the CX (10–15%); the bundle of His has a dual blood supply derived from the PDA and LAD. The anterior papillary muscle of the mitral valve also has a dual blood supply that is fed by diagonal branches of the LAD and marginal branches of the CX. In contrast, the posterior papillary of the mitral valve is usually supplied only by the PDA and is therefore much more vulnerable to ischemic dysfunction.

2. Determinants of Coronary Perfusion

Coronary perfusion is unique in that it is intermittent rather than continuous, as it is in other organs. During contraction, intramyocardial pressures in the left ventricle approach systemic arterial pressure. The force of left ventricular contraction almost completely occludes the intramyocardial part of the coronary arteries; in fact, blood flow may transiently reverse in epicardial vessels. Even during the latter part of diastole, left ventricular pressure eventually exceeds venous (right atrial) pressure. Thus, coronary perfusion pressure is usually determined by the difference between aortic pressure and ventricular pressure, and the left ventricle is perfused almost entirely during diastole. In contrast, the right ventricle is perfused during both systole and diastole (Figure 19–12). Moreover, arterial diastolic pressure is a more important determinant of myocardial blood flow than is mean arterial pressure:

$$\frac{\text{coronary perfusion}}{\text{pressure}} = \frac{\text{Arterial}}{\text{diastolic} - \text{LVEDP}}{\text{pressure}}$$

Decreases in aortic pressure or increases in ventricular end-diastolic pressure can reduce coronary perfusion pressure. Increases in heart rate also decrease coronary perfusion because of the disproportionately greater reduction in diastolic time as heart rate increases (Figure 19–13). Because it is subjected to the greatest intramural pressures during systole, the endocardium tends to be most vulnerable to ischemia during decreases in coronary perfusion pressure.

Control of Coronary Blood Flow

Coronary blood flow normally parallels myocardial metabolic demand. In the average adult man, coronary

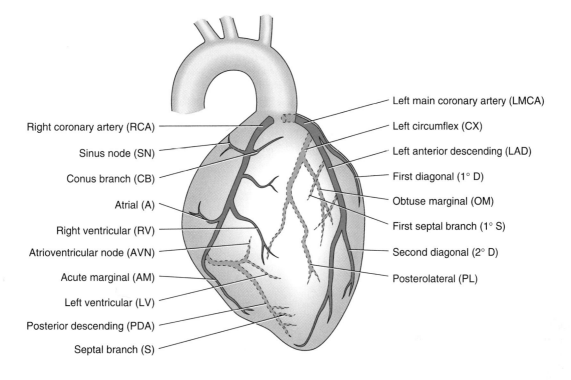

A. RIGHT ANTERIOR OBLIQUE VIEW

Right coronary artery (RCA)
Sinus node (SN)
Conus branch (CB)
Atrial (A)
Right ventricular (RV)
Atrioventricular node (AVN)
Acute marginal (AM)
Left ventricular (LV)
Posterior descending (PDA)
Septal branch (S)

Left main coronary artery (LMCA)
Left circumflex (CX)
Left anterior descending (LAD)
First diagonal (1° D)
Obtuse marginal (OM)
First septal branch (1° S)
Second diagonal (2° D)
Posterolateral (PL)

B. LEFT ANTERIOR OBLIQUE VIEW

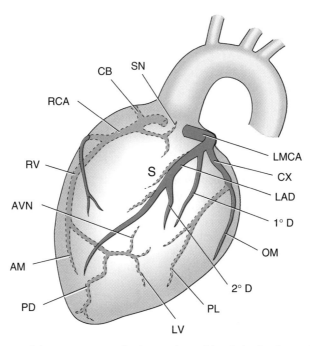

CB
SN
RCA
RV
AVN
AM
PD
S
LV
PL
2° D
OM
1° D
LAD
CX
LMCA

Figure 19–11. Anatomy of the coronary arteries in a patient with a right dominant circulation. *A:* Right anterior oblique view. *B:* Left anterior oblique view.

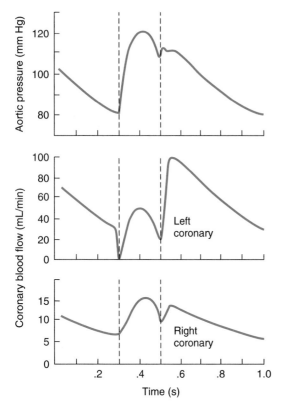

Figure 19–12. Coronary blood flow during the cardiac cycle. (Modified and reproduced, with permission, from Berne RM, Levy MD: *Cardiovascular Physiology,* 2nd ed. Mosby, 1972.)

blood flow is approximately 250 mL/min at rest. The myocardium regulates its own blood flow closely between perfusion pressures of 50 mm Hg and 120 mm Hg. Beyond this range, blood flow becomes increasingly pressure-dependent.

Under normal conditions, changes in blood flow are entirely due to variations in coronary arterial tone (resistance) in response to metabolic demand. Hypoxia—either directly, or indirectly through the release of adenosine—causes coronary vasodilation. Autonomic influences are generally weak. Both α_1- and β_2-adrenergic receptors are present in the coronary arteries. The α_1-receptors are primarily located on larger epicardial vessels, while β_2-receptors are mainly found on the smaller intramuscular and subendocardial vessels. Sympathetic stimulation generally increases myocardial blood flow because of an increase in metabolic demand and a predominance of β_2-receptor activation. Parasympathetic effects on the coronary vasculature are generally minor and are weakly vasodilatory.

3. Myocardial Oxygen Balance

Myocardial oxygen demand is normally the most important determinant of myocardial blood flow. Relative contributions to oxygen requirements include basal requirements (20%), electrical activity (1%), volume work (15%), and pressure work (64%). The myocardium normally extracts 65% of the oxygen in arterial blood, compared with 25% in most other tissues (see Chapter 22). Coronary sinus oxygen saturation is normally 30%. Therefore, the myocardium (unlike other tissues) cannot compensate for reductions in blood flow by extracting more oxygen from hemoglobin. Any increases in myocardial metabolic demand must be met by an increase in coronary blood flow. Table 19–6 lists the most important factors in myocardial oxygen demand and supply. Note that the heart rate and, to a lesser extent, ventricular end-diastolic pressure are important determinants of both supply and demand.

Effects of Anesthetic Agents

Most volatile anesthetic agents are coronary vasodilators. Their effect on coronary blood flow is variable because of their direct vasodilating properties, reduction of myocardial metabolic requirements (and secondary decrease due to autoregulation), and effects on arterial blood pressure. Although the mechanism is not clear, it may involve activation of ATP-sensitive K^+ channels and stimulation of adenosine (A_1) receptors. Halothane and isoflurane appear to have the greatest effect; the former primarily affects large coronary vessels, while the latter affects mostly smaller vessels. Vasodilation due to

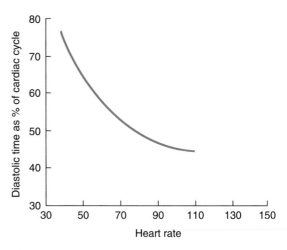

Figure 19–13. The relationship between diastolic time and heart rate.

Table 19–6. Factors affecting myocardial oxygen supply-demand balance.

Supply
Heart rate
Diastolic time
Coronary perfusion pressure
Aortic diastolic blood pressure
Ventricular end-diastolic pressure
Arterial oxygen content
Arterial oxygen tension
Hemoglobin concentration
Coronary vessel diameter
Demand
Basal requirements
Heart rate
Wall tension
Preload (ventricular radius)
Afterload
Contractility

---

desflurane appears to be primarily autonomically mediated, while sevoflurane appears to lack coronary vasodilating properties. Dose-dependent abolition of autoregulation may be greatest with isoflurane. Evidence that volatile anesthetics cause a coronary steal phenomena in humans is lacking.

Volatile agents appear to exert beneficial effects in the setting of myocardial ischemia and infarction. They not only reduce myocardial oxygen requirements but appear to be protective against reperfusion injury; these effects may also be mediated by activation of ATP-sensitive K$^+$ channels. Some evidence also suggests that volatile anesthetics enhance recovery of the "stunned"

myocardium. Moreover, even though they decrease myocardial contractility, they can potentially be beneficial in patients with heart failure because they decrease preload and afterload.

■ THE PATHOPHYSIOLOGY OF HEART FAILURE

Systolic heart failure exists when the heart is unable to pump a sufficient amount of blood to meet the body's metabolic requirements. Clinical manifestations usually reflect the effects of the low cardiac output on tissues (eg, fatigue, oxygen debt, acidosis), the damming-up of blood behind the failing ventricle (systemic or pulmonary venous congestion), or both. The left ventricle is most commonly involved, often with secondary involvement of the right ventricle. Isolated right ventricular failure can occur in the setting of advanced disease of the lung parenchyma or pulmonary vasculature. Left ventricular failure most commonly results from primary myocardial dysfunction (usually from coronary artery disease) but may also result from valvular dysfunction, arrhythmias, or pericardial disease.

Diastolic dysfunction can also cause symptoms of heart failure as a result of atrial hypertension (Figure 19–14). Common causes include hypertension, coronary artery disease, hypertrophic cardiomyopathy, and pericardial disease. Although diastolic dysfunction can cause symptoms of heart failure even in the presence of normal systolic function, systolic and diastolic dysfunction are commonly associated.

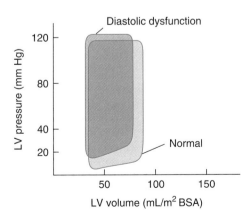
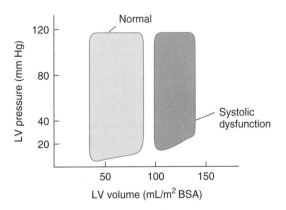

Figure 19–14. Ventricular pressure volume relationships in isolated systolic and diastolic dysfunction. (Modified and reproduced, with permission, from Zile MR: Mod Concepts Cardiovasc Dis 1990;59:1.)

Cardiac output is reduced in most forms of heart failure. Inadequate oxygen delivery to tissues is reflected by a low mixed venous oxygen tension and an increase in the arterial-venous oxygen content difference (see Chapter 22). In compensated heart failure, the arteriovenous difference may be normal at rest, but it rapidly widens during stress or exercise.

Heart failure is less commonly associated with an elevated cardiac output. This form of heart failure is most commonly seen with sepsis and other hypermetabolic states, which are typically associated with a low SVR.

COMPENSATORY MECHANISMS

Major compensatory mechanisms generally present in patients with heart failure include increased preload, increased sympathetic tone, activation of the renin-angiotensin-aldosterone system, release of AVP, and ventricular hypertrophy. Although these mechanisms can initially compensate for mild to moderate cardiac dysfunction, with increasing severity of dysfunction they may actually contribute to the cardiac impairment.

Increased Preload

An increase in ventricular size not only reflects an inability to keep up with venous return but also serves to maximize stroke volume by moving the heart up the Starling curve (see Figure 19–5). Even when EF is reduced, an increase in ventricular end-diastolic volume can maintain a normal stroke volume. Worsening venous congestion caused by the damming-up of blood behind the failing ventricle and excessive ventricular dilatation can rapidly lead to clinical deterioration. Left ventricular failure results in pulmonary vascular congestion and progressive transudation of fluid, first into the pulmonary interstitium and then into alveoli (pulmonary edema). Right ventricular failure leads to systemic venous hypertension, which results in peripheral edema, hepatic congestion and dysfunction, and ascites. Dilatation of the annulus of either AV valve leads to valvular regurgitation, further impairing ventricular output.

Increased Sympathetic Tone

Sympathetic activation increases norepinephrine release from nerve endings in the heart and the adrenal secretion of epinephrine into the circulation. Plasma catecholamine levels are generally directly proportional to the degree of left ventricular dysfunction. Although enhanced sympathetic outflow can initially maintain cardiac output by increasing heart rate and contractility, worsening ventricular function elicits increasing degrees of vasoconstriction in an effort to maintain arterial blood pressure. The associated increase in afterload, however, reduces cardiac output and exacerbates the ventricular failure.

Chronic sympathetic activation in patients with heart failure eventually decreases the response of adrenergic receptors to catecholamines (down-regulation), the number of receptors, and cardiac catecholamine stores. Nonetheless, the failing heart becomes increasingly dependent on circulating catecholamines. Abrupt withdrawal in sympathetic outflow or decreases in circulating catecholamine levels, such as can occur following induction of anesthesia, may lead to acute cardiac decompensation. A reduced density of M_2 receptors also decreases parasympathetic influences on the heart.

Sympathetic activation tends to redistribute systemic blood flow output away from the skin, gut, kidneys, and skeletal muscle to the heart and brain. Decreased renal perfusion together with β_1-adrenergic activity at the juxtaglomerular apparatus activate the renin-angiotensin-aldosterone axis (see Chapter 28), which leads to sodium retention and interstitial edema. Moreover, vasoconstriction secondary to elevated angiotensin II levels increases left ventricular afterload and causes further deterioration of systolic function. The latter accounts for the efficacy of angiotensin-converting enzyme inhibitors in heart failure. Symptoms may also improve in some patients with careful, low-dose β-adrenergic blockade.

Circulating AVP levels are often twice normal in patients with severe heart failure. Elevations in AVP also increase ventricular afterload and are responsible for a defect in free water clearance that is commonly associated with hyponatremia (see Chapter 28).

Atrial natriuretic peptide is found predominantly in atrial tissue. This hormone is released in response to atrial distention and has salutary effects in heart failure. It is a potent vasodilator and has properties that antagonize the effects of angiotensin, aldosterone, and AVP.

Ventricular Hypertrophy

Ventricular hypertrophy can occur with or without dilatation, depending on the type of stress imposed on the ventricle. When the heart is subjected to either pressure or volume overload, the initial response is to increase sarcomere length and optimally overlap actin and myosin. With time, ventricular muscle mass begins to increase in response to the abnormal stress.

In the volume-overloaded ventricle, the problem is an increase in diastolic wall stress. The increase in ventricular muscle mass is only sufficient to compensate for the increase in diameter: The ratio of the ventricular radius to wall thickness is unchanged. Sarcomeres replicate mainly in series, resulting in eccentric hypertrophy.

Although ventricular EF remains depressed, the increase in end-diastolic volume can maintain normal at-rest stroke volume (and cardiac output).

The problem in a pressure-overloaded ventricle is an increase in systolic wall stress. Sarcomeres in this case mainly replicate in parallel, resulting in concentric hypertrophy: The hypertrophy is such that the ratio of myocardial wall thickness to ventricular radius increases. As can be seen from Laplace's law, systolic wall stress can then be normalized. Ventricular hypertrophy, especially that caused by pressure overload, usually results in progressive diastolic dysfunction.

CASE DISCUSSION:
A PATIENT WITH A SHORT
P–R INTERVAL

A 38-year-old man is scheduled for endoscopic sinus surgery following a recent onset of headaches. He gives a history of having passed out at least once during one of these headaches. A preoperative electrocardiogram (ECG) is normal except for a P–R interval of 0.116 seconds with normal P-wave morphology.

What is the significance of the short P–R interval?

The P–R interval, which is measured from the beginning of atrial depolarization (P wave) to the beginning of ventricular depolarization (QRS complex), normally represents the time required for depolarization of both atria, the atrioventricular (AV) node, and the His-Purkinje system. Although the P–R interval can vary with the heart rate, it is normally 0.12–0.2 seconds in duration. Abnormally short P–R intervals can be seen with either low atrial (or upper AV junctional) rhythms or preexcitation phenomena. The two can usually be differentiated by P-wave morphology: With a low atrial rhythm, atrial depolarization is retrograde, resulting in an inverted P wave in leads II, III, and aVF; with preexcitation, the P wave is normal during sinus rhythm. If the pacemaker rhythm originates from a lower AV junctional focus, the P wave may be lost in the QRS complex or may follow the QRS.

What is preexcitation?

*Preexcitation usually refers to early depolarization of the ventricles by an abnormal conduction pathway from the atria. Rarely, more than one such pathway is present. The most common form of preexcitation is due to the presence of an accessory pathway (**bundle of Kent**) that connects one of the atria with one of the ventricles. This abnormal connection between the atria and ventricles allows electrical impulses to bypass the AV node (hence the term bypass tract). The ability to conduct impulses along the bypass tract can be quite variable and may be only intermittent or rate-dependent. Bypass tracts can conduct in both directions, retrograde only (ventricle to atrium) or, rarely, anterograde only (atrium to ventricle). The name **Wolff-Parkinson-White (WPW) syndrome** is often applied to ventricular preexcitation associated with tachyarrhythmias.*

How does preexcitation shorten the P–R interval?

In patients with preexcitation, the normal cardiac impulse originating from the sinoatrial (SA) node is conducted simultaneously through the normal (AV nodal) and anomalous (bypass-tract) pathways. Because conduction is more rapid in the anomalous pathway than in the AV nodal pathway, the cardiac impulse rapidly reaches and depolarizes the area of the ventricles where the bypass tract ends. This early depolarization of the ventricle is reflected by a short P–R interval and a slurred initial deflection (delta wave) in the QRS complex. The spread of the anomalous impulse to the rest of the ventricle is delayed because it must be conducted by ordinary ventricular muscle, not by the much faster Purkinje system. The remainder of the ventricle is then depolarized by the normal impulse from the AV node as it catches up with the preexcitation front. Although the P–R interval is shortened, the resulting QRS is slightly prolonged and represents a fusion complex of normal and abnormal ventricular depolarizations.

The P–R interval in patients with preexcitation depends on relative conduction times between the AV nodal pathway and the bypass pathway. If conduction through the former is fast, preexcitation (and the delta wave) is less prominent, and QRS will be relatively normal. If conduction is delayed in the AV nodal pathway, preexcitation is more prominent, and more of the ventricle will be depolarized by the abnormally conducted impulse. When the AV nodal pathway is completely blocked, the entire ventricle is depolarized by the bypass pathway, resulting in a very short P–R interval, a very prominent delta wave, and a wide, bizarre QRS complex. Other factors that can affect the degree of preexcitation include interatrial conduction time, the distance of the atrial end of the bypass tract from the SA node, and autonomic tone. The P–R interval is often normal or only slightly shortened with a left lateral bypass tract (the most common location). Preexcitation may be more apparent at fast heart rates because conduction slows through the AV node with increasing heart rates. Secondary ST-segment and T-wave changes are also common because of abnormal ventricular repolarization.

What is the clinical significance of preexcitation?

Preexcitation occurs in approximately 0.3% of the general population. An estimated 20–50% of affected persons develop paroxysmal tachyarrhythmias, typically paroxysmal supraventricular tachycardia (PSVT). Although most patients are otherwise normal, preexcitation can be associated with other cardiac anomalies, including Ebstein's anomaly, mitral valve prolapse, and cardiomyopathies. Depending on its conductive properties, the bypass tract in some patients may predispose them to tachyarrhythmias and even sudden death. Tachyarrhythmias include PSVT, atrial fibrillation, and, less commonly, atrial flutter. Ventricular fibrillation can be precipitated by a critically timed premature atrial beat that travels down the bypass tract and catches the ventricle at a vulnerable period. Alternatively, very rapid conduction of impulses into the ventricles by the bypass tract during atrial fibrillation can rapidly lead to myocardial ischemia, hypoperfusion, and hypoxia and culminate in ventricular fibrillation.

Recognition of the preexcitation phenomenon is also important because its QRS morphology on the surface ECG can mimic bundle branch block, right ventricular hypertrophy, ischemia, myocardial infarction, and ventricular tachycardia (during atrial fibrillation).

What is the significance of the history of syncope in this patient?

This patient should be evaluated preoperatively by a cardiologist for possible electrophysiologic studies, curative radiofrequency ablation of the bypass tract, and the need for perioperative drug therapy. Such studies can identify the location of the bypass tracts, reasonably predict the potential for malignant arrhythmias by programmed pacing, and assess the efficacy of antiarrhythmic therapy if curative ablation is not possible; ablation is reported to be curative in over 90% of patients. A history of syncope may be ominous because it may indicate the ability to conduct impulses very rapidly through the bypass tract, leading to systemic hypoperfusion and perhaps predisposing to sudden death.

Patients with only occasional asymptomatic tachyarrhythmias generally do not require investi-

gation or prophylactic drug therapy. Those with frequent episodes of tachyarrhythmias or arrhythmias associated with significant symptoms require drug therapy and close evaluation.

How do tachyarrhythmias generally develop?

Tachyarrhythmias develop as a result of either abnormal impulse formation or abnormal impulse propagation (reentry). Abnormal impulses result from enhanced automaticity, abnormal automaticity, or triggered activity. Normally, only cells of the SA node, specialized atrial conduction pathways, AV nodal junctional areas, and His-Purkinje system depolarize spontaneously. Because diastolic repolarization (phase 4) is fastest in the SA node, other areas of automaticity are suppressed. Enhanced or abnormal automaticity in other areas, however, can usurp pacemaker function from the SA node and lead to tachyarrhythmias. Triggered activity is the result of either early afterdepolarizations (phase 2 or 3) or delayed afterdepolarizations (after phase 3). It consists of small-amplitude depolarizations that can follow action potentials under some conditions in atrial, ventricular, and His-Purkinje tissue. If these afterdepolarizations reach threshold potential, they can result in an extrasystole or repetitive sustained tachyarrhythmias. Factors that can promote abnormal impulse formation include increased catecholamine levels, electrolyte disorders (hyperkalemia, hypokalemia, and hypercalcemia), ischemia, hypoxia, mechanical stretch, and drug toxicity (especially digoxin).

The most common mechanism for tachyarrhythmias is reentry. Four conditions are necessary to initiate and sustain reentry (Figure 19–15): (1) two areas in the myocardium that differ in conductivity or refractoriness and that can form a closed electrical loop; (2) unidirectional block in one pathway (Figures 19–15A and B); (3) slow conduction or sufficient length in the circuit to allow recovery of the conduction block in the first pathway (Figure 19–15C; and (4) excitation of the initially blocked pathway to complete the loop (Figure 19–15D). Reentry is usually precipitated by a premature cardiac impulse.

What is the mechanism of PSVT in patients with WPW syndrome?

If the bypass tract is refractory during anterograde conduction of a cardiac impulse, as during a critically timed atrial premature contraction (APC), and the impulse is conducted by the AV node, the same impulse can be conducted retrograde from

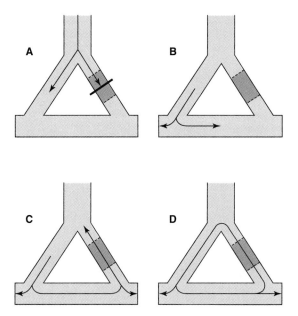

Figure 19–15. The mechanism of reentry. See text for description.

the ventricle back into the atria via the bypass tract. The retrograde impulse can then depolarize the atrium and travel down the AV nodal pathway again, establishing a continuous repetitive circuit (circus movement). The impulse reciprocates between the atria and ventricles and conduction alternates between the AV nodal pathway and the bypass tract. The term concealed conduction is often applied because the absence of preexcitation during this arrhythmia results in a normal QRS that lacks a delta wave.

The circus movement less commonly involves anterograde conduction through the bypass tract and retrograde conduction through the AV nodal pathway. In such instances, the QRS has a delta wave and is completely abnormal; the arrhythmia can be mistaken for ventricular tachycardia.

What other mechanisms may be responsible for PSVT?

In addition to WPW syndrome, PSVT can caused by AV reentrant tachycardia, AV nodal reentrant tachycardia, and SA node and atrial reentrant tachycardias. Patients with AV reentrant tachycardia have an extra-nodal bypass tract similar to those with WPW syndrome, but the bypass tract conducts only retrograde; preexcitation and a delta wave are absent. The PSVT may be initiated either by an APC or a ventricular premature con-

traction (VPC). A retrograde P wave is usually visible because atrial depolarization always follows ventricular depolarization.

Functional differences in conduction and refractoriness may occur within the AV node, SA node, or the atria; a large bypass tract is not necessary. Thus the circus movement may occur on a smaller scale within the AV node, SA node, or atria, respectively. PSVT is always induced during AV nodal reentry by an APC with a prolonged P–R interval; a retrograde P wave is either absent or buried in the QRS complex. Another APC may terminate the arrhythmia.

PSVT associated with SA node or atrial reentry is always triggered by an APC. The P wave is usually visible and has a prolonged P–R interval. Its morphology is normal with SA nodal reentry and abnormal with atrial reentry.

How does atrial fibrillation in patients with WPW syndrome differ from the arrhythmia in other patients?

Atrial fibrillation can occur when a cardiac impulse is conducted rapidly retrograde up into the atria and arrives to find different parts of the atria out of phase in recovery from the impulse. Once atrial fibrillation is established, conduction into the ventricles most commonly occurs through the bypass tract only; because of the accessory pathway's ability to conduct very rapidly (unlike the AV nodal pathway), the ventricular rate is typically very rapid (180–300 beats/min). The majority of QRS complexes are bizarre, but periodic conduction of an impulse through the AV nodal pathway results in occasional normal-looking QRS complexes. Less commonly, impulses during atrial fibrillation are conducted mainly through the AV nodal pathway (resulting in mostly normal QRS complexes) or through both the bypass tract and the AV nodal pathway (resulting in a mixture of normal, fusion, and bizarre QRS complexes). As stated previously, atrial fibrillation in patients with WPW syndrome is a very dangerous arrhythmia.

What anesthetic agents can safely be used in patients with preexcitation?

Few data are available comparing the use of different anesthetic agents or techniques in patients with preexcitation. Almost all the volatile and intravenous agents have been used with equal success. Volatile anesthetics increase antegrade refractoriness in both normal and accessory pathways (enflurane > isoflurane > halothane) and increase the coupling interval (a measure of the ability of an extrasystole to induce tachycardia). Propofol, opioids and benzodiazepines appear to have little electrophysiologic effect. Factors that tend to cause sympathetic stimulation and increased cardiac automaticity are undesirable. Premedication with a benzodiazepine helps reduce high sympathetic tone preoperatively. Agents that can increase sympathetic tone, such as ketamine and perhaps pancuronium in large bolus doses, should generally be avoided. Anticholinergics should be used cautiously; glycopyrrolate may be preferable to atropine (see Chapter 11). Endotracheal intubation should be carried out only after

the patient is deeply anesthetized (see Chapter 20); pretreatment with a β-adrenergic blocker such as esmolol may be useful. Light anesthesia, hypercapnia, acidosis, and even transient hypoxia will activate the sympathetic system and are to be avoided. A deep extubation and good postoperative analgesia (without respiratory acidosis) may also help prevent the onset of arrhythmias. When patients with preexcitation are anesthetized for electrophysiologic study and surgical ablation, opioids, propofol, and benzodiazepines may be the agents least likely to alter conduction characteristics.

Table 19–7. Classification of antiarrhythmic agents.

Class	Mechanism of Action	Agents	Intravenous Loading dose
I	Blocks fast sodium channels; decreases slope of phase 0 (V_{max})		
Ia	Moderate depression of V_{max}, prolongs ADP	Quinidine[1-3]	NR
		Procainamide[1,3]	5–10 mg/kg
		Disopyramide[1,3]	NA
Ib	Minimal effect on V_{max}, shorten ADP	Lidocaine	1–2 mg/kg
		Phenytoin	5–15 mg/kg
		Tocainide	NA
		Mexiletine	NA
		Moricizine	NA
Ic	Marked depression of V_{max}, minimal effect of ADP	Flecainide	NA
		Propafenone	NA
II	Blocks β-adrenergic receptors	Propranolol	1–3 mg
		Esmolol	0.5 mg/kg
		Metoprolol	5–10 mg
III	Prolongs repolarization	Amiodarone[4-6]	150 mg
		Bretylium[7]	5–10 mg/kg
		Sotalol[8]	NA
		Ibutilide	1 mg
		Dofetilide	NA
IV	Blocks slow calcium channels	Verapamil	2.5–10 mg
		Diltiazem	0.25–0.35 mg/kg
V	Various (miscellaneous agents)	Digoxin	0.5–0.75 mg
		Adenosine	6–12 mg

V_{max} = maximum velocity; ADP = action potential duration; NR = not recommended; NA = not available for IV use.
[1]Also has antimuscarinic (vagolytic activity).
[2]Also blocks α-adrenergic receptors.
[3]Also prolongs repolarization.
[4]Also binds inactivated fast sodium channels.
[5]Also causes noncompetitive α- and β-adrenergic blockade.
[6]Also blocks slow calcium channels.
[7]Transiently releases catecholamine stores from nerve endings.
[8]Also has nonselective β-adrenergic blocking activity.

How are antiarrhythmic agents selected for tachyarrhythmias?

Most antiarrhythmic agents act by altering myocardial cell conduction (phase 0), repolarization (phase 3), or automaticity (phase 4). Prolongation of repolarization increases the refractoriness of cells. Many antiarrhythmic drugs also exert direct or indirect autonomic effects. While antiarrhythmic agents are generally classified according to broad mechanisms of action or electrophysiologic effects (Table 19–7), the most commonly used classification system is not perfect because some agents have more than one mechanism of action. Moreover, newer agents have very specific and unique actions; for example, dofetilide acts on the delayed rectifying potassium channels.

Selection of an antiarrhythmic agent generally depends on whether the arrhythmia is ventricular or supraventricular and whether acute control or chronic therapy is required. Intravenous agents are usually employed in the acute management of arrhythmias, while oral agents are reserved for chronic therapy.

Which agents are most useful for tachyarrhythmias in patients with WPW syndrome?

Cardioversion (see Chapter 48) is the treatment of choice in hemodynamically compromised patients. Adenosine is the drug of choice for PSVT because of its short duration of action. Small of doses of phenylephrine (100 μg) together with vagal maneuvers (carotid massage) help support arterial blood pressure and may terminate the arrhythmia. The most useful pharmacologic agents are class Ia drugs, especially procainamide. These agents increase the refractory period and decrease conduction in the accessory pathway. Moreover, class Ia drugs frequently terminate and can suppress the recurrence of PSVT and atrial fibrillation. Class Ic drugs and amiodarone are also useful because they slow conduction and prolong refractoriness in both the AV node and the accessory pathway. β-Adrenergic blocking agents may also be useful, especially in controlling ventricular rate

once these rhythms are established. Verapamil and digoxin are contraindicated during atrial fibrillation or flutter in these patients because they can dangerously accelerate the ventricular response. Both types of agents decrease conduction through the AV node, favoring conduction of impulses down the accessory pathway. The bypass tract is capable of conducting impulses into the ventricles much faster than the AV nodal pathway. Digoxin may also increase the ventricular response by shortening the refractory period and increasing conduction in accessory pathways. Although verapamil can terminate PSVT, its use in this setting may be hazardous because patients can subsequently develop atrial fibrillation or flutter. Moreover, atrial fibrillation may not be readily distinguishable from ventricular tachycardia in these patients if wide-QRS tachycardia develops. Procainamide may be preferable to lidocaine in such instances, because the former is generally effective for both arrhythmias.

SUGGESTED READING

Balser JR: The rational use of intravenous amiodarone in the perioperative period. Anesthesiology 1997;86:974.

Colson P, Ryckwaert F, Coriat P: Renin angiotensin system antagonists and anesthesia. Anesth Analg 1999;89:1143.

Ganong WF: *Review of Medical Physiology,* 20th ed. McGraw-Hill, 2001.

Gomez MN: Magnesium and cardiovascular disease. Anesthesiology 1998;89:222.

Jacobsohn E, Chorn R, O'Connor M: The role of the vasculature in regulating venous return and cardiac output: Historical and graphical approach. Can J Anaesth 1997;44:849.

Ross S, Foex P: Protective effects of anaesthetics in reversible and irreversible ischemia-reperfusion injury. Br J Anaesth 1999;82:622.

Van Gelder IC, Tuinenburg AE, Schoonderwoerd BS, Tieleman RG, Crijns HJ: Pharmacologic versus direct-current electrical cardioversion of atrial flutter and fibrillation. Am J Card 1999;84:147R.

Yost CS: Potassium channels. Basic aspects, functional roles and medical significance. Anesthesiology 1999;90:1186.

Anesthesia for Patients With Cardiovascular Disease

20

KEY CONCEPTS

 Cardiovascular complications account for 25–50% of deaths following noncardiac surgery. Perioperative myocardial infarction (MI), pulmonary edema, congestive heart failure (CHF), arrhythmias, and thromboembolism are most commonly seen in patients with preexisting cardiovascular disease.

 The two most important preoperative risk factors are a history of recent MI (less than 1 month) and evidence of CHF. Generally accepted contraindications to elective noncardiac surgery include an MI less than 1 month prior to surgery, uncompensated heart failure, and severe aortic or mitral stenosis.

 Regardless of the level of preoperative blood pressure control, many patients with hypertension display an accentuated hypotensive response to induction of anesthesia, followed by an exaggerated hypertensive response to intubation. Hypertensive patients may display an exaggerated response to both endogenous catecholamines (from intubation or surgical stimulation) and exogenously administered sympathetic agonists.

 Patients with extensive (three-vessel or left main) coronary artery disease, a history of MI, or ventricular dysfunction are at greatest risk for cardiac complications. Recent data suggest the greatest risk is during the first month postinfarction. Moreover, the risk appears related to the amount of residual ischemia remaining (additional myocardium at risk of infarction). Mortality rates reported for perioperative infarcts are usually more than 50%.

 Holter monitoring, exercise electrocardiography, scintigraphy, and two-dimensional echocardiography are important in determining perioperative risk and the need for coronary angiography.

 Sudden withdrawal of antianginal medication perioperatively—especially β-blockers—can precipitate a sudden increase in ischemic episodes (rebound).

 Intraoperative detection of ischemia depends on recognition of electrocardiographic changes, hemodynamic manifestations, or regional wall motion abnormalities on transesophageal echocardiography. Down-sloping and horizontal ST depression are of greater specificity for ischemia than is up-sloping depression. New ST-segment elevations are rare during noncardiac surgery and are indicative of severe ischemia, vasospasm, or infarction.

 Patients with ischemic heart disease who have good ventricular function are generally managed with volatile anesthetic-based technique, while those with depressed ventricular function are often managed with an opioid-based anesthetic.

(continued)

(continued)

 The principal hemodynamic goals in managing mitral stenosis are to maintain a sinus rhythm (if present preoperatively) and to avoid tachycardia, large increases in cardiac output, and both hypovolemia and fluid overload by judicious fluid therapy.

 Anesthetic management should be tailored to the severity of mitral regurgitation as well as the underlying left ventricular function. Factors that exacerbate the regurgitation, such as slow heart rates (long systole) and acute increases in afterload, should be avoided. Excessive volume expansion can also worsen the regurgitation by dilating the left ventricle.

 Maintenance of normal sinus rhythm, heart rate, and intravascular volume is critical in patients with aortic stenosis. Loss of a normally timed atrial systole often leads to rapid deterioration, especially when associated with tachycardia. Spinal and epidural anesthesia are contraindicated in patients with severe aortic stenosis.

 Bradycardia and increase in systemic vascular resistance (SVR) increase the regurgitant volume in patients with aortic regurgitation, while tachycardia can contribute to myocardial ischemia. Excessive myocardial depression should also be avoided. The compensatory increase in cardiac preload should be maintained, but overzealous fluid replacement can readily result in pulmonary edema.

 In patients with congenital heart disease, an increase in SVR relative to pulmonary vascular resistance (PVR) favors left-to-right shunting, while an increase in PVR relative to SVR favors right-to-left shunting.

 The presence of shunt flow between the right and left hearts, regardless of the direction of blood flow, mandates the meticulous exclusion of air bubbles or clot from intravenous fluids to prevent paradoxical embolism into the cerebral or coronary circulations.

 The goals of anesthetic management in patients with tetralogy of Fallot should be to maintain intravascular volume and SVR. Increases in PVR, such as might occur from acidosis or excessive airway pressures, should be avoided. The right-to-left shunting tends to slow the uptake of inhalational anesthetics; in contrast, it may accelerate the onset of intravenous agents.

 The transplanted heart is totally denervated, so direct autonomic influences are absent. Moreover, the absence of reflex increases in heart rate can make patients especially sensitive to rapid vasodilation. Indirect vasopressors such as ephedrine and dopamine are less effective than direct-acting agents because of the absence of catecholamine stores in myocardial neurons.

Cardiovascular diseases—especially hypertensive, ischemic, and valvular heart disease—are the medical illnesses most frequently encountered in anesthetic practice and a major cause of perioperative morbidity and mortality. Management of patients with these diseases continues to challenge the ingenuity and resources of the anesthesiologist. The adrenergic response to surgical stimulation and the circulatory effects of anesthetic agents, endotracheal intubation, positive pressure ventilation, blood loss, fluid shifts, and alterations in body temperature impose additional burdens on an often already compromised cardiovascular system. Most anesthetic agents cause cardiac depression, vasodilation, or both. Even anesthetics that have no direct circulatory effects may cause apparent circulatory depression in severely compromised patients who are dependent on chronically enhanced sympathetic activity. Interruption of this activity by the anesthetized state can lead to acute circulatory decompensation.

Optimal anesthetic management of patients with cardiovascular disease requires a thorough knowledge of normal cardiac physiology (see Chapter 19), the circulatory effects of the various anesthetic agents (see Chapters 7 through 10), and the pathophysiology and treatment of these diseases. The same principles used in treating these diseases preoperatively should be applied intraoperatively. In most instances, the choice of anesthetic agent is not as important as how the agent is used and an understanding of the underlying pathophysiology.

■ CARDIAC RISK FACTORS

 Cardiovascular complications account for 25–50% of deaths following noncardiac surgery. Perioperative myocardial infarction, pulmonary edema, congestive heart failure, arrhythmias, and thromboembolism are most commonly seen in patients with preexisting cardiovascular disease. The incidence of postoperative cardiogenic pulmonary edema is approximately 2% in all patients over 40 years, but 6% in patients with a history of heart failure and 16% in patients with poorly compensated heart failure. The relatively high prevalence of cardiovascular disorders in surgical patients has given rise to attempts to define *cardiac risk* or the likelihood of intraoperative or postoperative fatal or life-threatening cardiac complications (Table 20–1). An American College of Cardiology/American Heart Association Task Force Report has divided clinical markers of increased cardiovascular risk into major, intermediate, and minor predictors (Table 20–2).

The two most important **preoperative risk factors** are a history of recent myocardial infarction (less than 1 month) and evidence of congestive heart failure. Identifying patients at greatest risk allows appropriate measures to be taken that may alter the outcome favorably. Indeed, some studies suggest that a lower complication rate is achieved when invasive monitoring and aggressive hemodynamic interventions (eg, vasodilators, adrenergic blockade) are employed for patients at high risk for cardiac complications. Generally accepted contraindications to elective noncardiac surgery include a myocardial infarction less than 1 month prior to surgery, uncompensated heart failure, and severe aortic or mitral stenosis.

The most important **intraoperative risk factor** appears to be the operative site, while the least consistent

Table 20–1. Factors associated with cardiac complications following noncardiac surgery.

Preoperative factors
Myocardial infarction within 6 months
Congestive heart failure
S_3 gallop
Elevated jugular venous pressure
Abnormal ECG
More than five premature ventricular contractions per minute
A rhythm other than sinus
Premature atrial contractions
Significant aortic stenosis
Patient older than 70 years
Poor general condition of the patient
Intraoperative factors
Emergency surgery
Intrathoracic, intraperitoneal, or aortic procedures
Operative time longer than 3 hours
Wide hemodynamic variations

Table 20–2. Predictors of increased cardiovascular risk following noncardiac surgery.[1]

Major predictors
    Unstable coronary syndromes
        Recent myocardial infarction with evidence of ischemia risk
        Severe or unstable angina
    Severe valvular heart disease
    Decompensated congestive heart failure
    Significant arrhythmias
        High-grade atrioventricular block
        Symptomatic arrhythmia with underlying heart disease
        Supraventricular arrhythmias with uncontrolled ventricular rate
Intermediate predictors
    Mild angina
    Compensated or prior congestive heart failure
    Diabetes mellitus
Minor predictors
    Advanced age
    Abnormal electrocardiogram
    Rhythm other than sinus
    Low functional capacity
    History of stroke
    Uncontrolled systemic hypertension

[1]Based on American College of Cardiology/American Heart Association Practice Guidelines.

factor is operative time. Other suggested factors include unintentional hypotension, unnecessary use of vasopressors, and a high rate-pressure product (heart rate × systolic blood pressure). Although poorly controlled hypertension is not clearly established as a risk factor for postoperative complications, it is frequently associated with wide intraoperative swings in blood pressure. Interestingly, intraoperative hypertension has been more closely linked than hypotension to cardiac morbidity.

While the superiority of regional anesthesia over general anesthesia for patients with cardiovascular disease might seem obvious, studies supporting this view are lacking. Moreover, the hemodynamic effects of spinal and epidural anesthesia (see Chapter 16) may be more detrimental than well-managed general anesthesia for some patients.

■ HYPERTENSION

Preoperative Considerations

Hypertension is a leading cause of death and disability in most Western societies and the most frequent preoperative abnormality in surgical patients, with an overall prevalence of 20–25%. Long-standing uncontrolled hypertension accelerates atherosclerosis and hypertensive organ damage. Hypertension is a major risk factor for cardiac, cerebral, renal, and vascular disease. Complications include myocardial infarction, congestive heart failure, stroke, renal failure, peripheral occlusive disease, and aortic dissection. The presence of left ventricular hypertrophy (LVH) in hypertensive patients may be an important predictor of cardiac mortality. Increased cardiac mortality has also been reported in patients with carotid bruits—even in the absence of symptoms.

Definitions

Blood pressure measurements are affected by many variables, including posture, time of day or night, emotional state, recent activity, and drug intake as well as the equipment and technique used. A diagnosis of hypertension cannot be made by one preoperative reading but requires confirmation by a history of consistently elevated measurements. While preoperative anxiety or pain often produces some degree of hypertension even in normal patients, patients with a history of hypertension generally exhibit greater preoperative elevations in blood pressure.

Epidemiologic studies demonstrate a direct and continuous correlation between both diastolic and systolic blood pressures and mortality rates. The definition of systemic hypertension is somewhat arbitrary but is generally considered to be a consistently elevated diastolic blood pressure greater than 90–95 mm Hg or a systolic pressure greater than 140–160 mm Hg. Borderline hypertension is said to exist when the diastolic pressure is 85–89 mm Hg or the systolic pressure is 140–159 mm Hg. Even patients with borderline hypertension appear to be at some increased for cardiovascular complications. Accelerated, or severe, hypertension is defined as a recent, sustained, and progressive increase in blood pressure, usually with diastolic blood pressures in excess of 110–115 mm Hg; renal dysfunction is often present. Malignant hypertension is a true medical emergency characterized by severe hypertension (> 200/140 mm Hg) associated with papilledema and, frequently, encephalopathy.

Pathophysiology

Hypertension can be either idiopathic (essential) or, less commonly, secondary to other medical conditions such as renal disease, primary hyperaldosteronism, Cushing's syndrome, acromegaly, pheochromocytoma, pregnancy, or estrogen therapy. Essential hypertension accounts for 80–95% of cases and may be associated with an abnormal baseline elevation of cardiac output, sys-

temic vascular resistance (SVR), or both. An evolving pattern is commonly seen over the course of the disease. Initially, cardiac output is elevated, but SVR appears to be in the normal range (in reality, it is inappropriately high). As the disease progresses, cardiac output returns to normal but SVR becomes abnormally high. Extracellular fluid volume and plasma renin activity (see Chapter 29) may be low, normal, or high. The chronic increase in cardiac afterload results in concentric LVH and altered diastolic function (see Chapter 19). Hypertension also alters cerebral autoregulation (see Chapter 25) so that normal cerebral blood flow is maintained in the face of high blood pressures; autoregulation limits may be in the range of mean blood pressures of 110–180 mm Hg.

The mechanisms responsible for the changes observed in hypertensive patients remain elusive but appear to involve vascular hypertrophy, hyperinsulinemia, abnormal increases in intracellular calcium, and increased intracellular sodium concentrations in vascular smooth muscle and renal tubular cells. The increased intracellular calcium presumably results in increased arteriolar tone, while the increased sodium concentration impairs renal excretion of sodium. Sympathetic nervous system overactivity and enhanced responses to sympathetic agonists are present in some patients. Hypertensive patients often display an exaggerated response to vasopressors. Overactivity of the renin-angiotensin-aldosterone system (see Chapter 29) appears to play an important role in patients with accelerated hypertension.

Long-Term Treatment

Drug therapy has been shown to reduce the progression of hypertension, and the incidence of stroke, congestive heart failure, coronary artery disease, and renal damage. Treatment can, however, reverse some of the concomitant pathophysiologic changes, such as LVH and altered cerebral autoregulation.

Most patients with mild hypertension require only single-drug therapy, which may consist of a β-adrenergic blocker, angiotensin-converting enzyme (ACE) inhibitor, calcium channel blocker, or diuretic. Concomitant illnesses that influence drug selection include bronchospastic pulmonary disease, coronary artery disease, congestive heart failure, diabetes, and hyperlipidemia. ACE inhibitors and β-adrenergic blockers are generally less effective in black patients. Also, therapy with β-adrenergic blockers alone may also be less effective in elderly patients.

Patients with moderate to severe hypertension often require a second or third drug. Diuretics are less commonly used as first-line agents because of concerns over electrolyte and metabolic side effects and increased fre-

Table 20–3. Oral antihypertensive agents.

Category	Class	Subclass	Agent
Diuretics	Thiazide-type		Chlorothiazide
			Chlorthalidone
			Hydrochlorothiazide
			Indapamide
			Metolazone
	Potassium-sparing		Spironolactone
			Triamterene
			Amiloride
	Loop		Bumetanide
			Ethacrynic acid
			Furosemide
			Torasemide
Sympatholytics	Adrenergic-receptor blockers	Beta	Acebutolol
			Atenolol
			Betaxolol
			Bisoprolol
			Carteolol
			Metoprolol
			Nadolol
			Penbutolol
			Pindolol
			Propranolol
			Timolol
		Alpha	α_1
			Doxazosin
			Prazosin
			Terazosin
			$\alpha_1 + \alpha_2$
			Phenoxybenzamine
		Alpha and beta	Labetalol
			Carvedilol
	Central α_2-agonists		Clonidine
			Guanabenz
			Guanfacine
			Methyldopa
	Postganglionic blockers	Guanadrel	Guanethidine
			Reserpine

(*continued*)

quency of arrhythmias. These agents are often used to supplement β-adrenergic blockers and ACE inhibitors when single drug therapy is ineffective. ACE inhibitors have been shown to prolong survival in patients with congestive heart failure or left ventricular dysfunction. In addition, these agents appear to preserve renal function in patients with diabetes and those with underlying renal disease. Familiarity with the names and mechanisms of action of commonly used antihypertensive agents is mandatory for anesthesiologists (Table 20–3).

PREOPERATIVE MANAGEMENT

A recurring question in anesthetic practice is the degree of preoperative hypertension that is acceptable for pa-

Table 20–3. Oral antihypertensive agents. (continued)

Category	Class	Subclass	Agent
Vasodilators	Calcium channel blockers	Benzothiazepine	
			Diltiazem
		Phenylalkylamines	
			Verapamil
		Dihydropyridines	
			Amlodipine
			Felodipine
			Isradipine
			Nicardipine
			Nifedipine
			Nisoldipine
	ACE inhibitors		Benazepril
			Captopril
			Enalapril
			Fosinopril
			Lisinopril
			Moexipril
			Perindopril
			Quinapril
			Ramipril
			Trandopril
	Angiotensin-receptor antagonists		Candesartan
			Eprosartan
			Irbesartan
			Losartan
			Telmisartan
			Valsartan
	Direct vasodilators		Hydralazine
			Minoxidil

tients scheduled for elective surgery. Except for optimally controlled patients, most hypertensive patients present to the operating room with some degree of hypertension. While data suggest that even moderate preoperative hypertension (diastolic < 90–110 mm Hg) is not clearly statistically associated with *postoperative* complications, other data indicate that the untreated or poorly controlled hypertensive patient is more apt to experience *intraoperative* episodes of myocardial ischemia, arrhythmias, or both hypertension and hypotension. Intraoperative adjustments in anesthetic depth and use of vasoactive drugs should reduce the incidence of postoperative complications referable to poor preoperative control of hypertension.

While patients should ideally undergo elective surgery only when rendered normotensive, this approach is not always feasible or necessarily desirable because of altered cerebral autoregulation. Excessive reductions in blood pressure can compromise cerebral perfusion. Moreover, the decision whether to delay or to proceed with surgery should be individualized, based on the severity of the preoperative blood pressure elevation; the likelihood of coexisting myocardial ischemia, ventricular dysfunction, or cerebrovascular or renal complications; and the surgical procedure (whether major surgically induced changes in cardiac preload or afterload are anticipated). In many instances, preoperative hypertension is due to the patient's noncompliance with the drug regimen. With rare exceptions, antihypertensive drug therapy should be continued up to the time of surgery. Some clinicians withhold ACE inhibitors on the morning of surgery because of their association with an increased incidence of intraoperative hypotension; however, withholding these agents increases the risk of marked perioperative hypertension and the need for parenteral antihypertensive agents. Surgical procedures on patients with sustained preoperative diastolic blood pressures higher than 110 mm

Hg—especially those with evidence of end-organ damage—should be delayed until blood pressure is better controlled over the course of several days.

History

The preoperative history should inquire into the severity and duration of the hypertension, the drug therapy currently prescribed, and the presence or absence of hypertensive complications. Symptoms of myocardial ischemia, ventricular failure, impaired cerebral perfusion, or peripheral vascular disease should be elicited, as well as the patient's record of compliance with the drug regimen. Questions should deal with chest pains, exercise tolerance, shortness of breath (especially at night), dependent edema, postural lightheadedness, syncope, amaurosis, and claudication. Adverse effects of current antihypertensive drug therapy (Table 20–4) should also be identified. Evaluating a history of a previous myocardial infarction is dealt with below; stroke is discussed in Chapter 27.

Physical Examination & Laboratory Evaluation

Ophthalmoscopy is probably the most useful examination in hypertensive patients (other than sphygmo-manometry), but unfortunately it is usually not done. Visible changes in the retinal vasculature usually parallel the severity and progression of arteriosclerosis and hypertensive damage in other organs. An S_4 cardiac gallop is common in patients with LVH. Other physical findings such as pulmonary rales and an S_3 cardiac gallop are late findings and indicate congestive heart failure. Blood pressure should be measured in both the supine and standing positions. Orthostatic changes can be due to volume depletion (see Chapter 29), excessive vasodilation, or sympatholytic drug therapy; preoperative fluid administration can prevent severe hypotension after induction of anesthesia in these patients. Although asymptomatic carotid bruits are usually hemodynamically insignificant (see Chapter 27), they are reflective of atherosclerotic vascular disease that may affect the coronary circulation.

The electrocardiogram (ECG) is often normal, but in patients with a long history of hypertension it often shows evidence of ischemia, conduction abnormalities, an old infarction, or left ventricular hypertrophy or strain. A normal ECG does not necessarily exclude coronary artery disease or LVH. Similarly, a normal heart size on a chest radiograph does not necessarily exclude ventricular hypertrophy. Echocardiography is a more sensitive test of LVH and can be used to evaluate

Table 20–4. Adverse effects of long-term antihypertensive therapy.

Class	Adverse Effects
Diuretics	
Thiazide	Hypokalemia, hyponatremia, hyperglycemia, hyperuricemia, hypomagnesemia, hyperlipidemia, hypercalcemia
Loop	Hypokalemia, hyperglycemia, hypocalcemia, hypomagnesemia, metabolic alkalosis
Potassium-sparing	Hyperkalemia
Sympatholytics	
β-Adrenergic blockers	Bradycardia, conduction blockade, myocardial depression, enhanced bronchial tone, sedation, fatigue, depression
α-Adrenergic blockers	Postural hypertension, tachycardia, fluid retention
Central α₂-agonists	Postural hypotension, sedation, dry mouth, depression, decreased anesthetic requirements, bradycardia, rebound hypertension, positive Coombs test and hemolytic anemia (methyldopa), hepatitis (methyldopa)
Ganglionic blockers	Postural hypotension, diarrhea, fluid retention, depression (reserpine)
Vasodilators	
Calcium channels blockers	Cardiac depression, bradycardia, conduction blockade (verapamil, diltiazem), peripheral edema (nifedipine), tachycardia (nifedipine), enhanced neuromuscular nondepolarizing blockade
ACE inhibitors	Cough, angioedema, reflex tachycardia, fluid retention, renal dysfunction, renal failure in bilateral renal artery stenosis, hyperkalemia, bone marrow depression (captopril)
Angiotensin-receptor antagonists	Hypotension, renal failure in bilateral renal artery stenosis, hyperkalemia
Direct vasodilators	Reflex tachycardia, fluid retention, headache, systemic lupus erythematosus-like syndrome (hydralazine), pleural or pericardial effusion (minoxidil)

ACE = angiotensin-converting enzyme.

ventricular systolic and diastolic functions in patients with symptoms of heart failure (see Chapter 19). Chest radiographs are usually unremarkable but may show a boot-shaped heart (suggestive of LVH), frank cardiomegaly, or pulmonary vascular congestion.

Renal function is best evaluated by measurement of serum creatinine and blood urea nitrogen levels (see Chapter 32). Serum electrolyte levels should be determined in patients taking diuretics or digoxin or those with renal impairment. Mild to moderate hypokalemia is often seen in patients taking diuretics (3–3.5 mEq/L) but usually does not appear to affect outcome adversely. Potassium replacement should probably be undertaken only in symptomatic patients or those who are also taking digoxin (see Chapter 28). Hypomagnesemia is also often present and may be an important cause of perioperative arrhythmias. Hyperkalemia may be encountered in patients—especially those with impaired renal function (see Chapter 29)—who are taking potassium-sparing diuretics or ACE inhibitors.

Premedication

Premedication reduces preoperative anxiety and is highly desirable in hypertensive patients. Mild to moderate preoperative hypertension often resolves following administration of an anxiolytic agent, such as midazolam. Preoperative antihypertensive agents should be continued as close to schedule as possible and can be given with a small sip of water. As mentioned earlier in this chapter, some clinicians withhold ACE inhibitors because of concerns over an increased incidence of intraoperative hypotension. Central α_2-adrenergic agonists can be useful adjuncts for premedicating hypertensive patients; clonidine (0.2 mg) augments sedation, decreases the intraoperative anesthetic requirement, and reduces perioperative hypertension. Unfortunately, preoperative clonidine administration has been associated with profound intraoperative hypotension and bradycardia.

INTRAOPERATIVE MANAGEMENT

Objectives

The overall anesthetic plan for a hypertensive patient is to maintain a stable blood pressure range appropriate for that patient. Patients with borderline hypertension may be treated as normotensive patients. Those with long-standing or poorly controlled hypertension, however, have altered autoregulation of cerebral blood flow; higher than normal mean blood pressures may be required to maintain adequate cerebral blood flow. Because most patients with long-standing hypertension must be assumed to have some element of coronary

artery disease and cardiac hypertrophy, excessive blood pressure elevations are undesirable. Hypertension, especially in association with tachycardia, can precipitate or exacerbate myocardial ischemia, ventricular dysfunction, or both. Arterial blood pressure should generally be kept within 10–20% of preoperative levels. If marked hypertension (> 180/120 mm Hg) is present preoperatively, arterial blood pressure should be maintained in the high-normal range (150–140/90–80 mm Hg).

Monitoring

Most hypertensive patients do not require special intraoperative monitors. Direct intra-arterial pressure monitoring should be reserved for patients with wide swings in blood pressure and for those undergoing major surgical procedures associated with rapid or marked changes in cardiac preload or afterload. Electrocardiographic monitoring should focus on detecting signs of ischemia. Urinary output should generally be closely monitored with an indwelling urinary catheter in patients with renal impairment who are undergoing procedures expected to last more than 2 hours. When invasive hemodynamic monitoring is used, reduced ventricular compliance (see Chapter 19) is often apparent in patients with ventricular hypertrophy; higher pulmonary capillary wedge pressures (12–18 mm Hg) may be required to maintain adequate left ventricular end-diastolic volume and cardiac output.

Induction

 Induction of anesthesia and endotracheal intubation are often a period of hemodynamic instability for hypertensive patients. Regardless of the level of preoperative blood pressure control, many patients with hypertension display an accentuated hypotensive response to induction of anesthesia, followed by an exaggerated hypertensive response to intubation. The hypotensive response at induction may reflect the additive circulatory depressant effects of anesthetic agents and antihypertensive agents (see Table 20–4). Many, if not most, antihypertensive agents and general anesthetics are vasodilators, cardiac depressants, or both. In addition, many hypertensive patients are already volume-depleted. Sympatholytic agents also attenuate the normal protective circulatory reflexes (see Chapter 19), reducing sympathetic tone and enhancing vagal activity.

Up to 25% of patients may exhibit severe hypertension following endotracheal intubation. The duration of laryngoscopy, which bears some relationship to the degree of hypertension, should be as short as possible. Moreover, intubation should generally be performed under deep anesthesia, (provided hypotension can be avoided). One of several techniques may be used before intubation to attenuate the hypertensive response:

- Deepening anesthesia with a potent volatile agent for 5–10 minutes
- Administering a bolus of an opioid (fentanyl, 2.5–5 μg/kg; alfentanil, 15–25 μg/kg; or sufentanil, 0.25–0.5 μg/kg; or remifentanil 0.5–1 μg/kg)
- Administering lidocaine, 1.5 mg/kg intravenously or intratracheally
- Achieving β-adrenergic blockade with esmolol, 0.3–1.5 mg/kg; propranolol, 1–3 mg; or labetalol, 5–20 mg
- Giving intravenous nitroprusside or nitroglycerin, 0.5–1 μg/kg
- Using topical airway anesthesia (see Chapter 5).

Choice of Anesthetic Agents

A. INDUCTION AGENTS:

The superiority of any one agent or technique over another has not been clearly established for hypertensive agents. Even following regional anesthesia, hypertensive patients frequently have more exaggerated reductions in blood pressure than do normotensive patients. Barbiturates, benzodiazepines, propofol, and etomidate are equally safe for inducing general anesthesia in most hypertensive patients. Ketamine by itself is contraindicated for elective procedures, because its sympathetic stimulation can precipitate marked hypertension (see Chapter 8); its sympathetic stimulating properties can be blunted or eliminated by the concomitant administration of a small doses of another agent, especially a benzodiazepine or propofol.

B. MAINTENANCE AGENTS:

Anesthesia may be safely continued with volatile agents (alone or with nitrous oxide), a balanced technique (opioid + nitrous oxide + muscle relaxant), or totally intravenous techniques. Regardless of the primary maintenance technique, addition of a volatile agent or intravenous vasodilator generally allows more satisfactory intraoperative blood pressure control. The vasodilation and relatively rapid and reversible myocardial depression afforded by volatile agents allows titration of their effects against arterial blood pressure. Some clinicians believe that, of the opioids, sufentanil may provide the

Table 20–5. Parenteral agents for the acute treatment of hypertension.

Agent	Dosage Range	Onset	Duration
Nitroprusside	0.5–10 μg/kg/min	30–60 sec	1–5 min
Nitroglycerin	0.5–10 μg/kg/min	1 min	3–5 min
Esmolol	0.5 mg/kg over 1 min; 50–300 μg/kg/min	1 min	12–20 min
Labetalol	5–20 mg	1–2 min	4–8 h
Propranolol	1–3 mg	1–2 min	4–6 h
Trimethaphan	1–6 mg/min	1–3 min	10–30 min
Phentolamine	1–5 mg	1–10 min	20–40 min
Diazoxide	1–3 mg/kg slowly	2–10 min	4–6 h
Hydralazine	5–20 mg	5–20 min	4–8 h
Nifedipine (sublingual)	10 mg	5–10 min	4 h
Methyldopa	250–1000 mg	2–3 h	6–12 h
Nicardipine	0.25–0.5 mg	1–5 min	3–4 h
Enalaprilat	0.625–1 mg	6–15 min	4–6 h
Fenoldopam	0.1–1.6 μg/kg/min	5 min	5 min

greatest autonomic suppression and control over blood pressure.

C. MUSCLE RELAXANTS:

With the possible exception of large boluses of pancuronium, any muscle relaxant (also called neuromuscular blocking agents) can be used routinely. Pancuronium-induced vagal blockade and neural release of catecholamines can exacerbate hypertension in poorly controlled patients. When pancuronium is given slowly in small increments, however, marked increases in heart rate or blood pressure are less likely. Moreover, pancuronium is useful in offsetting excessive vagal tone induced by opioids or surgical manipulations. Hypotension following large (intubating) doses of tubocurarine, metocurine, atracurium, or mivacurium (see Chapter 9) may be accentuated in hypertensive patients.

D. VASOPRESSORS:

 Hypertensive patients may display an exaggerated response to both endogenous catecholamines (from intubation or surgical stimulation) and exogenously administered sympathetic agonists. If a vasopressor is necessary to treat excessive hypotension, a small dose of a direct-acting agent such as phenylephrine (25–50 μg) may be preferable to an indirect agent. Nonetheless, small doses of ephedrine (5–10 mg) are more appropriate when vagal tone is high. Patients taking sympatholytics preoperatively may exhibit a decreased response to vasopressors, especially ephedrine.

Intraoperative Hypertension

Intraoperative hypertension not responding to an increase in anesthetic depth (especially with a volatile agent) can be treated with a variety of parenteral agents (Table 20–5). Readily reversible causes—such as inadequate anesthetic depth, hypoxemia, or hypercapnia—should always be excluded before initiating antihypertensive therapy. Selection of a hypotensive agent (see Chapter 13) depends on the severity, acuteness, and cause of hypertension, the baseline ventricular function, the heart rate, and the presence of bronchospastic pulmonary disease. β-Adrenergic blockade alone or as a supplement is a good choice for a patient with good ventricular function and an elevated heart rate but is contraindicated in those with bronchospastic disease. Nicardipine may be preferable for patients with bronchospastic disease. Reflex tachycardia following sublingual nifedipine has been associated with myocardial ischemia. Nitroprusside remains the most rapid and effective agent for the intraoperative treatment of moderate to severe hypertension. Nitroglycerin may be less effective but is also useful in treating or preventing myocardial ischemia. Fenoldopam

is also a useful agent and may improve or maintain renal function. Hydralazine provides sustained blood pressure control but has a delayed onset and is often associated with reflex tachycardia. The latter is not seen with labetalol because of combined α- and β-adrenergic blockade.

POSTOPERATIVE MANAGEMENT

Postoperative hypertension (see Chapter 49) is common and should be anticipated in patients who have poorly controlled hypertension. Close blood pressure monitoring should be continued in both the recovery room and the early postoperative period. In addition to myocardial ischemia and congestive heart failure, marked sustained elevations in blood pressure can contribute to the formation of wound hematomas and the disruption of vascular suture lines.

Hypertension in the recovery period is often multifactorial and enhanced by respiratory abnormalities, pain, volume overload, or bladder distention (see Chapter 49). Contributing causes should be corrected and parenteral antihypertensive agents given if necessary. Intravenous nicardipine is useful in controlling blood pressure in this setting, particularly if myocardial ischemia is suspected or bronchospasm is present. When the patient resumes oral intake, preoperative medications should be restarted.

ISCHEMIC HEART DISEASE

Preoperative Considerations

Myocardial ischemia is characterized by a metabolic oxygen demand that exceeds oxygen supply (see Chapter 19). Ischemia can therefore result from a marked increase in myocardial metabolic demand, a reduction in myocardial oxygen delivery, or a combination of both. Common causes include severe hypertension or tachycardia (especially in the presence of ventricular hypertrophy); coronary arterial vasospasm or anatomic obstruction; severe hypotension, hypoxemia, or anemia; and severe aortic stenosis or regurgitation.

By far the most common cause of myocardial ischemia is atherosclerosis of the coronary arteries. Coronary artery disease is responsible for well over one-third of all deaths in Western societies and is a major cause of perioperative morbidity and mortality. The overall incidence of coronary artery disease in surgical patients is estimated to be between 5% and 10%. Major risk factors for coronary artery disease include hyperlipidemia, hypertension, diabetes, cigarette smoking, increasing age, male sex, and a positive family history. Other risk factors include obesity, a history of cerebrovascular or peripheral vascular disease, menopause, use of high-estrogen oral contraceptives (in women who smoke), a sedentary life-style, and perhaps a coronary-prone behavior pattern. By age 65, the incidence of coronary artery disease is close to 37% for men, compared with 18% for women.

Coronary artery disease may be clinically manifested by symptoms of myocardial necrosis (infarction), ischemia (usually angina), arrhythmias (including sudden death), or ventricular dysfunction (congestive heart failure). When symptoms of congestive heart failure predominate, the term **ischemic cardiomyopathy** is often used. Three major clinical syndromes are generally recognized: myocardial infarction, unstable angina, and chronic stable angina. Acute myocardial infarction is discussed in Chapter 50.

Unstable Angina

This clinical entity is defined as (1) an abrupt increase in severity, frequency (more than three episodes per day) or duration of anginal attacks (**crescendo angina**), (2) angina at rest, or (3) new onset of angina (within the past 2 months) with severe or frequent episodes (> 3/day). The anginal episodes are often not related to any apparent precipitating factors. Unstable angina may also occur following myocardial infarction or be precipitated by noncardiac medical conditions (including severe anemia, fever, infections, thyrotoxicosis, hypoxemia, and emotional distress) in previously stable patients.

The importance of this syndrome, especially when it is associated with significant ST-segment changes at rest, is that it usually reflects severe underlying coronary disease and frequently precedes myocardial infarction. Plaque disruption with platelet aggregates or thrombi and vasospasm are frequent pathologic correlates. Critical stenosis in one or more major coronary arteries is present in over 80% of patients. Patients with unstable angina require admission to a coronary care unit for evaluation and treatment. Anticoagulation with heparin is usually instituted, together with aspirin, intravenous nitroglycerin, β-blockers and, possibly, calcium channel blockers. If the ischemia does not resolve within 24–48 hours, the patient is evaluated by coronary angiography for angioplasty or emergency surgical revascularization.

Chronic Stable Angina

Chest pains are most often substernal, exertional, radiating to the neck or arm, and relieved by rest or nitroglycerin. Variations are common, including epigastric, back, or neck pain or transient shortness of breath from ventricular dysfunction (**anginal equivalent**). Nonexertional ischemia and silent (asymptomatic) ischemia are recognized as fairly common occurrences. Diabetics have a relatively high incidence of silent ischemia.

Symptoms are generally absent until the atherosclerotic lesions cause 50–75% occlusions in the coronary circulation. When a stenotic segment reaches 70% occlusion, maximum compensatory dilatation is usually present distally: blood flow is generally adequate at rest but becomes inadequate with increased metabolic demand. An extensive collateral blood supply allows some patients to remain relatively asymptomatic in spite of severe disease. Coronary vasospasm is also a cause of transient transmural ischemia in some patients; 90% of vasospastic episodes occur at preexisting stenotic lesions in epicardial vessels and are often precipitated by a variety of factors, including emotional upset and hyperventilation (**Prinzmetal's angina**). Coronary spasm is most often observed in patients who have angina with varying levels of activity or with emotional stress (**variable-threshold**); it is least common with classic exertional (**fixed-threshold**) angina.

The overall prognosis of patients with coronary artery disease is related to both the number and severity of coronary obstructions as well as ventricular function.

Treatment of Ischemic Heart Disease

The general approach in treating patients with ischemic heart disease is 5-fold:

- Correction of coronary risk factors in the hope of slowing disease progression
- Modification of the patient's lifestyle to eliminate stress and improve exercise tolerance
- Correction of complicating medical conditions that can exacerbate ischemia, such as hypertension, anemia, hypoxemia, thyrotoxicosis, fever, infection, or adverse drug effects
- Pharmacologic manipulation of the myocardial oxygen supply-demand relationship (see Chapter 19)
- Correction of coronary lesions by percutaneous angioplasty (with or without stenting, atherectomy, or brachytherapy) or coronary artery bypass surgery.

With the exception of the first, these approaches are of direct relevance to anesthesiologists. The same principles should be applied in the care of these patients in both the operating room and the intensive care unit.

The most commonly used pharmacologic agents are nitrates, β-blockers, and calcium channel blockers. These drugs also have potent circulatory effects, which are compared in Table 20–6. Any of these agents can be used for mild angina. Calcium channel blockers are the drugs of choice for patients with predominantly vasospastic angina, while β-adrenergic blocking agents are usually used in patients with exertional angina and good ventricular function. Nitrates are good agents for both types of angina.

Table 20–6. Comparison of antianginal agents.

Cardiac Parameter	Nitrates	Calcium Channel Blockers			β-Blockers
		Verapamil	*Nifedipine Nicardipine Nimodipine*	*Diltiazem*	
Preload	↓↓	—	—	—	—/↑
Afterload	↓	↓	↓↓	↓	—/↓
Contractility	—	↓↓	—	↓	↓↓↓
SA node automaticity	↑/—	↓↓	↑/—	↓↓	↓↓↓
AV conduction	—	↓↓↓	—	↓↓	↓↓↓
Vasodilation					
Coronary	↑	↑↑	↑↑↑	↑↑	—/↓
Systemic	↑↑	↑	↑↑	↑	—/↓

SA = sinoatrial, AV = atrioventricular.
↑ = Increases.
— = No change.
↓ = Decreases.

A. NITRATES:

Nitrates relax all vascular smooth muscle but have a much greater effect on venous than on arterial vessels. Decreasing venous tone and reducing venous return to the heart (cardiac preload) reduces wall tension and afterload. These effects tend to reduce myocardial oxygen demand. The prominent venodilation makes nitrates excellent agents when congestive heart failure is also present.

Perhaps equally important, nitrates dilate the coronary arteries. Even minor degrees of dilation at stenotic sites may be sufficient to increase blood flow, because flow is inversely related to the fourth power of the radius. Nitrate-induced coronary vasodilation preferentially increases subendocardial blood flow in ischemic areas. This favorable redistribution of coronary blood flow to ischemic areas may be dependent on the presence of collaterals in the coronary circulation.

Nitrates can be used for both the treatment of acute ischemia and prophylaxis against frequent anginal episodes. Unlike β-blockers and calcium channel blockers, nitrates do not have a negative inotropic effect—a desirable feature in the presence of ventricular dysfunction. Intravenous nitroglycerin can also be used for controlled hypotensive anesthesia (see Chapter 13).

B. CALCIUM CHANNEL BLOCKERS:

The effects and uses of the most commonly used calcium channel blockers are shown in Tables 20–6 and 20–7. This group of agents reduces myocardial oxygen demand by decreasing cardiac afterload and augments

oxygen supply by increasing blood flow (coronary vasodilation). Verapamil and diltiazem also reduce demand by slowing the heart rate.

Nifedipine's potent effects on the systemic blood pressure may precipitate hypotension, reflex tachycardia, or both; its fast-onset preparations (eg, sublingual) has been associated with myocardial infarction in some patients. Its tendency to decrease afterload generally offsets any negative inotropic effect. The slow-release form of nifedipine is associated with much less reflex tachycardia and is more suitable than other agents for patients with ventricular dysfunction. Amlodipine, which has a similar profile to nifedipine but almost no effect on heart rate, is also used in patients with ventricular dysfunction. In contrast, verapamil and diltiazem have greater effects on cardiac contractility and atrioventricular (AV) conduction and therefore should be used cautiously, if at all, in patients with ventricular dysfunction, conduction abnormalities, or bradyarrhythmias. Diltiazem appears to be better tolerated than verapamil in patients with impaired ventricular function. Nicardipine and nimodipine generally have the same effects as nifedipine; nimodipine is primarily used in preventing cerebral vasospasm following subarachnoid hemorrhage, while nicardipine is used as an intravenous arterial vasodilator.

Calcium channel blockers can have significant interactions with anesthetic agents. All agents appear to potentiate both depolarizing and nondepolarizing neuromuscular blocking agents and the circulatory effects of volatile agents. Verapamil may also modestly decrease anesthetic requirements. Both verapamil and diltiazem

Table 20–7. Comparison of calcium channel blockers.

Agent	Route	Dosage[1]	Half-life	Clinical Use			
				Angina	Hypertension	Cerebral Vasospasm	Supraventricular Tachycardia
Verapamil	PO	40–240 mg	5 h	+	+		+
	IV	5–15 mg	5 h	+			+
Nifedipine	PO	30–180 mg	2 h	+	+		
	SL	10 mg	2 h	+	+		
Diltiazem	PO	30–60 mg	4 h	+	+		+
	IV	0.25–0.35 mg/kg	4 h	+			+
Nicardipine	PO	60–120 mg	2–4 h	+	+		
	IV	0.25–0.5 mg/kg	2–4 h	+	+		
Nimodipine	PO	240 mg	2 h			+	
Bepridil[2]	PO	200–400 mg	24 h	+	+		
Isradipine	PO	2.5–5.0 mg	8 h		+		
Felodipine	PO	5–20 mg	9 h		+		
Amlodipine	PO	2.5–10 mg	30–50 h	+	+		

SVT = supraventricular tachycardia.
[1]Total oral dose per day divided into three doses unless otherwise stated.
[2]Also possesses antiarrhythmic properties.

can potentiate depression of cardiac contractility and conduction in the AV node by volatile anesthetics. Nifedipine and similar agents can potentiate systemic vasodilation by volatile and intravenous agents.

C. β-ADRENERGIC BLOCKING AGENTS:

These drugs decrease myocardial oxygen demand by reducing heart rate and contractility and, in some cases, afterload (via their antihypertensive effect). Optimal blockade results in a resting heart rate between 50 and 60 beats/min and prevents appreciable increases with exercise (< 20 beats/min increase during exercise). Available agents differ in receptor selectivity, intrinsic sympathomimetic (partial agonist) activity, and membrane-stabilizing properties (Table 20–8). Membrane stabilization, often described as a quinidine-like effect, results in antiarrhythmic activity. Agents with intrinsic sympathomimetic properties are better tolerated by patients with mild to moderate ventricular dysfunction. Low doses of β-blockers have been shown to be beneficial in some patients with compensated congestive heart failure. Nonselective β-receptor blockade is contraindicated in patients with significant ventricular dysfunction, conduction abnormalities, or bronchospastic disease. Blockade of β$_2$-adrenergic receptors also can mask

hypoglycemic symptoms in awake diabetic patients, delay metabolic recovery from hypoglycemia, and impair the handling of large potassium loads (see Chapter 28). Nonselective blockers can also theoretically intensify coronary vasospasm in some patients and thus may be contraindicated in patients with predominantly vasospastic angina. Cardioselective (β$_1$-receptor specific) agents must still be used cautiously in patients with reactive airways, because the selectivity of these agents tends to be dose-dependent. Acebutolol may be most useful in patients with bronchospastic airway disease, because it is has both β$_1$-selectivity and intrinsic sympathomimetic activity.

D. OTHER AGENTS:

ACE inhibitors have been shown to prolong survival in patients with congestive heart failure or left ventricular dysfunction. Digoxin is beneficial for patients with atrial fibrillation who are capable of a rapid ventricular response and for patients with cardiomegaly, especially if symptoms of heart failure are present. Chronic aspirin therapy appears to reduce coronary events even in patients with asymptomatic coronary artery disease. Antiarrhythmic therapy in patients with complex ventricular ectopy who have significant coronary artery dis-

Table 20–8. Comparison of β-adrenergic blocking agents.

Agent	β₁-Receptor Selectivity	Half-life	Sympathomimetic	α-Receptor Blockade	Membrane Stabilizing
Acebutolol	+	2–4 h	+		+
Atenolol	++	5–9 h			
Betaxlol	++	14–22 h			
Esmolol	++	9 min			
Metoprolol	++	3–4 h			±
Bisoprolol	+	9–12 h			
Oxprenolol		1–2 h	+		+
Alprenolol		2–3 h	+		+
Pindolol		3–4 h	++		±
Penbutolol		5 h	+		+
Carteolol		6 h	+		
Labetalol		4–8 h		+	±
Propranolol		3–6 h			++
Timolol		3–5 h			
Sotalol¹		5–13 h			
Nadolol		10–24 h			
Carvedilol		6–8 h		+	±

¹Also possesses unique antiarrhythmic properties.

ease and left ventricular dysfunction should be guided by an electrophysiologic study. Patients with inducible sustained ventricular tachycardia or ventricular fibrillation are candidates for an automatic internal cardioverter-defibrillator. Treatment of ventricular ectopy (with the exception of sustained ventricular tachycardia) in patients with good ventricular function does not improve survival and may increase mortality.

E. COMBINATION THERAPY:

Moderate to severe angina frequently requires combination therapy with two or all three classes of agents. Patients with ventricular dysfunction may not tolerate the combined negative inotropic effect of a β-blocker and a calcium channel blocker together; an ACE inhibitor is better tolerated and appears to improve survival. Similarly, the additive effect of a β-blocker and a calcium channel blocker on the AV node may precipitate heart block in susceptible patients. The combination of amlodipine and a long-acting nitrate is generally well tolerated by patients with significant ventricular dysfunction but may cause excessive vasodilation in some patients.

PREOPERATIVE MANAGEMENT

The importance of ischemic heart disease—especially a history of myocardial infarction—as a risk factor for perioperative morbidity and mortality has been discussed above. Numerous investigations have been done to delineate more specific relationships between preoperative electrocardiographic changes, angina, a history of myocardial infarction, angiographic evidence of coronary occlusions, previous coronary artery bypass surgery, and outcome. Most studies confirm that perioperative outcome is related to both disease severity and ventricular function. Patients with extensive (three-vessel or left main) coronary artery disease, a history of myocardial infarction, or ventricular dysfunction are at greatest risk for cardiac complications. Chronic stable (mild to moderate) angina does not appear to increase perioperative risk substantially.

The most consistent finding relates to the incidence of perioperative myocardial infarction in patients with a previous myocardial infarction. The risk is the same whether the infarct was transmural or subendocardial. Older studies suggested that patients with myocardial infarction less than 6 months previously appear to be at greatest risk. Moreover, the mortality rates reported for such perioperative infarcts are usually more than 50%. More recent data suggest the greatest risk is during the first month postinfarction. Moreover, the risk appears related to the amount of residual ischemia remaining (additional myocardium at risk of infarction). A history of prior coronary artery bypass surgery or coronary angioplasty alone does not appear to increase perioperative risk. The use of invasive hemodynamic monitoring and aggressive intraoperative interventions, such as vasodilators and β-blockers, may substantially reduce the reinfarction rate in patients with a recent myocardial infarction.

History

The history is of prime importance in patients with ischemic heart disease. Questions should encompass symptoms, current and past treatment, complications, and the results of previous evaluations. This information alone is usually enough to provide some estimate of disease severity and ventricular function.

The most important symptoms to elicit include chest pains, dyspnea, poor exercise tolerance, syncope, or near-syncope. The relationship between symptoms and activity level should be established. Activity should be described in terms of everyday tasks such as walking or climbing stairs. Patients with severe disease may be relatively asymptomatic because of a very sedentary lifestyle. The patient's description of chest pains may suggest a major role for vasospasm (variable-threshold angina). Easy fatigability or shortness of breath suggests compromised ventricular function.

A history of unstable angina or myocardial infarction should include the time of its occurrence and whether it was complicated by arrhythmias, conduction disturbances, or heart failure. Patients with prior anterior infarctions tend to have more severe disease than do those with prior inferior infarctions. Localization of the areas of ischemia is invaluable in deciding which electrocardiographic leads to monitor intraoperatively. Arrhythmias and conduction abnormalities are more common in patients with previous infarction and those with poor ventricular function.

Physical Examination & Routine Laboratory Evaluation

Evaluation of patients with coronary artery disease is similar to that of patients with hypertension; indeed, both diseases are often simultaneously present in the same patient. Laboratory evaluation for patients who have a history compatible with recent unstable angina and are undergoing emergency procedures should also include serum cardiac enzymes. Serum levels of cardiac-specific troponins (T or I), creatine kinase (MB isoenzyme), and lactate dehydrogenase (type 1 isoenzyme) levels are useful in excluding myocardial infarction. Serum digoxin and other antiarrhythmic levels may also be useful in excluding drug toxicity.

The baseline ECG is normal in 25–50% of patients with coronary artery disease but no prior myocardial infarction. A very straight ST-segment has been associated with underlying coronary artery disease; the normal ST-segment gradually slopes away from the QRS complex and into the T wave. Electrocardiographic evidence of ischemia often becomes apparent only during chest pain. The most common baseline abnormalities are nonspecific ST-segment and T-wave changes. Prior infarction more often than not is manifested by Q waves or loss of R waves in the leads closest to the infarct. First-degree AV block, bundle-branch block, or hemiblock may be present. Persistent ST-segment elevation following myocardial infarction is often indicative of a left ventricular aneurysm. A long rate-corrected QT interval ($QT_c > 0.44$ sec) may reflect the underlying ischemia, drug toxicity (usually class Ia antiarrhythmic agents, antidepressants, or phenothiazines), electrolyte abnormalities (hypokalemia or hypomagnesemia), autonomic dysfunction, mitral valve prolapse or, less commonly, a congenital abnormality. Patients with a long QT interval are at risk for developing ventricular arrhythmias—especially polymorphic ventricular tachycardia (torsade de pointes), which can lead to ventricular fibrillation. The long QT interval reflects nonuniform prolongation of ventricular repolarization and predisposes patients to reentry phenomena (see Chapter 19). Elective surgery should be postponed until drug toxicity and electrolyte imbalances are excluded. In contrast to polymorphic ventricular arrhythmias with a normal QT interval, which respond to conventional antiarrhythmics (see Chapters 19 and 48), polymorphic tachyarrhythmias with a long QT interval generally respond best to pacing or magnesium. Patients with congenital prolongation generally respond to β-adrenergic blocking agents. Left stellate ganglion blockade (see Chapter 18) is also effective and suggests that autonomic imbalance plays an important role in this group of patients.

The chest film is a useful screening test in excluding cardiomegaly or pulmonary vascular congestion secondary to ventricular dysfunction. Rarely, calcification of the coronaries, aorta, or the aortic valve may be seen.

Specialized Studies

When used as screening tests for the general population, noninvasive stress tests have a low predictability in normal patients but are sufficiently reliable in patients with suspected coronary disease (Bayes' theorem). Correct preoperative interpretation of these tests is important, especially in patients in whom coronary artery disease is suspected. Holter monitoring, exercise electrocardiography, scintigraphy, and two-dimensional echocardiography are important in determining perioperative risk and the need for coronary angiography.

A. HOLTER MONITORING:

Continuous ambulatory electrocardiographic (Holter) monitoring is useful in evaluating arrhythmias, antiarrhythmic drug therapy, and the severity and frequency of ischemic episodes. Silent (asymptomatic) ischemic episodes are frequent findings in patients with coronary artery disease. Moreover, the preoperative occurrence of frequent ischemic episodes on Holter monitoring correlates well with intraoperative and postoperative ischemia. Holter monitoring may be a good screening test because it has an excellent negative predictive value for postoperative cardiac complications.

B. EXERCISE ELECTROCARDIOGRAPHY:

The usefulness of this test is limited in patients with baseline ST-segment abnormalities and those who are unable to increase their heart rate (> 85% of maximal predicted) because of fatigue, dyspnea, or drug therapy. Overall sensitivity is 65%, while specificity is 90%. The test is most sensitive (85%) in patients with three-vessel or left main coronary artery disease. Disease that is limited to the left circumflex artery may also be missed because ischemia in its distribution may not be evident on the standard surface ECG. A normal test does not necessarily exclude coronary artery disease but suggests that severe disease is not likely. The degree of ST-segment depression, its severity and configuration, the time of onset in the test, and the time required for resolution are important findings. Other significant findings include changes in blood pressure and the occurrence of arrhythmias. Exercise-induced ventricular ectopy frequently indicates severe coronary artery disease associated with ventricular dysfunction. The ischemia presumably leads to electrical instability in myocardial cells. Factors associated with severe multivessel disease are listed in Table 20–9.

C. THALLIUM IMAGING (SCINTIGRAPHY):

Thallium studies following exercise or injection of dipyridamole (a coronary vasodilator) have a high sensitivity but only fairly good specificity for detecting coronary artery disease. They are best for detecting two- or three-vessel disease. These scans can locate and quantitate areas of ischemia or scarring and differentiate between the two. Perfusion defects that fill in on the redistribution phase represent ischemia, not previous

Table 20–9. Factors associated with severe multivessel disease during exercise electrocardiography.

- More than 2 mm horizontal or down-sloping ST depression
- Early onset of ST depression with low workload
- Persistence of ST depression after exercise for 5 minutes or longer
- Sustained decrease ($\geq$ 10 mm Hg) in systolic blood pressure during exercise
- Failure to reach a maximum heart rate greater than 70% of predicted
- Frequent or complex ventricular dysrhythmias at a low heart rate

infarction. A dipyridamole-thallium study may be useful in patients with poor conditioning or peripheral vascular disease, because it obviates the need for exercise.

D. TWO-DIMENSIONAL ECHOCARDIOGRAPHY:

This technique provides information about both regional and global ventricular function, and may be carried at rest, following exercise, or with administration of dobutamine. Detectable regional wall motion abnormalities and the derived left ventricular ejection fraction have good correlation with angiographic findings. Moreover, dobutamine stress echocardiography appears to be a reliable predictor of adverse cardiac complications. New or worsening wall motion abnormalities following dobutamine infusion are indicative of significant ischemia. Patients with an ejection fraction less than 50% tend to have severe disease and have increased perioperative morbidity.

E. CORONARY ANGIOGRAPHY:

Coronary angiography remains the gold standard in evaluating coronary artery disease and is now associated with an acceptably low complication rate (< 1%). Nonetheless, coronary angiography should be performed only to determine if the patient may benefit from percutaneous coronary angioplasty or coronary artery bypass grafting prior to noncardiac surgery. The location and severity of occlusions can be defined, and coronary vasospasm may also be observed on angiography. In evaluating fixed stenotic lesions, occlusions greater than 50–75% are generally considered significant. Estimates of the percentage of occlusion can be misleading (especially when between 40% and 80%) because of differences among observers and the typical assumption that occlusions are concentric when they are often eccentric. The severity of disease is often expressed according to the number of major coronary vessels affected (one-, two-, or three-vessel disease). Significant stenosis of the left main coronary artery is ominous because it affects almost the entire left ventricle. Moreover, even 50–75% occlusions in the left main artery can be hemodynamically significant.

Ventriculography and measurement of intracardiac pressures also provide important information. The single most important measurement is the ejection fraction. Indicators of significant ventricular dysfunction include an ejection fraction less than 0.5, a left ventricular end-diastolic pressure greater than 18 mm Hg after injection of contrast, a cardiac index less than 2.2 L/min/m^2, and marked or multiple wall motion abnormalities.

Premedication

Allaying fear, anxiety, and pain preoperatively are desirable goals in patients with coronary artery disease. Satisfactory premedication prevents sympathetic activation, which adversely affects the myocardial oxygen supply-demand balance. Overmedication is equally detrimental, however, and should be avoided because it may result in hypoxemia, respiratory acidosis, and hypotension. A benzodiazepine, alone or in combination with a opioid, is most commonly used (see Chapter 8). Excellent results can also be obtained by a combination of morphine, 0.1–0.15 mg/kg, and scopolamine, 0.2–0.4 mg, intramuscularly. Concomitant administration of oxygen via nasal cannula helps avoid hypoxemia following premedication. Patients with poor ventricular function and those with coexistent lung disease should receive reduced doses. Preoperative medications should generally be continued up until the time of surgery. They may be given orally with a small sip of water, intramuscularly, intravenously, sublingually, or transdermally. Sudden withdrawal of antianginal medication perioperatively—especially β-blockers—can precipitate a sudden increase in ischemic episodes (rebound). Moreover, prophylactic β-adrenergic blockade has been shown to reduce the incidence of intraoperative and postoperative ischemic episodes and appears to be superior to prophylaxis with a calcium channel blocker alone. Many clinicians prophylactically administer nitrates intravenously or transdermally to patients with coronary artery disease in the perioperative period. Although this practice may be theoretically advantageous, its efficacy in patients not previously on long-term nitrate therapy is not well established.

INTRAOPERATIVE MANAGEMENT

The intraoperative period is regularly associated with factors and events that can adversely affect the myocardial oxygen demand and supply relationship. Activation of the sympathetic system plays a major role. Hypertension and enhanced contractility increase myocardial oxygen demand, while tachycardia increases demand and reduces supply (see Chapter 19). Although myocardial ischemia is commonly associated with tachycardia, it can occur even in the absence of any apparent hemodynamic derangement.

Objectives

The overwhelming priority in managing patients with ischemic heart disease is maintaining a favorable myocardial supply-demand relationship. Autonomic-mediated increases in heart rate and blood pressure should be controlled by deep anesthesia or adrenergic blockade, while excessive reductions in coronary perfusion pressure (see Chapter 19) or arterial oxygen content are to be avoided. Although exact limits are not predictable, diastolic arterial pressure should generally be maintained at 50 mm Hg or above. Higher diastolic pressures may be preferable in patients with high-grade coronary occlusions. Excessive increases—such as those caused by fluid overload—in left ventricular end-diastolic pressure should be avoided because they increase ventricular wall tension (afterload) and can reduce subendocardial perfusion (see Chapter 19). Adequate blood hemoglobin concentrations (> 9–10 mg/dL) and arterial oxygen tensions (> 60 mm Hg) should generally be maintained.

Monitoring

Intra-arterial pressure monitoring is advisable for all patients with severe coronary artery disease and those with major or multiple cardiac risk factors (see Tables 20–1 and 20–2). Central venous or pulmonary artery pressure monitoring should be used during prolonged or complicated procedures involving large fluid shifts or blood loss (see Chapter 6). Pulmonary artery pressure monitoring is highly desirable for patients with significant ventricular dysfunction (ejection fraction < 40–50%). Two-dimensional transesophageal echocardiography (TEE) also provides valuable information, both qualitative and quantitative, on contractility and ventricular chamber size (preload).

Intraoperative detection of ischemia depends on recognition of electrocardiographic changes, hemodynamic manifestations, or regional wall motion abnormalities on TEE. Doppler TEE also allows detection of the onset of mitral regurgitation caused by ischemic papillary muscle dysfunction.

A. Electrocardiography:

Early ischemic changes are subtle and can often be overlooked. They involve changes in T wave morphol-

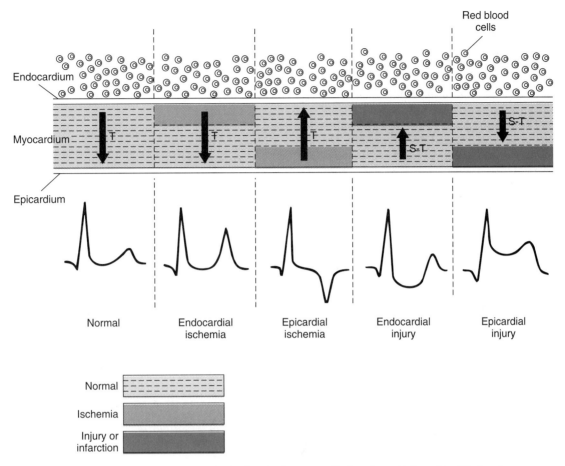

Figure 20–1. Electrocardiographic signs of ischemia. Patterns of ischemia and injury. (Modified and reproduced, with permission, from Schamroth L: *The 12 Lead Electrocardiogram.* Blackwell, 1989.)

ogy, including inversion, tenting, or both (Figure 20–1). More obvious ischemia may be seen in the form of progressive ST-segment depression. Downsloping and horizontal ST depression are of greater specificity for ischemia than is up-sloping depression. New ST-segment elevations are rare during noncardiac surgery and are indicative of severe ischemia, vasospasm, or infarction. It should be noted that isolated minor ST elevation in the mid-precordial leads (V_3 and V_4) can be a normal variant in young patients. Ischemia may also present as an unexplained intraoperative atrial or ventricular arrhythmia or the onset of a new conduction abnormality. The sensitivity of the ECG in detecting ischemia is related to the number of leads monitored. Studies suggest that the V_5, V_4, II, V_2, and V_3 leads (in decreasing sensitivity) are most useful. Ideally, at least two leads should be monitored simultaneously. Usually, lead II is monitored for inferior wall ischemia and arrhythmias and V_5 for anterior wall ischemia. An esophageal lead may also be useful in patients with posterior wall ischemia. When only one channel can be monitored, a modified V_5 lead provides the highest sensitivity (see Chapter 6).

B. HEMODYNAMIC MONITORING:

The most common hemodynamic abnormalities observed during ischemic episodes are hypertension and tachycardia. They are nearly always a cause rather than the result of ischemia. Hypotension is a late and ominous manifestation of progressive ventricular dysfunction. The most sensitive hemodynamic correlates are derived from pulmonary artery pressure monitoring. Ischemia is frequently, but not always, associated with an abrupt increase in pulmonary capillary wedge pressure. The sudden appearance of a prominent *v* wave on the wedge waveform is usually indicative of acute mitral regurgitation from ischemic papillary muscle dysfunction or acute left ventricular dilatation.

C. Two-Dimensional Transesophageal Echocardiography:

Two-dimensional transesophageal echocardiography can be extremely valuable in detecting both global and regional cardiac dysfunction as well as valvular function. Moreover, detection of new regional wall motion abnormalities is a rapid and more sensitive indicator of myocardial ischemia than is the ECG. In animal studies where coronary blood flow is gradually reduced, regional wall motion abnormalities develop before the ECG changes. Although the occurrence of new intraoperative abnormalities correlates with postoperative myocardial infarctions in some studies, not all such abnormalities are necessarily ischemic. Both regional and global abnormalities can be caused by changes in heart rate, preload, afterload, or drug-induced changes in contractility. Decreased systolic wall thickening may be a more reliable index for ischemia than is endocardial wall motion alone. Unfortunately, TEE requires expensive equipment and considerable familiarity with the technique in order to make correct—and rapid—interpretations intraoperatively.

Choice of Anesthesia

A. Regional Anesthesia:

Although studies documenting the superiority of regional over general anesthesia are lacking, the former is often a good choice for procedures involving the extremities, the perineum, and possibly the lower abdomen. Precipitous drops in blood pressure following spinal or epidural anesthesia should be rapidly treated with small doses (25–50 µg) of phenylephrine or a similar agent to preserve coronary perfusion pressure until sufficient intravenous fluid can be given. Small doses of ephedrine (5–10 mg) may be preferable in the presence of bradycardia. Marked hypotension can usually be avoided by prior volume loading (see Chapter 16). Hypotension not responding to phenylephrine or ephedrine may be treated with epinephrine (5–10 µg).

Patients with compensated congestive heart failure usually tolerate the sympathectomy surprising well and may not need preoperative volume loading. Patchy or incomplete surgical anesthesia or excessive sedation during regional anesthesia defeats the purpose of selecting a regional technique, unnecessarily stresses the patient, and may precipitate myocardial ischemia. Conversion of the regional anesthetic to a general anesthetic is appropriate in such instances and corrects the often-associated hypertension, tachycardia, hypoxia, or hypercapnia.

B. General Anesthesia:

1. Induction—The same general principles that apply to patients with hypertension also apply to most patients with ischemic heart disease. Many, if not most, patients with coronary artery disease have hypertension. The induction technique for patients with moderate to severe coronary artery disease (three-vessel disease, left main disease, or ejection fractions < 50%) requires some modification. The induction should have minimal hemodynamic effects, produce reliable loss of consciousness, and provide sufficient depth of anesthesia to prevent a vasopressor response to intubation (if intubation is required); although, in many cases, mild to moderate hypertension is better tolerated than hypotension. Regardless of the agent used, these objectives are most consistently achieved by a slow controlled technique. Induction with small incremental doses of the selected agent usually avoids the precipitous drops in blood pressure that can be seen following a large bolus. Titration of the induction agent—first against loss of consciousness, and then to an acceptable decrease in blood pressure—allows for individual variations in response. Moreover, sufficient anesthetic depth for endotracheal intubation can be achieved with less cardiovascular depression than that caused by the bolus technique. Administration of a muscle relaxant (as soon as the eyelid reflex is lost) and controlled ventilation ensure generally adequate oxygenation throughout induction. Hypercarbia is often associated with hypertension. Endotracheal intubation is performed once sufficient anesthetic depth is reached or arterial blood pressure reaches its lowest acceptable limit. Blood pressure, heart rate, and the ECG should be repeatedly assessed with each step during induction.

2. Choice of agents

a. Induction agents—Selection of a specific agent is not critical in most patients. Propofol, barbiturates, etomidate, benzodiazepines, opioids, and various combinations of these drugs are often used. Ketamine by itself is relatively contraindicated because its indirect sympathomimetic effects can adversely affect the myocardial oxygen demand-supply balance. When combined with a benzodiazepine or propofol, however, ketamine does not appreciably increase sympathetic activity and results in relatively stable hemodynamics with minimal myocardial depression. The combination of a benzodiazepine and ketamine may be most useful in patients with poor ventricular function.

High-dose opioid anesthesia has been widely advocated for patients with significant ventricular dysfunction. With the exception of meperidine (in large doses), opioids alone are generally associated with minimal or no cardiac depression. Combining them with other intravenous agents (particularly benzodiazepines), however, often results in significant, dose-dependent cardiac depression. Apparent cardiac depression may also occur with pure high-dose opioid inductions (see Chapter 21); this likely represents withdrawal of an elevated baseline sympathetic tone. Patients with poor ventricular function often rely on an elevated sympathetic tone to maintain their cardiac output (see Chapter 19) and may decompensate even with pure high-dose opioid anesthesia. Moreover, opioids used as sole agents may not be complete anesthetics because of an unacceptably high incidence of intraoperative awareness (recall) and hypertension (see Chapter 21); the prolonged respiratory depression following this technique is also unsuitable for most noncardiac operations. Most clinicians always use small supplemental doses of an intravenous agent or volatile anesthetic with high-dose opioid anesthesia.

Control of the adrenergic response to endotracheal intubation has been discussed in the section on hypertension.

 b. Maintenance agents—Patients with good ventricular function are generally managed with volatile anesthetic-based technique, while those with depressed ventricular function are often managed with an opioid-based anesthetic. Patients with ejection fractions less than 40–50% are often very sensitive to the depressant effects of the potent volatile agents. Nitrous oxide, especially in the presence of narcotics, can also produce significant cardiac depression.

The effects of the potent volatile agents on the coronary circulation are discussed in Chapter 19. All volatile agents generally have a favorable effect on myocardial oxygen balance, reducing demand more than supply. Isoflurane dilates intramyocardial arteries more than the larger epicardial vessels but there is little evidence that isoflurane causes an intracoronary steal phenomenon in clinical practice.

Detection of intraoperative ischemia should prompt a search for precipitating factors and initiation of interventions to correct it. Oxygenation should be checked and hemodynamic abnormalities (hypotension, hypertension, or tachycardia) corrected. Failure to identify a cause or to reverse the ischemic manifestations may be an indication for starting intravenous nitroglycerin. The latter optimally requires insertion of an arterial line and, in some patients (those with moderate to severe ventricular impairment), a pulmonary artery catheter. Nitroglycerin paste may be used if intravenous nitroglycerin is not possible, but it is associated with a delayed onset and variable absorption.

c. Muscle relaxants—Lack of significant circulatory side effects generally makes rocuronium, vecuronium, rapacuronium,* pipecuronium, and doxacurium good muscle relaxants for patients with ischemic heart disease. Severe bradycardia has been reported with vecuronium (and atracurium) on rare occasions, but in nearly all instances it has been associated with concomitant administration of a synthetic opioid. When used properly, other muscle relaxants (see Chapter 9) can also be safely administered to patients with coronary artery disease. Moreover, their circulatory side effects can be used to balance the side effects of other anesthetic agents—eg, the vagolytic properties of pancuronium can counteract the vagotonic effects of potent opioids (see Chapter 8). Atracurium in doses less than 0.4 mg/kg and mivacurium, up to 0.15 mg/kg, given slowly also generally have minimal hemodynamic effects. The circulatory effects of succinylcholine are primarily due to stimulation of autonomic ganglia and cardiac muscarinic receptors and can result in variable effects on heart rate and blood pressure (see Chapter 9). Its net effect is influenced by preexisting relative sympathetic and parasympathetic tone, premedication with an anticholinergic, and β-adrenergic blockade. Bradycardia may be seen following succinylcholine in patients taking β-adrenergic blocking agents.

Reversal of muscle paralysis with standard agents does not appear to have any detrimental effects in patients with coronary artery disease. Use of glycopyrrolate instead of atropine may lessen the likelihood of transient tachycardia (see Chapter 10).

POSTOPERATIVE MANAGEMENT

Recovery from anesthesia and the immediate postoperative period can continue to stress the myocardium. The patient should receive supplemental oxygen until adequate oxygenation is established. Shivering usually resolves following administration of meperidine, 20–30 mg intravenously; other reported treatments include clonidine, 75 μg, or butorphanol, 1–2 mg intravenously. Hypothermia should be corrected with a forced-air surface warmer. Postoperative pain should be controlled with generous analgesics or a regional anesthetic technique (see Chapter 18). If there is a suspicion of fluid overload or the patient has a history of poor ventricular function, a postoperative chest film is useful. Pulmonary congestion can be rapidly treated with furosemide, 20–40 mg intravenously, or intravenous vasodilator therapy (usually nitroglycerin).

---

* At the time of publication, rapacuronium had been voluntarily withdrawn by the manufacturer. See Chapter 9 for details.

The greatest risk to these patients postoperatively is unrecognized ischemia. While the majority of perioperative Q-wave myocardial infarctions occur within the first 3 days following surgery (usually after 24–48 hours), a significant number of non–Q-wave infarctions present in the first 24 hours. Because fewer than half of patients have chest pain, routine postoperative 12-lead ECGs may be necessary to detect such events. A common presentation is unexplained hypotension. Other presentations include congestive heart failure and altered mental status. Nearly all patients experiencing this complication are older than 50 years. The diagnosis is usually based on electrocardiographic findings and cardiac enzyme or, less commonly, radionuclide studies.

■ VALVULAR HEART DISEASE

1. General Evaluation of Patients

Regardless of the lesion or its cause, preoperative evaluation should be primarily concerned with determining the severity of the lesion and its hemodynamic significance, residual ventricular function, and the presence of secondary effects on pulmonary, renal, and hepatic function. Concomitant coronary artery disease should not be overlooked, especially in older patients and those with known risk factors (see above). Myocardial ischemia may also occur in the absence of significant coronary occlusion in patients with severe aortic stenosis or regurgitation.

History

The preanesthesia history should focus on symptoms related to ventricular function and should be correlated with laboratory data. Questions should concern exercise tolerance, fatigability, and pedal edema and shortness of breath in general (dyspnea), when lying flat (orthopnea), or at night (paroxysmal nocturnal dyspnea). The New York Heart Association functional classification of heart disease (Table 20–10) is useful for grading the clinical severity of heart failure, comparing patients, and estimating prognosis. Patients should also be questioned about chest pains and neurologic symptoms. Some valvular lesions are associated with thromboembolic phenomena. Prior procedures such as valvotomy or valve replacement and their effects should also be well documented.

A review of medications should evaluate efficacy and exclude serious side effects. Commonly used agents include digoxin, diuretics, vasodilators, ACE inhibitors, antiarrhythmics, and anticoagulants. Digoxin is gener-

Table 20–10. Modified New York Association functional classification of heart disease.

Class	Description
I	Asymptomatic except during severe exertion
II	Symptomatic with moderate activity
III	Symptomatic with minimal activity
IV	Symptomatic at rest

ally most effective for controlling the ventricular rate in patients with atrial fibrillation. The ventricular rate should be less than 80–90 beats/min at rest and should not exceed 120 beats/min with stress or exercise. Signs of digoxin toxicity are primarily cardiac (arrhythmias), gastrointestinal (nausea or vomiting), neurologic (confusion), or visual (altered color perception or scotomas). Arrhythmias caused by digoxin arise from a combination of enhanced automaticity and decreased conduction in specialized cells in the atria, ventricles, and AV and sinoatrial (SA) nodes. Preoperative vasodilator therapy may be used to decrease preload, afterload, or both. Excessive vasodilation worsens exercise tolerance and is often first manifested as postural hypotension.

Physical Examination

The most important signs to search for on physical examination are those of congestive heart failure. Left-sided (S_3 gallop or pulmonary rales) as well as right-sided signs (jugular venous distention, hepatojugular reflux, hepatosplenomegaly, or pedal edema) may be present. Auscultatory findings may confirm the valvular dysfunction (Table 20–11), but echocardiographic studies are generally more reliable. Neurologic deficits, which are usually secondary to embolic phenomena, should be documented.

Laboratory Evaluation

In addition to the laboratory studies discussed for patients with hypertension and coronary artery disease, liver function tests (see Chapter 34) are useful in assessing hepatic dysfunction caused by passive hepatic congestion in patients with severe or chronic right-sided failure. Arterial blood gases should be measured in patients with significant pulmonary symptoms. Reversal of anticoagulants should be documented with a prothrombin time and partial thromboplastin time prior to surgery.

Electrocardiographic findings are generally nonspecific. They may include T-wave or ST-segment changes, arrhythmias, conduction abnormalities, or QRS-axis deviation reflecting ventricular hypertrophy.

Table 20–11. Effects of diagnostic maneuvers on heart murmurs (variable effects omitted).

Maneuver	Systolic Murmurs							Diastolic Murmurs			
	PS	TR	HCM	MVP	MR	VSD	AS	PR	TS	AR	MS
Inspiration	↑	↑						↑	↑		
Valsalva	↑		↑	↑			↓	↑			↓
Standing			↑	↑	↓						
Squatting or handgrip			↓	↓	↑	↑	↓			↑	↑
Leg elevation			↑	↓	↓		↑				
Transient arterial occlusion					↑	↑				↑	
Amyl nitrite inhalation	↑	↑	↑	↑	↓	↓	↑	↑	↑	↓	↑

↑ = Increases
↓ = Decreases
PS = pulmonary stenosis; TR = tricuspid regurgitation; HCM = hypertrophic cardiomyopathy; MVP = mitral valve prolapse; MR = mitral regurgitation; VSD = ventricular septal defect; AS = aortic stenosis; PR = pulmonary regurgitation; TS = tricuspid stenosis; AR = aortic regurgitation; MS = mitral stenosis.

A prolonged P–R interval may suggest digoxin toxicity. Arrhythmias associated with digoxin toxicity include (in order of decreasing frequency) ventricular ectopy, paroxysmal atrial tachycardia with 2:1 AV block, AV block alone, marked sinus bradycardia, low atrial or AV junctional rhythms, and AV dissociation.

The chest film is invaluable in assessing cardiac size and pulmonary vascular congestion. Specific cardiac chamber enlargement may be apparent (Figure 20–2).

Special Studies

Echocardiography, radionuclide angiography, and cardiac catheterization provide important diagnostic and prognostic information about valvular lesions. More than one valvular lesion is often found. In many instances, noninvasive studies obviate the need for cardiac catheterization. Information from these studies is best reviewed with a cardiologist. The following questions must be answered:

- Which valvular abnormality is most important hemodynamically?
- What is the severity of that lesion?
- What degree of ventricular impairment is present?
- What is the hemodynamic significance of other identified abnormalities?
- Is there any evidence of coronary artery disease?

2. Premedication

Premedication with standard doses of any of the commonly used agents (see Chapter 8) is desirable and well tolerated in patients with normal or near-normal ventricular function. Patients with poor ventricular function, on the other hand, tend to be very sensitive to most agents, and premedication doses should be reduced in proportion to the severity of ventricular impairment. Patients should generally receive their usual medications on the morning of surgery. Supplemental oxygen may be desirable in patients with pulmonary hypertension or underlying pulmonary disease.

Antibiotic Prophylaxis

The risk of infective endocarditis in patients with valvular heart disease following bacteremic events—including dental, oropharyngeal or nasopharyngeal, gastrointestinal, or genitourinary surgery or any incision and drainage (I & D)—is well established. Prophylaxis is best accomplished according to the general guidelines originally recommended by the American Heart Association (Table 20–12).

Anticoagulation Management

Patients who are receiving anticoagulants can generally have their drug regimen interrupted for 1–3 days perioperatively without danger. The incidence of thromboembolic complications increases with a prior history of embolism and the presence of a thrombus, atrial fibrillation, or a prosthetic mechanical valve. The risk of thromboembolism is highest with a caged-ball mechanical (Starr-Edwards) prosthesis, especially in the mitral or tricuspid position; intermediate for tilting-disc (St.

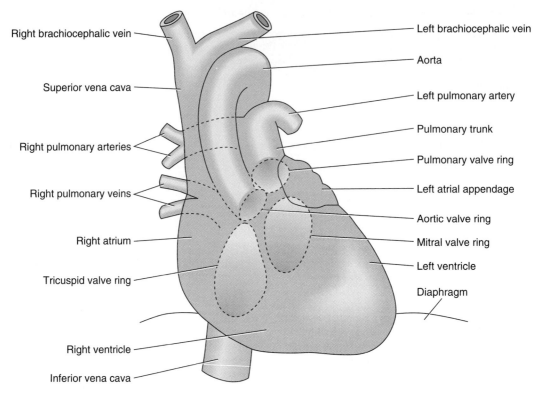

Figure 20–2. Radiologic localization of cardiac chambers and structures on the front chest film.

Jude) valves; and lowest for bioprostheses (porcine or bovine tissue valves). Most patients can safely have their warfarin stopped 3 days prior to surgery and restarted 2–3 days postoperatively. If the thromboembolic risk is deemed high, anticoagulation can be stopped the day before surgery and reversed with vitamin K or fresh frozen plasma; intravenous heparin therapy can then be initiated 12–24 hours postoperatively once surgical hemostasis is believed to be adequate.

Table 20–12. Antibiotic prophylaxis against endocarditis.

I. Dental, oral, nasal, pharyngeal, upper airway, and esophageal procedures
  A. Standard
    Adults
      Amoxicillin, 3 g orally, 1 hour before and 1.5 g, 6 hours after the procedure
      OR
      Ampicillin, 2 g IV or IM, 30 minutes before
    Children
      Amoxicillin, 50 mg/kg orally, 1 hour before and 25 mg/kg, 6 hours after the procedure
      Or
      Ampicillin, 50 mg/kg IV, 30 minutes before
  B. Penicillin allergy
    Adults
      Erythromycin, 1 g orally, 2 hours before and 500 mg, 6 hours afterward
      OR
      Azithromycin or clarithromycin, 500 mg orally before

(continued)

Table 20–12. Antibiotic prophylaxis against endocarditis. (continued)

OR
Clindamycin, 600 mg orally, 2 hours before and 300 mg, 6 hours afterward
OR
Clindamycin, 600 mg IV, 30 minutes before
OR
Cefazolin, 1 g IV or IM, 30 minutes before[1]
Children
Erythromycin, 20 mg/kg orally, 2 hours before and 10 mg/kg 6 hours afterward
OR
Clindamycin, 10 mg/kg orally, 2 hours before and 5 mg/kg, 6 hours afterward
OR
Clindamycin, 20 mg/kg IV, 30 minutes before and 5 mg/kg, 6 hours afterward
OR
Cefazolin, 25 mg/kg IV or IM, 30 minutes before and 25 mg/kg, 6 hours after the procedure[1]
  C. High risk (prosthetic valve or prior endocarditis)
Adults
Ampicillin, 2 g IV or IM, and gentamicin, 1.5 mg/kg (up to 80 mg) IV or IM, 30 minutes before; and amoxicillin, 1.5 g orally
6 hours afterward, or repeat IV regimen 8 hours later
Children
Ampicillin, 50 mg/kg IV or IM, and gentamicin, 2 mg/kg IV or IM, 30 minutes before; and amoxicillin, 50 mg/kg orally,
6 hours afterward, or repeat IV regimen 8 hours later
  D. High risk with penicillin allergy
Adults
Vancomycin, 1 g IV, 1 hour before (infuse over 1 hour)
Children
Vancomycin, 20 mg/kg IV, 1 hour before (infuse over 1 hour)
II. Genitourinary and gastrointestinal procedures
  A. Standard
Adults
Ampicillin, 2 g IV or IM, and gentamicin, 1.5 mg/kg (up to 80 mg) IV or IM, 30 minutes before; and amoxicillin, 1.5 g orally,
6 hours afterward
Children
Ampicillin, 50 mg/kg IV or IM, and gentamicin, 2 mg/kg IV or IM, 30 minutes before; and amoxicillin, 50 mg/kg orally,
6 hours afterward
  B. Penicillin allergy
Adults
Vancomycin, 1 g IV, 1 hour before (infuse over 1 hour) and gentamicin, 1.5 mg/kg (up to 80 mg) IV
Children
Vancomycin, 20 mg/kg IV, 1 hour before (infuse over 1 hour) and gentamicin, 2 mg/kg IV
  C. Low risk
Adults
Amoxicillin, 3 g orally, 1 hour before and 1.5 g, 6 hours after the procedure
Children
Amoxicillin, 50 mg/kg orally, 1 hour before and 25 mg/kg, 6 hours after the procedure

[1]Do not use with a history of immediate hypersensitivity-type allergy to penicillin.

3. Specific Valvular Disorders

MITRAL STENOSIS

Preoperative Considerations

Mitral stenosis nearly always occurs as a delayed complication of acute rheumatic fever. Two-thirds of patients with mitral stenosis are female. The stenotic process is estimated to begin after a minimum of 2 years following the acute disease and results from progressive fusion and calcification of the valve leaflets. Symptoms generally develop after 20–30 years, when the mitral valve orifice is reduced from its normal 4–6 cm^2 opening to less than 2 cm^2. Less than 50% of patients have isolated mitral stenosis; the remaining patients also have mitral regurgitation and up to 25% also have rheumatic involvement of the aortic valve (stenosis or regurgitation).

Pathophysiology

The rheumatic process causes the valve leaflets to thicken, calcify, and become funnel-shaped; annular calcification may also be present. The mitral commissures fuse, the chordae tendinae fuse and shorten, and the valve cusps become rigid; as a result, the valve leaflets typically display bowing or doming during diastole on echocardiography.

Significant restriction of blood flow through the mitral valve results in a transvalvular pressure gradient that depends on cardiac output, heart rate (diastolic time), and the presence or absence of a normal atrial kick. Increases in either cardiac output or heart rate (decreased diastolic time) necessitate higher flows across the valve and result in higher transvalvular pressure gradients. The left atrium is often markedly dilated and promotes supraventricular tachycardias, especially atrial fibrillation. Blood flow stasis in the atrium promotes the formation of thrombi, usually in the left atrial appendage. Loss of normal atrial systole (which is usually responsible for 20–30% of ventricular filling) necessitates even higher diastolic flow across the valve to maintain the same cardiac output and increases the transvalvular gradient.

Acute elevations in left atrial pressure are rapidly transmitted back to the pulmonary capillaries. If mean pulmonary capillary pressure acutely rises above 25 mm Hg, transudation of capillary fluid results in pulmonary edema. Chronic elevations in pulmonary capillary pressure are partially compensated by increases in pulmonary lymph flow but eventually result in pulmonary vascular changes leading to irreversible increases in pulmonary vascular resistance (PVR) and pulmonary hypertension. Reduced lung compliance and a secondary increase in the work of breathing contribute to chronic dyspnea. Right ventricular failure is frequently precipitated by acute or chronic elevations in right ventricular afterload. Marked dilatation of the right ventricle can result in tricuspid or pulmonary valve regurgitation.

Embolic events are common in patients with mitral stenosis and atrial fibrillation. Dislodgment of clots from the left atrium results in systemic emboli, most commonly to the cerebral circulation. Patients also have an increased incidence of pulmonary emboli, pulmonary infarction, hemoptysis, and recurrent bronchitis. Hemoptysis most commonly results from rupture of pulmonary-bronchial venous communications. Chest pain occurs in 10–15% of patients with mitral stenosis, even in the absence of coronary atherosclerosis; its etiology often remains unexplained but may be emboli in

the coronary circulation or acute right ventricular pressure overload. Patients may develop hoarseness as a result of compression of the left recurrent laryngeal nerve by the enlarged left atrium.

Left ventricular function is normal in the majority of patients with pure mitral stenosis (Figure 20–3), but impaired left ventricular function may be encountered in up to 25% of patients and presumably represents residual damage from rheumatic myocarditis or coexistent hypertensive or ischemic heart disease.

Calculating Mitral Valve Area & Transvalvular Gradient

The relationship between cardiac output, valvular area, and the transvalvular gradient can be expressed by the Gorlin equation:

$$\text{Valve area} = \frac{\text{Flow across valve}}{K \times \sqrt{\text{Mean transvalvular gradient}}}$$

where K is a hydraulic-pressure constant. When mitral valvular flow is expressed as mL/sec, pressure as mm Hg, and valve area as cm^2, K = 38. Mitral valve flow (MVF) can be estimated as follows:

$$\text{MVF} = \frac{\text{Cardiac output}}{\text{Diastolic filling period} \times \text{heart rate}}$$

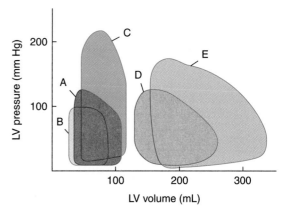

Figure 20–3. Pressure-volume loops in patients with valvular heart disease. A = normal; B = mitral stenosis; C = aortic stenosis; D = mitral regurgitation (chronic); E = aortic regurgitation (chronic). LV = left ventricular. (Reproduced, with permission, from Jackson JM, Thomas SJ, Lowenstein E: Anesthetic management patients with valvular heart disease. Semin Anesth 1982;1:239.)

Two-dimensional and Doppler echocardiography can be used to estimate both the pressure drop across a stenotic valve and the valve area. Based on the assumption that the velocity of blood flow is much greater distal than proximal to an obstruction, the Bernoulli equation can be simplified:

$$\Delta P = 4V^2$$

where ΔP is the pressure gradient (mm Hg) and V is blood flow velocity (m/sec) distal to the obstruction. Valve orifice can be estimated from the time it takes for the initial peak pressure gradient to fall to one-half its original value, the pressure half-time ($T\frac{1}{2}$). This relationship is approximated by:

$$A = \frac{220}{T_{1/2}}$$

where A is valve orifice (cm^2) and $T\frac{1}{2}$ is the time from peak flow velocity (V_{max}) to $V_{max}\sqrt{2}$ ($V_{max}/1.4$). This relationship is based on the observation that $T\frac{1}{2}$ remains relatively constant for a given orifice over a wide range of flows. A pressure half-time of 220 msec corresponds to a mitral valve area of 1 cm^2. Valve area can also be estimated by planimetry in a short-axis view of the left ventricle (see Chapter 21). In the absence of significant mitral regurgitation, mitral valve area (MVA) can additionally be derived from the continuity equation (see section on aortic stenosis):

$$MVA = SV_{mv} / VTI_{MS-jet}$$

where SV_{mv} is stroke volume (transmitral) and $VTI_{MS\text{-}jet}$ is the velocity time integral of the Doppler signal of the mitral stenosis jet; stroke volume can be calculated from measuring the cross-sectional area and Doppler velocity time integral in the left ventricular outflow tract (see section on aortic stenosis).

Mitral valve areas less than 1 cm^2 are typically associated with transvalvular gradients of 20 mm Hg at rest and dyspnea with minimal exertion; a mitral valve area less than 1 cm^2 is often referred to as critical mitral stenosis. Patients with valve areas between 1.5 cm^2 and 2.0 cm^2 are generally asymptomatic or have only mild symptoms with exertion. When the mitral valve area is between 1 cm^2 and 1.5 cm^2, most patients are symptomatic with mild to moderate exertion. Although cardiac output may be normal at rest, it fails to increase appropriately during exertion because of decreased left ventricular preload.

Treatment

The time from onset of symptoms to incapacitation averages 5–10 years. At that stage, most patients die within 2–5 years. Surgical correction (open valvuloplasty) is therefore usually undertaken once significant symptoms develop. Recurrent mitral stenosis following valvuloplasty is usually managed with valve replacement. Percutaneous transseptal balloon valvuloplasty may be used in selected young or pregnant patients as well as older patients who are poor surgical candidates. Medical management is primarily supportive and includes limitation of physical activity, sodium restriction, and diuretics. Digoxin is useful only in patients with atrial fibrillation and a rapid ventricular response. Small doses of a β-adrenergic blocking drug may also be useful in controlling heart rate in patients with mild to moderate symptoms. Patients with a history of emboli and those at high risk (older than 40 years; a large atrium with chronic atrial fibrillation) are usually anticoagulated.

Anesthetic Management

A. OBJECTIVES:

 The principal hemodynamic goals are to maintain a sinus rhythm (if present preoperatively) and to avoid tachycardia, large increases in cardiac output, and both hypovolemia and fluid overload by judicious fluid therapy.

B. MONITORING:

Full hemodynamic monitoring (of direct intra-arterial pressure and pulmonary artery pressure) is generally indicated for all major surgical procedures, especially those associated with large fluid shifts. Overzealous fluid replacement readily precipitates pulmonary edema in patients with severe disease. Pulmonary artery pressures should be monitored closely. Pulmonary capillary wedge pressure measurements in the presence of mitral stenosis reflect the transvalvular gradient and not necessarily left ventricular end-diastolic pressure. Prominent *a* waves and a decreased *y* descent are typically present on the pulmonary capillary wedge pressure waveform in patients who are in sinus rhythm. A prominent *cv* wave on the central venous pressure waveform is usually indicative of secondary tricuspid regurgitation. The ECG typically shows a notched P wave in patients who are in sinus rhythm.

C. CHOICE OF AGENTS:

Patients may be very sensitive to the vasodilating effects of spinal and epidural anesthesia. Epidural is preferable to spinal anesthesia because of the more gradual onset of sympathetic blockade. Ketamine by itself is generally a poor induction agent for general anesthesia because of its sympathetic stimulation. Similarly, pancuronium-induced tachycardia is to be avoided. In considering the type of agent to use, an opioid may be a better choice than a volatile agent. The latter can produce undesirable vasodilation or precipitate junctional rhythm with loss of an effective atrial kick. Of the volatile agents, halothane may be the most suitable because it decreases heart rate and is the least vasodilating, but other volatile agents have been used safely. Nitrous oxide should be used cautiously, since it can acutely increase PVR in some patients.

Intraoperative tachycardia may be controlled by deepening anesthesia with an opioid (excluding meperidine) or β-blocker (esmolol or propranolol). In the presence of atrial fibrillation, ventricular rate may be controlled with diltiazem or digoxin. Verapamil may be less desirable because of the associated vasodilation. Marked hemodynamic deterioration from sudden supraventricular tachycardia necessitates cardioversion. Phenylephrine is preferred over ephedrine as a vasopressor because the former lacks β-adrenergic agonist activity. Treatment of acute hypertension or afterload reduction with potent vasodilators should be undertaken only with full hemodynamic monitoring.

MITRAL REGURGITATION

Preoperative Considerations

Mitral regurgitation can develop acutely or insidiously as a result of a large number of disorders. Chronic mitral regurgitation is usually the result of rheumatic fever (often with concomitant mitral stenosis); congenital or developmental abnormalities of the valve apparatus; or dilation, destruction, or calcification of the mitral annulus. Acute mitral regurgitation is usually due to myocardial ischemia or infarction (papillary muscle dysfunction or rupture of a chorda tendinea), infective endocarditis, or chest trauma.

Pathophysiology

The principal derangement is a reduction in forward stroke volume due to backward flow of blood into the left atrium during systole. The left ventricle compensates by dilating and increasing end-diastolic volume (Figure 20–3). Regurgitation through the mitral valve reduces left ventricular afterload, which often initially enhances contractility. End-systolic volume thus remains normal but eventually increases as the disease progresses. By increasing end-diastolic volume, the volume-overloaded left ventricle can maintain a normal cardiac output even as ejection fraction decreases. With time, patients with chronic mitral regurgitation eventu-

ally develop eccentric left ventricular hypertrophy (see Chapter 19) and progressive impairment in contractility, as reflected by a decrease in ejection fraction (< 50%). In patients with severe mitral regurgitation, the regurgitant volume may exceed the forward stroke volume.

The regurgitant volume passing through the mitral valve is dependent on the size of the mitral valve orifice (which can vary with ventricular cavity size), the heart rate (systolic time), and the left ventricular-left atrial pressure gradient during systole. The last factor is affected by the relative resistances of the two outflow paths from the left ventricle, namely, SVR and left atrial compliance. Thus, a decrease in SVR or an increase in mean left atrial pressure will reduce the regurgitant volume. Atrial compliance also determines the predominant clinical manifestations. Patients with normal or reduced atrial compliance (acute mitral regurgitation) have mainly pulmonary vascular congestion and edema. Patients with increased atrial compliance (long-standing mitral regurgitation resulting in a large dilated left atrium) primarily show signs of a low cardiac output. Most patients are between the two extremes and exhibit symptoms of both pulmonary congestion and low cardiac output. Patients with a regurgitant fraction less than 30% of the total stroke volume generally have mild symptoms. Regurgitant fractions of 30–60% generally cause moderate symptoms, while fractions greater than 60% are associated with severe disease.

Echocardiography, especially TEE, is extremely useful in delineating the underlying pathophysiology of mitral regurgitation as well as in guiding treatment. Mitral valve leaflet motion is often described as normal, excessive (prolapsing), or restrictive (Figure 20–4). Excessive motion or prolapse is defined by systolic movement of a leaflet beyond the plane of the mitral valve and into the left atrium (see below section on mitral valve prolapse). Eccentric regurgitant jets on color-flow Doppler echocardiography is typical of a prolapsing valve, while central jets are more typical of regurgitation with normal or restricted valve motion.

Calculating Regurgitant Fraction

In order to calculate regurgitant fraction (RF), forward stroke volume (SV) and the regurgitant stroke volume (RSV) must be measured. Although they can both be estimated by catheterization data, pulsed Doppler echocardiography provides reasonably acute calculations. Stroke volume is measured at the left ventricular outflow tract (LVOT) and at the mitral valve (MV), where

$$\text{Stroke volume} = \text{cross sectional area (A)} \times \text{(TVI)}$$

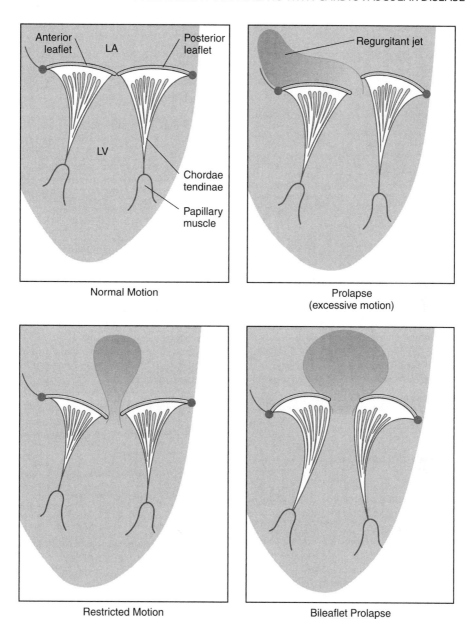

Figure 20–4. Classification of mitral valve leaflet motion (as seen from transesophageal echocardiography). Note that with prolapse, the free edge of the leaflet(s) extends beyond the plane of the mitral annulus producing an eccentric jet. With restricted motion, the leaflets fail to coapt resulting in a central jet.

The time velocity integral (TVI) is the area of velocity versus time signal obtained with pulsed Doppler (see Chapter 21). Thus,

$$RSV_{mitral\ regurgitation} = (A_{MV} \times VTI_{MV})$$
$$-(A_{LVOT} \times TVI_{LVOT}),$$

and,

$$RF = RSV/SV.$$

A RSV greater than 65 mL usually correlates with severe mitral regurgitation.

Treatment

Medical treatment includes digoxin, diuretics, and vasodilators—including ACE inhibitors. Afterload reduction is beneficial in nearly all patients and may even be lifesaving in patients with acute mitral regurgitation. Reduction of SVR increases forward SV and decreases the regurgitant volume. Surgical treatment is usually reserved for patients with moderate to severe symptoms. Surgical valvuloplasty is performed whenever possible to avoid the problems associated with valve replacement (eg, thromboembolism, hemorrhage, and prosthetic failure).

Anesthetic Management

A. OBJECTIVES:

Anesthetic management should be tailored to the severity of mitral regurgitation as well as the underlying left ventricular function. Factors that exacerbate the regurgitation, such as slow heart rates (long systole) and acute increases in afterload, should be avoided. Bradycardia can increase the regurgitant volume by increasing left ventricular end-diastolic volume and acutely dilating the mitral annulus. The heart rate should ideally be kept between 80 and 100 beats/min. Acute increases in left ventricular afterload, such as following endotracheal intubation and surgical stimulation, should be treated rapidly but without excessive myocardial depression. Excessive volume expansion can also worsen the regurgitation by dilating the left ventricle.

B. MONITORING:

Monitors are based on the severity of ventricular dysfunction as well as the procedure. Pulmonary artery pressure monitoring is extremely useful in patients with symptomatic disease. Intraoperative afterload reduction with a vasodilator requires full hemodynamic monitoring. Mitral regurgitation may be recognized on the pulmonary artery wedge waveform as a large v wave and a rapid y descent (Figure 20–5). The height of the v wave is inversely related to atrial and pulmonary vascular compliance but directly proportional to pulmonary blood flow and the regurgitant volume; thus the v wave may not be prominent in patients with chronic mitral regurgitation except during acute deterioration. Very large v waves are often apparent on the pulmonary artery pressure waveform even without wedging the catheter. Color-flow Doppler TEE can be invaluable in quantitating the severity of the regurgitation and guiding therapeutic interventions in patients with severe mitral regurgitation (Table 20–13). By definition, blood flow reverses in the pulmonary veins during systole with severe mitral regurgitation.

C. CHOICE OF AGENTS:

Patients with relatively well-preserved ventricular function tend to do well with most anesthetic techniques. Spinal and epidural anesthesia are well tolerated, provided bradycardia is avoided. Patients with moderate to severe ventricular impairment are often very sensitive to the depressant effects of volatile agents. A primarily opioid-based anesthetic may be more suitable for those patients—again, provided bradycardia is avoided. The selection of pancuronium as muscle relaxant with an opioid-based anesthetic may be useful in this regard.

MITRAL VALVE PROLAPSE

Preoperative Considerations

Mitral valve prolapse is classically characterized by a midsystolic click with or without a late apical systolic murmur on auscultation. It is a relatively common abnormality that is present in up to 5% of the general population, being most common in women (up to 15%). The diagnosis is based on auscultatory findings and confirmed by echocardiography, which shows systolic prolapse of mitral valve leaflets into the left atrium. Patients with the murmur often have some element of mitral regurgitation. The posterior mitral leaflet is more commonly affected than the anterior leaflet. The mitral annulus may also be dilated. Pathologically, most patients have redundancy or some myxomatous degeneration of the valve leaflets. Most cases of mitral valve prolapse are sporadic or familial, affecting otherwise normal persons. A high incidence of mitral valve prolapse is found in patients with connective tissue disorders (especially Marfan syndrome).

The overwhelming majority of patients with mitral valve prolapse are asymptomatic, but in a small percent-

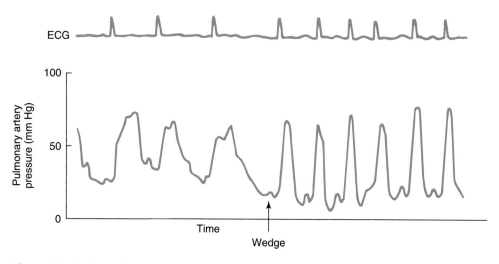

Figure 20–5. The pulmonary capillary wedge waveform in mitral regurgitation, demonstrating a large *v* wave.

age the myxomatous degeneration is progressive. Manifestations, when they occur, can include chest pains, arrhythmias, embolic events, florid mitral regurgitation, infective endocarditis and, rarely, sudden death. The diagnosis can made preoperatively by auscultation of the characteristic click but must be confirmed by echocardiography. The prolapse is accentuated by maneuvers that decrease ventricular volume (preload). The ECG is usually normal but in some patients often shows inverted or biphasic T waves or ST-segment changes inferiorly. Both atrial and ventricular arrhythmias are common. Although bradyarrhythmias also are reported, paroxysmal supraventricular tachycardia is the most commonly encountered sustained arrhythmia. An increased incidence of abnormal AV bypass tracts (see Chapter 19) is reported in patients with mitral valve prolapse.

Most patients have a normal life span. About 15% develop progressive mitral regurgitation. A smaller percentage develop embolic phenomena or infective endocarditis. Patients with both a click and a systolic murmur appear to be at greater risk for developing complications. Anticoagulation or antiplatelet agents may be used for patients with a history of emboli, while β-adrenergic blocking drugs are commonly employed for arrhythmias.

Anesthetic Management

The management of these patients is based on their clinical course. Most patients are asymptomatic and, except for antibiotic prophylaxis, do not require special care. Patients with a systolic murmur appear to be at greatest risk for infective endocarditis. Ventricular arrhythmias may occur intraoperatively, especially following sympathetic stimulation, and will generally respond to lidocaine or β-adrenergic blocking agents. Relatively deep anesthesia with a volatile agent usually lessens the

Table 20–13. Echocardiographic assessment of regurgitant lesions by color-flow Doppler.

Grade	Description	Criterion
0	None	No regurgitation into receiving chamber
1+	Mild	Regurgitant flow limited to area immediately near valve
2+	Mild to moderate	Regurgitant flow occupies up to 1/3 of receiving chamber
3+	Moderate to severe	Regurgitant flow occupies up to 2/3 of receiving chamber
4+	Severe	Regurgitant flow occupies most of receiving chamber and flow reversal is present[1]

[1]For atrioventricular valves flow reversal occurs proximally in the veins filling the atrium, while for semilunar valves flow reversal occurs distally in the great vessels.

likelihood of intraoperative arrhythmias. Mitral regurgitation caused by prolapse is generally exacerbated by decreases in ventricular size. Hypovolemia and factors that increase ventricular emptying—such as increased sympathetic tone or decreased afterload—should therefore be avoided. Vasopressors with pure α-adrenergic agonist activity (such as phenylephrine) may be preferable to those that are primarily β-adrenergic agonists (ephedrine).

AORTIC STENOSIS

Preoperative Considerations

Valvular aortic stenosis is the most common cause of obstruction to left ventricular outflow. Left ventricular outflow obstruction is less commonly due to **hypertrophic cardiomyopathy,** discrete congenital subvalvular stenosis or, rarely, supravalvular stenosis. Valvular aortic stenosis is nearly always congenital, rheumatic, or degenerative. Abnormalities in the number of cusps (most commonly a bicuspid valve) or in their architecture produce turbulence that traumatizes the valve and eventually leads to stenosis. Rheumatic aortic stenosis is rarely isolated; it is more commonly associated with aortic regurgitation or mitral valve disease. In the most common degenerative form, calcific aortic stenosis, wear and tear results in the buildup of calcium deposits on normal cusps, preventing them from opening completely.

Pathophysiology

In contrast to acute obstruction of left ventricular outflow, which rapidly dilates the ventricle and reduces SV (see Chapter 21), obstruction caused by valvular aortic stenosis is nearly always gradual, allowing the ventricle, at least initially, to compensate and maintain SV. Concentric ventricular hypertrophy enables the left ventricle to maintain SV by generating a significant transvalvular gradient and reduce ventricular wall stress (Figure 20–3).

Critical aortic stenosis is said to exist when the aortic valve orifice is reduced to 0.5–0.7 cm² (normal is 2.5–3.5 cm²). With this degree of stenosis, patients generally have a transvalvular gradient of approximately 50 mm Hg at rest (with a normal cardiac output) and are unable to increase cardiac output appreciably. Moreover, further increases in the transvalvular gradient do not significantly increase SV. Aortic valve areas between 0.7 and 0.9 cm² are generally associated with mild to moderate symptoms. With long-standing aortic stenosis, myocardial contractility progressively deteriorates and further compromises left ventricular function. Most patients with aortic stenosis have a long latency period of 30–60 years (depending on the cause) before significant symptoms develop.

Classically, patients with advanced aortic stenosis have the triad of dyspnea on exertion, angina, and orthostatic or exertional syncope. A prominent feature of aortic stenosis is a decrease in left ventricular compliance as a result of hypertrophy (see Chapter 19). Diastolic dysfunction is the result of an increase in ventricular muscle mass, fibrosis, or myocardial ischemia. In contrast to left ventricular end-diastolic volume, which remains normal until very late in the disease, left ventricular end-diastolic pressure is elevated early. The decreased diastolic pressure gradient between the left atrium and left ventricle impairs ventricular filling, which becomes quite dependent on a normal atrial contraction. Loss of atrial systole can precipitate congestive heart failure or hypotension in patients with aortic stenosis. Cardiac output may be normal in symptomatic patients at rest, but characteristically, it does not appropriately increase with exertion. Patients may experience angina even in the absence of coronary artery disease. Myocardial oxygen demand increases because of ventricular hypertrophy, while myocardial oxygen supply decreases as a result of the marked compression of intramyocardial coronary vessels caused by high intracavitary systolic pressures (up to 300 mm Hg). Exertional syncope or near-syncope is thought to be due to an inability to tolerate the vasodilation in muscle tissue during exertion. Arrhythmias leading to severe hypoperfusion may also account for syncope and sudden death in some patients. Calcium emboli may occasionally result in neurologic complications.

Calculating Aortic Valve Area & Transvalvular Gradient

As with mitral stenosis, valve area can be derived from catheterization data because the transvalvular gradient is proportionate to cardiac output. Using the Gorlin equation:

$$\text{Valve area} = \frac{\text{Flow across valve}}{K \times \sqrt{\text{mean transvalvular gradient}}}$$

Aortic valve flow is expressed as mL/sec, pressure as mm Hg, and valve area as cm²; K = 44. Aortic valve flow can be derived as follows:

$$\text{Aortic valve flow} = \frac{\text{Cardiac output}}{\text{Systolic ejection period} \times \text{heart rate}}$$

As with mitral stenosis, the pressure gradient across the aortic valve can be determined noninvasively using continuous wave Doppler echocardiography:

$$\Delta P = 4V^2$$

where ΔP is the peak pressure gradient (mm Hg) and V is peak blood flow velocity (m/sec) distal to the obstruction. Peak velocities greater than 4.5 m/sec are usually indicative of severe stenosis. Moreover, if the area proximal to the stenosis (LVOT) can be measured, the continuity equation can then be applied to estimate valve area. Either TVIs or maximum velocities can be used:

$$A_2 = \frac{A_1 V_1}{V_2}$$

where A_2 is valve area, A_1 is the cross-sectional area of the LVOT, V_1 is maximum blood flow velocity in LVOT, and V_2 is maximum flow velocity through the aortic valve. The presence of aortic regurgitation does not affect the accuracy of this calculation.

Treatment

Once significant symptoms develop, most patients die without surgical treatment within 2–5 years. Patients with congestive heart failure are treated with digoxin, sodium restriction, and small doses of diuretics. Percutaneous balloon valvuloplasty is generally used for younger patients with congenital aortic stenosis; it can also be used for elderly patients with calcific aortic stenosis who are poor candidates for aortic valve replacement. Its efficacy for the latter group is short-lived, however, and restenosis usually occurs within 6–12 months.

Anesthetic Management

A. OBJECTIVES:

 Maintenance of normal sinus rhythm, heart rate, and intravascular volume is critical in patients with aortic stenosis. Loss of a normally timed atrial systole often leads to rapid deterioration, especially when associated with tachycardia. The combination of the two (atrial fibrillation) seriously impairs ventricular filling and necessitates immediate cardioversion. The reduced ventricular compliance also makes the patient very sensitive to abrupt changes in intravascular volume. Many patients behave as though they have a fixed SV in spite of adequate hydration; under these conditions, cardiac output becomes very rate-dependent. Bradycardia (< 50 beats/min) is therefore poorly tolerated. Heart rates between 60 and 90 beats/min are optimal in most patients.

B. MONITORING:

Close monitoring of the ECG and blood pressure is crucial. Monitoring for ischemia is complicated by baseline ST-segment and T-wave abnormalities. Intra-arterial pressure monitoring is desirable in patients with severe aortic stenosis, since many of these patients do not tolerate even brief episodes of hypotension. Pulmonary artery catheterization is also useful, but data should be interpreted carefully; a higher than normal pulmonary capillary wedge pressure is often required to maintain adequate left ventricular end-diastolic volume and cardiac output. Prominent *a* waves are often visible on the pulmonary artery wedge pressure waveform. Vasodilators should generally only be employed when a pulmonary artery catheter is in place, because patients are often very sensitive to these agents. TEE can be useful in these patients for monitoring ischemia, ventricular preload, contractility, valvular function, and the effects of therapeutic interventions.

C. CHOICE OF AGENTS:

Patients with mild to moderate aortic stenosis (generally asymptomatic) may tolerate spinal or epidural anesthesia. These techniques should be employed very cautiously, however, because hypotension readily occurs as a result of reductions in preload, afterload, or both. Epidural anesthesia is preferable to spinal anesthesia because of the former's slower onset of hypotension, which allows more aggressive correction. Spinal and epidural anesthesia are contraindicated in patients with severe aortic stenosis.

The selection of general anesthetic agents is most critical in patients with symptomatic (moderate to severe) aortic stenosis. In these patients, a primarily opioid-based anesthetic technique generally results in minimal cardiac depression; suitable nonopioid induction agents include etomidate and the combination of ketamine and a benzodiazepine. If a volatile agent is used, the concentration should be carefully controlled to avoid excessive myocardial depression, vasodilation, or loss of normal atrial systole. Tachycardia and hypertension, which can precipitate ischemia, should be treated by increasing anesthetic depth. If a β-adrenergic blocking agent is used, esmolol may be preferable because of its short half-life. Most patients with aortic stenosis are extremely sensitive to vasodilators. Moreover, because of an already precarious myocardial oxygen demand-supply balance, they tolerate even mild degrees of hypotension poorly. Hypotension should generally be treated with small doses (25–50 µg) of phenylephrine. Intraoperative supraventricular tachycardias with hemodynamic compromise should be treated with immediate synchronized cardioversion. Frequent ventricular ectopy (which often reflects ischemia) is usually poorly tolerated hemodynamically and should be treated with intravenous lidocaine. Amiodarone is generally effective for both supraventricular and ventricular arrhythmias.

HYPERTROPHIC CARDIOMYOPATHY

Preoperative Considerations

Hypertrophic cardiomyopathy can be hereditary (usually with variable penetrance) or may occur sporadically. It has been called by many other names: idiopathic hypertrophic subaortic stenosis, asymmetric septal hypertrophy, hypertrophic obstructive cardiomyopathy, and muscular subaortic stenosis. It is characterized by heterogeneous left ventricular hypertrophy that is without any obvious cause. The hypertrophied muscle typically displays abnormal cellular architecture.

Affected patients characteristically display *diastolic dysfunction* that is reflected by elevated left ventricular end-diastolic pressures in spite of often hyperdynamic ventricular function. The diastolic stiffness is presumably due to the abnormal hypertrophied muscle, which tends to be located in the upper interventricular septum below the aortic valve; rarely, only the ventricular apex is involved. In about 25% of patients, the hypertrophy results in dynamic obstruction of left ventricular outflow during systole. Obstruction is the result of the narrowing in subaortic area caused by a systolic anterior motion (SAM) of the anterior mitral valve leaflet against the hypertrophied septum. SAM may be at least partly due to a Venturi effect drawing in the anterior leaflet during rapid ejection of the hypertrophied ventricle. In contrast to fixed obstruction (valvular aortic stenosis), the resulting obstruction (and pressure gradient) is dynamic and peaks in mid-to-late systole. Moreover, the degree of obstruction can vary from beat to beat. Factors that tend to worsen the obstruction include enhanced contractility, decreased ventricular volume, and decreased left ventricular afterload. Mitral regurgitation secondary to SAM is due to failure of mitral leaflets to normally coapt in late systole usually resulting in a posteriorly directed regurgitant jet. Anatomic studies also suggest that almost all patients have abnormalities of the mitral valve; the mitral leaflets, especially the anterior one, are frequently longer than normal.

Most patients are asymptomatic. Patients who are symptomatic generally complain of dyspnea on exertion, but they may also have fatigue, syncope, near-syncope, or angina. Symptoms do not necessarily correlate with the presence or severity of dynamic left ventricular outflow obstruction. Sudden cardiac death is often the first manifestation of the disorder in patients younger than 30 years and is the most common cause of death. Both supraventricular and ventricular arrhythmias are common. Patients with obstruction have a characteristic harsh systolic murmur (see Table 20–11). The ECG typically shows left ventricular hypertrophy and deep, broad Q waves. The diagnosis can be confirmed by echocardiography. Even asymptomatic patients may show myocardial perfusion defects on thallium-201 scans. The peak pressure gradient can be measured with Doppler echocardiography by determining peak velocity in the LVOT (see above section on aortic stenosis).

Treatment is with β-adrenergic and calcium channel blocking agents. Both agents decrease contractility and can prevent increases in the subaortic pressure gradient in patients with obstruction. Calcium channel blockers may also improve diastolic compliance (relaxation). Amiodarone is generally effective for both supraventricular and ventricular arrhythmias. Nitrates, digoxin, and diuretics are avoided because they can worsen left ventricular obstruction. Surgical myomectomy/myotomy is reserved for patients with moderate to severe symptoms; TEE is invaluable aid for such resections.

Anesthetic Management

Preoperative evaluation of patients with hypertrophic cardiomyopathy should focus on evaluating the potential for significant dynamic obstruction, malignant arrhythmias, and myocardial ischemia. The results of echocardiography (or angiography) and Holter monitoring should ideally be reviewed with a cardiologist. Anesthetic goals should be to minimize sympathetic activation, expand intravascular volume in order to avoid hypovolemia, and minimize decreases in left ventricular afterload.

Monitoring requirements are dictated by the severity of obstruction and the surgical procedure. Full hemodynamic monitoring is generally desirable to guide fluid therapy in the presence of abnormal ventricular compliance. The arterial pressure waveform in patients with obstruction may be bifid (bisferiens pulse): The initial rapid peak represents early unobstructed ventricular ejection, while the subsequent decrease and second peak are due to dynamic obstruction.

In patients with significant obstruction, some degree of myocardial depression is usually desirable and can be achieved by the use of volatile anesthetic agents, especially halothane and enflurane. β-Adrenergic agents are also useful in counteracting the effects of sympathetic activation and decreasing obstruction. Regional anesthesia may exacerbate left ventricular outflow obstruction by decreasing both cardiac preload and afterload. Phenylephrine and other pure α-adrenergic agonists are ideal vasopressors in these patients because they do not augment contractility but increase SVR (ventricular afterload).

AORTIC REGURGITATION

Preoperative Considerations

Aortic regurgitation usually develops slowly and is progressive (chronic), but it can also develop quickly (acute). Chronic aortic regurgitation may be caused by abnormalities of the aortic valve, the aortic root, or both. Abnormalities in the valve are usually congenital (bicuspid valve) or due to rheumatic fever. Diseases affecting the ascending aorta cause regurgitation by dilating the aortic annulus; they include syphilis, annuloaortic ectasia, cystic medial necrosis (with or without Marfan syndrome), ankylosing spondylitis, rheumatoid and psoriatic arthritis, and a variety of other connective tissue disorders. Acute aortic insufficiency most commonly follows infective endocarditis, trauma, or aortic dissection.

Pathophysiology

Regardless of the cause, aortic regurgitation produces volume overload of the left ventricle (Figure 20–3). The effective forward SV is reduced because of backward (regurgitant) flow of blood into the left ventricle during diastole. Systemic arterial diastolic pressure and SVR are typically low. The decrease in cardiac afterload helps facilitate ventricular ejection. Total SV is the sum of the effective stroke volume and the regurgitant volume. The regurgitant volume depends on the heart rate (diastolic time) and the diastolic pressure gradient across the aortic valve (diastolic aortic pressure minus left ventricular end-diastolic pressure). Slow heart rates increase regurgitation because of the associated disproportionate increase in diastolic time (see Chapter 19), while increases in diastolic arterial pressure favor regurgitant volume by increasing the pressure gradient for backward flow.

With chronic aortic regurgitation, the left ventricle progressively dilates and undergoes eccentric hypertrophy. Patients with severe aortic regurgitation have the largest end-diastolic volumes of any heart disease; the massively dilated heart is often referred to as **cor bovinum.** The resulting increase in end-diastolic volume maintains an effective SV because end-systolic volume is unchanged. Any increase in the regurgitant volume is compensated by an increase in end-diastolic volume. Left ventricular end-diastolic pressure is usually normal or only slightly elevated, because ventricular compliance initially increases. Eventually, as ventricular function deteriorates, the ejection fraction declines, and impaired ventricular emptying is manifested as gradual increases in left ventricular end-diastolic pressure and end-systolic volume.

Sudden incompetence of the aortic valve does not allow compensatory dilation or hypertrophy of the left ventricle. Effective SV rapidly declines because the normal-sized ventricle is unable to accommodate a sudden large regurgitant volume. The sudden rise in left ventricular end-diastolic pressure is transmitted back to the pulmonary circulation and causes acute pulmonary congestion.

Acute aortic regurgitation typically presents as the sudden onset of pulmonary edema and hypotension, while chronic regurgitation usually presents insidiously as congestive heart failure. Symptoms are generally minimal (in the chronic form) when the regurgitant volume remains under 40% of SV but become severe when it exceeds 60%. Angina can occur even in the absence of coronary disease. The myocardial oxygen demand is increased from muscle hypertrophy and dilation, while the myocardial blood supply is reduced by low diastolic pressures in the aorta as a result of the regurgitation.

Calculating Regurgitant Fraction & Other Measurements of Severity

As with mitral regurgitation, RSV and RF for aortic regurgitation can be estimated by pulsed Doppler echocardiography. Stroke volume is measured at the left ventricular outflow tract (LVOT) and at the mitral valve (MV).

Thus,

$$RSV_{\text{aortic regurgitation}} = (A_{LVOT} \times TVI_{LVOT}) \\ -(A_{MV} \times VTI_{MV})$$

and

$$RF = RSV/SV$$

Pressure half-time (T½, see Mitral Stenosis above) of the regurgitant jet is another useful echocardiographic parameter for clinically assessing the severity of aortic regurgitation. The shorter the half-time the more severe is the regurgitation; severe regurgitation rapidly raises left ventricular diastolic pressure and results in more rapid pressure equilibration. Unfortunately, T½ is affected not only by the regurgitant orifice area but also aortic and ventricular pressure. An aortic regurgitation jet with a T½ less than 240 msec is associated with severe regurgitation.

Treatment

Most patients with chronic aortic regurgitation remain asymptomatic for 10–20 years. Once significant symptoms develop, the expected survival time is about 5 years without valve replacement. Digitalis, diuretics, and afterload reduction, especially with ACE inhibitors, generally benefit patients with advanced chronic aortic regurgitation. The decrease in arterial blood pressure reduces the diastolic gradient for regurgitation. Patients with chronic aortic regurgitation should be operated on before irreversible ventricular dysfunction occurs.

Patients with acute aortic regurgitation typically require intravenous inotropic (dopamine or dobutamine) and vasodilator (nitroprusside) therapy. Early surgery is indicated for patients with acute aortic regurgitation: medical management alone is associated with a high mortality rate.

Anesthetic Management

A. OBJECTIVES:

 The heart rate should be maintained toward the upper limits of normal (80–100 beats/min). Bradycardia and increases in SVR increase the regurgitant volume in patients with aortic regurgitation, while tachycardia can contribute to myocardial ischemia. Excessive myocardial depression should also be avoided. The compensatory increase in cardiac preload should be maintained, but overzealous fluid replacement can readily result in pulmonary edema.

B. MONITORING:

Full hemodynamic monitoring should generally be employed for all patients with acute aortic regurgitation and those with severe chronic regurgitation. Premature closure of the mitral valve often occurs during acute aortic regurgitation and may cause pulmonary capillary wedge pressure to give a falsely high estimate of left ventricular end-diastolic pressure. The appearance of a large *v* wave suggests mitral regurgitation secondary to dilation of the left ventricle. The arterial pressure wave in patients with aortic regurgitation characteristically has a very wide pulse pressure. A bisferiens pulse may also be present in some patients and is thought to result from the rapid ejection of a large SV. Color-flow Doppler TEE can be invaluable in quantitating the severity of the regurgitation and guiding therapeutic interventions (see Table 20–13). By definition, some blood flow reversal is present in the aorta during all of diastole (holodiastolic) with severe aortic regurgitation; moreover, the further down the aorta that holodiastolic flow reversal is detected, the more severe the regurgitation.

C. CHOICE OF AGENTS:

Most patients tolerate spinal and epidural anesthesia, provided intravascular volume is maintained. When general anesthesia is required, isoflurane and desflurane may be ideal because of the associated vasodilation. A primarily opioid-based general anesthetic technique is more suitable for patients with depressed ventricular function. Pancuronium is a good choice as a muscle relaxant with the latter technique because it often prevents bradycardia. Intraoperative afterload reduction with nitroprusside optimally requires full hemodynamic monitoring. Ephedrine is generally the preferred vasopressor for the treatment of hypotension. Small doses of phenylephrine (25–50 μg) can be used when the hypotension is clearly due to excessive vasodilation, however. Large doses of phenylephrine can increase SVR (and arterial diastolic pressure) and may exacerbate the regurgitation.

TRICUSPID REGURGITATION

Preoperative Considerations

Up to 70–90% of patients have mild tricuspid regurgitation on echocardiography; the regurgitant volume in these cases is nearly always insignificant. Clinically significant tricuspid regurgitation, however, is most commonly due to dilation of the right ventricle from the pulmonary hypertension that is associated with chronic left ventricular failure. Tricuspid regurgitation can also follow infective endocarditis (usually in injecting drug abusers), rheumatic fever, carcinoid syndrome, or chest trauma or may be due to Ebstein's anomaly (downward displacement of the valve because of abnormal attachment of the valve leaflets).

Pathophysiology

Chronic left ventricular failure often leads to sustained increases in pulmonary vascular pressures. The chronic increase in afterload causes progressive dilation of the thin-walled right ventricle, and excessive dilation of the tricuspid annulus eventually results in regurgitation. An increase in end-diastolic volume allows the right ventricle to compensate for the regurgitant volume and maintain an effective forward flow. Because the right atrium and the vena cava are compliant and can usually accommodate the volume overload, mean right atrial and central venous pressures are generally only slightly elevated. Acute or marked elevations in pulmonary artery pressures increase the regurgitant volume and are reflected by an increase in central venous pressure. Moreover, sudden marked increases in right ventricular afterload sharply reduce the effective right ventricular output, reduce left ventricular preload, and can precipitate systemic hypotension.

Chronic venous hypertension leads to passive congestion of the liver and progressive hepatic dysfunction, which can eventually result in cardiac cirrhosis. Severe right ventricular failure with underloading of the left heart may also produce right-to-left shunting through an incompletely closed (or probe-patent) foramen ovale, which can result in marked hypoxemia.

Calculating Regurgitant Volume & Pulmonary Artery Pressure

To calculate the regurgitant volume, stroke volume is calculated at the tricuspid valve and at another (unaffected) site such as the LVOT or mitral valve (see above section on mitral regurgitation):

$$RSV_{tricuspid\ regurgitation} = (A_{TV} \times VTI_{TV})$$
$$-(A_{LVOT} \times TVI_{LVOT})$$

where A_{TV} is the area of tricuspid valve and VTI_{TV} is the time velocity integral of flow across the tricuspid valve. With severe tricuspid regurgitation the normal systolic inflow into the right atrium is reversed and the flow reversal is also observed in the hepatic veins.

Systolic pulmonary artery pressure (PAS) can be estimated from the peak velocity of the regurgitant:

$$\Delta P = 4 \times V^2$$

where ΔP is the systolic pressure gradient (mm Hg) between the right ventricle and right atrium and V is peak blood flow velocity (m/sec) of the regurgitant jet. If the central venous pressure (CVP) is known or assumed, then

$$PAS = CVP + \Delta P$$

Treatment

Tricuspid regurgitation is generally well tolerated by most patients. In the absence of pulmonary hypertension, many even tolerate complete surgical excision of the tricuspid valve. Because the underlying disorder is generally more important than the tricuspid regurgitation itself, treatment is aimed at the underlying disease process. With moderate to severe regurgitation, tricuspid annuloplasty may be performed in conjunction with replacement of another valve.

Anesthetic Management

A. OBJECTIVES:

Hemodynamic goals should be directed primarily toward the underlying disorder. Hypovolemia and factors that increase right ventricular afterload, such as hypoxia and acidosis, should be avoided to maintain effective right ventricular SV and left ventricular preload. Positive end-expiratory pressure and high mean airway pressures may also be undesirable during mechanical ventilation because they reduce venous return and increase right ventricular afterload.

B. MONITORING:

In these patients, monitoring of both central venous and pulmonary artery pressures is useful. The latter is not always possible, since a large regurgitant flow may make passage of a pulmonary artery catheter across the tricuspid valve difficult. Central venous pressure is extremely useful in following right ventricular function, while pulmonary artery pressures allow measurement of its afterload and left ventricular preload. Increasing central venous pressures imply worsening right ventricular dysfunction. The x descent is absent and a prominent cv wave is usually present on the central venous pressure waveform. Thermodilution cardiac output measurements are falsely elevated because of the tricuspid regurgitation. Color-flow Doppler TEE is useful in evaluating the severity of the regurgitation and other associated abnormalities.

C. CHOICE OF AGENTS:

The selection of anesthetic agents should be based on the underlying disorder. Most patients tolerate spinal and epidural anesthesia well. Coagulopathy secondary to hepatic dysfunction should be excluded prior to any regional technique. During general anesthesia, nitrous oxide may exacerbate the pulmonary hypertension and should be administered cautiously, if at all.

■ CONGENITAL HEART DISEASE

Preoperative Considerations

Congenital heart disease encompasses a seemingly endless list of abnormalities that may be detected in infancy, early childhood or, less commonly, adulthood. The incidence of congenital heart disease approaches 1% of all live births. The natural history of some defects is such that patients often survive to adulthood (Table 20–14). Moreover, the number of surviving adults with congenital heart disease appears to be steadily increasing, possibly as a result of advances in

Table 20–14. Common congenital heart defects in which patients typically survive to adulthood without treatment.

Bicuspid aortic valve
Coarctation of the aorta
Pulmonic valve stenosis
Ostium secundum atrial septal defect
Ventricular septal defect
Patent ductus arteriosus

medical treatment. An increasing number of patients with congenital heart disease may therefore be encountered during noncardiac surgery and obstetric deliveries.

The complex nature and varying pathophysiology of congenital heart defects makes classification difficult. A commonly used scheme is presented in Table 20–15. Most patients present with cyanosis, congestive heart failure, or an asymptomatic abnormality. Cyanosis is typically the result of an abnormal intracardiac communication that allows unoxygenated blood to reach the systemic arterial circulation (right-to-left shunting). Congestive heart failure is most prominent with defects that either obstruct left ventricular outflow or markedly increase pulmonary blood flow. The latter is usually due to an abnormal intracardiac communication that returns oxygenated blood to the right heart (left-to-right shunting). While right-to-left shunts generally decrease pulmonary blood flow, some complex lesions increase pulmonary blood flow—even in the presence of right-to-left shunting. In many cases, more than one lesion is present. In fact, survival with some anomalies (eg, transposition, total anomalous venous return, pulmonary atresia) depends on the simultaneous presence of another shunting lesion (eg, patent ductus arteriosus, patent foramen ovale, ventricular septal defect). Chronic hypoxemia in patients with cyanotic heart disease typically results in erythrocytosis. This increase in red cell mass, which is due to enhanced erythropoietin secretion from the kidneys, serves to restore tissue oxygen concentration to normal. Unfortunately, blood viscosity can also rise to the point where it may interfere with oxygen delivery. Moreover, iron deficiency exacerbates the hyperviscosity by making red cells more rigid and less deformable in the microcirculation. When tissue oxygenation is restored to normal, the hematocrit is stable (usually < 65%), and symptoms of the hyperviscosity syndrome are absent, the patient is said to have **compensated erythrocytosis.** Patients with uncompensated erythrocytosis do not establish this equilibrium; they have symptoms of hyperviscosity and may be at risk for thrombotic complications, especially stroke. The last is aggravated by dehydration and iron deficiency. Children younger than 4 years appear to be at greatest risk for stroke. Factors that may lead to stroke in adults are excessive phlebotomy and aspirin or anticoagulation therapy. Phlebotomy is generally not recommended if symptoms of hyperviscosity are absent and the hematocrit is < 65%.

Coagulation abnormalities are common in patients with cyanotic heart disease. Platelet counts tend to be low-normal, and many patients have subtle or overt defects in the coagulation cascade. Phlebotomy may improve hemostasis in some patients. Hyperuricemia often occurs because of increased urate reabsorption secondary to renal hypoperfusion. Gouty arthritis is uncommon, but the hyperuricemia can result in progressive renal impairment.

Preoperative Doppler echocardiography is invaluable in helping define the anatomy of the defect(s), confirm or exclude the existence of other lesions or complications, their physiologic significance, and the effects of any therapeutic interventions.

Anesthetic Management

This population of patients includes four groups: those who have undergone corrective cardiac surgery and re-

Table 20–15. Classification of congenital heart disease.

Lesions causing outflow obstruction
Left ventricle
Coarctation of the aorta
Aortic stenosis
Right ventricle
Pulmonic valve stenosis
Lesions causing left-to-right shunting
Ventricular septal defect
Patent ductus arteriosus
Atrial septal defect
Endocardial cushion defect
Partial anomalous pulmonary venous return
Lesions causing right-to-left shunting
With decreased pulmonary blood flow
Tetralogy of Fallot
Pulmonary atresia
Tricuspid atresia
With increased pulmonary blood flow
Transposition of the great vessels
Truncus arteriosus
Single ventricle
Double-outlet right ventricle
Total anomalous pulmonary venous return
Hypoplastic left heart

Table 20–16. Common problems in survivors of surgery for congenital heart defects.

Arrhythmias
Hypoxemia
Pulmonary hypertension
Existing shunts
Paradoxical embolism
Bacterial endocarditis

quire no further operations, those who have had only palliative surgery, those who have not yet undergone any cardiac surgery, and those whose conditions are inoperable and may be awaiting cardiac transplantation. While the management of the first group of patients may be the same as for normal patients (save for consideration of prophylactic antibiotic therapy (see Table 20–12), the care of others requires familiarity with the complex pathophysiology of these defects. Even patients that have had corrective surgery may be prone to development of perioperative problems (Table 20–16). Some surgical procedures eliminate the risk of endocarditis while others increase the risk through the use of prosthetic valves or conduits or the creation of new shunts. Patients with ostium secundum atrial septal defects and those with mild pulmonic stenosis appear to have the lowest risk.

The management of patients for cardiac surgery and during obstetric delivery is discussed in Chapters 21 and 43, respectively. The general management of the pediatric patient is discussed in Chapter 44.

For the purpose of anesthetic management, congenital heart defects may be divided into obstructive lesions, predominately left-to-right shunts, or predominately right-to-left shunts (see Table 20–15). In reality, shunts can also be bidirectional and may reverse under certain conditions.

1. Obstructive Lesions

Congenital aortic stenosis has already been discussed above (see section on aortic stenosis) and coarctation of the aorta is discussed in Chapter 21.

Pulmonic Stenosis

Pulmonary valve stenosis obstructs right ventricular outflow and causes concentric right ventricular hypertrophy. Severe obstruction presents in the neonatal period, while lesser degrees of obstruction may go undetected until adulthood. The valve is usually deformed, and either bicuspid or tricuspid. Valve leaflets are often partially fused and display systolic doming on echocar-

diography. The right ventricle undergoes hypertrophy and post-stenotic dilation of the pulmonary artery is often present. Symptoms are those of right ventricular heart failure (see Chapter 19). Symptomatic patients readily develop fatigue, dyspnea, and peripheral cyanosis with exertion as a result of the limited pulmonary blood flow and increased oxygen extraction by tissues. With severe stenosis, the pulmonic valve gradient exceeds 60–80 mm Hg, depending on the age of the patient. Right-to-left shunting may also occur in the presence of a patent foramen ovale or atrial septal defect. Cardiac output is very dependent on an elevated heart rate, but excessive increases in the latter can compromise ventricular filling. Percutaneous balloon valvuloplasty is generally considered the initial treatment of choice for most patients with symptomatic pulmonic stenosis. Anesthetic management for patients undergoing surgery should maintain a normal or slightly high heart rate, augment preload, and avoid factors that increase PVR (see Chapter 22).

2. Predominately Left-to-Right (Simple) Shunts

Simple shunts are isolated abnormal communications between the right and left sides of the heart. Since pressures are normally higher on the left side, blood usually flows across from left to right, and blood flow through the right heart and the lungs increases. Depending on the size and location of the communication, the right ventricle may also be subjected to the higher left-sided pressures, resulting in both pressure and volume overload. Right ventricular afterload is normally 1/20th that of the left ventricle, so even small left-to-right pressure gradients can produce large increases in pulmonary blood flow. The ratio of pulmonary to systemic blood flow can be calculated from oxygen saturations at the time of catheterization by the following equation:

$$\frac{\dot{Q}_P}{\dot{Q}_S} = \frac{C_{aO_2} - C_{\bar{v}O_2}}{C_{pvO_2} - C_{paO_2}}$$

where CaO_2 is systemic arterial, $C\bar{v}O_2$ is mixed venous, $C_{pv}O_2$ is oxygen content of pulmonary venous blood (ie, in pulmonary veins), and $C_{pa}O_2$ is oxygen content of pulmonary artery blood.

A ratio greater than 1 usually indicates a left-to-right shunt, while a ratio less than 1 indicates a right-to-left shunt. A ratio of 1 indicates either no shunting or a bidirectional shunt of opposing magnitudes.

Large increases in pulmonary blood flow produce pulmonary vascular congestion and increase extravascular lung water. The latter interferes with gas exchange, decreases lung compliance, and increases the work of breathing. Left atrial distention also compresses the left bronchus, while distention of pulmonary vessels compresses smaller bronchi.

Over the course of several years, chronic increases in pulmonary blood flow produce vascular changes that irreversibly increase PVR. Elevation of right ventricular afterload produces hypertrophy and progressively raises right-sided cardiac pressures. With advanced disease, the pressures within the right heart can exceed those within the left heart. Under these conditions, the intracardiac shunt reverses and becomes right-to-left (**Eisenmenger syndrome**).

When a communication is small, shunt flow depends primarily on the size of the communication (**restrictive shunt**). When the communication is large (**nonrestrictive shunt**), shunt flow depends on the relative balance between PVR and SVR. An increase in SVR relative to PVR favors left-to-right shunting, while an increase in PVR relative to SVR favors right-to-left shunting. Common chamber lesions (eg, single atrium, single ventricle, truncus arteriosus) represent the extreme form of nonrestrictive shunts; shunt flow with these lesions is bidirectional and totally dependent on relative changes in the ventricular afterload.

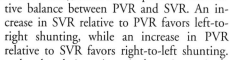

The presence of shunt flow between the right and left hearts, regardless of the direction of blood flow, mandates the meticulous exclusion of air bubbles or clot from intravenous fluids to prevent paradoxical embolism into the cerebral or coronary circulations.

Atrial Septal Defects

Ostium secundum atrial septal defects (ASDs) are the most common type and usually occur as isolated lesions in the area of the fossa ovalis. The defect is sometimes associated with partial anomalous pulmonary venous return, most commonly of the right upper pulmonary vein. A secundum ASD may result in single or multiple (fenestrated) openings between the atria. The less common sinus venosus, and ostium primum ASDs are typically associated with other cardiac abnormalities. Sinus venosus defects are located in the upper interatrial septum close to the superior vena cava; one or more of the right pulmonary veins often abnormally drains into the superior vena cava. In contrast, ostium primum ASDs are located in the lower interatrial septum and overlie the mitral and tricuspid valves; most patients also have cleft in the anterior leaflet of the mitral valve and some have an abnormal septal leaflet in the tricuspid valve.

Most children with ASDs are minimally symptomatic; some have recurrent pulmonary infections. Congestive heart failure and pulmonary hypertension are more commonly encountered in adults with ASDs. Patients with ostium primum defects often have large shunts and may also develop significant mitral regurgitation. In the absence of heart failure, anesthetic responses to inhalational and intravenous agents are generally not significantly altered in patients with ASDs. Increases in SVR should be avoided because they may worsen the left-to-right shunting.

Ventricular Septal Defects

Ventricular septal defect (VSD) is the most common congenital heart defect, accounting for up to 25–35% of congenital heart disease. The defect is most frequently in the membranous part of the interventricular septum (membranous or infracristal VSD) in a posterior position and anterior to the septal leaflet of the tricuspid valve. Muscular VSDs are the next most frequent type and are located in the mid or apical portion of the interventricular septum, where there may be a single defect or multiple openings (resembling Swiss cheese). Defects in the subpulmonary (supracristal) septum are often associated with aortic regurgitation because the right coronary cusp can prolapse into the VSD. Septal defects at the ventricular inlet are usually similar in development and location to AV septal defects (see next section).

The resulting functional abnormality of a VSD is dependent on the size of the defect, PVR, and the presence or absence of other abnormalities. Small VSDs, especially of the muscular type, often close during childhood. Restrictive defects are associated with only small left-to-right shunts (pulmonary-systemic blood flow ratios less than 1.75:1). Large defects produce large left-to-right shunts (shunts larger than 2:1) that vary directly with SVR and indirectly with PVR. Recurrent pulmonary infections and congestive heart failure are common with pulmonary-systemic flow ratios of 3–5:1. Patients with small VSDs are treated medically and followed by electrocardiography (for signs of right ventricular hypertrophy) and by echocardiography. Surgical closure is usually undertaken for patients with large VSDs, before pulmonary vascular disease and Eisenmenger physiology develop. As with atrial defects, in the absence of heart failure, anesthetic responses to inhalational and intravenous agents are generally not significantly altered. Similarly, increases in SVR worsen the left-to-right shunting. When right-to-left shunting is present, abrupt increases in PVR or decreases in SVR are poorly tolerated.

Atrioventricular Septal Defects

Endocardial cushion (AV canal) defects produce contiguous atrial and ventricular septal defects often with very abnormal AV valves. This is a common lesion in patients with Down syndrome (see Chapter 44). The defect can produce large shunts both at the atrial and ventricular levels. Mitral and tricuspid regurgitation exacerbate the volume overload on the ventricles. Initially, shunting is predominately left to right; however, with increasing pulmonary hypertension, Eisenmenger syndrome with obvious cyanosis develops.

Patent Ductus Arteriosus

Persistence of the communication between the main pulmonary artery and the aorta can produce restrictive or nonrestrictive left-to-right shunts. This abnormality is commonly responsible for the cardiopulmonary deterioration of premature infants, and occasionally presents later in life. Anesthetic goals should be similar to atrial and ventricular septal defects.

Partial Anomalous Venous Return

This defect is present when one or more pulmonary veins drains into the right side of the heart; the anomalous veins are usually from the right lung. Possible anomalous entry sites include the right atrium, superior or inferior vena cava, and the coronary sinus. The resulting abnormality produces a variable amount of left-to-right shunting. The clinical course and prognosis is usually excellent and similar to that with a secundum ASD. A very large coronary sinus on TEE suggests anomalous drainage into the coronary sinus, which may complicate the management of cardioplegia during cardiac surgery (see Chapter 21).

3. Predominately Right-to-Left (Complex) Shunts

Lesions within this group (some also called **mixing lesions**) often produce both ventricular outflow obstruction and shunting. The obstruction favors shunt flow toward the unobstructed side. When the obstruction is relatively mild, the amount of shunting is affected by the ratio of SVR to PVR, but increasing degrees of obstruction fix the direction and magnitude of the shunt. Atresia of any one of the cardiac valves represents the extreme form of obstruction. Shunting occurs proximal to the atretic valve and is completely fixed; survival depends on another distal shunt (usually a patent ductus arteriosus [PDA], patent foramen ovale, ASD, or VSD), where blood flows in the opposite direction. This group of defects may also be divided according to whether they increase or decrease pulmonary blood flow (see Table 20–15).

Tetralogy of Fallot

This tetralogy classically includes right ventricular obstruction, right ventricular hypertrophy, and a VSD with an overriding aorta. Right ventricular obstruction in most patients is due to infundibular stenosis, which is due to hypertrophy of the subpulmonic muscle (crista ventricularis). At least 20–25% of patients also have pulmonic stenosis, and a small percentage have some element of supravalvular obstruction. The pulmonic valve is often bicuspid or less commonly atretic. Infundibular obstruction may be increased by sympathetic tone and therefore dynamic; this obstruction is likely responsible for the hypercyanotic spells observed in very young patients. The combination of right ventricular obstruction and a VSD results in ejection of unoxygenated right ventricular blood as well as oxygenated left ventricular into the aorta. The right-to-left shunting across the VSD has both fixed and variable components. The fixed component is determined by the severity of the right ventricular obstruction, while the variable component depends on SVR and PVR.

Neonates with severe right ventricular obstruction may deteriorate quickly as pulmonary blood flow decreases when a PDA starts to close. Intravenous prostaglandin E_1 (0.05–0.2 μg/kg/min) is used to prevent ductal closure in such instances. Surgical palliation with a left-to-right systemic shunt or complete correction is then usually undertaken. For the former, a modified Blalock-Taussig (left subclavian-pulmonary artery) shunt is most often used to increase pulmonary blood flow. In this procedure, a synthetic graft is anastomosed between a subclavian artery and an ipsilateral pulmonary artery. Complete correction involves closure of the VSD, removal of obstructing infundibular muscle, and pulmonic valvulotomy or valvuloplasty, when necessary.

 The goals of anesthetic management in patients with tetralogy of Fallot should be to maintain intravascular volume and SVR. Increases in PVR, such as might occur from acidosis or excessive airway pressures, should be avoided. Ketamine (intramuscular or intravenous) is a commonly used induction agent because it maintains or increases SVR and therefore does not aggravate the right-to-left shunting. Patients with milder degrees of shunting generally tolerate inhalational induction with halothane. The right-to-left shunting tends to slow the uptake of inhalational anesthetics (see Chapter 7); in contrast, it may accelerate the onset of intravenous agents. Oxygenation often improves following induction of anesthesia. Muscle relaxants that release histamine should be avoided. Hypercyanotic spells may be treated with intravenous fluid and phenylephrine (5 μg/kg). Propranolol (0.1 μg/kg) may also be effective in relieving infundibular spasm. Sodium bicarbonate, to correct the resulting metabolic acidosis, may also be helpful when the hypoxemia is severe and prolonged.

Tricuspid Atresia

With tricuspid atresia, blood can only flow out of the right atrium via a patent foramen ovale (or an ASD). Moreover, a PDA (or VSD) is necessary for blood to flow from the left ventricle into the pulmonary circulation. Cyanosis is usually evident at birth and its severity depends on the amount of pulmonary blood flow that is achieved. Early survival is dependent on prostaglandin E_1 infusion with or without a percutaneous, Rashkind balloon atrial septostomy. Severe cyanosis requires a modified Blalock-Taussig early in life. The preferred surgical management is a modified Fontan procedure, where the right atrium is anastomosed to the right pulmonary artery. In some centers a superior vena cava to the main pulmonary artery (bidirectional Glenn) shunt may be employed before or instead of a Fontan procedure. With both procedures, blood from the systemic veins flows to the left atrium entirely as a result of a pressure gradient. Success of the procedure depends on a high systemic venous pressure and maintaining both low PVR and a low left atrial pressure. Heart transplantation may be necessary for a failed Fontan procedure.

Transposition of the Great Arteries

In patients with transposition of the great arteries (TGA), pulmonary and systemic venous return flow normally back to the right and left atrium, respectively, but the aorta arises from the right ventricle and the pulmonary artery arises from the left ventricle. Thus, deoxygenated blood returns back into the systemic circulation, while oxygenated blood returns back to the lungs. Survival is only possible through mixing of oxygenated and deoxygenated blood across the foramen ovale and a PDA. The presence of a VSD increases mixing and reduces the level of hypoxemia. Prostaglandin E_1 infusion is usually necessary. Rashkind septostomy may be necessary if surgical correction is delayed. Corrective surgical treatment involves an arterial switch procedure, where the aorta is divided and reanastomosed to the left ventricle and the pulmonary artery is divided and reanastomosed to the right ventricle. The coronary arteries must also be reimplanted into the old pulmonary artery root. A VSD, if present, is closed. Less commonly, an atrial switch (Senning) procedure may be carried out if an arterial switch is not possible. In this latter procedure, an intra-atrial baffle is created from the atrial wall and blood from the pulmonary veins flows across an ASD to the right ventricle, from where it is ejected into the systemic circulation.

Transposition of the great vessels may occur with a VSD and pulmonic stenosis. This combination of defects mimics tetralogy of Fallot; however, the obstruction affects the left ventricle not the right ventricle. Corrective surgery involves patch closure of the VSD, directing left ventricular outflow into the aorta, ligation of the proximal pulmonary artery, and connecting the right ventricular outflow to the pulmonary artery with a valved conduit (Rastelli procedure).

Total Anomalous Venous Return

The absence of a direct connection between the pulmonary veins and the left atrium results in total anomalous venous return. Mixing of deoxygenated and oxygenated blood occurs at or before the right atrial level because the pulmonary veins usually drain into the superior or inferior vena cava, coronary sinus, or ductus venosus. Blood usually reaches the left atrium via the foramen ovale or an ASD. Obstruction of the pulmonary venous return, which may occur when the blood drains into the ductus venous and it begins to close, results in severe pulmonary congestion. Surgical correction involves reanastomosing the common pulmonary venous trunk directly into the left atrium and closure of any ASD.

Truncus Arteriosus

With a truncus arteriosus defect, a single arterial trunk supplies the pulmonary and systemic circulation. The truncus always overrides a VSD, allowing both ventricles to eject into it. As PVR gradually decreases after birth, pulmonary blood flow increases greatly resulting in heart failure. If left untreated, PVR increases and cyanosis develops again along with Eisenmenger physiology. Surgical correction closes the VSD, separates the pulmonary artery from the truncus, and the right ventricle is connected to the pulmonary artery with a conduit (Rastelli repair).

Hypoplastic Left Heart Syndrome

This syndrome describes a group of defects characterized by marked underdevelopment of the left ventricle. It is often associated with other major noncardiac congenital anomalies. The right ventricle is the main pumping chamber for both systemic and pulmonary circulations. It ejects normally into the pulmonary artery and all (or nearly all) blood flow entering the aorta is usually derived from a PDA. Surgical treatment options are either palliation with the very complicated Norwood procedure or cardiac transplantation. The Norwood procedure is typically carried out in three stages.

■ THE PATIENT WITH A TRANSPLANTED HEART

Preoperative Considerations

The number of patients with cardiac transplants is increasing because of both the increasing frequency of transplantation and improved survival rates. These patients may present to the operating room early in the postoperative period for mediastinal exploration or retransplantation, or they may appear later for incision and drainage of infections, orthopedic surgery, or unrelated procedures.

The transplanted heart is totally denervated, so direct autonomic influences are absent. Cardiac impulse formation and conduction are normal, but the absence of vagal influences causes a relatively high resting heart rate (100–120 beats/min). Although sympathetic fibers are similarly interrupted, the response to circulating catecholamines is normal or even enhanced because of denervation sensitivity (increased receptor density). Partial reinnervation may occur in some patients after some time. Cardiac output tends to be low-normal and increases relatively slowly in response to exercise because the response is dependent on an increase in circulating catecholamines. Because the Starling relationship between end-diastolic volume and cardiac output (see Chapter 19) is normal, the transplanted heart is also often said to be *preload-dependent.* Coronary autoregulation is preserved.

Preoperative evaluation should focus on evaluating the functional status of the transplanted organ and detecting complications of immunosuppression. The highest incidence of rejection occurs within the first 3 months; thereafter rejection rates are about one per patient-year. Rejection may be heralded by arrhythmias (in the first 6 months) or decreased exercise tolerance from a progressive deterioration of myocardial performance. Periodic echocardiographic evaluations are commonly used to monitor for rejection, but the most reliable technique is endomyocardial biopsy. Accelerated atherosclerosis in the graft is a very common and serious problem that limits the life of the transplant. Moreover, myocardial ischemia and infarction are al-

most always silent because of the denervation. Because of this, patients must undergo periodic evaluations, including angiography, for coronary atherosclerosis.

Immunosuppressive therapy usually includes cyclosporine, azathioprine, and prednisone. Important side effects include nephrotoxicity, bone marrow suppression, hepatotoxicity, opportunistic infections, and osteoporosis. Hypertension and fluid retention are common and typically require treatment with a diuretic and an ACE inhibitor. Stress doses of corticosteroids are needed when patients undergo major procedures (see Chapter 36).

Anesthetic Management

Nearly all anesthetic techniques, including regional anesthesia have been used successfully for transplanted patients. The preload-dependent function of the graft makes maintenance of a normal or high cardiac preload desirable. Moreover, the absence of reflex increases in heart rate can make patients especially sensitive to rapid vasodilation. Indirect vasopressors such as ephedrine and dopamine are less effective than direct-acting agents because of the absence of catecholamine stores in myocardial neurons (see Chapter 12). Isoproterenol or dilute epinephrine (10 µg/mL) should be readily available to increase the heart rate if necessary. Bradycardia secondary to opioids and cholinesterase inhibitors is absent. Similarly, increases in heart rate are not seen following anticholinergics, pancuronium, or meperidine. An anticholinergic must still be given to reverse muscle relaxants in order to block the noncardiac muscarinic effects of acetylcholine.

Careful electrocardiographic monitoring for ischemia is necessary. The ECG usually demonstrates two sets of P waves, one representing the recipient's own SA node (which is left intact) and the other representing the donor's SA node. The recipient's SA node may still be affected by autonomic influences, but it does not affect cardiac function. Direct arterial, central venous, and pulmonary artery pressure monitoring should be used for major operations; strict asepsis should be observed during placement.

CASE DISCUSSION:
HIP FRACTURE IN AN ELDERLY
WOMAN WHO FELL

A 71-year-old woman presents for open reduction and internal fixation of a left hip fracture. She gives a history of two episodes of lightheadedness several days prior to her fall today. When questioned about her fall, she can only recall standing in her bathroom while brushing her teeth and then awakening on the floor with hip pain. The preoperative ECG shows a sinus rhythm with a P–R interval of 220 msec and a right bundle-branch block (RBBB) pattern.

Why should the anesthesiologist be concerned about a history of syncope?

A history of syncope in elderly patients should always raise the possibility of arrhythmias and underlying organic heart disease. Although arrhythmias can occur in the absence of organic heart disease, the two are commonly related. Cardiac syncope usually results from an abrupt arrhythmia that suddenly compromises cardiac output and impairs cerebral perfusion. Lightheadedness, presyncope, may reflect lesser degrees of cerebral impairment. Both bradyarrhythmias and tachyarrhythmias (see Chapter 19) can produce syncope. Table 20–17 lists other cardiac and noncardiac causes of syncope.

How do bradyarrhythmias commonly arise?

Bradyarrhythmias may arise from either sinoatrial (SA) node dysfunction or abnormal atrioventricular (AV) conduction of the cardiac impulse. A delay or block of the impulse can occur anywhere between the SA node and the distal His–Purkinje system (see Chapter 19). Reversible abnormalities may be due to abnormal vagal tone, electrolyte abnormalities, drug toxicity, hypothermia, or myocardial ischemia. Irreversible abnormalities, which initially may be only intermittent before they become permanent, reflect either isolated conduction system abnormalities or underlying heart disease (most commonly hypertensive, coronary artery, or valvular heart disease).

What is the pathophysiology of sinus node dysfunction?

*Patients with sinus node dysfunction may have a normal baseline 12-lead electrocardiogram (ECG) but abrupt pauses in SA node activity (sinus arrest) or intermittent block of conduction of the SA impulse to the surrounding tissue (exit block). Symptoms are usually present when pauses are prolonged (> 3 seconds) or the effective ventricular rate is less than 40 beats/min. Patients may experience intermittent dizziness, syncope, confusion, fatigue, or shortness of breath. Symptomatic SA node dysfunction, or **sick sinus syndrome,** is often unmasked by β-adrenergic blocking agents, calcium channel blockers, digoxin, or quinidine. The term **bradycardia-tachycardia syndrome** is often used when patients experience paroxysmal*

Table 20–17. Causes of syncope.

Cardiac
  Arrhythmias
    Tachyarrhythmias (usually > 180 beats/min)
    Bradyarrhythmias (usually < 40 beats/min)
  Impairment of left ventricular ejection
    Aortic stenosis
    Hypertrophic cardiomyopathy
    Massive myocardial infarction
    Atrial myxoma
  Impairment of right ventricular output
    Tetralogy of Fallot
    Primary pulmonary hypertension
    Pulmonary embolism
    Pulmonic valve stenosis
  Biventricular impairment
    Cardiac tamponade
    Massive myocardial infarction
Noncardiac
  Accentuated reflexes
    Vasodepressor reflex (ie, vasovagal syncope)
    Carotid sinus hypersensitivity
    Neuralgias
  Postural hypotension
    Hypovolemia
    Sympathectomy
    Autonomic dysfunction
  Sustained Valsalva maneuver
  Cerebrovascular disease
  Seizures
  Metabolic
    Hypoxia
    Marked hypocapnia
    Hypoglycemia

tachyarrhythmias (usually atrial flutter or fibrillation) followed by sinus pauses or bradycardia. The latter, bradycardia, probably represents failure of the SA node to recover normal automaticity following suppression by the tachyarrhythmia. The diagnosis must be based on electrocardiographic recordings made during symptoms (Holter monitoring) or after provocative tests (carotid baroreceptor stimulation or rapid atrial pacing).

How are AV conduction abnormalities manifested on the surface 12-lead ECG?

AV conduction abnormalities are usually manifested by abnormal ventricular depolarization (bundle-branch block), prolongation of the P–R interval (first-degree AV block), failure of some atrial impulses to depolarize the ventricles (second-degree AV block), or AV dissociation (third-degree AV block; also called complete heart block).

What determines the significance of these conduction abnormalities?

The significance of a conduction system abnormality depends on its location, its likelihood for progression to complete heart block, and the likelihood that a more distal pacemaker site will be able to maintain a stable and adequate escape rhythm (> 40 beats/min). The His bundle is normally the lowest area in the conduction system that can maintain a stable rhythm (usually 40–60 beats/min). When conduction fails anywhere above it, a normal His bundle can take over the pacemaker function of the heart and maintain a normal QRS complex unless a distal intraventricular conduction defect is present. When the escape rhythm arises farther down in the His-Purkinje system, the rhythm is usually slower (< 40 beats/min) and often unstable; it results in a wide QRS complex.

What is the significance of isolated bundle-branch block with a normal P–R interval?

A conduction delay or block in the right bundle-branch results in a typical RBBB QRS pattern on the surface ECG (M-shape or rSR' in V_1) and may represent a congenital abnormality or underlying organic heart disease. In contrast, a delay or block in the main left bundle-branch results in a left bundle-branch block (LBBB) QRS pattern (wide R with a delayed upstroke in V_5) and nearly always represents underlying heart disease. The term hemiblock is often used if only one of the two fascicles of the left bundle-branch is blocked (left anterior or left posterior hemiblock). When the P–R interval is normal—and in the absence of an acute myocardial infarction—a conduction block in either the left or right bundle rarely leads to complete heart block.

Can the site of AV block always be determined from a 12-lead ECG?

No. A first-degree AV block (P–R interval > 200 msec) can reflect abnormal conduction anywhere between the atria and the distal His-Purkinje system. Mobitz type I second-degree AV block, which is characterized by progressive lengthening of the P–R interval before a P wave is not conducted (a QRS does not follow the P wave), is usually due to a block in the AV node itself; progression to third-degree AV block is uncommon.

In patients with Mobitz type II second-degree AV block, atrial impulses are periodically not conducted into the ventricle without progressive prolongation of the P–R interval. The conduction block is nearly always in or below the His bundle

and frequently progresses to complete (third-degree) AV block, especially following an acute anteroseptal myocardial infarction. The QRS is typically wide.

In patients with third-degree AV block, the atrial rate and ventricular depolarization rates are independent (AV dissociation) because atrial impulses completely fail to reach the ventricles. If the site of the block is in the AV node, a stable His bundle rhythm will result in a normal QRS complex and the ventricular rate will often increase following administration of atropine. If the block involves the His bundle, the origin of the ventricular rhythm is more distal, resulting in wide QRS complexes. A wide QRS complex does not necessarily exclude a normal His bundle, as it may represent a more distal block in one of the bundle branches.

Can AV dissociation occur in the absence of AV block?

Yes. AV dissociation is common during anesthesia with volatile agents in the absence of AV block and results from sinus bradycardia or an accelerated AV junctional rhythm. During isorhythmic dissociation, the atria and ventricles beat independently at nearly the same rate. The P wave often just precedes or follows the QRS complex, and their relationship is generally maintained. In contrast, interference AV dissociation results from a junctional rhythm that is faster than the sinus rate—such that sinus impulses always find the AV node refractory.

How do bifascicular and trifascicular blocks present?

A bifascicular block exists when two of the three major His bundle-branches (right, left anterior, or left posterior) are partially or completely blocked. If one fascicle is completely blocked and the others are only partially blocked, a bundle-branch block pattern will be associated with either first-degree or second-degree AV block. If all three are affected, a trifascicular block is said to exist. A delay or partial block in all three fascicles results in either a prolonged P–R interval (first-degree AV block) or alternating LBBB and RBBB. Complete block in all three fascicles results in third-degree AV block.

What is the significance of the electrocardiographic findings in this patient?

The electrocardiographic findings (first-degree AV block plus RBBB) suggest a bifascicular block. Extensive disease of the conduction system is likely. Moreover, the patient's syncopal and near-

syncopal episodes suggest that she may be at risk for life-threatening bradyarrhythmias (third-degree AV block). Intracardiac electrocardiographic recordings would be necessary to confirm the site of the conduction delay.

How do intracardiac electrophysiologic studies help in localizing conduction abnormalities and determining the need for preoperative pacing?

Placing a multipolar catheter across the tricuspid valve allows electrical activity in the His bundle to be directly recorded. The interval from depolarization of the atrium adjacent to the His bundle to the beginning of depolarization in the His bundle is called the AH interval, is normally 60–125 msec, and represents conduction time in the AV node. The interval between the beginning of electrical activity in the His bundle and the beginning of ventricular depolarization on the surface ECG is the HV interval; it is normally 35–55 msec and represents conduction time in the His-Purkinje system. Patients with HV intervals greater than 100 msec are at relatively high risk for developing complete heart block with an inadequate escape rhythm; they should have a permanent pacemaker—or at least a temporary pacemaker prior to surgery.

What is appropriate management for this patient?

Cardiologic evaluation is required because of the symptomatic bifascicular block. One of two approaches can be recommended, depending on the urgency of the surgery. If the surgery is truly emergent, a temporary transvenous pacing catheter is indicated prior to induction of general or regional anesthesia. If the surgery can be postponed 24–48 hours (as in this case), continuous electrocardiographic monitoring, serial 12-lead ECGs, and measurements of cardiac isoenzymes are required to exclude myocardial ischemia or infarction and to try to record findings during symptoms. Moreover, a brief intracardiac His bundle study can be useful in determining the need for a permanent pacemaker. If the HV interval is greater than 100 msec, the patient needs a pacemaker prior to surgery (see above). If the HV interval is normal or 60–100 msec, permanent pacing may not necessarily be indicated, but central (internal jugular) venous access and ready access to pacing equipment are still advisable because of the history of syncope.

What are general perioperative indications for temporary pacing?

Suggested indications include the following: any documented symptomatic bradyarrhythmia; a new bundle-branch block, second-degree (type II) AV block, or third-degree AV block associated with myocardial infarction; bifascicular block in a comatose patient (controversial); and refractory supraventricular tachyarrhythmias.

The first three indications generally require ventricular pacing, while the fourth requires atrial pacing electrodes and a programmable rapid atrial pulse generator.

How can temporary cardiac pacing be established?

Pacing can be established by transvenous, transcutaneous, epicardial, or transesophageal electrodes. The most reliable method is generally via a transvenous pacing electrode in the form of a pacing wire or a balloon-tipped pacing catheter. A pacing wire should always be positioned fluoroscopically, but a flow-directed pacing catheter can also be placed in the right ventricle under pressure monitoring. A pacing wire must be used when blood flow has ceased. If the patient has a rhythm, intracardiac electrocardiographic recording showing ST-segment elevation when the electrode comes in contact with the right ventricular endocardium confirms placement of either type of electrode. Specially designed pulmonary artery catheters have an extra port for passage of a right ventricular pacing wire. These catheters are especially useful in patients with LBBB, who can develop complete heart block during catheter placement. Transcutaneous ventricular pacing is also possible via large stimulating adhesive pads placed on the chest and should be used whenever transvenous pacing is not readily available. Epicardial electrodes are usually used during cardiac surgery. Pacing the left atrium via an esophageal electrode is a simple, relatively noninvasive technique, but it is useful only for symptomatic sinus bradycardias and for terminating some supraventricular tachyarrhythmias.

Once positioned, the pacing electrodes are attached to an electrical pulse generator that periodically delivers an impulse at a set rate and magnitude. Most pacemaker generators can also sense the heart's spontaneous (usually ventricular) electrical activity: when activity is detected, the generator suppresses its next impulse. By altering the generator's sensing threshold, the pacemaker generator can function in a fixed (asynchronous) mode or in a demand mode (by increasing sensitivity). The lowest current through the electrode that can depolarize the myocardium is called the threshold current (usually < 2 mA for transvenous electrodes). An LBBB pattern is observed when the pacing electrode is within the right ventricle, because the right ventricle is depolarized directly, while the left ventricle is depolarized (later) by conduction across the myocardium, not the normal conducting system.

What is AV sequential pacing?

Ventricular pacing often reduces cardiac output because the atrial contribution to ventricular filling is lost. When the AV conducting system is diseased, atrial contraction can still be maintained by sequential stimulation by separate atrial and ventricular electrodes. The P–R interval can be varied by adjusting the delay between the atrial and ventricular impulses (usually set at 150–200 msec).

How are pacemakers classified?

Pacemakers are categorized by a five-letter code, according to the chambers paced, chambers sensed, response to sensing, programmability, and arrhythmia function (Table 20–18). The two most commonly used pacing modes are VVI and DDD (the last two letters are frequently omitted).

If a pacemaker is placed in this patient, how can its function be evaluated?

If the patient's underlying rhythm is slower than the rate of a demand pacemaker, pacing spikes should be seen on the ECG. The spike rate should be identical to the programmed (permanent pacemaker—usually 72/min) or set (temporary) pacemaker rate; a slower rate may indicate a low battery. Every pacing spike should be followed by a QRS complex (100% capture). Moreover, every impulse should be followed by a palpable arterial pulse. If the patient has a temporary pacemaker, the escape rhythm can be established by temporarily slowing the pacing rate or decreasing the current output.

When the patient's heart rate is faster than the set pacemaker rate, pacing spikes should not be observed if the generator is sensing properly. In this instance, ventricular capture cannot be evaluated unless the pacemaker rate increases or the spontaneous heart rate decreases. The latter may be accomplished by transiently increasing vagal tone (Valsalva maneuver or carotid stimulation). Fortunately, when the battery is low, sensing is generally affected before pacing output decreases. A chest radiograph is useful in excluding fracture or displacement of pacing leads. If pacemaker malfunction is suspected, cardiologic consultation is essential.

What intraoperative conditions may cause the pacemaker to malfunction?

Electrical interference from surgical electrocautery units can be interpreted as myocardial electrical activity and can suppress the pacemaker generator. Problems with electrocautery may be minimized by limiting its use to short bursts, limiting its power output, placing its grounding plate as far from the pacemaker generator as possible, and using bipolar cautery. Moreover, continuous monitoring of an arterial pulse wave (pressure, plethysmogram, or oximetry signal) is mandatory to ensure continuous perfusion during electrocautery. Accentuated myopotentials associated with succinylcholine-induced fasciculations or postoperative shivering can similarly suppress the pacemaker generator.

Table 20–18. Classification of pacemakers.

Chamber-paced	Chamber-sensed	Response to sensing	Programmability	Antitachyarrhythmia function
O = none	O = none	O = none	O = none	O = none
A = atrium	A = atrium	T = triggered	P = simple	P = pacing
V = ventricle	V = ventricle	I = inhibited	M = multi-programmable	S = shock
D = dual (atrium and ventricle)	D = dual (atrium and ventricle)	D = dual (triggered and inhibited)	C = communicating	D = dual (pacing and shock)
			R = rate modulation	

Both hypokalemia and hyperkalemia can alter the pacing electrodes' threshold for depolarizing the myocardium and can result in failure of the pacing impulse to depolarize the ventricle. Myocardial ischemia, infarction, or scarring can also increase the electrodes' threshold and cause failure of ventricular capture.

What are appropriate measures if a pacemaker fails intraoperatively?

If a temporary pacemaker fails intraoperatively, the inspired oxygen concentration should be increased to 100%. All connections and the generator battery should be checked. Most units have a battery-level indicator and a light that flashes with every impulse. The generator should be set into the asynchronous mode, and the ventricular output should be set on maximum. Failure of a temporary transvenous electrode to capture the ventricle is usually due to displacement of the electrode away from the ventricular endocardium; careful slow advancement of the catheter or wire while pacing often results in capture. Pharmacologic management (atropine, isoproterenol, or epinephrine) may be useful until the problem is resolved. If an adequate arterial blood pressure cannot be maintained with adrenergic agonists, cardiopulmonary resuscitation should be instituted until another pacing electrode is placed or a new generator box is obtained.

If a permanent pacemaker malfunctions (as with electrocautery), it should generally be converted to an asynchronous mode. Some units will automatically reprogram themselves to the asynchronous mode if malfunction is detected. Other pacemaker units must be reprogrammed by placing either an external magnet or, preferably, a programming device over the generator. The effect of an external magnet on some pacemakers—especially during electrocautery—may be unpredictable and should generally be determined prior to surgery.

Which anesthetic agents are appropriate for patients with pacemakers?

All anesthetic agents have been safely used in patients who already have pacemakers. Even volatile agents appear to have no effect on pacing electrode thresholds. Local anesthesia with light intravenous sedation is usually used for placement of permanent pacemakers.

When permanent transvenous pacemaker leads are placed, how is their function assessed?

The function of the permanent leads in their final position is analyzed by an external testing device that measures voltage threshold, lead impedance, and the amplitude of the sensed potentials. With an initial voltage output of 5 V and a pulse duration of 0.5 msec, the pacing rate is increased until 100% capture occurs. At that point, the voltage output is slowly decreased to determine the minimum voltage that results in 100% capture (voltage threshold). The ventricular voltage threshold should be ≤ 0.8 V, while the atrial voltage threshold should be ≤ 1.5 V. Lead impedance should be 250–1000 ohms at a nominal output of 5 V. The amplitude of the sensed potentials is usually > 6 mV and > 2 mV for ventricular and atrial electrodes, respectively.

SUGGESTED READING

Balser JR: The rational use of intravenous amiodarone in the perioperative period. Anesthesiology 1997;86:974.

Bannister J: *Anaesthesia for Vascular Surgery.* Oxford University Press, 2000.

Braunwald E, Zipes DP, Libby P: *Heart Disease,* 6th ed. WB Saunders and Company, 2001.

Estafanous FG, Barash PG, Reves JG: *Cardiac Anesthesia: Principles and Clinical Practice.* 2nd ed. Lippincott, 2001.

Executive summary of the ACC/AHA Task Force Report: Guidelines for Perioperative Cardiovascular Evaluation for Noncardiac Surgery. Anesth Analg 1996;82:854.

Goldman L: Cardiac risk in noncardiac surgery: An update. Anesth Analg 1995;80:810.

Kaplan JA, Reich DL, Kronstadt SN: *Cardiac Anesthesia,* 4th ed. WB Saunders and Company, 1999.

Lake CL: *Pediatric Cardiac Anesthesia,* 3rd ed. McGraw-Hill, 1998.

Otto CM: *Textbook of Clinical Echocardiography.* 2nd ed. WB Saunders and Company, 2000.

Otto CM: *Valvular Heart Disease.* WB Saunders and Company, 1999.

Poortmanns G, Schupfer G, Roosens C, Poelaert J: Transesophageal echocardiographic evaluation of left ventricular function. J Cardiothorac Vasc Anesth 1999;14:588.

Ross S, Foex P: Protective effects of anaesthetics in reversible and irreversible ischemia-reperfusion injury. Br J Anaesth 1999;82:622.

Thys D: *Textbook of Cardiothoracic Anesthesia.* McGraw-Hill, 2001.

Zaidan JR: Implantable cardioverter-defibrillators. J Cardiothorac Vasc Anesth 1999;13:475.

Anesthesia for Cardiovascular Surgery

21

KEY CONCEPT

 1 Cardiopulmonary bypass (CPB) diverts venous blood away from the heart, adds oxygen, removes CO_2, and returns the blood to a large artery (usually the aorta). As a result, nearly all blood flow through the heart and most of that through the lungs ceases.

2 The fluid level in the reservoir of the CPB machine is critical: If the reservoir is allowed to empty, air can enter the main pump and cause fatal air embolism.

3 Initiation of CPB is associated with a marked increase in stress hormones, including catecholamines, cortisol, arginine vasopressin, and angiotensin.

4 Establishing the adequacy of cardiac reserve must be based on exercise (activity) tolerance, measurements of myocardial contractility such as ejection fraction, the severity and location of coronary stenoses, ventricular wall motion abnormalities, cardiac end-diastolic pressures, cardiac output, and valvular areas and gradients.

5 Blood should be available for immediate transfusion if the patient has already had a midline sternotomy (a "redo"); in these cases, the right ventricle or coronary grafts may be adherent to the sternum and may be inadvertently entered during the repeat sternotomy.

 6 In general, pulmonary artery catheterization should be used in patients with compromised ventricular function (ejection fraction < 40–50%) or pulmonary hypertension and in those undergoing complicated procedures.

 7 Transesophageal echocardiography (TEE) provides valuable information about cardiac anatomy and function during surgery. Two-dimensional, multiplane TEE can detect regional and global ventricular abnormalities, chamber dimensions, valvular anatomy, and the presence of intracardiac air.

8 The severity of regional wall motion abnormalities can be classified into three categories: hypokinesis (reduced wall motion, which can be further classified into mild, moderate, and severe); akinesis (no wall motion); and dyskinesis (paradoxical wall motion).

 9 It should be emphasized that anesthetic dose requirements are extremely variable and generally inversely related to ventricular function. Severely compromised patients should be given anesthetic agents slowly and in small increments.

10 Anticoagulation must be established before CPB to prevent acute disseminated intravascular coagulation and formation of clots in the CPB pump.

(continued)

(continued)

Aprotinin therapy should be considered for patients who are undergoing a repeat operation, especially myocardial revascularization; for those who refuse blood products, such as Jehovah's Witnesses; and for those who are at high risk for postoperative bleeding because of recent aspirin ingestion, coagulopathy, and possibly long and complicated procedures involving the heart and aorta.

Hypotension from impaired ventricular filling often occurs during manipulation of the venae cavae and the heart.

Hypothermia itself is usually anesthetic, but reports of awareness during CPB are common, especially during rewarming.

Protamine administration can result in a number of adverse hemodynamic effects, which appear to be either immune or idiosyncratic nonimmune reactions. Although protamine given slowly usually has minimal effects, hypotension from acute systemic vasodilation or marked pulmonary hypertension may be seen.

Persistent bleeding following bypass may be due to inadequate surgical control of bleeding sites, inadequate reversal of heparin, reheparinization, thrombocytopenia, platelet dysfunction, hypothermia, undiagnosed preoperative hemostatic defects, or newly acquired defects. If oozing continues despite adequate surgical hemostasis and the activated clotting time (ACT) is normal or the heparin-protamine titration assay shows no residual heparin, thrombocytopenia or platelet dysfunction is most likely.

Chest tube drainage in the first 2 hours of more than 250–300 mL/hour (10 mL/kg/hour)—in the absence of a hemostatic defect—is excessive and often requires surgical reexploration. Intrathoracic bleeding at a site not adequately drained causes cardiac tamponade, which necessitates immediate reopening of the chest.

Factors known to increase pulmonary vascular resistance (PVR) such as acidosis, hypercapnia, hypoxia, enhanced sympathetic tone, and high mean airway pressures are to be avoided for patients with right-to-left shunting; hyperventilation (hypocapnia) with 100% oxygen is usually effective in lowering PVR. Conversely, patients with left-to-right shunting benefit from systemic vasodilation and increases in PVR, although specific hemodynamic manipulation is generally not attempted.

Induction of general anesthesia in patients with cardiac tamponade is extremely hazardous and may precipitate cardiac arrest. The anesthetic technique should maintain a high sympathetic tone until the tamponade is relieved. Avoid cardiac depression, vasodilation, and slowing of the heart rates. Ketamine is the induction and maintenance agent of choice until the tamponade is relieved.

The sudden increase in left ventricular afterload after application of the aortic cross-clamp during aortic surgery may precipitate acute left ventricular failure, and myocardial ischemia, especially in patients with underlying ventricular dysfunction or coronary disease. The greatest period of hemodynamic instability is following release of the aortic cross-clamp; the abrupt decrease in afterload together with bleeding and the release of vasodilating acid metabolites from the ischemic lower body can precipitate severe systemic hypotension. Decreasing anesthetic depth, volume loading, and partial or slow release of the cross-clamp are helpful in avoiding severe hypotension.

The emphasis of anesthetic management during caroid surgery is on maintaining adequate cerebral perfusion without stressing the heart. Regardless of the anesthetic agents selected, mean arterial blood pressure should be maintained at—or slightly above—the patient's usual range.

Anesthesia for cardiovascular surgery requires a precise understanding of circulatory physiology, pharmacology, and pathophysiology as well as thorough familiarity with cardiopulmonary bypass (CPB), transesophageal echocardiography (TEE), myocardial preservation, and surgical techniques. Because surgical manipulations often have a profound impact on circulatory function, the anesthesiologist must follow the progress of the surgery intently and anticipate problems associated with each step.

This chapter presents an overview of cardiovascular anesthesia and of the principles, techniques, and physiology of CPB. Surgery on the aorta, carotid arteries, and the pericardium presents problems that also require special anesthetic considerations.

■ CARDIOPULMONARY BYPASS

 CPB is a technique that diverts venous blood away from the heart, adds oxygen, removes CO_2, and returns the blood to a large artery (usually the aorta). As a result, nearly all blood flow through the heart and most of that through the lungs ceases. When CPB is fully established, the extracorporeal circuit is in series with the systemic circulation and provides both artificial ventilation and perfusion. Unfortunately, this technique is entirely nonphysiologic, because arterial pressure is typically below normal and blood flow is usually nonpulsatile. To minimize organ damage during this stressful period,

systemic hypothermia (20–32 °C) is usually employed. Topical hypothermia (an ice-slush solution) and cardioplegia (a chemical solution for arresting myocardial electrical activity) are also used to protect the heart.

Operation of the CPB machine is a complex task requiring the uninterrupted attention of a perfusionist—a highly specialized technician. Optimal results with CPB require close cooperation and communication between the surgeon, anesthesiologist, and perfusionist.

BASIC CIRCUIT

The CPB machine has five basic components: a venous reservoir, an oxygenator, a heat exchanger, a main pump, and an arterial filter (Figure 21–1). Modern machines use a single disposable unit with the reservoir, oxygenator, and heat exchanger built in. Most machines also have separate accessory pumps that can be used for blood salvage (cardiotomy suction), venting (draining) the left ventricle, and cardioplegia. A number of other filters, alarms, and in-line pressure, oxygen-saturation, and temperature monitors are also typically used.

Prior to use, the CPB circuit must be primed with fluid (1200–1800 mL for adults) that is devoid of bubbles. A balanced salt solution, such as Plasmalyte-A, is generally used, but other components are frequently added, including colloid (albumin or hetastarch), mannitol (for renal protection), heparin (500–5000 units), bicarbonate, and potassium (if cardioplegia will not be used). At the onset of bypass, hemodilution usually decreases the hematocrit to about 22–25% in most pa-

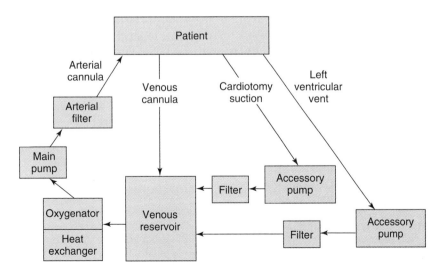

Figure 21–1. The basic design of cardiopulmonary bypass machines.

tients. Blood is used as a priming solution for small pediatric and severely anemic adult patients to prevent severe hemodilution.

Reservoir

The reservoir of the CPB machine receives blood from the patient via one or two venous cannulas in the right atrium or the superior and inferior vena cava. Blood flows to the reservoir by gravity drainage. Because venous pressure is normally low, the driving force is directly proportional to the difference in height between the patient and the reservoir but inversely proportional to the resistance of the cannulas and tubing. Priming the machine creates a siphon effect. Entrainment of air can produce an air lock that may prevent blood flow.

 The fluid level in the reservoir is critical: If the reservoir is allowed to empty, air can enter the main pump and cause fatal air embolism. A low reservoir level alarm is typically present.

Oxygenator

Blood is drained by gravity from the bottom of the venous reservoir into the oxygenator, which contains a blood gas interface that allows blood to equilibrate with the gas mixture (primarily oxygen). A volatile anesthetic is also frequently added at the oxygenator gas inlet. The blood-gas interface in a modern, membrane-type oxygenator is a very thin, gas-permeable silicone membrane. Arterial oxygenation is generally inversely related to the thickness of the blood film in contact with the membrane, while arterial CO_2 tension during CPB is dependent on total gas flow. Because the inspired oxygen concentration can be varied, a membrane oxygenator allows independent control of PaO_2 and $PaCO_2$. In the older bubble-type oxygenators, tiny bubbles (foam) are formed as the oxygen passed through small holes at the base of a blood column. The tiny bubbles provide a large surface area for blood to equilibrate with the inflow gases; the bubbles are then removed by passing the blood across a defoaming agent (a charged silicone polymer). A major disadvantage of bubble oxygenators was trauma to the formed elements in blood, which became more significant for procedures requiring more than 2 hours of CPB.

Heat Exchanger

Blood from the oxygenator enters the heat exchanger. The blood is then either cooled or warmed, depending on the temperature of the water flowing through the exchanger (4–42 °C); heat transfer occurs by conduction. Because gas solubility decreases as blood temperature rises, a filter is built into the unit to catch any bubbles that may form during rewarming.

Main Pump

Modern CPB machines use either an electrically driven double-arm roller (positive displacement) or a centrifugal pump to propel blood through the CPB circuit.

A. ROLLER PUMPS:

Roller pumps produce flow by compressing large-bore tubing in the main pumping chamber as the heads turn. Subtotal occlusion of the tubing prevents excessive red cell trauma. The constant speed of the rollers pumps blood regardless of the resistance encountered, and produces a continuous nonpulsatile flow. Flow is directly proportional to the number of revolutions per minute. In some pumps, an emergency back-up battery provides power in case of an electrical power failure. All roller pumps have a hand crank to allow manual pumping.

B. CENTRIFUGAL PUMPS:

Centrifugal pumps consist of a series of cones in a plastic housing. As the cones spin, the centrifugal forces created propel the blood from the centrally located inlet to the periphery. In contrast to roller pumps, blood flow with centrifugal pumps is pressure-sensitive and must be monitored by an electromagnetic flowmeter. Increases in distal pressure will decrease flow and must be compensated by increasing the pump speed. Because these pumps are nonocclusive, they are less traumatic to blood than roller pumps. Unlike roller pumps which are placed after the oxygenator (Figure 21–1), centrifugal pumps are normally between the venous reservoir and the oxygenator.

C. PULSATILE FLOW:

Pulsatile blood flow is possible with some roller pumps. Pulsations can be produced by instantaneous variations in the rate of rotation of the roller heads; they can also be added after flow is generated. Pulsatile flow is not available with centrifugal pumps. Although the matter is controversial, some clinicians feel that pulsatile flow improves tissue perfusion, enhances oxygen extraction, attenuates the release of stress hormones, and results in lower systemic vascular resistances (SVRs) during CPB. These observations are supported by experimental studies suggesting improved renal and cerebral blood flow during pulsatile perfusion in animals.

Arterial Filter

Particulate matter (eg, thrombi, fat globules, calcium, tissue debris) enters the CPB circuit with alarming regularity. Although filters are often used at other locations, a final, in-line, arterial filter (27–40 μm) is mandatory to prevent systemic embolism. Once filtered, the propelled blood returns to the patient, usually via a cannula in the ascending aorta. A normally functioning aortic valve prevents blood from entering the left ventricle.

The filter is always constructed with a (normally clamped) bypass limb in case it becomes clogged or develops high resistance. For the same reason, arterial inflow pressure is measured before the filter. The filter is also designed to trap air, which can be bled out through a built-in stopcock.

Accessory Pumps & Devices

A. Cardiotomy Suction:

The cardiotomy suction pump aspirates blood from the surgical field during CPB and returns it to the main pump reservoir. A cell-saver suction device may also be used, but that blood is returned to a separate reservoir. At the end of the procedure, the cell-saver blood is centrifuged, washed, and given back to the patient. Excessive suction pressure contributes to red cell trauma. Moreover, excessive use of cell-saver suction (instead of cardiotomy suction) during bypass depletes CPB circuit volume. The high negative pressure of ordinary wall suction produces excessive red cell trauma and precludes blood salvage from that source.

B. Left Ventricular Vent:

With time, even after institution of total bypass, blood reaccumulates in the left ventricle as a result of residual pulmonary flow from the bronchial arteries (which arise directly from the aorta or the intercostal arteries) or thebesian vessels (see Chapter 19) or as a result of aortic regurgitation. Aortic regurgitation can occur as a result of either structural valvular abnormalities or surgical manipulation of the heart (functional). Distention of the left ventricle compromises myocardial preservation (see below) and requires decompression (venting). In most centers, this is accomplished by a catheter inserted into the left ventricle via the right superior pulmonary vein and left atrium. Venting is less commonly accomplished through a catheter in the left ventricular apex or through the aortic valve. The blood aspirated by the vent pump normally passes through a filter and is returned to the venous reservoir.

C. Cardioplegia Pump:

Cardioplegia is most often administered via an accessory pump on the CPB machine. This technique allows optimal control over the infusion pressure, rate, and temperature (see below). A separate heat exchanger ensures control of the cardioplegia solution's temperature. Alternatively, cardioplegia may be infused from a cold intravenous fluid bag given under pressure or by gravity.

D. Ultrafilter:

Ultrafiltration can be used during CPB to increase the patient's hematocrit without transfusion. Hemultrafilters consist of hollow capillary fibers that can function as membranes, allowing separation of the aqueous phase of blood from its cellular and proteinaceous elements. Blood can be diverted to pass through the fibers either from the arterial side of the main pump or from the venous reservoir using an accessory pump. Hydrostatic pressure forces water and electrolytes across the fiber membrane. Effluents of up to 40 mL/min may be removed.

SYSTEMIC HYPOTHERMIA

Intentional hypothermia is routinely used following the initiation of CPB. Core body temperature is usually reduced to 20–32 °C. Metabolic oxygen requirements are generally halved with each reduction of 10 °C in body temperature. At the end of the surgical procedure, rewarming via the heat exchanger restores normal body temperature.

Profound hypothermia to temperatures of 15–18 °C allows total circulatory arrest for complex repairs for up to 60 minutes. During that time, both the heart and the CPB machine are stopped.

The adverse effects of hypothermia are platelet dysfunction; potentiation of citrate toxicity, which leads to reduction in serum ionized calcium; reversible coagulopathy; and depression of myocardial contractility.

MYOCARDIAL PRESERVATION

Optimal results in cardiac surgery not only require perfect surgical repair of cardiac pathology but also prevention of myocardium damage and maintenance of normal cellular integrity and function during CPB. Nearly all patients sustain some myocardial damage during cardiac surgery. With proper preservation techniques, however, most of the damage is usually reversible. Although myocardial injury can be related to the anesthetic or surgical technique, it most commonly appears to be related to suboptimal myocardial preservation during CPB. The common denominator in most instances is an imbalance between myocardial oxygen demand and supply, resulting in cell ischemia, injury, or death. Patients at greatest risk are those in New York Heart Association (NYHA) functional class IV (see Table 20–10) and those who have ventricular hypertrophy or severe coronary artery disease. Inadequate myocardial preservation is usually manifested at the end of bypass as a persistently low cardiac output, electrocardiographic signs of myocardial ischemia, or cardiac arrhythmias.

Aortic cross-clamping during CPB completely abolishes coronary blood flow. While estimates of a safe cross-clamping period are not valid because of differing vulnerabilities between patients, CPB times longer than 120 minutes are generally considered undesirable. Myocardial ischemia during bypass can also occur before and after release of the cross-clamp. Low arterial pressures, coronary embolism (from thrombi, platelets, air, fat, or calcium), coronary or graft vasospasm, and excessive surgical manipulation of the heart—causing compression or distortion of the coronary vessels—are all contributory. Areas of myocardium distal to a high-grade coronary obstruction are at greatest risk.

Ischemia causes depletion of high-energy phosphate compounds and an accumulation of intracellular calcium. The latter, through its action on contractile proteins, further depletes energy supplies (see Chapter 19). Maintenance of normal cellular integrity and function during CPB depends on reducing energy expenditure and preserving the availability of high-energy phosphate compounds. When coronary blood flow ceases, creatine phosphate and anaerobic metabolism become the principal sources of cellular energy; fatty acid oxidation is impaired. Unfortunately, these energy stores rapidly become depleted, and the progressive acidosis that develops limits glycolysis. While measures directed at increasing or replenishing energy substrates in the form of glucose or glutamate infusions are used, the emphasis of myocardial preservation has been on reducing cellular energy requirements to minimal levels. This is accomplished by systemic and topical cardiac hypothermia (ice slush) and the use of potassium cardioplegia (below). The former reduces basal metabolic oxygen consumption, while the latter abolishes the energy expenditure associated with both electrical and mechanical activity. Myocardial temperature can be monitored directly; 10–15 °C is usually considered desirable.

Ventricular fibrillation and distention are important causes of myocardial damage. Fibrillation can double myocardial oxygen consumption, while distention not only increases oxygen demand but also reduces oxygen supply by interfering with subendocardial blood flow. The combination of the two is especially detrimental. Other factors that might contribute to myocardial damage include the use of inotropes and excessive administration of calcium.

Potassium Cardioplegia

The most widely used method of arresting myocardial electrical activity is the administration of potassium-rich crystalloid or blood. Following initiation of CPB,

induction of hypothermia, and aortic cross-clamping, the coronary circulation is perfused with cold cardioplegia. The resulting increase in extracellular potassium concentration reduces the transmembrane potential (less negative inside). The latter progressively interferes with the normal sodium current during depolarization, decreasing the rate of rise, amplitude, and conduction velocity of subsequent action potentials (see Chapter 19). Eventually, the sodium channels are completely inactivated, action potentials are abolished, and the heart is arrested in diastole. Usually, cold cardioplegia must be repeated several times (about every 30 minutes) because of gradual washout and rewarming of the myocardium. Washout occurs as a result of persistence of noncollateral coronary blood flow derived from pericardial vessels, which are branches of intercostal arteries. Moreover, multiple doses of cardioplegia solutions may improve myocardial preservation by preventing the excessive build-up of metabolites that inhibit anaerobic metabolism. Preferential warming of the posterior ventricular wall can also occur as a result of direct contact with warmer blood in the descending aorta.

Typical components of potassium cardioplegia are given in Table 21–1. Although the exact composition varies from center to center, the essential elements of cardioplegia are the same. Potassium concentration is kept below 50 mEq/L, because higher levels can be associated with a paradoxic increase in myocardial energy requirements and excessive potassium loads. Sodium concentration in cardioplegia solutions is less than that in plasma because ischemia tends to increase intracellular sodium content. A small amount of calcium is needed to maintain cellular integrity, while magnesium appears to control an excessive influx of calcium intracellularly. A buffer—most commonly bicarbonate—is necessary to prevent excessive build-up of acid metabo-

Table 21–1. Typical components of cardioplegia solutions.

Potassium	15–40 mEq/L
Sodium	100–120 mEq/L
Chloride	110–120 mEq/L
Calcium	0.7 mEq/L
Magnesium	15 mEq/L
Glucose	28 mmol/L
Bicarbonate	27 mmol/L

lites; in fact, alkalotic perfusates are reported to produce better myocardial preservation. Alternative buffers include histidine and tromethamine (also known as THAM). Other components may include hypertonic agents to control cellular edema (mannitol), glucocorticoids (for their membrane-stabilizing effect), prostacyclin (for its antiplatelet effect), calcium channel or β-adrenergic blockers (to reduce metabolic demand), and free-radical scavengers (mannitol). Energy substrates may be provided as glucose, glutamate, or aspartate. The question of whether to use crystalloid or blood as a vehicle for achieving cardioplegia remains controversial. Evidence suggests that at least some groups of high-risk patients may do better with blood cardioplegia. Certainly, oxygenated blood cardioplegia has the added benefit of delivering more oxygen than does crystalloid cardioplegia.

Because cardioplegia may not reach areas distal to high-grade coronary obstructions (the areas that need it most), many surgeons also administer cardioplegia retrogradely through a coronary sinus catheter. Continuous normothermic cardioplegia has been promoted by some groups. While some evidence suggests this technique may be superior to intermittent hypothermic cardioplegia for myocardial preservation, the absence of a bloodless field complicates surgery. Moreover, warm cardiac surgery raises additional concerns about loss of the potentially protective effects of hypothermia, especially on cerebral function.

When ischemic damage to the myocardium is prolonged, reperfusion of myocardium can be associated with extensive cell injury, rapid accumulation of intracellular calcium, and potentially irreversible cellular necrosis. Oxygen-derived free radicals may play an important role on reperfusion injury; free radical scavengers, such as with mannitol therapy, may help decrease reperfusion injury. Several steps may help limit reperfusion injury. During the first 10 minutes of reperfusion, the heart should be arrested by cardioplegia to minimize metabolic requirement, and hypercalcemia should be avoided. Then, the heart should be in an empty and beating state for an additional 10–30 minutes before weaning the patient from CPB, to further minimize metabolic requirement. Acidosis and hypoxia should be corrected.

Excessive cardioplegia can result in an absence of electrical activity, atrioventricular conduction block, or a poorly contractile heart at the end of bypass. Persistent systemic hyperkalemia may also result. Although calcium administration partially offsets these effects, excessive calcium can enhance myocardial damage. Myocardial performance generally improves with time as the contents of the cardioplegia are cleared from the heart.

PHYSIOLOGIC EFFECTS OF CARDIOPULMONARY BYPASS

Hormonal & Humoral Responses

 Initiation of CPB is associated with a marked increase in stress hormones, including catecholamines, cortisol, arginine vasopressin, and angiotensin. This phenomenon is at least partly due to decreased metabolism secondary to hypothermia and exclusion of the pulmonary circulation, where many of these substances are normally broken down. Anesthetic agents may only partially suppress the hormonal stress response to CPB.

Multiple humoral systems are also activated, including complement, coagulation, fibrinolysis, and the kallikrein system. Contact of blood with the internal surfaces of the CPB system activates complement via the alternate pathway (C3) as well as the classic pathway through activation of Hageman factor (XII); the latter also activates the coagulation cascade, platelets, plasminogen, and kallikrein. Mechanical trauma also appears to activate platelets and neutrophils. A systemic inflammatory response syndrome similar to that seen with sepsis and trauma can develop (see Chapter 50). When this response is intense or prolonged, patients can develop the same complications, including generalized edema, the acute respiratory distress syndrome, and acute renal failure.

CPB also alters and depletes glycoprotein receptors on the surface of platelets. The resulting platelet dysfunction increases perioperative bleeding and potentiates other coagulation abnormalities (activation of plasminogen and the inflammatory response described above).

Altered Pharmacokinetics

Plasma and serum concentrations of most drugs acutely decrease at the onset of CPB but the unbound fraction may remain unaltered for some drugs. The effects of CPB are complex because of the sudden increase in volume of distribution with hemodilution, decreased protein binding, and changes in perfusion and redistribution between peripheral and central compartments. Some drugs, such as opioids, also bind CPB components. Heparin potentially alters protein binding by releasing and activating lipoprotein lipase, which hydrolyzes plasma triglycerides into free fatty acids; the latter can competitively inhibit drug binding to plasma proteins. With the possible exception of propofol, constant infusion of a drug during CPB generally causes progressively higher blood levels as a result of reduced hepatic and renal perfusion (reduced elimination) and hypothermia (reduced metabolism). Alterations in α_1-acid-glycoprotein, which increases after CPB, can also affect drug binding in the postoperative period.

ANESTHETIC MANAGEMENT OF CARDIAC SURGERY

ADULTS

The preoperative evaluation and anesthetic management of common cardiovascular diseases are discussed in Chapter 20. The same principles apply whether these patients are undergoing cardiac or noncardiac surgery. An important distinction is that patients undergoing cardiac procedures generally have more advanced disease, and the importance of establishing the adequacy of cardiac reserve cannot be overemphasized. This information must be based on exercise (activity) tolerance, measurements of myocardial contractility such as ejection fraction, the severity and location of coronary stenoses, ventricular wall motion abnormalities, cardiac end-diastolic pressures, cardiac output, and valvular areas and gradients (see Chapter 20). Fortunately, unlike noncardiac surgery, cardiac surgery improves cardiac function in the majority of patients. Preoperative evaluation should also focus on pulmonary, neurologic, and renal function, since impairment of these organ systems predisposes patients to postoperative complications.

1. Preinduction Period

Premedication

The prospect of heart surgery is frightening. Relatively heavy premedication is generally desirable, particularly for patients with coronary artery disease (see Chapter 20). Conversely, light premedication is more appropriate in frail patients with valvular disease, who are often physiologically dependent on enhanced sympathetic tone. Habitus, age, and physiologic status should be considered in selecting agents and doses.

Benzodiazepine sedative-hypnotics (midazolam, 5–10 mg IM; diazepam, 5–10 mg PO; or lorazepam, 2–4 mg PO), alone or in combination with an opioid (morphine, 5–10 mg IM), are most often used. Alternatively, the time-honored combination of intramuscular morphine, 0.1–0.15 mg/kg, and scopolamine, 0.2–0.3 mg, also provides excellent sedation, analgesia, and amnesia. Doses should be reduced in patients with poor cardiac reserve and those with underlying pulmonary disease. Scopolamine should generally be avoided in patients older than 70 years because it is associated with a

high incidence of confusion in this group. Supplemental oxygen (2–3 L/min via nasal cannula) is useful in avoiding hypoxemia following premedication.

Preparation

Formulation of a clear anesthetic plan and adequate preparations are essential for cardiac anesthesia. Many patients are critically ill, and there is little time intraoperatively to debate the merits of one technique over another or to search for drugs and equipment. At the same time, the anesthetic plan should not be too rigid; if problems are encountered with one technique, the anesthesiologist should be ready to change to another without delay. Organization and meticulous attention to detail are crucial in dealing with intraoperative problems. The anesthesia machine, monitors, infusion pumps, and blood warmer should all be checked before the patient arrives. Drugs—including anesthetic and vasoactive agents—should be immediately available. Many clinicians prepare one vasodilator and one inotropic infusion solutions for use before the start of the procedure.

Venous Access

Cardiac surgery is commonly associated with large and rapid fluid shifts, often with the need for multiple drug infusions. Ideally, two large-bore (16-gauge or larger) intravenous catheters should be placed. One of these should be in a large central vein, usually the internal jugular vein, although the subclavian and external jugular veins are suitable alternatives. Entry into the superior vena cava is not always possible with the external jugular vein; nonetheless, it serves as a good site for an extra peripheral intravenous line. Central venous cannulations may be accomplished while the patient is awake but sedated or after induction of anesthesia. Small doses of an opioid or midazolam can be used for sedation. Supplemental oxygen via face mask helps avoid hypoxemia during catheterization.

Drug infusions should ideally be given into a central catheter, preferably directly into the catheter or into the injection port closest to the catheter (to minimize dead space). Multilumen central venous and pulmonary artery catheters facilitate multiple drug infusions and allow simultaneous measurement of vascular pressures. One intravenous port should be dedicated for drug infusions and nothing else, and another port should be used for drug and fluid boluses. The side port of the introducer sheath used for a pulmonary catheter can be used for drug infusions but serves better as a fluid bolus line when a large-bore introducer (9F) is used.

Blood should be available for immediate transfusion if the patient has already had a midline sternotomy (a "redo"); in these cases, the right ventricle or coronary grafts may be adherent to the sternum and may be inadvertently entered during the repeat sternotomy.

Monitoring

In addition to all basic monitoring, arterial cannulation is generally performed prior to induction of anesthesia, as this period represents one of the major hemodynamic stresses of the procedure. Depending on the patient, central venous cannulation may be done before or after induction of anesthesia.

A. ELECTROCARDIOGRAPHY:

The electrocardiogram (ECG) is continuously monitored with two leads, usually leads II and V_5. Baseline tracings of all leads may be recorded on paper for further reference. The advent of monitors with computerized ST-segment analysis and the use of additional monitoring leads (V_4, aVF, and V_{4R}) have greatly improved detection of ischemic episodes.

B. ARTERIAL BLOOD PRESSURE:

Arterial blood pressure should generally be directly monitored by catheterization of the radial artery in the nondominant hand. Radial arterial catheters, especially on the left side, may occasionally give falsely low readings following sternal retraction as a result of compression of the subclavian artery between the clavicle and the first rib. The radial artery on the side of a brachial artery cutdown (for cardiac catheterization) should not be used, because doing so is associated with a high incidence of arterial thrombosis and wave distortion. Other useful catheterization sites include the ulnar, brachial, femoral, and axillary arteries. A backup manual or automatic blood pressure cuff should also be placed on the opposite side for comparison with direct measurements.

C. CENTRAL VENOUS AND PULMONARY ARTERY PRESSURE:

Central venous pressure should be monitored in all patients. The decision whether or not to use a pulmonary artery catheter is based on the patient, the procedure, and the preferences of the surgical team. Routine use of a pulmonary artery catheter is controversial. Left ventricular filling pressures can be measured with a left atrial pressure line inserted by the surgeon during bypass. In general, pulmonary artery catheterization should be used in patients with compromised ventricular function (ejection fraction < 40–50%) or pulmonary hypertension and in those undergoing complicated procedures. The most

useful data are pulmonary artery pressures, the wedge pressure, and thermodilution cardiac outputs (see Chapter 6). Specialized catheters provide extra infusion ports, continuous measurements of mixed venous oxygen saturation and cardiac output, and the capability for right ventricular or atrioventricular sequential pacing.

The internal jugular vein is the preferred approach for central venous cannulation (see Chapter 6). Catheters placed through the subclavian or external jugular veins, especially on the left side, may be prone to kinking following sternal retraction (above).

Pulmonary artery catheters often migrate distally during CPB and may spontaneously wedge without balloon inflation. Inflation of the balloon under these conditions can rupture a pulmonary artery and cause lethal pulmonary hemorrhage. When a pulmonary artery catheter is used, it should be routinely pulled back slightly (2–3 cm) during CPB and the balloon subsequently inflated slowly. If the catheter wedges with less than 1.5 mL of air in the balloon, it should be pulled back farther.

D. URINARY OUTPUT:

Once the patient is asleep, an indwelling urinary catheter is placed to monitor the hourly output. Bladder temperature is often monitored but may be affected by low urinary flow. The sudden appearance of red urine may indicate excessive red hemolysis caused by CPB or a transfusion reaction.

E. TEMPERATURE:

Multiple temperature monitors are usually placed once the patient is anesthetized. Bladder or rectal, esophageal, and pulmonary artery (blood) temperatures are usually simultaneously monitored. Because of the heterogeneity of readings during cooling and rewarming, bladder and rectal readings are generally taken to represent an average body temperature, while esophageal and, to a lesser extent, pulmonary artery values represent core temperature. Nasopharyngeal and tympanic probes may be most reflective of brain temperature. Myocardial temperature is often measured directly during CPB.

F. LABORATORY PARAMETERS:

Intraoperative laboratory monitoring is mandatory during cardiac surgery. Blood gases, hematocrit, serum potassium, ionized calcium, and glucose measurements should be immediately available. Serum magnesium measurements may also be useful. The **activated clotting time (ACT)** is used to monitor anticoagulation; some centers also use heparin assays. The role of thromboelastography is not well defined during CPB.

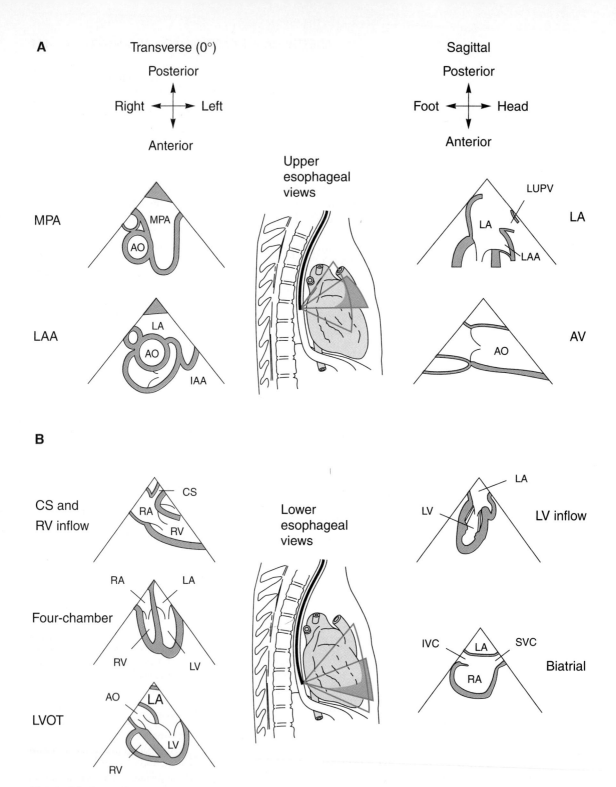

Figure 21–2. Useful views during transesophageal echocardiography from the upper esophagus (**A**), lower esophagus (**B**),

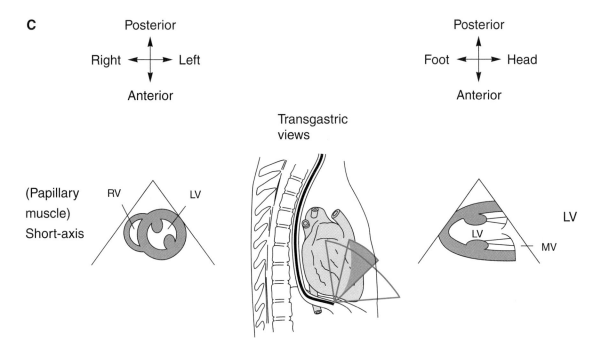

AO = aorta; AV = aortic valve; CS = coronary sinus; IVC = inferior vena cava; LA = left atrium; LAA = left atrial appendage; LUPV = left upper pulmonary vein; LV = left ventricle; LVOT = left ventricular outflow tract; MPA = main pulmonary artery; MV = mitral valve; RA = right atrium; RV = right ventricle; SVC = superior vena cava.

Figure 21–2. (continued) and transgastric position (**C**). Note that different views can be obtained in each of these positions. In the transverse plane (0°), the tip of the probe is tilted either upward (anteflexion) or backward (retroflexion), while in the sagittal (90°) plane the probe is rotated from left to right. The transverse views in each of the three positions are shown in order as the probe is tilted from upward to backward; sagittal views are shown as the probe is rotated from left to right. (Modified and reproduced, with permission, from Richardson SG et al: Biplane transesophageal echocardiography utilizing transverse and sagittal imaging planes. Echocardiography 1991;8:293.)

G. SURGICAL FIELD:

One of the most important intraoperative monitors is the surgical field. Once the sternum is opened, lung expansion can be seen through the pleura. When the pericardium is opened, the heart (primarily the right ventricle) is visible, so that cardiac rhythm, volume, and contractility can often be judged visually. Blood loss and surgical maneuvers must be closely watched and related to changes in hemodynamics and rhythm.

H. TRANSESOPHAGEAL ECHOCARDIOGRAPHY:

TEE provides extremely valuable information about cardiac anatomy and function during surgery. Two-dimensional, multiplane TEE can detect regional and global ventricular abnormalities, chamber dimensions, valvular anatomy, and the presence of intracardiac air. It can also be helpful for confirming cannulation of the coronary sinus for cardioplegia. Multiple views can be obtained from the upper esophagus, lower esophagus, and transgastric positions in the transverse, sagittal, and in-between planes (Figure 21–2A–C). The two most commonly used views during cardiac surgery are the transverse four-chamber view (Figure 21–3) and the transgastric (short-axis) view (Figure 21–4). Unfortunately, the cost, together with the training required to correctly interpret data from this sophisticated monitor, limit its widespread use.

The most important applications for intraoperative TEE are assessing ventricular function, assessing valvular function, examining for residual air, and assessing other cardiac structures and abnormalities.

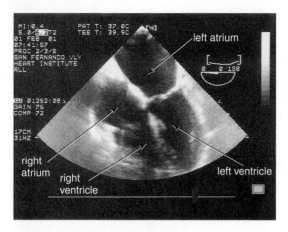

Figure 21–3. Transesophageal echocardiogram of the midesophageal four-chamber view, showing the right and left atria and ventricles.

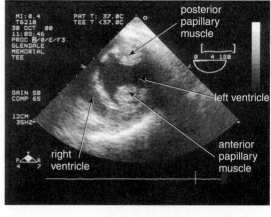

Figure 21–4. Transesophageal echocardiogram at the lower esophageal/transgastric level looking up at the left ventricle at the level of the papillary muscles.

1. Assessing ventricular function–Ventricular function can be assessed by global systolic function, determined by ejection fraction and left ventricular end-diastolic volume; diastolic function (ie, looking for abnormal relaxation and restrictive diastolic pattern by checking mitral flow velocity); and regional systolic function, by assessing wall motion and thickening abnormalities. Regional wall abnormalities following myocardial ischemia often appear before ECG changes. The severity of regional wall motion abnormalities can be classified into three categories (Figure 21–5): hypokinesis (reduced wall motion, which can be further classified into mild, moderate, and severe); akinesis (no wall motion); and dyskinesis (paradoxical wall motion). Left ventricular myocardium is supplied by three major arteries: the left anterior descending artery, the left circumflex artery, and the right coronary artery (Figure 21–6A-C). The ventricular short-axis mid view at mid papillary muscle level contains all three blood supplies from the major coronary arteries (see Figure 21–4).

2. Assessing valvular function–Valvular morphology can be assessed by multiplane TEE. Pressure gra-

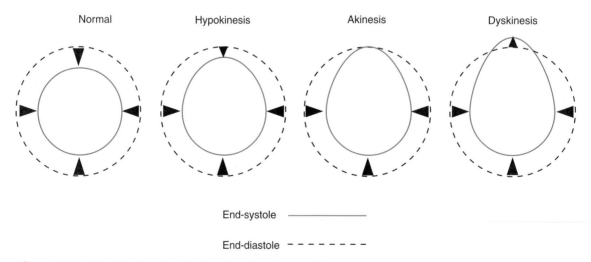

Normal   Hypokinesis   Akinesis   Dyskinesis

End-systole ————

End-diastole – – – – – – –

Figure 21–5. Classification of regional wall motion abnormalities.

A B C

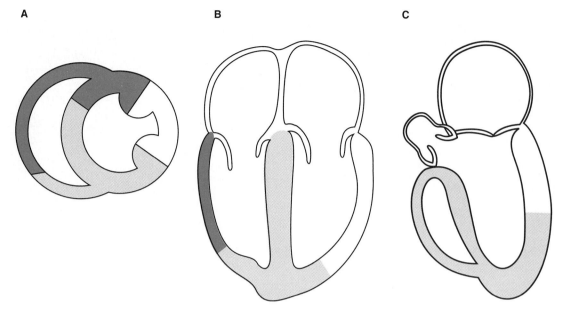

Figure 21–6. Coronary artery supply of the left and right ventricles in three views: short-axis view (***A***), the four-chamber view (***B***), and the three-chamber view (***C***). Dark blue = RCA; light blue = LAD; white = CX.

dients, stenotic valve area, severity of stenosis, and severity of valvular regurgitation can be assessed reliably by Doppler echocardiography and color-flow imaging (Figure 21–7A–B). Colors are usually adjusted so that flow toward the probe is red, while flow in the opposite direction is blue. TEE also can detect prosthetic valve dysfunction, such as obstruction, regurgitation, and endocarditis.

The TEE images in the upper esophagus at 40–60° and 110–130° are most useful for examining the aortic valve and ascending aorta (Figure 21–8A–B). The valve annular diameter can also be estimated with reasonable accuracy. Doppler flow across the aortic valve must be measured looking up from the transgastric view (Figure 21–9). The mitral valve is examined from the

A

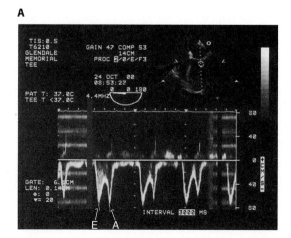

B

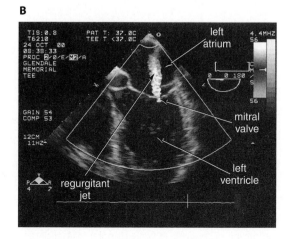

Figure 21–7. Transesophageal echocardiography Doppler and color-flow imaging. Pulse-wave Doppler recording of mitral valve inflow showing two phases, E (early filling) and A (atrial filling) (***A***). Color-flow demonstrates backward flow (regurgitant jet) across the mitral valve during systole (mitral regurgitation) (***B***).

A

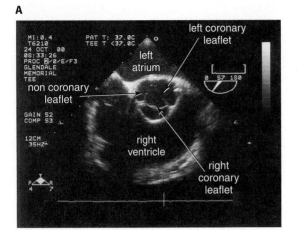

B

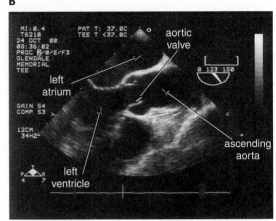

Figure 21–8. Two views of the aortic valve. Between 40 and 60 degrees, all three leaflets are usually visualized (**A**). Between 110 and 130 degrees, the left ventricular outflow, aortic valve, and ascending aorta are clearly visualized (**B**).

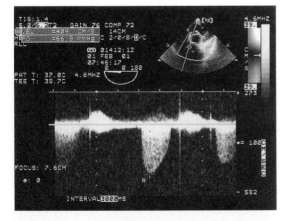

Figure 21–9. Transesophageal echocardiographic recording of continuous wave Doppler from the transgastric view looking up at the aortic valve, demonstrating severe aortic stenosis. Peak velocity of 409 cm/sec indicates a gradient of 66.9 mm Hg.

midesophageal position, looking at the mitral valve apparatus with and without color in the 0° through 150° views (Figure 21–10A–D). TEE is an invaluable aid in mitral valve repair surgery.

3. Examination for residual air–Air is introduced into the heart during all open-heart procedures. Residual amounts of air often remain even after the best de-airing maneuvers. TEE is very helpful in detecting residual air, so that additional, surgi-cal maneuvers are undertaken to help avoid cerebral or coronary embolism.

4. Assessment of other cardiac structures and abnormalities–TEE also can detect congenital heart diseases such as a patent foramen ovale, atrial septal defect, ventricular septal defect; pericardial diseases such as pericardial tamponade and constrictive pericarditis; and cardiac tumors. Doppler color-flow imaging helps delineate abnormal intracardiac blood flows and shunts. TEE is used to assess the extent of myomectomy in patients with hypertrophic cardiomypathy (idiopathic hypertrophic subaortic stenosis). It is also extremely valuable in diagnosing aortic disease processes such as aortic dissection, aortic aneurysm, and atheroma. The extent of dissections in the ascending and descending aorta can be accurately assessed; airway structures prevent adequate visualization of the aortic arch. The presence of protruding atheroma in the ascending aorta significantly increases the risk of postoperative stroke and may prompt the use of an alternate arterial cannulation site.

I. ELECTROENCEPHALOGRAPHY:

Computer-processed electroencephalographic (EEG) recordings can be useful in assessing anesthetic depth during cardiac surgery and, perhaps more importantly, ensuring complete electrical silence prior to circulatory arrest. However, the usefulness of these recordings in detecting neurologic insults during CPB is limited by the combined effects of anesthetic agents, hypothermia,

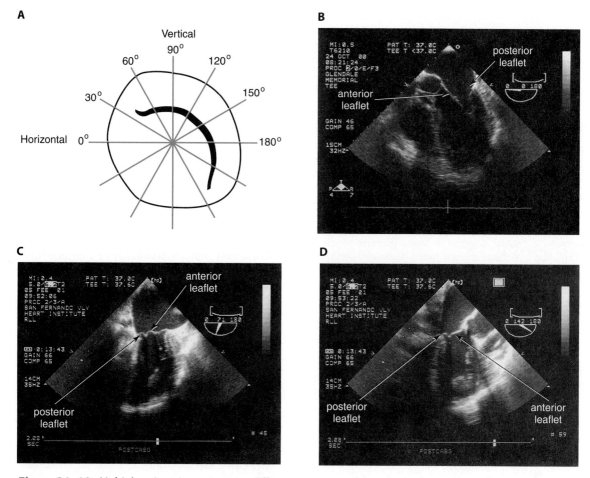

Figure 21–10. Multiplane imaging cuts across different segments of the mitral valve apparatus between 0 and 180 degrees (***A***). Images of the mitral valve at 0, 71, and 142 degrees (***B, C, D,*** respectively). AL= anterior leaflet. PL = posterior leaflet.

and hemodilution. Progressive hypothermia is typically associated with electroencephalographic slowing, burst suppression, and finally an isoelectric recording. Moreover, most strokes during CPB are due to small emboli and are not likely to be detected on the EEG. Artifacts from the CPB roller pump may be seen on the raw EEG but can usually be identified as such by computer processing.

J. TRANSCRANIAL DOPPLER (TCD):

This modality provides noninvasive measurements of blood flow velocity in the basal arteries of the brain (usually the middle cerebral artery) through the temporal bone. While studies have not shown these flow velocities to correlate reliably with other measurements of cerebral blood flow, TCD appears to be useful for de-

tecting cerebral emboli. Preliminary evidence suggests that emboli detected by TCD are often associated with postoperative neuropsychological changes.

Induction of Anesthesia

Cardiac operations require general anesthesia, endotracheal intubation, and controlled ventilation. For elective procedures, induction should generally be performed in a slow, smooth, controlled fashion often referred to as a **cardiac induction.** The principles are discussed in Chapter 20. Selection of anesthetic agents (see below) is generally less important than the way they are used. It should be emphasized that dose requirements are extremely variable and generally inversely related to ventricular function. Severely compromised patients should be given anesthetic agents slowly and in small increments. A series of challenges may be used to judge when anesthetic depth will allow intubation without a marked vasopressor response or excessive hypotension. Blood pressure and heart rate are continuously evaluated following unconsciousness (loss of the eyelid reflex), insertion of a nasal or oral airway, urinary catheterization, and intubation. A sudden increase in heart rate or blood pressure indicates light anesthesia and the need for more anesthetic prior to the next challenge, while a decrease or no change suggests that the patient is ready for the subsequent stimulus. Muscle relaxant is given as soon as consciousness is lost. Blood pressure reductions greater than 20% generally call for administration of a vasopressor (see below).

The period following intubation is often characterized by a gradual decrease in blood pressure resulting from the anesthetized state (often associated with vasodilation and decreased sympathetic tone) and a lack of surgical stimulation. Patients are often volume-depleted from preoperative fasting or diuretic therapy and usually respond to fluid boluses. Colloid boluses are in most cases more effective than crystalloid boluses in rapidly expanding intravascular volume (see Chapter 29). In the absence of bleeding, the administration of large amounts of intravenous fluids prior to the bypass accentuates the hemodilution associated with CPB (below). Small doses of phenylephrine (25–50 μg) or ephedrine (5–10 mg) may be necessary to avoid excessive hypotension. Following intubation and controlled ventilation, hemodynamic measurements are usually repeated; the baseline ACT (normal < 130 seconds), arterial blood gases, hematocrit, and serum potassium concentration are measured.

Choice of Anesthetic Agents

Although the choice of anesthesia is often thought of as total intravenous versus inhalational, the two are most often used in combination. Total intravenous techniques are generally most suitable for patients with severely compromised ventricular function, while predominantly inhalational techniques are reserved for patients with relatively good ventricular function (ejection fraction 40–50% or more). In either case, a muscle relaxant must be used to facilitate endotracheal intubation and retraction of the chest and to prevent patient movement and shivering.

A. PREDOMINANTLY INHALATIONAL TECHNIQUES:

Inhalational anesthesia is, in almost all cases, preceded by intravenous induction. Barbiturates (eg, thiopental, thiamylal, methohexital), benzodiazepines (eg, diazepam, midazolam), opioids, etomidate, propofol, or ketamine, alone or in combination, can be used. Fol-

lowing loss of consciousness, the muscle relaxant is given and a volatile agent is added; its concentration is slowly increased and carefully titrated to the blood pressure. The patient is intubated when anesthetic depth is judged to be sufficient. The major advantage of volatile agents is the ability to change the anesthetic concentration rapidly. Their principal disadvantage is dose-dependent direct cardiac depression. In spite of a few reports suggesting a potential for inducing intracoronary steal (see Chapter 20), isoflurane remains the most commonly used volatile agent. Nitrous oxide is generally not used because of its tendency to expand any intravascular air bubbles that may form during CPB. If nitrous oxide is used, it should be discontinued 15–20 minutes prior to CPB.

B. PREDOMINANTLY INTRAVENOUS TECHNIQUES:

1. High-dose opioid techniques—Pure high-dose, opioid anesthesia is rarely used in adults because of two major potential disadvantages: patient awareness (recall) during surgery and prolonged respiratory depression postoperatively. High-dose opioids also fail to consistently control the hypertensive response to stimulation, which is most common in patients with good ventricular function; it is least likely to be seen in those receiving β-adrenergic blockers or those who have marked ventricular dysfunction. Addition of a vasodilator (nitroglycerin or nitroprusside), a β-blocker (propranolol or esmolol), or a volatile agent may be necessary during periods of increased stimulation to prevent hypertension. The concomitant use of a benzodiazepine or a low dose of volatile agent diminishes the likelihood of awareness. Hemodynamic changes do not reliably correlate with awareness.

High doses of fentanyl and sufentanil are *generally* associated with minimal cardiac depression and relatively stable hemodynamics when given alone. When combined with small doses of other intravenous agents, such as benzodiazepines or barbiturates, however, hypotension caused by vasodilation and cardiac depression may be seen. Sufentanil may be more likely than fentanyl to cause hemodynamic compromise, especially in elderly patients and those with poor ventricular function; a decrease in sympathetic tone may be responsible. High-dose alfentanil is generally not used because of its cost and reports that it provides less hemodynamic stability than do fentanyl and sufentanil. Experience with remifentanil is limited. Opioid-induced bradycardia and muscle rigidity can occur with any of these agents following rapid administration (see Chapter 8). To prevent rigidity, a muscle relaxant should be given as soon as consciousness is lost. Administration of a small dose of a nondepolarizing muscle relaxant, such as pancuronium (1 mg), prior to induction helps attenuate any rigidity. Patients anesthetized with high-dose sufentanil (continuous infusion technique) generally regain consciousness sooner and can often be extubated earlier than those anesthetized with high-dose fentanyl.

The opioid may be administered in boluses or as a loading dose followed by a continuous infusion. Fentanyl is given as a slow bolus of 15–40 µg/kg for induction and intubation; maintenance anesthesia is provided by additional boluses of 3–5 µg/kg as needed or by a continuous infusion of 0.3–1.0 µg/kg/min. The total dose of fentanyl used is generally 50–100 µg/kg. The same technique using sufentanil generally employs 5–10 µg/kg for induction and intubation, followed by 1 µg/kg boluses or 0.075 µg/kg/min as a continuous infusion. The total dose of sufentanil is generally 15–30 µg/kg.

2. Other techniques—The combination of ketamine with midazolam for induction and maintenance of anesthesia is also associated with relatively stable hemodynamics, good amnesia and analgesia, and minimal postoperative respiratory depression. Ketamine and midazolam have similar pharmacokinetic profiles, are compatible in solution, and may be mixed together in the same syringe or infusion bag in a 20:1 ratio. For induction, ketamine, 1–2 mg/kg, with midazolam, 0.05–0.1 mg/kg, is given as a slow intravenous bolus. Anesthesia can then be maintained by infusion of ketamine, 1.4 mg/kg/hour, and midazolam, 0.07 mg/kg/hour. Significant hypertension following intubation or surgical stimulation requires additional use of small doses of propofol, an opioid, volatile agent, or a vasodilator. This technique is especially useful for patients with poor ventricular function. Combining ketamine with diazepam also results in stable hemodynamics with minimal side effects.

C. MUSCLE RELAXANTS:

Unless airway difficulties are expected, intubation is usually performed with a nondepolarizing muscle relaxant. The choice of muscle relaxant is based chiefly on the desired hemodynamic response. Ideally, in most instances, the agent should be devoid of significant circulatory effects. Rocuronium and vecuronium are most commonly used. Vecuronium, however, has been reported to markedly enhance opioid-induced bradycardia. Pancuronium may be the best choice with high-dose opioid anesthesia because its vagolytic effects offset opioid-induced bradycardia. Succinylcholine should be considered for endotracheal intubation if the potential for a difficult airway exists (see Chapter 5).

2. Prebypass Period

Following induction and intubation, the anesthetic course is typically characterized by an initial period of minimal stimulation (skin preparation and draping) that is frequently associated with hypotension, followed by discrete periods of intense stimulation that can produce tachycardia and hypertension. These periods of stimulation include the skin incision, sternotomy and sternal retraction, opening the pericardium and, sometimes, aortic dissection. The anesthetic agent should be adjusted appropriately in anticipation of these events.

Accentuated vagal responses resulting in marked bradycardia and hypotension may occur during sternal retraction or opening of the pericardium. This response may be more pronounced in patients who have been taking β-adrenergic blocking agents, diltiazem, or verapamil. Deeply anesthetized patients frequently have a progressive decline in cardiac output after the chest is opened. The reduction in cardiac output is probably due to decreased venous return as the normally negative intrathoracic pressure becomes atmospheric. Intravenous fluid administration at least partially reverses this effect.

Myocardial ischemia in the prebypass period is often but not always associated with hemodynamic perturbations such as tachycardia, hypertension, or hypotension. Although controversial, prophylactic infusion of nitroglycerin (1–2 µg/kg/min) intraoperatively may reduce the incidence of ischemic episodes.

Anticoagulation

 Anticoagulation must be established prior to CPB to prevent acute disseminated intravascular coagulation and formation of clots in the CPB pump. Moreover, the adequacy of anticoagulation must be confirmed with determination of the ACT. An ACT longer than 400–450 seconds is considered safe at most centers. Heparin, 300–400 U/kg, is usually given while the aortic purse-string sutures are placed during cannulation. Many surgeons prefer to give the heparin themselves directly into the right atrium. If heparin is administered by the anesthesiologist, it should be given through a central line, and the ACT should be measured after 3–5 minutes. If the ACT is less than 400 seconds, additional heparin 100 U/kg is given. When aprotinin is used, a kaolin-ACT rather than celite-ACT should be used to guide heparin therapy. If kaolin-ACTs are not available, heparin therapy should be given as a fixed-dose regimen based on the patient's weight and the duration of CPB. Heparin concentration assays (see Reversal of Anticoagulation, below) measure heparin levels and not necessarily effect; these assays are therefore not reliable for measuring the degree of anticoagulation. The high-dose thrombin time (HiTT) is unaffected by aprotinin but is more complicated to perform than a kaolin-ACT. HiTT cannot provide a preheparin control and does not provide an index for the adequacy of reversal with protamine (below).

Heparin resistance is occasionally encountered; most patients have antithrombin III deficiency (acquired or congenital). Antithrombin III is a circulating serine protease that irreversibly binds and inactivates thrombin (as well as the activated forms of factors X, XI, XII, and XIII). When heparin complexes with antithrombin III, the latter's anticoagulant activity is enhanced 1000-fold. Patients with antithrombin III deficiency will achieve adequate anticoagulation following infusion of 2 U of fresh frozen plasma, antithrombin III concentrate, or synthetic antithrombin III.

Patients with a history of heparin-induced thrombocytopenia (HIT) require special consideration. These patients produce heparin-dependent antibodies that agglutinate platelets and produce thrombocytopenia with or without thromboembolic phenomena. If the history of HIT is remote and antibodies can no longer be demonstrated, heparin may safely be used but only for CPB. When significant antibody titers are detected, plasmapheresis may be used to eliminate them transiently, allowing normal heparinization. Alternative anticoagulants include hirudin and ancrod, but experience with them is limited. Inactivation of platelets prior to heparinization with aspirin, dipyridamole, or iloprost, a prostacyclin analog, has also been used in emergency cardiac surgery for patients with HIT.

Bleeding Prophylaxis

Bleeding prophylaxis with antifibrinolytic agents may be initiated before or after anticoagulation. Some clinicians prefer to administer antifibrinolytic agents after heparinization to possibly reduce the incidence of thrombotic complications; delayed administration may reduce their efficacy. Aprotinin therapy should be considered for patients who are undergoing a repeat operation (especially myocardial revascularization); for those who refuse blood products (such as Jehovah's Witnesses); and for those who are at high risk for postoperative bleeding because of recent aspirin ingestion, coagulopathy, and possibly long and complicated procedures involving the heart and aorta. Although its exact mechanism is not known, aprotinin is an inhibitor of serine proteases, such as plasmin, kallikrein, and trypsin. Its most important action, however, may be to preserve platelet function (adhesiveness and aggregation). Aprotinin therapy is highly effective in reducing perioperative blood loss and transfusion requirements (by 40–80%). It also appears to blunt the intense inflammatory response associated with CPB. Serious allergic reactions, including anaphylaxis (< 0.5%) may be encountered with aprotinin. Reactions are more likely to occur upon repeat exposure. A test dose of 1.4 mg (10,000 KIU) is given prior to a loading dose of 280 mg (2 million KIU) over 20–30 minutes via a central venous catheter. The drug is then infused at 70 mg/hour (500,000 KIU/hour) for the duration of the surgery. The CPB pump is also primed 280 mg (2 million KIU). The celite-ACT should not be used because it is artificially prolonged by aprotinin in the presence of heparin; the latter can potentially lead to inadequate coagulation during CPB. The kaolin-ACT is less affected by aprotinin therapy; it appears that the kaolin activator adsorbs aprotinin from blood.

Although possibly less effective, ε-aminocaproic acid 5–10 g followed by 1 g/hour or tranexamic acid 10 mg/kg followed by 1 mg/kg/hour can be used instead of aprotinin. ε-Aminocaproic acid and tranexamic acid do not effect the ACT and are less likely to induce allergic reactions. Unlike aprotinin, they do not appear to preserve platelet function. Intraoperative collection of platelet-rich plasma by pheresis prior to CPB is employed by some centers; reinfusion following bypass may decrease bleeding and reduce transfusion requirements.

Cannulation

Cannulation for CPB is a critical time. *After heparinization,* aortic cannulation is usually done first because of the hemodynamic problems frequently associated with venous cannulation. Moreover, rapid fluid infusions can be given through the aortic cannula if necessary. The ascending aorta is most often used. The small opening of most arterial cannulas produces a jet stream that, if not positioned properly, can cause aortic dissection or preferential flow of blood to the innominate artery during CPB. Reduction of systemic arterial pressure (to 90–100 mm Hg systolic) facilitates placement of the aortic cannula. Bubbles should be completely removed from the arterial cannula, and backflow of blood into the arterial line must be demonstrated before bypass is initiated. Failure to remove all the bubbles results in air emboli, usually into the coronary or cerebral circulations, while failure to enter the aorta properly results in aortic dissection. Some clinicians advocate temporary compression of the carotid arteries during aortic cannulation to decrease the likelihood of cerebral emboli.

One or two venous cannulas are placed in the right atrium, usually through the right atrial appendage. One cannula is usually adequate for most coronary artery bypass and aortic valve operations. The single cannula used often has two ports (two-stage) such that when it is properly positioned, one is in the right atrium and the other is in the inferior vena cava.

⑫ Separate caval cannulas are used for open-heart procedures. Hypotension from impaired ventricular filling often occurs during manipulation of the venae cavae and the heart. Venous cannulation also frequently precipitates atrial or, less commonly, ventricular arrhythmias. Premature atrial contractions and transient bursts of a supraventricular tachycardia are common. Sustained paroxysmal atrial tachycardia or atrial fibrillation frequently leads to hemodynamic deterioration, which must be treated pharmacologically, electrically, or by immediate anticoagulation and initiation of bypass. Malpositioning of the venous cannulas can interfere with venous return or impede venous drainage from the head and neck (superior vena cava syndrome). Upon initiation of CPB, the former is manifested as poor venous return to the reservoir, while the latter produces edema of the head and neck. Under these circumstances, central venous pressure increases only if the tip of the catheter is high in the vena cava.

3. Bypass Period

Initiation

Once the cannulas are properly placed and secured, the ACT is acceptable, and the perfusionist is ready, CPB is initiated. The clamps placed across cannulas during insertion are removed (venous first, then arterial), and the main CPB pump is started. Establishing the adequacy of venous return to the pump reservoir is critical. Normally, the reservoir level rises and CPB pump flow is gradually increased. If venous return is poor, as shown by a decreasing reservoir level, the pump prime will quickly empty and air can enter the pump circuit. The cannulas should be checked for proper placement, forgotten clamps, kinks, or an air lock. Under these circumstances, pump flow should be slowed until the problem is resolved. Adding volume (blood or colloid) to the reservoir may be necessary. With full CPB, the heart should gradually empty; failure to do so or progressive distention implies malpositioning of the venous cannula or aortic regurgitation. In the latter instance, immediate aortic cross-clamping and cardioplegia are necessary.

Flow & Pressure

Systemic arterial pressure is closely monitored as pump flow is gradually increased to 2–2.5 L/min/m². At the onset of CPB, systemic arterial pressure usually decreases abruptly. Initial mean systemic arterial (radial) pressures of 30–40 mm Hg are not unusual. This decrease is usually attributed to abrupt hemodilution, which reduces blood viscosity and effectively lowers SVR. The effect is partially compensated by subsequent hypothermia, which tends to raise blood viscosity again.

Persistent and excessive decreases (< 30 mm Hg) should prompt a search for unrecognized aortic dissection. If dissection is present, CPB must be temporarily stopped until the aorta is recannulated distally. Other possible causes include poor venous return, pump malfunction, or pressure-transducer error. Factitious hypertension can occur when the right radial artery is used for monitoring and the aortic cannula is directed toward the innominate artery.

The relationship between pump flow, SVR, and mean systemic arterial blood pressure may be conceptualized as follows:

$$\text{Mean arterial pressure} = \text{Pump flow} \times \text{SVR}$$

Consequently, with a constant SVR, mean arterial pressure is proportional to pump flow. Similarly, at any given pump flow, mean arterial pressure is proportional to SVR. The general conduct of CPB should be such as to maintain both adequate arterial pressures and blood flows by manipulating pump flow and SVR. Although some controversy still surrounds this issue, most centers strive for blood flows of 2–2.5 L/min/m² (50–60 mL/kg/min) and mean arterial pressures between 50 mm Hg and 80 mm Hg. Flow requirements are generally proportional to core body temperature. Evidence also suggests that during deep hypothermia (20–25 °C), mean blood pressures as low as 30 mm Hg may still provide adequate cerebral blood flow. SVR can be increased with phenylephrine or methoxamine.

High systemic arterial pressures (> 150 mm Hg) are also deleterious and may promote aortic dissection or cerebral hemorrhage. Generally, when mean arterial pressure exceeds 100 mm Hg, hypertension is said to exist and is treated by decreasing pump flow or adding isoflurane to the oxygenator inflow gas. If the hypertension is refractory to these maneuvers or if pump flow is already low, a vasodilator, such as nitroprusside, is used.

Monitoring

Additional monitoring during CPB includes the pump flow rate, venous reservoir level, arterial inflow line pressure (see above), blood (perfusate and venous) and myocardial temperatures, and in-line (arterial and venous) oxygen saturations. In-line pH, CO_2 tension, and oxygen tension sensors are also available. Blood gas tensions and pH should be confirmed by direct measurements (see below). In the absence of hypoxemia, low venous oxygen saturations (< 70%), a progressive metabolic acidosis, or low urinary output are indicative of inadequate flow rates.

During bypass, arterial inflow line pressure is nearly always higher than the systemic arterial pressure recorded from a radial artery or even an aortic catheter. The difference in pressure represents the pressure drop across the arterial filter, the arterial tubing, and the narrow opening of the aortic cannula. Nonetheless, monitoring this pressure is important in detecting problems with an arterial inflow line. Inflow pressures should remain below 300 mm Hg; higher pressures may indicate a clogged arterial filter, obstruction of the arterial tubing or cannula, or aortic dissection.

Serial ACT, hematocrit, and potassium measurements are necessary during CPB. The ACT is measured immediately after bypass and then every 20–30 minutes thereafter. Cooling generally increases the half-life of heparin and prolongs its effect. A heparin dose-response curve is often used to facilitate calculation of subsequent heparin doses and protamine reversal (Figure 21–11). Although the relationship does not always conform to a linear function, it remains clinically useful. The hematocrit is usually kept between 20% and 25%. Red cell transfusions into the pump reservoir may be necessary. Marked increases in serum potassium concentrations (secondary to cardioplegia) are usually treated with furosemide.

Hypothermia & Cardioplegia

Moderate (26–32 °C) or deep (20–25 °C) hypothermia is used routinely for most procedures. The lower the temperature, the longer the time necessary for cooling and rewarming. Low temperatures, however, allow lower CPB flows. At a temperature of 20 °C, flows as low as 1.2 L/min/m² may be adequate.

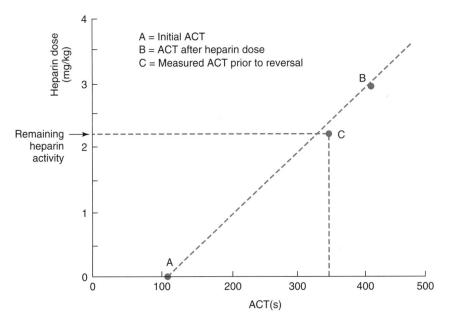

Figure 21–11. Heparin dose-response curve. Activated clotting time (ACT) in seconds versus total heparin dose in milligrams per kilogram.
1. Plot the initial ACT on the *x* axis.
2. Plot the ACT after heparinization.
3. Draw the line defined by these two points.
4. If additional anticoagulation is needed, find the desired ACT on that line. The amount of additional heparin needed is the difference on the *y* axis between the present ACT and the desired ACT.
5. If the third point does not lie on the original line, a new line is drawn originating from the baseline ACT and passing midway between the other two points.
6. For reversal of anticoagulation, the protamine dose is based on the remaining heparin activity, estimated to be the heparin dose corresponding to the latest ACT on the dose-response line.

Ventricular fibrillation often occurs as the heart is cooled below 28–29 °C. Cardioplegia should established immediately, since fibrillation rapidly consumes high-energy phosphates and jeopardizes myocardial preservation. Cardioplegia is achieved by cross-clamping the ascending aorta proximal to the aortic inflow cannula and infusing cardioplegia solution through a small catheter proximal to the cross-clamp; alternatively, it can be given directly into the coronary ostia if the aorta is opened. Many surgeons routinely employ retrograde cardioplegia via a catheter in the coronary sinus (see above). During aortocoronary bypass grafting, cardioplegia solution may also be given through the graft if the surgeon elects to do the distal anastomosis first.

Ventilation

Ventilation of the lungs is usually continued until adequate pump flows are reached and the heart stops ejecting blood. Following institution of full CPB, ventricular ejection continues briefly until left ventricular volume reaches a critical low level. Discontinuing ventilation prematurely causes any remaining pulmonary blood flow to act as a right-to-left shunt that can promote hypoxemia (see Chapter 22). The importance of this mechanism depends on the relative ratio of remaining pulmonary blood flow to pump flow. At some centers, once ventilation is stopped, oxygen flow is continued in the anesthesia circuit with a small amount of positive end-expiratory pressure (5 cm H_2O) to prevent postoperative pulmonary dysfunction. Most centers stop all gas flow or continue a low flow of oxygen (1–2 L/min) in the anesthesia circuit. Ventilation is resumed at the conclusion of CPB when the heart begins to eject blood.

Management of Respiratory Gases

There is some controversy about whether to use corrected or uncorrected arterial blood gas tensions during hypothermic CPB. The controversy stems from the fact that the solubility of a gas increases with hypothermia. As a result, although total content does not change (in a closed system), the partial pressure of the gas will decrease as blood temperature drops. The problem is most significant for arterial CO_2 tension because of its effect on arterial pH and cerebral blood flow. As temperature decreases, plasma bicarbonate concentration does not change, but the decrease in arterial CO_2 tension tends to increase pH and make blood alkalotic (by normothermic definitions). Blood with a CO_2 tension of 40 mm Hg and a pH of 7.40 at 37 °C, when cooled to 25 °C will have a CO_2 tension of about 23 mm Hg and a pH of 7.60.

Normally—regardless of the patient's temperature—blood samples are heated to 37 °C in blood gas analyzers before gas tensions are measured. If a temper-ature-corrected reading is desired, a table or a program in the blood gas machine can be used to estimate gas tension and pH at the patient's temperature. The practice of temperature-correcting gas tensions and maintaining a "normal" CO_2 tension of 40 mm Hg and a pH of 7.40 during hypothermia is referred to as **pH-stat management** and has come into question. During hypothermic CPB, pH-stat management, which may require adding CO_2 to oxygenator gas inflow, increases total blood CO_2 content. Under these conditions, cerebral blood flow becomes more dependent on CO_2 tension and mean arterial blood pressure than on oxygen consumption (see Chapter 25).

The use of uncorrected gas tensions during hypothermia—**α-stat management**—is more common. The basis of this approach is that preservation of normal protein function depends on maintaining a constant state of intracellular electroneutrality (the balance of charges on proteins). At physiologic pH, these charges are primarily located on the imidazole rings of histidine residues (referred to as **α residues**). Moreover, as temperature decreases, K_w—the dissociation constant for water—also decreases (pK_w increases). Therefore, at lower temperatures, the electroneutrality of aqueous solutions, where $[H^+] = [OH^-]$, corresponds to a lower $[H^+]$ (a higher pH). Hypothermic alkalosis thus does not necessarily reflect $[OH^-] > [H^+]$ but rather an absolute decrease in $[H^+]$. Hypothermic CPB with α-stat management usually does not require addition of CO_2 to the oxygenator: the total CO_2 content of blood and electroneutrality are unchanged. In contrast to pH-stat management, α-stat management appears to preserve cerebral autoregulation of blood flow and may improve myocardial preservation. Despite the theoretical and observed differences, comparisons between the two techniques fail to reveal appreciable differences in patient outcome.

Anesthesia

 Hypothermia itself is usually anesthetic, but reports of awareness during CPB are common, especially during rewarming. Failure to give anesthetic agents during CPB frequently results in light anesthesia and contributes to awareness. Hypertension often develops and, if muscle paralysis is also allowed to wear off, patient may begin to move. Additional doses of muscle relaxants and anesthetic agents may be necessary during CPB. Low concentrations of a volatile agent (isoflurane) via the oxygenator are frequently used. The volatile agent, however, should generally be discontinued just prior to termination of bypass to avoid residual myocardial depression. Patients with poor left ventricular function may be very sensitive to the combined residual effects of cardioplegia and a volatile agent. Additional doses of a narcotic or small doses of a benzodiazepine are preferable for these patients. Many clinicians routinely administer a benzodiazepine (eg, midazolam, 5–10 mg intravenously) or scopolamine (0.2–0.4 mg) when rewarming is initiated. Alternatively, opioid or ketamine-midazolam infusions may be continued during CPB. Sweating during rewarming is common and does not necessarily reflect light anesthesia but rather a hypothalamic response to perfusion with blood that is often at 39 °C.

Cerebral Protection

Neurologic complications following CPB may be as high as 40%. Fortunately, in most instances, they consist of transient neuropsychiatric dysfunction (ranging from subtle cognitive and intellectual changes to delirium and organic brain syndromes). More serious complications such as strokes are less common (2–5%). Factors that have been associated with neurologic sequelae include intracardiac (valvular) procedures, advanced age, and preexisting cerebrovascular disease. While embolic phenomena appear responsible for most neurologic deficits, the contribution of cerebral hypoperfusion remains unclear. Although controversial, prophylactic thiopental infusions (completely suppressing electroencephalographic activity) immediately prior to and during intracardiac (open ventricle) procedures have been reported to decrease the incidence and severity of neurologic deficits. They may, however, increase the need for inotropic support upon termination of CPB. Prior to circulatory arrest with very deep hypothermia, corticosteroid (methylprednisolone 30 mg/kg), mannitol (0.5 g/kg), and phenytoin 10–15 mg/kg) are also usually administered. The head is also covered with ice bags (avoiding the eyes). Studies suggest that magnesium may also be beneficial. The role of calcium channel blockers (nimodipine and nicardipine) and N-methyl-D-aspartate (NMDA) antagonists (ketamine) remains largely investigational.

4. Termination of CPB

Discontinuation of bypass is accomplished by a series of necessary procedures and conditions:

1. Rewarming must be completed.
2. Air must be evacuated from the heart and any bypass grafts.
3. The aortic cross-clamp must be removed.
4. Lung ventilation must be resumed.

The surgeon's decision about when to rewarm is critical; adequate rewarming requires time, but rewarming too soon removes the protective effects of hypother-

mia. Rapid rewarming often results in large temperature gradients between well-perfused organs and peripheral vasoconstricted tissues; subsequent equilibration following separation from CPB decreases core temperature again. Infusion of a vasodilator drug (nitroprusside or nitroglycerin) by allowing higher pump flows often speeds the rewarming process and decreases large temperature gradients. Moreover, rapid rewarming can result in the formation of gas bubbles in the bloodstream as the solubility of gases rapidly decreases. If the heart fibrillates during rewarming, defibrillation (5–10 joules) may be necessary. Administration of lidocaine 100–200 mg and magnesium sulfate 1–2 g prior to removal of the aortic cross-clamping may lessen the likelihood of fibrillation. Many clinicians advocate a head-down position while intracardiac air is being evacuated to lessen the likelihood of cerebral emboli. Lung inflation facilitates expulsion of (left-sided) intracardiac air by squeezing pulmonary vessels and returning blood into the left heart. TEE is extremely useful in detecting residual intracardiac air. Reinflation of the lungs requires temporarily higher than normal airway pressure and should generally be done with direct visualization (or through the pleura) because overzealous lung expansion can interfere with internal mammary artery grafts.

General guidelines for separation from CPB include the following:

- Core body temperature should be at least 37 °C.
- A stable rhythm (preferably sinus) must be present. Atrioventricular pacing may be necessary and confers the benefit of a properly timed atrial systole. Persistence of atrioventricular block should prompt measurement of serum potassium concentration. If hyperkalemia is present, it can be treated with calcium, $NaHCO_3$, furosemide, or glucose and insulin (see Chapter 28).
- The heart rate must be adequate (generally 80–100 beats/min). Slow heart rates are generally more of a problem than rapid ones and are best treated by pacing. Inotropic agents are useful in increasing heart rate. Supraventricular tachycardias generally require cardioversion.
- Laboratory values must be within acceptable limits. Significant acidosis (pH < 7.20), hypocalcemia (ionized), and hyperkalemia (> 5.5 mEq/L) should be treated; the hematocrit should be at least 22–25%. When CPB reservoir volume and flow are adequate, ultrafiltration may be used to increase the hematocrit (see above).
- Adequate ventilation with 100% oxygen must have been resumed.
- All monitors should be rechecked for proper function and recalibrated if necessary.

Weaning from CPB

Discontinuation of CPB should be gradual as systemic arterial pressure, ventricular volumes and filling pressures, and cardiac output (if available) are assessed. Central aortic pressure is often measured directly and should be correlated with the radial artery pressure and cuff pressure (if necessary). A reversal of the normal systolic pressure gradient, with aortic pressure becoming higher than radial pressure (see Chapter 6) between these two sites is often seen. Central aortic root pressure can also be estimated by palpation by the surgeon. Ventricular volume and contractility can be estimated visually, while filling pressures are measured directly by central venous, pulmonary artery, or left atrial catheters. Cardiac output is measured by thermodilution. TEE also provides invaluable information about chamber volumes, contractility, and valvular function.

Weaning is accomplished by releasing any tapes around the vena cava and progressively clamping the venous return line (tubing). As the beating heart fills, ventricular ejection resumes. Pump flow is gradually decreased as arterial pressure rises. Once the venous line is completely occluded and systolic arterial pressure is judged adequate (> 80–90 mm Hg), pump flow is stopped and the patient is evaluated. Most patients fall into one of four groups when coming off bypass (Table 21–2). Patients with good ventricular function are usu-

ally quick to develop good blood pressure and cardiac output and can be separated from CPB immediately. Hyperdynamic patients can also be rapidly weaned. These patients emerge from CPB with a very low SVR, demonstrating good contractility and adequate volume, but have low arterial pressure; their hematocrit is usually very low (< 22%). The diagnosis is confirmed by measuring cardiac output. Ultrafiltration (off CPB) or red blood cell transfusions increase arterial blood pressure.

Hypovolemic patients are a mixed group that includes both patients with normal ventricular function and those with varying degrees of impairment. Those with preserved myocardial function quickly respond to 100-mL aliquots of pump blood infused via the aortic cannula. Blood pressure and cardiac output rise with each bolus, and the increase becomes progressively more sustained. Most of these patients maintain good blood pressure and cardiac output with a left ventricular filling pressure below 10–15 mm Hg. Ventricular impairment should be suspected in hypovolemic patients whose filling pressures rise during volume infusion without appreciable changes in blood pressure or cardiac output or in those who require filling pressures above 10–15 mm Hg.

Patients with pump failure emerge from CPB with a sluggish, poorly contracting heart that progressively distends. In such cases, CPB is reinstituted while inotropic therapy is initiated. If SVR is high, afterload reduction

Table 21–2. Post-CPB hemodynamic subgroups.

	Group I: Vigorous	Group II: Hypovolemic	Group IIIA: LV Pump Failure	Group IIIB: RV Pump Failure	Group IV: Vasodilated (Hyperdynamic)
Blood pressure	Normal	Low	Low	Low	Low
Central venous pressure	Normal	Low	Normal or high	High	Normal or low
Pulmonary artery pressure	Normal	Low	High	Normal or high	Normal or low
Pulmonary wedge pressure	Normal	Low	High	Normal or low	Normal or low
Cardiac output	Normal	Low	Low	Low	High
Systemic vascular resistance	Normal	Normal or high	High	Normal or high	Low
Treatment	None	Volume	Inotrope; reduce afterload, IABP, LVAD	Pulmonary vasodilator; RVAD	Increase hematocrit

CPB = cardiopulmonary bypass; LV = left ventricular; RV = right ventricular; IABP = intra-aortic balloon pump; LVAD = left ventricular assist device; RVAD = right ventricular assist device.

with nitroprusside or an inodilator (eg, milrinone) can be tried. The patient should be evaluated for unrecognized ischemia (kinked graft or coronary vasospasm), valvular dysfunction, shunting, or right ventricular failure (the distention is primarily right-sided). TEE may facilitate the diagnosis in these cases. If inotropes and afterload reduction fail, **intra-aortic balloon pump (IABP)** is initiated before another attempt is made to wean the patient. The efficacy of IABP is critically dependent on proper timing of inflation and deflation of the balloon. The balloon is ideally inflated just after the dicrotic notch to augment diastolic blood pressure and coronary flow. Maximum deflation should be timed just prior to left ventricular ejection to decrease its afterload. Use of partial bypass, in the form of a left or right ventricular assist device (LVAD or RVAD, respec-

tively) may be necessary for patients with refractory pump failure; sufficient recovery of contractile function may allow complete weaning after 12–48 hours in some patients. Circulatory assist devices, such as the Abiomed and HeartMate, can be used as bridge to cardiac transplantation; the former can be used for several days while the latter device can be left in place for up to several months.

Many clinicians feel that inotropes should not be used routinely in patients coming off CPB because they increase myocardial oxygen demand. The routine use of calcium similarly has the potential to worsen ischemic injury and may contribute to coronary spasm (especially in patients who were taking calcium channel blockers preoperatively). Commonly used inotropes and vasopressors are listed in Table 21–3. Dopamine

Table 21–3. Vasopressors and inotropic agents.

	Bolus	Infusion	Adrenergic Activity			Phosphodiesterase inhibition
			Alpha	*Beta*	*Indirect*	
Epinephrine	2–10 μg	1–2 μg/min	+	+++	0	0
		2–10 μg/min	++	+++	0	0
		>10 μg/min	+++	++	0	0
		(0.01–0.1 μg/kg/min)				
Norepinephrine		1–16 μg/min	+++	++	0	0
		(0.01–0.1 μg/kg/min)				
Isoproterenol	1–4 μg	1–5 μg/min	0	+++	0	0
		(0.01–0.1 μg/kg/min)				
Dobutamine		2–20 μg/kg/min	0	++	0	0
Dopamine		2–10 μg/kg/min	+	++	+	0
		10–20 μg/kg/min	++	++	+	0
		>20 μg/kg/min	+++	++	+	0
Ephedrine	5–25 mg		+	++	+	0
Metaraminol	50–100 μg	40–400 μg/min	+++	++	+	0
Phenylephrine	50–200 μg	10–50 μg/min	+++	0	0	0
Methoxamine	2–10 mg		+++	0	0	0
Amrinone	0.5–1.5 mg/kg	5–10 μg/kg/min	0	0	0	++
Milrinone	50 μg/kg	0.375–0.75 μg/kg/min	0	0	0	++
T3		0.12 μg/kg/min	0	0	0	0
Arginine vasopressin		2–8 μ/h	0	0	0	0

+ = mild activity
++ = moderate activity
+++ = marked activity

and dobutamine are the most commonly used agents. Dobutamine, unlike dopamine, does not increase filling pressures and may be associated with less tachycardia; unfortunately, cardiac output often increases without significant changes in blood pressure. On the other hand, dopamine specifically improves renal blood flow (in low doses; see Chapter 12) and is often more effective in raising blood pressure than in raising cardiac output. Clinically, epinephrine is the most potent inotrope and is usually effective in increasing both cardiac output and systemic blood pressure when others agents have failed. In lower doses, it has predominantly β-agonist activity. Amrinone and milrinone, both selective phosphodiesterase type III inhibitors, are inotropes with significant arterial and venodilator properties; milrinone may be less likely than amrinone to decrease the platelet count. Unlike other inotropes, these two inodilators may not appreciably increase myocardial oxygen consumption because they decrease left ventricular afterload and do not directly increase heart rate. The combination of an inodilator and a β-adrenergic agonist results in synergistic inotropic effects. Norepinephrine is useful for increasing SVR, but high doses compromise renal blood flow. Some clinicians use norepinephrine in combination with phosphodiesterase inhibitors to prevent excessive reductions in systemic arterial pressure. Arginine vasopressin may be used in patients with refractory hypotension, a low SVR, and resistance to norepinephrine. Inhaled nitric oxide and prostaglandin E$_1$ may also be helpful for refractory pulmonary hypertension and right ventricular failure (Table 21–4); nitric oxide has the added advantage of not decreasing systemic arterial pressure. The role of additional inotropic support in the form of thyroid hormone (T$_3$) and glucose-insulin-potassium infusions is not well defined.

5. Postbypass Period

During the postbypass period, bleeding is controlled, bypass cannulas are removed, anticoagulation is reversed, and the chest is closed. Systolic arterial pressure is generally maintained at 90–110 mm Hg to minimize bleeding. Checking for bleeding, especially from the posterior surface of the heart, requires lifting the heart, which can cause severe hypotension. If it does, the surgeon should be informed of the extent and duration of the hypotension. Atrial cannulas are removed before the aortic cannula in case the latter must be used to rapidly administer volume to the patient. Most patients need additional blood volume subsequent to termination of bypass. Administration of blood, colloids, and crystalloid fluid is guided by filling pressures and the postbypass hematocrit. A final hematocrit of 25–30% is generally desirable. Blood remaining in the CPB reservoir can be transfused via the aortic cannula (if still in place) or processed by a cell saver device and given intravenously. Frequent ventricular ectopy may reflect electrolyte disturbances or residual ischemia and should be treated with lidocaine, procainamide, or amiodarone; hypokalemia or hypomagnesemia should be corrected. Ventricular arrhythmias in this setting can rapidly deteriorate into ventricular tachycardia and fibrillation.

Reversal of Anticoagulation

Once hemostasis is judged acceptable and the patient continues to be stable, heparin activity is reversed with protamine. **Protamine** is a highly positively charged protein that binds and effectively inactivates heparin (a highly negatively charged polysaccharide). Heparin-protamine complexes are then removed by the reticuloendothelial system. Several protamine dosing techniques of varying sophistication can be used, but all are empiric and should be checked for adequacy by repeating the ACT 3–5 minutes after reversal. Additional increments of protamine may be necessary.

The simplest technique bases the protamine dose on the amount of heparin initially required to produce the desired ACT; the protamine is then given in a ratio of 1–1.3 mg of protamine per 100 U of heparin. Another approach calculates the protamine dose based on the heparin dose-response curve (Figure 21–11). Automated heparin-protamine titration assays effectively measure residual heparin concentration and can also be used to calculate the protamine dose. This methodology is based on the observation that when protamine is given in excess it has anticoagulant activity (1/100 that of heparin). Premeasured amounts of protamine are therefore added in varying quantities to several wells, each containing a blood sample. The well whose protamine concentration best matches the heparin concentration will clot first. Clotting will be prolonged in wells containing either too much or too little protamine. The protamine dose can then be estimated by multiplying the concentration in the tube that clots first by the patient's calculated blood volume.

Table 21–4. Vasodilators.

Fenoldopam	0.03–0.6 µg/kg/min
Nitroglycerin	0.5–10 µg/kg/min
Nitroprusside	0.5–10 µg/kg/min
Nitric oxide	10–60 ppm (inhaled)
Nicardipine	2.5–10 mg/h
Prostaglandin E$_1$	0.01–0.2 µg/kg/min

Protamine administration can result in a number of adverse hemodynamic effects, which appear to be either immune or idiosyncratic nonimmune reactions (see Chapter 47). Although protamine given slowly usually has minimal effects, hypotension from acute systemic vasodilation or marked pulmonary hypertension may be encountered. Diabetics previously maintained on protamine-containing insulin may be at increased risk for allergic reactions.

Persistent Bleeding

Persistent bleeding following bypass often follows long bypass periods (> 2 hours) and in most instances is due

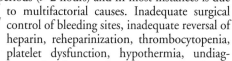

to multifactorial causes. Inadequate surgical control of bleeding sites, inadequate reversal of heparin, reheparinization, thrombocytopenia, platelet dysfunction, hypothermia, undiagnosed preoperative hemostatic defects, or newly acquired defects may be responsible. The absence of clot formation may be noted. The ACT should return to baseline following protamine; additional protamine (25–50 mg) doses may be necessary. Reheparinization (heparin rebound) after apparent adequate reversal may be explained by a redistribution either of protamine to peripheral compartments or of peripherally bound heparin to the central compartment. Hypothermia (< 35 °C) accentuates hemostatic defects and should be corrected. The administration of platelets and coagulation factors should generally be guided by additional coagulation studies, but empiric therapy may be necessary when such tests are not readily available as well as following massive transfusion (see Chapter 29).

If oozing continues despite adequate surgical hemostasis and the ACT is normal or the heparin-protamine titration assay shows no residual heparin, thrombocytopenia or platelet dysfunction is most likely. Both defects are recognized complications of CPB. Platelet transfusion may be necessary and should be given to maintain the platelet count above 100,000/μL. Significant depletion of coagulation factors, especially factors V and VIII, during CPB is less commonly responsible for bleeding but should be treated with fresh frozen plasma; both the prothrombin time and partial thromboplastin time are usually prolonged in such instances. Hypofibrinogenemia (fibrinogen level < 100 mg/dL or a prolonged thrombin time without residual heparin) should be treated with cryoprecipitate. The role of aprotinin for prophylaxis against excessive bleeding has already been discussed above. Desmopressin (DDAVP), 0.3 μg/kg (IV over 20 minutes), can increase factors VIII and XII and the von Willebrand factor activities by releasing them from vascular endothelium. DDAVP may be effective in reversing qualitative platelet defects in some

patients but is not recommended for routine use. Accelerated fibrinolysis may occasionally be encountered following CPB and should be treated with ε-aminocaproic acid (5 g followed by 1 g/hour) or tranexamic acid (10 mg/kg), if not already being given; the diagnosis should be confirmed by elevated fibrin degradation products (> −32 mg/mL), or evidence of clot lysis on thromboelastography.

Anesthesia

Unless a continuous intravenous infusion technique is used, additional anesthetic agents are necessary following CPB; the choice is often determined by the hemodynamic response of the patient following CPB. Unstable patients usually receive small amounts of an opioid, benzodiazepine, or scopolamine, while hyperdynamic patients tolerate anesthetic doses of a volatile agent. Hypertension not responding to boluses of a narcotic or the addition of a volatile agent should be treated with nitroglycerin or nitroprusside (Table 21–4). Fenoldopam may also be used and has the added benefit of increasing renal blood flow and possibly improving creatinine clearance in the early postoperative period.

Even if a volatile agent is used following CPB, an opioid is usually given to provide sedation during transfer to the intensive care unit and analgesia during emergence.

Transportation

Transporting patients from the operating room to the intensive care unit is a hazardous process that is complicated by the possibilities of a complete monitoring blackout, overdosing with or interruption of drug infusions, and hemodynamic instability en route. Portable monitoring equipment, infusion pumps, and a full oxygen cylinder with a self-inflating bag for ventilation should be readied prior to the end of the operation. Minimum monitoring during transportation includes the ECG, arterial blood pressure, and pulse oximetry. An extra pressure channel for central pressures is also desirable. An endotracheal tube, laryngoscope, succinylcholine, and emergency resuscitation drugs should also accompany the patient. Upon arrival in the ICU, the patient should be attached to the ventilator, breath sounds should be checked, and an orderly transfer of monitors and infusions (one at a time) should follow. The ICU staff should be given a brief summary of the procedure, intraoperative problems, current drug therapy, and any expected difficulties.

6. Postoperative Period

Depending on the patient, the type of surgery, and local practices, most patients remain on mechanical ventilation for 2–12 hours postoperatively. Sedation may be accomplished by small doses of morphine (2–3 mg) or a propofol infusion (20–30 μg/kg/min). The emphasis in the first few postoperative hours should be on maintaining hemodynamic stability and monitoring for excessive postoperative bleeding. Chest tube drainage in the first 2 hours of more than 250–300 mL/hour (10 mL/kg/hour)—in the absence of a hemostatic defect—is excessive and often requires surgical reexploration. Subsequent drainage that exceeds 100 mL/hour is also worrisome. Intrathoracic bleeding at a site not adequately drained causes cardiac tamponade, which necessitates immediate reopening of the chest.

Hypertension that is unresponsive to analgesics or sedation is a common postoperative problem and should generally be treated aggressively so as not to exacerbate bleeding or myocardial ischemia. Nitroprusside or nitroglycerin is generally used. Longer-acting agents or β-blockade may be suitable for patients with good ventricular function.

Fluid replacement should be guided by filling pressures. Most patients continue to require volume for several hours following operation. Hypokalemia and hypomagnesemia (from intraoperative diuretics) often develop and require replacement therapies.

Extubation should be considered only when muscle paralysis has worn off and the patient is hemodynamically stable. Caution should be exercised in obese and elderly patients and those with underlying pulmonary disease. Thoracic procedures are typically associated with marked decreases in functional residual capacity and postoperative diaphragmatic dysfunction (see Chapter 23). Most patients can be extubated by the following morning.

■ OFF-PUMP CORONARY ARTERY BYPASS SURGERY

The development of advanced epicardial stabilizing devices, such as the Octopus (Figure 21–12) has allowed coronary artery bypass grafting without the use of CPB, also known as off-pump CAB (OPCAB). This type of retractor uses suction to stabilize and lift the anastomotic site rather than compress it down; this feature allows for greater hemodynamic stability. β-Adrenergic blockade is not required to slow the heart rate as with older OPCAB techniques. Full or half (CPB) dose heparinization is usually given and the CPB machine is usually primed and immediately available if needed.

Intravenous fluid loading together with intermittent or low-dose infusion of a vasopressor may be necessary during the distal anastomosis. In contrast, a vasodilator is usually required to reduce the systolic pressure to 90–100 mm Hg during partial clamping of the aorta for the proximal anastomosis. Although the technique was initially developed for one or two vessel bypass grafting on patients with good left ventricular function,

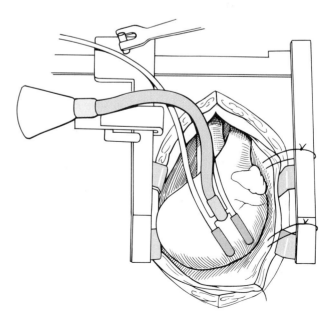

Figure 21–12. Schematic illustration of the Octopus retractor for off-pump coronary artery bypass surgery.

careful application of the technique has allowed it to be used routinely for multi-graft surgery, redo-operations, and patients with compromised left ventricular function. Long-term graft patency appears to be similar to procedures done with CPB. Moreover, OPCAB may reduce the incidence of postoperative neurologic and pulmonary complications.

PEDIATRIC PATIENTS

Cardiovascular function in young children differs from that in adults (see Chapter 44). The Starling relationship (see Chapter 19) plateaus early. Stroke volume is relatively fixed, so that cardiac output is primarily dependent on heart rate. The relatively immature hearts of neonates and infants often poorly tolerate pressure or volume overload. Furthermore, the functions of both ventricles are more interdependent, so that failure of one ventricle often precipitates failure of the other (**biventricular heart failure**). Transition of the neonate from the fetal to the adult circulation is discussed in Chapter 42.

Preoperative Evaluation

The complex nature of these lesions and their operative repair requires close communication between the anesthesiologist, cardiologist, and surgeon. The full hemodynamic significance of the lesion and the surgical plan must be clear preoperatively. Moreover, the patient's condition must be optimized to the maximum extent possible. Congestive heart failure and pulmonary infections should be controlled. Prostaglandin E_1 infusion (0.05–0.1 μg/kg/min) is used preoperatively to prevent closure of the ductus arteriosus in patients dependent on ductal flow for survival. Indications for operation include severe hypoxemia, excessive increases in pulmonary blood flow, refractory congestive heart failure, severe left ventricular obstruction, and preservation of ventricular function.

Assessment of disease severity relies on both clinical and laboratory evaluation. Deterioration in infants is manifested by increasing tachypnea, cyanosis, or sweating, especially during feeding. Older children may complain of easy fatigability. Body weight is generally a good indication of overall disease severity. Signs of congestive heart failure include tachycardia, an S_3 gallop, weak pulses, tachypnea, pulmonary rales, bronchospasm, and hepatomegaly. Cyanosis may be noted, but hypoxemia is best assessed by arterial blood gas measurements and the hematocrit. In the absence of iron deficiency, the degree of polycythemia is directly related to the severity and duration of hypoxemia. Clubbing of the fingers is frequently noted in children with cyanotic defects. The evaluation should also search

for other congenital abnormalities, which are present in up to 30% of patients with congenital heart disease.

The results of echocardiography, heart catheterization, electrocardiography, and chest radiography should be reviewed. Laboratory evaluation should include a complete blood cell count, platelet count, coagulation studies, electrolytes, blood urea nitrogen, and serum creatinine. Ionized calcium and glucose determinations are also useful in neonates and critically ill children.

Preinduction Period

A. FASTING:

Fasting requirements vary according to the patient's age (see Chapter 44). Patients younger than 1 year should have their last feeding 4 hours prior to surgery and may be given clear liquids until 2 hours prior to surgery. Patients between 1 and 2 years of age should have their last feeding 6 hours prior to surgery and may receive clear liquids up to 4 hours before induction. Patients older than 2 years can generally fast for 8 hours. A preoperative intravenous infusion that provides maintenance fluid requirements should be used in patients susceptible to dehydration or with severe polycythemia and when excessive delays occur prior to surgery.

B. PREMEDICATION:

Premedication varies according to age and cardiac and pulmonary reserves. Atropine, 0.02 mg/kg intramuscularly (minimum dose: 0.15 mg), is usually given to all pediatric cardiac patients to counteract enhanced vagal tone. Neonates and infants under 6 months of age are given only atropine. Sedation is desirable in older patients, especially with cyanotic lesions (tetralogy of Fallot), as agitation and crying worsen right-to-left shunting. Some clinicians additionally administer pentobarbital 2 mg/kg IM or 2–4 mg/kg PO to patients 6 months to 1 year of age. Patients older than 1 year are usually given morphine, 0.1 mg/kg, and pentobarbital, 2–3 mg/kg, intramuscularly in addition to atropine. Alternatively, midazolam can be used orally (0.5–0.6 mg/kg) or intramuscularly (0.08 mg/kg).

Induction of Anesthesia

A. HEMODYNAMIC ANESTHETIC GOALS:

1. Obstructive lesions—Anesthetic management should strive to avoid hypovolemia, bradycardia, tachycardia, and myocardial depression. The optimal heart rate should be selected according to age (see Chapter 44); slow rates decrease cardiac output, while fast rates can impair ventricular filling. Some cardiac depression may be desirable in hyperdynamic patients with coarctation of the aorta.

2. Shunts—A favorable ratio of pulmonary vascular resistance (PVR) to SVR should be maintained in the presence of shunting. Factors known to increase pulmonary vascular resistance (PVR) such as acidosis, hypercapnia, hypoxia, enhanced sympathetic tone, and high mean airway pressures are to be avoided for patients with right-to-left shunting; hyperventilation (hypocapnia) with 100% oxygen is usually effective in lowering PVR. Specific pulmonary vasodilators are not available; alprostadil (prostaglandin E_1) or nitroglycerin may be tried but often causes systemic hypotension. Systemic vasodilation also worsens right-to-left shunting and should be avoided; phenylephrine may be used to raise SVR. Inhaled nitric oxide has no effect on systemic arterial pressure. Conversely, patients with left-to-right shunting benefit from systemic vasodilation and increases in PVR, although specific hemodynamic manipulation is generally not attempted.

B. MONITORING:

Standard intraoperative monitors are generally used until the patient is anesthetized. A large discrepancy between end-tidal and arterial CO_2 tensions should be anticipated in patients with large right-to-left shunts because of increased dead space. Following induction, intra-arterial and central venous pressure monitoring are employed for thoracotomies and all procedures employing CPB. A 20- or 22-gauge catheter is used to enter the radial artery; 24-gauge catheters may be more appropriate for small neonates and premature infants. A cutdown may be necessary in some instances. The internal or external jugular vein is generally used for central venous cannulation; if unsuccessful, the central venous catheter may be placed intraoperatively by the surgeon. Pulmonary artery catheterization is much less commonly used in pediatric patients; 7F catheters may be used for patients weighing more than 25 kg, while those 7–25 kg require a 5F catheter.

TEE can be invaluable in pediatric patients, especially for assessing the surgical repair following CPB. It is generally most useful in patients over 12 kg because the probes required for smaller patients have less resolution. Probes are available for patients as small as 3 kg. Intraoperative epicardial echocardiography is commonly used either in addition to or instead of TEE.

C. VENOUS ACCESS:

Venous access is desirable but not always necessary for induction. The use of EMLA (eutectic [easily melted] mixture of local anesthetic) cream (see Chapter 14) can greatly facilitate placement of a venous cannula prior to induction. Agitation and crying are especially undesirable in patients with cyanotic lesions because they can increase right-to-left shunting. Intravenous access can be established after induction but before intubation in most patients. Subsequently, at least two intravenous fluid infusions are required; one is typically via a central venous catheter. Extreme caution is necessary to avoid even the smallest air bubbles. Shunting lesions allow the passage of venous air into the arterial circulation; paradoxical embolism can occur through the foramen ovale even in patients without obvious right-to-left shunting (see Chapter 26). Aspiration prior to each injection prevents dislodgment of any trapped air at the injection port.

D. ROUTE OF INDUCTION:

In premature infants and young neonates, the trachea is usually intubated while the patient is awake and after adequate preoxygenation. In older patients, inhalational, intravenous, or intramuscular induction is necessary prior to intubation. To a major extent, the effect of premedication and the presence of venous access determine the induction technique. Intubation is facilitated by a nondepolarizing agent (rocuronium 1.2 mg/kg or pancuronium, 0.1 mg/kg) or, less commonly, succinylcholine, 1.5–2 mg/kg (see Chapter 44). Pancuronium's vagolytic effects are especially useful in pediatric patients.

1. Intravenous—Thiopental, 3–5 mg/kg; propofol 2–3 mg/kg, ketamine, 1–2 mg/kg; fentanyl, 25–50 μg/kg; or sufentanil, 5–15 μg/kg, can be used for intravenous induction. High-dose opioids may be suitable for very small and critically ill patients when postoperative ventilation is planned. The onset of intravenous agents may be more rapid in patients with right-to-left shunting; drug boluses should be given slowly to avoid transiently high arterial blood levels. In contrast, recirculation in patients with large left-to-right shunts dilutes arterial blood concentration and can delay the onset of intravenous agents.

2. Intramuscular—Ketamine, 4–10 mg/kg, is most commonly used, and onset of anesthesia is within 5 minutes. Preoperative atropine helps prevent excessive secretions. Ketamine is a good choice for agitated and uncooperative patients as well as patients with decreased cardiac reserve. Its safety with cyanotic lesions is well established. Ketamine does not appear to increase PVR in children.

3. Inhalational—Halothane is the most commonly used volatile agent. The technique is the same as that for noncardiac surgery (see Chapter 44), except that the concentration is increased slowly to avoid excessive cardiac depression. Halothane and sevoflurane are most suitable for patients with good cardiac reserve. Halothane's safety in patients with cyanotic heart disease and good cardiac reserve is also well established; systemic arterial vasodilation is generally minimal. Halothane induction should not be used in very young patients and those with low cardiac outputs. Nitrous oxide is typically used with inhalational inductions; its concentration should be limited to 50% in patients with cyanotic lesions. Nitrous oxide does not appear to increase PVR in pediatric patients. The uptake of inhalational agents, especially less soluble agents, such as nitrous oxide, may be slowed in patients with right-to-left shunts; in contrast, no significant effect on uptake is generally observed with left-to-right shunting.

Maintenance Anesthesia

Following induction, opioids or inhalational anesthetics are used for maintenance. Fentanyl and sufentanil are the most commonly used intravenous agents, while halothane, isoflurane, sevoflurane, and nitrous oxide are the most commonly used inhalational agents. The choice of agent should be modified according to the patient's hemodynamic response. Isoflurane and sevoflurane may be more suitable than halothane in some cases; in equivalent anesthetic doses, they causes less myocardial depression, less slowing of the heart rate, and more vasodilation than does halothane. Nitrous oxide can cause cardiac depression in patients with poor cardiac reserve. Moreover, it should probably be discontinued in all patients well before bypass to lessen the likelihood of expansion of intravascular air bubbles (see above).

Cardiopulmonary Bypass

The circuit and technique used are the same as for adults. Since the smallest circuit volume used is still about three times their blood volume, blood is used to prime the machine for neonates and infants to prevent excessive hemodilution. CPB may be complicated by intracardiac and extracardiac shunts and a very compliant arterial system (in very young patients); both tend to lower mean arterial pressure (20–50 mm Hg) and can impair systemic perfusion. Shunts should be controlled as much as possible at the start of bypass. High flow rates (up to 200 mL/kg/min) may be necessary to ensure adequate perfusion in very young patients. Some evidence suggests that pH-stat management during CPB may be associated with better neurologic outcome in children. Weaning from CPB is generally not a problem in pediatric patients if the surgical repair is adequate; primary pump failure is unusual. Difficulty in weaning should prompt the surgeon to check the repair and search for undiagnosed lesions. Intraoperative echocardiography, together with measurement of the pressure and oxygen saturation within the various chambers, usually reveals the problem. Inotropic support may be provided by any of the agents used for adults. Calcium chloride is useful in

critically ill young patients, who often have impaired calcium homeostasis; ionized calcium measurements are invaluable in such cases. Close monitoring of glucose is required because both hyperglycemia and hypoglycemia may be observed. Dopamine and epinephrine are the most commonly used inotropes in pediatric patients. Addition of a phosphodiesterase inhibitor is also useful when PVR or SVR is increased. Hypocapnia, systemic alkalosis, and a high inspired oxygen concentration should also be used to decrease PVR in patients with pulmonary hypertension (see Chapter 22); additional pharmacologic adjuncts may include prostaglandin E_1 (0.05–0.1 µg/kg/min), or prostacyclin (1–40 µg/kg/min). Inhalational nitric oxide may also be helpful for refractory pulmonary hypertension.

Children appear to have a very intense inflammatory response during CPB that may be related to their blood being exposed to very large artificial surfaces relative to their size. Corticosteroids are often given to suppress this response. Many centers use modified ultrafiltration after weaning from CPB to not only partially correct the hemodilution but remove inflammatory vasoactive substances (cytokines); the technique takes blood from the aortic cannula and venous reservoir, passes it through an ultrafilter, and returns it to the right atrium.

Surgical correction of complex congenital lesions sometimes requires complete circulatory arrest under deep hypothermia (**hypothermic circulatory arrest**). Following institution of CPB, cooling is accomplished by the combination of surface cooling and a cold perfusate. At a core temperature of 15 °C, up to 60 minutes of complete circulatory arrest may be safe. Ice packing around the head is used for surface cooling of the brain. Pharmacologic brain protection is also usually attempted with methylprednisolone, 30 mg/kg; mannitol, 0.5 g/kg; and phenytoin, 10 mg/kg. Following the repair, CPB flow is restarted, and rewarming takes place.

Postbypass Period

Because of the large priming volumes used (often 200–300% of the patient's blood volume), hemostatic defects from dilution of clotting factors and platelets are commonly seen after CPB in infants; in addition to heparin reversal, administration of fresh frozen plasma and platelets is often necessary. The use of fresh whole blood transfusions instead of packed red blood cells may decrease the need for platelets and clotting factors.

All patients younger than 6 months should generally remain intubated, as should all other patients undergoing extensive or complicated procedures. Extubation may be considered for older, relatively healthy patients undergoing simple procedures such as closure of a small patent ductus or atrial septal defect or repair of a coarctation.

■ CARDIAC TRANSPLANTATION

Preoperative Considerations

Cardiac transplantation is the treatment of choice for patients with end-stage heart disease who are unlikely to survive the next 6–12 months. The procedure is generally associated with 80–90% postoperative survival at 1 year, and 60–90% survival at 5 years. Moreover, transplantation significantly improves the quality of life and many, if not most, patients are able to resume a relatively normal lifestyle. Unfortunately, the number of cardiac transplants performed is limited by the supply of donor hearts, which are obtained from brain-dead patients (see Chapter 50), most commonly following head trauma.

Patients with intractable heart failure have an ejection fraction of less than 20% and fall into NYHA functional class IV (see Chapter 20). For most patients, the primary diagnosis is either a cardiomyopathy or coronary artery disease. Others may have a severe congenital lesion, a prior transplantation, or valvular heart disease. Medical therapy has usually consisted of diuretics, vasodilators, and even oral inotropes; oral anticoagulation with warfarin may also be necessary. Patients may become dependent on intravenous dopamine or dobutamine while awaiting transplantation. Intra-aortic balloon counterpulsation, a LVAD, or even a total mechanical heart may also be necessary.

Transplant candidates must not have suffered extensive end-organ damage or have other major systemic illnesses. Reversible renal and hepatic dysfunction are common because of chronic hypoperfusion and venous congestion. PVR must be normal or at least responsive to oxygen or vasodilators. Irreversible pulmonary vascular disease is usually associated with a PVR of more than 6–8 Wood units (1 Wood unit = 80 dyne·sec·cm^{-5}), and is a contraindication to orthotopic cardiac transplantation because right ventricular failure is a major cause of early postoperative mortality. Patients with long-standing pulmonary hypertension may, however, be candidates for combined heart-lung transplantation.

Tissue cross-matching is generally not performed. Donor-recipient compatibility is based on size, ABO blood-group typing, and cytomegalovirus serology. Donor organs from patients with hepatitis B or C, or HIV infection are excluded.

ANESTHETIC MANAGEMENT

Proper timing and coordination are necessary between the donor organ retrieval team and the transplant center. Premature induction of anesthesia unnecessarily prolongs CPB, while delaying induction jeopardizes graft function by prolonging the period of ischemia.

Patients may receive little advance warning of the availability of a suitable organ. Many—if not most—will have eaten a recent meal, and should be considered to have a full stomach. Oral cyclosporine must be given preoperatively. Administration of a clear antacid (sodium citrate), a histamine H$_2$-receptor blocker, and metoclopramide should be considered. Patients are typically very sensitive to premedication, which may be best accomplished intravenously and judiciously.

Monitoring is similar to that for other cardiac procedures and is generally established prior to induction. Strict asepsis should be observed during invasive procedures. Use of the right internal jugular vein for central access does not appear to compromise its future use for postoperative endomyocardial biopsies. A pulmonary artery catheter is routinely used in many centers. Placement is often complicated by tricuspid regurgitation, a tendency to coil in the right ventricle, and ventricular irritability.

Unfortunately, patients usually do not tolerate a rapid-sequence induction. Slight head-up positioning and maintenance of cricoid pressure during induction may decrease the risk of aspiration. The principal objective of anesthetic management is to maintain organ perfusion until the patient is on CPB. Induction may be carried out with small doses of opioids (fentanyl, 5–10 μg/kg) with or without etomidate (0.2–0.3 mg/kg). A low-dose ketamine-midazolam technique (above) may also be suitable. Succinylcholine, 1.5 mg/kg, or rocuronium, 1 mg/kg, can be used to intubate the trachea rapidly. Many clinicians prefer pancuronium (0.1 mg/kg) because it counteracts any opioid-induced bradycardia. Additional boluses or an infusion of an opioid are usually used for maintenance of anesthesia. A TEE probe is placed following induction, and an intravenous infusion of azathioprine is given. Hypotension following induction is relatively common and requires the judicious use of inotropes, vasopressors, and fluids.

Sternotomy and cannulation for CPB typically require 1–2 hours and are complicated by prior cardiac operations. Aprotinin can be used to decrease postoperative bleeding. CPB is initiated following cannulation of the aorta and both cavae. If a pulmonary artery catheter was placed, it must be withdrawn completely out of the heart and into the introducer sheath. It must remain in its sterile, protective sheath if it is to be refloated again into the pulmonary artery following CPB. The recipient's heart is then excised, allowing the posterior wall of both atria (with the caval and pulmonary vein openings) to remain. The atria of the donor heart are anastomosed to the recipient's atrial remnants (left side first). The aorta and then the pulmonary artery are anastomosed end-to-end. The heart is then flushed with saline and intracardiac air is evacuated. Methylprednisolone is given before the aortic cross-clamp is released.

Inotropic support (isoproterenol) is usually started prior to separation from CPB. Prolonged graft ischemia may result in transient myocardial depression. Slow junctional rhythms are common and may require epicardial pacing. Although the transplanted heart is totally denervated and direct autonomic influences are absent, its response to circulating catecholamines is usually normal (see Chapter 20). The pulmonary artery catheter can be refloated into position after CPB and is used in conjunction with TEE to evaluate the patient. The most common post-CPB problem is right ventricular failure from pulmonary hypertension, which should be treated with hyperventilation, prostaglandin E_1 (0.025–0.2 μg/kg/min), nitric oxide (10–60 ppm), and a RVAD, if necessary. Bleeding is a common problem because of extensive suture lines and preoperative hemostatic defects.

Patients remain intubated as with other major cardiac operations. The postoperative course is frequently complicated by acute rejection, renal and hepatic dysfunction, and infections.

PERICARDIAL DISEASE

The parietal pericardium is a fairly stiff fibrous membrane surrounding the heart. The negative pericardial pressure following cardiac systole helps promote diastolic ventricular filling. The pericardium encompasses a relatively fixed intrapericardiac volume that includes the pericardial sac, the pericardial fluid (20–50 mL in adults), the heart, and blood. As a result, the pericardium normally limits acute dilatation of the ventricles and promotes diastolic coupling of the two ventricles (distention of one ventricle interferes with filling of the other). The latter effect is also due to the interventricular septal wall they share. Moreover, diseases affecting the pericardium or pericardial fluid volume can seriously impair ventricular function.

1. Cardiac Tamponade

Preoperative Considerations

Cardiac tamponade exists when an increase in pericardial pressure impairs diastolic filling of the heart. Cardiac filling is ultimately related to the diastolic transmural (distending) pressure across each chamber. The transmural pressure across a chamber is the pressure within, minus the pericardial pressure. Consequently, any increase in pericardial pressure relative to the pressure within reduces filling. Although pericardial pressure is equally applied to each chamber, the thin-walled atria and the right ventricle appear to be most affected.

Pericardial pressure is normally similar to the pleural pressure (see Chapter 22), varying with respiration between −4 and +4 mm Hg. Elevations in pericardial pressure are most commonly due to increases in pericardial fluid volume (as a consequence of effusions or bleeding). The magnitude of the increase depends on the rate of fluid accumulation; sudden increases exceeding 100–200 mL precipitously increase pericardial pressure, while very slow accumulations up to 1000 mL allow the pericardium to stretch with minimal increases in pericardial pressure.

The principal hemodynamic feature of cardiac tamponade is a decrease in cardiac output from a reduced stroke volume with an increase in central venous pressure. In the absence of severe left ventricular dysfunction, equalization of diastolic pressure occurs throughout the heart (right atrial pressure [RAP] = right ventricular end-diastolic pressure [RVEDP] = left atrial pressure [LAP] = left ventricular end-diastolic pressure [LVEDP]).

The central venous pressure waveform (see Chapter 19) is characteristic in cardiac tamponade. Impairment of both diastolic filling and atrial emptying abolishes the y descent; the x descent (systolic atrial filling) is normal or even accentuated. Reflex sympathetic activation is a prominent compensatory response in cardiac tamponade. Increases in heart rate and contractility help maintain cardiac output. Arterial vasoconstriction (increased SVR) supports systemic blood pressure, while venoconstriction augments the venous return to the heart. Because stroke volume remains relatively fixed, cardiac output becomes primarily dependent on heart rate.

Acute cardiac tamponade usually presents as sudden hypotension, tachycardia, and tachypnea. Physical signs include jugular venous distention, a narrowed arterial pulse pressure, and muffled heart sounds. A friction rub may be audible. A prominent pulsus paradoxus (a cyclic inspiratory decrease in systolic blood pressure of more than 10 mm Hg) is typically present. The latter actually represents exaggeration of a normal phenomenon related to inspiratory decreases in intrathoracic pressure. Each decrease augments venous return and increases right ventricular end-diastolic volume (preload) but reduces left ventricular end-diastolic volume. The latter is probably due to a right ventricular distention and rightward shift of the interventricular septum. A marked pulsus paradoxus may also be seen with severe airway obstruction and right ventricular infarction. The heart may be normal or enlarged on a chest radiograph. Electrocardiographic signs are generally nonspecific and often limited to decreased voltage in all leads and nonspecific ST-segment and T-wave abnormalities. Electrical alternans (cyclic alteration in magnitude of the P waves, QRS complex, and T waves) may be seen with large pericardial effusions and is thought to be due to pendular swinging of the heart within the pericardium. Generalized ST-segment elevation may also be seen in two or three limb leads as well as V_2 to V_6 in the early phase of pericarditis. Echocardiography is invaluable in diagnosing pericardial effusions and cardiac tamponade and as an aid to pericardiocentesis. Two-dimensional echocardiography is especially accurate in estimating effusion size. Signs of tamponade include diastolic compression or collapse of the right atrium and right ventricle, leftward displacement of the ventricular septum, and an exaggerated increase in right ventricular size with a reciprocal decrease in left ventricular size during inspiration.

Large pericardial effusions may develop slowly without overt signs of tamponade. Some patients may have "low pressure tamponade" in which pericardial pressure is only slightly elevated and central venous pressure is normal. These patients may complain of weakness or dyspnea on exertion.

Pericardial effusions may be due to viral, bacterial, or fungal infections; malignancies or surgery; trauma; uremia; myocardial infarction; aortic dissection; hypersensitivity or autoimmune disorders; drugs; or myxedema.

Anesthetic Considerations

Cardiac tamponade requires expeditious evacuation of the pericardial fluid, either surgically or by pericardiocentesis. The latter is associated with a significant risk of lacerating the heart or coronary arteries and of pneumothorax. Traumatic postoperative (following thoracotomy) cardiac tamponade is always treated surgically (a second thoracotomy), while tamponade from other causes may be treated by either route. Surgical treatment is also often undertaken for large recurrent pericardial effusions (infectious, malignant, autoimmune, uremic, or radiation-induced) to prevent tamponade. Simple drainage of pericardial fluid may be achieved through a subxiphoid approach, while drainage combined with pericardial biopsy or pericardiectomy may be performed via a left anterior thoracotomy or median sternotomy. Drainage and biopsies can also be accomplished through left-sided thoracoscopy (see Chapter 24).

The anesthetic approach must be tailored to the clinical setting. For the still intubated postoperative cardiac patient in extremis, the chest may be reopened immediately in the intensive care unit without the benefit of anesthesia (at least initially). For awake conscious patients undergoing left thoracotomy or median sternotomy, general anesthesia and endotracheal intubation are necessary. Local anesthesia is often used for patients undergoing simple drainage through a subxiphoid approach. Premedication with atropine is often recommended to prevent reflex bradycardia during pericardial manipulation. Small doses of ketamine also provide excellent supplemental analgesia.

 Induction of general anesthesia in patients with cardiac tamponade is extremely hazardous and may precipitate cardiac arrest. Pericardiocentesis or subxiphoid drainage under local anesthesia prior to induction is often advisable. Removal of even a small volume of fluid may be sufficient to greatly improve cardiac output and allow safe induction of general anesthesia.

Large-bore intravenous access is mandatory. Monitoring of intra-arterial and central venous pressures is desirable, but placement of these monitors should not delay pericardial drainage if the patient is unstable. The anesthetic technique should maintain a high sympathetic tone until the tamponade is relieved. Cardiac depression, vasodilation, and slowing of the heart rates are to be avoided. Similarly, increases in mean airway pressures can seriously jeopardize venous return. Awake intubation with maintenance of spontaneous ventilation are theoretically desirable, but coughing, straining, hypoxemia, and respiratory acidosis are equally detrimental and should be avoided. Thoracoscopy generally requires one-lung anesthesia (see Chapter 24).

Ketamine is the induction and maintenance agent of choice until the tamponade is relieved. Pancuronium's circulatory effects also make it the muscle relaxant of choice, but succinylcholine can be used initially for intubation. Small doses of epinephrine (10 μg) may be useful as a temporary inotrope and chronotrope. Generous intravenous fluid administration is useful in maintaining venous return.

2. Constrictive Pericarditis
Preoperative Considerations

Constrictive pericarditis may develop as a sequela of acute or recurrent pericarditis. Pathologically, the pericardium is thickened, fibrotic, and often calcified. The parietal pericardium is typically adherent to the heart, often obliterating the pericardial space. The very stiff pericardium limits diastolic filling of the heart, allowing it to fill only to a fixed volume. In contrast to acute cardiac tamponade, diastolic filling does occur, but to a limited extent; in fact, filling during early diastole is typically accentuated and manifested by a prominent *y* descent on the central venous pressure waveform.

Patients with constrictive pericarditis display jugular venous distention, hepatomegaly, and often ascites. Abnormal liver function may be present. In contrast to acute tamponade, constrictive pericarditis prevents respiratory fluctuations in pericardial pressure; because venous return to the heart does not increase during inspiration, a pulsus paradoxus is uncommon. In fact, venous pressure does not fall or may paradoxically rise during inspiration (Kussmaul's sign). The heart may be large or small on a chest radiograph, which often reveals pericardial calcification. Low QRS voltage and diffuse T-wave abnormalities are usually present on the ECG. Atrial fibrillation and conduction blocks may be present. Echocardiography may be helpful in making the diagnosis but confirmation requires computed tomography or magnetic resonance imaging.

Anesthetic Considerations

Pericardiectomy is usually reserved for patients with moderate to severe disease. The procedure is usually performed through a median sternotomy. It is complicated by the necessity for extensive manipulations of the heart that interfere with cardiac filling and ejection, induce frequent arrhythmias, and risk cardiac perforation. CPB facilitates management, but the need for heparinization increases blood loss. The pericardium is generally dissected away from the left ventricle first; freeing the right ventricle first has occasionally resulted in pulmonary edema.

Selection of anesthetic agents is generally not as critical as avoiding excessive cardiac depression, vasodilation, and bradycardia. Cardiac output is generally very rate dependent. Adequate large-bore intravenous access and direct arterial and central venous pressure monitoring are mandatory. Antiarrhythmic therapy (generally lidocaine) is often necessary. Although cardiac function usually improves immediately following pericardiectomy, some patients display a persistently low cardiac output and require temporary postoperative inotropic support.

■ ANESTHETIC MANAGEMENT OF VASCULAR SURGERY

ANESTHESIA FOR SURGERY ON THE AORTA

Preoperative Considerations

Surgery on the aorta represents one of the greatest challenges for anesthesiologists. Regardless of which part of the vessel is involved, the procedure is complicated by

the need to cross-clamp the aorta and by the potential for large intraoperative blood losses. Aortic cross-clamping without CPB acutely increases left ventricular afterload and severely compromises organ perfusion distal to the point of occlusion. Severe hypertension, myocardial ischemia, left ventricular failure, or aortic valve regurgitation may be precipitated. Interruption of blood flow to the spinal cord and kidneys can produce paraplegia and renal failure, respectively. Moreover, emergency aortic surgery is frequently necessary in critically ill patients who are acutely hypovolemic and have a high incidence of coexistent cardiac, renal, and pulmonary disease; hypertension; and diabetes.

Indications for aortic surgery include aortic dissections, aneurysms, occlusive disease, trauma, and coarctation. Lesions of the ascending aorta are those between the aortic valve and the innominate artery, while those of the aortic arch lie between the innominate and left subclavian arteries. Disease distal to the left subclavian artery but above the diaphragm involves the descending thoracic aorta; lesions below the diaphragm involve the abdominal aorta.

SPECIFIC LESIONS OF THE AORTA

Aortic Dissection

In an aortic dissection an intimal tear allows blood to be forced into the aortic wall (the media) or hemorrhage in the aortic media extends and disrupts the aortic intima. In either case, a primary degenerative process called **medial cystic necrosis** is necessary for dissection to occur. Propagation of the dissection is thought to occur as a result of hemodynamic shear forces acting on the intimal tear; indeed, hypertension is a common finding in patients with aortic dissection. Patients with hereditary connective tissue defects such as Marfan syndrome and Ehlers-Danlos syndrome eventually develop medial cystic necrosis and are at risk for aortic dissection. Dissection can also occur from hemorrhage into an atheromatous plaque or at the cannulation site following cardiac surgery.

Dissection along the aortic media may occlude the opening of any artery arising directly from the aorta; may extend into the aortic root, producing incompetence of the aortic valve; or may rupture into the pericardium or pleura, producing cardiac tamponade or hemothorax, respectively. TEE plays an important role in diagnosing aortic dissections. Dissections are most commonly of the proximal type (Stanford type A, De Bakey types I and II) involving the ascending aorta. Type II dissections do not extend beyond the innominate artery. Distal dissections (Stanford type B, De Bakey type III) originate beyond the left subclavian artery and propagate only distally. Proximal dissections are nearly always treated surgically, while distal dissections may be treated medically. In either case, from the time the diagnosis is suspected, measures to reduce systolic blood pressure (usually to 90–120 mm Hg) and aortic wall stress are initiated. This usually includes intravenous nitroprusside and β-adrenergic blockade (esmolol). The latter is important in reducing the shear forces related to the rate of rise of aortic pressure (dP/dt); dP/dt may actually rise with nitroprusside alone. Alternatively, trimethaphan or labetalol can be used (see Chapter 13).

Aortic Aneurysms

Aneurysms most commonly involve the abdominal aorta but may involve any part of the aorta. The vast majority of aortic aneurysms are due to atherosclerosis; medial cystic necrosis is also an important cause of thoracic aortic aneurysms. Syphilitic aneurysms characteristically involve the ascending aorta. Other etiologies include rheumatoid arthritis, spondyloarthropathies, and trauma. Dilatation of the aortic root often produces aortic regurgitation. Expanding aneurysms of the upper thoracic aorta can also cause tracheal or bronchial compression or deviation, hemoptysis, and superior vena cava syndrome. Compression of the left recurrent laryngeal nerve produces hoarseness and left vocal cord paralysis. Distortion of normal anatomy may also complicate endotracheal or endobronchial intubation or cannulation of the internal jugular and subclavian veins.

The greatest danger from aneurysms is rupture and exsanguination. A pseudoaneurysm forms when the intima and media are ruptured and only adventia or blood clot forms the outer layer. Acute expansion (from leaking), manifested as sudden severe pain, may herald rupture. The likelihood of catastrophic rupture is related to size. The data are least equivocal for abdominal aortic aneurysms; rupture occurs in 50% of patients within 1 year when an aneurysm is 6 cm or more in diameter. The normal aorta in adults varies from 2 cm to 3 cm in width (it is wider cephalad). Elective resection is generally performed in most patients with aneurysms greater than 4 cm. A prosthetic graft is usually used, and the aneurysm may be completely excised or left in place around the graft. The operative mortality rate is about 2–5% in good-risk patients and exceeds 50% if leaking or rupture has already occurred.

Occlusive Disease of the Aorta

Thromboembolic obliteration of the aorta is most commonly atherosclerotic in origin and occurs at the aortic bifurcation (**Leriche's syndrome**). Occlusion results from a combination of atherosclerotic plaque and thrombosis. The atherosclerotic process is usually generalized and affects other parts of the arterial system, including the cerebral and coronary arteries (see Chapters 20 and 27). Surgical treatment consists of an aortobifemoral bypass with a synthetic graft; proximal thromboendarterectomy may also be necessary.

Aortic Trauma

Aortic trauma may be penetrating or nonpenetrating. Both types of injuries can result in massive hemorrhage and require immediate operation. While penetrating injuries are usually obvious, blunt aortic trauma may be easily overlooked if not suspected and sought. Nonpenetrating aortic trauma typically results from sudden high-speed decelerations such as those caused by automobile accidents and falls. The injury can vary from a partial tear to a complete aortic transection. Because the aortic arch is relatively fixed while the descending aorta is relatively mobile, the shear forces are greatest and the site of injury most common just distal to the subclavian artery (aortic isthmus). The most consistent finding is a wide mediastinum on a chest film.

Coarctation of the Aorta

This lesion is usually considered a congenital heart defect. Two types are generally recognized and classified according to the position of the narrowed segment relative to the position of the ductus arteriosus. In the preductal (infantile) type, the narrowing occurs proximal to the opening of the ductus. This lesion, which is often associated with other congenital heart defects, is recognized in infancy because of a marked difference in perfusion between the upper and lower halves of the body; the lower half is cyanotic. Perfusion to the upper body is derived from the aorta, while perfusion to the lower is primarily from the pulmonary artery. Postductal coarctation of the aorta may be not recognized until adulthood. The symptoms and hemodynamic significance of this lesion depend on the severity of the narrowing and the extent of collateral circulation that develops to the lower body (internal mammary, subscapular, and lateral thoracic to intercostal arteries). Hypertension in the upper body, with or without left ventricular failure, is usually present.

ANESTHETIC MANAGEMENT

Surgery on the Ascending Aorta

Surgery on the ascending aorta routinely uses median sternotomy and cardiopulmonary bypass. The conduct of anesthesia is similar to that for cardiac operations involving CPB, but the intraoperative course may be complicated by aortic regurgitation, long aortic cross-clamp times, and large intraoperative blood losses; TEE monitoring is extremely useful. Blood loss can be reduced by aprotinin administration (discussed earlier). Concomitant aortic valve replacement and coronary reimplantation are often necessary (Bentall procedure). The left radial artery should be used to monitor arterial blood pressure, because clamping of the innominate artery may be necessary during the procedure; the femoral and dorsalis pedis arteries are suitable alternatives. Nitroprusside for precise blood pressure control is generally used. β-Adrenergic blockade (esmolol) should also be employed in the presence of an aortic dissection. Bradycardia worsens aortic regurgitation and should be avoided (see Chapter 20). The arterial inflow cannula for CPB is placed in a femoral artery for patients with dissections. In the event that sternotomy may rupture an aneurysm, prior establishment of partial CPB (using the femoral artery and femoral vein) should be considered.

Surgery Involving the Aortic Arch

These procedures are usually performed through a median sternotomy with deep hypothermic circulatory arrest (following institution of CPB). Additional considerations focus on achieving optimal cerebral protection with systemic and topical hypothermia (above). Hypothermia to 15 °C, thiopental infusion to maintain a flat EEG, methylprednisolone or dexamethasone, mannitol, and phenytoin are also commonly used. The necessarily long rewarming periods probably contribute to the large intraoperative blood loss commonly observed after CPB. The safety of aprotinin in this setting is not well established.

Surgery Involving the Descending Thoracic Aorta

Surgery limited to the descending thoracic aorta is typically performed through a left thoracotomy without CPB; a thoracoabdominal incision is necessary for lesions that also involve the abdominal aorta. One-lung anesthesia (see Chapter 24) greatly facilitates surgical exposure and reduces pulmonary trauma from retractors. Correct positioning of the endobronchial tube may be difficult because of distortion of the anatomy; a flexible pediatric fiberoptic bronchoscope can be invaluable in this case. A right-sided double-lumen tube or a regular endotracheal tube with a bronchial blocker may be necessary.

The aorta must be cross-clamped above and below the lesion. Acute hypertension develops above the clamp, with hypotension below. Arterial blood pressure should be monitored from the right radial artery, since clamping of the left subclavian artery may be necessary.

 The sudden increase in left ventricular afterload after application of the aortic cross-clamp during aortic surgery may precipitate acute left ventricular failure, and myocardial ischemia, especially in patients with underlying ventricular dysfunction or coronary disease; it can also exacerbate pre-existing aortic regurgitation. Cardiac output falls while left ventricular end-diastolic pressure and volume rise. The magnitude of these changes is inversely related to ventricular function. Moreover, these effects become less pronounced as the clamp is applied more distally. A nitroprusside infusion is almost always needed to prevent excessive increases in blood pressure and decreases in cardiac output. In patients with good ventricular function, increasing anesthetic depth just prior to cross-clamping may also be helpful.

A major problem in management during these procedures is excessive intraoperative bleeding. Prophylaxis with aprotinin may be helpful. A blood scavenging device (cell saver) for autotransfusion is routinely used. Adequate venous access and intraoperative monitoring are critical. Multiple large-bore (14-gauge) intravenous catheters (preferably with two blood warmers) are mandatory. Pulmonary artery catheterization is invaluable for guiding intraoperative fluid replacement and following cardiac function, especially in conjunction with TEE. The latter is additionally a very useful monitor for myocardial ischemia (see Chapter 20). The greatest period of hemodynamic instability is following release of the aortic cross-clamp (**release hypotension**); the abrupt decrease in afterload together with bleeding and the release of vasodilating acid metabolites from the ischemic lower body can precipitate severe systemic hypotension. Decreasing anesthetic depth, volume loading, and partial or slow release of the cross-clamp are helpful in avoiding severe hypotension. A small dose of a vasopressor may be necessary. Sodium bicarbonate should be used for persistent severe metabolic acidosis (pH < 7.20) in association with hypotension. Calcium chloride may be necessary following massive transfusion of citrated blood products (see Chapter 29).

PARAPLEGIA:

A major complication of clamping the thoracic aorta is spinal cord ischemia and paraplegia. The incidence of transient postoperative deficits and postoperative paraplegia are 11% and 6%, respectively. Higher rates are associated with cross-clamping periods longer than 30 minutes, extensive surgical dissections, and emergency procedures. The classic deficit is that of an anterior spinal artery syndrome with loss of motor function and pinprick sensation but preservation of vibration and proprioception. Anatomic variations in spinal cord blood supply are responsible for the unpredictable occurrence of deficits. The spinal cord receives its blood supply from the vertebral arteries and from the thoracic and abdominal aorta. One anterior and two posterior arteries descend along the cord. Intercostal arteries feed the anterior and posterior arteries in the upper thoracic aorta, while in the lower thoracic and lumbar cord the anterior spinal artery is supplied by the thoracolumbar artery of Adamkiewicz. This artery has a variable origin from the aorta, arising between T5 and T8 in 15%, between T9 and T12 in 60%, and between L1 and L2 in 25% of individuals; it nearly always arises on the left side. It may be damaged during surgical dissection or occluded by the aortic cross-clamping. Monitoring somatosensory evoked potentials (SSEP; see Chapters 6 and 25) may be useful in preventing paraplegia, but false-positive and false-negative responses are reported.

Use of a temporary heparin-coated shunt or partial CPB with hypothermia maintains distal perfusion and decreases the incidence of paraplegia, hypertension, and ventricular failure. Partial CPB is generally not used because heparinization increases blood loss. Using a heparin-coated shunt may preclude the need for heparinization. It is usually placed proximally in the ascending aorta, left subclavian artery, or left ventricular apex and positioned distally in a common femoral artery. Other therapeutic measures that may be protective of the spinal cord include methylprednisolone, mild hypothermia, mannitol, and drainage of cerebrospinal fluid (CSF); magnesium is also protective in some animal models. Mannitol's efficacy appears related to its ability to lower CSF pressure by decreasing its production. Spinal cord perfusion pressure is mean arterial blood pressure minus CSF pressure; the rise in CSF pressure following experimental cross-clamping of the aorta may explain how mannitol can increase spinal cord perfusion pressure. Drainage of CSF via a lumbar catheter may have a similar mechanism.

The use of nitroprusside to control the hypertensive response to cross-clamping has been implicated as a contributing factor in spinal cord ischemia, since its hypotensive actions also occur distal to the cross-clamp. Excessive blood pressure reduction above the cross-clamp should therefore be avoided to prevent excessive hypotension below it.

RENAL FAILURE:

An increased incidence of renal failure following aortic surgery is reported after emergency procedures, prolonged cross-clamping periods, and prolonged hypotension, especially in patients with preexisting renal disease. Infusion of mannitol (0.5 g/kg) prior to cross-clamping may decrease the incidence of renal failure. Low (renal)-dose dopamine is not as effective but may be used as an adjunct for a persistently low urinary output after the cross-clamp is released. Fenoldopam

infusion appears to preserve renal blood flow and may help reduce postoperative renal impairment. Maintenance of adequate cardiac function (preload, contractility, and systemic perfusion pressure) is also mandatory.

Surgery on the Abdominal Aorta

Either an anterior transperitoneal or an anterolateral retroperitoneal approach can be used for access to the abdominal aorta. Depending on the location of the lesion, the cross-clamp can be applied to the supraceliac, suprarenal, or infrarenal aorta. Heparinization prior to occlusion is necessary. Intra-arterial blood pressure can be monitored from either upper extremity. In general, the farther distally the clamp is applied, the less the effect on left ventricular afterload. In fact, occlusion of the infrarenal aorta in patients with good ventricular function frequently results in minimal hemodynamic changes. In contrast, release of the clamp frequently produces hypotension; the same techniques to prevent release hypotension (see above) should be used. The large incision and extensive retroperitoneal surgical dissection significantly increase fluid requirements (up to 10–12 mL/kg/hour) beyond intraoperative blood loss. A combination of colloid and crystalloid fluids is generally used (see Chapter 29). Fluid replacement should be guided by central venous or pulmonary artery pressure monitoring, using the latter for all patients with ventricular dysfunction or significant coronary artery disease. TEE should also be considered for this group of patients.

Renal prophylaxis with mannitol should be considered, especially in patients with preexisting renal impairment. Clamping of the infrarenal aorta has been shown to significantly decrease renal blood flow, which may contribute to postoperative renal failure. The decrease in renal blood flow is not prevented by epidural anesthesia or blockade of the renin-angiotensin system.

Some centers use continuous epidural anesthesia—in addition to general anesthesia—for abdominal aortic surgery. This combined technique decreases the general anesthetic requirement and appears to suppress the release of stress hormones. It also provides an excellent route for administering postoperative epidural analgesia. Unfortunately, systemic heparinization during surgery introduces the risk of paraplegia secondary to an epidural hematoma. Some studies suggest that careful placement of the epidural catheter prior to heparinization—and removal only when coagulation function is normal—lowers the risk of an epidural hematoma.

Postoperative Considerations

Most patients undergoing surgery on the ascending aorta, arch, or the thoracic aorta should remain intubated and ventilated for 2–24 hours postoperatively. As with cardiac surgery, the initial emphasis in their postoperative care should be on maintaining hemodynamic stability and monitoring for postoperative bleeding. Patients undergoing abdominal aortic surgery are often extubated at the end of the procedure. All patients typically continue to require a marked increase in maintenance fluids for several hours postoperatively.

ANESTHESIA FOR CAROTID ARTERY SURGERY

Preoperative Considerations

Ischemic cerebrovascular disease accounts for 80% of strokes; the remaining 20% are due to hemorrhage (see Chapter 27). Ischemic strokes are usually the result of either thrombosis or embolism in one of the blood vessels supplying the brain; vasospasm can also be responsible (see Chapter 26). By convention, a stroke is defined as a neurologic deficit that lasts more than 24 hours; its pathologic correlate is typically focal infarction of brain. **Transient ischemic attacks (TIAs)**, on the other hand, are neurologic deficits that resolve within 24 hours; they may be due to a low-flow state at a tightly stenotic lesion or to emboli that arise from an extracranial vessel or the heart. When a stroke results in progressive worsening of signs and symptoms, it is frequently termed a **stroke in evolution.** A second distinction is also often made between complete and incomplete strokes, based on whether the involved territory is completely affected or additional brain remains at risk for focal ischemia (for example, hemiplegia versus hemiparesis). These distinctions are potentially important in the treatment of stroke.

The origin of the internal carotid artery is the most common site of atherosclerosis leading to TIA or stroke. The mechanism may be embolization of platelet-fibrin or plaque material; stenosis; or complete occlusion. The last may be the result of thrombosis or hemorrhage into a plaque. Symptoms depend on the adequacy of collateral circulation (see Chapter 25). The majority of thrombotic strokes are preceded by TIAs or by a minor stroke that later evolves into a major stroke. Emboli distal to areas of collateral blood flow are more likely to produce symptoms. Small emboli in the ophthalmic branches can cause transient monocular blindness (**amaurosis fugax**). Larger emboli usually enter the middle cerebral artery, producing contralateral motor and sensory deficits that primarily affect the arm and face. Aphasia also develops if the dominant hemisphere is affected. Emboli in the anterior cerebral artery territory typically result in contralateral motor and sensory deficits that are worse in the leg.

Indications for carotid endarterectomy include TIAs associated with ipsilateral severe carotid stenosis (> 70% occlusion), severe ipsilateral stenosis in a patient with a minor (incomplete) stroke, and 30–70% occlusion in a patient with ipsilateral symptoms (usually an ulcerated plaque). Some surgeons also advocate carotid endarterectomy for asymptomatic but significantly stenotic lesions (> 60%). Operative mortality is 1–4% and is primarily due to cardiac complications (myocardial infarction). Perioperative morbidity is 4–10% and principally neurologic; it is highest in patients with preexisting neurologic deficits. Studies suggest that age greater than 75 years, symptomatic lesions, uncontrolled hypertension, angina, carotid thrombus and occlusions near the carotid siphon increase operative risk.

Preoperative Anesthetic Evaluation and Management

Most patients undergoing carotid endarterectomy are elderly and hypertensive, with generalized arteriosclerosis. A significant number are also diabetic. Preoperative evaluation and management should focus on defining preexisting neurologic deficits as well as optimizing the patient's clinical status in terms of coexisting diseases. Although most postoperative neurologic deficits appear to be related to surgical technique, uncontrolled preoperative hypertension increases the incidence of new deficits following surgery. Uncontrolled hyperglycemia can also increase morbidity by enhancing ischemic cerebral injury (see Chapter 25).

With the possible exception of diuretics, patients should receive their usual medications on schedule until the time of surgery. Blood pressure and the plasma-glucose concentration should be well controlled preoperatively. Angina should be stable and controlled, and signs of overt congestive heart failure should be absent. Premedication is tailored to each patient's needs. Alleviation of anxiety to prevent hypertension and tachycardia is desirable. Since most patients are elderly, enhanced sensitivity to premedication should be expected.

General Anesthesia

The emphasis of anesthetic management during carotid surgery on maintaining adequate cerebral perfusion without stressing the heart. Traditionally, this is accomplished by close regulation of arterial blood pressure and avoidance of tachycardia. Intra-arterial pressure monitoring is therefore mandatory. Electrocardiographic monitoring should include the V_5 lead to detect ischemia. Continuous computerized ST-segment analysis is desirable. Additional hemodynamic monitoring should be based primarily on underlying cardiac function, since carotid endarterectomy is not usually associated with significant blood loss or fluid shifts.

Regardless of the anesthetic agents selected, mean arterial blood pressure should be maintained at—or slightly above—the patient's usual range. Thiopental, propofol, and etomidate are the most popular choices for induction because of their favorable cerebral effects, reducing cerebral metabolic rate proportionately more than cerebral blood flow (see Chapter 25). Propofol and etomidate appear to lack the same protective effects as thiopental in focal ischemia, but propofol allows more rapid awakening. Small doses of an opioid or β-adrenergic blocker can be used to blunt the hypertensive response to endotracheal intubation (see Chapter 20). Isoflurane may be the volatile agent of choice because it appears to provide the greatest protection against cerebral ischemia (see Chapter 25). Desflurane qualitatively has similar cerebral effects but may not be as effective as isoflurane; however, desflurane is very useful in accelerating awakening and allowing immediate neurologic assessment in the operating room. Some clinicians also use remifentanil as the opioid for the same reasons.

Intraoperative hypertension is common and usually necessitates the use of an intravenous vasodilator. Nitroglycerin is usually a good choice for mild to moderate hypertension because of its beneficial effects on the coronary circulation. Marked hypertension requires a more potent agent, such as nitroprusside. β-Adrenergic blockade facilitates management of the hypertension and prevents tachycardia but should be used cautiously. Intravenous nicardipine (see Chapter 20) may be a good alternative because of its possible protective effect in focal ischemia. Hypotension should be treated with judicious amounts of intravenous fluid and/or vasopressors. Some clinicians consider phenylephrine the vasopressor of choice; if selected, it should be administered in 25-μg increments to prevent excessive hypertension.

Pronounced or sustained reflex bradycardia or heart block caused by manipulation of the carotid baroreceptor should be treated with atropine. To prevent this response, some surgeons infiltrate the area of the carotid sinus with lidocaine, but the infiltration itself can induce bradycardia. Arterial CO_2 tension should be routinely measured because end-tidal measurements are not sufficiently reliable (see Chapter 6). Hypercapnia can induce intracerebral steal (see Chapter 25) while excessive hypocapnia decreases cerebral perfusion. Ventilation should be adjusted to maintain normocapnia. Intravenous fluids should generally consist of glucose-free solutions because of the potentially adverse effects of hyperglycemia. Heparin (5000–7,500 units IV) is necessary prior to occlusion of the carotid artery. Some clinicians also routinely administer thiopental, 4–6 mg/kg, just prior to carotid cross-clamping for cerebral protection, but the routine use of a shunt (below) may

obviate the need. Protamine, 50–150 mg, is usually given for reversal prior to skin closure.

Although rapid emergence from anesthesia is desirable because it allows immediate neurologic assessment, it frequently results in hypertension and tachycardia requiring a vasodilator or β-adrenergic blocker. Postoperative hypertension may be related to surgical denervation of the ipsilateral carotid baroreceptor. Denervation of the carotid body blunts the ventilatory response to hypoxemia. Following extubation, patients should be observed closely for the development of a wound hematoma, which can rapidly compromise the airway. Transient postoperative hoarseness and ipsilateral deviation of the tongue may be noted; they are due to surgical retraction of the recurrent laryngeal and hypoglossal nerves, respectively.

Monitoring Cerebral Function

Unless regional anesthesia is used (below), indirect methods must be relied upon to assess the adequacy of cerebral perfusion during carotid cross-clamping. Many surgeons routinely use a shunt, but this practice may increase the incidence of postoperative neurologic deficits; shunt insertion can dislodge emboli. Carotid stump pressure distal to the cross-clamp, EEG, and SSEPs have been used by some centers to determine the need for a shunt; a distal stump pressure < 50 mm Hg has traditionally been used as an indication for a shunt. Electrophysiologic signs of ischemia after cross-clamping dictate the use of a shunt; changes lasting more than 10 minutes may be associated with a new postoperative neurologic deficit. Although multichannel recordings and computer processing can enhance the sensitivity of the EEG, neither EEG nor SSEP monitoring is sufficiently sensitive or specific to reliably predict the need for shunting or the occurrence of postoperative deficits. Other techniques, including measurements of regional cerebral blood flow with radioactive xenon 133, transcranial Doppler measurement of middle cerebral artery flow velocity, cerebral oximetry, jugular venous oxygen saturation, and transconjunctival oxygen tension, are also not sufficiently reliable.

Regional Anesthesia

Carotid surgery may be performed under regional anesthesia. Superficial and deep cervical plexus blocks (see Chapter 17) effectively block the C2–C4 nerves and allow the patient to remain comfortably awake during surgery. The principal advantage of regional anesthesia is that the patient can be examined intraoperatively; thus, the need for a temporary shunt can be assessed and any new neurologic deficits diagnosed during surgery. In fact, intraoperative neurologic examination may be the most reliable method for assessing the adequacy of cerebral perfusion during carotid cross-clamping. The examination minimally consists of level of consciousness, speech, and contralateral handgrip. Some studies also suggest that, when compared with general anesthesia, regional anesthesia results in more stable hemodynamics but outcomes appear similar. Unfortunately, regional anesthesia requires the full cooperation of the patient. Moreover, the airway is not secured, and access to it is difficult once the operation begins. Cervical plexus block and the surgery itself may result in ipsilateral phrenic nerve paralysis; it usually is well tolerated and transient.

CASE DISCUSSION: A PATIENT FOR CARDIOVERSION

A 55-year-old man with new-onset atrial fibrillation is scheduled for elective cardioversion.

What are the indications for an elective cardioversion?

Direct current cardioversion may be used to terminate supraventricular and ventricular tachyarrhythmias caused by reentry. It is not effective for arrhythmias from enhanced automaticity (multifocal atrial tachycardia) or triggered activity (digitalis toxicity). By simultaneously depolarizing the entire myocardium and possibly prolonging the refractory period, DC cardioversion can terminate atrial fibrillation and flutter, atrioventricular nodal reentry, reciprocating tachycardias from preexcitation syndromes, and ventricular tachycardia or fibrillation.

Specific indications for patients with atrial fibrillation include symptomatic fibrillation of less than 12 months' duration, a history of embolism, recent onset, and no response to medications. Patients with long-standing fibrillation, a large atrium, chronic obstructive lung disease, congestive heart failure, and mitral regurgitation have a high recurrence rate.

Emergency cardioversion is indicated for any tachyarrhythmia associated with significant hypotension, congestive heart failure, or angina (see Chapter 19).

How is cardioversion performed?

Although usually performed by cardiologists, the need for immediate cardioversion may arise in the operating room, intensive care unit, or during cardiopulmonary resuscitation (see Chapter 48). Anesthesiologists must therefore be familiar with the technique. Following heavy sedation or light general anesthesia, DC shock is applied by either self-adhesive pads or 8–13-cm paddles. Larger paddles help reduce any shock-induced myocardial necrosis by distributing the current over a wider area. The energy output should be kept to the minimally effective level to prevent myocardial damage. Placement of the electrodes can be anterolateral or anteroposterior. In the first position, one electrode is placed on the right second intercostal space next to the sternum and the other is placed on the left fifth intercostal space in the midclavicular line. When pads are used for the amteroposterior technique, one is placed anteriorly over the ventricular apex in the fifth intercostal space and the other underneath the patient in the left infrascapular region.

For supraventricular tachycardias, with the notable exception of atrial fibrillation, energy levels of 25–50 joules can successfully reestablish normal sinus rhythm. Synchronized shocks should be used for all tachyarrhythmias except ventricular fibrillation. Synchronization times the delivery so that it is given during the QRS complex. If the shock occurs in the ST segment or the T wave (unsynchronized), it can precipitate a more serious arrhythmia, including ventricular fibrillation. All medical personnel should stand clear of the patient and the bed during the shock.

Atrial fibrillation usually requires a minimum of 50–100 joules. Hemodynamically stable ventricular tachycardia can often be terminated with 25–50 joules, but ventricular fibrillation and unstable ventricular tachycardia require 200–400 joules (see Chapter 48). Regardless of the arrhythmia, a higher energy level is necessary when the first shock is ineffective. If ventricular arrhythmias develop following the initial shock, lidocaine should be given prior to the next one.

The cardiologist wants to do the cardioversion in the recovery room. Is this an appropriate place for cardioversion?

Elective cardioversion can be performed in any setting where full provisions for cardiopulmonary resuscitation, including cardiac pacing capabilities, are immediately available. A physician skilled in airway management should be in attendance. Cardioversions are most commonly performed in an intensive care unit, emergency room, recovery room, or cardiac catheterization suite.

How would you evaluate this patient?

The patient should be evaluated and treated as though he were receiving a general anesthetic in the operating room. Patients should fast for 6–8 hours prior to the procedure to decrease the risk of aspiration; airway reflexes will be depressed by sedatives and anesthetic agents. A 12-lead ECG is performed immediately before the procedure to confirm that the arrhythmia is still present; another one is performed immediately afterwards to confirm the new rhythm. Preoperative laboratory values should be within normal limits because metabolic disorders, especially electrolyte and acid-base abnormalities, may contribute to the arrhythmia; if not corrected preoperatively, they can reinitiate the tachycardia following cardioversion. Withholding digitalis in a patient without evidence of toxicity is not necessary. Quinidine or another antiarrhythmic is often started in patients with atrial fibrillation 1–2 days prior to the procedure to help maintain normal sinus rhythm. Patients may also be anticoagulated with warfarin for 1–2 weeks prior to cardioversion. A TEE may be performed immediately before to rule out an atrial thrombus.

What are the minimum monitors and anesthetic equipment required?

Minimum monitoring consists of the ECG, blood pressure, and pulse oximetry. A precordial stethoscope is useful for monitoring breath sounds. It is essential to monitor the patient's level of consciousness; maintaining continuous verbal contact with the patient may the best method.

In addition to a DC defibrillator capable of delivering up to 400 joules (synchronized or unsynchronized) and transcutaneous pacing, the minimum equipment should include the following:

- Reliable intravenous access
- A functional bag-mask device capable of delivering 100% oxygen (see Chapter 3)
- An oxygen source from a wall outlet or a full tank
- An airway kit with oral and nasal airways and appropriate laryngoscopes and endotracheal tubes
- A functional suction apparatus
- An anesthetic drug kit that includes at least one sedative-hypnotic as well as succinylcholine
- A crash cart that includes all necessary drugs and equipment for cardiopulmonary resuscitation (see Chapter 48).

What anesthetics techniques would be appropriate?

Premedication is not necessary. Only very brief (1–2 minutes) amnesia or light general anesthesia is required. A short-acting barbiturate (methohexital), propofol, etomidate, or a benzodiazepine (eg, midazolam, diazepam) can be used. Following preoxygenation with 60–100% oxygen for 3–5 minutes, the sedative-hypnotic is given in small increments (eg, methohexital, 20 mg) every 2–3 minutes (if necessary) while maintaining verbal contact with the patient. The shock is delivered when the patient is no longer able to respond verbally; some clinicians use loss of the eyelid reflex as an end point. The shock usually arouses the patient. Transient airway obstruction or apnea may be observed, especially if more than one shock is necessary.

What are complications of cardioversion?

Complications include transient myocardial depression, postshock arrhythmias, and arterial embolism. Arrhythmias are usually due to inadequate synchronization, but even a properly timed cardioversion can occasionally result in ventricular fibrillation. Most arrhythmias are transient and resolve spontaneously. Although patients may develop ST-segment elevation, serum creatine phosphokinase levels (MB fraction) are usually normal. Embolism may be responsible for delayed awakening.

How should the patient be cared for following cardioversion?

Although recovery of consciousness is usually very rapid, patients should be treated like others receiving general anesthesia (see Chapter 49). Recovery also specifically includes monitoring for both recurrence of the arrhythmia and signs of cerebral embolism.

SUGGESTED READING

Ackerstaff RG, van de Vlasakker CJ: Monitoring brain function during carotid endarterectomy: an analysis of contemporary methods. J Cardiothorac Vasc Anesth 1998;12:341.

Aronson S, Blumenthal R: Perioperative renal dysfunction and cardiovascular anesthesia: Concerns and controversies. J Cardiothorac Vasc Anesth 1998;12:567.

Arrowsmith JE, Grocott HP, Reves JG, Newman MF: Central nervous system complications of cardiac surgery. Br J Anaesth 2000;84:378.

Balser JR: The rational use of intravenous amiodarone in the perioperative period. Anesthesiology 1997;86:974.

Bannister J: *Anaesthesia for Vascular Surgery.* Oxford University Press, 2000.

Beique FA, Joffe D, Tousignant G, Konstadt S: Echocardiography-based assessment and management of atherosclerotic disease of the thoracic aorta. J Cardiothorac Vasc Anesth 1998;12: 206.

Cook DJ: Changing temperature management for cardiopulmonary bypass. Anesth Analg 1999;88:1254.

Davies LK: Cardiopulmonary bypass in infants and children: How is it different? J Cardiothorac Vasc Anesth 1999;13:330.

Despotis GJ, Gravlee G, Filos K: Anticoagulation monitoring during cardiac surgery. Anesthesiology 1999;91:1122.

Dinardo J: *Anesthesia for Cardiac Surgery.* McGraw-Hill, 1998.

Estafanous FG, Barash PG, Reves JG: *Cardiac Anesthesia: Principles and Clinical Practice.* 2nd ed. Lippincott, 2001.

Gomez MN: Magnesium and cardiovascular disease. Anesthesiology 1998;89:222.

Gothard JW: *Essentials of Cardiac and Thoracic Anaesthesia.* Butterworth-Heinemann, 1999.

Gravlee G: *Cardiopulmonary Bypass.* Lippincott Williams & Wilkins, 2000.

Hensley FA, Martin DE: *A Practical Approach to Cardiac Anesthesia.* 2nd ed. Little Brown and Company, 1995.

Higgens TL: Quantifying risk and assessing outcome in cardiac surgery. J Cardiothorac Vasc Anesth 1998;12:330.

Izzat MB, Sanderson JE, Sutton MG: *Echocardiography in Adult Cardiac Surgery.* Isis Medical Media, 1999.

Kaplan JA, Reich DL, Kronstadt SN: *Cardiac Anesthesia,* 4th ed. WB Saunders and Company, 1999.

Kohrs R, Durieux M: Ketamine: Teaching an old drug new tricks. Anesth Analg 1998;87:1186.

Lake CL: *Pediatric Cardiac Anesthesia,* 3rd ed. McGraw-Hill, 1998.

Ling E, Arellano R: Systematic overview of the evidence supporting the use of cerebrospinal fluid drainage in the thoracoabdominal aneurysm surgery for prevention of paraplegia. Anesthesiology 2000;93:1115.

Martlew VJ: Perioperative management of patients with coagulation disorders. Br J Anaesth 2000;85:446.

Mets B: Anesthesia for left ventricular assist device placement. J Cardiothorac Vasc Anesth 2000;14:316.

Muhiudeen Russell IA, Miller-Hance WC, Silverman NH: Intraoperative transesophageal echocardiography for pediatric patients with congenital heart disease. Anesth Analg 1998; 87:1058.

Nanda NC, Domanski MJ: *Atlas of Transesophageal Echocardiography.* Williams & Wilkins, 1998.

Otto CM: *Textbook of Clinical Echocardiography.* 2nd ed. WB Saunders and Company, 2000.

Otto CM: *The Practice of Clinical Echocardiography.* WB Saunders and Company, 1997.

Otto CM: *Valvular Heart Disease.* WB Saunders and Company, 1999.

Poelaert J, Skarvan K: *Transesophageal Echocardiography in Anaesthesia.* BMJ Publishing, 2000.

Poortmanns G, Schupfer G, Roosens C, Poelaert J: Transesophageal echocardiographic evaluation of left ventricular function. J Cardiothorac Vasc Anesth 1999;14:588.

Pua HL, Bissonnette B: Cerebral physiology in paediatric cardiopulmonary bypass. Can J Anaesth 1998;45:960.

Slaughter TF, Green berg CS: Heparin-associated thrombocytopenia and thrombosis. Anesthesiology 1997;87:667.

Steudel W, Hurford WE, Zapol WM: Inhaled nitric oxide: Basic biology and clinical application. Anesthesiology 1999;91: 1090.

Stoneham MD, Knighton JD: Regional anaesthesia for carotid endarterectomy. Br J Anaesth 1999;82:910.

Stump DA, Jones TJ, Rorie KD: Neurophysiologic monitoring and outcomes in cardiovascular surgery. J Cardiothorac Vasc Anesth 1999;13:600.

Suriani RJ: Transesophageal echocardiography during organ transplantation. J Cardiothorac Vasc Anesth 1998;12:686.

Tempe DK, Siddiquie RA: Awareness during cardiac surgery. J Cardiothorac Vasc Anesth 1999;13:214.

Thys D: *Textbook of Cardiothoracic Anesthesia.* McGraw-Hill, 2001.

Weissman C: Pulmonary function after cardiac and thoracic surgery. Anesth Analg 1999;88:1272.

Willens HJ, Kessler KM: Transesophageal echocardiography in the diagnosis of diseases of the thoracic aorta: Part II—Atherosclerotic and traumatic diseases of the aorta. Chest 2000; 117:233.

Youngberg JA, Lake CL, Roizen MF, Wilson RS: *Cardiac, Vascular, and Thoracic Anesthesia.* Churchill Livingstone, 1999.

Zaidan JR: Implantable cardioverter-defibrillators. J Cardiothorac Vasc Anesth 1999;13:475.

Respiratory Physiology & Anesthesia

KEY CONCEPTS

 General anesthesia typically reduces both $\dot{V}O_2$ and $\dot{V}CO_2$ by about 15%.

 At end-expiration, intrapleural pressure normally averages about −5 cm H_2O and since alveolar pressure is 0 (no flow), transpulmonary pressure is +5 cm H_2O.

 The lung volume at the end of a normal exhalation is called functional residual capacity (FRC).

 Closing capacity is normally well below FRC, but it rises steadily with age. This increase is probably responsible for the normal age-related decline in arterial oxygen tension.

 While both forced expiratory volume in 1 second and forced vital capacity are effort-dependent, forced midexpiratory flow ($FEF_{25–75\%}$) is effort-independent and may be a more reliable measure of obstruction.

 Induction of anesthesia consistently produces an additional 15–20% reduction in FRC (400 mL in most patients) beyond that which occurs with the supine position alone.

 Hypoxia is a powerful stimulus for pulmonary vasoconstriction (the opposite of its systemic effect).

 Ventilation/perfusion for individual lung units (each alveolus and its capillary) can range from 0 (no ventilation) to infinity (no perfusion); the former is referred to as intrapulmonary shunt, while the latter constitutes alveolar dead space.

 Shunting denotes the process whereby desaturated, mixed venous blood from the right heart returns to the left heart without being resaturated with oxygen in the lungs.

 General anesthesia commonly increases venous admixture to 5–10%, probably as a result of atelectasis and airway collapse in dependent areas of the lung.

 Large increases in $PaCO_2$ (> 75 mm Hg) readily produce hypoxia (PaO_2 < 60 mm Hg) at room air but not at high inspired-oxygen concentrations.

 The binding of oxygen to hemoglobin appears to be the principal rate-limiting factor in the transfer of oxygen from alveolar gas to blood.

 The greater the shunt, the less likely the possibility that an increase in the fraction of inspired oxygen will prevent hypoxemia.

(continued)

(continued)

 A rightward shift in the oxygen-hemoglobin dissociation curve lowers oxygen affinity, displaces oxygen from hemoglobin, and makes more oxygen available to tissues; a leftward shift increases hemoglobin's affinity for oxygen, reducing its availability to tissues.

 As a result of a reaction between H_2O and CO_2, bicarbonate represents the largest fraction of CO_2 in blood.

 Central chemoreceptors are thought to lie on the anterolateral surface of the medulla and respond primarily to changes in cerebrospinal fluid $[H^+]$. This mechanism is effective in regulating $PaCO_2$, because the blood-brain barrier is permeable to dissolved CO_2 but not to bicarbonate ions.

 With increasing depth of anesthesia, the slope of the $PaCO_2$/minute ventilation curve decreases and the apneic threshold increases.

The importance of pulmonary physiology to anesthetic practice is obvious. The most commonly used anesthetics—the inhalational agents—depend on the lungs for uptake and elimination. The most important side effects of both inhalational and intravenous anesthetics are primarily respiratory. Moreover, muscle paralysis, unusual positioning during surgery, and techniques such as one-lung anesthesia and cardiopulmonary bypass profoundly alter normal respiratory physiology.

Much of modern anesthetic practice is based on a thorough understanding of pulmonary physiology and may be considered applied pulmonary physiology. This chapter reviews the basic respiratory concepts necessary for understanding and applying anesthetic techniques. Although the respiratory effects of each of the various anesthetic agents are discussed elsewhere in the book, this chapter also reviews the overall effects of general anesthesia on lung function.

CELLULAR RESPIRATION

The principal function of the lungs is to allow gas exchange between blood and inspired air. This need arises as a direct result of cellular aerobic metabolism, which creates a constant demand for uptake of oxygen and elimination of CO_2.

1. Aerobic Metabolism

Normally, nearly all human cells derive energy aerobically, ie, by using oxygen. Carbohydrates, fats, and proteins are metabolized to two-carbon fragments (acetyl-coenzyme A [acetyl-CoA]) that enter the citric acid cycle within mitochondria (see Chapter 34). As the acetyl-CoA is metabolized to CO_2, energy is derived and stored in nicotine adenine dinucleotide (NAD),

flavin adenine dinucleotide (FAD), and guanosine triphosphate (GTP). That energy is subsequently transferred to adenosine triphosphate (ATP) through a process called **oxidative phosphorylation.** Oxidative phosphorylation accounts for more than 90% of total body oxygen consumption and involves a series of enzyme-mediated (cytochrome) electron transfers that are coupled to ATP formation. In the last step, molecular oxygen is reduced to water.

For glucose, an important cellular fuel, the overall reaction is as follows:

$$C_6H_{12}O_6 + 6 O_2 \rightarrow 6 CO_2 + 6 H_2O + Energy$$

The energy generated (approximately 1200 kJ per mole of glucose) is actually stored in the third phosphate bond on ATP:

$$Energy + ADP + P \rightarrow ATP$$

For every molecule of glucose oxidized, up to a total of 38 molecules of ATP can be produced. Once formed, the energy stored in ATP can be used for ion pumps, muscle contraction, protein synthesis, or cellular secretion; in the process, the adenosine diphosphate (ADP) is regenerated:

$$ATP \rightarrow ADP + P + Energy$$

Cells maintain a ratio of ATP to ADP of 10:1.

Note: ATP cannot be stored but must be continually formed requiring a constant supply of metabolic substrates and oxygen.

The ratio of total CO_2 production ($\dot{V}CO_2$) to oxygen consumption ($\dot{V}O_2$) is referred to as the **respiratory quotient (RQ)** and is generally indicative of the primary type of fuel being utilized. The respiratory quotients for carbohydrates, lipids, and proteins are 1.0, 0.7, and 0.8, respectively. $\dot{V}CO_2$ is normally about 200 mL/min, while $\dot{V}O_2$ is approximately 250 mL/min. Because proteins are generally not used as a primary fuel source, the normal respiratory quotient of 0.8 probably reflects utilization of a combination of both fats and carbohydrates. An RQ of > 1 is seen with lipogenesis (overfeeding), and an RQ of 0.7 implies lipolysis (fasting or starvation). Oxygen consumption can also be estimated based on a patient's weight in kilograms (see Chapter 7):

$$\dot{V}O_2 = 10 \ (weight)^{3/4}$$

2. Anaerobic Metabolism

Compared with aerobic metabolism, anaerobic metabolism produces a very limited amount of ATP. In the absence of oxygen, ATP can be produced only from the conversion of glucose to pyruvate to lactic acid. The anaerobic metabolism of each molecule of glucose yields a net of only two ATP molecules (61˙kJ) (compared with 38 ATP molecules formed aerobically). Moreover, the progressive lactic acidosis that develops severely limits the activity of the enzymes involved. When oxygen tension is restored to normal, lactate is reconverted to pyruvate and aerobic metabolism is resumed.

3. Effects of Anesthesia on Cell Metabolism

 General anesthesia typically reduces both $\dot{V}O_2$ and $\dot{V}CO_2$ by about 15%. Additional reductions are often seen as a result of hypothermia (see Chapter 21). The greatest reductions are in cerebral and cardiac oxygen consumption.

FUNCTIONAL RESPIRATORY ANATOMY

1. Rib Cage & Muscles of Respiration

The rib cage contains the two lungs, each surrounded by its own pleura. The apex of the chest is small, allowing only for entry of the trachea, esophagus, and blood vessels, while the base is formed by the diaphragm. Contraction of the diaphragm—the principal respiratory muscle—causes the base of the thoracic cavity to descend 1.5–7 cm and its contents (the lungs) to expand. Diaphragmatic movement normally accounts for 75% of the change in chest volume. Accessory respiratory muscles also increase chest volume (and lung expansion) by their action on the ribs. Each rib (except for the last two) articulates posteriorly with a vertebra

and is angulated downward as it attaches anteriorly to the sternum. Upward and outward rib movement expands the chest.

During normal breathing, the diaphragm and, to a lesser extent, the external intercostal muscles are responsible for inspiration; expiration is generally passive. With increasing respiratory effort, the sternocleidomastoid, scalene, and pectoralis muscles can be recruited during inspiration. The sternocleidomastoids assist in elevating the rib cage, while the scalene muscles prevent inward displacement of the upper ribs during inspiration. The pectoralis muscles can assist chest expansion when the arms are placed on a fixed support. Expiration is normally passive in the supine position but becomes active in the upright position and with increased respiratory effort. Exhalation is facilitated by muscles—including the abdominal muscles (rectus abdominis, external and internal oblique, and transversus) and perhaps the internal intercostals—aiding the downward movement of the ribs.

Although not usually considered respiratory muscles, some pharyngeal muscles are important in maintaining the patency of the airway (see Chapter 5). Tonic and reflex inspiratory activity in the genioglossus keeps the tongue away from the posterior pharyngeal wall. Tonic activity in the levator palati, tensor palati, palatopharyngeus, and palatoglossus prevents the soft palate from falling back against the posterior pharynx, especially in the supine position.

2. Tracheobronchial Tree

Humidification and filtering of inspired air is a function of the upper airway (nose, mouth, and pharynx). The function of the tracheobronchial tree is to conduct gas flow to and from the alveoli. Dichotomous division (each branch dividing into two smaller branches), starting with the trachea and ending in alveolar sacs, is estimated to involve 23 divisions, or generations (Figure 22–1). With each generation, the number of airways is approximately doubled. Each alveolar sac contains, on average, 17 alveoli. An estimated 300 million alveoli provide an enormous membrane (50–100 m²) for gas exchange in the average adult.

With each successive division, the mucosal epithelium and supporting structures of the airways gradually change. The mucosa makes a gradual transition from ciliated columnar to cuboidal and finally to flat alveolar epithelium. Gas exchange can occur only across the flat epithelium, which begins to appear on respiratory bronchioles (generations 17–19). The wall of the airway gradually loses its cartilaginous support (at the bronchioles) and then its smooth muscle. Loss of cartilaginous support causes the patency of smaller airways to become dependent on radial traction by the elastic

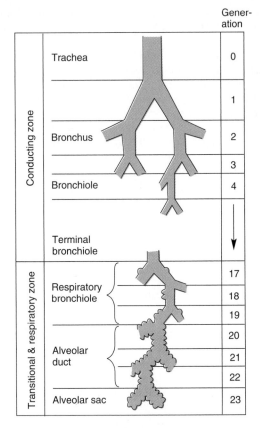

		Generation
Conducting zone	Trachea	0
		1
	Bronchus	2
		3
	Bronchiole	4
	Terminal bronchiole	
Transitional & respiratory zone	Respiratory bronchiole	17
		18
		19
		20
	Alveolar duct	21
		22
	Alveolar sac	23

Figure 22–1. Dichotomous division of the airways. (Reproduced, with permission from: Guyton AC: *Textbook of Medical Physiology*, 7th ed. WB Saunders and Company, 1986, p 111.)

recoil of the surrounding tissue; as a corollary, airway diameter becomes dependent on total lung volume (see below).

Cilia on the columnar and cuboidal epithelium normally beat in a synchronized fashion such that the mucus produced by the secretory glands lining the airway (and any associated bacteria or debris) moves up toward the mouth.

Alveoli

Alveolar size is a function of both gravity and lung volume. The average diameter of an alveolus is thought to be 0.05–0.33 mm. In the upright position, the largest alveoli are at the pulmonary apex, while the smallest tend to be at the base. With inspiration, discrepancies in alveolar size diminish.

Each alveolus is in close contact with a network of pulmonary capillaries. The walls of each alveolus are asymmetrically arranged (Figure 22–2). On the thin side, where gas exchange occurs, the alveolar epithelium and capillary endothelium are separated only by their respective cellular and basement membranes; on the thick side, where fluid and solute exchange occurs, the pulmonary interstitial space separates alveolar epithelium from capillary endothelium. The pulmonary interstitial space contains mainly elastin, collagen, and perhaps nerve fibers. Gas exchange occurs primarily on the thin side of the alveolocapillary membrane, which is less than 0.4 μm thick. The thick side (1–2 μm) provides structural support for the alveolus.

The respiratory epithelium contains at least two cell types. Type I pneumocytes are flat and form tight (1-nm) junctions with one another. These tight junctions are important in preventing the passage of large oncotically active molecules such as albumin into the alveolus. Type II pneumocytes, which are more numerous than type I pneumocytes (but because of their shape occupy less than 10% of the alveolar space), are round cells that contain prominent cytoplasmic inclusions (lamellar bodies). These inclusions contain surfactant, an important substance necessary for normal pulmonary mechanics (see below). Unlike type I cells, type II pneumocytes are capable of cell division and can produce type I pneumocytes if the latter are destroyed. They are also resistant to oxygen toxicity.

Other cell types present in the lower airways include pulmonary alveolar macrophages, mast cells, lymphocytes, and APUD (amino precursor uptake and decarboxylation) cells. Neutrophils are also typically present in smokers and in patients with acute lung injury.

3. Pulmonary Circulation & Lymphatics

The lungs are supplied by two circulations, pulmonary and bronchial. The bronchial circulation arises from the left heart and sustains the metabolic needs of the tracheobronchial tree down to the level of the respiratory bronchioles. Below that level, lung tissue is supported by a combination of the alveolar gas and the pulmonary circulation.

The pulmonary circulation normally receives the total output of the right heart via the pulmonary artery, which divides into right and left branches to supply each lung. Deoxygenated blood passes through the pulmonary capillaries, where oxygen is taken up and CO_2 is eliminated. The oxygenated blood is then returned to the left heart by four main pulmonary veins (two from each lung). Although flows through the systemic and pulmonary circulations are equal, the lower pulmonary vascular resistance results in pulmonary vascular pres-

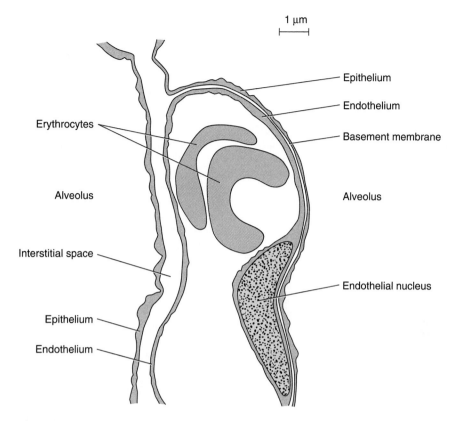

Figure 22–2. The pulmonary interstitial space, with a capillary passing between the two alveoli. The capillary is incorporated into the thin (gas-exchanging) side of the alveolus on the right. The interstitial space is incorporated into the thick side of the alveolus on the left. (Redrawn and reproduced, with permission from: Nunn JF: *Applied Physiology,* 4th ed. Butterworth, 1993, p 14.)

sures one-sixth as great as those in the systemic circulation; as a result, both pulmonary arteries and veins normally have thinner walls with less smooth muscle.

There are connections between the bronchial and the pulmonary circulations. Direct pulmonary arteriovenous communications, bypassing the pulmonary capillaries, are normally insignificant but may become important in certain pathologic states (see Chapters 26 and 35). The importance of the bronchial circulation in contributing to the normal venous admixture is discussed below.

Pulmonary Capillaries

Pulmonary capillaries are incorporated into the walls of alveoli. The average diameter of these capillaries (about 10 μm) is barely enough to allow passage of a single red cell. Because each capillary network supplies more than

one alveolus, blood may pass through several alveoli before reaching the pulmonary veins. Because of the relatively low pressure in the pulmonary circulation, the amount of blood flowing through a given capillary network is affected by both gravity and alveolar size. Large alveoli have a smaller capillary cross-sectional area and consequently increased resistance to blood flow. In the upright position, apical capillaries tend to have reduced flows, while basal capillaries have higher flows.

The pulmonary capillary endothelium has relatively large junctions, 5-nm wide, allowing the passage of large molecules such as albumin. As a result, pulmonary interstitial fluid is relatively rich in albumin. Circulating macrophages and neutrophils are able to pass through the endothelial as well as the smaller alveolar epithelial junctions with relative ease. Pulmonary macrophages are commonly seen in the interstitial space and inside alveoli; they serve to prevent bacterial infection and to scavenge foreign particles.

Pulmonary Lymphatics

Lymphatic channels in the lung originate in the interstitial spaces of large septa. Because of the large endothelial junctions, pulmonary lymph has a relatively high protein content, and total pulmonary lymph flow is normally as much as 20 mL/hour. Large lymphatic vessels travel upward alongside the airways, forming the tracheobronchial chain of lymph nodes. Lymphatic drainage channels from both lungs communicate along the trachea. Fluid from the left lung drains primarily into the thoracic duct while that from the right lung empties into the right lymphatic duct.

4. Innervation

The diaphragm is innervated by the phrenic nerves, which arise from the C3–C5 nerve roots. Unilateral phrenic nerve block or palsy only modestly reduces most indices of pulmonary function (about 25%). Although bilateral phrenic nerve palsies produce more severe impairment, accessory muscle activity may maintain adequate ventilation in some patients. Intercostal muscles are innervated by their respective thoracic nerve roots. Cervical cord injuries above C5 are incompatible with spontaneous ventilation because both phrenic and intercostal nerves are affected.

The vagus nerves provide sensory innervation to the tracheobronchial tree. Both sympathetic and parasympathetic autonomic innervation of bronchial smooth muscle and secretory glands is present. Vagal activity mediates bronchoconstriction and increases bronchial secretions via muscarinic receptors. Sympathetic activity (T1–T4) mediates bronchodilation and also decreases secretions via β_2-receptors. α_1-Adrenergic receptor stimulation decreases secretions but may cause bronchoconstriction. A nonadrenergic, noncholinergic bronchodilator system is also present; vasoactive intestinal peptide is its putative neurotransmitter. The nerve supply of the larynx is reviewed in Chapter 5.

Both α- and β-adrenergic receptors are present in the pulmonary vasculature but the sympathetic system normally has little effect on pulmonary vascular tone. α_1-Activity causes vasoconstriction; β_2-activity mediates vasodilation. Parasympathetic vasodilatory activity appears to be mediated via the release of nitric oxide.

BASIC MECHANISM OF BREATHING

The periodic exchange of alveolar gas with the fresh gas from the upper airway reoxygenates desaturated blood and eliminates CO_2. This exchange is brought about by small cyclic pressure gradients established within the airways. During spontaneous ventilation, these gradients are secondary to variations in intrathoracic pressure; during mechanical ventilation they are produced by intermittent positive pressure in the upper airway.

Spontaneous Ventilation

Normal pressure variations during spontaneous breathing are shown in Figure 22–3. The pressure within alveoli is always greater than the surrounding (intrathoracic) pressure unless the alveoli are collapsed. Alveolar pressure is normally atmospheric (zero for reference) at end-inspiration and end-expiration. By convention in respiratory physiology, pleural pressure is used as a measure of intrathoracic pressure. Although it may not be entirely correct to refer to the pressure in a potential space, the concept allows the calculation of transpulmonary pressure. Transpulmonary pressure, or $P_{transpulmonary}$, is then defined as follows:

$$P_{transpulmonary} = P_{alveolar} - P_{intrapleural}$$

 At end-expiration, intrapleural pressure normally averages about −5 cm H_2O and since alveolar pressure is 0 (no flow), transpulmonary pressure is +5 cm H_2O.

Diaphragmatic and intercostal muscle activation during inspiration expands the chest and decreases intrapleural pressure from −5 cm H_2O to −8 or 9 cm H_2O. As a result, alveolar pressure also decreases (between −3 and −4 cm H_2O), and an alveolar-upper airway gradient is established; gas flows from the upper airway into alveoli. At end-inspiration (when gas inflow has ceased), alveolar pressure returns to zero, but intrapleural pressure remains decreased; the new transpulmonary pressure (5 cm H_2O) sustains lung expansion.

During expiration, diaphragmatic relaxation returns intrapleural pressure to −5 cm H_2O. Now the transpulmonary pressure does not support the new lung volume, and the elastic recoil of the lung causes a reversal of the previous alveolar-upper airway gradient; gas flows out of alveoli, and original lung volume is restored.

Mechanical Ventilation

Most forms of mechanical ventilation intermittently apply positive airway pressure at the upper airway. During inspiration, gas flows into alveoli until alveolar pressure reaches that in the upper airway. During the expiratory phase of the ventilator, the positive airway pressure is removed or decreased; the gradient reverses, allowing gas flow out of alveoli.

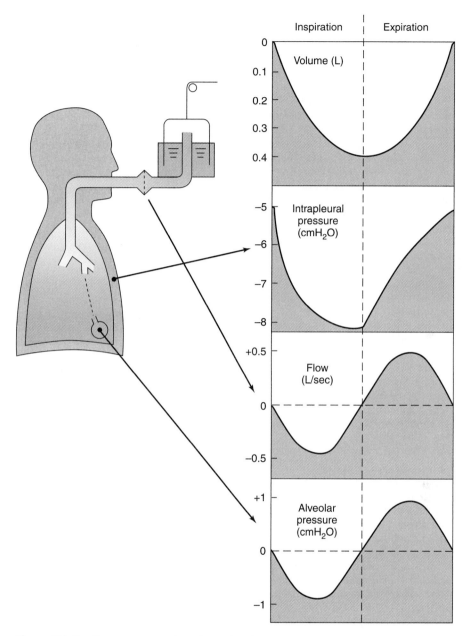

Figure 22–3. Changes in intrapleural and alveolar pressures during normal breathing. Note that at maximal tidal volume, flow is zero and alveolar pressure is atmospheric. (Adapted from: West JB: *Respiratory Physiology—The Essentials,* 3rd ed. Williams & Wilkins, 1985, p 102.)

Effects of Anesthesia on Respiratory Pattern

The effects of anesthesia on breathing are complex and relate to both changes in position and anesthetic agents. When a patient is placed supine from an upright or sitting position, the proportion of breathing from rib-cage excursion decreases; abdominal breathing predominates. The diaphragm's higher position in the chest (about 4 cm) allows it to contract more effectively than when the patient is upright. Similarly, in the lateral decubitus position, ventilation favors the dependent lung because the dependent hemidiaphragm takes a higher position in the chest (see Chapter 24).

Regardless of the agent used, light anesthesia often results in irregular breathing patterns; breath holding is common. Breaths become regular with deeper levels of anesthesia. Inhalational agents generally produce rapid, shallow breaths, while nitrous-narcotic techniques result in slow, deep breaths.

Interestingly, induction of anesthesia activates expiratory muscles; expiration becomes active. The latter regularly necessitates paralysis during abdominal surgery. Inspiratory muscle activity may also be altered. Most of the volatile anesthetics cause dose-dependent decreases in thoracic chest excursion; intercostal muscle activity is gradually lost with increasing anesthetic depth. This relative preservation of diaphragmatic function further favors abdominal over thoracic chest excursion. The latter effect may not be as prominent with ketamine and methohexital.

MECHANICS OF VENTILATION

The movement of the lungs is passive and determined by the impedance of the respiratory system, which can be divided into the elastic resistance of tissues and the gas-liquid interface, and nonelastic resistance to gas flow. The former governs lung volume and the associated pressures under static conditions (no gas flow). The latter relates to frictional resistance to airflow and tissue deformation. The work necessary to overcome elastic resistance is stored as potential energy, but that necessary to overcome nonelastic resistance is lost as heat.

1. Elastic Resistance

Both the lungs and the chest have elastic properties. The chest has a tendency to expand outward, while the lungs have a tendency to collapse. When the chest is exposed to atmospheric pressure (open pneumothorax), it usually expands about 1 L in adults. In contrast, when the lung is exposed to atmospheric pressure, it collapses completely and all the gas within it is expelled. The re-

coil properties of the chest are due to structural components that resist deformation and probably include chest wall muscle tone. The elastic recoil of the lungs is due to their high content of elastin fibers and, even more important, the surface tension forces acting at the air-fluid interface in alveoli.

Surface Tension Forces

The gas-fluid interface lining the alveoli causes them to behave as bubbles. Surface tension forces tend to reduce the area of the interface and favor alveolar collapse. Laplace's law can be used to quantify these forces:

$$Pressure = \frac{2 \times Surface\ tension}{Radius}$$

The pressure derived from the equation is that within the alveolus. Alveolar collapse is therefore directly proportional to surface tension but inversely proportional to alveolar size. Collapse is more likely when surface tension increases or alveolar size decreases. Fortunately, pulmonary surfactant (see above) decreases alveolar surface tension. Moreover, surfactant's ability to lower surface tension is directly proportional to its concentration within the alveolus. As alveoli become smaller, the surfactant within becomes more concentrated, and surface tension is more effectively reduced. Conversely, when alveoli are overdistended, surfactant becomes less concentrated, and surface tension increases. The net effect is to stabilize alveoli; small alveoli are prevented from getting smaller, while large alveoli are prevented from getting larger.

Compliance

Elastic recoil is usually measured in terms of compliance (C), which is defined as the change in volume divided by the change in distending pressure. Compliance measurements can be obtained for either the chest, the lung, or both together (Figure 22–4). In the supine position, chest wall (Cw) compliance is reduced because of the weight of the abdominal contents against the diaphragm. Measurements are usually obtained under static conditions, ie, at equilibrium. (Dynamic lung compliance [Cdyn,L], which is measured during rhythmic breathing, is also dependent on airway resistance.) **Lung compliance (CL)** is defined as:

$$C_L = \frac{Change\ in\ lung\ volume}{Change\ in\ transpulmonary\ pressure}$$

A UPRIGHT

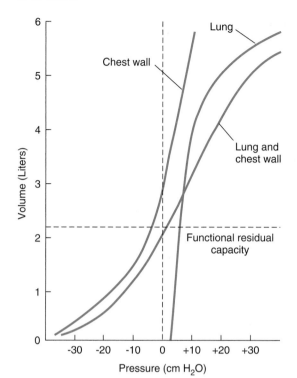

B SUPINE

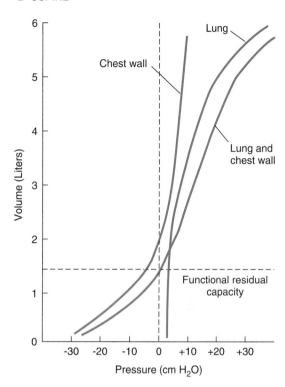

Figure 22–4. The pressure-volume relationship for the chest wall, lung, and both together in the upright (**A**) and supine (**B**) positions. (Modified and reproduced, with permission from: Scurr C, Feldman S: *Scientific Foundations of Anesthesia,* Heinemann, 1982, p 203.)

C_L is normally 150–200 mL/cm H_2O. A variety of factors, including lung volume, pulmonary blood volume, extravascular lung water, and such pathologic processes as inflammation and fibrosis (see Chapter 23), affect C_L.

$$\frac{\text{Chest wall}}{\text{compliance (Cw)}} = \frac{\text{Change in chest volume}}{\text{Change in transthoracic pressure}}$$

where transthoracic pressure equals atmospheric pressure minus intrapleural pressure.

Normal chest wall compliance is 200 mL/cm H_2O. Total compliance (lung and chest wall together) is 100 mL/cm H_2O and is expressed by the following equation:

$$\frac{1}{C_{\text{total}}} = \frac{1}{Cw} + \frac{1}{C_L}$$

2. Lung Volumes

Lung volumes are important parameters in respiratory physiology and clinical practice (Table 22–1 and Figure 22–5). The sum of all the named lung **volumes** equals the maximum to which the lung can be inflated. Lung **capacities** are clinically useful measurements that represent a combination of two or more volumes.

Functional Residual Capacity

The lung volume at the end of a normal exhalation is called **functional residual capacity** (**FRC**). At this volume, the inward elastic recoil of the lung approximates the outward elastic recoil of the chest (including resting diaphragmatic tone). Thus, the elastic properties of both chest and lung define the point from which normal breathing takes place. Functional residual capacity can be measured by nitrogen wash-out or helium wash-in technique or by body plethysmography. Factors known to alter the FRC include the following:

Table 22–1. Lung volumes and capacities.

Measurement	Definition	Average Adult Values (mL)
Tidal volume (V_T)	Each normal breath	500
Inspiratory reserve volume (IRV)	Maximal additional volume that can be inspired above V_T	3000
Expiratory reserve volume (ERV)	Maximal volume that can be expired below V_T	1100
Residual volume (RV)	Volume remaining after maximal exhalation	1200
Total lung capacity (TLC)	RV + ERV + V_T + IRV	5800
Functional residual capacity (FRC)	RV + ERV	2300

- **Body habitus:** FRC is directly proportional to height. Obesity, however, can markedly decrease FRC (primarily as a result of reduced chest compliance).
- **Sex:** FRC is reduced by about 10% in females compared with males.
- **Posture:** FRC decreases as a patient is moved from an upright to a supine or prone position. This is the result of reduced chest compliance as the abdominal contents push up against the diaphragm. The greatest change occurs between 0 and 60 degrees of inclination. No further decrease is observed with a head-down position of up to 30 degrees.

- **Lung disease:** Decreased compliance of the lung, chest, or both is characteristic of restrictive pulmonary disorders (see Chapter 23), all of which are necessarily associated with a low FRC.
- **Diaphragmatic tone:** This normally contributes to FRC.

Closing Capacity

As described above (see Functional Respiratory Anatomy), small airways lacking cartilaginous support depend on radial traction caused by the elastic recoil of surrounding tissue to keep them open; patency of

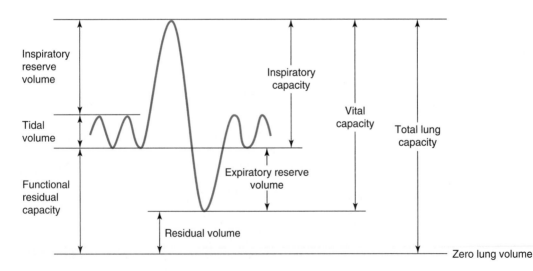

Figure 22–5. Spirogram showing static lung volumes. (Reproduced, with permission, from: Nunn JF: *Applied Respiratory Physiology,* 5th ed. Lumb A (editor), Butterworth-Heinemann, 2000.)

these airways, especially in basal areas of the lung, is highly dependent on lung volume. The volume at which these airways begin to close in dependent parts of the lung is called the **closing capacity.** At lower lung volumes, alveoli in dependent areas continue to be perfused but are no longer ventilated; **intrapulmonary shunting** of deoxygenated blood promotes hypoxemia (see below).

Closing capacity is usually measured using a tracer gas (xenon 133), which is inhaled near residual volume and then exhaled from total lung capacity. Closing capacity is normally well below FRC (Figure 22–6), but it rises steadily with age (Figure 22–7). This increase is probably responsible for the normal age-related decline in arterial oxygen tension. At an average age of 44 years, closing capacity equals FRC in the supine position; by age 66, closing capacity equals or exceeds FRC in the upright position in most individuals. Unlike FRC, closing capacity is unaffected by posture.

Vital Capacity

Vital capacity (VC) is the maximum volume of gas that can be exhaled following maximal inspiration. In addition to body habitus, VC is also dependent on respiratory muscle strength and chest-lung compliance. Normal VC is about 60–70 mL/kg.

3. Nonelastic Resistances

Airway Resistance to Gas Flow

Gas flow in the lung is a mixture of laminar and turbulent flow. Laminar flow can be thought of as consisting of concentric cylinders of gas flowing at different velocities; velocity is highest in the center and decreases toward the periphery. During laminar flow,

$$\text{Flow} = \frac{\text{Pressure gradient}}{\text{Raw}}$$

where Raw is airway resistance.

$$\text{Raw} = \frac{8 \times \text{Length} \times \text{Gas viscosity}}{\pi \times (\text{Radius})^4}$$

Turbulent flow is characterized by random movement of the gas molecules down the air passages. Mathematical description of turbulent flow is considerably more complex

$$\text{Pressure gradient} \approx \text{Flow}^2 \times \frac{\text{Gas density}}{\text{Radius}^5}$$

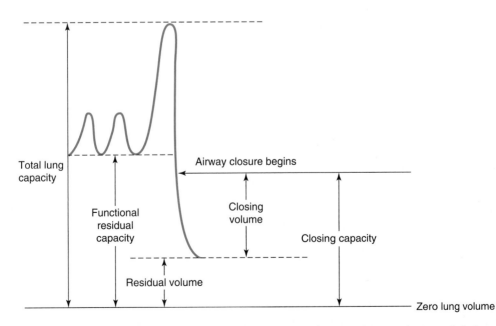

Figure 22–6. The relationship between functional residual capacity, closing volume, and closing capacity. (Reproduced, with permission from: Nunn JF: *Applied Respiratory Physiology,* 5th ed. Lumb A (editor), Butterworth-Heinemann, 2000.)

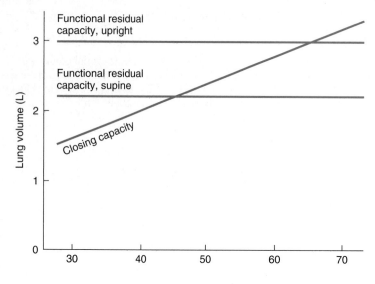

Figure 22–7. The effect of age on closing capacity and its relationship to functional residual capacity (FRC). Note that FRC does not change. (Reproduced, with permission, from: Nunn JF: *Applied Respiratory Physiology*, 5th ed. Lumb A (editor), Butterworth-Heinemann, 2000.)

Resistance is not constant but increases in proportion to gas flow. Moreover, resistance is directly proportional to gas density and inversely proportional to the fifth power of the radius. As a result, turbulent gas flow is extremely sensitive to airway caliber.

Turbulence generally occurs at high gas flows, at sharp angles or branching points, and in response to abrupt changes in airway diameter. Whether turbulent or laminar flow occurs can be predicted by the Reynolds number, which is arrived at by the following equation.

$$\text{Reynolds number} = \frac{\text{Linear velocity} \times \text{Diameter} \times \text{Gas density}}{\text{Gas viscosity}}$$

A low Reynolds number (< 1000) is associated with laminar flow, whereas a high value (> 1500) produces turbulent flow. Laminar flow normally occurs only distal to small bronchioles (< 1 mm). Flow in larger airways is probably turbulent. Of the gases used clinically, only helium has a significantly lower density-to-viscosity ratio, making it useful clinically during severe turbulent flow (as caused by upper airway obstruction). A helium-oxygen mixture not only is less likely to cause turbulent flow but also reduces airway resistance when turbulent flow is present (Table 22–2).

Normal total airway resistance is about 0.5–2 cm $H_2O/L/s$, with the largest contribution coming from medium-sized bronchi (before the seventh generation). Resistance in large bronchi is low because of their large diameters, while resistance in small bronchi is low because of their large total cross-sectional area. The most important causes of increased airway resistance include bronchospasm, secretions, and mucosal edema (see Chapter 23), as well as volume-related and flow-related airway collapse.

Table 22–2. Physical properties of several gas mixtures.

Mixture	Viscosity	Density	Density/Viscosity
Oxygen (100%)	1.11	1.11	1.00
N_2O/O_2	0.89	1.41	1.49
Helium/O_2 (80:20)	1.08	0.33	0.31

Viscosities and densities are expressed relative to air. (Reproduced with permission from: Nunn JF: *Applied Respiratory Physiology*, 5th ed. Lumb A (editor), Butterworth-Heineman, 2000.)

A. VOLUME-RELATED AIRWAY COLLAPSE:

At low lung volumes, loss of radial traction increases the contribution of small airways to total resistance; airway resistance becomes inversely proportional to lung volume (Figure 22–8). Increasing lung volume up to normal with positive end-expiratory pressure (PEEP) can reduce airway resistance.

B. FLOW-RELATED AIRWAY COLLAPSE:

During forced exhalation, reversal of the normal transmural airway pressure can cause collapse of these airways (dynamic airway compression). Two contributing factors are responsible: generation of a positive pleural pressure and a large pressure drop across intrathoracic airways as a result of increased airway resistance. The latter is in turn due to high (turbulent) gas flow and the reduced lung volume. The terminal portion of the flow/volume curve is therefore termed effort-independent (Figure 22–9).

The point along the airways where dynamic compression occurs is called the **equal pressure point**. It is normally beyond the eleventh generation of bronchioles where cartilaginous support is absent (see above). The equal pressure point moves toward smaller airways as lung volume decreases. Emphysema or asthma predisposes patients to dynamic airway compression. Emphysema destroys the elastic tissues that normally support smaller airways. In patients with asthma, bronchoconstriction and mucosal edema intensify airway collapse and promote reversal of transmural pressure gradients across airways. Patients may terminate exhalation prematurely or purse their lips to increase expiratory resistance at the mouth; both maneuvers help prevent reversal of transmural pressure gradients and lessen the trapping of air. Premature termination of exhalation also increases FRC above normal (auto PEEP).

C. FORCED VITAL CAPACITY:

Measuring vital capacity as an exhalation that is as hard and as rapid as possible (Figure 22–10) provides important information about airway resistance. The ratio of the forced expiratory volume in 1 second (FEV_1) to the total forced vital capacity (FVC) is proportional to the degree of airway obstruction. Normally, FEV_1/FVC

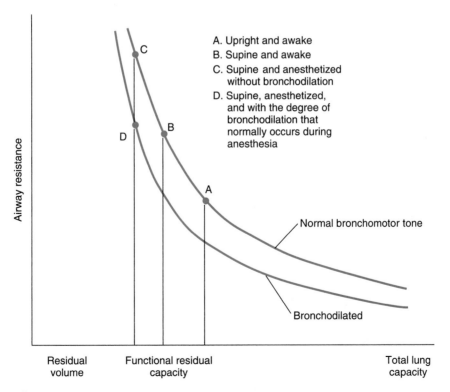

Figure 22–8. The relationship between airway resistance and lung volume. (Modified and reproduced, with permission, from: Nunn JF: *Applied Respiratory Physiology*, 5th ed. Lumb A (editor), Butterworth-Heinemann, 2000.)

A

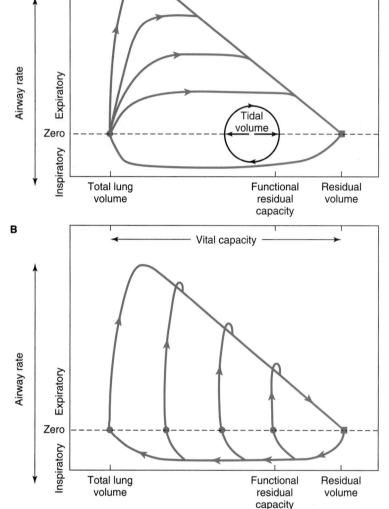

Figure 22–9. Gas flow (**A**) during forced exhalation from total lung capacity with varying effort and (**B**) with maximal effort from different lung volumes. Note that regardless of initial lung volume or effort, terminal expiratory flows are effort-independent. (Reproduced, with permission, from: Nunn JF: *Applied Respiratory Physiology,* 5th ed. Lumb A (editor), Butterworth-Heinemann, 2000.)

is ≥80%. While both FEV_1 and FVC are effort-dependent, forced midexpiratory flow ($FEF_{25-75\%}$) is effort-independent and may be a more reliable measurement of obstruction.

Tissue Resistance

This component of nonelastic resistance is generally underestimated and often overlooked, but may account for up to half of total airway resistance. It appears to be primarily due to viscoelastic (frictional) resistance of tissues to gas flow.

4. Work of Breathing

Because expiration is normally entirely passive, both the inspiratory and the expiratory work of breathing is performed by the inspiratory muscles (primarily the diaphragm). Three factors must be overcome during ventilation: the elastic recoil of the chest and lung, frictional resistance to gas flow in the airways, and tissue frictional resistance.

Respiratory work can be expressed as the product of volume and pressure (Figure 22–11). During inhalation, both inspiratory airway resistance and pulmonary

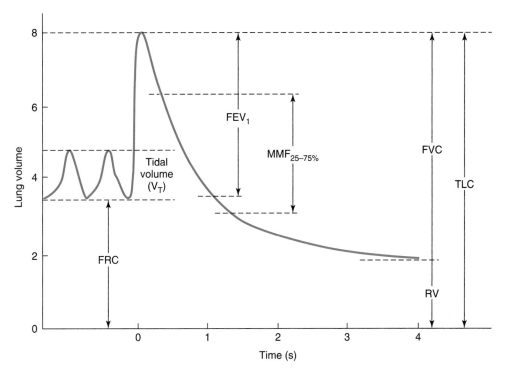

Figure 22–10. The normal forced exhalation curve. FEF$_{25-75\%}$, also called the maximum midexpiratory flow rate (MMF$_{25-75\%}$). FRC = functional residual capacity; FEV$_1$ = forced expiratory volume in 1 second; FVC = forced vital capacity; RV = residual volume; TLC = total lung capacity.

elastic recoil must be overcome; nearly 50% of the energy expended is stored pulmonary elastic recoil. During exhalation, the stored potential energy is released and overcomes expiratory airway resistance. Increases in either inspiratory or expiratory resistance are compensated by increased inspiratory muscle effort. When expiratory resistance increases, the normal compensatory response is to increase lung volume such that tidal breathing occurs at an abnormally high FRC. The greater elastic recoil energy stored at a higher lung volume overcomes the added expiratory resistance. Excessive amounts of expiratory resistance also activate expiratory muscles (see above).

Respiratory muscles normally account for only 2–3% of oxygen consumption but operate at about 10% efficiency. Ninety percent of the work is dissipated as heat (due to elastic and airflow resistance). In pathologic conditions that increase the load on the diaphragm, muscle efficiency usually progressively decreases and contraction may become uncoordinated with increasing ventilatory effort; moreover, a point is reached whereby any increase in oxygen uptake (because of augmented ventilation) is consumed by the respiratory muscles themselves.

The work required to overcome elastic resistance increases as tidal volume increases, while the work required to overcome airflow resistance increases as respiratory rate (and, necessarily, expiratory flow) increases. Faced with either condition, patients minimize the work of breathing by altering respiratory rate and tidal volume (Figure 22–12). Patients with reduced compliance tend to have rapid, shallow breaths, whereas those with increased airflow resistance have a slow, deep breathing pattern.

5. Effects of Anesthesia on Pulmonary Mechanics

Effects on Lung Volumes & Compliance

Induction of anesthesia consistently produces an additional 15–20% reduction in FRC (400 mL in most patients) beyond that which occurs with the supine position alone. Loss of normal end-expiratory diaphragmatic tone allows the abdominal contents to rise farther up against the diaphragm (Figure 22–13). The higher position of the diaphragm decreases lung volume and reduces both chest

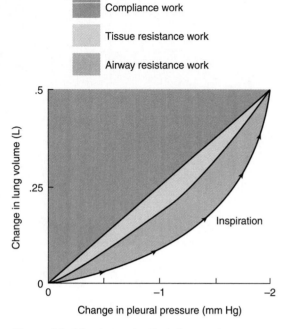

Figure 22–11. The work of breathing and its components during inspiration. (Reproduced, with permission, from: Guyton AC: *Textbook of Medical Physiology,* 7th ed. WB Saunders and Company, 1986, p 469.)

and lung compliance. This decrease in FRC is not related to anesthetic depth and may persist for several hours following anesthesia. Steep head-down (Trendelenburg) position (> 30 degrees) may reduce FRC even further as intrathoracic blood volume increases. In contrast, induction of anesthesia in the sitting position appears to have little effect on FRC. Muscle paralysis does not appear to change FRC significantly when the patient is already anesthetized.

The effects of anesthesia on closing capacity are more variable. Both FRC and closing capacity, however, are generally reduced to the same extent under anesthesia. Thus, the risk of increased intrapulmonary shunting under anesthesia is similar to that in the conscious state; it is greatest in the elderly, in obese patients, and in those with underlying pulmonary disease.

Effects on Airway Resistance

The reduction in FRC associated with general anesthesia would be expected to increase airway resistance. Increases in resistance are not usually observed, however, because of the bronchodilating properties of the volatile inhalational anesthetics. Increased airway resistance is more commonly due to pathologic factors (posterior

displacement of the tongue; laryngospasm; bronchoconstriction; or secretions, blood, or tumor in the airway) or equipment problems (small endotracheal tubes or connectors, malfunction of valves, or obstruction of the breathing circuit).

Effects on the Work of Breathing

Increases in the work of breathing under anesthesia are most often secondary to reduced lung and chest wall compliance and, less commonly, increases in airway resistance (see above). The problems of increased work of breathing are usually circumvented by controlled mechanical ventilation.

VENTILATION/PERFUSION RELATIONSHIPS

1. Ventilation

Ventilation is usually measured as the sum of all exhaled gas volumes in 1 minute (minute ventilation, or $\dot{V}$). If tidal volume is constant,

$$\text{Minute ventilation} = \text{Respiratory rate} \times \text{Tidal volume}$$

For the average adult at rest, minute ventilation is about 5 L/min.

Not all the inspired gas mixture reaches alveoli; some of it remains in the airways and is exhaled without being exchanged with alveolar gases. That part of the tidal volume (V_T) not participating in alveolar gas exchange is known as dead space (V_D). Alveolar ventilation ($\dot{V}_A$) is the volume of inspired gases actually taking part in gas exchange in 1 minute.

$$\dot{V}_A = \text{Respiratory rate} \times V_T - V_D$$

Dead space is actually composed of gases in nonrespiratory airways (anatomic dead space) as well as in alveoli that are not perfused (alveolar dead space). The sum of the two is referred to as **physiologic dead space.** In the upright position, dead space is normally about 150 mL for most adults (approximately 2 mL/kg) and is nearly all anatomic. The weight of an individual in pounds is roughly equivalent to dead space in milliliters. Dead space can be affected by a variety of factors (Table 22–3).

Since tidal volume in the average adult is approximately 450 mL (6 mL/kg), V_D/V_T is normally 33%. This ratio can be derived by the Bohr equation:

$$\frac{V_D}{V_T} = \frac{Pa_{CO_2} - Pe_{CO_2}}{Pa_{CO_2}}$$

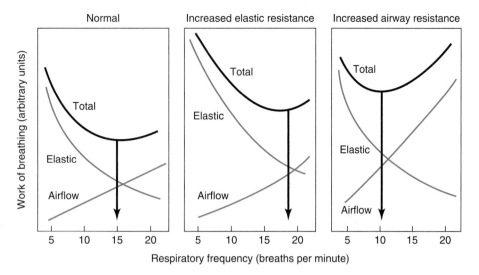

Figure 22–12. The work of breathing in relation to respiratory rate for normal individuals, patients with increased elastic resistance, and patients with increased airway resistance. (Reproduced, with permission, from: Nunn JF: *Applied Respiratory Physiology,* 5th ed. Lumb A (editor), Butterworth-Heinemann, 2000.)

where P_{ACO_2} is the alveolar CO_2 tension and P_{ECO_2} is the mixed expired CO_2 tension. This equation is useful clinically if arterial CO_2 tension (P_{aCO_2}) is used to approximate the alveolar concentration and the CO_2 tension in expired air gases is the average measured over several minutes.

Distribution of Ventilation

Regardless of body position, alveolar ventilation is unevenly distributed in the lungs. The right lung receives more ventilation than the left one (53% versus 47%), and lower (dependent) areas of both lungs tend to be better ventilated than do the upper areas because of a gravitationally induced gradient in intrapleural pressure (and necessarily transpulmonary pressure). Pleural pressure decreases about 1 cm H_2O (becomes less negative) per 3 cm decrease in lung height. This difference places alveoli from different areas at different points on the pulmonary compliance curve (Figure 22–14). Because of a higher transpulmonary pressure, alveoli in upper lung areas are near-maximally inflated and relatively noncompliant, and they undergo little more expansion during inspiration. In contrast, the smaller alveoli in dependent areas have a lower transpulmonary pressure, are more compliant, and undergo greater expansion during inspiration.

Airway resistance can also contribute to regional differences in pulmonary ventilation. Final alveolar inspi-

ratory volume is solely dependent on compliance only if inspiratory time is unlimited. In reality, inspiratory time is necessarily limited by the respiratory rate and the time necessary for expiration; consequently, an excessively short inspiratory time will prevent alveoli from reaching the expected change in volume. Moreover, alveolar filling follows an exponential function that is dependent on both compliance and airway resistance. Therefore, even with a normal inspiratory time, abnormalities in either compliance or resistance can prevent complete alveolar filling.

Time Constants

Lung inflation can be described mathematically by the time constant, τ.

$$\tau = \text{Total compliance} \times \text{Airway resistance}$$

Regional variations in resistance or compliance not only interfere with alveolar filling but can cause asynchrony in alveolar filling during inspiration; some alveolar units may continue to fill as others empty.

Variations in time constants within the normal lung can be demonstrated in normal individuals breathing spontaneously during abnormally high respiratory rates. Rapid shallow breathing reverses the normal distribu-

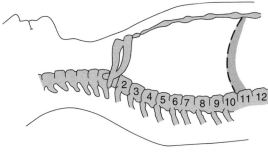

Awake spontaneous

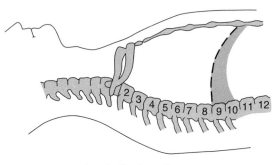

Anesthetized spontaneous

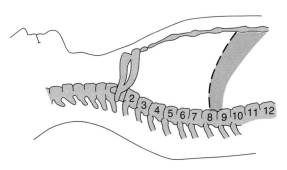

Anesthetized paralyzed

Figure 22–13. The end-expiratory position of the diaphragm (broken line) in an awake spontaneously ventilating patient, an anesthetized spontaneously ventilating patient, and a paralyzed patient. The shaded area shows diaphragmatic excursion. (Modified and reproduced, with permission, from: Froese AB, Bryan AC: Effects of anesthesia and paralysis on diaphragmatic mechanics in man. Anesthesiology 1974;41:242-243.)

tion of ventilation, preferentially favoring upper (nondependent) areas of the lung over the lower areas.

2. Pulmonary Perfusion

Of the approximately 5 L/min of blood flowing through the lungs, only about 70–100 mL at any one time are within the pulmonary capillaries undergoing gas exchange. At the alveolar-capillary membrane, this small volume forms a 50–100 m^2 sheet of blood approximately one red cell thick. Moreover, to ensure optimal gas exchange, each capillary perfuses more than one alveolus.

Although capillary volume remains relatively constant, total pulmonary blood volume can vary between 500 mL and 1000 mL. Large increases in either cardiac output or blood volume are tolerated with little change in pressure as a result of passive dilation of open vessels and perhaps some recruitment of collapsed pulmonary vessels. Small increases in pulmonary blood volume normally occur during cardiac systole and with each normal (spontaneous) inspiration. A shift in posture from supine to erect decreases pulmonary blood volume (up to 27%); Trendelenburg positioning has the opposite effect. Changes in systemic capacitance also influence pulmonary blood volume: systemic venoconstriction shifts blood from the systemic to the pulmonary circulation, while vasodilation causes a pulmonary-to-systemic redistribution. In this way, the lung acts as a reservoir for the systemic circulation.

Table 22–3. Factors affecting dead space.

Factor	Effect
Posture	
Upright	↑
Supine	↓
Position of airway	
Neck extension	↑
Neck flexion	↓
Age	↑
Artificial airway	↓
Positive pressure ventilation	↑
Drugs—Anticholinergic	↑
Pulmonary perfusion	
Pulmonary emboli	↑
Hypotension	↑
Pulmonary vascular disease	
Emphysema	↑

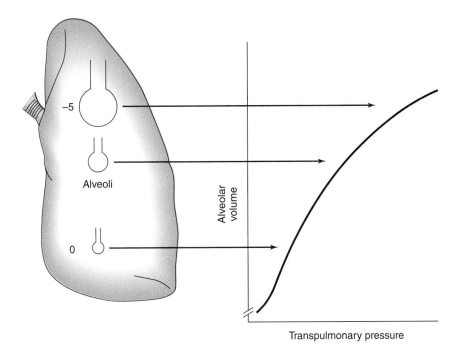

Figure 22–14. The effect of gravity on alveolar compliance in the upright position.

Local factors are more important than the autonomic system in influencing pulmonary vascular tone (above). Hypoxia is a powerful stimulus for pulmonary vasoconstriction (the opposite of its systemic effect). Both pulmonary arterial (mixed venous) and alveolar hypoxia induce vasoconstriction, but the latter is a more powerful stimulus. This response appears to be due to either the direct effect of hypoxia on the pulmonary vasculature or increased production of leukotrienes relative to vasodilatory prostaglandins. Inhibition of nitric oxide production may also play a role. Hypoxic pulmonary vasoconstriction is an important physiologic mechanism in reducing intrapulmonary shunting and preventing hypoxemia (see below). Hyperoxia has little effect on the pulmonary circulation in normal individuals. Hypercapnia and acidosis have a constrictor effect, while hypocapnia causes pulmonary vasodilation.

Distribution of Pulmonary Perfusion

Pulmonary blood flow is also not uniform. Regardless of body position, lower (dependent) portions of the lung receive greater blood flow than upper (nondependent) areas. This pattern is the result of a gravitational gradient of 1 cm H_2O/cm lung height. The normally low pressures in the pulmonary circulation (see Chapter

19) allow gravity to exert a significant influence on blood flow.

For simplification, each lung can be divided into three zones, based on alveolar (PA), arterial (Pa), and venous (Pv) pressures (Figure 22–15). Zone 1 is the upper zone and represents alveolar dead space because alveolar pressure continually occludes the pulmonary capillaries. In the middle zone (zone 2), pulmonary capillary flow is intermittent and varies during respiration according to the arterial-alveolar pressure gradient. Pulmonary capillary flow is continuous in zone 3 and is proportional to the arterial-venous pressure gradient.

Ventilation/Perfusion Ratios

Since alveolar ventilation ($\dot{V}A$) is normally about 4 L/min and pulmonary capillary perfusion ($\dot{Q}$) is 5 L/min, the overall $\dot{V}/\dot{Q}$ ratio is about 0.8. $\dot{V}/\dot{Q}$ for individual lung units (each alveolus and its capillary) can range from 0 (no ventilation) to infinity (no perfusion); the former is referred to as **intrapulmonary shunt,** while the latter constitutes alveolar dead space. $\dot{V}/\dot{Q}$ normally ranges between 0.3 and 3.0, with the majority of lung areas being close to 1.0 (Figure 22–16A). Because perfusion increases at a greater rate than ventilation, nondependent (apical)

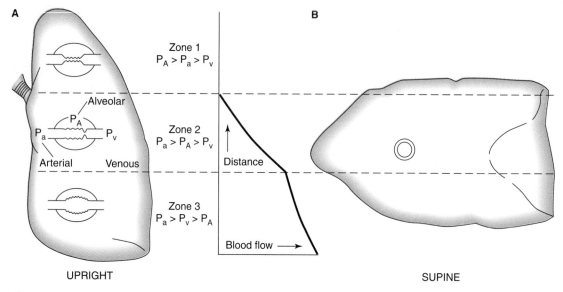

A

Zone 1
$P_A > P_a > P_v$

Alveolar

P_A

P_a — — — P_v

Arterial   Venous

Zone 2
$P_a > P_A > P_v$

Distance

Zone 3
$P_a > P_v > P_A$

Blood flow →

UPRIGHT

B

SUPINE

Figure 22–15. The three-zone model of the lung. ***A:*** Upright position. ***B:*** Supine position.

areas tend to have higher $\dot{V}/\dot{Q}$ ratios than do dependent (basal) areas (Figure 22–16B).

The importance of $\dot{V}/\dot{Q}$ ratios relates to the efficiency with which lung units resaturate venous blood with oxygen and eliminate CO_2. Pulmonary venous blood (the effluent) from areas with low $\dot{V}/\dot{Q}$ ratios has a low O_2 tension and high CO_2 tension—similar to systemic mixed venous blood. Blood from these units tends to depress arterial oxygen tension and elevate arterial CO_2 tension. Their effect on arterial oxygen tension is much more profound than that on CO_2 tension; in fact, arterial CO_2 tension often decreases from a hypoxemia-induced reflex increase in alveolar ventilation. An appreciable compensatory increase in oxygen uptake cannot take place in remaining areas where $\dot{V}/\dot{Q}$ is normal, because pulmonary end-capillary blood is usually already maximally saturated with oxygen (see below).

3. Shunts

Shunting denotes the process whereby desaturated, mixed venous blood from the right heart returns to the left heart without being resaturated with oxygen in the lungs (Figure 22–17). The overall effect of shunting is to decrease (dilute) arterial oxygen content; this type of shunt is referred to as *right-to-left*. Left-to-right shunts (in the absence of pulmonary congestion), however, do not produce hypoxemia.

Intrapulmonary shunts are often classified as absolute or relative. **Absolute shunt** refers to anatomic shunts and

lung units where $\dot{V}/\dot{Q}$ is zero. A **relative shunt** is an area of the lung with a low but finite $\dot{V}/\dot{Q}$ ratio. Clinically, hypoxemia from a relative shunt can usually be partially corrected by increasing the inspired oxygen concentration; that caused by an absolute shunt cannot.

Venous Admixture

This term refers to a concept rather than an actual physiologic entity. **Venous admixture** is the amount of mixed venous blood that would have to be mixed with pulmonary end-capillary blood to account for the difference in oxygen tension between arterial and pulmonary end-capillary blood. Pulmonary end-capillary blood is considered to have the same concentrations as alveolar gas. Venous admixture ($\dot{Q}s$) is usually expressed as a fraction of total cardiac output ($\dot{Q}T$). The equation for $\dot{Q}s/\dot{Q}T$ may be derived with the law for the conservation of mass for oxygen across the pulmonary bed:

$$\dot{Q}T \times CaO_2 = (\dot{Q}s \times C\bar{v}O_2) + (\dot{Q}\acute{c} \times C\acute{c}O_2)$$

where

$\dot{Q}\acute{c}$ = Blood flow across normally ventilated pulmonary capillaries,

$\dot{Q}T = \dot{Q}\acute{c} + \dot{Q}s$,

$C\acute{c}O_2$ = oxygen content of ideal pulmonary end-capillary blood,

CaO_2 = arterial oxygen content, and

$C\bar{v}O_2$ = mixed venous content.

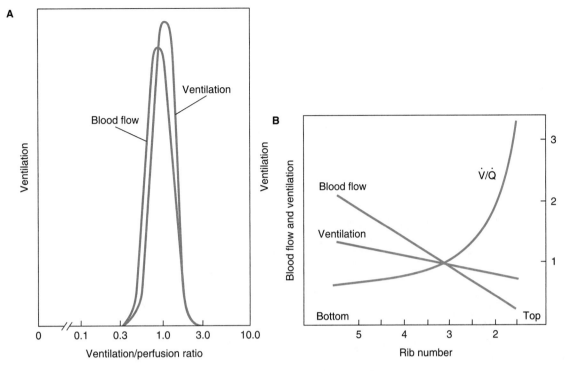

Figure 22–16. The distribution of $\dot{V}/\dot{Q}$ ratios for the whole lung (***A***) and according to height (***B***) in the upright position. Note that blood flow increases more rapidly than ventilation in dependent areas. (Reproduced, with permission, from: West JB: *Ventilation/Blood Flow and Gas Exchange,* 3rd ed. Blackwell, 1977.)

The simplified equation is

$$\dot{Q}s/\dot{Q}_T = \frac{Cc'O_2 - CaO_2}{Cc'O_2 - C\bar{v}O_2}$$

The formula for calculating the oxygen content of blood is given below.

$\dot{Q}s/\dot{Q}_T$ can be calculated clinically by obtaining mixed venous and arterial blood gas measurements; the former requires a pulmonary artery catheter. The alveolar gas equation is used to derive pulmonary end-capillary oxygen tension. Pulmonary capillary blood is usually assumed to be 100% saturated for an $FiO_2 \geq 0.21$.

The calculated venous admixture assumes that all shunting is intrapulmonary and is due to absolute shunts ($\dot{V}/\dot{Q} = 0$). In reality, neither is ever the case; nonetheless, the concept is extremely useful clinically. Normal $\dot{Q}s/\dot{Q}_T$ is primarily due to communication between deep bronchial veins and pulmonary veins, the thebesian circulation in the heart, and areas of low but finite $\dot{V}/\dot{Q}$ in the lungs (Figure 22–18). The venous ad-

mixture in normal individuals (physiologic shunt) is typically less than 5%.

4. Effects of Anesthesia on Gas Exchange

Abnormalities in gas exchange during anesthesia are common. They include increased dead space, hypoventilation, and increased intrapulmonary shunting. There is increased scatter of $\dot{V}/\dot{Q}$ ratios. Increases in alveolar dead space are most commonly seen during controlled ventilation, but may also occur during spontaneous ventilation. General anesthesia commonly increases venous admixture to 5–10%, probably as a result of atelectasis and airway collapse in dependent areas of the lung. Inhalational agents, including nitrous oxide, also can inhibit **hypoxic pulmonary vasoconstriction** in high doses; for volatile agents, the ED_{50} is about 2 MAC. Elderly patients appear to have the largest increases in $\dot{Q}s/\dot{Q}_T$. Inspired oxygen tensions of 30–40% usually prevent hypoxemia suggesting anesthesia increases relative shunt. PEEP is often effective in reducing venous admixture and preventing hypoxemia during general anesthesia as long as cardiac

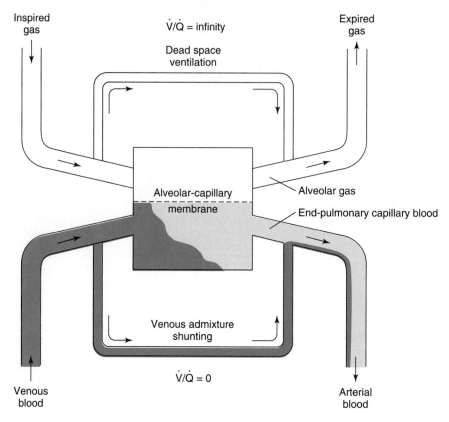

Figure 22–17. A three-compartment model of gas exchange in the lungs, showing dead space ventilation, normal alveolar-capillary exchange, and shunting (venous admixture). (Modified and reproduced, with permission from: Nunn JF: *Applied Respiratory Physiology*, 5th ed. Lumb A (editor), Butterworth-Heinemann, 2000.)

output is maintained (see Chapter 50). Prolonged administration of high inspired oxygen concentrations (> 50%) may be associated with increases in absolute shunt. In these instances, complete collapse of alveoli with previously low $\dot{V}/\dot{Q}$ ratios is thought to occur once all the oxygen within is absorbed (**absorption atelectasis**).

ALVEOLAR, ARTERIAL, & VENOUS GAS TENSIONS

When dealing with gas mixtures, each gas is considered to contribute separately to total gas pressure, and its partial pressure is directly proportional to its concentration. Air has an oxygen concentration of approximately 21%; therefore, if the barometric pressure is 760 mm Hg (sea level), the partial pressure of oxygen (PO_2) in air is normally 159.6 mm Hg:

$$760 \text{ mm Hg} \times 0.21 = 159.6 \text{ mm Hg}$$

In its general form, the equation may be written as follows:

$$PIO_2 = P_B \times FIO_2$$

where P_B = barometric pressure and FIO_2 = the fraction of inspired oxygen.

Two rules of thumb can also be used:

- Partial pressure in millimeters of mercury approximates the percentage × 7.
- Partial pressure in kilopascals is approximately the same as the percentage.

1. Oxygen

Alveolar Oxygen Tension

With every breath, the inspired gas mixture is humidified at 37 °C in the upper airway. The inspired tension

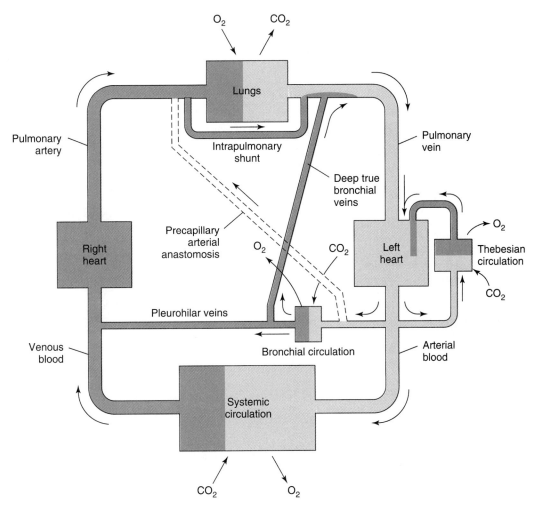

Figure 22–18. Components of the normal venous admixture. (Reproduced, with permission, from: Nunn JF: *Applied Respiratory Physiology,* 5th ed. Lumb A (editor), Butterworth-Heinemann, 2000.)

of oxygen (PIO_2) is therefore reduced by the added water vapor. Water vapor pressure is dependent only on temperature, being 47 mm Hg at 37 °C. In humidified air, the normal partial pressure of oxygen at sea level is 149.7 mm Hg:

$$(760 - 47) \times 0.21 = 149.7 \text{ mm Hg}$$

The general equation is:

$$PIO_2 = (P_B - P_{H_2O}) \times FIO_2$$

where P_{H_2O} = the vapor pressure of water at body temperature.

In alveoli, the inspired gases are mixed with residual alveolar gas from previous breaths, oxygen is taken up, and CO_2 is added. The final alveolar oxygen tension (PAO_2) is therefore dependent on all these factors and can be estimated by the following equation:

$$PAO_2 = PIO_2 - \frac{PaCO_2}{R_Q}$$

where $PaCO_2$ = arterial CO_2 tension and R_Q = respiratory quotient.

R_Q is usually not measured. Note that large increases in $PaCO_2$ (> 75 mm Hg) readily produce hypoxia (PaO_2 < 60 mm Hg) at room air but not at high inspired-oxygen concentrations.

A yet simpler method of approximating PAO_2 in millimeters of mercury is to multiply the percentage of inspired oxygen concentration by 6. Thus, at 40%, PAO_2 is 6 × 40, or 240 mm Hg.

Pulmonary End-Capillary Oxygen Tension

For all practical purposes, pulmonary end-capillary oxygen tension ($Pc'O_2$) may be considered identical to PAO_2; the PAO_2-$Pc'O_2$ gradient is normally minute. $Pc'O_2$ is dependent on the rate of oxygen diffusion across the alveolar-capillary membrane as well as on pulmonary capillary blood volume and transit time. The large capillary surface area in alveoli and the 0.4–0.5 μm thickness of the alveolar-capillary membrane greatly facilitate oxygen diffusion. Enhanced oxygen binding to hemoglobin at saturations above 80% also augments oxygen diffusion (see below). Capillary transit time can be estimated by dividing pulmonary capillary blood volume by cardiac output (pulmonary blood flow); thus, normal capillary transit time is 70 mL ÷ 5000 mL/min (0.8 sec). Maximum $Pc'O_2$ is usually attained after only 0.3 seconds, providing a large safety margin.

The binding of oxygen to hemoglobin appears to be the principal rate-limiting factor in the transfer of oxygen from alveolar gas to blood. Therefore, pulmonary diffusing capacity reflects not only the capacity and permeability of the alveolar-capillary membrane but also pulmonary blood flow. Moreover, oxygen uptake is normally limited by pulmonary blood flow not oxygen diffusion across the alveolar-capillary membrane; the latter may become significant during exercise in normal individuals at high altitudes and in patients with extensive destruction of the alveolar-capillary membrane.

Oxygen transfer across the alveolar-capillary membrane is expressed as oxygen diffusing capacity (DLO_2):

$$DLO_2 = \frac{Oxygen\ uptake}{PAO_2 - Pc'O_2}$$

Since $Pc'O_2$ cannot be measured accurately, measurement of carbon monoxide diffusion capacity ($DLCO$) is used instead to assess gas transfer across the alveolar-capillary membrane. Because carbon monoxide has a very high affinity for hemoglobin, there is little or no CO in pulmonary capillary blood so that even when it is administered at low concentration, $Pc'CO$ can be considered zero. Therefore,

$$DLCO = \frac{Carbon\ monoxide\ uptake}{PACO}$$

Reductions in $DLCO$ imply an impediment in gas transfer across the alveolar-capillary membrane. Such impediments may be due to abnormal $\dot{V}/\dot{Q}$ ratios, extensive destruction of the gas alveolar-capillary membrane, or very short capillary transit times. Abnormalities are accentuated by increases in oxygen consumption and cardiac output, such as occurs during exercise.

Arterial Oxygen Tension

PaO_2 cannot be calculated like PAO_2 but must be measured at room air. The alveolar-to-arterial oxygen partial pressure gradient (A-a gradient) is normally less than 15 mm Hg, but progressively increases with age up to 20–30 mm Hg. Arterial oxygen tension can be approximated by the following formula (in mm Hg):

$$PaO_2 = 102 - \frac{Age}{3}$$

The range is 60–100 mm Hg (8–13 kPa). Decreases are probably the result of a progressive increase in closing capacity relative to FRC (see above). Table 22–4 lists the mechanisms of hypoxemia (PaO_2 < 60 mm Hg).

The most common mechanism for hypoxemia is an increased **alveolar-arterial gradient.** The A-a gradient for oxygen depends on the amount of right-to-left shunting, the amount of $\dot{V}/\dot{Q}$ scatter, and the **mixed venous oxygen tension** (see below). The last depends

Table 22–4. Mechanisms of hypoxemia.

Low alveolar oxygen tension
  Low inspired oxygen tension
    Low fractional inspired concentration
    High altitude
  Alveolar hypoventilation
  Third gas effect (diffusion hypoxia)
  Increased oxygen consumption
Increased alveolar-arterial gradient
  Right-to-left shunting
  Increased areas of low $\dot{V}/\dot{Q}$ ratios
  Low mixed venous oxygen tension
    Decreased cardiac output
    Increased oxygen consumption
    Decreased hemoglobin concentration

$\dot{V}/\dot{Q}$ = ventilation/perfusion.

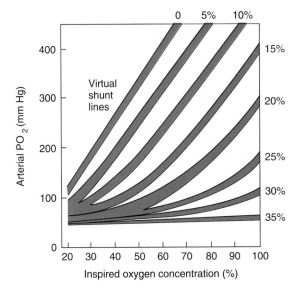

Figure 22–19. Isoshunt curves showing the effect of varying amounts of shunt on PaO_2. Note that there is little benefit in increasing inspired oxygen concentration in patients with very large shunts. (Modified and reproduced with permission from: Benatar SR, Hewlett AM, Nunn JF: The use of isoshunt lines for control of oxygen therapy. Br J Anaesth 1973;45:711.

on cardiac output, oxygen consumption, and hemoglobin concentration.

The A-a gradient for oxygen is directly proportional to shunt but inversely proportional to mixed venous oxygen tension. The effect of each variable on PaO_2 (and consequently the A-a gradient) can be determined only when the other variables are held constant. Figure 22–19 shows the effect of different degrees of shunting on PaO_2. It should also be noted that the greater the shunt, the less likely the possibility that an increase in FIO_2 will prevent

hypoxemia. Moreover, isoshunt lines appear to be most useful for oxygen concentrations between 35% and 100%. Lower oxygen concentrations require modification of isoshunt lines to account for the effect of $\dot{V}/\dot{Q}$ scatter.

The effect of cardiac output on the A-a gradient (Figure 22–20) is due not only to its secondary effects on mixed venous oxygen tension (see Chapter 19), but also to a direct relationship between cardiac output and intrapulmonary shunting. As can be seen, a low cardiac output tends to accentuate the effect of shunt on PaO_2. A reduction in venous admixture is usually observed with low cardiac outputs secondary to accentuated pulmonary vasoconstriction from a lower mixed venous oxygen tension. On the other hand, high cardiac outputs can increase venous admixture by elevating mixed venous oxygen tension; the latter inhibits hypoxic pulmonary vasoconstriction.

Oxygen consumption and hemoglobin concentration can also affect PaO_2 through their secondary effects on mixed venous oxygen tension (below). High oxygen consumption rates and low hemoglobin concentrations can increase the A-a gradient and depress PaO_2.

Mixed Venous Oxygen Tension

Normal mixed venous oxygen tension ($P\bar{v}O_2$) is about 40 mm Hg and represents the overall balance between oxygen consumption and oxygen delivery (Table 22–5; see below). A true mixed venous blood sample contains venous drainage from the superior vena cava, the inferior vena cava, and the heart; it must therefore be obtained from a pulmonary artery catheter (see Chapter 6).

2. Carbon Dioxide

Carbon dioxide is a by-product of aerobic metabolism in mitochondria. There are therefore small continuous gradients for CO_2 tension from mitochondria to cell

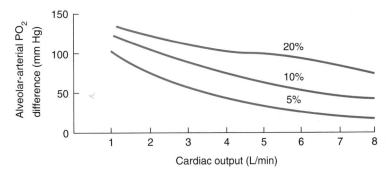

Figure 22–20. The effect of cardiac output on the alveolar-arterial PO_2 difference with varying degrees of shunting. ($\dot{V}O_2 = 200$ mL/min and $PaO_2 = 180$ mm Hg.) (Modified and reproduced, with permission, from: Nunn JF: *Applied Respiratory Physiology*, 5th ed. Lumb A (editor), Butterworth-Heinemann, 2000.)

Table 22–5. Alterations in mixed venous oxygen tension (and saturation).

Decreased $P\bar{v}O_2$
  Increased O_2 consumption
    Fever
    Shivering
    Exercise
    Malignant hyperthermia
    Thyroid storm
  Decreased O_2 delivery
    Hypoxia
    Decreased cardiac output
    Decreased hemoglobin concentration
    Abnormal hemoglobin
Increased $P\bar{v}O_2$
  Left-to-right shunting
  High cardiac output
  Impaired tissue uptake
    Cyanide poisoning
  Decreased oxygen consumption
    Hypothermia
  Combined mechanisms
    Sepsis
  Sampling error
    Wedged pulmonary artery catheter

cytoplasm, extracellular fluid, venous blood, and alveoli, where the CO_2 is finally eliminated.

Mixed Venous Carbon Dioxide Tension

Normal mixed venous CO_2 tension ($P\bar{v}CO_2$) is about 46 mm Hg and is the end result of mixing of blood from tissues of varying metabolic activity. Venous CO_2 tension is lower in tissues with low metabolic activity (eg, skin) but higher in blood from those with relatively high activity (eg, heart).

Alveolar Carbon Dioxide Tension

Alveolar CO_2 tension ($PACO_2$) is generally considered to represent the balance between total CO_2 production ($\dot{V}CO_2$) and alveolar ventilation (elimination):

$$PaCO_2 = \frac{\dot{V}CO_2}{\dot{V}A}$$

where $\dot{V}A$ is alveolar ventilation (Figure 22–21). In reality, $PACO_2$ is related to CO_2 elimination rather than production. Although the two are equal in a steady state, an imbalance occurs during periods of acute hypoventilation or hypoperfusion and the excess CO_2 increases total body CO_2 content. Clinically, $PACO_2$ is

more dependent on alveolar ventilation than is $\dot{V}CO_2$, because CO_2 output does not vary appreciably under most circumstances. Moreover, the body's large capacity to store CO_2 (see below) buffers acute changes in $\dot{V}CO_2$.

Pulmonary End-Capillary Carbon Dioxide Tension

Pulmonary end-capillary CO_2 tension ($PćCO_2$) is virtually identical to $PACO_2$ for the same reasons as those discussed in the section about oxygen. In addition, the diffusion rate for CO_2 across the alveolar-capillary membrane is 20 times that of oxygen.

Arterial Carbon Dioxide Tension

Arterial CO_2 tension ($PaCO_2$), which is readily measurable, is identical to $PćCO_2$ and, necessarily, $PACO_2$. Normal $PaCO_2$ is 38 + 4 mm Hg (5.1 + 0.5 kPa); in practice, 40 mm Hg is usually considered normal.

Although low $\dot{V}/\dot{Q}$ ratios tend to increase $PaCO_2$ while high $\dot{V}/\dot{Q}$ ratios tend to decrease it (in contrast to the case for oxygen [see above]), significant arterial-to-alveolar gradients for CO_2 develop only in the presence of marked $\dot{V}/\dot{Q}$ abnormalities (> 30% venous admixture); even then the gradient is relatively small (2–3 mm Hg). Moreover, small increases in the gradient appreciably increase CO_2 output into alveoli with relatively normal $\dot{V}/\dot{Q}$. Even moderate to severe disturbances usually fail to appreciably alter arterial CO_2 because of a reflex increase in ventilation from concomitant hypoxemia.

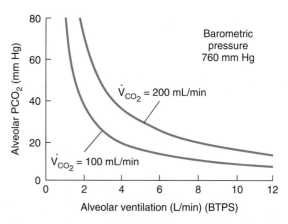

Figure 22–21. The effect of alveolar ventilation on alveolar PCO_2 at two rates of CO_2 production. (Modified and reproduced, with permission from: Nunn JF: *Applied Respiratory Physiology*, 5th ed. Lumb A (editor), Butterworth-Heinemann, 2000.)

End-Tidal Carbon Dioxide Tension

Because end-tidal gas is primarily alveolar gas and $PaCO_2$ is virtually identical to $PaCO_2$, end-tidal CO_2 tension ($PETCO_2$) is used clinically as an estimate of $PaCO_2$ (see Chapter 6). The $PaCO_2$-$PETCO_2$ gradient is normally less than 5 mm Hg and represents dilution of alveolar gas with CO_2-free gas from nonperfused alveoli (alveolar dead space).

TRANSPORT OF RESPIRATORY GASES IN BLOOD

1. Oxygen

Oxygen is carried in blood in two forms: dissolved in solution and in reversible association with hemoglobin.

Dissolved Oxygen

The amount of oxygen dissolved in blood can be derived from **Henry's law,** which states that the concentration of any gas in solution is proportional to its partial pressure. The mathematical expression is as follows:

$$\text{Gas concentration} = \alpha \times \text{Partial pressure}$$

where α = the gas solubility coefficient for a given solution at a given temperature.

The solubility coefficient for oxygen at normal body temperature is 0.003 mL/dL/mm Hg. Even with a PaO_2 of 100 mm Hg, the maximum amount of oxygen dissolved in blood is very small (0.3 mL/dL) compared with that bound to hemoglobin.

Hemoglobin

Hemoglobin is a complex large molecule consisting of four heme and four protein subunits. Heme is an iron-porphyrin compound that is an essential part of the oxygen-binding sites; only the divalent form (+2 charge) of iron can bind oxygen. The normal hemoglobin molecule (hemoglobin A_1) consists of two α and two β chains (subunits); the four subunits are held together by weak bonds between the amino acid residues. Each gram of hemoglobin can theoretically carry up to 1.39 mL of oxygen.

Hemoglobin Dissociation Curve

Each hemoglobin molecule binds up to four oxygen molecules. The complex interaction between the hemoglobin subunits results in nonlinear (an elongated S shape) binding with oxygen (Figure 22–22). Hemoglobin saturation is the amount of oxygen bound as a percentage of its total oxygen-binding capacity. Four separate chemical reactions are involved in binding each of the four oxygen molecules. The change in molecular

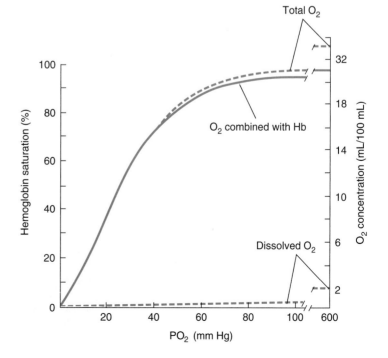

Figure 22–22. The normal adult hemoglobin-oxygen dissociation curve. (Modified with permission from: West JB: *Respiratory Physiology—The Essentials,* 3rd ed. Williams & Wilkins, 1985, p 69.)

conformation induced by the binding of the first three molecules greatly accelerates binding of the fourth oxygen molecule. The last reaction is responsible for the accelerated binding between 25% and 100% saturation. At about 90% saturation, the decrease in available oxygen receptors flattens the curve until full saturation is reached.

Factors Influencing the Hemoglobin Dissociation Curve

Clinically important factors altering oxygen binding include hydrogen ion concentration; CO_2 tension; temperature; and 2,3-diphosphoglycerate (2,3-DPG) concentration. Their effect on hemoglobin-oxygen interaction can be expressed by P_{50}, the oxygen tension at which hemoglobin is 50% saturated (Figure 22–23). Each factor shifts the dissociation curve either to the right (increasing P_{50}) or to the left (decreasing P_{50}). A rightward shift lowers oxygen affinity, displaces oxygen from hemoglobin, and makes more oxygen available to tissues; a leftward shift increases hemoglobin's affinity for oxygen, reducing its availability to tissues. The normal P_{50} in adults is 26.6 mm Hg (3.4 kPa).

An increase in blood hydrogen ion concentration reduces oxygen binding to hemoglobin (**Bohr effect**). Because of the shape of the **hemoglobin dissociation curve,** the effect is more important in venous blood than arterial blood (Figure 22–23); the net result is facilitation of oxygen release to tissue with little impairment in oxygen uptake (unless severe hypoxia is present).

The influence of CO_2 tension on hemoglobin's affinity for oxygen is important physiologically and is secondary to the associated rise in hydrogen ion concentration when CO_2 tension increases. The high CO_2 content of venous capillary blood, by decreasing hemoglobin's affinity for oxygen, facilitates the release of oxygen to tissues; conversely, the lower CO_2 content in pulmonary capillaries increases hemoglobin's affinity for oxygen again, facilitating oxygen uptake from alveoli.

2,3-DPG is a by-product of glycolysis (the Rapoport-Luebering shunt) and accumulates during anaerobic metabolism. Although its effects on hemoglobin under these conditions are theoretically beneficial, its physiologic importance normally appears minor. 2,3-DPG levels may, however, play an important compensatory role in patients with chronic anemia

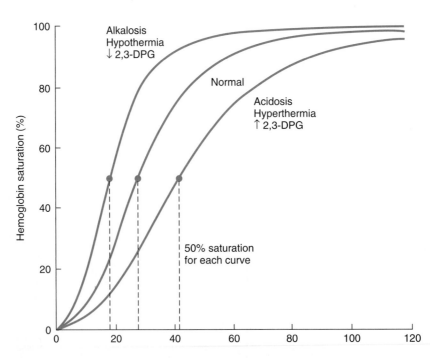

Figure 22–23. The effects of changes in acid-base status, body temperature, and 2,3-DPG concentration on the hemoglobin-oxygen dissociation curve.

and may significantly affect the oxygen-carrying capacity of blood transfusions (see Chapter 29).

Abnormal Ligands & Abnormal Forms of Hemoglobins

Carbon monoxide, cyanide, nitric acid, and ammonia can combine with hemoglobin at oxygen-binding sites. They can displace oxygen and shift the saturation curve to the left. Carbon monoxide is especially potent, having 200–300 times the affinity of oxygen for hemoglobin, combining with it to form carboxyhemoglobin. Carbon monoxide decreases hemoglobin's oxygen-carrying capacity and impairs the release of oxygen to tissues.

Methemoglobin results when the iron in heme is oxidized to its trivalent (+3) form. Nitrates, nitrites, sulfonamides, and other drugs can rarely result in significant methemoglobinemia. Methemoglobin cannot combine with oxygen unless reconverted by the enzyme methemoglobin reductase; methemoglobin also shifts the normal hemoglobin saturation curve to the left. Methemoglobinemia, like carbon monoxide poisoning, therefore decreases the oxygen-carrying capacity as well as impairing the release of oxygen. Reduction of methemoglobin to normal hemoglobin is facilitated by such agents as methylene blue or ascorbic acid.

Abnormal hemoglobins can also result from variations in the protein subunit composition. Each variant has its own oxygen-saturation characteristics. These include fetal hemoglobin, hemoglobin A_2, and sickle hemoglobin (see Chapter 29).

Oxygen Content

The total oxygen content of blood is the sum of that in solution plus that carried by hemoglobin. In reality, oxygen binding to hemoglobin never achieves the theoretical maximum (see above) but is closer to 1.31 mL O_2/dL blood/mm Hg. Total oxygen content is expressed by the following equation:

$$\text{Oxygen content} = ([0.003 \text{ mL } O_2/\text{dL blood/mm Hg}] \times PO_2) + (SO_2 \times Hb \times 1.31 \text{ mL/dL blood})$$

where Hb is hemoglobin concentration in g/dL blood and SO_2 is hemoglobin saturation at the given PO_2.

Using the above formula and a hemoglobin of 15 g/dL, the normal oxygen content for both arterial and mixed venous blood and the arteriovenous difference can be calculated:

$$CaO_2 = (0.003 \times 100) + (0.975 \times 15 \times 1.31)$$
$$= 19.5 \text{ mL/dL blood}$$
$$C\bar{v}O_2 = (0.003 \times 40) + (0.75 \times 15 \times 1.31)$$
$$= 14.8 \text{ mL/dL blood}$$
$$(CaO_2 - C\bar{v}O_2) = 4.7 \text{ mL/dL blood}$$

Oxygen Transport

Oxygen transport is dependent on both respiratory and circulatory function (see Chapter 19). Total oxygen delivery ($\dot{D}O_2$) to tissues is the product of arterial oxygen content and cardiac output:

$$\dot{D}O_2 = CaO_2 \times \dot{Q}T$$

Note that arterial oxygen content is dependent on PaO_2 as well as hemoglobin concentration. As a result, deficiencies in oxygen delivery may be due to a low PaO_2, a low hemoglobin concentration, or an inadequate cardiac output. Normal oxygen delivery can be calculated as follows:

$$\text{Oxygen delivery} = 20 \text{ mL } O_2/\text{dL blood} \times 50 \text{ dL/min} = 1000 \text{ mL } O_2/\text{min}$$

The **Fick equation** expresses the relationship between oxygen consumption, oxygen content, and cardiac output:

$$\text{Oxygen consumption} = \dot{V}O_2 = \dot{Q}T \times (CaO_2 - C\bar{v}O_2)$$

Rearranging the equation:

$$CaO_2 = \frac{\dot{V}O_2}{\dot{Q}T} + C\bar{v}O_2$$

Consequently, the arteriovenous difference is a good measure of the overall adequacy of oxygen delivery.

With a normal oxygen consumption of approximately 250 mL/min and a cardiac output of 5000 mL/min, the normal arteriovenous difference by this equation again calculates to be about 5 mL O_2/dL blood. Note that the normal extraction fraction for oxygen $[(CaO_2 - C\bar{v}O_2)/CaO_2]$ is 5 mL ÷ 20 mL, or 25%; thus, the body normally consumes only 25% of the oxygen carried on hemoglobin. When oxygen demand exceeds supply, the extraction fraction exceeds 25%. Conversely, if oxygen supply exceeds demand, the extraction fraction falls below 25%.

When $\dot{D}O_2$ is even moderately reduced, $\dot{V}O_2$ usually remains normal because of increased oxygen extraction (mixed venous oxygen saturation decreases); $\dot{V}O_2$ remains independent of delivery. With further reductions in $\dot{D}O_2$, however, a critical point is reached beyond which $\dot{V}O_2$ becomes directly proportional to $\dot{D}O_2$. This state of supply-dependent oxygen is typically associated with progressive lactic acidosis (see Chapter 30) caused by cellular hypoxia.

Oxygen Stores

The concept of oxygen stores is important in anesthesia. When the normal flux of oxygen is interrupted by apnea, existing oxygen stores are consumed by cellular metabolism; if stores are depleted, hypoxia and eventual cell death follow. Theoretically, normal oxygen stores in adults are about 1500 mL. This amount includes the oxygen remaining in the lungs, that bound to hemoglobin (and myoglobin), and that dissolved in body fluids. Unfortunately, hemoglobin's high affinity for oxygen (myoglobin's affinity is even higher) and the very limited quantity of oxygen in solution restrict the availability of these stores. The oxygen contained within the lungs at FRC (initial lung volume during apnea), therefore, becomes the most important source of oxygen. Of that volume, however, probably only 80% is usable.

Apnea in a patient previously breathing room air leaves approximately 480 mL of oxygen in the lungs. (If FIO_2 = 0.21 and FRC = 2300 mL, oxygen content = FIO_2 × FRC.) The metabolic activity of tissues rapidly depletes this reservoir (presumably at a rate equivalent to $\dot{V}O_2$); severe hypoxemia usually occurs within 90 seconds. The onset of hypoxemia can be delayed by increasing the FIO_2 prior to the apnea. Following ventila-

tion with 100% O_2, FRC contains about 2300 mL of oxygen; this delays hypoxemia following apnea for 4–5 minutes. This concept is the basis for preoxygenation prior to induction of anesthesia (see Chapter 5).

2. Carbon Dioxide

Carbon dioxide is transported in blood in three forms: dissolved in solution, as bicarbonate, and with proteins in the form of carbamino compounds (see Table 22–6). The sum of all three forms is the total CO_2 content of blood (routinely reported with electrolyte measurements).

Dissolved Carbon Dioxide

Carbon dioxide is more soluble in blood than oxygen, with a solubility coefficient of 0.031 mmol/L/mm Hg (0.067 mL/dL/mm Hg) at 37 °C.

Bicarbonate

In aqueous solutions, CO_2 slowly combines with water to form carbonic acid and bicarbonate, according to the following reaction:

$$H_2O + CO_2 \leftrightarrow H_2CO_3 \leftrightarrow H^+ + HCO_3^-$$

In plasma, although less than 1% of the dissolved CO_2 undergoes this reaction, the presence of the enzyme carbonic anhydrase within erythrocytes and endothe-

Table 22–6. Contributions to carbon dioxide transport in 1 L of whole blood.

Form	Plasma	Erythrocytes	Combined	Contribution (%)
Mixed venous whole blood				
Dissolved CO_2	0.76	0.51	1.27	5.5
Bicarbonate	14.41	5.92	20.33	87.2
Carbamino CO_2	Negligible	1.70	1.70	7.3
Total CO_2	15.17	8.13	23.30	
Arterial whole blood				
Dissolved CO_2	0.66	0.44	1.10	5.1
Bicarbonate	13.42	5.88	19.30	89.9
Carbamino CO_2	Negligible	1.10	1.10	5.1
Total CO_2	14.08	7.42	21.50	

Values are expressed in mmol, except where indicated otherwise. (Modified with permission from: Nunn JF: *Applied Respiratory Physiology*, 5th ed. Lumb A. (editor), Butterworth-Heinemann, 2000.)

lium greatly accelerates the reaction. As a result, bicarbonate represents the largest fraction of the CO_2 in blood (Table 22–6). Administration of acetazolamide, a carbonic anhydrase inhibitor, can impair CO_2 transport between tissues and alveoli.

On the venous side of systemic capillaries, CO_2 enters red blood cells and is converted to bicarbonate, which diffuses out of red cells into plasma; chloride ions move from plasma into red cells to maintain electrical balance. In the pulmonary capillaries, the reverse occurs: chloride ions move out of red cells as bicarbonate ions reenter them for conversion back to CO_2, which diffuses out into alveoli. This sequence is referred to as the **chloride** or **Hamburger shift.**

Carbamino Compounds

Carbon dioxide can react with amino groups on proteins as shown by the following equation:

$$R\text{-}NH_2 + CO_2 \rightarrow RNH - CO_2^- + H^+$$

At physiologic pH, only a small amount of CO_2 is carried in this form, mainly as carbamino-hemoglobin. Deoxygenated hemoglobin (deoxyhemoglobin) has a greater affinity (3.5 times) for CO_2 than does oxyhemoglobin. As a result, venous blood carries more CO_2 than arterial blood does (**Haldane effect;** see Table 22–6). PCO_2 normally has little effect on the fraction of CO_2 carried as carbamino-hemoglobin.

Effects of Hemoglobin Buffering on Carbon Dioxide Transport

The buffering action of hemoglobin (see Chapter 30) also accounts for part of the Haldane effect. Hemoglobin can act as a buffer at physiologic pH because of its high content of histidine. Moreover, the acid-base behavior of hemoglobin is influenced by its oxygenation state:

$$H^+ + HbO_2 \rightarrow HbH^+ + O_2$$

Removal of oxygen from hemoglobin in tissue capillaries causes the hemoglobin molecule to behave more like a base; by taking up hydrogen ions, hemoglobin shifts the CO_2-bicarbonate equilibrium in favor of greater bicarbonate formation:

$$CO_2 + H_2O + HbO_2 \rightarrow HbH^+ + HCO_3^- + O_2$$

As a direct result, deoxyhemoglobin also increases the amount of CO_2 that is carried in venous blood as bicarbonate. As CO_2 is taken up from tissue and converted to bicarbonate, the total CO_2 content of blood increases (Table 22–6).

In the lungs, the reverse is true. Oxygenation of hemoglobin favors its action as an acid, and the release of hydrogen ions shifts the equilibrium in favor of greater CO_2 formation:

$$O_2 + HCO_3^- + HbH^+ \rightarrow H_2O + CO_2 + HbO_2$$

Bicarbonate concentration decreases as CO_2 is formed and eliminated, so that the total CO_2 content of blood decreases in the lungs. Note that there is a difference between CO_2 content (concentration per liter) of whole blood (Table 22–6) and plasma (Table 22–7).

Carbon Dioxide Dissociation Curve

A CO_2 dissociation curve can be constructed by plotting the total CO_2 content of blood against PCO_2. The contribution of each form of CO_2 can also be quantified in this manner (Figure 22–24).

Carbon Dioxide Stores

Carbon dioxide stores in the body are large (approximately 120 L in adults) and primarily in the form of dissolved CO_2 and bicarbonate. When an imbalance occurs between production and elimination, establishing a new CO_2 equilibrium requires 20–30 minutes (compared with less than 4–5 minutes for oxygen; see above). Carbon dioxide stores may be classified as rapid, intermediate, and slow equilibrating compartments. Because of the larger capacity of the intermediate and slow compartments, the rate of rise in arterial CO_2 tension is generally slower than its fall following acute changes in ventilation.

CONTROL OF BREATHING

Spontaneous ventilation is the result of rhythmic neural activity in respiratory centers within the brain-

Table 22–7. Carbon dioxide content of plasma (mmol/L).

	Arterial	Venous
Dissolved CO_2	1.2	1.4
Bicarbonate	24.4	26.2
Carbamino CO_2	Negligible	Negligible
Total CO_2	25.6	27.6

Values are expressed in mmol, except where indicated otherwise. (Modified with permission from: Nunn JF: *Applied Respiratory Physiology*, 5th ed. Lumb A (editor), Butterworth-Heinemann, 2000.)

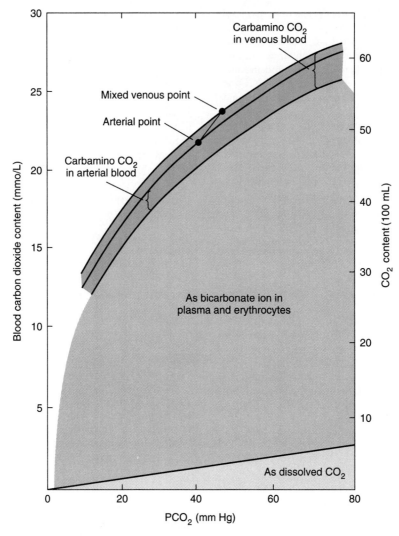

Figure 22–24. The CO_2 dissociation curve for whole blood. (Reproduced, with permission from: Nunn JF: *Applied Respiratory Physiology,* 5th ed. Lumb A (editor), Butterworth-Heinemann, 2000.)

stem. This activity regulates respiratory muscles to maintain normal tensions of oxygen and CO_2 in the body. The basic neuronal activity is modified by inputs from other areas in the brain, volitional and autonomic, as well as various central and peripheral receptors (sensors).

1. Central Respiratory Centers

The basic respiratory rhythm originates in the medulla. Two medullary groups of neurons are generally recognized: a dorsal respiratory group, which is primarily ac-

tive during inspiration; and a ventral respiratory group, which is active during expiration. Although not firmly established, the origin of the basic rhythm is due to either intrinsic spontaneous discharge activity in the dorsal group or reciprocating activity between the dorsal and ventral groups. The close association of the dorsal respiratory group of neurons with the tractus solitarius may explain reflex changes in breathing from vagal or glossopharyngeal nerve stimulation.

Two pontine areas influence the dorsal (inspiratory) medullary center. A lower pontine (apneustic) center is excitatory, while an upper pontine (pneumotaxic) center is inhibitory. The pontine centers appear to fine-tune respiratory rate and rhythm.

2. Central Sensors

The most important of these sensors are chemoreceptors that respond to changes in hydrogen ion concentration. Central chemoreceptors are thought to lie on the anterolateral surface of the medulla and respond primarily to changes in cerebrospinal fluid $[H^+]$. This mechanism is effective in regulating $PaCO_2$, because the blood-brain barrier (see Chapter 25) is permeable to dissolved CO_2 but not to bicarbonate ions. Acute changes in $PaCO_2$ but not in arterial $[HCO_3^-]$ are reflected in cerebrospinal fluid (CSF); thus, a change in CO_2 must result in a change in $[H^+]$:

$$CO_2 + H_2O \leftrightarrow H^+ + HCO_3^-$$

Over the course of a few days, cerebrospinal fluid $[HCO_3^-]$ can compensate to match any change in arterial $[HCO_3^-]$.

Increases in $PaCO_2$ elevate CSF hydrogen ion concentration and activate the chemoreceptors. Secondary stimulation of the adjacent respiratory medullary centers increases alveolar ventilation (Figure 22–25) and reduces $PaCO_2$ back to normal. Conversely, decreases in CSF hydrogen ion concentration secondary to reductions in $PaCO_2$ reduce alveolar ventilation and elevate $PaCO_2$. Note that the relationship between $PaCO_2$ and minute volume is nearly linear. Also note that very high arterial $PaCO_2$ tensions depress the ventilatory response (CO_2 narcosis). The $PaCO_2$ at which ventilation is zero (*x*-intercept) is known as the **apneic threshold.** Spontaneous respirations are typically absent under anesthesia when $PaCO_2$ falls below the apneic threshold. (In the awake state, cortical influences prevent apnea, so apneic thresholds are not ordinarily seen.) In contrast to peripheral chemoreceptors (see below), central chemoreceptor activity is depressed by hypoxia.

3. Peripheral Sensors

Peripheral Chemoreceptors

Peripheral chemoreceptors include the carotid bodies (at the bifurcation of the common carotid arteries) and the aortic bodies (surrounding the aortic arch). The carotid bodies are the principal peripheral chemoreceptors in humans and are sensitive to changes in PaO_2, $PaCO_2$, pH, and arterial perfusion pressure. They interact with central respiratory centers via the glossopharyngeal nerves, producing reflex increases in alveolar

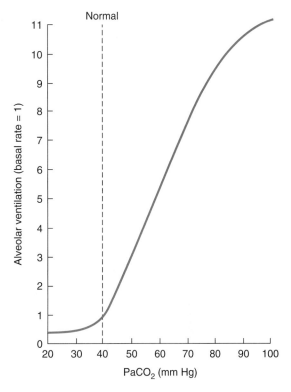

Figure 22–25. The relationship between $PaCO_2$ and minute ventilation. (Reproduced, with permission from: Guyton AC: *Textbook of Medical Physiology*, 7th ed. WB Saunders and Company, 1986, p 508.)

ventilation in response to reductions in PaO_2, arterial perfusion or elevations in $[H^+]$ and $PaCO_2$. Peripheral chemoreceptors are also stimulated by cyanide, doxapram, and large doses of nicotine. In contrast to central chemoreceptors, which respond primarily to $PaCO_2$ (really $[H^+]$), the carotid bodies are most sensitive to PaO_2 (Figure 22–26). Note that receptor activity does not appreciably increase until PaO_2 decreases below 50 mm Hg. Cells of the carotid body (glomus cells) are thought to be primarily dopaminergic neurons. Antidopaminergic drugs (such as phenothiazines), most commonly used anesthetics, and bilateral carotid surgery abolish the peripheral ventilatory response to hypoxemia.

Lung Receptors

Impulses from these receptors are carried centrally by the vagus nerve. Stretch receptors are distributed in the smooth muscle of airways; they are responsible for inhibition of inspiration when the lung is inflated to exces-

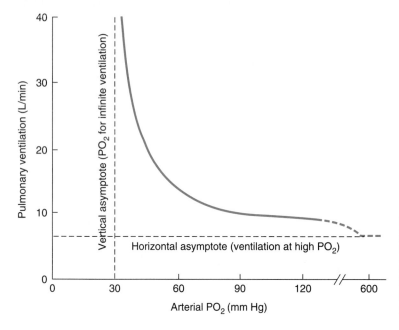

Figure 22–26. The relationship between PaO$_2$ and minute ventilation at rest and with a normal PaO$_2$. (Reproduced, with permission from: Nunn JF: *Applied Respiratory Physiology,* 5th ed. Lumb A (editor), Butterworth-Heinemann, 2000.)

sive volumes (**Hering-Breuer inflation reflex**) and shortening of exhalation when the lung is deflated (**deflation reflex**). Stretch receptors normally play a minor role in humans. In fact, bilateral vagal nerve blocks have a minimal effect on the normal respiratory pattern.

Irritant receptors in the tracheobronchial mucosa react to noxious gases, smoke, dust, and cold gases; activation produces reflex increases in respiratory rate, bronchoconstriction, and coughing. J (juxtacapillary) receptors are located in the interstitial space within alveolar walls; these receptors induce dyspnea in response to expansion of interstitial space volume and various chemical mediators following tissue damage.

Other Receptors

These include various muscle and joint receptors on respiratory muscles and the chest wall. Input from these sources is probably important during exercise and in pathologic conditions associated with decreased lung or chest compliance.

4. Effects of Anesthesia on the Control of Breathing

The most important effect of most general anesthetics on breathing is a tendency to promote hypoventilation. The mechanism is probably dual: central depression of the chemoreceptor, and depression of external intercostal muscle activity. The magnitude of the hypoventilation is generally proportional to anesthetic depth. 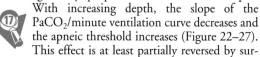 With increasing depth, the slope of the PaCO$_2$/minute ventilation curve decreases and the apneic threshold increases (Figure 22–27). This effect is at least partially reversed by surgical stimulation.

The peripheral response to hypoxemia is even more sensitive to anesthetics than the central CO$_2$ response and is nearly abolished by even subanesthetic doses of most inhalational agents (including nitrous oxide) and many intravenous agents. Anesthetic agents may also impair the peripheral stimulatory response of doxapram, but its central actions appear to be preserved (see Chapter 15). The respiratory effects of individual agents are discussed in Chapters 7 and 8.

NONRESPIRATORY FUNCTIONS OF THE LUNG

Filtration & Reservoir Function

A. FILTRATION:

The unique in-series position of the pulmonary capillaries within the circulation allows them to act as a filter for debris in the bloodstream. The lungs' high content of heparin and plasminogen activator facilitates the breakdown of entrapped fibrin debris. Although pulmonary capillaries have an average diameter of 7 μm,

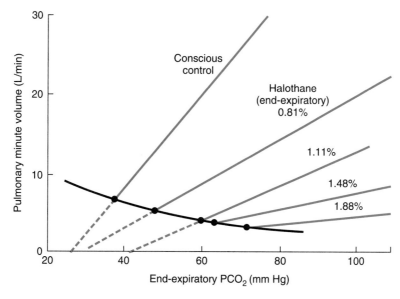

Figure 22–27. The effect of volatile agents (halothane) on the PetCO$_2$-ventilation response curve (see text). (Modified and reproduced, with permission from: Nunn JF: *Applied Respiratory Physiology*, 5th ed. Lumb A (editor), Butterworth-Heinemann, 2000.)

larger particles have been shown to pass through to the left heart.

B. Reservoir Function:

The role of the pulmonary circulation as a reservoir for the systemic circulation was discussed above.

Metabolism

The lungs are metabolically very active organs. In addition to surfactant synthesis, pneumocytes account for a major portion of extrahepatic mixed-function oxidation. Neutrophils and macrophages in the lung produce oxygen-derived free radicals in response to infection (and systemic inflammatory responses; see Chapter 50). The pulmonary endothelium metabolizes a variety of vasoactive compounds, including norepinephrine, serotonin, bradykinin, and a variety of prostaglandins and leukotrienes. Histamine and epinephrine are generally not metabolized in the lungs; in fact the lungs can be a major site of histamine synthesis and release during allergic reactions.

The lungs are also responsible for converting angiotensin I to its physiologically active form, angiotensin II. The enzyme responsible, angiotensin-converting enzyme, is bound on the surface of the pulmonary endothelium.

CASE DISCUSSION: UNILATERALLY DIMINISHED BREATH SOUNDS DURING GENERAL ANESTHESIA

A 67-year-old man with carcinoma is undergoing colon resection under general anesthesia. His history includes an old anterior myocardial infarction and compensated congestive heart failure. Arterial and pulmonary artery catheters are placed preoperatively for monitoring during surgery. Following a smooth thiopental-fentanyl induction and an atraumatic intubation with succinylcholine, anesthesia is maintained with 60% nitrous oxide in oxygen, isoflurane, and vecuronium. One-half hour into the operation, the surgeon asks for the Trendelenburg position to facilitate surgical exposure. The pulse oximeter, which had been reading 99% saturation, suddenly drops and remains at 93%. The pulse oximeter's signal strength and waveform are unchanged. Auscultation of the lungs reveals diminished breath sounds over the left lung.

What is the most likely explanation?

Unilaterally diminished breath sounds under anesthesia are most commonly caused by inad-

vertent placement or migration of the endotracheal tube into one of the two main bronchi. As a result, only one lung is ventilated. Other causes of unilaterally diminished breath sounds (such as pneumothorax, a large mucus plug, lobar atelectasis, or an undiagnosed mediastinal mass) are less easily diagnosed but are fortunately less common during anesthesia.

The Trendelenburg (head-down) position typically causes the tip of the endotracheal tube to advance 1–2 cm relative to the carina. In this case, the tube was apparently placed just above the carina with the patient in the supine position but migrated into the right bronchus when the Trendelenburg position was imposed. The diagnosis is confirmed by drawing the tube back 1–2 cm at a time while the chest is auscultated. Breath sounds will become equal again when the tip of the tube reenters the trachea. Following initial placement, endotracheal tubes should be routinely checked for correct positioning by auscultating the chest, ascertaining depth of tube insertion by the markings on the tube (normally 20–24 cm at the teeth for an adult), and feeling for the cuff in the suprasternal notch. Tube position can also be quickly confirmed with a flexible fiberoptic bronchoscope.

Are endotracheal tubes just as likely to enter either main bronchus?

In most cases of unintentional endobronchial intubation, the endotracheal tube enters the right bronchus because the latter diverges away from the trachea at a less acute angle than does the left bronchus (see Chapter 24).

Why did hemoglobin saturation decrease?

Failure to ventilate one lung while it continues to be perfused creates a large intrapulmonary shunt. Venous admixture increases and tends to depress PaO_2 and hemoglobin saturation.

Does a saturation of 93% exclude endobronchial intubation?

No; if both lungs continued to have equal blood flow, venous admixture should have theoretically increased to 50%, resulting in severe hypoxemia and very low hemoglobin saturation. Fortunately, hypoxic pulmonary vasoconstriction is a powerful compensatory response that tends to reduce flow to the hypoxic lung and reduces the expected venous admixture. In fact, if the patient has

been receiving a higher inspired oxygen concentration (50–100%), the drop in arterial tension may not be detectable by the pulse oximeter owing to the characteristics of the normal hemoglobin saturation curve. For example, endobronchial intubation in a patient inspiring 50% oxygen might drop PaO_2 from 250 mm Hg to 95 mm Hg; the resulting change in pulse oximeter readings (100–99 to 98–97) would hardly be noticeable.

Arterial and mixed venous blood gas tensions are obtained with the following results:

PaO_2 = 69 mm Hg; $PaCO_2$ = 42 mm Hg; SaO_2 = 93%; $P\bar{v}O_2$ = 40 mm Hg; and $S\bar{v}O_2$ = 75%. Hemoglobin concentration is 15 g/dL.

What is the calculated venous admixture?

In this case, $Pc'O_2 = PaO_2 = ([760 – 47] \times 0.4) – 42 = 243$ mm Hg. Therefore, $Cc'O_2 = (15 \times 1.31 \times 1.0) + (243 \times 0.003) = 20.4$ mL/dL.
$CaO_2 = (15 \times 1.31 \times 0.93) + (69 \times 0.003) = 18.5$ mL/dL
$C\bar{v}O_2 = (15 \times 1.31 \times 0.75) + (40 \times 0.003) = 14.8$ mL/dL
$\dot{Q}s/\dot{Q}T = (20.4 – 18.5) / (20.4 – 14.8) = 32\%$

How does endobronchial intubation affect arterial and end-tidal O_2 tensions?

$PaCO_2$ is typically not appreciably altered as long as the same minute ventilation is maintained (see One-Lung Anesthesia, Chapter 24). Clinically, the $PaCO_2$–$P_{ET}CO_2$ gradient often widens, possibly because of increased alveolar dead space (overdistension of the ventilated lung). Thus, $P_{ET}CO_2$ may decrease or remain unchanged.

SUGGESTED READING

Ganong WF: *Review of Medical Physiology*, 20th ed. McGraw-Hill, 2001.

Guyton AC: *Textbook of Medical Physiology*, 10th ed. WB Saunders and Company, 2000.

Nunn JF: *Applied Respiratory Physiology*, 5th ed. Lumb A (editor), Butterworth-Heinemann, 2000.

West JB: *Respiratory Physiology—The Essentials*, 6th ed. Lippincott Williams & Wilkins, 2000.

Anesthesia for Patients with Respiratory Disease

23

KEY CONCEPTS

 In a patient with an acute asthma attack, a normal or high $PaCO_2$ indicates that the patient can no longer maintain the work of breathing and is often a sign of impending respiratory failure. A pulsus paradoxus and electrocardiographic signs of right ventricular strain (ST-segment changes, right-axis deviation, and right bundle branch block) are also indicative of severe airway obstruction.

 Whenever possible, patients who have asthma with active bronchospasm who are presenting for emergency surgery should undergo intensive treatment. Supplemental oxygen, aerosolized β_2-agonists, and intravenous glucocorticoids can dramatically improve lung function in a few hours.

 Intraoperative bronchospasm is usually manifested as wheezing, increasing peak inflation pressures (plateau pressure should remain unchanged), decreasing exhaled tidal volumes, or a slowly rising waveform on the capnograph.

 If wheezing does not resolve after deepening the anesthetic, other causes should be considered before starting other drug therapy. Obstruction of the endotracheal tube from kinking, secretions, or an overinflated balloon; endobronchial intubation; active expiratory efforts (straining) because of light anesthesia; pulmonary edema or embolism; and pneumothorax can all simulate bronchospasm.

 In patients with chronic obstructive pulmonary disease, chronic hypoxemia leads to erythrocytosis, pulmonary hypertension, and eventually right ventricular failure (cor pulmonale).

 Oxygen therapy can dangerously elevate $PaCO_2$ in patients with CO_2 retention; elevating PaO_2 above 60 mm Hg can precipitate respiratory failure in these patients.

 Preoperative interventions aimed at correcting hypoxemia, relieving bronchospasm, mobilizing and reducing secretions, and treating infections may decrease the incidence of postoperative pulmonary complications in patients with chronic obstructive pulmonary disease. Patients at greatest risk for complications are those with preoperative pulmonary function measurements less than 50% of predicted.

 In restrictive pulmonary diseases, lung volumes are reduced, with preservation of normal expiratory flow rates. Thus, both forced expiratory volume in 1 second (FEV_1) and forced vital capacity (FVC) are reduced, but the FEV_1/FVC ratio is normal.

 Intraoperative pulmonary embolism usually presents as unexplained sudden hypotension, hypoxemia, or bronchospasm. A decrease in end-tidal CO_2 concentration is also suggestive but not specific.

The impact of preexisting pulmonary disease on respiratory function during anesthesia and in the postoperative period is predictable: Greater degrees of preoperative pulmonary impairment are associated with more marked intraoperative alterations in respiratory function (see Chapter 22) and higher rates of postoperative pulmonary complications. Failure to recognize patients who are at increased risk is a frequent contributory factor. This chapter examines pulmonary risk in general and then reviews the anesthetic approach to patients with the most common types of respiratory disease.

PULMONARY RISK FACTORS

Pulmonary dysfunction is the most common postoperative complication. The incidence of **atelectasis, pneumonia,** pulmonary embolism, and respiratory failure following surgery varies widely (from 6% to 60%) depending on the patient population studied and the surgical procedures performed. Six risk factors are generally cited (Table 23–1). With the exception of the operative site and the duration of the procedure, most appear related to preoperative pulmonary dysfunction. The two strongest predictors of complications appear to be operative site and a history of dyspnea, which correlates with the degree of preexisting pulmonary disease. The least consistent factor is the duration of surgery.

The association between smoking and respiratory disease is well established; abnormalities in maximal midexpiratory flow (MMEF) rates are often demonstrable well before symptoms of chronic obstructive pulmonary disease (COPD) appear. Even in normal individuals, advancing age is associated with an increasing prevalence of pulmonary disease and an increase in closing capacity. Obesity decreases functional residual capacity (FRC), increases the work of breathing, and predisposes patients to deep venous thrombosis.

Thoracic and upper abdominal surgical procedures can have marked effects on pulmonary function. Operations near the diaphragm often result in diaphragmatic dysfunction and a restrictive ventilatory defect (see below). Upper abdominal procedures consistently decrease FRC (60–70%); the effect is maximal on the first postoperative day and usually lasts 7–10 days. Vertical incisions produce greater impairment than do horizontal incisions. Rapid shallow breathing with an ineffective cough caused by pain (splinting), a decrease in the number of sighs, and impaired mucociliary clearance lead to microatelectasis and loss of lung volume. Intrapulmonary shunting promotes hypoxemia (see Chapter 22). Residual anesthetic effects, the recumbent position, sedation from opioids, abdominal distention, and restrictive dressings may also be contributory. Complete relief of pain with regional anesthesia can lessen but does not completely reverse these abnormalities. Persistent microatelectasis and retention of secretions favor the development of postoperative pneumonia.

While many adverse effects of general anesthesia on pulmonary function are described (see Chapter 22), the superiority of regional over general anesthesia for patients with pulmonary impairment is not firmly established.

■ OBSTRUCTIVE PULMONARY DISEASE

Obstructive lung diseases are the most common form of pulmonary dysfunction. They include asthma, emphysema, chronic bronchitis, cystic fibrosis, bronchiectasis, and bronchiolitis. The hallmark of these disorders is resistance to airflow. Characteristically, both forced expiratory volume in 1 second (FEV_1) and the FEV_1/FVC (forced vital capacity) ratio are less than 70% of the predicted values. An MMEF of < 70% (forced expiratory flow [$FEF_{25-75\%}$]; see Chapter 22) is often the only abnormality early in the course of these disorders. Values for $FEF_{25-75\%}$ in adult males and females are normally > 2.0 and > 1.6 L/sec, respectively.

Elevated airway resistance and air trapping increases the work of breathing; respiratory gas exchange is impaired because of ventilation/perfusion ($\dot{V}/\dot{Q}$) imbalance. The predominance of expiratory airflow resistance results in air trapping; residual volume and total lung capacity (TLC) increase. Wheezing is a common finding and represents turbulent airflow. It is often absent with mild obstruction that may be manifested initially only by prolonged exhalation. Progressive obstruction typically results first in expiratory wheezing only, and then in both inspiratory and expiratory wheezing. With marked obstruction, wheezing may be absent when airflow has nearly ceased.

Table 23–1. Risk factors for postoperative pulmonary complications.

Preexisting pulmonary disease
Thoracic or upper abdominal surgery
Smoking
Obesity
Age (> 60 years)
Prolonged general anesthesia (> 3 hours)

ASTHMA

Preoperative Considerations

Asthma is a common disorder affecting 5–7% of the population. Its hallmark is airway (bronchiolar) inflammation and hyperreactivity in response to a variety of stimuli. Clinically, asthma is manifested by episodic attacks of dyspnea, cough, and wheezing. Airway obstruction, which is generally reversible, is the result of bronchial smooth muscle constriction, edema, and increased secretions. Classically, the obstruction is precipitated by a variety of airborne substances, including pollens, animal danders, dusts, pollutants, and various chemicals. Some patients also develop bronchospasm following ingestion of aspirin, nonsteroidal anti-inflammatory agents, sulfiting agents, or tartrazine and other dyes. Exercise, emotional excitement, and viral infections also precipitate bronchospasm in many patients.

The terms **extrinsic (allergic) asthma** (attacks related to environmental exposures) and **intrinsic (idiosyncratic) asthma** (attacks usually occur without provocation) were used in the past but these classifications were imperfect; many patients show features of both forms. Moreover, overlap with chronic bronchitis (see below) also occurs. Asthma is now classified as **acute** or **chronic.** The latter is further classified as mild intermittent and mild, moderate, and severe persistent disease.

PATHOPHYSIOLOGY:

The pathophysiology of asthma involves the local release of various chemical mediators in the airway, and possibly overactivity of the parasympathetic nervous system. Inhaled substances can initiate bronchospasm through both specific and nonspecific immune mechanisms by degranulating bronchial mast cells. In classic allergic asthma, antigen binding to IgE on the surface of mast cells causes degranulation; bronchoconstriction is the result of the subsequent release of histamine; bradykinin; leukotrienes C, D, and E; platelet-activating factor; prostaglandins (PG) PGE_2, $PGF_{2\alpha}$, and PGD_2; and neutrophil and eosinophil chemotactic factors. The role of serotonin, a potent bronchoconstrictor, is uncertain in humans. The parasympathetic nervous system plays a major role in maintaining normal bronchial tone (see Chapter 22); a normal diurnal variation in tone is recognized with peak airway resistance at about 6:00 AM. Vagal afferents in the bronchi are sensitive to histamine and multiple noxious stimuli, including cold air, inhaled irritants, and instrumentation (eg, endotracheal intubation). Reflex vagal activation results in bronchoconstriction, which is mediated by an increase in intracellular cyclic guanosine monophosphate (cGMP).

During an asthma attack, bronchoconstriction, mucosal edema, and secretions increase resistance to gas flow at all levels of the lower airways. As an attack resolves, airway resistance normalizes first in the larger airways (main-stem, lobar, segmental and subsegmental bronchi), and then in more peripheral airways. Consequently, expiratory flow rates are initially decreased throughout a forced vital capacity procedure but during resolution of the attack the expiratory flow rate is reduced only at low lung volumes. TLC, residual volume (RV), and FRC are all increased. In acutely ill patients, RV and FRC are often increased by more than 400% and 100%, respectively. Prolonged or severe attacks markedly increase the work of breathing and can fatigue respiratory muscles. The number of alveolar units with low V/Q ratios increases, resulting in hypoxemia. Tachypnea is likely due to stimulation of bronchial receptors and typically produces hypocapnia (see Chapter 22). A normal or high $PaCO_2$ indicates that the patient can no longer maintain the work of breathing and is often a sign of impending respiratory failure. A pulsus paradoxus (see Chapter 21) and electrocardiographic signs of right ventricular strain (ST-segment changes, right-axis deviation, and right bundle branch block) are also indicative of severe airway obstruction.

TREATMENT:

Drugs used to treat asthma include **β-adrenergic agonists,** methylxanthines, **glucocorticoids,** anticholinergics, leukotriene blockers, and mast cell stabilizing agents; with the exception of the last, these drugs may be used for either acute or chronic treatment of asthma. Cromolyn sodium and nedocromil are effective only for preventing bronchospasm in patients with extrinsic asthma and in some with intrinsic asthma. Although devoid of any bronchodilating properties, both agents block the degranulation of mast cells.

Sympathomimetic agents (Table 23–2) are the most useful and most commonly used agents. They produce bronchodilation via β₂-agonist activity. Activation of β₂-adrenergic receptors on bronchiolar smooth muscle in turn activates adenylate cyclase, which results in the formation of intracellular cyclic adenosine monophosphate (cAMP). These agents are usually administered via a metered-dose inhaler or by aerosol. Use of more selective β₂-agonists, such as terbutaline or albuterol, may decrease the incidence of undesirable β₁ cardiac effects but are often not that selective in high doses.

Methylxanthines traditionally are thought to produce bronchodilation by inhibiting phosphodiesterase, the enzyme responsible for the breakdown of cAMP. Their pulmonary effects appear much more complex and include catecholamine release, blockade of histamine release, and diaphragmatic stimulation. Oral

Table 23–2. A comparison of commonly used bronchodilators.

Agent	Adrenergic Activity	
	β_1	β_2
Albuterol (Ventolin)	+	—
Bitolterol (Tornalate)	+	++++
Epinephrine (Various)	++++	++
Isoetharine (Bronkosol)	++	+++
Isoproterenol (Isuprel)	++++	—
Metaproterenol (Alupent)	+	+
Pirbuterol (Maxair)	+	++++
Salmeterol (Serevent)	+	++++
Terbutaline (Brethaire)	+	+++

+ Indicates level of activity.

long-acting theophylline preparations are used for patients with nocturnal symptoms. Unfortunately, theophylline has a narrow therapeutic range; therapeutic blood levels are considered to be 10–20 μg/mL. Lower levels, however, may be effective. Aminophylline is the only available intravenous theophylline preparation.

Glucocorticoids are used for both acute treatment and maintenance therapy of patients with asthma because of their anti-inflammatory and membrane-stabilizing effects. Beclomethasone, triamcinolone, flunisolide, and budesonide are synthetic steroids commonly used in metered-dose inhalers for maintenance therapy. Although they are associated with a low incidence of undesirable systemic effects, their use does not necessarily prevent adrenal suppression. Intravenous hydrocortisone or methylprednisolone is used acutely for severe attacks, followed by tapering doses of oral prednisone. Glucocorticoids usually require several hours to become effective.

Anticholinergic agents produce bronchodilation through their antimuscarinic action and may block reflex bronchoconstriction. Ipratropium, a congener of atropine that can be given by a metered-dose inhaler or aerosol, is a moderately effective bronchodilator without appreciable systemic anticholinergic effects.

Anesthetic Considerations

PREOPERATIVE MANAGEMENT:

The emphasis in evaluating patients with asthma should be on determining the recent course of the disease (review **peak flow diary** if available) and whether the patient has ever been hospitalized for an acute asthma attack as well as on ascertaining that the patient is in optimal condition. The difference between anesthetizing an asthmatic patient who has recently been hospitalized or who has clearly audible preoperative wheezing and one without such a history or finding on examination may be a potentially life-threatening anesthetic experience versus a totally uneventful one.

The clinical history is of critical importance. No or minimal dyspnea, wheezing, or cough is optimal. Complete resolution of recent exacerbations should be confirmed by chest auscultation. Patients with frequent or chronic bronchospasm should be placed on an optimal bronchodilating regimen, including β_2-adrenergic agonists; glucocorticoids should also be considered. Pulmonary function testing—particularly expiratory airflow measurements such as FEV_1, FEV_1/FVC, and peak expiratory flow rate (PEFR)—should be used to confirm clinical impressions. Comparisons with previous measurements are invaluable. FEV_1 values are normally more than 3 L for men and 2 L for women. FEV_1/FVC should normally be > 70%. Normal PEFR values exceed 200 L/min (often > 500 L/min in young adult males). An FEV_1, FEV_1/FVC, or PEFR less than 50% of normal is indicative of moderate to severe asthma. A chest radiograph may be useful in assessing air trapping; hyperinflation results in a flattened diaphragm, a small-appearing heart, and hyperlucent lung fields.

Asthmatic patients with active bronchospasm presenting for emergency surgery should undergo a period of intensive treatment whenever possible. Supplemental oxygen, aerosolized β_2-agonists, and intravenous glucocorticoids can dramatically improve lung function in a few hours. Arterial blood gases may be useful in severe cases. Hypoxemia and hypocapnia are typical of moderate and severe disease; even slight hypercapnia is indicative of severe air trapping and may be a sign of impending respiratory failure (see above). An FEV_1 below 40% of normal may also be predictive of respiratory failure.

Some degree of preoperative sedation is desirable in asthmatic patients presenting for elective surgery—especially in patients whose disease has an emotional component. In general, benzodiazepines are the most satisfactory agents for premedication. Anticholinergic agents are not customarily given unless very copious secretions are present or if ketamine is to be used for induction of anesthesia. In typical intramuscular doses, anticholinergics are not effective in preventing reflex bronchospasm following intubation. The use of an H_2-blocking agent (such as cimetidine or ranitidine) is theoretically detrimental, since H_2-receptor activation normally produces bronchodilation; in the event of histamine release, unopposed H_1 activation with H_2 blockade may accentuate bronchoconstriction.

Bronchodilators should be continued up to the time of surgery; in order of effectiveness, they are β-agonists, inhaled glucocorticoids, leukotriene blockers, chromones, theophyllines, and anticholinergics. Patients who have been receiving long-term glucocorticoid therapy should be given supplemental doses to compensate for adrenal suppression. Hydrocortisone (50–100 mg preoperatively and 100 mg q8h for 1 to 3 postoperative days, depending on the degree of surgical stress) is most commonly used.

INTRAOPERATIVE MANAGEMENT:

The most critical time for asthmatic patients undergoing anesthesia is during instrumentation of the airway. General anesthesia by mask or regional anesthesia will circumvent this problem but neither necessarily eliminates the possibility of bronchospasm. In fact, some clinicians believe that high spinal or epidural anesthesia may aggravate bronchoconstriction by blocking sympathetic tone to the lower airways (T_1–T_4) and allowing unopposed parasympathetic activity. Pain, emotional stress, or stimulation during light general anesthesia can precipitate bronchospasm. Drugs often associated with histamine release (eg, curare, atracurium, mivacurium, morphine, meperidine) should be avoided or given very slowly when used. The goal of any general anesthetic is a smooth induction and emergence, with anesthetic depth adjusted to stimulation.

Which induction agent is chosen is not as important as achieving deep anesthesia before intubation and surgical stimulation. Thiopental is most commonly used for adults but occasionally can induce bronchospasm as a result of exaggerated histamine release. Propofol and etomidate are suitable alternatives and, in fact, are preferred by some clinicians. Ketamine, the only intravenous agent with bronchodilating properties, is a good choice for patients who are also hemodynamically unstable. Ketamine should probably not be used in patients with high theophylline levels, as the combined actions of the two drugs can precipitate seizure activity. Halothane usually provides the smoothest inhalation induction with bronchodilation in asthmatic children. Isoflurane and desflurane can provide equal bronchodilation but must be increased slowly because they exert a mild irritant effect on the airways.

Reflex bronchospasm can be blunted before intubation by an additional dose of thiopental (1–2 mg/kg), ventilating the patient with 2–3 minimum alveolar concentration (MAC) of a volatile agent for 5 minutes, or administering intravenous or intratracheal lidocaine (1–2 mg/kg). Note that intratracheal lidocaine itself can initiate bronchospasm if an inadequate induction dose of thiopental is used. A large dose of an anticholinergic (atropine, 2 mg, or glycopyrrolate, 1 mg) can also block reflex bronchospasm but causes excessive tachycardia. Although succinylcholine may on occasion induce marked histamine release, it can generally be safely used in most asthmatic patients. In the absence of capnography, confirmation of correct endotracheal placement by chest auscultation can be difficult in the presence of marked bronchospasm.

Volatile anesthetics are most often used for maintenance of anesthesia to take advantage of their potent bronchodilating properties. Halothane can sensitize the heart to aminophylline and β-adrenergic agonists administered during anesthesia; for that reason—together with concern over hepatotoxicity—halothane is generally avoided in adults. Ventilation should be controlled with warmed humidified gases whenever possible. Airflow obstruction during expiration is apparent on capnography as a delayed rise of the end-tidal CO_2 value (Figure 23–1); the severity of obstruction is generally inversely related to the rate of rise in end-tidal CO_2. Severe bronchospasm is manifested by rising peak inspiratory pressures and incomplete exhalation. In the past, tidal volumes of 10–12 mL/kg with ventilatory rates of 8–10 breaths/min were considered desirable. Currently, minimizing the tidal volume ($\leq$ 10 mL/kg) with prolongation of the expiratory time may allow more uniform distribution of gas flow to both lungs, and may help avoid air trapping. The $PaCO_2$ may increase, which is acceptable if there is no contraindication from a cardiovascular or neurologic perspective.

Intraoperative bronchospasm is usually manifested as wheezing, increasing peak inflation pressures (plateau pressure should remain unchanged), decreasing exhaled tidal volumes, or a slowly rising waveform on the capnograph. It should be treated by increasing the concentration of the volatile agent (deepening the anesthetic). If the wheezing does not resolve, less common causes should always be considered before administering more specific phar-

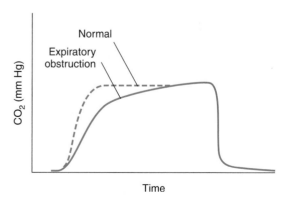

Figure 23–1. Capnograph of a patient with expiratory airway obstruction.

macologic treatment. Obstruction of the endotracheal tube from kinking, secretions, or an overinflated balloon; endobronchial intubation; active expiratory efforts (straining) because of light anesthesia; pulmonary edema or embolism; and pneumothorax can all simulate bronchospasm.

Bronchospasm should be treated with a β-adrenergic agonist delivered either by aerosol or a metered-dose inhaler into the inspiratory limb of the breathing circuit. (The carrier gas used in metered-dose inhalers can interfere with mass spectrometer readings.) Intravenous hydrocortisone (1.5–2 mg/kg) can be given, especially in patients with a history of glucocorticoid therapy.

At the completion of surgery, the patient should ideally be free of wheezing. Reversal of nondepolarizing neuromuscular blocking agents with anticholinesterase agents does not precipitate bronchoconstriction if preceded by the appropriate dose of an anticholinergic (see Chapter 10). Deep extubation (before airway reflexes return) prevents bronchospasm on emergence. Lidocaine as a bolus (1.5–2 mg/kg) or a continuous infusion (1–2 mg/min) may help obtund airway reflexes during emergence.

CHRONIC OBSTRUCTIVE PULMONARY DISEASE

Preoperative Considerations

COPD is the most common pulmonary disorder encountered in anesthetic practice. Its prevalence increases with age, it is strongly associated with cigarette smoking, and it has a male predominance (affecting up to 20% of men). The overwhelming majority of patients are asymptomatic or only mildly symptomatic but show expiratory airflow obstruction upon pulmonary function testing. In many patients, the obstruction has an element of reversibility, presumably from bronchospasm (as shown by improvement in response to bronchodilator administration). With advancing disease, maldistribution of both ventilation and pulmonary blood flow results in areas of low $\dot{V}/\dot{Q}$ ratios (intrapulmonary shunt) as well as areas of high $\dot{V}/\dot{Q}$ ratios (dead space). Traditionally, patients have been classified as having chronic bronchitis or emphysema (Table 23–3); most patients, however, have features of both.

CHRONIC BRONCHITIS:

The clinical diagnosis of chronic bronchitis is defined by the presence of a productive cough on most days of 3 consecutive months for at least 2 consecutive years. In addition to cigarette smoking, air pollutants, occupational exposure to dusts, recurrent pulmonary infec-

Table 23–3. Signs and symptoms of chronic obstructive pulmonary disease.

Feature	Chronic Bronchitis	Emphysema
Cough	Frequent	With exertion
Sputum	Copious	Scant
Hematocrit	Elevated	Normal
PaCO$_2$ (mm Hg)	Often elevated (> 40)	Usually normal or < 40
Chest radiograph	Increased lung markings	Hyperinflation
Elastic recoil	Normal	Decreased
Airway resistance	Increased	Normal to slightly increased
Cor pulmonale	Early	Late

tions, and familial factors may be responsible. Secretions from hypertrophied bronchial mucous glands and mucosal edema from inflammation of the airways produce airflow obstruction. The term **chronic asthmatic bronchitis** may be used when bronchospasm is a major feature. Recurrent pulmonary infections (viral and bacterial) are common and often associated with bronchospasm. RV is increased but TLC is often normal. Intrapulmonary shunting is prominent, and hypoxemia is common.

Chronic hypoxemia leads to erythrocytosis, pulmonary hypertension, and eventually right ventricular failure (cor pulmonale); this combination of findings is often referred to as the **blue bloater syndrome,** but < 5% of patients with COPD fit this description. In the course of disease progression, patients gradually develop chronic CO$_2$ retention; the normal ventilatory drive becomes less sensitive to arterial CO$_2$ tension and may be depressed by oxygen administration (below).

EMPHYSEMA:

Emphysema is a pathologic disorder with irreversible enlargement of the airways distal to terminal bronchioles and destruction of alveolar septa. The diagnosis can be reliably made with computed tomography (CT) of the chest. Mild apical emphysematous changes are a normal but clinically insignificant consequence of aging. Significant emphysema is nearly always related to cigarette smoking. Less commonly, emphysema occurs at an early age and is associated with a homozygous deficiency of α_1-antitrypsin. This is a protease inhibitor that prevents excessive activity of proteolytic enzymes (mainly elastase) in the lungs; these enzymes are produced by pulmonary neutrophils and macrophages in response to infection and pollutants. Emphysema associated with smoking may similarly be due to a relative imbalance between protease and antiprotease activities in susceptible individuals. Loss of the elastic recoil that normally supports small airways by radial traction allows premature collapse during exhalation (dynamic airway collapse). Patients characteristically have increases in RV, FRC, TLC, and the RV/TLC ratio.

Destruction of pulmonary capillaries in the alveolar septa decreases carbon monoxide diffusion capacity (see Chapter 22) and inevitably leads to pulmonary hypertension in the terminal stages of the disease. Large cystic areas, or bullae, develop in some patients. Increased dead space is a prominent feature of emphysema. Arterial oxygen tensions are usually normal or only slightly reduced; CO_2 tension is also typically normal. When dyspneic, patients with emphysema often purse their lips to delay closure of the small airways (see Chapter 22)—which accounts for the term *pink puffers* that is often used. The majority of patients, though, have a combination of bronchitis and emphysema and carry the diagnosis of COPD.

TREATMENT:

Treatment for COPD is primarily supportive. The most important intervention is cessation of smoking. Patients demonstrating a reversible element in airway obstruction (> 15% improvement in FEV_1 following administration of a bronchodilator) should be started on long-term bronchodilator therapy. Inhaled β_2-adrenergic agonists, glucocorticoids, and ipratropium are very useful; ipratropium has more of a role in the management of these patients than in patients with asthma. Even patients who do not show improvement in their pulmonary function tests from the use of bronchodilators may improve clinically with bronchodilator therapy. Exacerbations are often related to bouts of bronchitis, heralded by a change in sputum; frequent treatment with broad-spectrum antibiotics (eg, ampicillin, tetracycline, sulfamethoxazole-trimethoprim) may be necessary. Hypoxemia should be treated carefully with supplemental oxygen. Patients with chronic hypoxemia (PaO_2 < 55 mm Hg) and pulmonary hypertension require low-flow oxygen therapy (1–2 L/min).

Oxygen therapy can dangerously elevate $PaCO_2$ in patients with CO_2 retention; elevating PaO_2 above 60 mm Hg can precipitate respiratory failure in these patients. Abolition of a hypoxic respiratory drive or, more likely, a release of hypoxic vasoconstriction that results in greater blood flow to areas of low V̇/Q̇ may well be responsible (see Chapter 22). When cor pulmonale is present, diuretics are used to control peripheral edema; beneficial effects

from digoxin and vasodilators are inconsistent. Physical conditioning has no effect on pulmonary function tests but has been shown to improve symptoms. Some studies even suggest the ability to increase oxygen consumption during exercise is inversely related to postoperative complications.

Anesthetic Considerations

PREOPERATIVE MANAGEMENT:

Patients with COPD should be optimally prepared prior to elective surgical procedures in the same way as patients with asthma (above). They should be questioned about recent changes in dyspnea, sputum, and wheezing. Patients with a FEV_1 less than 50% of predicted (1.2–1.5 L) usually have dyspnea on exertion, while those with a FEV_1 less than 25% (< 1 L for men) typically have dyspnea with minimal activity. The latter finding, in patients with predominantly chronic bronchitis, is also often associated with CO_2 retention and pulmonary hypertension. Pulmonary function studies, chest radiographs, and arterial blood gas measurements should be reviewed carefully. The presence of bullous changes on the radiograph should be noted. Many patients have concomitant cardiac disease and should also receive a careful cardiovascular evaluation (see Chapter 20).

In contrast to asthma, only limited improvement in respiratory function may be seen after a short period of intensive preoperative preparation. Nonetheless, preoperative interventions aimed at correcting hypoxemia, relieving bronchospasm, mobilizing and reducing secretions, and treating infections may decrease the incidence of postoperative pulmonary complications. Patients at greatest risk for complications are those with preoperative pulmonary function measurements less than 50% of predicted. The possibility that postoperative ventilation may be necessary in high-risk patients should be discussed with both the patient and the surgeon.

Smoking should be discontinued for at least 6–8 weeks before the operation to decrease secretions and to reduce pulmonary complications. Cigarette smoking increases mucus production and decreases clearance. Both gaseous and particulate phases of cigarette smoke can deplete glutathione and vitamin C and may promote oxidative injury to tissues. Carbon monoxide increases carboxyhemoglobin levels, while breakdown products of nitric oxide and nitrogen dioxide can increase methemoglobin levels. Cessation of smoking for as little as 24 hours therefore has theoretically beneficial effects on the oxygen-carrying capacity of hemoglobin, but this has not been borne out with clinical studies. Preoperative chest physiotherapy (chest percussion and postural drainage) and antibiotics for patients with a change in sputum are beneficial in reducing secretions. Bronchospasm should be treated with bronchodilators. Patients with moderate to severe disease may benefit from a perioperative course of glucocorticoids. Those with malnutrition should receive nutritional supplementation before major surgery. Pulmonary hypertension should be treated by optimizing oxygenation. Perioperative digitalization may be useful in patients with cor pulmonale, especially if right ventricular failure is also present.

INTRAOPERATIVE MANAGEMENT:

Although regional anesthesia is often considered preferable to general anesthesia, high spinal or epidural anesthesia can decrease lung volumes, restrict the use of accessory respiratory muscles, and produce an ineffective cough, leading to dyspnea and retention of secretions. Loss of proprioception from the chest and unusual positioning, such as lithotomy or the lateral decubitus position, often accentuate dyspnea in awake patients.

Preoxygenation prior to induction of general anesthesia prevents the rapid oxygen desaturation often seen in these patients. The selection of anesthetic agents and general intraoperative management are similar to those for asthmatic patients (see above). Unfortunately, the use of bronchodilating anesthetics improves only the reversible component of airflow-obstruction bronchospasm; significant expiratory obstruction is still often present even under deep anesthesia. Enhanced respiratory depression from anesthetics is often seen with moderate to severe disease. As with asthmatic patients, ventilation should be controlled with small to moderate tidal volumes and slow rates to avoid air trapping. Humidified gases should be used if significant bronchospasm is present and for long procedures (> 2 hours). Nitrous oxide should be avoided in patients with bullae and in those who have pulmonary hypertension. Pneumothorax from expansion can occur with the former, while further elevations in pulmonary artery pressures may be seen with the latter. Inhibition of hypoxic pulmonary vasoconstriction by inhalational anesthetics is usually not clinically significant at the usual doses (see Chapter 22).

Measurement of arterial blood gases is desirable for prolonged peripheral, extensive intra-abdominal, and all thoracic procedures. Although pulse oximetry accurately detects significant arterial desaturation, direct measurement of arterial oxygen tensions may be necessary to detect more subtle changes in intrapulmonary shunting. Moreover, arterial CO_2 measurements should be used to guide ventilation because increased dead space widens the normal arterial to end-tidal CO_2 gradient. Ventilation should be adjusted to maintain a normal arterial pH. Normalization of $PaCO_2$ in patients with preoperative CO_2 retention results in alkalo-

sis (see Chapter 30). Hemodynamic monitoring should be dictated by any underlying cardiac dysfunction as well as the extent of the surgery. In patients with pulmonary hypertension, central venous pressure measurements reflect right ventricular function rather than intravascular volume.

At the end of surgery, the timing of extubation should balance the risk of bronchospasm with that of pulmonary insufficiency, but evidence suggests that early extubation (in the operating room) is beneficial. An awake extubation allows a more accurate assessment of immediate postoperative pulmonary function but risks bronchospasm; deep extubation lessens the risk of reflex bronchospasm but assumes that the patient will be able to maintain adequate ventilation. Patients with an FEV_1 below 50% are most likely to require a period of postoperative ventilation, especially following upper abdominal and thoracic operations. General criteria for extubation are discussed in Chapters 5 and 50.

■ RESTRICTIVE PULMONARY DISEASE

Restrictive pulmonary diseases are characterized by decreased lung compliance. Lung volumes are typically reduced, with preservation of normal expiratory flow rates. Thus, both FEV_1 and FVC are reduced, but the FEV_1/FVC ratio is normal.

Restrictive pulmonary diseases include many acute and chronic intrinsic pulmonary disorders as well as extrinsic (extrapulmonary) disorders involving the pleura, chest wall, diaphragm, or neuromuscular function. Reduced lung compliance increases the work of breathing, resulting in a characteristic rapid but shallow breathing pattern. Respiratory gas exchange is usually maintained until the disease process is advanced.

ACUTE INTRINSIC PULMONARY DISORDERS

These disorders include pulmonary edema (including the acute respiratory distress syndrome [ARDS]), infectious pneumonia, and aspiration pneumonitis.

Preoperative Consideration

Reduced lung compliance in these disorders is primarily due to an increase in extravascular lung water, from either an increase in pulmonary capillary pressure or an increase in pulmonary capillary permeability (see Chapter 50). Increased pressure occurs with left ventricular failure and fluid overload, while increased permeability is present with ARDS. Localized or generalized increases in permeability also occur following aspiration or infectious pneumonitis.

Anesthetic Considerations

PREOPERATIVE MANAGEMENT:

Patients with acute pulmonary disease should be spared elective surgery. In preparation for emergency procedures, oxygenation and ventilation should be optimized preoperatively to the greatest extent possible. Fluid overload should be treated with diuretics; heart failure may also require vasodilators and inotropes. Drainage of large pleural effusions should be considered. Similarly, massive abdominal distention should be relieved by nasogastric compression or drainage of ascites. Persistent hypoxemia may require positive pressure ventilation and positive end-expiratory pressure (PEEP). Associated systemic disturbances such as hypotension or infection should be aggressively treated.

INTRAOPERATIVE MANAGEMENT:

Selection of anesthetic agents should be tailored to each patient. Surgical patients with acute pulmonary disorders, such as ARDS, cardiogenic pulmonary edema, or pneumonia, are critically ill; anesthetic management should be a continuation of their preoperative intensive care. Anesthesia is most often provided with a combination of intravenous and inhalational agents together with a neuromuscular blocking agent. High inspired oxygen concentrations and PEEP may be required. The decreased lung compliance results in high peak inspiratory pressures during positive pressure ventilation, and increases the risk of barotrauma and volutrauma. Tidal volumes for these patients should be reduced to 4–8 mL/kg, with a compensatory increase in the ventilatory rate (14–18 breaths/min), even if the result is an increase in end-tidal CO_2. Airway pressure should generally not exceed 30 cm H_2O. The ventilator on the anesthesia machine may prove inadequate for patients with severe ARDS because of its limited gas flow capabilities, low pressure-limiting settings, and the absence of certain ventilatory modes (see Chapter 50); a more sophisticated intensive care unit ventilator should be used in such instances. Aggressive hemodynamic monitoring is recommended.

CHRONIC INTRINSIC PULMONARY DISORDERS

This group of disorders is also often referred to as **interstitial lung diseases.** Regardless of etiology, the disease process is generally characterized by an insidious onset, chronic inflammation of alveolar walls and peri-

alveolar tissue, and progressive pulmonary fibrosis. The latter can eventually interfere with gas exchange and ventilatory function. The inflammatory process may be primarily confined to the lungs or may be part of a generalized multiorgan process. Causes include hypersensitivity pneumonitis from occupational and environmental pollutants), drug toxicity (bleomycin and nitrofurantoin), radiation pneumonitis, idiopathic pulmonary fibrosis, autoimmune diseases, and sarcoidosis. Chronic pulmonary aspiration, oxygen toxicity, and severe ARDS can also produce chronic fibrosis.

Preoperative Considerations

Patients typically present with dyspnea on exertion and sometimes a nonproductive cough. Symptoms of cor pulmonale are present only with advanced disease. Physical examination may reveal fine (dry) crackles over the lung bases and, in late stages, evidence of right ventricular failure. The chest radiograph progresses from a "ground glass" appearance to prominent reticulonodular markings, and finally to a "honey-comb" appearance. Arterial blood gases usually show mild hypoxemia with normocarbia. Pulmonary function tests are typical of a restrictive ventilatory defect (see above), and carbon monoxide diffusing capacity is reduced 30–50%.

Treatment is directed at abating the disease process and preventing further exposure to the causative agent (if known). Glucocorticoid and immunosuppressive therapy may be used for idiopathic pulmonary fibrosis, autoimmune disorders, and sarcoidosis. If the patient has chronic hypoxemia, oxygen therapy may be started to prevent, or attenuate, right ventricular failure.

Anesthetic Considerations

PREOPERATIVE MANAGEMENT:

Preoperative evaluation should focus on determining the degree of pulmonary impairment as well as the underlying disease process. The latter is important in determining the potential involvement of other organs. A history of **dyspnea on exertion** (or at rest) should be evaluated further with pulmonary function tests and arterial blood gas analysis. A vital capacity less than 15 mL/kg is indicative of severe dysfunction (normal is > 70 mL/kg). A chest radiograph is helpful in assessing disease severity.

INTRAOPERATIVE MANAGEMENT:

The management of these patients is complicated by a predisposition to hypoxemia and the need to control ventilation to ensure optimum gas exchange; anesthetic drug selection is generally not critical. The reduction in FRC (and oxygen stores) predisposes these patients to rapid hypoxemia following induction of anesthesia (see

Chapter 22); their uptake of inhalational anesthetics may also be accelerated. Because these patients may be more susceptible to oxygen-induced toxicity, especially patients who have received **bleomycin,** the inspired fractional concentration of oxygen should be kept to the minimum concentration compatible with acceptable oxygenation (SpO_2 of > 88–92%). High peak inspiratory pressures during mechanical ventilation increase risk of pneumothorax and should prompt smaller than normal tidal volumes with a faster rate.

EXTRINSIC RESTRICTIVE PULMONARY DISORDERS

These disorders alter gas exchange by interfering with normal lung expansion. They include **pleural effusions, pneumothorax,** mediastinal masses, **kyphoscoliosis,** pectus excavatum, **neuromuscular disorders,** and increased intra-abdominal pressure from ascites, pregnancy, or bleeding. Marked obesity also produces a restrictive ventilatory defect (see Chapter 36). Anesthetic considerations are similar to those discussed above for intrinsic restrictive disorders.

■ PULMONARY EMBOLISM

Preoperative Considerations

Pulmonary embolism results from the entry of **blood clots,** fat, tumor cells, **air, amniotic fluid,** or foreign material into the venous system. Clots from the lower extremities (nearly always above the knee), pelvic veins, or, less commonly, the right side of the heart are usually responsible. Venous stasis or hypercoagulability is often contributory in such cases (Table 23–4). Pulmonary embolism can also occur intraoperatively in normal individuals undergoing certain procedures. Fat embolism is discussed in Chapter 40; air embolism is discussed in Chapter 26.

PATHOPHYSIOLOGY:

Embolic occlusions in the pulmonary circulation increase dead space, and if minute ventilation does not change, this increase in dead space should theoretically increase $PaCO_2$. However, in practice, hypoxemia is more often seen. Pulmonary emboli acutely increase pulmonary vascular resistance by reducing the cross-sectional area of the pulmonary vasculature causing reflex and humoral vasoconstriction. Localized or generalized reflex bronchoconstriction further increases areas with low $\dot{V}/\dot{Q}$ ratios. The net effect is an increase in pulmonary shunt and hypoxemia. The affected area loses its surfactant within hours and may become at-

Table 23–4. Factors associated with deep venous thrombosis and pulmonary embolism.

Prolonged bed rest
Postpartum state
Fracture of the lower extremities
Surgery on the lower extremities
Carcinoma
Heart failure
Obesity
Surgery lasting more than 30 minutes
Hypercoagulability
Antithrombin III deficiency
Protein C deficiency
Protein S deficiency
Plasminogen-activator deficiency

electatic within 24–48 hours. Pulmonary infarction occurs if the embolus involves a large vessel and collateral blood flow from the bronchial circulation is insufficient for that part of the lung (incidence < 10%). In previously healthy persons, occlusion of more than 50% of the pulmonary circulation (massive pulmonary embolism) is necessary before sustained pulmonary hypertension is seen. Patients with preexisting cardiac or pulmonary disease can develop acute pulmonary hypertension with occlusions of lesser magnitude. A sustained increase in right ventricular afterload can precipitate acute right ventricular failure. If the patient survives acute pulmonary thromboembolism, the thrombus usually begins to resolve within 1 to 2 weeks.

DIAGNOSIS:

Clinical manifestations of pulmonary embolism include sudden tachypnea, dyspnea, chest pain, or hemoptysis. The latter generally implies infarction. Symptoms are often absent or mild and nonspecific unless massive embolism has occurred. Wheezing may be present on auscultation. Arterial blood gas analysis typically shows mild hypoxemia with respiratory alkalosis (the latter due to an increase in ventilation). The chest radiograph is commonly normal but may show an area of oligemia (radiolucency), a wedge-shaped density with an infarct, atelectasis with an elevated diaphragm, or an asymmetrically enlarged proximal pulmonary artery with acute pulmonary hypertension. Cardiac signs include tachycardia and wide fixed splitting of the second heart sound; hypotension with elevated central venous pressure is usually indicative of right ventricular failure. The electrocardiogram frequently shows tachycardia and may show signs of acute cor pulmonale, such as new right axis deviation, right bundle branch block, and tall peaked T waves. Impedance plethysmography is also helpful in demonstrating deep venous thrombosis above the knee. The diagnosis of embolism is more difficult to make intraoperatively (see below).

Pulmonary angiography is the most accurate means of diagnosing a pulmonary embolism, but noninvasive pulmonary perfusion and ventilation scans using gamma-emitting radionucleotides may be helpful and are widely used. A normal perfusion scan virtually excludes significant embolism. An abnormal perfusion scan is diagnostic only if perfusion defects are present in areas with normal ventilation. Helical CT scanning is increasingly used in large medical centers to diagnose pulmonary embolism.

TREATMENT:

The best treatment for pulmonary embolism is prevention. Minidose heparin (5000 U q12h begun preoperatively or immediately postoperatively in high-risk patients), oral anticoagulation (warfarin), aspirin, or dextran therapy together with early ambulation can decrease the incidence of postoperative emboli. The use of high elastic stockings and pneumatic compression of the legs may also decrease the incidence of venous thrombosis in the legs but not in the pelvis or the heart.

Systemic anticoagulation prevents the formation of new blood clots or the extension of existing clots. Heparin therapy is begun with the goal of achieving an activated partial thromboplastin time of 1.5 to 2.4 times normal. Low molecular weight heparin (LMWH) is as effective and is given subcutaneously at a fixed dose (based on body weight) without laboratory monitoring. LMWH is more expensive than unfractionated heparin but is more cost-effective. All patients should start warfarin therapy concurrent with starting heparin therapy and the two should overlap for 4–5 days. The international normalized ratio should be within the therapeutic range on two consecutive measurements at least 24 hours apart before the heparin is stopped. Warfarin should be continued for 3–12 months. Thrombolytic therapy with tissue plasminogen activator or streptokinase is indicated for patients with massive pulmonary embolism or circulatory collapse. Recent surgery and active bleeding are contraindications to anticoagulation and thrombolytic therapy. In these cases, an inferior vena cava umbrella filter may be placed to prevent recurrent pulmonary emboli. Pulmonary embolectomy may be indicated for patients with massive embolism in whom thrombolytic therapy is contraindicated.

Anesthetic Considerations

PREOPERATIVE MANAGEMENT:

Patients with acute pulmonary embolism may present in the operating room for placement of a caval filter or, rarely, for pulmonary embolectomy. In most instances,

the patient will have a history of pulmonary embolism and presents for unrelated surgery; in this group of patients, the risk of interrupting anticoagulant therapy perioperatively is unknown. If the acute episode is more than 1 year old, the risk of temporarily stopping anticoagulant therapy is probably small. Moreover, except in the case of chronic recurrent pulmonary emboli, pulmonary function has usually returned to normal. The emphasis in the perioperative management of these patients should be in preventing new episodes of embolism (see above).

INTRAOPERATIVE MANAGEMENT:

Vena cava filters are usually placed percutaneously under local anesthesia with sedation. Patients may display enhanced sensitivity to the circulatory effects of most anesthetic agents. Decreased venous return during placement of the device can precipitate hypotension.

Although no definite recommendations can be made regarding the choice of anesthesia for patients with a history of pulmonary embolism, studies suggest that regional anesthesia for some procedures (eg, hip surgery) decreases the incidence of postoperative deep venous thrombosis and pulmonary embolism. The use of regional anesthesia is contraindicated in patients with residual anticoagulation or a prolonged bleeding time. When general anesthesia is selected, the use of short-acting agents may allow early postoperative ambulation.

Patients presenting for pulmonary embolectomy are critically ill. They are usually already intubated but tolerate positive pressure ventilation poorly. Inotropic support is necessary until the clot is removed. They also tolerate all anesthetic agents very poorly. Small doses of an opioid, etomidate, or ketamine may be used, but the latter can theoretically increase pulmonary artery pressures. Cardiopulmonary bypass may be necessary.

INTRAOPERATIVE PULMONARY EMBOLISM:

Significant pulmonary embolism is a rare occurrence during anesthesia. Diagnosis requires a high index of suspicion. Air emboli are common but are often overlooked unless large amounts are entrained (see Chapter 26). Fat embolism can occur during orthopedic procedures (see Chapter 40), while amniotic fluid embolism is a rare, unpredictable—and often fatal—complication of obstetrical delivery (see Chapter 43). Thromboembolism may occur intraoperatively during prolonged procedures. The clot may have been present prior to surgery or may form intraoperatively; surgical manipulations or a change in the patient's position may then dislodge the venous thrombus. Manipulation of tumors with intravascular extension can similarly produce pulmonary embolism. Intraoperative pulmonary embolism usually presents as unexplained sudden hypotension, hypoxemia, or bronchospasm. A decrease in end-tidal CO_2 concentration is also suggestive but not specific. Invasive monitoring may reveal elevated central venous and pulmonary arterial pressures. Depending on the type and location of an embolism, a transesophageal echocardiogram may be helpful. If air is identified in the right atrium, or if it is suspected, emergent central vein cannulation and aspiration of the air may be lifesaving. For all other emboli, treatment is supportive, with intravenous fluids and inotropes. Placement of a vena cava filter should be considered postoperatively.

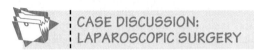

CASE DISCUSSION: LAPAROSCOPIC SURGERY

A 45-year-old woman is scheduled for a laparoscopic cholecystectomy. Known medical problems include obesity and a smoking history.

What are the advantages of laparoscopic cholecystectomy compared with open cholecystectomy?

Laparoscopic techniques have rapidly increased in popularity because of the multiple benefits associated with much smaller incisions than traditional open techniques. These benefits include decreased postoperative pain, less postoperative pulmonary impairment, a reduction in postoperative ileus, shorter hospital stays, earlier ambulation, and smaller surgical scars. Thus, laparoscopic surgery can provide substantial medical and economic advantages.

How does laparoscopic surgery affect intraoperative pulmonary function?

The hallmark of laparoscopy is the creation of a pneumoperitoneum with pressurized CO_2. The resulting increase in intra-abdominal pressure displaces the diaphragm cephalad, causing a decrease in lung compliance and an increase in peak inspiratory pressure. Atelectasis, diminished functional residual capacity (FRC), ventilation/perfusion mismatch, and pulmonary shunting contribute to a decrease in arterial oxygenation. One would expect these changes to be exaggerated in this obese patient with a long history of tobacco use.

The high solubility of CO_2 increases systemic absorption by the vasculature of the peritoneum. This, combined with smaller tidal volumes because of poor lung compliance, leads to increased arterial CO_2 levels and decreased pH.

Why does patient position affect oxygenation?

A head-down position (Trendelenburg position) is commonly requested during insertion of the Veress needle and cannula. This position causes a cephalad shift in abdominal viscera and the diaphragm. FRC, total lung volume, and pulmonary compliance will be decreased. Although these changes are usually well tolerated by healthy patients, this patient's obesity and presumed preexisting lung disease increase the likelihood for hypoxemia. A head-down position also tends to shift the trachea upward, so that an endotracheal tube anchored at the mouth may migrate into the right main-stem bronchus. This tracheobronchial shift may be exacerbated during insufflation of the abdomen.

After insufflation, the patient's position is usually changed to a steep head-up position (reverse Trendelenburg) to facilitate surgical dissection. The respiratory effects of the head-up position are the opposite of the head-down position: FRC increases and the work of breathing decreases.

Does laparoscopic surgery affect cardiac function?

Moderate insufflation pressures usually leave heart rate, central venous pressure, and cardiac output unchanged or slightly elevated. This appears to result from increased effective cardiac filling because blood tends to be forced out of the abdomen and into the chest. Higher insufflation pressures (> 25 cm H_2O, or 18 mm Hg), however, tend to collapse the major abdominal veins (particularly the inferior vena cava), which decreases venous return and leads to a drop in preload and cardiac output in some patients.

Hypercarbia, if allowed to develop, will stimulate the sympathetic nervous system and thus increase blood pressure, heart rate, and the risk of dysrhythmias. Attempting to compensate by increasing the tidal volume or respiratory rate will increase the mean intrathoracic pressure, further hindering venous return and increasing mean pulmonary artery pressures. These effects can prove especially challenging in patients with restrictive lung disease, impaired cardiac function, or intravascular volume depletion.

Although the Trendelenburg position increases preload, mean arterial pressure and cardiac output usually either remain unchanged or decrease. These seemingly paradoxical responses may be explained by carotid and aortic baroreceptor-medi-

ated reflexes. The reverse Trendelenburg position decreases preload, cardiac output, and mean arterial pressure.

Describe the advantages and disadvantages of alternative anesthetic techniques for this patient.

Anesthetic approaches to laparoscopic surgery include infiltration of local anesthetic with an intravenous sedative, epidural or spinal anesthesia, or general anesthesia. Experience with local anesthesia has been largely limited to brief gynecologic procedures (laparoscopic tubal sterilization, intrafallopian transfers) in young, healthy, and motivated patients. Although postoperative recovery is rapid, patient discomfort and suboptimal visualization of intra-abdominal organs precludes the use of this local anesthesia technique for laparoscopic cholecystectomy.

Epidural or spinal anesthesia represent another alternative for laparoscopic surgery. A high level is required for complete muscle relaxation and to prevent diaphragmatic irritation caused by gas insufflation and surgical manipulations, however. An obese patient with lung disease may not be able to increase spontaneous ventilation to maintain normocarbia in the face of a high (T2 level) regional block during insufflation and a 20-degree Trendelenburg position. Another disadvantage of a regional technique is the occasional occurrence of referred shoulder pain from diaphragmatic irritation. General anesthesia would therefore be the preferred technique for this patient.

Does a general anesthetic technique require endotracheal intubation?

Endotracheal intubation with positive pressure ventilation is usually favored for many reasons: the risk of regurgitation from increased intra-abdominal pressure during insufflation; the necessity for controlled ventilation to prevent hypercapnia; the relatively high peak inspiratory pressures required because of the pneumoperitoneum; the need for muscle paralysis during surgery to allow lower insufflation pressures, provide better visualization, and prevent unexpected patient movement; and the placement of a nasogastric tube and gastric decompression to minimize the risk of visceral perforation during trocar introduction and optimize visualization. The obese patient presented here would benefit from intubation to lessen the likelihood of hypoxemia, hypercarbia, and aspiration.

What special monitoring should be considered for this patient?

Monitoring end-tidal CO_2 normally provides an adequate guide for determining the minute ventilation required to maintain normocarbia. This assumes a constant gradient between arterial CO_2 and end-tidal CO_2, which is generally valid in healthy patients undergoing laparoscopy. This assumption would not apply if alveolar dead space changes during surgery. For example, any significant reduction in lung perfusion increases alveolar dead space, dilutes expired CO_2, and thereby lessens end-tidal CO_2 measurements. This may occur during laparoscopy if cardiac output drops because of high inflation pressures, the reverse Trendelenburg position, or gas embolism. Furthermore, abdominal distention lowers pulmonary compliance. Large tidal volumes are usually avoided because they are associated with high peak inspiratory pressures and can cause considerable movement of the surgical field. The resulting choice of lower tidal volumes and higher respiratory rates may lead to poor alveolar gas sampling and erroneous end-tidal CO_2 measurements. In fact, end-tidal CO_2 values have been found to be particularly unreliable in patients with significant cardiac or pulmonary disease undergoing laparoscopy. Thus, placement of an arterial catheter should be considered in patients with cardiopulmonary disease.

What are some possible complications of laparoscopic surgery?

Surgical complications include hemorrhage if a major abdominal vessel is lacerated or peritonitis if a viscus is perforated during trocar introduction. Significant intraoperative hemorrhage may go unrecognized because of the limitations of laparoscopic visualization. Fulguration has been associated with bowel burns and bowel gas explosions. The use of pressurized gas introduces the possibility of extravasation of CO_2 along tissue planes, resulting in subcutaneous emphysema, pneumomediastinum, or pneumothorax. Nitrous oxide should be discontinued and insufflating pressures decreased as much as possible. Patients with this complication may benefit from the continuation of mechanical ventilation into the immediate postoperative period.

Venous CO_2 embolism resulting from unintentional insufflation of gas into an open vein may lead to hypoxemia, pulmonary hypertension, pulmonary edema, and cardiovascular collapse. Un-

like air embolism, end-tidal CO_2 may transiently increase during CO_2 gas embolism. Treatment includes immediate release of the pneumoperitoneum, discontinuation of nitrous oxide, insertion of a central venous catheter for gas aspiration, and placement of the patient in a head-down left lateral decubitus position.

Vagal stimulation during trocar insertion, peritoneal insufflation, or manipulation of viscera can result in bradycardia and even sinus arrest. Although this usually resolves spontaneously, elimination of the stimulus (eg, deflation of the peritoneum) and administration of a vagolytic drug (eg, atropine sulfate) should be considered. Intraoperative hypotension may be more common during laparoscopic cholecystectomy than during cholecystectomy by laparotomy. Preoperative fluid loading has been recommended to avoid this complication.

Even though laparoscopic procedures are associated with less muscle trauma and incisional pain than is open surgery, pulmonary dysfunction can persist for at least 24 hours postoperatively. For example, forced expiratory volume, forced vital capacity, and forced expiratory flow are reduced by approximately 25% following laparoscopic cholecystectomy as opposed to a 50% reduction following open cholecystectomy. The cause of this dysfunction may be related to diaphragmatic tension during the pneumoperitoneum.

Nausea and vomiting are common following laparoscopic procedures, despite routine emptying of the stomach with a nasogastric tube. Pharmacologic prophylaxis is recommended.

SUGGESTED READING

Benumof J: *Anesthesia and Uncommon Diseases.* 4th ed. WB Saunders and Company, 1998.

Hurford WE: The bronchospastic patient. *Int Anesthesiol Clin* 2000; 38:77.

Lumb A, Nunn JF: *Nunn's Applied Respiratory Physiology.* 5th ed. Butterworth-Heinemann, 2000.

Reilly JJ Jr: Evidence-based preoperative evaluation candidates for thoracotomy. *Chest* 1999; 116:474.

Anesthesia for Thoracic Surgery 24

KEY CONCEPTS

 Mixing of unoxygenated blood from the collapsed upper lung with oxygenated blood from the still ventilated dependent lung widens the alveolar-to-arterial oxygen gradient and can result in hypoxemia.

 Malpositioning of a double-lumen endotracheal tube is usually indicated by poor lung compliance and low exhaled tidal volume.

 If intraspinal opioids are to be used postoperatively, their intravenous use should be limited during surgery to prevent excessive postoperative respiratory depression.

 Postoperative hemorrhage complicates about 3% of thoracotomies and may be associated with up to 20% mortality; signs include increased chest tube drainage (> 200 mL/hour), hypotension, tachycardia, and a falling hematocrit.

 Bronchopleural fistula presents as a sudden large air leak from the chest tube that may be associated with an increasing pneumothorax and partial lung collapse.

 Acute herniation of the heart into the operative hemithorax can occur through the pericardial defect left following a radical pneumonectomy.

 Nitrous oxide is contraindicated in patients with pulmonary cysts and bullae because it can expand the air space and cause rupture, which may be signaled by sudden hypotension, bronchospasm, or an abrupt rise in peak inflation pressure, and requires immediate placement of a chest tube.

 Following lung transplantation, peak inspiratory pressures should be kept to the minimum compatible with good lung expansion and the inspired oxygen concentration is kept < 60%.

 Regardless of the procedure, the major anesthetic consideration for patients with esophageal disease is the risk of pulmonary aspiration.

 During the transhiatal approach, substernal and diaphragmatic retractors can interfere with cardiac function.

Indications and techniques for thoracic surgery have continually evolved since its origins. Common indications are no longer restricted to complications of tuberculosis and suppurative pneumonitis but now include thoracic malignancies (mainly of the lungs and esophagus), chest trauma, esophageal disease, and mediastinal tumors. Diagnostic procedures such as bronchoscopy, mediastinoscopy, and open lung biopsies are also common. Anesthetic techniques for separating the ventilation to each lung have allowed the refinement of surgical techniques to the point that many procedures are increasingly performed thoracoscopically. High frequency jet ventilation and cardiopulmonary bypass now allow complex procedures such as tracheal resection and lung transplantation, respectively. Anesthetic management of cardiac surgery is considered in Chapter 21. Anesthesia for thoracic aortic aneurysms is also discussed in Chapter 21, while that for thoracic trauma is reviewed in Chapter 41.

■ PHYSIOLOGIC CONSIDERATIONS DURING THORACIC ANESTHESIA

Thoracic surgery presents a unique set of physiologic problems for the anesthesiologist that requires special consideration. These include physiologic derangements caused by placing the patient with one side down (lateral decubitus position), opening the chest (open **pneumothorax**), and the frequent need for **one-lung ventilation.**

THE LATERAL DECUBITUS POSITION

The lateral decubitus position provides optimal access for most operations on the lungs, pleura, esophagus, the great vessels, other mediastinal structures, and vertebrae. Unfortunately, this position has the potential to significantly alter the normal pulmonary ventilation/perfusion relationships (see Chapter 22). These de-

rangements are further accentuated by induction of anesthesia, initiation of mechanical ventilation, muscle paralysis, opening the chest, and surgical retraction. Although perfusion continues to favor the dependent (lower) lung, ventilation progressively favors the less perfused upper lung. The resulting mismatch markedly increases the risk of hypoxemia.

The Awake State

When a supine patient assumes the lateral decubitus position, ventilation/perfusion matching is preserved during spontaneous ventilation. The lower lung receives more perfusion and more ventilation than does the upper lung. The former is the effect of gravity, while the latter is because:

- contraction of the dependent hemidiaphragm is more efficient as it assumes a higher position in the chest (compared with the upper hemidiaphragm) due to its disproportionate share in supporting the weight of abdominal contents;
- the dependent lung is on a more favorable part of the compliance curve (Figure 24–1).

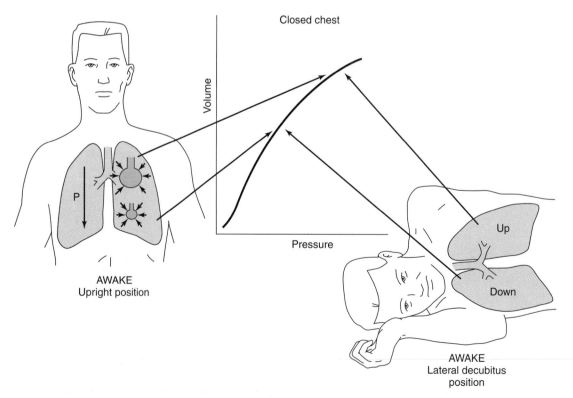

Figure 24–1. The effect of the lateral decubitus position on lung compliance.

Induction of Anesthesia

The decrease in functional residual capacity (FRC) with induction of general anesthesia (see Chapter 22) moves the upper lung to a more favorable part of the compliance curve, but moves the lower lung to a less compliant position (Figure 24–2). As a result, the upper lung is ventilated more than the dependent lung; ventilation/perfusion mismatching occurs because the dependent lung continues to have greater perfusion.

Positive Pressure Ventilation

Controlled positive pressure ventilation favors the upper lung in the lateral position because the upper lung is more compliant than the lower one. Muscle paralysis enhances this effect by allowing the abdominal contents to rise up further against the dependent hemidiaphragm and impede ventilation of the lower lung. Using a rigid "bean bag" to maintain the patient in the lateral decubitus position further restricts movement of the dependent hemithorax. Finally, opening the nondependent side of the chest further accentuates differences in compliances between the two sides because the upper lung now is less restricted in movement. All these effects worsen ventilation/perfusion mismatching and predispose to hypoxemia.

THE OPEN PNEUMOTHORAX

The lungs are normally kept expanded by a negative pleural pressure—the net result of the tendency of the lung to collapse and the chest wall to expand (see Chapter 22). When one side of the chest is opened, the negative pleural pressure is lost and the elastic recoil of the lung on that side tends to collapse it. Spontaneous ventilation with an open pneumothorax in the lateral position results in paradoxical respirations and mediastinal shift. These two phenomena can cause progressive hypoxemia and hypercapnia, but fortunately, their effects are overcome by the use of positive pressure ventilation during general anesthesia.

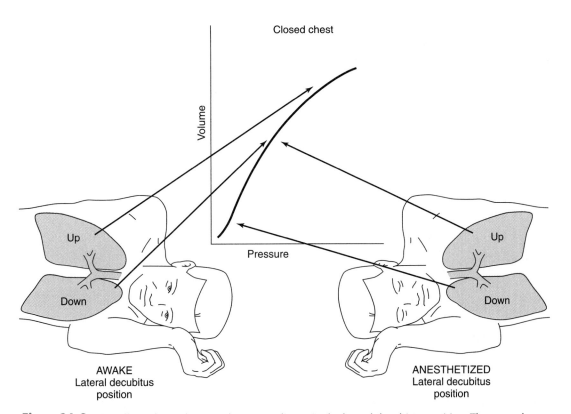

Figure 24–2. The effect of anesthesia on lung compliance in the lateral decubitus position. The upper lung assumes a more favorable position, while the lower lung becomes less compliant.

Mediastinal Shift

During spontaneous ventilation in the lateral position, inspiration causes pleural pressure to become more negative on the dependent side but not on the side of the open pneumothorax. This results in a downward shift of the mediastinum during inspiration and an upward shift during expiration (Figure 24–3). The major effect of mediastinal shift is to decrease the contribution of the dependent lung to the tidal volume.

PARADOXICAL RESPIRATIONS:

Spontaneous ventilation in a patient with an open pneumothorax also results in to-and-fro gas flow between the dependent and nondependent lungs (paradoxical respiration [pendeluft]). During inspiration, the pneumothorax increases and gas flows from the upper lung across the carina to the dependent lung. During expiration, the gas flow reverses and moves from the dependent to the upper lung (Figure 24–4).

ONE-LUNG VENTILATION

Intentional collapse of the lung on the operative side facilitates most thoracic procedures but greatly complicates anesthetic management. Since the collapsed lung continues to be perfused and is deliberately no longer ventilated, the patient develops a large right-to-left intrapulmonary shunt (20–30%). Mixing of unoxygenated blood from the collapsed upper lung with oxygenated blood from the still ventilated dependent lung widens the P_A–a (alveolar-to-arterial) O_2 gradient and can result in hypoxemia. Fortunately, blood flow to the nonventilated lung is decreased by hypoxic pulmonary vasoconstriction (HPV—see Chapter 22) and possibly surgical compression of the upper lung.

Factors known to inhibit HPV and thus worsen the right-to-left shunting include: (1) very high or very low pulmonary artery pressures; (2) hypocapnia; (3) high or very low mixed venous PO_2; (4) vasodilators such as nitroglycerin, nitroprusside, β-adrenergic agonists (including dobutamine and salbutamol) and calcium channel blockers; (5) pulmonary infection; and (6) inhalation anesthetics (see Chapter 22).

Factors that decrease blood flow to the ventilated lung can be equally detrimental; they counteract the effect of HPV by indirectly increasing blood flow to the collapsed lung. Such factors include: (1) high mean airway pressures in the ventilated lung due to high positive end-expiratory pressure (PEEP), hyperventilation, or high peak inspiratory pressures; (2) a low FIO_2, which produces hypoxic pulmonary vasoconstriction in the ventilated lung; (3) vasoconstrictors that may have a greater effect on normoxic vessels than hypoxic ones; and (4) intrinsic PEEP that develops due to inadequate expiratory times.

Carbon dioxide elimination is usually not affected by one-lung ventilation provided minute ventilation is unchanged and preexisting CO_2 retention was not present while ventilating both lungs; arterial CO_2 tension is usually not appreciably altered.

INSPIRATION

Pneumothorax

EXPIRATION

Pneumothorax

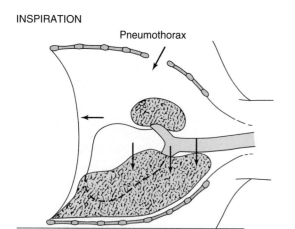
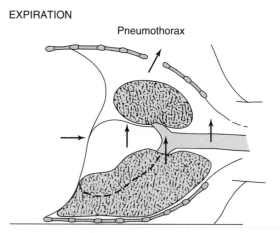

Figure 24–3. Mediastinal shift in a spontaneously breathing patient in the lateral decubitus position (Reproduced, with permission, from Tarhan S, Moffitt EA: Principles of thoracic anesthesia. Surg Clin North Am 1973;53:813.)

INSPIRATION

Pneumothorax

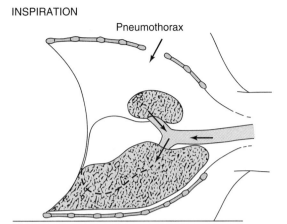

EXPIRATION

Pneumothorax

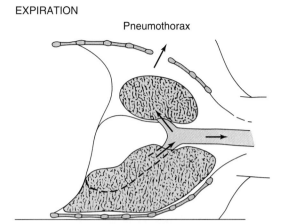

Figure 24–4. Paradoxical respiration in spontaneously breathing patients on their side (Reproduced, with permission, from Tarhan S, Moffitt EA: Principles of thoracic anesthesia. Surg Clin North Am 1973;53:813.)

■ TECHNIQUES FOR ONE-LUNG VENTILATION

One-lung ventilation can also be utilized to isolate a lung or to facilitate ventilatory management under certain conditions (Table 24–1). Three techniques can be employed: (1) placement of a double-lumen endobronchial tube; (2) use of a single-lumen endotracheal tube in conjunction with a bronchial blocker; or (3) use

Table 24–1. Indications for one-lung ventilation.

Patient-Related
   Confine infection to one lung
   Confine bleeding to one lung
   Separate ventilation to each lung
      Bronchopleural fistula
      Tracheobronchial disruption
      Large lung cyst or bulla
   Severe hypoxemia due to unilateral lung disease
Procedure-Related
   Repair of thoracic aortic aneurysm
   Lung resection
      Pneumonectomy
      Lobectomy
      Segmental resection
   Thoracoscopy
   Esophageal surgery
   Single lung transplantation
   Anterior approach to the thoracic spine
   Bronchoalveolar lavage

of a single-lumen endobronchial tube. Double-lumen tubes are most often used.

DOUBLE-LUMEN ENDOBRONCHIAL TUBES

The principal advantages of double-lumen tubes are relative ease of placement, the ability of ventilating either or both lungs, and the ability to suction either lung.

All double-lumen tubes (Table 24–2) share the following characteristics:

- A longer bronchial lumen which enters either the right or left main bronchus and another shorter tracheal lumen which remains in the lower trachea;
- A preformed curve that allows preferential entry into either bronchus;
- A bronchial cuff; and
- A tracheal cuff.

Ventilation can be delivered to only one lung by clamping either the bronchial or tracheal lumen with

Table 24–2. Types of double-lumen tubes.

Name	Bronchus Intubated	Carinal Hook	Shape of Lumen
Carlens	Left	Yes	Oval
White	Right	Yes	Oval
Robert-Shaw	Right or left	No	D-shaped

both cuffs inflated; opening the port on the appropriate connector allows the ipsilateral lung to collapse. Because of differences in bronchial anatomy between the two sides, tubes are designed specifically for either the right or left bronchus.

The most commonly used double-lumen tubes are of the Robert-Shaw type. They are available in sizes 35, 37, 39, and 41F (internal diameters of about 5.0, 5.5, 6.0, and 6.5 mm, respectively). A 39F tube is used for most men, while a 37F tube is selected for most women.

Anatomic Considerations

The adult trachea is 11–13 cm long. It begins at the level of the cricoid cartilage (C6) and bifurcates behind the sternomanubrial joint (T5). Major differences between the right and left main bronchi are as follows: (1) the wider right bronchus diverges away from the trachea at a 25-degree angle, while the left bronchus diverges at a 45-degree angle (Figure 24–5); (2) the right bronchus has upper, middle, and lower lobe branches, while the left bronchus divides into only upper and lower lobe branches; and (3) the orifice of the right upper lobe bronchus is about 1–2.5 cm from the carina, while that of the left upper lobe is about 5 cm distal to the carina.

Right-sided endobronchial tubes must have a slit in the bronchial cuff for ventilating the right upper lobe (Figure 24–6). Anatomic variations between individuals in the distance between the right upper lobe orifice and the carina often result in difficulties in ventilating that lobe with right-sided tubes. Right-sided tubes were designed for left thoracotomies, while left-sided tubes were designed for right thoracotomies. Most anesthetists, however, use a left-sided tube regardless of the operative side; for left-sided surgery, the tube can be withdrawn into the trachea prior to clamping of the left bronchus, if necessary.

Some tubes have carinal hooks (eg, Carlens and White), but the difficulties often encountered in placing them through the larynx have caused many clinicians to abandon them. The most widely used double-lumen tubes are disposable versions of the Robert-Shaw tube.

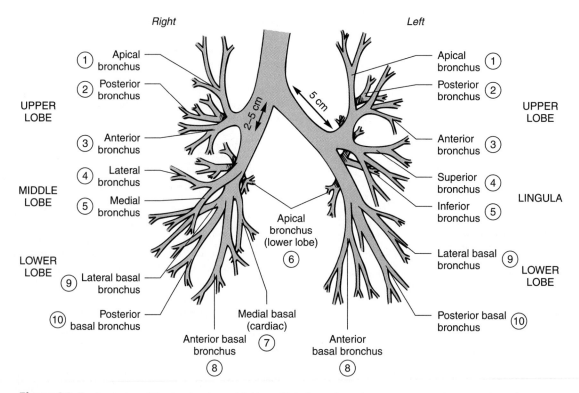

Figure 24–5. Anatomy of the tracheobronchial tree. Note bronchopulmonary segments as numbered. (Adapted and reproduced, with permission, from Gothard JWW, Branthwaite MA: *Anesthesia for Thoracic Surgery.* Blackwell, 1982.)

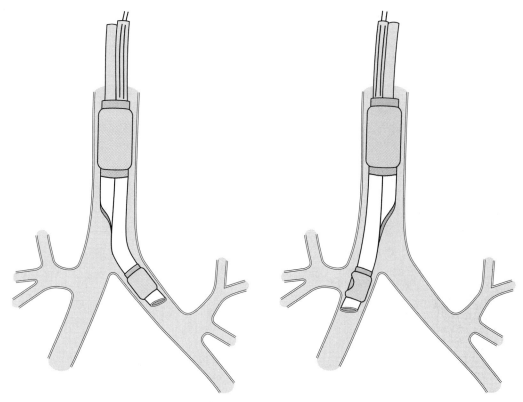

Figure 24–6. Correct position of a right- and left-sided double-lumen tube.

Placement of Double-Lumen Tubes

Laryngoscopy with a curved (MacIntosh) blade usually provides better visualization than a straight blade; the latter may be more useful if the larynx is anterior (see Chapter 5). The double-lumen tube is passed with the distal curvature concave anteriorly and is rotated 90 degrees (toward the side of the bronchus to be intubated) after the tip enters the larynx (Figure 24–7). It is advanced until resistance is felt; the average depth of insertion is about 29 cm (at the teeth). Correct tube placement should be established using a preset protocol (Figure 24–8 and Table 24–3), and confirmed by flexible fiberoptic bronchoscopy. When problems are encountered in intubating the patient with the double-lumen tube, placement of a smaller (6.0-7.0 ID) regular tube should attempted; once positioned in the trachea, the latter can be exchanged for the double-lumen tube by utilizing a specially designed catheter guide ("tube exchanger").

Most double-lumen tubes easily accommodate bronchoscopes with a 3.6–4.2 mm outer diameter. When the bronchoscope is introduced into the tracheal lumen and advanced to the tracheal orifice, the carina should be visible (Figure 24–9) and the bronchial tip of the tube should be seen entering the left bronchus; additionally, the top of the bronchial cuff (usually colored blue) should be visible but should not extend above the carina. If the bronchial cuff of a left-sided double-lumen tube is not visible, it may be low enough to obstruct the orifice of the left lower lobe (below); the tube should be withdrawn until the cuff becomes visible. The bronchial cuff should ideally be inflated only to the point at which the audible leak from the open tracheal lumen disappears while ventilating only through the bronchial lumen. Tube position should be reconfirmed after the patient is positioned for surgery because the tube may move relative to the carina as the patient is turned into the lateral decubitus position.

Malpositioning of a double-lumen tube is usually indicated by poor lung compliance and low exhaled tidal volume. Problems with left-sided double-lumen tubes are usually related to one of three possibilities: (1) the tube is too deep; (2) it is not deep enough; or (3) it entered the

A

B

C

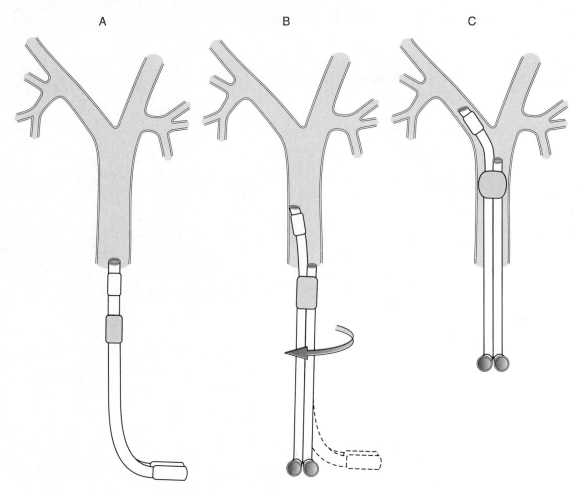

Figure 24–7. Placement of a left-sided double-lumen tube. Note that the tube is turned 90 degrees as soon as it enters the larynx. ***A:*** Initial position. ***B:*** Rotated 90 degrees. ***C:*** Final position.

right bronchus (the wrong side). If the tube is too deep, (as can occur when using a smaller tube in a tall person), the bronchial cuff can obstruct the left upper or the left lower lobe orifice with the opening of the bronchial lumen in the left lower or left upper lobe bronchus, respectively. When the tube is not advanced far enough, the bronchial cuff can occlude the right bronchus. In both instances, deflation of the bronchial cuff improves ventilation to the affected lung and helps identify the problem. It is possible in some patients for the bronchial lumen to be within the left upper or left lower lobe bronchus, but with the tracheal opening remaining above the carina; this situation is suggested by collapse of only one of the left lobes when the bronchial lumen is clamped. Worse, if the surgical procedure is in

the right thorax, when the tracheal lumen is clamped, only the left upper or left lower lobe will be ventilated; hypoxia usually develops rapidly.

Problems with right-sided double-lumen tubes arise because the orifice of the right upper lobe is close (≤1 cm) to the carina. It is very easy to occlude the right upper lobe orifice with the bronchial tube cuff and, hence, the preference for using left-sided double-lumen tubes.

If the tube inadvertently enters the wrong bronchus, the fiberoptic bronchoscope can be used to reposition it into the correct side: (1) the bronchoscope is passed through the bronchial lumen to the tip of the tube; (2) under direct vision the tube and the bronchoscope are withdrawn together into the trachea just above the ca-

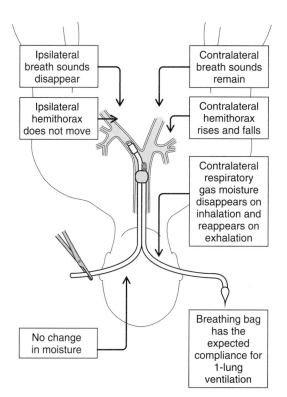

Figure 24–8. Results of unilateral clamping of the endotracheal tube when the double-lumen tube is in the correct position.

Table 24–3. Protocol for checking placement of a left-sided double-lumen tube.

1. Inflate the tracheal cuff (5–10 mL of air).
2. Check for bilateral breath sounds. Unilateral breath sounds indicate that the tube is too far down (tracheal opening is endobronchial).
3. Inflate the bronchial cuff (1–2 mL).
4. Clamp the tracheal lumen.
5. Check for unilateral left-sided breath sounds.
   a. Persistence of right-sided breath sounds indicates that the bronchial opening is still in the trachea (tube should be advanced).
   b. Unilateral right-sided breath sounds indicate incorrect entry of the tube in the right bronchus.
   c. Absence of breath sounds over the entire right lung and the left upper lobe indicates the tube is too far down the left bronchus.
6. Unclamp the tracheal lumen and clamp the bronchial lumen.
7. Check for unilateral right breath sounds. Absence or diminution of breath sounds indicates that the tube is not far enough down and the bronchial cuff is occluding the distal trachea.

rina; (3) the bronchoscope alone is then advanced into the correct bronchus; and (4) the double-lumen tube is gently advanced over the bronchoscope which functions as a stylet to guide the bronchial lumen into the correct bronchus.

Complications of Double-Lumen Tubes

Major complications of double-lumen tubes include (1) hypoxemia due to tube malplacement or occlusion; (2) traumatic laryngitis (especially with tubes that have a carinal hook); (3) tracheobronchial rupture resulting from overinflation of the bronchial cuff, and (4) inadvertent suturing of the tube to a bronchus during surgery (detected as inability to withdraw the tube during attempted extubation).

SINGLE-LUMEN ENDOTRACHEAL TUBES WITH A BRONCHIAL BLOCKER

Bronchial blockers are inflatable devices that are passed alongside or through a single-lumen endotracheal tube to selectively occlude a bronchial orifice. A single-lumen endotracheal tube with a built-in side channel for a retractable bronchial blocker is commercially available (Univent tube; Vitaid; Lewiston, NY). The tube is placed with the blocker fully retracted; its natural curve is such that turning the tube with the curve concave toward the right preferentially directs the bronchial blocker toward the right bronchus; turning the tube such that the curve is concave to the left usu-

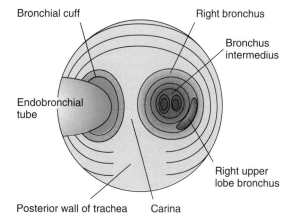

Figure 24–9. The view of the carina looking down the tracheal lumen of a properly positioned left double-lumen endobronchial tube.

ally directs the blocker toward the left bronchus. The bronchial blocker must be advanced, positioned, and inflated under direct visualization via a flexible bronchoscope. The latter is passed through an adapter with a self-sealing diaphragm that allows uninterrupted ventilation. The cuff of the blocker is a high pressure-low volume cuff (see Chapter 5), so the minimum volume that prevents a leak should be used. A channel within the blocker allows the lung to deflate (though slowly) and can be used for suctioning or insufflating oxygen (below). The major advantage of this tube is that, unlike a double-lumen tube, it does not need to be replaced with a regular endotracheal tube if the patient is to be left intubated postoperatively (below). Its major disadvantage is that the "blocked" lung collapses slowly (and sometimes incompletely) because of the small size of the channel within the blocker.

An inflatable (Fogarty) catheter (3 mL) can be used as a bronchial blocker in conjunction with a regular endotracheal tube (inside or alongside); a guidewire in the catheter can be used to facilitate placement. This technique is being used with increased frequency. It also does not allow suctioning or ventilation of the isolated lung, and the catheter is easily dislodged. Nonetheless, bronchial blockers may be useful for one-lung anesthesia in pediatric patients and for tamponading endobronchial bleeding in adult patients (see below).

SINGLE-LUMEN ENDOBRONCHIAL TUBES

Single-lumen endobronchial tubes are now rarely used. The Gordon-Green tube is a right-sided single-lumen tube which can be used for left thoracotomies; it has both tracheal and bronchial cuffs as well as a carinal hook. Inflating the bronchial cuff isolates and allows ventilation of only the right lung. When the bronchial cuff is deflated and the tracheal cuff is inflated, both lungs can be ventilated. A much larger slit in the bronchial cuff (compared with right-sided double-lumen tubes) results in a high success rate for ventilating the right upper lobe. The principal disadvantages of the Gordon-Green tube are the hazards of a carinal hook and the inability to suction the left lung. An ordinary, uncut single-lumen endotracheal tube may be used as an endobronchial tube in an emergency situation (unilateral pulmonary hemorrhage). The tube can usually be advanced blindly into the right bronchus if the source of the hemorrhage is the left lung; unfortunately, the right upper lobe may not be ventilated (see above). Positioning the tube blindly into the left bronchus is more difficult (advancing the tube with its convexity posteriorly while turning the head to the right) and should be guided by bronchoscopy, whenever possible.

■ ANESTHESIA FOR LUNG RESECTION

PREOPERATIVE CONSIDERATIONS

Lung resections are usually carried out for the diagnosis and treatment of pulmonary tumors, and less commonly for complications of necrotizing pulmonary infections and bronchiectasis.

1. Tumors

Pulmonary tumors may be either obviously benign or malignant, or can have an intermediate nature. This distinction often cannot be made until the time of surgery. Hamartomas account for 90% of benign pulmonary tumors; they are usually peripheral pulmonary lesions, and represent disorganized normal pulmonary tissue. Bronchial adenomas are usually central pulmonary lesions that are typically benign but occasionally may be locally invasive and rarely can metastasize. These tumors include pulmonary carcinoids, cylindromas, and mucoepidermoid adenomas. They often obstruct the bronchial lumen and cause recurrent pneumonia distal to the obstruction in the same area. Pulmonary carcinoids are derived from APUD cells and may secrete multiple hormones, including adrenocorticotropic hormone (ACTH) and arginine vasopressin; manifestations of the carcinoid syndrome are uncommon and are more likely with hepatic metastases (see Chapter 36).

Malignant pulmonary tumors are divided into small ("oat") cell (20% of tumors with a 5–10% 5-year survival) and non–small cell carcinomas (80% of tumors with a 15–20% 5-year survival). The latter includes squamous cell (epidermoid) tumors, adenocarcinomas, and large cell (anaplastic) carcinomas. All types are most commonly encountered in smokers, but adenocarcinoma also occurs in nonsmokers. Epidermoid and small cell carcinomas usually present as central masses with endobronchial lesions, while adenocarcinoma and large cell carcinomas are more typically peripheral lesions that often involve the pleura.

Clinical Manifestations

Symptoms may include cough, hemoptysis, dyspnea, wheezing, weight loss, fever, or productive sputum. The latter two suggest a postobstructive pneumonia. Pleuritic chest pain or pleural effusion suggests pleural extension. Involvement of mediastinal structures is suggested by hoarseness that results from compression of the recurrent laryngeal nerve, a Horner's syndrome (see

Chapter 18) caused by involvement of the sympathetic chain, an elevated hemidiaphragm caused by compression of the phrenic nerve, dysphagia from compression of the esophagus, or the superior vena cava syndrome. Pericardial effusion or cardiomegaly suggests cardiac involvement. Extension of apical (superior sulcus) tumors can result in either shoulder or arm pain or both because of involvement of the C7–T2 roots of the brachial plexus (Pancoast syndrome). Distant metastases most commonly involve the brain, bone, liver, and adrenal glands.

Lung carcinomas—especially small cell—can produce remote effects that are not related to malignant spread (paraneoplastic syndromes). Mechanisms include ectopic hormone production and immunologic cross-reactivity between the tumor and normal tissues. Cushing's syndrome, hyponatremia, and hypercalcemia may be encountered, resulting from secretion of ACTH, arginine vasopressin and parathyroid hormone, respectively (see Chapter 36). Lambert-Eaton (myasthenic) syndrome is characterized by a proximal myopathy in which muscle strength increases with repeated effort (in contrast to myasthenia gravis—see Chapter 37). Other paraneoplastic syndromes include hypertrophic osteoarthropathy, cerebellar degeneration, peripheral neuropathy, polymyositis, migratory thrombophlebitis, and nonbacterial endocarditis.

Treatment

Surgery is the treatment of choice for the curative treatment of lung cancer. Surgical resection is attempted for non–small cell carcinomas in the absence of advanced lymph node involvement, direct extension into mediastinal structures, or distant metastases. In contrast, small cell carcinomas are infrequently treated surgically because they nearly always have already metastasized by the time the diagnosis is made; these cancers are treated with chemotherapy or chemotherapy and radiation.

RESECTABILITY AND OPERABILITY:

Resectability is determined by the anatomic stage of the tumor, while operability is also dependent on the extent of the procedure and the physiologic status of the patient. Anatomic staging includes chest radiography, computed tomography (CT), bronchoscopy, and mediastinoscopy (below). Patients with ipsilateral peribronchial or ipsilateral hilar lymph node metastases are considered resectable. Resection of lesions with ipsilateral mediastinal or subcarinal lymph node metastases, however, is controversial. Lesions associated with scalene, supraclavicular, contralateral mediastinal, or contralateral hilar lymph node metastases are usually considered unresectable. In the absence of mediastinal metastases, some centers also perform en bloc resections

of tumors involving the chest wall; similarly, in the absence of mediastinal metastases, superior sulcus tumors may be resected after preoperative radiotherapy.

The extent of the surgery should maximize the chances for a cure but still allow for adequate residual pulmonary function postoperatively. Lobectomy via a posterior thoracotomy, through the fifth or sixth intercostal space, is the procedure of choice for most lesions. Segmental or wedge resections may be performed in patients with small peripheral lesions and poor pulmonary reserve. Pneumonectomy is necessary for curative treatment of lesions involving the left or right main bronchus or when the tumor extends to the hilum. Operative criteria for pneumonectomy are discussed below. A sleeve resection may be employed for patients with proximal lesions and limited pulmonary reserve as an alternative to pneumonectomy; in such instances, the involved lobar bronchus together with part of the right or left main bronchus is resected and the distal bronchus is reanastomosed to the proximal bronchus or the trachea. Sleeve pneumonectomy may be considered for tumors involving the trachea. The mortality for pneumonectomy is generally 5–7%, compared with 2–3% for a lobectomy. Mortality is higher for right-sided pneumonectomy compared to left pneumonectomy possibly because of greater loss of lung tissue. Most postoperative deaths result from cardiac causes.

Operative Criteria for Pneumonectomy

Operability is ultimately a clinical decision, but pulmonary function tests offer useful preliminary guidelines. The degree of preoperative impairment—as measured by routine pulmonary function tests—is directly related to operative risk. Standard preliminary criteria for operability are set forth in Table 24–4. Failure to

Table 24–4. Preoperative laboratory criteria for pneumonectomy.

Test	High-Risk Patients
Arterial blood gas	$PaCO_2 > 45$ mm Hg (on room air) $PaO_2 < 50$ mm Hg
FEV_1 (Predicted postoperative FEV_1)	<2 L <0.8 L or <40% of predicted
FEV_1/FVC	<50% of predicted
Maximum breathing capacity	<50% of predicted
Maximum $\dot{V}O_2$	<10 mL/kg/min

FEV_1 = forced expiratory volume in 1 second; FVC = forced vital capacity.

meet any one of these criteria necessitates split lung function tests if pneumonectomy is still contemplated. The most commonly used criterion for operability is a predicted postoperative FEV_1 greater than 800 mL. The percentage contribution of each lung to total FEV_1 is assumed to be proportionate to the percentage of the total pulmonary blood flow it receives as determined by radioisotopic scanning (133Xe or 99Tc).

$$\text{Postoperative } FEV_1 = \% \text{ blood flow to remaining lung} \times \text{total } FEV_1$$

Removal of extensively diseased lung (nonventilated but perfused) may not adversely affect pulmonary function and may actually improve oxygenation. If the predicted postoperative FEV_1 is less than 800 mL but resection is still considered, the ability of the remaining pulmonary vasculature to tolerate total blood flow can be tested but is rarely done. The main pulmonary artery on the diseased side is occluded with a balloon catheter; if the mean pulmonary artery pressure exceeds 40 mm Hg or PaO_2 decreases to < 45 mm Hg, the patient is not a candidate for pneumonectomy.

The two greatest risks to lung resection involve the pulmonary and cardiac systems. It makes sense, therefore, to test both systems. Patients capable of climbing two to three flights of stairs without becoming too winded often tolerate surgery relatively well without further testing. Maximum oxygen consumption ($\dot{V}O_2$) during exercise also appears to be useful predictor of postoperative morbidity and mortality. Patients with $\dot{V}O_2 > 20$ mL/kg have low complication rates, while those with $\dot{V}O_2 < 10$ mL/kg have unacceptably high morbidity and mortality.

2. Infection

Pulmonary infections may present as a solitary nodule or cavitary lesion (necrotizing pneumonitis). An exploratory thoracotomy may be carried out to exclude malignancy and diagnose the infectious agent. Lung resection is also indicated for cavitary lesions that are refractory to antibiotic treatment, are associated with refractory empyema, or result in massive hemoptysis. Responsible organisms include both bacteria (anaerobes, Mycoplasma, *Mycobacterium tuberculosis, Nocardia,* and a variety of enteric and nonenteric pyogenic species) and fungi (*Histoplasma, Coccidioides, Cryptococcus, Blastomyces, Mucor,* and *Aspergillus*).

3. Bronchiectasis

Bronchiectasis is a permanent dilation of bronchi. It is usually the end result of severe or recurrent inflammation and obstruction of bronchi. Causes include a vari-

ety of viral, bacterial, and fungal pathogens, as well as inhalation of toxic gases, aspiration of gastric acid, and defective mucociliary clearance (cystic fibrosis and disorders of ciliary dysfunction). Bronchial muscle and elastic tissue is typically replaced by very vascular fibrous tissue. The latter predisposes to bouts of hemoptysis. Pulmonary resection is usually indicated for massive hemoptysis when conservative measures have failed and the disease is localized. Patients with diffuse disease have a significant chronic obstructive ventilatory defect (see Chapter 23).

ANESTHETIC CONSIDERATIONS

1. Preoperative Management

The majority of patients undergoing pulmonary resections have underlying lung disease. Preoperative assessment of such patients is discussed in detail in Chapter 23. It should be emphasized that smoking is a risk factor for both chronic obstructive pulmonary disease and coronary artery disease (see Chapter 20); both disorders commonly coexist in patients presenting for thoracotomy. Echocardiography is very useful for assessing baseline cardiac function and may suggest evidence of cor pulmonale (right ventricular enlargement or hypertrophy). Dobutamine stress echocardiography may be useful in detecting occult coronary artery disease (see Chapter 20).

Patients with tumors should be evaluated for complications related to local extension of the tumor and paraneoplastic syndromes (above). Preoperative chest radiographs and CT and magnetic resonance imaging scans should be reviewed carefully. Tracheal or bronchial deviation can complicate endotracheal intubation or proper positioning of endobronchial tubes. Moreover, airway compression can lead to difficulty in ventilating the patient following induction of anesthesia. Pulmonary consolidation, atelectasis, and large pleural effusions predispose to hypoxemia. The location of any bullous cysts or abscesses should be noted.

Patients undergoing thoracic procedures are at increased risk for postoperative pulmonary and cardiac complications (see Chapter 23). Good preoperative preparation may reduce pulmonary complications in high-risk patients. Perioperative arrhythmias, especially supraventricular tachycardias, are thought to result from surgical manipulations or distention of the right atrium following reduction of the pulmonary vascular bed. The incidence of arrhythmias increases with age and with the amount of pulmonary resection.

Premedication

Patients with moderate to severe respiratory compromise should receive little or no sedative premedication.

Although anticholinergics (atropine, 0.5 mg IM or IV, or glycopyrrolate, 0.1–0.2 mg IM or IV) can theoretically inspissate secretions and increase dead space, clinically they are very useful in reducing copious secretions. The latter improves visualization during repeated laryngoscopies and facilitates the use of a fiberoptic bronchoscope.

2. Intraoperative Management

Preparation

As with anesthesia for cardiac surgery, optimal preparation may help prevent potentially catastrophic problems. The frequent presence of poor pulmonary reserve, anatomic abnormalities or compromise of the airways, and the need for one-lung anesthesia predisposes these patients to the rapid onset of hypoxemia. A clear and well thought-out plan to deal with potential difficulties is necessary. Moreover, in addition to items for basic airway management (see Chapter 5), specialized and properly functioning equipment—such as multiple sizes of single- and double-lumen tubes, a flexible (pediatric) fiberoptic bronchoscope, a small diameter "tube exchanger," a continuous positive airway pressure (CPAP) delivery system, and an anesthesia circuit adapter for administering bronchodilators—should be immediately available.

When epidural opioids are to be used for postoperative analgesia (below), consideration should be given to placing the catheter prior to induction of anesthesia while the patient is still awake. This practice can facilitate placement and may decrease the incidence of neurologic complications (see Chapter 16).

Venous Access

At least one large-bore intravenous line (14- or 16-gauge) is mandatory for all thoracic surgical procedures. Central venous access (preferably on the side of the thoracotomy), a blood warmer, and a rapid infusion device are also desirable if extensive blood loss is anticipated.

Monitoring

Direct arterial pressure monitoring is indicated for one-lung anesthesia (below), for resections of large tumors especially those with mediastinal or chest wall extension, for any procedure in patients with limited pulmonary reserve or significant cardiovascular disease. Central venous access with central venous pressure (CVP) monitoring is highly desirable for pneumonectomies and resections of large tumors. CVP reflects the net effect of venous capacitance, blood volume, and right ventricular function; consequently, it is only a rough guide to fluid management. Pulmonary artery

catheterization is indicated in patients with pulmonary hypertension, cor pulmonale, or left ventricular dysfunction; radiographic confirmation of the position of the catheter is useful in ascertaining that the pulmonary artery catheter (PAC) is not in a lung segment to be resected. When the PAC tip is in the nondependent (upper) lung and that lung is collapsed, cardiac output and mixed venous oxygen tension may be falsely depressed during one-lung ventilation. The balloon of a PAC should be inflated carefully following pneumonectomy because the remaining pulmonary vasculature has a significantly reduced cross-sectional area; balloon inflation can acutely increase right ventricular afterload and can lower left ventricular preload.

Induction of Anesthesia

After adequate preoxygenation, an intravenous anesthetic is used for induction of most patients. The selection of an induction agent should be based on the patient's preoperative status. Direct laryngoscopy should generally be performed only after deep anesthesia to prevent reflex bronchospasm and to obtund the cardiovascular pressor response. This may be accomplished by incremental doses of the induction agent, an opioid, or both (see Chapter 20). Deepening anesthesia with a volatile inhalational agent may be preferable in patients with reactive airways.

Endotracheal intubation is facilitated with succinylcholine or a nondepolarizing agent; the former may be more appropriate if difficult laryngoscopy is anticipated. Most thoracotomies can be performed with an ordinary endotracheal tube, but techniques for one-lung ventilation (above) greatly facilitate most thoracic operations. Use of a single-lumen endotracheal may be necessary, however, if the surgeon performs diagnostic bronchoscopy (below) prior to surgery; once the bronchoscopy is completed, the single-lumen tube can be replaced with a double-lumen endobronchial tube (above). Controlled positive pressure ventilation helps prevent atelectasis, paradoxical breathing, and mediastinal shift; it also allows control of the operative field to facilitate the surgery.

Positioning

Following induction, intubation, and confirmation of correct endotracheal or endobronchial tube position, additional venous access and monitoring may be secured before the patient is positioned for surgery. Most lung resections are performed via posterior thoracotomy with the patient in the lateral decubitus position. Proper positioning is critical to avoid injuries and to facilitate surgical exposure. The lower arm is flexed while the upper arm is extended in front of the head,

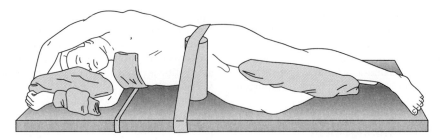

Figure 24–10. Proper positioning for a lateral thoracotomy (Reproduced, with permission, from Gothard JWW, Branthwaite MA: *Anesthesia for Thoracic Surgery.* Blackwell, 1982.)

pulling the scapula away from the operative field (Figure 24–10). Pillows are placed between the arms and legs, and an axillary roll is positioned just beneath the dependent axilla to avoid injury to the brachial plexus; care is taken to avoid pressure on the eyes and the dependent ear.

Maintenance of Anesthesia

All current anesthetic techniques have been successfully used for thoracic surgery, but the combination of a potent halogenated agent (halothane, isoflurane, sevoflurane or desflurane) with an opioid is preferred by most clinicians. Advantages of the former halogenated agents include: (1) potent dose-related bronchodilation; (2) depression of airway reflexes; (3) the ability to use a high inspired oxygen concentration (FiO_2); (4) the capability for relatively rapid adjustments in anesthetic depth; and (5) minimal effects on hypoxic pulmonary vasoconstriction (see below). Halogenated agents generally have minimal effects on HPV in doses < 1 minimum alveolar concentration (MAC) (see Chapter 22). Advantages of an opioid include: (1) generally minimal hemodynamic effects; (2) depression of airway reflexes;

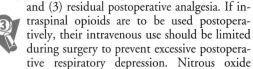

and (3) residual postoperative analgesia. If intraspinal opioids are to be used postoperatively, their intravenous use should be limited during surgery to prevent excessive postoperative respiratory depression. Nitrous oxide (N_2O) is generally not used because of the obligatory decrease in FiO_2. Like volatile agents, nitrous oxide can also inhibit hypoxic pulmonary vasoconstriction and additionally can exacerbate pulmonary hypertension in some patients.

Maintenance of muscle paralysis with a nondepolarizing neuromuscular blocking agent (also called muscle relaxants) during surgery facilitates rib spreading as well as anesthetic management. Maximal anesthetic depth is required when the ribs are spread apart. Sustained vagally mediated bradycardia due to surgical manipula-

tions should be treated with intravenous atropine. Venous return decreases when the chest is opened because negative pleural (intrathoracic) pressure is lost on the operative side. This effect may be reversed with an intravenous fluid bolus.

Intravenous fluids should generally be restricted in patients undergoing pulmonary resections. Fluid management only consists of basic maintenance requirements and replacement of blood loss (see Chapter 29); colloid or blood is usually used for the latter. Excessive fluid administration in the lateral decubitus position may promote a "lower lung syndrome," ie, gravity-dependent transudation of fluid into the dependent lung. The latter increases intrapulmonary shunting and promotes hypoxemia especially during one-lung ventilation. Moreover, the collapsed lung is also prone to edema following reexpansion as a result of surgical retraction.

During lung resections, the bronchus (or remaining lung tissue) is usually divided with an automated stapling device. The bronchial stump is then tested for an air leak under water by transiently sustaining 30 cm of positive pressure to the airway. During rib approximation, hand ventilation is helpful in avoiding injury to lung parenchyma from suture needles following lobectomy or wedge resection if a single-lumen tube is being used. Prior to completion of chest closure, all remaining lung segments should be fully expanded manually under direct vision. Controlled mechanical ventilation is then resumed and continued until chest tubes are connected to suction. Chest tubes are not needed following pneumonectomy.

Management of One-Lung Ventilation

The greatest risk of one-lung ventilation is hypoxemia. To reduce this risk, the period of one-lung ventilation should be kept to a minimum and 100% oxygen should be used. Major adjustments in ventilation are usually not necessary. If peak airway pressures rise excessively (> 30 cm H_2O), tidal volume may be reduced to 6–10 mL/kg and the ventilatory rate increased to maintain the same minute ventilation. Close monitoring of the pulse oximeter is mandatory. Periodic arterial blood gas analysis is helpful to ensure adequate ventilation. End-tidal carbon dioxide measurement may not be reliable (see Chapter 6).

Hypoxemia during one-lung anesthesia requires one or more of the following interventions:

Consistently effective measures:

(1) Periodic inflation of the collapsed lung with oxygen.
(2) Early ligation or clamping of the ipsilateral pulmonary artery (during pneumonectomy).
(3) 5–10 cm H_2O of CPAP to the collapsed lung; this is most effective when there is partial reexpansion of the lung which unfortunately can interfere with surgery.

Marginally effective measures:

(1) 5–10 cm H_2O of PEEP to the ventilated lung.
(2) Continuous insufflation of oxygen into the collapsed lung.
(3) Changing the tidal volume and ventilatory rate.

Persistent hypoxemia requires immediate reexpansion of the collapsed lung. The endobronchial tube (or bronchial blocker) position relative to the carina can change as a result of surgical manipulations or traction; repeat fiberoptic bronchoscopy through the tracheal lumen can quickly exclude this problem. Both lumens of the tube should also be suctioned to exclude excessive secretions or obstruction as a factor. If blood is present in the airway, instillation of 3–5 mL of sodium bicarbonate into the tube may help facilitate the removal of clots. Pneumothorax on the dependent, ventilated side should also be considered; the latter may be more likely to occur following extensive mediastinal dissection or with high peak inspiratory pressures.

Alternatives to One-Lung Ventilation

Ventilation can be stopped for short periods if 100% oxygen is insufflated at a rate greater than oxygen consumption (**apneic oxygenation**). Adequate oxygenation can often be maintained for prolonged periods, but progressive respiratory acidosis limits the use of this technique to 10–20 minutes in most patients. Arterial PCO_2 rises 6 mm Hg in the first minute, followed by a rise of 3–4 mm Hg during each subsequent minute.

High-frequency positive pressure ventilation and high-frequency jet ventilation (see Chapter 50) have been used during thoracic procedures as alternatives to one-lung ventilation. A standard endotracheal tube may be used with either technique. Small tidal volumes (< 2 mL/kg) allow decreased lung excursion, which may facilitate the surgery but still allow ventilation of both lungs. Unfortunately, mediastinal "bounce"—a to-and-fro movement—often interferes with the surgery.

3. Postoperative Management

General Care

Most patients are extubated early to decrease the risk of pulmonary barotrauma (particularly blowout of the bronchial suture line) and pulmonary infection. Patients with marginal pulmonary reserve should be left intubated until standard extubation criteria are met (see Chapter 50); if a double-lumen tube was used for one-lung ventilation, it must be replaced with a regular single lumen tube at the end of surgery. A catheter guide ("tube exchanger") should be used if the original laryngoscopy was difficult (above).

Patients are observed carefully in the postanesthesia care unit (PACU) and, in most instances, at least overnight or longer in an intensive care unit (ICU) or intermediate care unit. Postoperative hypoxemia and respiratory acidosis are common. These effects are largely caused by atelectasis from surgical compression of the lungs and "shallow breathing ('splinting')" due to incisional pain. Gravity-dependent transudation of fluid into the dependent lung (above) may also be contributory. Reexpansion edema of the collapsed, nondependent lung can also occur and may be more likely to occur with rapid reinflation of the lung.

 Postoperative hemorrhage necessitating reexploration complicates about 3% of thoracotomies and may be associated with up to 20% mortality. Signs of hemorrhage include increased chest tube drainage (> 200 mL/hour), hypotension, tachycardia, and a falling hematocrit. Postoperative supraventricular tachyarrhythmias are common and should be treated aggressively (see Chapters 19 and 48). Acute right ventricular failure is suggested by a low cardiac output, elevated CVP, oliguria, and a normal pulmonary capillary occlusion pressure (see Chapter 21).

Routine postoperative care should include maintenance of a semiupright (> 30 degrees) position, supplemental oxygen (40–50%), incentive spirometry, close electrocardiographic and hemodynamic monitoring, a postoperative radiograph, and aggressive pain relief.

Postoperative Analgesia

The balance between comfort and respiratory depression in patients with marginal lung function is difficult to achieve with parenteral opioids alone. Patients who have undergone thoracotomy clearly benefit from the use of other techniques described below which may obviate the need for any parenteral opioids. If parenteral opioids are used alone, small intravenous doses are superior to large intramuscular doses and probably best administered via a patient-controlled analgesia (PCA) device (see Chapter 18).

A long-acting agent such as 0.5% ropivacaine (4–5 mL), injected two levels above and below the thoracotomy incision, typically provides excellent pain relief. These blocks may be done under direct vision intraoperatively or via the standard technique (see Chapter 17) postoperatively. Intercostal blocks have been shown to improve arterial blood gases and pulmonary function tests, and shorten hospital stay. Alternatively, a cryoanalgesia probe may be used intraoperatively to freeze the intercostal nerves (cryoneurolysis) and produce long-lasting anesthesia; unfortunately, maximum analgesia may not be achieved until 24–48 hours after the cryoanalgesia procedure. Nerve regeneration is reported to occur approximately 1 month after the cryoneurolysis.

Epidural opioids with or without a local anesthetic can also provide excellent analgesia (see Chapter 18). Equally satisfactory analgesia may be obtained with either a lumbar or thoracic epidural catheter when morphine is used. Injection of morphine 5–7 mg in 10–15 mL of saline usually provides 6–24 hours of analgesia without autonomic, sensory, or motor blockade. The lumbar route may be safer because it is less likely to traumatize the spinal cord or puncture the dura, but the latter is more of a theoretical concern because it uncommonly occurs during cautious and correct placement of a thoracic epidural. Epidural injections of a lipophilic opioid, such as fentanyl, may be more effective via a thoracic catheter than a lumbar catheter (see Chapter 18). Some clinicians prefer epidural fentanyl because it is less likely to cause delayed respiratory depression. In either case, patients should be closely monitored for this complication.

Some studies suggest interpleural analgesia, also called intrapleural analgesia (see Chapter 18), can provide good analgesia following thoracotomy. Unfortunately, clinical experience has provided inconsistent results, possibly because of the necessary use of thoracostomy tubes and the presence of blood within the pleura.

Postoperative Complications

Postoperative complications following thoracotomy are relatively common, but fortunately most are minor and resolve uneventfully. Blood clots and thick secretions readily obstruct the airways and result in atelectasis; aggressive but gentle suctioning may be necessary. Significant atelectasis is suggested by tracheal deviation and shifting of the mediastinum to the operative side following segmental or lobar resections. Therapeutic bronchoscopy should be considered for persistent atelectasis, especially when associated with thick secretions. Air leaks from the operative hemithorax are common following segmental and lobar resections because fissures are usually incomplete; resection therefore often leaves open the small channels responsible for collateral ventilation.

 Most air leaks stop after a few days. Bronchopleural fistula presents as a sudden large air leak from the chest tube that may be associated with an increasing pneumothorax and partial lung collapse. When it occurs within the first 24–72 hours, it is usually the result of inadequate surgical closure of the bronchial stump. Delayed presentation is usually due to necrosis of the suture line associated with inadequate blood flow or infection.

Some complications are rare but deserve special consideration because they can be life-threatening, require a high index of suspicion, and may require immediate exploratory thoracotomy. Postoperative bleeding was discussed above. Torsion of a lobe or segment can occur as the remaining lung on the operative side expands to occupy the hemithorax. The torsion usually occludes the pulmonary vein to that part of the lung, causing venous outflow obstruction. Hemoptysis and infarction can rapidly follow. The diagnosis is suggested by an enlarging homogenous density on the chest radiograph and a closed lobar orifice on bronchoscopy. Acute herniation of the heart into the operative hemithorax can occur through the pericardial defect left following a radical pneumonectomy. A large pressure differential between the two hemithoraxes is thought to trigger this catastrophic event. Herniation into the right hemithorax results in sudden severe hypotension with an elevated CVP because of torsion of the central veins. Herniation into the left hemithorax following left pneumonectomy results in sudden compression of the heart at the atrioventricular groove, resulting in hypotension, ischemia and infarction. A chest radiograph shows a shift of the cardiac shadow into the operative hemithorax.

Extensive mediastinal dissections can injure the phrenic, vagus, and left recurrent laryngeal nerves. Postoperative phrenic nerve palsy presents as elevation of the ipsilateral hemidiaphragm together with difficulty in weaning the patient from the ventilator. Large en block chest wall resections may also involve part of the diaphragm causing a similar problem, in addition to a flail chest (see Chapter 41). Paraplegia can rarely follow thoracotomy for lung resection. Sacrificing the left lower intercostal arteries can produce spinal cord ischemia (see Chapter 21). Alternately, an epidural hematoma may form if the surgical dissection enters the epidural space through the chest cavity.

SPECIAL CONSIDERATIONS FOR PATIENTS UNDERGOING LUNG RESECTION

Massive Pulmonary Hemorrhage

Massive hemoptysis is usually defined as > 500–600 mL of blood loss from the tracheobronchial tree within 24 hours. It complicates only 1–2% of all cases of hemoptysis and is usually the result of tuberculosis, bronchiectasis, or a neoplasm, or follows transbronchial biopsies. Emergency surgical management with lung resection is reserved for "potentially lethal" massive hemoptysis. In most cases surgery is usually carried out on a semi-elective rather than on a true emergent basis whenever possible; even then, operative mortality may exceed 20% (compared with > 50% for medical management). Embolization of the involved bronchial arteries may be attempted. The most common cause of death is asphyxia secondary to blood in the airway. Patients may be brought to the operating room for rigid bronchoscopy when localization is not possible with fiberoptic flexible bronchoscopy. A bronchial blocker or Fogarty catheter (above) may be placed to tamponade the bleeding, or laser coagulation may be attempted (see Chapter 39).

The patient should be maintained in the lateral position as much as possible with the affected lung in a dependent position to tamponade the bleeding. Multiple large-bore intravenous catheters should be placed. Premedication should not be given to awake patients because they are usually already hypoxic; 100% oxygen should be given continuously. If the patient is already intubated and has bronchial blockers in place, sedation is helpful to prevent coughing. Moreover, the bronchial blocker should be left in position until the lung is resected. When the patient is not intubated, an awake intubation is preferable but rapid sequence induction (ketamine or etomidate with succinylcholine) is often necessary. Patients usually swallow a large amount of blood and should be considered to have a full stomach; a semi-upright position and cricoid pressure should therefore be maintained during induction of anesthesia. A large double-lumen endobronchial tube is ideal for protecting the normal lung from blood and for suctioning each lung separately. If any difficulty is encountered in placing the double-lumen tube or its relatively small lumens occlude easily, a large (> 8.0 mm ID) single-lumen tube may be safer; a single-lumen endotracheal tube with a built-in side channel for a retractable bronchial blocker (Univent) should be considered.

Sodium bicarbonate can be used to facilitate the suctioning of large clots from the airways (above).

Pulmonary Cysts & Bullae

Pulmonary cysts or bullae may be congenital or acquired as a result of emphysema. Large bullae can impair ventilation by compressing the surrounding lung. These air cavities often behave as if they have a one-way valve, predisposing them to progressively enlarge. Lung resection may be undertaken for progressive dyspnea or recurrent pneumothorax. The greatest risk of anesthesia is rupture of the air cavity during positive pressure ventilation, resulting in tension pneumothorax; the latter may occur on either side prior to thoracotomy or on the nonoperative side during the lung resection. Induction of anesthesia with maintenance of spontaneous ventilation is desirable until the side with the cyst or bullae is isolated with a double-lumen tube or until a chest tube is placed; most patients have a large increase in dead space, so assisted ventilation is necessary to 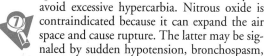 avoid excessive hypercarbia. Nitrous oxide is contraindicated because it can expand the air space and cause rupture. The latter may be signaled by sudden hypotension, bronchospasm, or an abrupt rise in peak inflation pressure, and requires immediate placement of a chest tube.

Lung Abscess

Lung abscesses result from a primary pulmonary infections, obstructing pulmonary neoplasms (above), or rarely, hematogenous spread of systemic infections. Anesthetic management emphasizes isolating the two lungs early to prevent soiling of the healthy one with pus. A rapid-sequence intravenous induction with endotracheal intubation with a double-lumen tube is generally recommended while the patient is in a semi-upright position with the affected lung in a dependent position; the latter helps prevent soiling of the healthy lung. As soon as the double-lumen tube is placed, both bronchial and tracheal cuffs are inflated. The bronchial cuff should make a tight seal before the patient is turned into the lateral decubitus position, with the diseased lung in a nondependent position. The diseased lung should be frequently suctioned during the procedure to lessen the likelihood of contaminating the healthy lung.

Bronchopleural Fistula

Bronchopleural fistulae occur following lung resection (usually pneumonectomy), rupture of a pulmonary abscess into a pleural cavity, pulmonary barotrauma, or spontaneous rupture of bullae. The majority of patients

A NORMAL

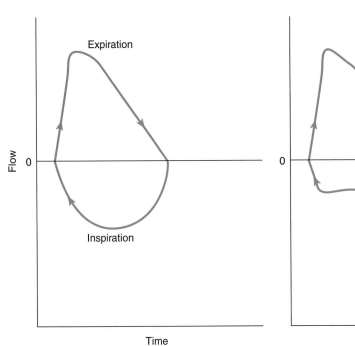

B VARIABLE EXTRATHORACIC OBSTRUCTION

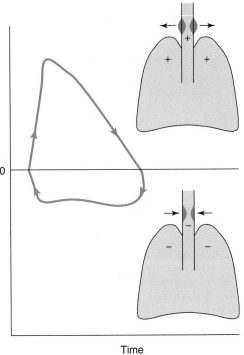

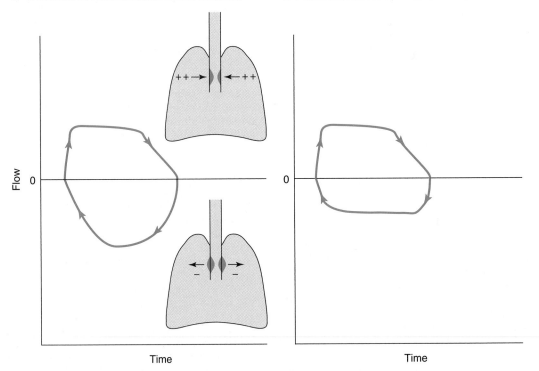

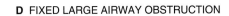

Figure 24–11. Flow-volume loops.

are treated (and cured) conservatively; patients come to surgery after conservative treatment with chest tube drainage and antibiotics has failed. Anesthetic management may be complicated by the inability to effectively ventilate the patient with positive pressure because of a large air leak, the potential for a tension pneumothorax, and the risk of contaminating the other lung if empyema is present. The empyema is usually drained as much as possible preoperatively, prior to closure of the fistula.

Some clinicians recommend an awake intubation with a double-lumen tube in the presence of a large air leak. Alternatively, a rapid sequence intravenous induction with endobronchial intubation may also be utilized. The double-lumen tube greatly simplifies anesthetic management by isolating the fistula and allowing one-lung ventilation to the healthy side. The patient should be extubated after the repair whenever possible.

■ ANESTHESIA FOR TRACHEAL RESECTION

Preoperative Considerations

Tracheal resection is most commonly performed for tracheal stenosis, tumors, or less commonly congenital abnormalities. Tracheal stenosis can follow penetrating or blunt trauma as well as endotracheal intubation and tracheostomy. Squamous cell and adenoid cystic carcinomas account for the majority of tumors. Compromise of the tracheal lumen results in progressive dyspnea. Wheezing or stridor may be evident only with exertion. The dyspnea may be worse when the patient is lying down with progressive airway obstruction. Hemoptysis can also complicate tracheal tumors. Computerized tomography is valuable in localizing the lesion. Measurement of flow-volume loops confirms the location of the obstruction and aids the clinician in evaluating its severity (Figure 24–11).

Anesthetic Considerations

Little or no premedication is given, since most patients presenting for tracheal resection have moderate to severe airway obstruction. Use of an anticholinergic agent to dry secretions is controversial because of the theoretical risk of inspissation. Monitoring should include direct arterial pressure measurements. The left radial artery is preferred for lower tracheal resections because a potential for compression of the innominate artery.

A slow inhalation induction (in 100% oxygen) is carried out for patients with severe obstruction. Halothane may be the preferred agent because it is least irritating to the airway and causes less respiratory depression compared to other volatile agents (see Chapter 7). Spontaneous ventilation is maintained throughout induction. Neuromuscular blocking agents are generally avoided because of the potential for complete airway obstruction following paralysis. Laryngoscopy is performed only when the patient is judged to be under deep anesthesia. Intravenous lidocaine (1–2 mg/kg) can deepen the anesthesia without depressing respirations. The surgeon may then perform rigid bronchoscopy to evaluate and possibly dilate the lesion. Following bronchoscopy the patient is intubated with a sufficiently small endotracheal tube that can be passed distal to the obstruction whenever possible.

A collar incision is utilized for high tracheal lesions. The surgeon divides the trachea in the neck and advances a sterile armored tube into the distal trachea passing off a sterile connecting hose to the anesthesiologist for ventilation during the resection. Following the resection and completion of the posterior part of the reanastomosis, the armored tube is removed and the original endotracheal tube is advanced distally past the anastomosis (Figure 24–12). Alternatively, high-frequency jet ventilation may be employed during the anastomosis by passing the jet cannula past the obstruction and into the distal trachea (Figure 24–13). Return of spontaneous ventilation and early extubation at the end of the procedure are desirable. Patients should be positioned with the neck flexed immediately postoperatively after the operation to minimize tension on the suture line (Figure 24–14).

Surgical management of low tracheal lesions requires a median sternotomy or right posterior thoracotomy. Anesthetic management is similar but more regularly requires more complicated techniques such as high-frequency ventilation or even cardiopulmonary bypass (the latter for complex congenital cases).

■ ANESTHESIA FOR THORACOSCOPIC SURGERY

Thoracoscopy is no longer only a diagnostic procedure, but is increasingly used for up to one third to one half of many thoracic surgical procedures that previously required open thoracotomy. The increasing list of procedures includes lung biopsy, segmental and lobar resections, pleurodesis, esophageal procedures (such as myomectomy) and even pericardectomy (see Chapter 21). Most procedures are performed through three or more small incisions in the chest with the patient in the lateral decubitus position.

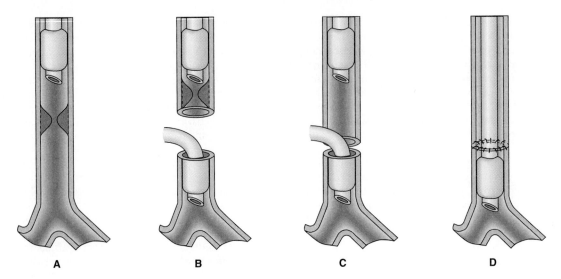

Figure 24–12. Airway management of a high tracheal lesion.

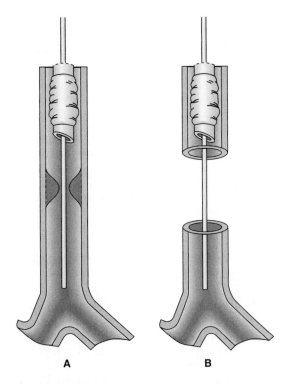

Figure 24–13. Tracheal resection using high-frequency jet ventilation. ***A:*** Catheter is advanced past obstruction and cuff is deflated when jet ventilation is initiated. ***B:*** Catheter is advanced distally by surgeon. Jet ventilation can be continued without interruption during resection and reanastomosis.

Anesthetic management is similar to that for open procedures (above) with the exception that one-lung ventilation is mandatory for all but the most minor procedures. Some centers may use only local anesthesia with spontaneous ventilation for minor procedures, but patient discomfort can be considerable. Opening one of the portals to the atmosphere allows the lung on the operative side to collapse; unlike laparoscopy, insufflation of gas is not only unnecessary but hazardous.

■ ANESTHESIA FOR DIAGNOSTIC THORACIC PROCEDURES

Bronchoscopy

Topical and local anesthesia for flexible bronchoscopy is discussed in Chapter 5. Rigid bronchoscopy for removal of foreign bodies or for tracheal dilatation is usually performed under general anesthesia. These procedures are complicated by the need to share the airway with the surgeon or pulmonologist; fortunately, they are often of short duration (5–10 minutes). After a standard intravenous induction, anesthesia is usually maintained with a potent inhalational agent in 100% oxygen and a short- or intermediate-acting neuromuscular blocking agent. Total intravenous anesthesia (such as with propofol) can also be used.

One of three techniques can then be used during rigid bronchoscopy: (1) apneic oxygenation with a small catheter alongside the bronchoscope (above); (2)

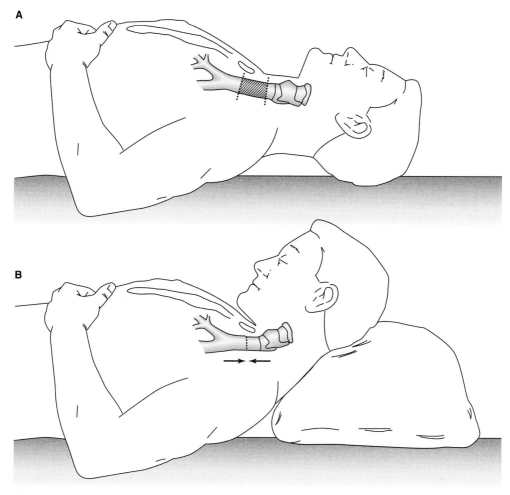

Figure 24–14. Position of the patient before (**A**) and after (**B**) tracheal resection and reanastomosis with the patient's neck flexed for the first 24–48 hours.

conventional ventilation through the side arm of a ventilating bronchoscope (when the proximal window of this instrument is opened for suctioning or biopsies, ventilation must be interrupted); or (3) high-frequency ventilation through an injector-type bronchoscope. In the latter instance, a narrow cannula (16- to 18-gauge) in the proximal end of the bronchoscope is used to inject oxygen at high pressures; the Venturi effect created proximally entrains an air-oxygen mixture down the trachea.

Mediastinoscopy

Mediastinoscopy provides access to the mediastinal lymph nodes and is used to establish either the diagnosis or the resectability of intrathoracic malignancies (above). Preoperative computerized tomography is es-

sential for evaluating tracheal distortion or compression.

Mediastinoscopy is performed under general endotracheal anesthesia with a muscle relaxant. Venous access with a large-bore intravenous catheter (14- to 16-gauge) is mandatory because of the risk of excessive bleeding and the difficulty in controlling bleeding when it occurs. Because the innominate artery may be compressed during the procedure, blood pressure should be measured in the left arm.

Complications associated with mediastinoscopy include: (1) vagally mediated reflex bradycardia from compression of the trachea or the great vessels; (2) excessive hemorrhage (see above); (3) cerebral ischemia from compression of the innominate artery (detected with a plethysmograph or pulse oximeter on the right hand); (4) pneumothorax (usually presents postoperatively); (5) air embolism (because of 30-degree head elevation, the risk being greatest during spontaneous ventilation); (6) recurrent laryngeal nerve damage; and (7) phrenic nerve injury.

Bronchoalveolar Lavage

This procedure may be employed for patients with pulmonary alveolar proteinosis. These patients produce excessive quantities of surfactant and fail to clear it. They present with dyspnea and bilateral consolidation on the chest radiograph. Bronchoalveolar lavage may be indicated for severe hypoxemia or worsening dyspnea. Often, one lung is lavaged, allowing the patient to recover for a few days before the other lung is lavaged; the worst lung is therefore done first. Increasingly, both lungs are lavaged during the same procedure, creating unique challenges to ensure adequate oxygenation during lavage of the second lung.

Unilateral bronchoalveolar lavage is performed under general anesthesia with a double-lumen endobronchial tube. The cuffs on the tube should be properly positioned and should make a water-tight seal to prevent spillage of fluid into the other side. The procedure is normally done in the supine position; although lavage with the lung in a dependent position helps minimize soiling of the other lung, this position can cause severe $\dot{V}/\dot{Q}$ mismatch. Warm normal saline is infused into the lung to be treated and is drained by gravity; treatment continues until the fluid returning is clear (about 10–20 L). At the end of the procedure, both lungs are well suctioned, and the double-lumen endotracheal tube is replaced with a single-lumen endotracheal tube.

■ ANESTHESIA FOR LUNG TRANSPLANTATION

PREOPERATIVE CONSIDERATIONS

Lung transplantation is indicated for end-stage pulmonary parenchymal disease or pulmonary hypertension. Candidates are functionally incapacitated by dyspnea and have a poor prognosis. Criteria vary according to the primary disease process. Common etiologies are listed in Table 24–5. The number of transplants is limited by the availability of suitable organs. Patients typically have dyspnea at rest or with minimal activity, and resting hypoxemia ($PaO_2 < 50$ mm Hg) with increasing oxygen requirements. Progressive CO_2 retention is also very common. Patients may be ventilator-dependent. Cor pulmonale does not necessarily require combined heart-lung transplantation, because right ventricular

Table 24–5. Indications for lung transplantation.

Infectious
  Cystic fibrosis
  Bronchiectasis
Obstructive
  Chronic obstructive pulmonary disease
  α_1-Antitrypsin deficiency
  Pulmonary lymphangiomatosis
Restrictive
  Idiopathic pulmonary fibrosis
Vascular
  Primary pulmonary hypertension
  Eisenmenger syndrome (congenital heart disease)

function may recover when pulmonary artery pressures normalize. Patients should have normal left ventricular function and be free of coronary artery disease as well as other serious health problems.

Single lung transplantation may be performed for selected patients with chronic obstructive pulmonary disease, while double lung transplantation is typically performed for patients with cystic fibrosis, bullous emphysema, or vascular diseases. Younger patients are more likely to receive bilateral lung transplants. Patients with Eisenmenger syndrome require combined heart-lung transplantation (see Chapter 21).

Organ selection is based on size and ABO compatibility. Cytomegalovirus serology matching may also be attempted.

ANESTHETIC CONSIDERATIONS

1. Preoperative Management

Effective coordination between the organ retrieval team and the transplant team minimizes graft ischemia time and avoids unnecessary prolongation of pre-transplant anesthesia time. These procedures are performed on an emergency basis so patients may have little time to fast for surgery. Oral cyclosporine also may be given preoperatively. Administration of a clear antacid, an H_2 blocker, or metoclopramide should be considered. Patients are very sensitive to sedatives, so premedication is usually administered only in the operating room in direct attendance with the patient. Intravenous azathioprine may also be administered just prior to induction.

2. Intraoperative Management

Monitoring

Strict asepsis should be observed for invasive monitoring procedures, which are similar to cardiac surgery (see

Chapter 21). Because of tricuspid regurgitation, difficulty may be encountered in floating a PAC. Central venous access might be accomplished only after induction of anesthesia because patients may not be able to lie flat while awake. The PAC must, however, be withdrawn into its sterile protective sheath just prior to lung resection (if it floats to the operative side); it may be refloated back into the pulmonary artery after transplantation. Care must be taken to avoid air bubbles or clots in the intravenous fluids; patients with a patent foramen ovale are at risk for paradoxical embolism because of high right atrial pressures.

Induction & Maintenance of Anesthesia

A modified rapid-sequence induction with moderate head-up position is utilized. A slow induction with ketamine, etomidate, and/or an opioid is employed to avoid precipitous drops in blood pressure. Succinylcholine or a nondepolarizing neuromuscular blocking agent is used to facilitate laryngoscopy. Cricoid pressure is maintained throughout induction until the airway is secured with an endotracheal or endobronchial tube (below). Hypoxemia and hypercarbia must be avoided to prevent further increases in pulmonary artery pressure. Hypotension should be treated with vasopressors (dobutamine) instead of large fluids boluses (below).

Anesthesia is usually maintained with an opioid infusion with or without a low dose of a volatile agent. Intraoperative difficulties in ventilation are not uncommon. Progressive carbon dioxide retention can continue to be a problem intraoperatively. Ventilation should be adjusted to maintain a normal arterial pH to limit metabolic alkalosis (see Chapter 30). Patients with cystic fibrosis have copious secretions and require frequent suctioning.

Single Lung Transplantation

Single lung transplantation is often attempted without cardiopulmonary bypass (CPB). The procedure is performed through a posterior thoracotomy. A left-sided double-lumen tube or single-lumen tube with a built-in bronchial blocker must be used for one-lung ventilation in such instances. The decision of whether to employ CPB during one lung transplantation is based on the patient's response to collapsing the lung to be replaced and clamping its pulmonary artery. Persistent arterial hypoxemia ($SpO_2 < 88\%$) or a sudden increase in pulmonary artery pressures necessitates CPB. Prostaglandin E_1, amrinone (or milrinone), nitroglycerin, and dobutamine, may be utilized to control pulmonary hypertension and prevent right ventricular failure. Inotropic support with dopamine may be necessary. When CPB is necessary femoral vein to femoral artery bypass

is employed during left thoracotomy, while right atrium to aorta bypass is used during right thoracotomy.

After the recipient lung is resected, the pulmonary artery, left atrial cuff (with the pulmonary veins) and bronchus of the donor lung are anastomosed. An omental flap may be mobilized to wrap around the bronchial anastomosis (omentopexy), to promote revascularization and help prevent ischemic break-down. Flexible bronchoscopy is used to examine the bronchial suture line after its completion.

Double Lung Transplantation

A "clamshell" transverse sternotomy is used for double-lung transplantation. The procedure is occasionally performed with normothermic CPB; sequential double-lung transplantation without CPB is more common. Normothermia increases the risk of awareness during CPB (see Chapter 21) and does not provide any cerebral protection. Severe metabolic alkalosis can develop in patients with marked chronic CO_2 retention if the CO_2 is normalized; administration of intravenous hydrochloric acid may be necessary (see Chapter 30).

Post-Transplantation Management

Following anastomosis of the donor organ or organs, ventilation to both lungs is resumed. Peak inspiratory pressures should be kept to the minimum compatible with good lung expansion and the inspired oxygen concentration is kept < 60%. Methylprednisolone is usually given prior to release of vascular clamps. Hyperkalemia may occur as the preservative fluid (Euro-Collins) is washed out of the donor organ. The patient is separated from CPB if the latter is employed, and the PAC is refloated into the main pulmonary artery. Pulmonary vasodilators and inotropes (above) may be necessary. Transesophageal echocardiography is very helpful in differentiating between right and left ventricular dysfunction as well as in evaluating blood flow in the pulmonary vessels before and after transplantation.

Transplantation disrupts the neural innervation, lymphatic drainage, and bronchial circulation of the transplanted lung. Respiratory pattern is unaffected but the cough reflex is abolished below the carina. Bronchial hyperreactivity is described in some patients. Hypoxic pulmonary vasoconstriction remains normal. Loss of lymphatic drainage increases extravascular lung water and predisposes the transplanted lung to pulmonary edema. Intraoperative fluid replacement must therefore be kept to a minimum. Loss of the bronchial circulation predisposes to ischemic breakdown of the bronchial suture line.

3. Postoperative Management

Patients are left intubated after surgery for 24–72 hours. A thoracic or lumbar epidural catheter may be employed for postoperative analgesia when coagulation studies are normal. The postoperative course is often complicated by acute rejection, infections, and renal and hepatic dysfunction. Deteriorating lung function may result from rejection or reperfusion injury. Occasionally, temporary extracorporeal membrane oxygenation may be necessary. Frequent bronchoscopy with transbronchial biopsies and lavage are necessary to differentiate between rejection and infection. Nosocomial gram-negative bacteria, cytomegalovirus, *Candida,* and *Aspergillus* and *Pneumocystis carinii* are common pathogens. Other postoperative surgical complications include damage to the phrenic, vagus, and left recurrent laryngeal nerves.

■ ANESTHESIA FOR ESOPHAGEAL SURGERY

PREOPERATIVE CONSIDERATIONS

Common indications for esophageal surgery include tumors, gastroesophageal reflux, and motility disorders (achalasia). Surgical procedures include simple endoscopy, esophageal dilatation, cervical esophagomyotomy, open or thoracoscopic distal esophagomyotomy, blunt esophagectomy, as well as and en block esophageal resections.

Squamous cell carcinomas account for a majority of esophageal tumors; adenocarcinomas are less common while benign tumors (leiomyomas) are rare. Most tumors occur in the distal esophagus. Operative treatment may be palliative or curative. Although the prognosis is generally poor, surgical therapy offers the only hope of a cure. After the esophageal resection, the stomach is pulled-up into the neck or the esophagus is functionally replaced with part of the colon (interposition).

Gastroesophageal reflux is treated surgically when the esophagitis is refractory to medical management or results in complications such as stricture, recurrent pulmonary aspiration, or Barrett's esophagus (columnar epithelium). A variety of antireflux operations may be performed (Nissen, Belsey, Hill, or Collis-Nissen) via thoracic or abdominal approaches, often laparoscopically. They all involve wrapping part of the stomach around the esophagus.

Achalasia and systemic sclerosis (scleroderma) account for the majority of surgical procedures performed for motility disorders. The former usually occurs as an isolated finding while the latter is part of a generalized collagen-vascular disorder. Cricopharyngeal muscle dysfunction can be associated with a variety of neurogenic or myogenic disorders and often results in a Zenker's diverticulum.

ANESTHETIC CONSIDERATIONS

Regardless of the procedure, the major anesthetic consideration for patients with esophageal disease is the risk of pulmonary aspiration. This may result from obstruction, altered motility, or abnormal sphincter function. In fact, most patients typically complain of dysphagia, heartburn, regurgitation, coughing and/or wheezing when lying flat. Dyspnea on exertion may also be prominent when chronic aspiration results in pulmonary fibrosis (see Chapter 23). Patients with malignancies may additionally present with anemia and weight loss. A history of heavy smoking is common, so patients should be evaluated for coexisting chronic obstructive pulmonary disease and coronary artery disease. Patients with systemic sclerosis (scleroderma) should be evaluated for involvement of other organs, especially the kidneys, heart, and lungs; Raynaud's phenomena is also common.

Consideration should be given to administering metoclopramide, an H_2 blocker, or a parietal cell, proton-pump inhibitor preoperatively; awake nasogastric suctioning may also be helpful in decreasing the risk of aspiration. With the patient in a semi-upright position, a rapid-sequence induction with cricoid pressure is used. Awake fiberoptic intubation should be considered in patients with systemic sclerosis when a difficult laryngoscopy appears likely. A double-lumen tube is used for procedures involving thoracoscopy or thoracotomy. The anesthesiologist may be asked to pass a large-diameter bougie into the esophagus as part of the surgical procedure; great caution must be exercised to help avoid pharyngeal or esophageal injury.

Transhiatal (blunt) and en block thoracic esophagectomies deserve special consideration. These procedures often involve considerable blood loss. The former requires an upper abdominal incision and a left cervical incision, while the latter requires posterior thoracotomy, a large abdominal incision, and finally, a left cervical incision. Arterial and central venous pressure monitoring are indicated. A PAC should also be used for patients with significant cardiac disease. Multiple large-bore intravenous access, fluid warmers, and a forced-air body warmer are advisable. During the transhiatal approach, substernal and diaphragmatic retractors can interfere with cardiac function. Moreover, as the esophagus is freed-up blindly from the posterior mediastinum by blunt dissection, the surgeon's hand transiently interferes with cardiac filling and produces profound hypotension. The dissection can also induce marked vagal stimulation.

Colonic interposition involves forming a pedicle graft of the colon and passing it through the posterior mediastinum up to the neck to take the place of the esophagus. This procedure is lengthy and involves considerable fluid shifts. Maintenance of an adequate blood pressure, cardiac output, and hemoglobin concentration is necessary to ensure graft viability. Graft ischemia may be heralded by a progressive metabolic acidosis. For relatively minor procedures, the patient should be extubated on the operating room table or in the postanesthesia recovery unit. Although usually in most cases the risk of aspiration likely diminishes following surgery, patients should generally be extubated only when fully awake. Postoperative ventilation should be considered for patients undergoing esophagectomy. Postoperative surgical complications include damage to the phrenic, vagus, and left recurrent laryngeal nerves.

ANESTHESIA FOR LUNG VOLUME REDUCTION SURGERY

Many patients with severe chronic obstructive pulmonary disease are being treated with lung volume reduction surgery (LVRS), either as part of a National Emphysema Treatment Trial (NETT), a multicenter randomized clinical trial of usual medical therapy versus usual medical therapy plus LVRS, or as part of routine clinical care. The NETT was discontinued because of a lack of efficacy of LVRS but some surgeons and patients are convinced of the efficacy of the technique.

PREANESTHETIC EVALUATION

It is imperative that patients be seen by the anesthesiologist prior to surgery, at which time a careful history and physical examination must be done. During the evaluation, information that must be obtained includes a history of previous anesthetics, whether or not the patient has a difficult airway, and possible abnormal emergence. The baseline breathing and respiratory capacity should be reviewed.

It is important for the patient and any family members to understand that the procedure is lengthy and includes the placement of intravascular lines, induction of anesthesia, placement of an endotracheal tube, initiation of mechanical ventilation, positioning of the patient, and emergence (and possible extubation) with recovery initially in the PACU or in an ICU. The risks associated with general anesthesia, endotracheal intubation, mechanical ventilation, and one-lung ventilation need to be addressed.

The anesthesiologist should use this opportunity to describe the use and importance of epidural analgesia to the patient, preferably allowing the patient an opportunity to become familiar with the PCA device that could be used either with the epidural or intravenous route of opioid administration. At this time, the anesthesiologist should also discuss the needs and techniques for placement of arterial lines and central venous lines, including a PAC.

Patients should continue all medications right up to and including the morning of surgery including cardiac (β-blockers, calcium channel blockers) and pulmonary (bronchodilators) medications.

The importance of incentive spirometry, coughing, and deep breathing postoperatively should be stressed. The correct use of inhalers at appropriate intervals should be reviewed.

ANESTHETIC CONSIDERATIONS

The assessment of the airway, the degree of respiratory failure with particular reference to the bullous disease component, degree of hyperinflation, oxygen requirement, and degree of resting hypercapnia are of particular importance to the anesthesiologist. Any cardiac disease with particular reference to ischemic coronary disease, left and right ventricular function and pulmonary vascular disease should also be reviewed. Anyone caring for such a patient should be well-trained in one-lung ventilation, fiberoptic bronchoscopy, hemodynamic monitoring, cardiopulmonary bypass, and postoperative analgesia.

Prior to induction, the anesthesiologist should also ensure that the ventilator on the anesthetic machine (see Chapter 50) is capable of several different ventilator modes, all capable of achieving long expiratory times, high gas flows, and pressure-controlled ventilation. A fiberoptic bronchoscope must be available.

All preoperative medications are continued as already discussed, and sedative drugs are avoided or given in minimal dose and appropriately monitored. Although one must guard against overly aggressive fluid resuscitation, many of these patients may benefit from a fluid bolus before induction of general anesthesia, especially if an epidural catheter with local anesthetic has been placed. Prophylactic antibiotics, deep venous thrombosis prophylaxis, and corticosteroids for those patients receiving steroids preoperatively should be also administered.

In terms of monitors, peripheral arterial catheterization and central venous catheterization—with or without a PAC—should be performed prior to induction or immediately afterwards. Transesophageal echocardiography should be considered if the transthoracic echocardiogram was not adequate and in all hemodynamically unstable patients.

There are no specific induction agents that have demonstrated superiority for LVRS. The choice of agents should be guided by the patient's medical condition. Doses should be reduced in those patients who are hypovolemic or who have significant cardiac disease. Following intubation, the ventilator should be adjusted to limit the degree of positive pressure ventilation (< 30 cm H_2O peak inspiratory pressure) and to prolong expiratory time. During induction, if there is sudden hemodynamic collapse, a tension pneumothorax must be ruled out, although the diagnosis may be very difficult because of the masking of physical signs by the preexisting pulmonary disease. Double-lumen tubes are strongly recommended to improve surgical exposure and allow selective lung ventilation. Position of the tube should be confirmed by fiberoptic bronchoscopy.

MAINTENANCE OF ANESTHESIA

Maintenance of anesthesia is often achieved either with inhalational or intravenous agents. Total intravenous anesthesia is particularly useful, especially if propofol or other short-acting agents are used to allow for a rapid postoperative extubation. Neuromuscular blocking agents that are easily and reliably reversed are recommended. Neuromuscular blocking agents that cause histamine release should be avoided. Minimal intravenous opioid use is recommended, again to allow early postoperative extubation. One must pay particular attention to maintaining core temperature; postoperative hypothermia leads to shivering, increased oxygen consumption, and perioperative adverse events.

Patients should be extubated at the conclusion of surgery or shortly thereafter. For those who require continued mechanical ventilation, the double-lumen endotracheal tube should be replaced with a single-lumen endotracheal tube. The FiO_2 needs to be decreased to maintain SpO_2 at around 88–90%. Corticosteroids, along with bronchodilators, should be administered to reduce airway inflammation and edema and to promote bronchodilation.

POSTOPERATIVE MANAGEMENT

Patients having LVRS should be cared for in a location with appropriate monitoring and personnel immediately available, ie, either a PACU or ICU. For those patients who have been extubated, noninvasive ventilation with BiPAP (bilevel positive airway pressure) should be considered for patients with a $PaCO_2$ > 70 mm Hg. Inotropes should be considered for treatment of hypotension that may develop in patients secondary to their

epidural anesthetic. Thoracic epidural analgesia is strongly recommended for patients having LVRS. Alternatives to the use of epidural analgesia include intercostal or paravertebral nerve blocks and the use of intravenous opioids either by PCA or through intermittent bolus with conversion to oral opioids within the first 24–72 hours postoperatively.

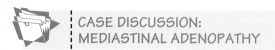

CASE DISCUSSION: MEDIASTINAL ADENOPATHY

A 9-year-old boy with mediastinal lymphadenopathy seen on a chest radiograph presents for biopsy of a cervical lymph node.

What is the most important preoperative consideration?

Is there any evidence of airway compromise? Tracheal compression may produce dyspnea (proximal obstruction) or a nonproductive cough (distal obstruction). Asymptomatic compression is also common and may only be evident as tracheal deviation on physical or radiographic examinations. A CT scan of the chest provides invaluable information about the presence, location, and severity of airway compression. Flow-volume loops will also detect subtle airway obstruction and provide important information regarding its location and functional importance (above).

Does the absence of any preoperative dyspnea make severe intraoperative respiratory compromise less likely?

No. Severe airway obstruction can occur following induction of anesthesia in these patients even in the absence of any preoperative symptoms. This fact mandates that the chest radiograph and CT scan be reviewed for evidence of asymptomatic airway obstruction. The point of obstruction is typically distal to the tip of the endotracheal tube. Moreover, loss of spontaneous ventilation can precipitate complete airway obstruction.

What is the superior vena cava syndrome?

Superior vena cava syndrome is the result of progressive enlargement of a mediastinal mass and compression of mediastinal structures, especially the vena cava. Lymphomas are most commonly responsible, but primary pulmonary or mediastinal neoplasms can also produce the syndrome. Superior vena cava syndrome is often associated with severe airway obstruction and cardiovascular collapse on induction of general anesthesia. The caval compression produces ve-

nous engorgement and edema of the head, neck, and arms. Direct mechanical compression as well as mucosal edema severely compromise airflow in the trachea. Most patients favor an upright posture, since recumbency worsens the airway obstruction. Cardiac output may be severely depressed owing to impeded venous return from the upper body, direct mechanical compression of the heart, and (with malignancies) pericardial invasion. An echocardiogram is useful in evaluating cardiac function and detecting pericardial fluid.

What is the anesthetic of choice for a patient with superior vena cava syndrome?

The absence of signs or symptoms of airway compression or superior vena cava syndrome does not preclude potentially life-threatening complications following induction of general anesthesia. Therefore, biopsy of a peripheral node (usually cervical or scalene) under local anesthesia is safest whenever possible. Although establishing a diagnosis is of prime importance, the presence of significant airway compromise or the superior vena cava syndrome may dictate empiric treatment with corticosteroids prior to tissue diagnosis at surgery (cancer is the most common cause); preoperative radiation therapy or chemotherapy may also be considered. The patient can usually safely undergo surgery with general anesthesia once airway compromise and other manifestations of the superior vena cava syndrome are alleviated.

General anesthesia may be indicated for establishing a diagnosis in young or uncooperative patients who have no evidence of airway compromise or the superior vena cava syndrome, and rarely, for patients unresponsive to steroids, radiation, and chemotherapy.

How does the presence of airway obstruction and the superior vena cava syndrome influence management of general anesthesia?

(1) Premedication: Only an anticholinergic should be given. The patient should be transported to the operating room in a semiupright position with supplemental oxygen.

(2) Monitoring: In addition to standard monitors, an arterial line is mandatory, but it should be placed after induction in young patients. At least one large-bore intravenous catheter should be placed in a lower extremity, since venous drainage from the upper body may be unreliable.

(3) Airway management: Difficulties with ventilation and intubation should be anticipated. Fol-

lowing preoxygenation, awake intubation with an armored endotracheal tube may be safest in a cooperative patient. Use of a flexible bronchoscope is advantageous in the presence of airway distortion and will define the site and degree of obstruction. Coughing or straining, however, may precipitate complete airway obstruction, because the resultant positive pleural pressure increases intrathoracic tracheal compression. Passing the armored tube beyond the area of compression may obviate this problem. Uncooperative patients require a careful slow inhalation induction.

(4) Induction: The goal should be a smooth induction maintaining spontaneous ventilation and hemodynamic stability. The ability to ventilate the patient with a good airway should be established prior to use of a muscle relaxant. Using 100% oxygen, one of three induction techniques can be used: (a) intravenous ketamine (because it results in greater hemodynamic stability in patients with reduced cardiac output); (b) inhalational induction with a volatile agent (usually halothane); or (c) incremental small doses of thiopental, propofol or etomidate.

Positive pressure ventilation can precipitate severe hypotension, and volume loading prior to induction may partly offset impaired ventricular filling secondary to caval obstruction.

(5) Maintenance of anesthesia: The technique selected should be tailored to the patient's hemodynamic status. Following intubation, paralysis prevents coughing or straining.

(6) Extubation: At the end of the procedure, patients should be left intubated until the airway obstruction has resolved, as determined by flexible bronchoscopy or the presence of an air leak around the endotracheal tube when the tracheal cuff is deflated.

SUGGESTED READING

Benumof JL: Anesthesia for Thoracic Surgery. 2nd ed. WB Saunders and Company, 1995.

Cohen E: The Practice of Thoracic Anesthesia. Lippincott, 1995.

Ghosh S, Latimer RD: Thoracic Anaesthesia: Principles and Practice. Butterworth Heineman, 1999.

Reilly JJ Jr: Evidence-based preoperative evaluation of candidates for thoracotomy. Chest 1999;116:474S.

Youngberg JA: Cardiac, Vascular, and Thoracic Anesthesia. Churchill Livingstone, 2000.

Neurophysiology & Anesthesia

KEY CONCEPTS

 1 Cerebral perfusion pressure (CPP) is the difference between mean arterial pressure and intracranial pressure (ICP) (or cerebral venous pressure, whichever is greater).

 2 The cerebral autoregulation curve is shifted to the right in patients with chronic arterial hypertension.

 3 The movement of a given substance across the blood-brain barrier is governed simultaneously by its size, charge, lipid solubility, and degree of protein binding in blood.

 4 The blood-brain barrier may be disrupted by severe hypertension, tumors, trauma, strokes, infection, marked hypercapnia, hypoxia, and sustained seizure activity.

 5 To prevent a rise in ICP, any increase in one of the three components of the cranial vault (brain, blood, and cerebrospinal fluid) must be offset by an equivalent decrease in another.

 6 With the exception of ketamine, all intravenous agents either have little effect on or reduce cerebral metabolic rate and cerebral blood flow (CBF).

 7 With normal autoregulation and an intact blood-brain barrier, vasopressors increase CBF only when mean arterial blood pressure is below 50–60 mm Hg or above 150–160 mm Hg.

 8 The brain is very vulnerable to ischemic injury because of its relatively high oxygen consumption and near total dependence on aerobic glucose metabolism.

 9 Hypothermia is the most effective method for protecting the brain during focal and global ischemia.

 10 Both animal and human data suggest that barbiturates are effective for brain protection in the setting of focal ischemia.

The anesthetic care of patients who undergo neurosurgery requires a basic understanding of the physiology of the central nervous system (CNS). The effects of anesthetic agents on cerebral metabolism, blood flow, cerebrospinal fluid (CSF) dynamics, and intracranial volume and pressure are often profound. In some instances, these alterations are deleterious, while in others they may actually be beneficial. This chapter reviews important physiologic concepts in anesthetic practice and then discusses the effects of commonly used anesthetics on cerebral physiology. While most of the discussion focuses on the brain, the same concepts also apply, at least qualitatively, to the spinal cord.

■ CEREBRAL PHYSIOLOGY

CEREBRAL METABOLISM

The brain is normally responsible for 20% of total body oxygen consumption. Most of cerebral oxygen consumption (60%) is used in generating adenosine triphosphate (ATP) to support neuronal electrical activity (Figure 25–1). The **cerebral metabolic rate (CMR)** is usually expressed in terms of oxygen consumption ($CMRO_2$), which averages 3–3.8 mL/100 g/min (50

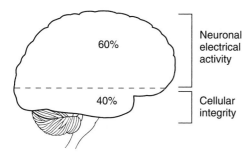

Neuronal electrical activity

Cellular integrity

Figure 25–1. Normal brain oxygen requirements.

mL/min) in adults. CMRO$_2$ is greatest in the gray matter of the cerebral cortex and generally parallels cortical electrical activity. Because of the relatively high oxygen consumption and the absence of significant oxygen reserves, interruption of cerebral perfusion usually results in unconsciousness within 10 seconds as oxygen tension rapidly drops below 30 mm Hg. If blood flow is not reestablished within minutes (3–8 minutes under most conditions), ATP stores are depleted and irreversible cellular injury begins to occur. The hippocampus and cerebellum appear to be most sensitive to hypoxic injury.

Neuronal cells normally utilize glucose as their primary energy source. Brain glucose consumption is approximately 5 mg/100 g/min, of which over 90% is metabolized aerobically. CMRO$_2$ therefore normally parallels glucose consumption. This relationship does not hold during starvation, when ketone bodies (acetoacetate and β-hydroxybutyrate) also become major energy substrates. Although the brain can also take up and metabolize some lactate, cerebral function is normally dependent on a continuous supply of glucose. Acute sustained hypoglycemia is equally as devastating as hypoxia. Paradoxically, hyperglycemia can exacerbate global hypoxic brain injury by accelerating cerebral acidosis and cellular injury; its effect on focal cerebral ischemia is less clear.

CEREBRAL BLOOD FLOW

Cerebral blood flow (CBF) varies with metabolic activity. It is most commonly measured with a gamma-emitting isotope such as xenon (^{133}Xe). Following systemic injection, detectors placed around the brain measure the rate of radioactive decay, which is directly proportionate to CBF. Newer techniques employing positron emission tomography (PET) in conjunction with short-lived isotopes such as ^{11}C and ^{15}O also allow measurement of CMR (for glucose and oxygen, respectively). Such studies confirm that regional CBF paral-

lels metabolic activity and can vary from 10 to 300 mL/100 g/min. For example, motor activity of a limb is associated with a rapid increase in regional CBF of the corresponding motor cortex. Similarly, visual activity is associated with an increase in regional CBF of the corresponding occipital visual cortex.

Although total CBF averages 50 mL/100 g/min, flow in gray matter is about 80 mL/100 g/min while that in white matter is estimated to be 20 mL/100 g/min. Total CBF in adults averages 750 mL/min (15–20% of cardiac output). Flow rates below 20–25 mL/100 g/min are usually associated with cerebral impairment, as evidenced by slowing on the electroencephalogram (EEG). CBF rates between 15 and 20 mL/100 g/min typically produce a flat (isoelectric) EEG, while values below 10 mL/100 g/min are usually associated with irreversible brain damage.

REGULATION OF CEREBRAL BLOOD FLOW

1. Cerebral Perfusion Pressure

Cerebral perfusion pressure (CPP) is the difference between mean arterial pressure (MAP) and intracranial pressure (ICP) (or cerebral venous pressure, whichever is greater). When cerebral venous pressure is significantly greater than ICP, perfusion pressure becomes the difference between MAP and cerebral venous pressure. Because ICP and cerebral venous pressure are normally within a few millimeters of mercury of each other and the former is easier to measure, CPP is expressed by the equation: CPP = MAP − ICP. CPP is normally 80 to 100 mm Hg. Moreover, since ICP is normally less than 10 mm Hg, CPP is primarily dependent on MAP.

Moderate to severe increases in ICP (> 30 mm Hg) can significantly compromise CPP and CBF even in the presence of a normal MAP. Patients with CPP values less than 50 mm Hg often show slowing on the EEG, while those with a CPP between 25 and 40 mm Hg typically have a flat EEG. Sustained perfusion pressures less than 25 mm Hg result in irreversible brain damage.

2. Autoregulation

Like the heart and kidneys, the brain normally tolerates wide swings in blood pressure with little change in blood flow. The cerebral vasculature rapidly (10 to 60 sec) adapts to changes in CPP, but abrupt changes in MAP will lead to transient changes in CBF even when autoregulation is intact. Decreases in CPP result in cerebral vasodilation, while elevations induce vasoconstriction. In normal individuals, CBF remains nearly

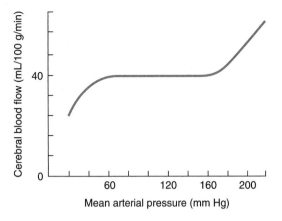

Figure 25–2. Cerebral autoregulation curve.

constant between mean arterial blood pressures of about 60 and 160 mm Hg (Figure 25–2). Beyond these limits, blood flow becomes pressure-dependent. Pressures above 150–160 mm Hg can disrupt the blood-brain barrier (see below) and may result in cerebral edema and hemorrhage.

 The **cerebral autoregulation curve** (Figure 25–2) is shifted to the right in patients with chronic arterial hypertension. Both upper and lower limits are shifted. Flow becomes more pressure-dependent at low "normal" arterial pressures in return for cerebral protection at higher arterial pressures. Studies suggest that long-term antihypertensive therapy can restore cerebral autoregulation limits toward normal.

Both myogenic and metabolic mechanisms have been proposed to explain cerebral autoregulation. The former involves an intrinsic response of smooth muscle cells in cerebral arterioles to changes in MAP. The latter theory holds that cerebral metabolic demands determine arteriolar tone. Thus, when tissue demand exceeds blood flow, the release of tissue metabolites causes vasodilation and increases flow. While hydrogen ions were previously thought to mediate this response, other metabolites are probably involved, including nitric oxide, adenosine, prostaglandins, and perhaps ionic (electrolyte) concentration gradients.

3. Extrinsic Mechanisms

Respiratory Gas Tensions

The most important extrinsic influences on CBF are respiratory gas tensions—especially $PaCO_2$. CBF is directly proportionate to $PaCO_2$ between tensions of 20 and 80 mm Hg (Figure 25–3). Blood flow changes approximately 1–2 mL/100 g/min per mm Hg change in

$PaCO_2$. This effect is almost immediate and is thought to be secondary to changes in the pH of CSF and cerebral tissue. Because ions do not readily cross the blood-brain barrier (see below) but CO_2 does, acute changes in $PaCO_2$ but not HCO_3^- affect CBF. Thus, acute metabolic acidosis has little effect on CBF because hydrogen ions (H^+) cannot readily cross the blood-brain barrier. After 24–48 hours, CSF HCO_3^- concentration adjusts to compensate for the change in $PaCO_2$, so that the effects of hypocapnia and hypercapnia are diminished. Marked hyperventilation ($PaCO_2 < 20$ mm Hg) shifts the oxygen-hemoglobin dissociation curve to the left, and with changes in CBF, may result in EEG changes suggestive of cerebral impairment even in normal individuals.

Only marked changes in PaO_2 alter CBF. While hyperoxia may be associated with only minimal decreases (–10%) in CBF, severe hypoxemia ($PaO_2 < 50$ mm Hg) profoundly increases CBF (Figure 25–3).

Temperature

CBF changes 5–7% per °C. Hypothermia decreases both CMR and CBF, while pyrexia has the reverse effect. At 20 °C, the EEG is isoelectric, but further decreases in temperature continue to reduce CMR throughout the brain. Above 42 °C, oxygen activity begins to decrease and may reflect cell damage.

Viscosity

Normally, changes in blood viscosity do not appreciably alter CBF. The most important determinant of blood viscosity is hematocrit. A decrease in hematocrit decreases viscosity and can improve CBF; unfortunately, a reduction in hematocrit also decreases oxygen

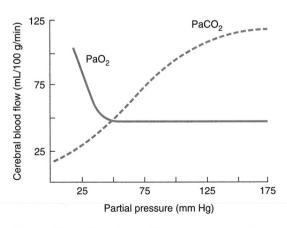

Figure 25–3. The relationship between cerebral blood flow and arterial respiratory gas tensions.

carrying capacity and thus can potentially impair oxygen delivery. Elevated hematocrits, as may be seen with marked polycythemia, increase blood viscosity and can reduce CBF. Some studies suggest that optimal cerebral oxygen delivery may occur at hematocrits between 30% and 34%.

Autonomic Influences

Intracranial vessels are innervated by sympathetic (vasoconstrictive), parasympathetic (vasodilatory), and noncholinergic nonadrenergic fibers; serotonin and vasoactive intestinal peptide appear to be the neurotransmitters for the latter. The normal physiologic function of this innervation is uncertain but it may play an important role in some pathologic states. This is especially true for the innervation of large cerebral vessels by sympathetic fibers originating in the superior cervical sympathetic ganglia. Intense sympathetic stimulation induces marked vasoconstriction in these vessels, which can limit CBF. Autonomic innervation may also play an important role in cerebral vasospasm following brain injury and stroke.

BLOOD-BRAIN BARRIER

Cerebral blood vessels are unique in that the junctions between vascular endothelial cells are nearly fused. The paucity of pores is responsible for what is termed the **blood-brain barrier.** This lipid barrier allows the passage of lipid-soluble substances but restricts the movement of those that are ionized or have large molecular weights. Thus, the movement of a given substance across the blood-brain barrier is governed simultaneously by its size, charge, lipid solubility, and degree of protein binding in blood. Carbon dioxide, oxygen, and lipid-soluble substances (such as most anesthetics) freely enter the brain, whereas most ions, proteins, and large substances such as mannitol penetrate poorly.

Water moves freely across the blood-brain barrier as a consequence of bulk flow, whereas movement of even small ions is impeded to some extent (the equilibration half-life for sodium is 2–4 hours). As a result, rapid changes in plasma electrolyte concentrations (and, secondarily, osmolality) produce a transient osmotic gradient between plasma and the brain. Acute hypertonicity of plasma results in net movement of water out of the brain, while acute hypotonicity causes a net movement of water into the brain. These effects are short-lived, since equilibration eventually occurs, but when marked they can cause rapid fluid shifts in the brain. Thus, marked abnormalities in serum sodium or glucose concentrations should generally be corrected slowly (see Chapters 28 and 36). Mannitol, an osmot-

ically active substance that does not normally cross the blood-brain barrier, causes a sustained decrease in brain water content and is often used to decrease brain volume.

The blood-brain barrier may be disrupted by severe hypertension, tumors, trauma, strokes, infection, marked hypercapnia, hypoxia, and sustained seizure activity. Under these conditions, fluid movement across the blood-brain barrier becomes dependent on hydrostatic pressure rather than osmotic gradients.

CEREBROSPINAL FLUID

CSF is found in the cerebral ventricles and cisterns and in the subarachnoid space surrounding the brain and spinal cord. Its major function is to protect the CNS against trauma.

Most of the CSF is formed by the choroid plexuses of the cerebral (mainly lateral) ventricles. Smaller amounts are formed directly by their ependymal cell linings and yet smaller quantities from fluid leaking into the perivascular spaces surrounding cerebral vessels (blood-brain barrier leakage). In adults, normal total CSF production is about 21 mL/h (500 mL/d), yet total CSF volume is only about 150 mL. CSF flows from the lateral ventricles through the interventricular foramina (of Monro) into the third ventricle, through the cerebral aqueduct (of Sylvius) into the fourth ventricle, and through the median aperture of the fourth ventricle (foramen of Magendie) and the lateral aperture of the fourth ventricle (foramina of Luschka) into the cerebellomedullary cistern (cisterna magna) (Figure 25–4). From the cerebellomedullary cistern, CSF enters the subarachnoid space, circulating around the brain and spinal cord before being absorbed in arachnoid granulations over the cerebral hemispheres.

CSF formation involves active secretion of sodium in the choroid plexuses. The resulting fluid is isotonic with plasma despite lower potassium, bicarbonate, and glucose concentrations. Its protein content is limited to the very small amounts that leak into perivascular fluid. Carbonic anhydrase inhibitors (acetazolamide), corticosteroids, spironolactone, furosemide, isoflurane, and vasoconstrictors decrease CSF production.

CSF absorption involves the translocation of fluid from the arachnoid granulations into the cerebral venous sinuses. Smaller amounts are absorbed at nerve root sleeves and by meningeal lymphatics. Although the mechanism remains unclear, absorption appears to be directly proportionate to ICP and inversely proportionate to cerebral venous pressure. Since the brain and spinal cord lack lymphatics, CSF absorption is also the principal means by which perivascular and interstitial protein is returned to blood.

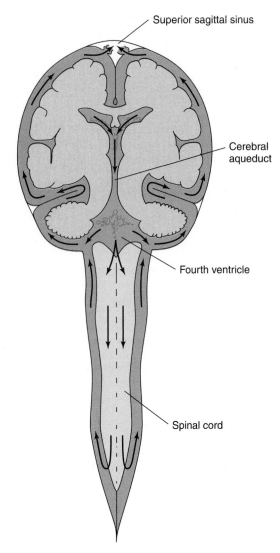

Figure 25–4. The flow of cerebrospinal fluid in the central nervous system (Reproduced, with permission, from Waxman SG: *Correlative Neuroanatomy,* 24th ed. McGraw-Hill, 2000).

INTRACRANIAL PRESSURE

The cranial vault is a rigid structure with a fixed total volume, consisting of brain (80%), blood (12%), and CSF (8%). Any increase in one component must be offset by an equivalent decrease in another to prevent a rise in ICP. ICP by convention means supratentorial CSF pressure measured in the lateral ventricles or over the cerebral cortex and is normally 10 mm Hg or less. Minor variations may occur depending on the site measured, but in the lateral recumbent position lumbar CSF pressure normally approximates supratentorial pressure.

Intracranial compliance is determined by measuring the change in ICP in response to a change in the intracranial volume. Normally, increases in volume are initially well-compensated (Figure 25–5). A point is eventually reached, however, at which further increases produce precipitous rises in ICP. Major compensatory mechanisms include (1) an initial displacement of CSF from the cranial to the spinal compartment, (2) an increase in CSF absorption, (3) a decrease in CSF production, and (4) a decrease in total cerebral blood volume (primarily venous).

The concept of total intracranial compliance is useful clinically even though compliance probably varies in the different compartments of the brain and is affected by arterial blood pressure and $PaCO_2$. Increases in blood pressure can reduce cerebral blood volume because autoregulation induces vasoconstriction in order to maintain CBF. In contrast, hypotension can increase cerebral blood volume as cerebral vessels dilate to maintain blood flow. Cerebral blood volume is estimated to increase 0.05 mL/100 g of brain per 1 mm Hg increase in $PaCO_2$.

Compliance can be determined in patients with intraventricular catheters by injecting sterile saline. An increase in ICP greater than 4 mm Hg following injection of 1 mL of saline indicates poor compliance. At that point, compensatory mechanisms have been exhausted and CBF is progressively compromised as ICP rises further. Sustained elevations in ICP can lead to catastrophic herniation of the brain. Herniation may occur at one of four sites (Figure 25–6): (1) the cingulate gyrus under the falx cerebri, (2) the uncinate gyrus

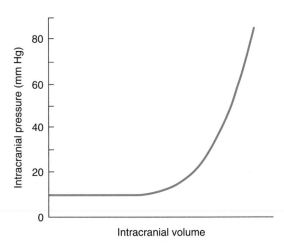

Figure 25–5. Normal intracranial compliance.

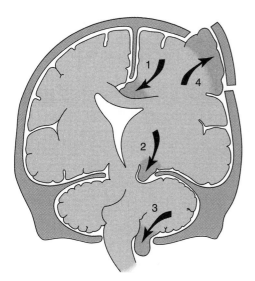

Figure 25–6. Potential sites of brain herniation. (Reproduced, with permission, from Fishman RA: Brain edema. N Engl J Med 1975;293:706.)

through the tentorium cerebelli, (3) the cerebellar tonsils through the foramen magnum, or (4) any area beneath a defect in the skull (transcalvarial).

■ EFFECT OF ANESTHETIC AGENTS ON CEREBRAL PHYSIOLOGY

Overall, most general anesthetics have a favorable effect on the CNS by reducing electrical activity. Carbohydrate metabolism decreases, while energy stores in the form of ATP, adenosine diphosphate, and phosphocreatine increase. Determination of the effects of the specific agents are complicated by the concomitant administration of other drugs, surgical stimulation, intracranial compliance, blood pressure, and CO_2 tension. For example, hypocapnia or prior administration of thiopental blunts the increases in CBF and ICP that usually occur with ketamine and volatile agents.

This section describes the changes generally associated with each drug when given alone. Table 25–1 summarizes and compares the effects of the various anesthetics. The effects of vasoactive agents and neuromuscular blocking agents (also called muscle relaxants) are also discussed.

EFFECT OF INHALATIONAL AGENTS

1. Volatile Anesthetics

Cerebral Metabolic Rate

Halothane, enflurane, desflurane, sevoflurane, and isoflurane produce dose-dependent decreases in CMR. Isoflurane and enflurane produce the greatest depression (up to 50% reduction), while halothane has the least effect (< 25% reduction). The effects of desflurane and sevoflurane appear to be similar to the first two agents. Unlike hypothermia, no further reduction in metabolic rate is observed once the EEG is isoelectric. Moreover, the reduction is not uniform throughout the brain; isoflurane reduces metabolic rate mainly in the neocortex. Enflurane's depression of CMR is reversed when it precipitates seizure activity on the EEG (see below); in fact, CMR increases with frank seizure activity.

Cerebral Blood Flow & Volume

Volatile anesthetics dilate cerebral vessels and impair autoregulation in a dose-dependent manner (Figure 25–7). Halothane has the greatest effect on CBF; at concentrations greater than 1%, it nearly abolishes cerebral autoregulation. Moreover, the increase in blood flow is generalized throughout all parts of the brain. At an equivalent minimum alveolar concentration (MAC) and blood pressure, halothane increases CBF up to 200%, compared with 40% and 20% for enflurane and isoflurane, respectively. Unlike halothane, isoflurane increases blood flow primarily in subcortical areas and the hindbrain. Qualitatively and quantitatively desflurane and sevoflurane may be closest to isoflurane. The effect of volatile agents on CBF also appears to be time-dependent, because with continued administration (2–5 hours) blood flow begins to return to normal.

The response of the cerebral vasculature to CO_2 is generally retained with all volatile agents. Hyperventilation (hypocapnia) can therefore abolish or blunt their initial effects on CBF. The timing of the hyperventilation is important because this effect is only observed if hyperventilation is initiated prior to halothane and enflurane. In contrast, simultaneous hyperventilation with administration of either isoflurane or sevoflurane can prevent increases in ICP. Hypocapnia may be less effective in decreasing ICP with desflurane compared with other volatile agents.

Increases in cerebral blood volume (10–12%) generally parallel increases in CBF, but the relationship is not necessarily linear. Expansion of cerebral blood volume can markedly elevate ICP in patients with reduced intracranial compliance. Studies indicate that cerebral blood volume increases to the same extent with all

Table 25–1. Comparative effects of anesthetic agents on cerebral physiology.

Agent	CMR	CBF	CSF Production	CSF Absorption	CBV	ICP
Halothane	↓↓	↑↑↑	↓	↓	↑↑	↑↑
Enflurane	↓↓	↑↑	↑	↓	↑↑	↑↑
Isoflurane	↓↓↓	↑	±	↑	↑↑	↑
Desflurane	↓↓↓	↑	↑	↓	?	↑↑
Sevoflurane	↓↓↓	↑	?	?	?	↑↑
Nitrous oxide	↓	↑	±	±	±	↑
Barbiturates	↓↓↓↓	↓↓↓	±	↑	↓↓	↓↓↓
Etomidate	↓↓↓	↓↓	±	↑	↓↓	↓↓
Proprofol	↓↓↓	↓↓↓↓	?	?	↓↓	↓↓
Benzodiazepines	↓↓	?	±	↑	↓	↓
Ketamine	±	↑↑	±	↓	↑↑	↑↑
Opioids	±	±	±	↑	±	±
Lidocaine	↓↓	↓↓	?	?	↓↓	↓↓

↑ = increase; ↓ = decrease; ± = little or no change; ? = unknown; CMR = cerebral metabolic rate; CBF = cerebral blood flow; CSF = cerebrospinal fluid; CBV = cerebral blood volume, ICP = intracranial pressure.

volatile agents, suggesting that each affects cerebral venous capacitance to a variable degree. Moreover, these studies demonstrate that hypocapnia most effectively blunts the increase in cerebral blood volume during isoflurane anesthesia.

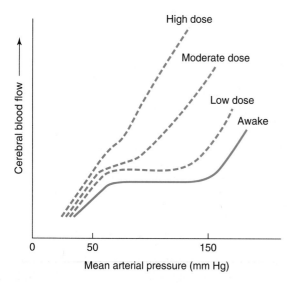

Figure 25–7. Dose-dependent depression of cerebral autoregulation by the volatile anesthetics.

Altered Coupling of Cerebral Metabolic Rate & Blood Flow

As is apparent from the discussion above, volatile agents alter but do not uncouple the normal relationship of CBF and CMR. The combination of a decrease in neuronal metabolic demand with an increase in CBF (metabolic supply) has been termed **luxury perfusion.** This state may be desirable during induced hypotension and support the use of a volatile agent, particularly isoflurane, during this technique. In contrast to this potentially beneficial effect during potential global ischemia, a detrimental circulatory steal phenomenon is possible with volatile anesthetics in the setting of focal ischemia. Volatile agents can increase blood flow in normal areas of the brain but not in ischemic areas, where arterioles already are maximally vasodilated. The end result may be a redistribution of blood flow away from ischemic to normal areas.

Cerebrospinal Fluid Dynamics

Volatile anesthetics affect both CSF formation and absorption. Enflurane is unique in its ability to increase CSF formation and retard absorption; both effects tend to elevate ICP in patients with reduced intracranial compliance. Halothane impedes CSF absorption but only minimally retards formation. Isoflurane, on the other hand, facilitates absorption and is therefore the only volatile agent with favorable effects on CSF dynamics.

Intracranial Pressure

The net effect of volatile anesthetics on ICP is the result of immediate changes in cerebral blood volume, delayed alterations on CSF dynamics, and arterial CO_2 tension. Based on these factors, isoflurane appears to be the volatile agent of choice in patients with decreased intracranial compliance. Animal studies suggest that desflurane may increase ICP more than other volatile agents.

Seizure Activity

In doses of 1.5–2 MAC, enflurane can cause seizure patterns (spike and wave activity) on the EEG, particularly during hypocapnia. Auditory stimuli are said to precipitate this type of activity. Although spike activity may also occasionally be associated with isoflurane prior to electrical silence, it does not progress to seizures.

2. Nitrous Oxide

The effects of nitrous oxide are generally mild and easily overcome by other agents or changes in CO_2 tension. Thus when combined with intravenous agents, nitrous oxide has minimal effects on CBF, metabolic rate, and ICP. Adding this agent to a volatile anesthetic, however, can further increase CBF. When given alone, nitrous oxide causes mild cerebral vasodilation and can potentially increase ICP.

EFFECT OF INTRAVENOUS AGENTS

1. Induction Agents

With the exception of ketamine, all intravenous agents either have little effect on or reduce CMR and CBF. Moreover, with some exceptions, changes in blood flow generally parallel those in metabolic rate. Cerebral autoregulation and CO_2 responsiveness are preserved with all agents.

Barbiturates

Barbiturates have four major actions on the CNS: (1) hypnosis, (2) depression of CMR, (3) reduction of CBF due to increased cerebral vascular resistance, and (4) anticonvulsant activity. These properties make barbiturates, especially thiopental, the most commonly used induction agents in neuroanesthesia.

Barbiturates produce dose-dependent decreases in CMR and CBF until the EEG becomes isoelectric. At that point, maximum reductions of nearly 50% are ob-

served; additional barbiturate does not further reduce metabolic rate. Unlike isoflurane, however, barbiturates reduce metabolic rate uniformly throughout the brain. CMR is depressed slightly more than CBF, such that metabolic supply exceeds metabolic demand (as long as CPP is maintained). Because barbiturate-induced cerebral vasoconstriction occurs only in normal areas, these agents tend to redistribute blood flow from normal to ischemic areas in the brain (**Robin Hood, or reverse steal phenomenon**). The cerebral vasculature in ischemic areas remains maximally dilated and is unaffected by the barbiturate because of ischemic vasomotor paralysis.

Barbiturates also appear to facilitate CSF absorption. The resultant reduction in CSF volume, combined with decreases in CBF and cerebral blood volume, make barbiturates highly effective in lowering ICP. Their anticonvulsant properties are also advantageous in neurosurgical patients who are at increased risk for seizures. The metabolic demand imposed by seizure activity promotes secondary injury in ischemic areas. Small doses of methohexital can activate seizure foci in patients with epilepsy, but higher doses are anticonvulsant like other barbiturates.

Other possible actions of barbiturates include blockade of sodium channels, reducing intracellular calcium influx, scavenging or suppression of free radical formation, and retardation of cerebral edema following ischemic brain injury. All these actions represent the theoretic justification for the controversial use of barbiturates for cerebral protection (below). Studies suggest that barbiturate prophylaxis is effective in preventing brain injury during focal ischemia but not global ischemia.

Opioids

All opioids generally have minimal effects on CBF, CMR, and ICP, unless $PaCO_2$ rises secondary to respiratory depression. Increases in ICP have been reported in some patients with intracranial tumors following sufentanil administration and to a lesser degree following alfentanil. The mechanism appears to be a precipitous drop in blood pressure; reflex cerebral vasodilation likely increases intracranial blood volume and potentially ICP. Although hypotension may be more likely with sufentanil and alfentanil than with fentanyl, significant decreases in blood pressure can adversely affect CPP regardless of the opioid selected. In addition, small doses of alfentanil (< 50 $\mu g/kg$) can activate seizure foci in patients with epilepsy. Morphine is generally not considered optimal in neuroanesthesia due to poor lipid solubility. The latter results in slow CNS penetration and prolonged sedative effects. Potential accumulation of normeperidine and cardiac depression limit the use of meperidine.

Etomidate

Etomidate decreases the CMR, CBF, and ICP in somewhat the same way as thiopental. Its effect on CMR is nonuniform, affecting the cortex more than the brainstem. Its limited effect on the brainstem may be responsible for greater hemodynamic stability in unstable patients when compared with barbiturates. Etomidate also decreases CSF production and enhances absorption. Unfortunately, concern over adrenal suppression limits its long-term use (see Chapter 8).

Induction with etomidate is associated with a relatively high incidence of myoclonic movements, but these movements are not associated with seizure activity on the EEG in normal individuals. The drug has been used to treat seizures, but reports of seizure activity following etomidate in patients with a history of epilepsy suggest that the drug is best avoided in those patients. In fact, small doses of etomidate can activate seizure foci in patients with epilepsy.

Propofol

Propofol reduces CBF and CMR similar to barbiturates and etomidate; however, the decrease in CBF may exceed that in metabolic rate. The drug also appears to be useful in lowering ICP. Although it has been associated with dystonic and choreiform movements, propofol appears to have significant anticonvulsant activity. Moreover, its short elimination half-life (see Chapter 8) makes it a useful agent for neuroanesthesia. Unfortunately, excessive hypotension and cardiac depression in elderly or unstable patients, can compromise CPP.

Benzodiazepines

Benzodiazepines lower CBF and CMR but to a lesser extent than barbiturates, etomidate, and propofol. Benzodiazepines also have useful anticonvulsant properties. Midazolam is the benzodiazepine of choice because of its short half-life. Midazolam induction frequently causes significant decreases in CPP in elderly and unstable patients and may prolong emergence in some instances.

Ketamine

Ketamine is the only intravenous anesthetic that dilates the cerebral vasculature and increases CBF (50–60%). Selective activation of certain areas (limbic and reticular) is partially offset by depression of other areas (somatosensory and auditory) such that total CMR does not change. Seizure activity in thalamic and limbic areas is also described. Ketamine also may impede CSF absorption without affecting formation. Increases in

CBF, cerebral blood volume, and CSF volume can potentially increase ICP markedly in patients with decreased intracranial compliance.

2. Anesthetic Adjuncts

Intravenous lidocaine decreases CMR, CBF, and ICP but to a lesser degree than other agents. Its principal advantage is that it decreases CBF (by increasing cerebral vascular resistance) without causing other significant hemodynamic effects. The risks of systemic toxicity and seizures, however, limit the usefulness of repeated dosing.

Droperidol has little or no effect on cerebral metabolism and minimally reduces blood flow. When used with an opioid as part of a neuroleptic technique, droperidol may cause undesirable prolonged sedation. Reversal of opioids or benzodiazepines with naloxone or flumazenil, respectively, can reverse any beneficial reductions in CBF and metabolic rate. Severe hypertension may also follow naloxone but not flumazenil.

3. Vasopressors

With normal autoregulation and an intact **blood-brain barrier,** vasopressors increase CBF only when mean arterial blood pressure is below 50–60 mm Hg or above 150–160 mm Hg. In the absence of autoregulation, vasopressors increase CBF by their effect on CPP. Changes in CMR generally parallel those in blood flow. β-Adrenergic agents seem to have a greater effect on the brain when the blood-brain barrier is disrupted; central β₁-receptor stimulation increases CMR and blood flow. β-Adrenergic blockers generally have no direct effect on metabolic rate or blood flow, while α₂-adrenergic agonists produce cerebral vasoconstriction. Excessive blood pressure elevations with any agent can disrupt the blood-brain barrier.

4. Vasodilators

In the absence of hypotension, most vasodilators induce cerebral vasodilation and increase CBF in a dose-related fashion. When these agents decrease blood pressure, CBF is usually maintained and may even increase. The resultant increase in cerebral blood volume can significantly elevate ICP in patients with decreased intracranial compliance. Of this group of drugs, only trimethaphan has little or no effect on CBF and cerebral blood volume; because it constricts pupils, trimethaphan may complicate the neurologic examination. Trimethaphan is no longer available in the United States, but it is available in Europe.

5. Neuromuscular Blocking Agents

Neuromuscular blocking agents lack direct action on the brain but can have important secondary effects. Hypertension and histamine-mediated cerebral vasodilation increase ICP, while systemic hypotension (from histamine release or ganglionic blockade) lower CPP. Succinylcholine can increase ICP, possibly as a result of cerebral activation associated with enhanced muscle spindle activity; but the increase is generally minimal if an adequate dose of thiopental is given and hyperventilation is initiated at induction. Moreover, a small (defasciculating) dose of a nondepolarizing relaxant appears to blunt the increase, at least partially. Agents that are likely to release histamine include tubocurarine, atracurium, metocurine, and mivacurium. Tachycardia and hypertension may follow large doses of pancuronium while ganglionic blockade may be seen following tubocurarine.

In the majority of instances, increases in ICP following administration of neuromuscular blocking agents are the result of a hypertensive response due to light anesthesia during laryngoscopy and endotracheal intubation. Acute elevations in ICP will also be seen if hypercapnia or hypoxemia results from prolonged apnea.

■ PHYSIOLOGY OF BRAIN PROTECTION

PATHOPHYSIOLOGY OF CEREBRAL ISCHEMIA

The brain is very vulnerable to ischemic injury because of its relatively high oxygen consumption and near total dependence on aerobic glucose metabolism (above). Interruption of cerebral perfusion, metabolic substrate (glucose), or severe hypoxemia rapidly results in functional impairment; reduced perfusion also impairs clearance of potentially toxic metabolites. If normal oxygen tension, blood flow, and glucose supply is not reestablished within 3–8 minutes under most conditions, ATP stores are depleted and irreversible neuronal injury begins. During ischemia, intracellular K^+ decreases and intracellular Na^+ increases (see Chapter 19). More important, intracellular Ca^{++} increases because of failure of ATP-dependent pumps to either extrude the ion extracellularly or into intracellular cisterns, increased intracellular Na^+ concentration (see Chapter 19), and release of the excitatory neurotransmitter glutamate (see Chapter 18).

Sustained increases in intracellular Ca^{++} activate lipases and proteases, which initiate and propagate structural damage to neurons. Increases in free fatty acid concentration and cyclooxygenase and lipoxygenase activities result in the formation of prostaglandins and leukotrienes, some of which are potent mediators of cellular injury. Accumulation of toxic metabolites such as lactic acid also impairs cellular function and interferes with repair mechanisms. Lastly, reperfusion of ischemic tissues can cause additional tissue damage due to the formation of oxygen-derived free radicals.

STRATEGIES FOR BRAIN PROTECTION

Ischemic brain injury is usually classified as focal (incomplete) or global (complete). On one hand, this convention may be somewhat artificial in that differences may be more in severity rather than mechanism. On the other hand, this classification is useful in defining clinical settings. **Global ischemia** includes total circulatory arrest as well as global hypoxia. Cessation of perfusion may be caused by cardiac arrest or deliberate circulatory arrest (see Chapter 21), while global hypoxia may be caused by severe respiratory failure, drowning, and asphyxia (including anesthetic mishaps). **Focal ischemia** includes embolic, hemorrhagic, and atherosclerotic strokes as well as blunt, penetrating, and surgical trauma.

In some instances, interventions aimed at restoring perfusion and oxygenation are possible; these include reestablishing an effective circulation, normalizing arterial oxygenation and oxygen carrying capacity, or reopening an occluded vessel. With focal ischemia, the brain tissue surrounding a severely damaged area may suffer marked functional impairment but still remain viable. Such areas are thought to have very marginal perfusion (< 15 mL/100 g/min), but if further injury can be limited and normal flow is rapidly restored these areas (the "ischemic penumbra") may recover completely. When the above interventions are not applicable or available, the emphasis must be on limiting the extent of brain injury.

From a practical point of view, efforts aimed at preventing or limiting neuronal tissue damage are often the same whether the ischemia is focal or global. Clinical goals are usually to optimize CPP, decrease metabolic requirements (basal and electrical), and possibly block mediators of cellular injury. Clearly, the most effective strategy is prevention, because once injury has occurred measures aimed at cerebral protection become less effective.

Hypothermia

Hypothermia is the most effective method for protecting the brain during focal and global ischemia. Indeed, profound hypothermia is often used for up to 1 hour of total circulatory arrest with little evidence of neurologic impairment (see Chapter 21). Unlike anesthetic agents, hypothermia decreases both basal and electrical metabolic requirements throughout the brain; metabolic requirements continue to decrease even after complete electrical silence. Even mild degrees of hypothermia (33–35 °C) appear to have some protective effects. Moreover, mild hypothermia has fewer adverse effects than more profound reductions in temperature (see Chapter 6).

Anesthetic Agents

Barbiturates, etomidate, propofol, and isoflurane can produce complete electrical silence of the brain and eliminate the metabolic cost of electrical activity; unfortunately, they have no effect on basal energy requirements. Furthermore, with the exception of barbiturates, their effects are nonuniform, affecting different parts of the brain to variable extents. Lastly, barbiturates can also produce inverse steal, reduce cerebral edema and calcium influx, inhibit free radical formation, and blockade of sodium channels (above).

 Both animal and human data suggest that barbiturates are effective for brain protection in the setting of focal ischemia. Although some animal data suggest that etomidate, propofol, and possibly isoflurane may be protective, the results are conflicting and clinical experience with these agents is limited. Ketamine may also have a protective effect because of its ability to block the actions of glutamate at the NMDA receptor (see Chapter 8), but animal studies for this agent are also conflicting.

No anesthetic agent has consistently been shown to be protective against global ischemia.

Specific Adjuncts

The calcium channel blockers, nimodipine and nicardipine, may be beneficial in reducing neurologic injury following hemorrhagic and ischemic strokes. Both agents have cerebral vasodilating properties; unfortunately, in some studies they improve CBF but not neurologic outcome. Methylprednisolone has been shown to reduce neurologic deficits following spinal cord injury if given within 8 hours. The nonglucocorticoid steroid, tirilazad improves neurologic outcome following subarachnoid hemorrhage. Acadesine, an adenosine modulating agent, has been reported to decrease the incidence of stroke following coronary artery surgery. Other agents that may prove to be beneficial include magnesium, dexmedetomidine (an α_2-adrenergic agonist that also interacts with NMDA receptors), dextromethorphan (a noncompetitive NMDA blocker), NBQX (an α-amino-3-hydroxy-5-methyl-4-isoxazole-

propionic acid (AMPA)–receptor blocker), and vitamin E (an antioxidant).

General Measures

Maintenance of an optimal CPP is critical. Thus arterial blood pressure should be normal or slightly elevated, and increases in venous and ICP should be avoided. Oxygen carrying capacity should ideally be maintained with a hematocrit of at least 30–34% and normal arterial oxygen tension. Hyperglycemia has been reported to aggravate neurologic injuries following either focal or global ischemia; although this association might be a secondary phenomena, it seems prudent to avoid excessive hyperglycemia (> 180 mg/dL). Normocarbia should be maintained as both hyper- and hypocarbia have no beneficial effect in the setting of ischemia and could prove detrimental; hypocarbia-induced cerebral vasoconstriction may aggravate the ischemia, while hypercarbia may induce a steal phenomena (with focal ischemia) or worsen intracellular acidosis.

■ EFFECT OF ANESTHESIA ON ELECTROPHYSIOLOGIC MONITORING

Electrophysiologic monitoring attempts to assess the functional integrity of the CNS. The most commonly used monitors for neurosurgical procedures are the EEG and evoked potentials. Proper application of these monitoring modalities is critically dependent on monitoring the specific area at risk and recognizing anesthetic-induced changes. Both monitoring modalities are described in Chapter 6.

The effects of anesthetic agents on the EEG and evoked potentials are summarized in Tables 25–2 and 25–3. Correct interpretation of changes requires correlation with anesthetic depth- and dose-related changes and with physiologic variables such as blood pressure, body temperature, and respiratory gas tensions. EEG slowing associated with relative hypotension is of greater concern during light anesthesia and intense surgical retraction than during deep anesthesia without stimulation. Regardless of the technique employed, recordings should be bilateral (for comparison) and correlated with the intraoperative course of events.

ELECTROENCEPHALOGRAPHY

EEG monitoring is most useful for assessing the adequacy of cerebral perfusion during carotid endarterectomy and controlled hypotension as well as assessing

Table 25–2. Electroencephalographic changes during anesthesia.

Activation	Depression
Inhalational agents (subanesthetic)	Inhalational agents (1–2 MAC)
Barbiturates (small doses)	Barbiturates
Benzodiazepines (small doses)	Opioids
Etomidate (small doses)	Propofol
Nitrous oxide	Etomidate
Ketamine	Hypocapnia
Mild hypercapnia	Marked hypercapnia
Sensory stimulation	Hypothermia
Hypoxia (early)	Hypoxia (late) Ischemia

anesthetic depth. EEG changes can be simplistically described as either activation or depression. EEG activation (a shift to predominantly high-frequency and low-voltage activity) is seen with light anesthesia and surgical stimulation, while EEG depression (a shift to predominantly low-frequency and high-voltage activity) occurs with deep anesthesia or cerebral compromise. Most anesthetics produce a biphasic pattern on the EEG consisting of an initial activation (at subanesthetic doses) followed by dose-dependent depression.

Inhalational Anesthetics

Clinically, halothane produces a typical biphasic pattern. Isoflurane is the only volatile anesthetic that can produce an isoelectric EEG at high clinical doses (1–2

Table 25–3. Effect of anesthetic agents on evoked potentials.

	SSEP		VER		BAER	
Agent	Amp	Lat	Amp	Lat	Amp	Lat
Nitrous oxide	↓	±	↓	↑	±	±
Halothane	↓	↑	±	↑	±	↑
Enflurane	↓	↑	↓	↑	±	↑
Isoflurane	↓	↑	↓	↑	±	↑
Barbiturates	±	±	↓	↑	±	±
Opioids*	±	±	±	±	±	±
Etomidate	↑	↑				
Propofol	↓	↑			↓	↑
Benzodiazepines	↓	±				
Ketamine	±	↑				

*At very high doses, can decrease the latency and decrease the amplitude of SSEP, ↑ = increase; ↓ = decrease; ± = little or no change; SSEP = somatosensory evoked potentials; VER = visual evoked response; BAER = brainstem auditory evoked response; Amp = amplitude; Lat = latency.

MAC). Desflurane and enflurane produce a burst suppression pattern at high doses (> 1.2 and > 1.5 MAC, respectively) but not electrical silence. Spike (seizure-like) activity may also be observed with enflurane. Nitrous oxide is also unusual in that it increases both frequency and amplitude (high amplitude activation).

Intravenous Agents

Benzodiazepines produce the typical biphasic pattern. Barbiturates, etomidate, and propofol produce a typical biphasic pattern and are the only intravenous agents capable of producing burst suppression and electrical silence at high doses. In contrast, opioids characteristically produce only a monophasic, dose-dependent depression of the EEG. Lastly, ketamine produces an unusual activation consisting of rhythmic high amplitude θ activity followed by very high amplitude δ and low amplitude β activities.

EVOKED POTENTIALS

Somatosensory evoked potentials (SSEPs) test the integrity of the dorsal spinal columns and the sensory cortex and may be useful during resection of spinal tumors, instrumentation of the spine, carotid endarterectomy, and aortic surgery. The adequacy of perfusion of the spinal cord during aortic surgery is probably better assessed with motor evoked potentials. Brainstem auditory evoked potentials test the integrity of the eighth cranial nerve and the auditory pathways above the pons, and are used for surgery in the posterior fossa. Visual evoked potentials may be used to monitor the optic nerve and upper brainstem during resections of large pituitary tumors.

Interpretation of evoked potentials is more complicated than that of the EEG. Evoked potentials have poststimulus latencies that are described as short, intermediate, and long. Short-latency evoked potentials arise from the nerve stimulated or from the brainstem. Intermediate- and long-latency evoked potentials are primarily of cortical origin. In general, short-latency potentials are least affected by anesthetic agents, while long-latency potentials are affected by even subanesthetic levels of most agents. Consequently, only short and intermediate potentials are monitored intraoperatively. Visual evoked potentials are most affected by anesthetics, while brainstem auditory evoked potentials are least affected.

Inhalational Anesthetics

Volatile anesthetics have the greatest effect of all anesthetics on evoked potentials, causing dose-dependent decreases in wave amplitude and increases in latencies.

To minimize anesthetic-induced changes, some authors recommend limiting isoflurane and enflurane concentrations to 0.5 MAC and halothane to 1 MAC. Nitrous oxide decreases wave amplitude but has no effect on latencies.

Intravenous Anesthetics

Intravenous agents in clinical doses generally have less effects on evoked potential compared with volatile agents, but in high doses can also decrease amplitude and increase latencies. It should be noted that evoked potentials are often preserved with barbiturates even when they produce an isoelectric EEG. Etomidate increases latencies of SSEP but can increase wave amplitude. Although most opioids produce dose-dependent increases in SSEP latencies and more variable decreases in wave amplitude, meperidine may increase amplitude. Ketamine has also been reported to increase SSEP wave amplitude.

CASE DISCUSSION:
POSTOPERATIVE HEMIPLEGIA

A 62-year-old man is undergoing radical neck dissection for a malignant parotid tumor on the right side. Anesthesia is induced with etomidate and maintained with enflurane plus 70% nitrous oxide in oxygen. The tumor was found to extend into the carotid sheath, and during the dissection the carotid artery was injured. The internal carotid artery had to be cross-clamped to control the bleeding and allow repair with a patch graft.

Describe the blood supply of the brain as it relates to this case.

The internal carotid and vertebral arteries from each side supply nearly the entire blood flow to the brain (Figure 25–8). The internal carotid artery arises at the bifurcation of the common carotid artery in the neck and enters the cranium through the temporal bone. The vertebral artery is a branch of the subclavian artery and ascends through the transverse processes of the cervical vertebrae (starting at C6), entering the skull through the foramen magnum. Anastomotic connections between the contralateral vessels and between the internal carotid and vertebral systems form a complete arterial circuit at the base of the brain (circle of Willis). These anastomoses can provide collateral blood flow and protect the brain from ischemia should blood flow cease in one of these vessels proximal to the circle of Willis.

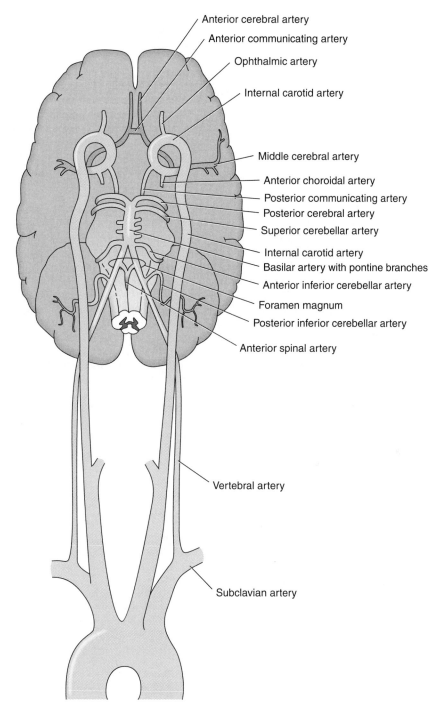

Figure 25–8. The cerebral circulation.

Additional collateral flow may also be available through anastomotic connections between branches of the internal carotid and external carotid arteries. Although the internal carotid artery does not have any major extracranial branches, its ophthalmic branch anastomoses with branches of the facial artery (a tributary of the external carotid artery) in the orbit. Ligation of both internal carotid arteries without neurologic sequelae has been reported in a few patients.

What is the anatomic basis of a hemispheric cerebral infarct occurring in this setting?

The anastomotic vessels completing the circle of Willis (anterior and posterior communicating arteries) are not always well developed. Variations in the size of these vessels are very common, and one or both posterior communicating arteries may be absent. Moreover, the incidence of significant atherosclerotic lesions in the cerebral circulation increases with age (6–8% in patients 60–70 years old). While moderate to severe stenoses or even complete occlusions may be asymptomatic under normal conditions, when cerebral blood flow (CBF) is compromised these lesions not only predispose to ischemia distally but also limit collateral blood flow to other areas of the brain.

When the surgeon clamps the right internal carotid artery, continued blood flow through the right middle and anterior cerebral arteries (branches of the internal carotid artery) becomes dependent on flow from (1) the left carotid system via the anterior communicating artery, (2) the vertebral-basilar system via the right posterior communicating artery, and (3) anastomoses between the internal and external carotid vessels around the right orbit. The presence of developmental abnormalities or acquired occlusive disease in these vessels would predispose this patient to a cerebral infarct.

What measures, if any, might protect against cerebral ischemia?

Use of a temporary shunt by the surgeon would be highly effective but has its own risks (see Chapter 21). Moreover, placement of a shunt in this case may not be technically feasible, or the surgeon may not be prepared to use a shunt.

At least theoretically, manipulation of respiratory gas tensions, arterial blood pressure, and anesthetic agents could also influence the outcome. Hyperventilation vasoconstricts the cerebral vasculature, limiting collateral blood flow, and should therefore be avoided. Hypercapnia may also be detrimental if it induces a cerebral steal phenomena. Consequently, a normal or slightly elevated arterial CO_2 tension is optimal.

Nitrous oxide should be discontinued and the inspired oxygen concentration increased to 100%. Although the resulting increase in dissolved oxygen is small compared with that carried on hemoglobin (see Chapter 22), it may theoretically be enough to partially ameliorate ischemia or reduce the amount of infarcted tissue.

Because volatile anesthetics produce cerebral vasodilation and favor pressure-dependent CBF (see Figure 25–7), arterial blood pressure should be maintained at normal or high normal levels (140–150 mm Hg systolic).

Consideration should be given to substituting isoflurane for enflurane. In clinically used doses, isoflurane produces less cardiovascular depression and greater depression of cerebral metabolic rate (above).

Lastly, prophylaxis with mild hypothermia and possibly thiopental for cerebral protection may be indicated. While ideally the thiopental should be administered until the EEG is isoelectric, it should be given empirically in this setting (500–1500 mg total dose) in small increments (50 mg) to prevent hypotension.

SUGGESTED READING

Albin M: *Textbook of Neuroanesthesia with Neurosurgical and Neuroscience Perspectives.* McGraw-Hill, 1997.

Cottrell JE, Smith DS: *Anesthesia and Neurosurgery,* 3rd ed. Mosby Year Book, 1994.

Cucchiara RF, Black S, Michenfelder JD: *Clinical Neuroanesthesia.* Churchill Livingstone, 2nd ed. 1998.

Newfield P, Cottrell JE: *Handbook of Neuroanesthesia,* 3rd ed. Lippincott Williams & Wilkins, 1999.

Schubert A: *Clinical Neuroanesthesia.* Butterworth-Heinemann, 1997.

Stone DJ, Sperry RJ: *The Neuroanesthesia Handbook.* Mosby, 1996.

Walters FJM, Ingram GS, Jenkinson JL: *Anaesthesia and Intensive Care for the Neurosurgical Patient.* Blackwell, 1994.

Anesthesia for Neurosurgery

26

KEY CONCEPTS

 In the preoperative management of patients with mass lesions, computed tomography and magnetic resonance imaging scans should be reviewed for evidence of brain edema, a midline shift greater than 0.5 cm, and ventricular size.

 Intracranial compliance can be improved by osmotic diuresis, steroids, or removal of cerebrospinal fluid (CSF) via a ventriculostomy immediately prior to induction. The goal is to induce anesthesia and intubate the trachea in a slow, controlled fashion without increasing intracranial pressure (ICP) or compromising cerebral blood flow (CBF).

 Operations in the posterior fossa can injure vital circulatory and respiratory brainstem centers as well as cranial nerves or their nuclei.

 Venous air embolism can occur when the pressure within an open vein is subatmospheric. These conditions may exist in any position (and during any procedure) whenever the wound is above the heart.

 Optimal recovery of air following venous air embolism is provided by a multi-orificed catheter positioned high in the atrium at its junction with the superior vena cava. Confirmation of correct positioning is important and is accomplished by intravascular electrocardiography or by transesophageal echocardiography.

 In patients with head trauma, correction of hypotension and control of any bleeding take precedence over radiographic studies and definitive neurosurgical treatment because systolic arterial blood pressures of less than 80 mm Hg correlate with a poor outcome.

 Minor bleeding from a ruptured aneurysm may predispose patients to delayed complications, such as cerebral vasospasm. The only therapy proven useful for symptomatic vasospasm is intravascular volume expansion and induced hypertension (triple H therapy: hypervolemia, hemodilution, and hypertension).

 Hyperventilation is avoided to prevent decreases in CBF, especially in patients with vasospasm.

 Massive blood loss from aortic or vena caval injury can occur intraoperatively or postoperatively with thoracic or lumbar procedures and is often initially occult. In suitable candidates, elective hypotension or infiltration of the wound with a weak epinephrine solution may decrease intraoperative blood loss.

Harvey Cushing, one of the founders of neurosurgery, is largely responsible for the development of the anesthesia record. Out of concern for the safety of his patients, he came to emphasize the need to record the surgical patient's pulse, respiratory rate, temperature, and blood pressure intraoperatively. A better understanding of the effects of anesthesia on the central nervous system (CNS) (see Chapter 25) and improvements in anesthetic techniques have similarly contributed to the improved outcomes seen in modern neurosurgery. Sophisticated monitoring techniques and improved operating conditions under anesthesia have allowed increasingly difficult procedures to be performed on patients previously deemed inoperable.

Anesthetic techniques must be modified in the presence of intracranial hypertension and marginal cerebral perfusion. In addition, many neurosurgical procedures require unusual patient positions—eg, sitting, prone—further complicating management. This chapter applies the principles developed in Chapter 25 to the anesthetic care of neurosurgical patients.

■ INTRACRANIAL HYPERTENSION

Intracranial hypertension is defined as a sustained increase in intracranial pressure (ICP) above 15 mm Hg. Uncompensated increases in the tissue or fluid within the rigid cranial vault produce sustained ICP elevations (see Chapter 25). Intracranial hypertension may result from an expanding tissue or fluid mass, interference with normal cerebrospinal fluid (CSF) absorption, excessive cerebral blood flow (CBF), or systemic disturbances promoting brain edema (see below). Multiple factors are often simultaneously present. For example, tumors in the posterior fossa are not only usually associated with some degree of brain edema, but they also readily obstruct CSF flow by compressing the fourth ventricle (obstructive hydrocephalus).

Although many patients are initially asymptomatic, all eventually develop characteristic symptoms and signs, including headache, nausea, vomiting, papilledema, focal neurologic deficits, and altered consciousness. When ICP exceeds 30 mm Hg, CBF progressively decreases and a vicious circle is established: ischemia causes brain edema, which in turn increases ICP, resulting in more ischemia. If left unchecked, this cycle continues until the patient dies of progressive neurologic damage or catastrophic herniation (see Chapter 25). Periodic increases in arterial blood pressure with reflex slowing of the heart rate (**Cushing response**) are often observed and can be correlated with abrupt increases in ICP (plateau or A waves) lasting 1–15 minutes. This phenomena is the result of autoregulatory mechanisms periodically decreasing cerebral vascular resistance in response to cerebral ischemia; unfortunately, the latter further increases ICP as cerebral blood volume increases. Eventually, severe ischemia and acidosis completely abolish autoregulation (vasomotor paralysis) and both ICP and CBF become passive to arterial blood pressure.

CEREBRAL EDEMA

An increase in brain water content can be produced by several mechanisms. Disruption of the blood-brain barrier (vasogenic edema) is most common and allows the entry of plasma-like fluid into the brain. Increases in blood pressure enhance the formation of this type of edema. Common causes of vasogenic edema include mechanical trauma, inflammatory lesions, brain tumors, hypertension, and infarction. Cerebral edema following metabolic insults (cytotoxic edema), such as hypoxemia or ischemia, results from failure of brain cells to actively extrude sodium and progressive cellular swelling. Interstitial cerebral edema is the result of obstructive hydrocephalus and entry of CSF into brain interstitium. Lastly, cerebral edema can also be the result of intracellular movement of water secondary to acute decreases in serum osmolality (water intoxication).

TREATMENT

Treatment of intracranial hypertension and cerebral edema is ideally directed at the underlying cause. Metabolic disturbances are corrected and operative intervention is undertaken whenever possible. Vasogenic edema—especially that associated with tumors—often responds to corticosteroids (dexamethasone), which appear to promote repair of the blood-brain barrier. Regardless of the cause, fluid restriction, osmotic agents, and loop diuretics are usually effective in temporarily decreasing brain edema and lowering ICP until more definitive measures can be undertaken. Diuresis lowers ICP chiefly by removing intracellular water from normal brain tissue. Moderate hyperventilation ($PaCO_2$ 25–30 mm Hg) is often very helpful in reducing CBF (see Chapter 25) and normalizing ICP but may aggravate ischemia in patients with focal ischemia.

Mannitol, in doses of 0.25–0.5 g/kg, is especially effective in rapidly decreasing ICP. Its efficacy is primarily related to its effect on serum osmolality (see Chapter 26); a serum osmolality of 300–315 mOsm/L is generally considered desirable. Mannitol can transiently decrease blood pressure by virtue of its weak vasodilating properties, but its principal disadvantage is a transient increase in intravascular volume, which can precipitate pulmonary edema in patients with borderline cardiac or renal function. Mannitol should generally not be used in patients with intracranial aneurysms, arteriovenous malformations (AVMs), or intracranial hemorrhage until the cranium is opened. Osmotic diuresis in such instances can expand a hematoma as the volume of the normal brain tissue around it decreases. Rapid osmotic diuresis in elderly patients can also occasionally cause a subdural hematoma due to rupture of fragile bridging veins entering the sagittal sinus. Rebound edema may follow the use of mannitol; thus, its use is limited to procedures (such as a craniotomy for tumor resection) in which intracranial volume will be reduced.

Use of a loop diuretic (furosemide), although less effective and requiring up to 30 minutes, may have the additional advantage of directly decreasing CSF formation. The combined use of mannitol and furosemide may be synergistic but requires close monitoring of the serum potassium concentration (see Chapter 28).

■ ANESTHESIA AND CRANIOTOMY FOR PATIENTS WITH MASS LESIONS

Intracranial masses may be congenital, neoplastic (benign or malignant), infectious (abscess or cyst), or vascular (hematoma or arteriovenous malformation). Craniotomy is commonly undertaken for primary and metastatic neoplasms of the brain. Primary tumors usually arise from glial cells (astrocytoma, oligodendroglioma, or glioblastoma), ependymal cells (ependymoma), or supporting tissues (meningioma, schwannoma, or choroidal papilloma). Childhood tumors include medulloblastoma, neuroblastoma, and chordoma.

Regardless of the cause, intracranial masses present according to growth rate, location, and ICP. Slowly growing masses are frequently asymptomatic for long periods, whereas rapidly growing ones usually present acutely. Common presentations include headache, seizures, a general decline in cognitive or specific neurologic functions, and focal neurologic deficits. Supratentorial masses typically present as seizures, hemiplegia, or aphasia, while infratentorial masses more commonly present as cerebellar dysfunction (ataxia, nystagmus, and dysarthria) or brainstem compression (cranial nerve palsies, altered consciousness, or abnormal respiration). As ICP increases, frank signs of intracranial hypertension also develop (above).

PREOPERATIVE MANAGEMENT

Preanesthetic evaluation should attempt to establish the presence or absence of intracranial hypertension. Computed tomographic (CT) and magnetic resonance imaging (MRI) scans should be reviewed for evidence of brain edema, a midline shift greater than 0.5 cm, and ventricular size. Examination should include a neurologic assessment documenting mental status and any existing sensory or motor deficits. Medications should be reviewed with special reference to corticosteroid, diuretic, and anticonvulsant therapy. Laboratory evaluation should rule out corticosteroid-induced hyperglycemia and electrolyte disturbances due to diuretics or abnormalities in antidiuretic hormone secretion (see Chapter 28). Anticonvulsant levels should be checked, especially when seizures are not well controlled.

Premedication

Premedication is best avoided when intracranial hypertension is suspected. Hypercapnia secondary to respiratory depression increases ICP and may be lethal. Patients with normal ICP are usually given a benzodiazepine (diazepam orally or midazolam intravenously or intramuscularly). Corticosteroids and anticonvulsant therapy should be continued up until the time of surgery.

INTRAOPERATIVE MANAGEMENT

Monitoring

In addition to standard monitors, direct intra-arterial pressure monitoring and bladder catheterization are mandatory for most patients undergoing craniotomy. Rapid blood pressure changes during induction, hyperventilation, intubation, positioning, surgical manipulation, and emergence necessitate continuous blood pressure monitoring to ensure optimal cerebral perfusion. Moreover, arterial blood gas measurements are necessary to closely regulate $PaCO_2$. Many neuroanesthesiologists zero the arterial pressure transducer at the level of the head (external auditory meatus)—instead of the right atrium—to facilitate calculation of cerebral perfusion pressure (CPP). End-tidal CO_2 measurements alone cannot be relied upon for precise regulation of ventilation; the arterial to end-tidal CO_2 gradient must be determined. Central venous access and pressure monitoring should be considered for patients requiring vasoactive drugs. Use of the internal jugular vein for access is somewhat controversial because of the risk of carotid puncture and concern that the catheter might interfere with venous drainage from the brain. Many clinicians avoid this issue by passing a long catheter centrally through the median basilic vein. The external jugular and subclavian veins may be suitable alternatives. A urinary catheter is necessary because of the frequent use of diuretics, the long duration of most neurosurgical procedures, and its utility in guiding fluid therapy. Neuromuscular function should be monitored on the unaffected side in patients with hemiparesis (see Chapter 27) because the twitch response is often abnormally resistant on the affected side. Monitoring visual evoked potentials may be useful in preventing optic nerve damage during resections of large pituitary tumors. Additional monitors for surgery in the posterior fossa are described below.

Management of patients with intracranial hypertension is greatly facilitated by monitoring ICP periop-

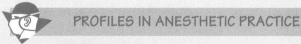

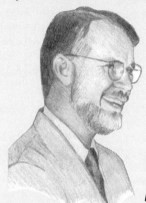

Robert F. Bedford, MD

ANESTHESIA FOR NEURONAVIGATION

Traditionally, anesthesia for neurosurgical resection of intracranial lesions has centered around the 4 Hs: hyperventilation, hypocarbia, hypothermia, and hypotension. Over the past 30 years, neuroanesthesiologists have tended to be obsessed with the adverse effect of inhalational anesthetics on cerebral blood flow (CBF), and its attendant increase in brain bulk. This effect, prior to craniotomy, can result in potentially dangerous increases in intracranial pressure or, during craniotomy, can make brain retraction and surgical intervention more difficult as the brain herniates through the incision or around retractors. Thus has developed the obsession with the so-called slack brain, produced by reductions in CBF resulting from hypocarbia or hypothermia, administration of mannitol to decrease brain water, or drainage of cerebrospinal fluid.[1]

In recent years, however, the world of neuronavigation has revolutionized neurosurgical intervention, particularly for small, deep-seated lesions that traditionally carried a high degree of morbidity and consequent mortality. In essence, neuronavigation relies on imaging technology and remote spatial orientation to guide slender devices for probing the brain and finding and resecting small lesions

through small incisions (Figure 1). Except in rare instances where intraoperative magnetic resonance imaging (MRI) is available, these techniques rely on preoperative scans to determine the lesion's coordinates within the skull and to direct the localizing and therapeutic probes, biopsy needles, endoscopes, resection devices, etc. For a successful outcome it is crucial that, during the operation, the patient's intracranial contents retain the identical spatial relationships that existed at the time the preoperative scan was performed.

During neuronavigation, the shift in brain substance that can be induced by an acute decrease in CBF or brain bulk is an anathema. Even an intracranial shift of 5 to 10 mm may result in a biopsy needle missing its mark in a deep-seated lesion (Figure 2). Worse yet, such a shift in brain substance may cause a resecting probe to miss the bulk of a lesion, conceivably resulting in resection of normal, functional brain tissue. During neuronavigation procedures,

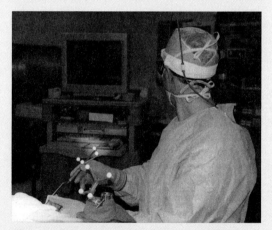

Figure 1. Who's watching the patient? The neurosurgeon is relying on yesterday's MRI scan to orient the brain biopsy probe during neuronavigation-guided procedure.

eratively. A ventriculostomy or subdural bolt is most commonly employed and is usually placed by the neurosurgeon preoperatively under local anesthesia. Electronic ICP monitoring is possible utilizing saline-filled tubing with a pressure transducer. The transducer should be zeroed to the same reference level as the arterial pressure transducer (usually the external auditory meatus; see above). A ventriculostomy has the added advantage of allowing removal of CSF to decrease ICP.

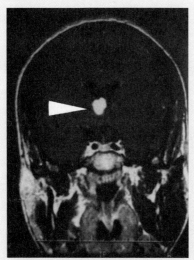

Figure 2. Small, deep-seated lesion (central white mass) unsupported by nearby bony structures. Significant movement of the mass may occur with a decrease in brain bulk, resulting in a probe missing the mark.

traditional neuroanesthetic approaches are avoided as the anesthesiologist attempts to minimize movement of intracranial contents. Normocarbia is highly desirable, despite the potentially adverse consequences of inhalational anesthetics. If inhalational agents are to be used, only mild hypocarbia (PaCO$_2$ ~ 35 mm Hg) is induced to counteract anesthetic-induced cerebral vasodilatation. Propofol, while expensive, may be the hypnotic or maintenance agent of choice because of its negligible effects on CBF during normocarbia. Judicious administration of opioids may be useful early to prevent hemodynamic responses to endotracheal intubation, but once the dura has been entered, analgesic requirements are negligible. Liberal use of local anesthetics for skull block works well to minimize hemodynamic responses to head-pinning and burr-hole placement.[2] On the other hand, there also is a need for complete paralysis to obviate the risk of coughing and cervical spine injury while the head is immobilized.

Finally, loss of cerebrospinal fluid from the incision may cause settling of brain contents and shift of intracranial lesions. Accordingly, the burr hole and dural incision should be placed in as nondependent a position as possible, occasionally resulting in some interesting positional challenges for the neuroanesthesia team.

The good news for the neuroanesthesiologist is the knowledge that an alert, oriented patient with an intracranial mass lesion (even a large one, if it is slow growing) is not likely to sustain a pathologic increase in intracranial pressure from a well-managed anesthetic as described above. Anesthetic management for neuronavigation is entirely different from caring for a patient with acute head trauma or an intracranial hemorrhage resulting in preoperative coma or stupor.

There is an additional caveat to observe during the patient's emergence from neuronavigation procedures. With only biopsy or mini-resection of a small lesion, there is minimal intracranial space to compensate for postoperative brain swelling. Occasionally the repeated passage of probes and endoscopes may initiate a process of reactive brain edema near the site of lesion resection. This, in turn, may cause pathologic increases in intracranial pressure and postoperative coma. If a patient fails to awaken to the point of eye opening on command in 15–20 minutes, it is imperative to rule out serious brain swelling or a postoperative hematoma by promptly performing a CT scan of the head. Occasionally, it is necessary to return these patients to the operating room for emergency intracranial decompression. At this time, all the old rules of minimizing intracranial pressure during craniotomy become paramount.

1. Bedford, RF: Supratentorial masses: anesthetic considerations. In Cottrell JE, Smith DS (editors): *Anesthesia and Neurosurgery.* 3rd ed. Mosby, 1994, pp. 307–21.
2. Pinosky ML, Fishman RL, Reeves ST, et al: The effect of bupivacaine skull block on the hemodynamic response to craniotomy. Anesth Analg 1996;83:1256–61.

Induction

Induction of anesthesia and endotracheal intubation are critical periods for patients with compromised intracranial compliance or an already elevated ICP. Intracranial compliance can be improved by osmotic diuresis, steroids, or removal of CSF via a ventriculostomy immediately prior to induction. The goal of any technique should be to induce anesthesia and intubate the trachea in a slow,

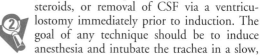

controlled fashion without increasing ICP or compromising CBF. Arterial hypertension during induction increases cerebral blood volume and promotes cerebral edema. Marked or sustained hypertension can lead to marked increases in ICP that can decrease CPP and risk herniation (see Chapter 25). Excessive decreases in arterial blood pressure can be equally detrimental by compromising CPP.

The most common induction technique employs thiopental or propofol together with hyperventilation to lower ICP and blunt the noxious effects of laryngoscopy and intubation. Cooperative patients can be asked to hyperventilate during preoxygenation. All patients are hyperventilated with controlled ventilation once the thiopental or propofol is injected. A neuromuscular blocking agent (also called muscle relaxant)is given to facilitate ventilation and prevent straining or coughing, both of which can abruptly increase ICP. An intravenous opioid—eg, fentanyl, 5–10 μg/kg—just prior to thiopental blunts the sympathetic response, especially in young patients. Esmolol, 0.5–1.0 mg/kg, is effective in preventing tachycardia in hypertensive patients.

The actual induction technique can be varied according to individual patient responses and coexisting diseases. Use of propofol has the added benefit of a very short recovery time, while substitution of etomidate for thiopental may provide greater protection against circulatory depression. The combination of a small dose of fentanyl, 5 μg/kg, with etomidate, 6–8 mg, is also useful in unstable patients. Conversely, for patients with reactive airways (bronchospastic disease), the combination of incremental doses of thiopental and low dose isoflurane with hyperventilation may be preferable.

A nondepolarizing neuromuscular blocking agent is generally given at induction to facilitate controlled ventilation and tracheal intubation. Rocuronium, vecuronium, pipecuronium, and doxacurium provide the greatest hemodynamic stability (see Chapter 9). Succinylcholine may increase ICP, especially if intubation is attempted prior to the establishment of deep thiopental anesthesia and hyperventilation (see Chapter 25). Succinylcholine, however, may be the agent of choice in patients at increased risk for aspiration or with a potentially difficult airway because hypoxemia and hypercarbia are even more detrimental. Significant muscle wasting is a relative contraindication to succinylcholine because of the risk of hyperkalemia.

Hypertension during induction should be treated with esmolol or by deepening the anesthetic with additional thiopental or propofol, or by hyperventilation with low doses (< 1 minimum alveolar concentration [MAC]) of isoflurane. Because of their potentially deleterious effect on cerebral blood volume and ICP (see Chapter 25), vasodilators (such as nitroprusside, nitroglycerin, calcium channel blockers and hydralazine)

should generally be avoided until the dura is opened. Transient hypotension should generally be treated with incremental doses of vasopressors (ephedrine or phenylephrine) rather than intravenous fluids.

Positioning

Frontal, temporal, and parieto-occipital craniotomies are performed in the supine position. The head is elevated 15–30 degrees to facilitate venous and CSF drainage. The head may also be turned to the side to facilitate exposure. Excessive flexion or rotation of the neck impedes jugular venous drainage and can increase ICP. During positioning, the endotracheal tube (ETT) should be well secured and all breathing circuit connections checked. The risk of unrecognized disconnections may be increased because the patient's airway is not easily assessible; the operating table is usually turned 90 or 180 degrees away from the anesthesiologist, and both the patient and the breathing circuit are almost completely covered by surgical drapes.

Maintenance of Anesthesia

Anesthesia is usually maintained with a nitrous-opioid-muscle relaxant technique. Any opioid may be used (see Chapter 25). Persistent hypertension requires the use of low-dose (< 1 MAC) isoflurane, sevoflurane, or desflurane. Alternatively, a combination of an opioid and low-dose inhalational agent, or a total intravenous technique may be used. Even though periods of stimulation are fairly limited, complete paralysis is recommended—unless electromyography is used—to prevent straining, bucking, or movement. Increased anesthetic requirements can be expected during the most stimulating periods: laryngoscopy-intubation, skin incision, dural opening, periosteal manipulations, and closure.

Hyperventilation should be continued intraoperatively to maintain $PaCO_2$ between 25 mm Hg and 30 mm Hg. Lower $PaCO_2$ tensions provide little additional benefit and may be associated with cerebral ischemia and impaired oxygen dissociation from hemoglobin. Positive end-expiratory pressure (PEEP) and ventilatory patterns resulting in high mean airway pressures (a low rate with large tidal volumes) should be avoided because of a potentially adverse effect on ICP by increasing central venous pressure.

Intravenous fluid replacement should be limited to glucose-free isotonic crystalloid (lactated Ringer's or normal saline) or colloid solutions. Hyperglycemia is common in neurosurgical patients (corticosteroid effect) and has been implicated in increasing ischemic brain injury (see Chapter 25). While controversy still surrounds the choice between crystalloid and colloid solutions, large amounts of hypotonic crystalloid solutions clearly can worsen brain edema. Colloid solutions should generally be used to restore intravascular volume deficits, while isotonic crystalloid solutions are used for maintenance fluid requirements. Intraoperative fluid replacement should be below calculated maintenance requirements (see Chapter 29) for patients with severe brain edema or increased ICP. Neurosurgical procedures result in minimal redistributive fluid losses but are often associated with "occult" blood loss (underneath surgical drapes or on the floor). Medical judgment should be used for making decisions on blood transfusions (see Chapter 29).

Emergence

Most patients undergoing craniotomy can be extubated at the end of the procedure as long as neurologic function is intact. Patients left intubated should remain sedated, paralyzed, and hyperventilated. Extubation in the operating room requires special handling during emergence. Straining or bucking on the ETT may precipitate intracranial hemorrhage or worsen cerebral edema. Like induction, emergence must be slow and controlled. As the skin is being closed, attempts should be made to have the patient breath spontaneously. After the head dressing is applied and full access to the patient is regained (the table is turned back to its original position as at induction), anesthetic gases are completely discontinued, and the neuromuscular blocking agent is reversed. Many anesthesiologists give intravenous lidocaine, 1.5 mg/kg, or a small dose of propofol (20–30 mg) or thiopental (25–50 mg) just before suctioning to try to suppress coughing prior to extubation. Rapid awakening facilitates immediate neurologic assessment and can generally be expected following a careful anesthetic. Delayed awakening may be seen following opioid overdose or prolonged administration of the volatile agent. Opioid overdosing is manifested by small pupils and slow respirations (< 12/min). In this circumstance, naloxone can be given in 0.04-mg increments, but it must be titrated carefully because if too much is given, the results can be dangerous. Most patients are taken to the intensive care unit postoperatively for close monitoring of neurologic function. Patients generally have minimal pain.

◼ ANESTHESIA FOR SURGERY IN THE POSTERIOR FOSSA

Craniotomy for a mass in the posterior fossa presents a unique set of potential problems: obstructive hydrocephalus, possible injury to vital brainstem centers, unusual positioning, pneumocephalus, postural hypotension, and **venous air embolism.**

Obstructive Hydrocephalus

Infratentorially located masses can obstruct CSF flow at the level of the fourth ventricle or the cerebral aqueduct. Even small but critically located lesions can markedly increase ICP. In such cases, a ventriculostomy is often performed under local anesthesia to decrease ICP prior to induction of general anesthesia.

Brainstem Injury

Operations in the posterior fossa can injure vital circulatory and respiratory brainstem centers as well as cranial nerves or their nuclei. Such injuries occur as a result of direct surgical trauma, retraction, or ischemia. Damage to respiratory centers is said to be nearly always associated with circulatory changes, so that abrupt changes in blood pressure, heart rate, or rhythm should alert the anesthesiologist to the possibility of such an injury. Communication of such changes to the surgeon is critical. Rarely, isolated damage to respiratory centers without premonitory circulatory signs has occurred during operations in the floor of the fourth ventricle; historically, spontaneous ventilation was used during these procedures to offer an additional monitor of function. At completion of the surgery, brainstem injuries often present as an abnormal respiratory pattern or as an inability to maintain a patent airway following extubation. Monitoring brainstem auditory evoked potentials may be useful in preventing eighth nerve damage during resections of acoustic neuromas. Electromyography is also used to avoid injury to the facial nerve, but the latter requires incomplete muscle paralysis.

Positioning

Although most posterior fossa explorations can be performed with the patient in either a modified lateral or prone position, the sitting position may be preferred by many surgeons. (See chapter 47, Profiles in Anesthetic Practice: The Seated Position—Gone Forever?) Regardless of position, the head is always elevated above the heart. The lateral position is discussed in Chapter 24, while the prone position is discussed below under spinal surgery.

The patient is actually semirecumbent in the standard sitting position (Figure 26–1); the back is elevated to 60 degrees, while the legs are elevated with the knees flexed. The head is fixed in a three-point holder with the neck flexed, while the arms remain at the sides with the hands resting on the lap.

Careful positioning helps avoid injuries. Pressure points such as the elbows, ischial spines, heels, and forehead must be protected. Excessive neck flexion has been

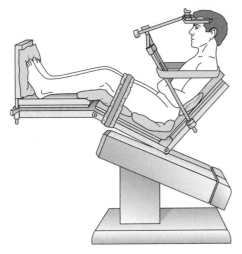

Figure 26-1. The sitting position for craniotomy.

associated with swelling of the upper airway (due to venous obstruction) and, rarely, quadriplegia (due to compression of the cervical spinal cord). Preexisting cervical spinal stenosis probably predisposes patients to the latter injury.

Pneumocephalus

The sitting position increases the likelihood of significant pneumocephalus. In this position, air readily enters the subarachnoid space as CSF is lost during surgery. In patients with cerebral atrophy, CSF drainage is marked; air can replace CSF on the surface of the brain and in the lateral ventricles. Expansion of a pneumocephalus following dural closure can compress the brain. Postoperative pneumocephalus can cause delayed awakening and continued impairment of neurologic function. Because of these concerns, some neuroanesthesiologists advocate not using nitrous oxide for sitting craniotomies (see also below).

Venous Air Embolism

Venous air embolism can occur when the pressure within an open vein is subatmospheric. These conditions may exist in any position (and during any procedure) whenever the wound is above the level of the heart. The incidence of venous air embolism is highest during sitting craniotomies (20–40%). Low pressure in veins and large cerebral venous sinuses increase the risk.

The physiologic consequences of venous air embolism depend on the volume as well as the rate of air entry, and whether the patient has a probe-patent fora-

men ovale (10–25% incidence). The latter is important because it can facilitate passage of air into the arterial circulation (**paradoxical air embolism**). Air bubbles entering the venous system ordinarily lodge in the pulmonary circulation, where their gases eventually diffuse into the alveoli and are exhaled. Small bubbles are well tolerated by most patients. When the amount entrained exceeds the rate of pulmonary clearance, pulmonary artery pressure progressively rises. Eventually, cardiac output decreases in response to increases in right ventricular afterload. Preexisting cardiac or pulmonary disease enhances the effects of venous air embolism; relatively small amounts of air may produce marked hemodynamic changes. Nitrous oxide, by increasing the volume of the entrained air, can markedly accentuate the effects of even small amounts of air. The dose for lethal venous air embolism in animals receiving nitrous oxide anesthesia is one-third to one-half that of control animals. Many clinicians are convinced that nitrous oxide should not be used for surgery on patients in the sitting position. Others continue to use it but in a concentration of 50% instead of 70%, and discontinue it if venous air embolism is detected.

Clinically, signs of venous air embolism are often not apparent until large amounts of air have been entrained. A decrease in end-tidal CO_2 or arterial oxygen saturation might be noticed. Arterial blood gas values may show only slight increases in $PaCO_2$ as a result of increased pulmonary dead space (areas with normal ventilation but decreased perfusion). Major hemodynamic manifestations such as sudden hypotension can occur well before hypoxemia is noted. Moreover, rapid entrainment of large amounts of air can produce sudden circulatory arrest by obstructing right ventricular outflow when intracardiac air impairs tricuspid and pulmonic valve function or blocks pulmonary arterioles.

Paradoxical air embolism can result in a stroke or coronary occlusion, which may only be apparent postoperatively. Paradoxic air emboli are more likely to occur in patients with probe-patent foramen ovale, especially when the normal transatrial (left > right) pressure gradient is reversed. Reversal of this gradient is favored by hypovolemia and perhaps by PEEP. Some studies suggest that a right > left pressure gradient can develop at some time during the cardiac cycle even when the overall mean gradient remains left > right. Transpulmonary passage of venous air into the arterial system has also been demonstrated and suggests that even small bubbles in intravenous infusions should be avoided in all patients.

A. CENTRAL VENOUS CATHETERIZATION:

Central venous access frequently allows aspiration of entrained air. Many clinicians consider right atrial catheterization mandatory for sitting craniotomies. Optimal recovery of air following venous air embolism is provided by a multi-orificed catheter positioned high in the atrium at its junction with the superior vena cava. Confirmation of correct positioning is important and is accomplished by intravascular electrocardiography or by transesophageal echocardiography (TEE). During intravascular electrocardiography, a high atrial position is indicated by appearance of a biphasic P wave. If the catheter is advanced too far, the P wave changes from a negative to a positive deflection, and a right ventricular waveform may also be observed when the pressure is transduced (see Chapter 6).

B. MONITORING FOR VENOUS AIR EMBOLISM:

The most sensitive monitors available should be used. Detecting even small amounts of venous air embolism is important because it allows surgical control of the entry site before additional air is entrained. Currently, the most sensitive intraoperative monitors are TEE and precordial Doppler sonography. These monitors can detect air bubbles as small as 0.25 mL. TEE has the added benefit of detecting the amount of the bubbles and their transatrial passage, as well as evaluating cardiac function. Doppler methods employ a probe over the right atrium (usually to the right of the sternum and between the third and sixth ribs). Interruption of the regular swishing of the Doppler signal by sporadic roaring sounds indicates venous air embolism. Changes in end-tidal respiratory gas concentrations and in pulmonary artery pressure are less sensitive but important monitors that can also detect venous air embolism before overt clinical signs are present. Venous air embolism causes a sudden decrease in end-tidal CO_2 tension in proportion to the increase in pulmonary dead space; unfortunately, such decreases can also be seen with hemodynamic changes unrelated to venous air embolism. A reappearance (or increase) of nitrogen in expired gases may also be seen with venous air embolism. Mean pulmonary artery pressure increases in direct proportion to the amount of air entrained. Changes in blood pressure and heart sounds (mill wheel murmur) are late manifestations of venous air embolism.

C. TREATMENT OF VENOUS AIR EMBOLISM:

1. The surgeon should be notified so that the surgical field can be flooded with saline or packed and bone wax applied to the skull edges until the entry site is identified.
2. Nitrous oxide (if used) should be discontinued and the inhalational agent delivered in 100% oxygen.
3. The central venous catheter should be aspirated in an attempt to retrieve the entrained air.

4. Intravascular volume infusion should be given to increase central venous pressure.
5. Vasopressors should be given to treat hypotension.
6. Bilateral jugular vein compression, by increasing cerebral venous pressure, may slow air entrainment and cause back bleeding, which might help the surgeon identify the source of the embolus.
7. Some authors advocate PEEP in an effort to increase cerebral venous pressure; however, reversal of the normal transatrial pressure gradient may promote paradoxic embolism.
8. If the above measures fail, the patient should be placed in the head-down position and the wound closed quickly.
9. Persistent circulatory arrest necessitates the supine position and institution of resuscitation efforts by cardiac compression.

ANESTHESIA FOR STEREOTACTIC SURGERY

Stereotactic procedures are used for the treatment of involuntary movement disorders, intractable pain, and epilepsy and in the diagnosis and treatment of deeply situated brain tumors.

These procedures are often performed under local anesthesia to allow periodic evaluation of the patient. Propofol infusion may be used for sedation and amnesia. Sedation should be omitted, however, if the patient already has increased ICP. The ability to rapidly provide controlled ventilation and general anesthesia for emergency craniotomy is mandatory but is complicated by the platform and localizing frame that is attached to the patient's head for the procedure. Although mask ventilation or ventilation through a laryngeal mask airway (LMA) or orotracheal intubation might be readily accomplished in an emergency, awake intubation with a fiberoptic bronchoscope may be the safest approach when intubation is necessary for a patient whose head is in a stereotactic head frame (see Chapter 5).

ANESTHESIA FOR HEAD TRAUMA

Head injuries are a contributory factor in up to 50% of deaths due to trauma. Most patients with head trauma are young, and many (10–40%) have associated intra-abdominal injuries, long bone fractures, or both. A general discussion of the trauma patient is found in Chapter 41. The significance of a head injury is dependent not only on the extent of the irreversible neuronal damage at the time of injury but also on the occurrence of any secondary insults. These additional insults include: (1) systemic factors such as hypoxemia, hypercapnia, or hypotension; (2) formation and expansion of an epidural, subdural, or intracerebral hematoma; and (3) sustained intracranial hypertension. Surgical and anesthetic management of these patients is directed at preventing these secondary insults. The **Glasgow Coma Scale (GCS) score** (Table 26–1) generally correlates well with the severity of injury and outcome. A GCS score of 8 or less is associated with approximately 35% mortality. Evidence of more than a 5-mm midline shift, a lesion larger than 25 mL, and ventricular compression on the CT scan are associated with substantially increased morbidity.

Specific lesions include skull fractures, subdural and epidural hematomas, brain concussions and contusions (including intracerebral hemorrhages), penetrating head injuries, and traumatic vascular occlusions and dissections. The presence of a skull fracture greatly increases the likelihood of a significant intracranial lesion. Linear skull fractures are commonly associated with subdural or epidural hematomas. Basilar skull fractures may be associated with CSF rhinorrhea, pneumocephalus, cranial nerve palsies, or even a cavernous

Table 26–1. Glasgow Coma Scale

Category	Score
Eye opening	
Spontaneous	4
To speech	3
To pain	2
Nil	1
Best motor response	
To verbal command	
Obeys	6
To pain	
Localizes	5
Withdraws	4
Decorticate flexion	3
Extensor response	2
Nil	1
Best verbal response	
Oriented	5
Confused conversation	4
Inappropriate words	3
Incomprehensible sounds	2
Nil	1

sinus-carotid artery fistula. Depressed skull fractures often present with an underlying brain contusion. Contusions may be limited to the surface of the brain or may involve hemorrhage in deeper hemispheric structures or the brainstem. Deceleration injuries often produce both coup and contrecoup lesions. Subdural and epidural hematomas can occur as isolated lesions as well as in association with cerebral contusions.

Operative treatment is usually elected for depressed skull fractures, evacuation of epidural, subdural, and some intracerebral hematomas, and debridement of penetrating injuries.

ICP monitoring is usually indicated for patients with significant contusions, intracerebral hemorrhage, or tissue shifts. Intracranial hypertension should be treated with hyperventilation, mannitol, barbiturates, or propofol (see Chapter 25). Studies suggest that sustained increases in ICP greater than 60 mm Hg result in irreversible brain edema. Unlike treatment following spinal cord trauma, the early use of large doses of glucocorticoids does not clearly improve outcome in patients with head trauma. ICP monitoring should also be considered for patients with signs of intracranial hypertension who are undergoing nonneurologic procedures.

PREOPERATIVE MANAGEMENT

Anesthetic care of patients with severe head trauma ideally begins in the emergency department. Measures to ensure the patency of the airway, the adequacy of ventilation and oxygenation, and correction of systemic hypotension should go forward simultaneously with neurologic evaluation. Airway obstruction and hypoventilation are common. Up to 70% of such patients have hypoxemia, which may be complicated by pulmonary contusion, fat emboli, or neurogenic pulmonary edema. The latter is the result of marked systemic and pulmonary hypertension secondary to intense sympathetic nervous system activity. Supplemental oxygen should be given to all patients while the airway and ventilation are evaluated. All patients must be assumed to have a cervical spine injury (up to 10% incidence) until the contrary is proven radiographically. In-line stabilization should be used during airway manipulation to maintain the head in neutral position (see Chapter 41). Patients with obvious hypoventilation, an absent gag reflex, or a persistent total score below 8 on the GCS (Table 26–1) require tracheal intubation and hyperventilation. All other patients should be carefully observed for deterioration.

Intubation

All patients should be regarded as having a full stomach and should have cricoid pressure applied during ventilation and intubation. Following adequate preoxygenation and hyperventilation by mask, the adverse effects of intubation on ICP are blunted by prior administration of thiopental, 2–4 mg/kg or propofol, 1.5–3.0 mg/kg and a short-acting neuromuscular blocking agent. If the patient is hypotensive (systolic blood pressure < 100 mm Hg), either a smaller dose of thiopental or propofol should be used or etomidate or lidocaine should be substituted. The use of succinylcholine in closed head injury is controversial because of its potential for increasing ICP and the rare occurrence of hyperkalemia in these patients; rapacuronium* or mivacurium is a suitable alternative. If a difficult intubation is anticipated, awake intubation, fiberoptic techniques, or tracheostomy may be necessary. Blind nasal intubation is contraindicated in the presence of a basilar skull fracture, which is suggested by CSF rhinorrhea or otorrhea, hemotympanum, or ecchymosis into periorbital tissues (raccoon sign) or behind the ear (Battle's sign).

Hypotension

Hypotension in the setting of head trauma is nearly always related to other associated injuries (usually intra-abdominal). Bleeding from scalp lacerations may be responsible in children. Hypotension may be seen with spinal cord injuries because of the sympathectomy associated with spinal shock. Correction of hypotension and control of any bleeding take precedence over radiographic studies and definitive neurosurgical treatment because systolic arterial blood pressures of less than 80 mm Hg correlate with a poor outcome. Fluid resuscitation with primarily colloid solutions and blood may be more advantageous than crystalloid solutions in preventing brain edema; temporary infusion of a vasopressor (dopamine) is often necessary for severe hypotension. Glucose-containing or hypotonic solutions should not be used (see above). The hematocrit should be maintained above 30%. Invasive monitoring of intra-arterial pressure, central venous or pulmonary artery pressure, and ICP are extremely valuable but should not delay diagnosis and treatment. Dysrhythmias and electrocardiographic abnormalities in the T wave, U wave, ST segment, and QT interval are common following head injuries but are not necessarily associated with cardiac injury; they likely represent altered autonomic function.

Diagnostic Studies

The choice between operative and medical management of head trauma is based on radiographic as well as clinical findings. Patients should be stabilized prior to any CT or angiographic studies. Critically ill patients should be closely monitored during such studies. Restless or uncooperative patients may additionally require general anesthesia. Sedation without control of the airway should generally be avoided because of the risk of further increases in ICP from hypercapnia or hypoxemia. In the event of neurologic deterioration prior to completion of these studies, intravenous mannitol should be considered.

INTRAOPERATIVE MANAGEMENT

Anesthetic management is generally similar to that for other mass lesions associated with intracranial hypertension. Management of the airway is discussed above. Intra-arterial and central venous (or pulmonary artery) pressure monitoring should be established if not already present but should not delay surgical decompression in a rapidly deteriorating patient.

A barbiturate-opioid-nitrous oxide-muscle relaxant technique is commonly used. Nitrous oxide should be avoided when air is entrapped within the cranium and during periods of hypotension. Hypotension may occur after induction of anesthesia as a result of the combined effects of vasodilation and hypovolemia and should be treated with α-adrenergic agents and volume infusion if necessary. Subsequent hypertension is common with surgical stimulation but may also occur with acute ICP elevations. The latter is often associated with bradycardia (Cushing phenomenon).

Hypertension is best treated by additional doses of thiopental, hyperventilation, and administration of an inhalational anesthetic agent. Excessive hyperventilation should be avoided in trauma patients to avoid excessive decreases in CBF. β-Adrenergic blockade is usually effective in controlling hypertension associated with tachycardia. CPP should be maintained between 70 and 110 mm Hg. Vasodilators should be avoided until the dura is opened. Excessive vagal tone should be treated with atropine.

Disseminated intravascular coagulation (DIC) may be seen with severe head injuries. Such injuries cause release of large amounts of brain thromboplastin and may also be associated with the acute respiratory distress syndrome (ARDS) (see Chapter 50). DIC should be diagnosed by coagulation testing and treated with platelets, fresh-frozen plasma, and cryoprecipitate, while ARDS may require mechanical ventilation with PEEP. Pulmonary aspiration and neurogenic pulmonary edema also may be responsible for deteriorating lung function. PEEP should only be applied with ICP monitoring or when the dura is opened. Diabetes insipidus, characterized by copious dilute urine, is frequently seen following injuries to the pituitary stalk.

---

* At the time of publication, rapacuronium had been voluntarily withdrawn by the manufacturer. See Chapter 9 for details.

Other likely causes of polyuria should be excluded and the diagnosis confirmed by measurement of urine and serum osmolality prior to treatment with vasopressin (see Chapter 28). Gastrointestinal hemorrhage may complicate management after several days; it is usually due to stress ulceration.

The decision whether to extubate the trachea at the conclusion of the surgical procedure depends on the severity of the injury, the presence of concomitant abdominal or thoracic injuries, preexisting illnesses, and the preoperative level of consciousness. Young patients who were conscious preoperatively may be extubated following the removal of a localized lesion, whereas patients with diffuse brain injury should be left intubated. Moreover, persistent intracranial hypertension requires continued paralysis, sedation, hyperventilation, and perhaps a pentobarbital infusion postoperatively.

■ ANESTHESIA & CRANIOTOMY FOR INTRACRANIAL ANEURYSMS & ARTERIOVENOUS MALFORMATIONS

Saccular aneurysms and AVMs are common causes of nontraumatic intracranial hemorrhages. Surgical treatment may be undertaken either electively to prevent hemorrhage, or emergently to prevent further complications once hemorrhage has taken place. Other causes of nontraumatic hemorrhage, including hypertensive and spontaneous lobar hemorrhages, are usually treated medically.

CEREBRAL ANEURYSMS

Preoperative Considerations

Cerebral aneurysms typically occur at the bifurcation of the large arteries at the base of the brain; the vast majority are located in the anterior circle of Willis. Approximately 10–30% of patients have more than one aneurysm. The general incidence of saccular aneurysms in some estimates is reported to be 5%, but only a minority of individuals suffer complications. Rupture of a saccular aneurysm is the most common cause of subarachnoid hemorrhage. The acute mortality following rupture is approximately 10%. Of those that survive the initial hemorrhage, about 25% subsequently die within 3 months from delayed complications. Moreover, up to one-half of survivors are left with significant neurologic deficits. As a result, the emphasis in manage-

ment is on prevention of rupture. Although anatomic correlates for the probability of rupture are not established, those larger than 7 mm are usually considered for surgical obliteration. Unfortunately, most patients present only after rupture has already occurred.

Unruptured Aneurysms

Patients often present with prodromal symptoms and signs suggesting progressive enlargement. The most common symptom is headache, and the most common sign is a third-nerve palsy. Other manifestations might include brainstem dysfunction, visual field defects, trigeminal neuralgia, cavernous sinus syndrome, seizures, and hypothalamic-pituitary dysfunction. The most commonly used techniques to diagnose an aneurysm are angiography, MRI angiography, and helical CT angiography. Following diagnosis, patients are brought to the operating room for elective clipping or obliteration of the aneurysm. Most patients are in the 40- to 60-year age group and in otherwise good health.

Ruptured Aneurysms

Ruptured aneurysms usually present acutely as subarachnoid hemorrhage, and less commonly they hemorrhage into the epidural space or the brain. Patients typically complain of a sudden severe headache without focal neurologic deficits, but often associated with nausea and vomiting. Transient loss of consciousness may occur and may result from a sudden rise in ICP and precipitous drop in CPP. If ICP does not decrease rapidly after the initial sudden increase, death usually follows. Large blood clots can cause focal neurologic signs in some patients. Minor bleeding may cause only a mild headache, vomiting, and nuchal rigidity. Unfortunately, even minor bleeding in the subarachnoid space appears to predispose to delayed complications.

Delayed complications include cerebral vasospasm, rerupture, and hydrocephalus. Cerebral vasospasm occurs in 30% of patients (usually after 4–14 days) and is the major cause of morbidity and mortality. The mechanism is unknown but is related to the presence of blood clot around cerebral vessels. Manifestations, which are principally due to cerebral ischemia and infarction, may vary and depend on the severity and distribution of the involved vessels. The calcium channel antagonists nimodipine and nicardipine may be useful in preventing vasospasm, but are usually ineffective once it is established. The only therapy proven useful for symptomatic vasospasm is intravascular volume expansion and induced hypertension (triple H therapy: hypervolemia, hemodilution, and hypertension). Dopamine is usually used to induce mild hypertension because marked hypertension can increase the risk of rebleeding. Glucocorticoids do not reduce cerebral edema following rupture. Cerebral edema should be managed as it is in patients with head trauma; ICP monitoring is often indicated.

Neurosurgical management of patients surviving a ruptured aneurysm is complicated by the risk of rebleeding and vasospasm. The incidence of rerupture is 10–30%. Early surgical obliteration of the aneurysm (within 24–72 hrs) is usually recommended for stable patients because rerupture carries a 60% mortality rate. Emergency surgical intervention is also indicated for neurologic deterioration associated with a subdural or intracerebral hematoma. Acute hydrocephalus requires emergency ventricular drainage, while chronic hydrocephalus requires delayed ventricular shunting.

PREOPERATIVE MANAGEMENT

Preanesthetic evaluation should determine whether rupture has occurred; signs of intracranial hypertension (above) should be sought. Generally, most patients have normal ICP by the time they come for surgery. A small group of patients, however, may have persistent ICP elevation. Hydrocephalus develops in these patients as a result of interference with CSF absorption and is usually evidenced by ventricular enlargement on the CT scan. In addition to neurologic findings, evaluation should include a search for coexisting diseases that may modify the use of elective hypotension intraoperatively. Preexisting hypertension and renal, cardiac, or ischemic cerebrovascular disease are relative contraindications to controlled hypotension. Electrocardiographic abnormalities are commonly seen in patients with subarachnoid hemorrhage but do not necessarily reflect underlying heart disease. Most conscious patients with normal ICP are sedated following rupture to prevent rebleeding; such sedation should be continued until induction of anesthesia. Patients with persistent ICP elevation should receive little or no premedication to avoid hypercapnia.

INTRAOPERATIVE MANAGEMENT

Aneurysm surgery can result in exsanguinating hemorrhage as a consequence of rupture or rebleeding. Blood should be available prior to the start of these operations.

Regardless of the anesthetic technique employed, anesthetic management should focus on preventing rupture (or rebleeding) and avoiding factors that promote cerebral ischemia or vasospasm. Intra-arterial and central venous (or pulmonary artery) pressure monitoring are mandatory. Sudden increases in blood pressure with tracheal intubation or surgical stimulation should be avoided. Judicious intravascular volume loading, guided by the central venous pressure, allows surgical

levels of anesthesia without excessive decreases in blood pressure. Because calcium channel blockers cause systemic vasodilation and reduce systemic vascular resistance, patients receiving these agents preoperatively may be especially prone to hypotension. Hyperventilation is avoided to prevent decreases in CBF, especially in patients with vasospasm.

Once the dura is opened, mannitol is often given to facilitate surgical exposure and reduce tissue trauma from surgical retraction. Rapid decreases in ICP prior to dural opening may promote rebleeding by removing a tamponading effect on the aneurysm.

Elective (controlled) hypotension is useful in aneurysm surgery. Decreasing mean arterial blood pressure reduces the transmural tension across the aneurysm, making rupture (or rebleeding) less likely and facilitating surgical clipping. Controlled hypotension can also decrease blood loss and improve surgical visualization in the event of bleeding. The combination of a slightly head-up position with a volatile anesthetic (isoflurane) enhances the effects of any of the commonly used hypotensive agents (see Chapter 13). Technical improvements in temporary vascular clips have enabled surgeons to use them more often to interrupt blood flow during aneurysm surgery; use of these clips has obviated the need for controlled hypotension and has made normotension or even mild hypertension at least theoretically possible for protecting cerebral perfusion during aneurysm clipping. Thiopental administration and mild hypothermia may protect the brain during periods of prolonged or excessive hypotension or vascular occlusion. Rarely, hypothermic circulatory arrest is used for large basilar artery aneurysms.

Depending on neurologic condition, most patients should be extubated at the end of surgery. Extubation should be handled similarly to other craniotomies (see above). A rapid awakening allows neurologic evaluation in the operating room prior to transfer to the intensive care unit.

ARTERIOVENOUS MALFORMATION

AVMs cause intracerebral hemorrhage more often than subarachnoid hemorrhage. These lesions are developmental abnormalities that result in arteriovenous fistulas; they typically grow in size with time. AVMs may present at any age but bleeding is most common between 10–30 years of age. Other common presentations include headache and seizures. The combination of high blood flow with low vascular resistance can rarely result in high output cardiac failure. When embolization and radiation are not successful or available, surgical excision may be undertaken.

Anesthetic management of patients with AVMs is often complicated by extensive blood loss. Venous access with multiple large-bore cannulas and direct arterial pressure monitoring is necessary. Embolization may be carried out prior to surgery in an attempt to reduce operative blood loss. Hyperventilation and mannitol may be used to facilitate surgical access. Pharmacologic brain protection should be considered for large lesions. Hyperemia and swelling can develop following resection possibly because of altered autoregulation in the remaining normal brain. Blood pressure must therefore be controlled carefully (usually with β-blockers) so as not to aggravate this problem.

ANESTHESIA FOR SURGERY ON THE SPINE

Spinal surgery is most often performed for symptomatic nerve root or cord compression secondary to degenerative disorders. Compression may occur from protrusion of an intervertebral disk or osteophytic bone (spondylosis) into the spinal canal (or an intervertebral foramen). Herniation of an intervertebral disk usually occurs at either the fourth or fifth lumbar or the fifth or sixth cervical levels in patients 30–50 years old. Spondylosis tends to affect the lower cervical spine more than lumbar spine and typically afflicts older patients. Spinal surgery may also be undertaken to correct deformities (scoliosis), decompress the cord, and fuse the spine following spinal trauma or to resect a tumor, a vascular malformation, or an abscess.

PREOPERATIVE MANAGEMENT

Preoperative evaluation should focus on any existing ventilatory impairment and the airway. Anatomic abnormalities and limited neck movements due to disease, traction, or braces complicate airway management and necessitate special techniques (see Chapter 5). Neurologic deficits should be documented. Most patients with degenerative disease have considerable pain preoperatively and should be given an opioid with premedication. Conversely, premedication should be used sparingly in patients with difficult airways or ventilatory impairment.

INTRAOPERATIVE MANAGEMENT

Anesthetic management is complicated primarily by the prone position. Spinal operations involving multiple levels, fusion, and instrumentation are also complicated by the potential for large intraoperative blood losses; a red cell salvage device is often used. Excessive distraction during spinal instrumentation (Harrington rod or pedicle screw fixation) can additionally injure the spinal

cord. A transthoracic approach to the spine requires one-lung ventilation (see Chapter 24).

Positioning

Most surgical procedures are carried out in the prone position. Use of the supine position (with head traction) for an anterior approach to the cervical spine facilitates anesthetic management but may be associated with injuries to the trachea, esophagus, recurrent laryngeal nerve, sympathetic chain, carotid artery, or jugular vein. A sitting or lateral decubitus position may occasionally be used. (See chapter 47, Profiles in Anesthetic Practice: The Seated Position—Gone Forever?)

Following induction of anesthesia and endotracheal intubation in the supine position, the patient is turned prone as a single unit (requiring at least four people). Care must be taken to maintain the neck in neutral position. Once in the prone position, the head may be turned to the side (not exceeding the patient's normal range of motion) or can remain face down on a cushioned holder. Extreme caution is necessary to avoid corneal abrasions or retinal ischemia from pressure on either globe or pressure necrosis of the nose, ears, forehead, breasts (females), or genitalia (males). The chest should rest on parallel rolls (foam) or special supports—if a frame is used—to facilitate ventilation. The arms should be at the sides in a comfortable position with the elbows flexed (avoiding excessive abduction at the shoulder).

Turning the patient prone is a critical maneuver. Monitor disconnects are hard to avoid and are often complicated by hypotension resulting from blunted postural sympathetic reflexes. Abdominal compression, especially in obese patients, may impede venous return and contributes to excessive intraoperative blood loss from engorgement of epidural veins. The use of specially designed frames that allow the abdomen to hang free may alleviate these problems.

Monitoring

When significant blood loss is anticipated or the patient has preexisting cardiac disease, intra-arterial and possibly central venous pressure monitoring should be undertaken prior to "positioning" or "turning." In suitable candidates, elective hypotension or infiltration of the wound with a weak epinephrine solution may decrease intraoperative blood loss. Massive blood loss from aortic or vena caval injury can occur intraoperatively or postoperatively with thoracic or lumbar procedures and is often initially occult.

Instrumentation of the spine requires the ability to intraoperatively detect spinal cord injury from excessive distraction. Intraoperative wake-up techniques, employing balanced or total intravenous anesthesia, allow testing of motor function following distraction. Once preservation of motor function is established, the patient's anesthetic is deepened. Monitoring somatosensory evoked potentials and motor evoked potentials (see Chapter 6) may be alternately used and avoids the problems associated with intraoperative awakening.

CASE DISCUSSION: RESECTION OF A PITUITARY TUMOR

A 41-year-old woman presents to the operating room for resection of a 10-mm pituitary tumor. She had complained of amenorrhea and had started noticing some decrease in visual acuity.

What hormones does the pituitary gland normally secrete?

Functionally and anatomically, the pituitary is divided into two parts: anterior and posterior. The latter is part of the neurohypophysis, which also includes the pituitary stalk and the median eminence.

The anterior pituitary is composed of several cell types, each secreting a specific hormone. Anterior pituitary hormones include adrenocorticotropic hormone (ACTH); thyroid-stimulating hormone (TSH); growth hormone (GH); the gonadotropins, follicle-stimulating hormone (FSH) and luteinizing hormone (LH); and prolactin (PRL). Secretion of each of these hormones is regulated by hypothalamic peptides (releasing hormones) that are transported to the adenohypophysis by a capillary portal system. The secretion of FSH, LH, ACTH, TSH, and their respective releasing hormones is also under negative feedback control by the products of their target organs. For example, an increase in circulating thyroid hormone inhibits the secretion of TSH releasing factor and TSH.

The posterior pituitary secretes antidiuretic hormone (ADH, also called vasopressin) and oxytocin. These hormones are actually formed in supraoptic and paraventricular neurons, respectively, and are transported down axons that terminate in the posterior pituitary. Hypothalamic osmoreceptors and, to a lesser extent, peripheral vascular stretch receptors regulate ADH secretion (see Chapter 28).

What is the function of these hormones?

ACTH stimulates the adrenal cortex to secrete glucocorticoids. Unlike mineralocorticoid production, glucocorticoid production is dependent on ACTH secretion. TSH accelerates the synthesis and release of thyroid hormone (thyroxine). Normal thyroid function is dependent on TSH production.

The gonadotropins FSH and LH are necessary for normal testosterone production and spermatogenesis in males and cyclic ovarian function in females. GH promotes tissue growth and increases protein synthesis as well as fatty acid mobilization. Its effects on carbohydrate metabolism are to decrease cellular glucose uptake and utilization and increase insulin secretion. PRL functions to support breast development during pregnancy. Dopamine receptor antagonists are known to increase PRL secretion.

Through its effect on water permeability in renal collecting ducts, ADH regulates extracellular osmolarity and blood volume (see Chapter 28). Oxytocin acts on areolar myoepithelial cells as part of the milk letdown reflex during suckling and enhances uterine activity during labor.

What factors will determine the surgical approach in this patient?

The pituitary gland is attached to the brain by a stalk and extends downward to lie in the sella turcica of the sphenoid bone. Anteriorly, posteriorly, and inferiorly, it is bordered by bone. Laterally it is bordered by the cavernous sinus, which contains cranial nerves III, IV, V_1, and VI as well as the cavernous portion of the carotid artery. Superiorly, the diaphragma sella, a thick dural reflection, usually tightly encircles the stalk and forms the roof of the sella turcica. In close proximity to the stalk lie the optic nerves and chiasm. In continuity and superior to the stalk lies the hypothalamus.

Tumors under 10 mm in diameter are usually approached via the transsphenoidal route, whereas tumors larger than 20 mm in diameter and with significant suprasellar extension are approached via a bifrontal craniotomy. With use of prophylactic antibiotics, morbidity and mortality rates are significantly less with the transsphenoidal approach; the operation is carried out with the aid of a microscope through an incision in the gingival mucosa beneath the upper lip. The surgeon enters the nasal cavity, dissects through the nasal septum, and finally penetrates the roof of the sphenoid sinus to enter the floor of the sella turcica.

What are the major problems associated with the transsphenoidal approach?

Problems include: (1) the need for mucosal injections of epinephrine-containing solution to reduce bleeding, (2) the accumulation of blood and tissue debris in the pharynx and stomach, (3) the risks of hemorrhage from inadvertent entry into the cavernous sinus or the internal carotid artery, (4) cranial nerve damage, and (5) pituitary hypo-

function. Prophylactic glucocorticoid administration is routinely used in most centers. Diabetes insipidus (see Chapter 29) develops postoperatively in up to 40% of patients but is usually transient. Less commonly, the diabetes insipidus presents intraoperatively. The supine and slightly head-up position used for this procedure may also predispose to venous air embolism.

What type of tumor does this patient have?

Tumors in or around the sella turcica account for 10–15% of intracranial neoplasms. Pituitary adenomas are most common, followed by craniopharyngiomas and then parasellar meningiomas. Primary malignant pituitary and metastatic tumors are rare. Pituitary tumors that secrete hormones (functional tumors) usually present early when they are still relatively small (< 10 mm). Other tumors present late with signs of increased ICP (headache, nausea and vomiting) or compression of contiguous structures (visual disturbances or pituitary hypofunction). Compression of the optic chiasm classically results in bitemporal hemianopia. Compression of normal pituitary tissue produces progressive endocrine dysfunction. Failure of hormonal secretion usually progresses in the order of gonadotropins, GH, ACTH, and TSH. Diabetes insipidus can also be seen preoperatively. Rarely, hemorrhage into the pituitary results in acute panhypopituitarism (pituitary apoplexy) with signs of a rapidly expanding mass, hemodynamic instability, and hypoglycemia.

This patient has the most common type of secretory adenoma—that producing hyperprolactinemia. Women with this tumor typically have amenorrhea, galactorrhea, or both. Men with prolactin-secreting adenomas may have galactorrhea or infertility but more commonly present with symptoms of an expanding mass.

What other types of secretory hormones are seen?

Adenomas secreting ACTH (Cushing's disease) produce classic manifestations of Cushing's syndrome: truncal obesity, moon facies, abdominal striae, proximal muscle weakness, hypertension, and osteoporosis (see Chapter 36). Glucose tolerance is typically impaired, but frank diabetes is less common (< 20%). Hirsutism, acne, and amenorrhea are also commonly seen in women.

Adenomas that secrete GH are often large and result in either gigantism (prepubertal patients) or acromegaly (adults). Excessive growth prior to epiphyseal fusion results in massive growth of the entire skeleton. After epiphyseal closure, the abnormal growth is limited to soft tissues and acral parts: hands, feet, nose, and mandible. Patients develop osteoarthritis, which often affects the temporomandibular joint and spine. Diabetes, myopathies, and neuropathies are common. Cardiovascular complications include hypertension, premature coronary disease, and cardiomyopathy in some patients. The most serious anesthetic problem encountered in these patients is difficulty in intubating the trachea.

Are any special monitors required for transsphenoidal surgery?

Monitoring should be carried out in somewhat the same way as for craniotomies. Visual evoked potentials may be employed with large tumors that involve the optic nerves. A precordial Doppler may be used for detecting venous air embolism. Venous access with large-bore catheters is desirable in the event of massive hemorrhage.

What modifications, if any, are necessary in the anesthetic technique?

The same principles discussed for craniotomies apply, especially if the patient has evidence of increased ICP. Intravenous antibiotic prophylaxis and glucocorticoid coverage (hydrocortisone, 100 mg) are usually given prior to induction. Many clinicians avoid nitrous oxide to prevent problems with a postoperative pneumocephalus (see above). Intense muscle paralysis is important to prevent movement while the surgeon is using the microscope. In some circumstances, the surgeon may request placement of a lumbar intrathecal catheter to drain CSF, thereby facilitating surgical exposure. The management of diabetes insipidus is discussed in Chapter 28.

SUGGESTED READING

Albin M: *Textbook of Neuroanesthesia with Neurosurgical and Neuroscience Perspectives.* McGraw-Hill, 1997.

Cottrell JE, Smith DS: *Anesthesia and Neurosurgery,* 3rd ed. Mosby Year Book, 1994.

Cucchiara RF, Black S, Michenfelder JD: *Clinical Neuroanesthesia,* 2nd ed. Churchill Livingstone, 1998.

Newfield P, Cottrell JE: *Handbook of Neuroanesthesia,* 3rd ed. Lippincott Williams & Wilkins, 1999.

Schubert A: *Clinical Neuroanesthesia.* Butterworth-Heinemann, 1997.

Stone DJ, Sperry RJ: *The Neuroanesthesia Handbook.* Mosby, 1996.

Walters FJM, Ingram GS, Jenkinson JL: *Anaesthesia and Intensive Care for the Neurosurgical Patient.* Blackwell, 1994.

Anesthesia for Patients With Neurologic & Psychiatric Diseases

27

KEY CONCEPTS

1 An asymptomatic cervical bruit does not appear to increase the risk of stroke following surgery but increases the likelihood of coexisting coronary artery disease.

2 Resistance to neuromuscular blockade—as assessed by train-of-four monitoring—may be observed in paretic extremities; neuromuscular blockade should therefore be monitored on the nonparetic side. Succinylcholine should be avoided in patients with a history of recent stroke as well as in those with extensive muscle wasting because of the risks of hyperkalemia.

3 If a seizure occurs, maintaining an open airway and adequate oxygenation take first priority. Intravenous thiopental (50–100 mg), phenytoin (500–1000 mg slowly), or diazepam (5–10 mg) can be used to terminate the seizure.

4 Induction of anesthesia in patients receiving long-term levodopa therapy (such as those patients with Parkinson's disease) may result in either marked hypotension or hypertension.

5 Increases in body temperature cause exacerbation of multiple sclerosis symptoms, presumably by decreasing nerve conduction.

6 The major risk in patients with autonomic dysfunction is severe hypotension, compromising cerebral and coronary blood flow.

7 Patients with high transections of the spinal cord often have impaired airway reflexes and are further predisposed to hypoxemia by a decrease in functional residual capacity. Hypotension and bradycardia are often present prior to induction.

8 Autonomic hyperreflexia should be expected in patients with lesions above T6 and can be precipitated by surgical manipulations.

9 During anesthesia, the most important interaction with tricyclic antidepressants is an exaggerated response to both indirect-acting vasopressors and sympathetic stimulation.

10 Opioids should generally be used with caution in patients receiving monoamine oxidase inhibitors, since rare but serious reactions to opioids have been reported. Most serious reactions are associated with meperidine, resulting in hyperthermia, seizures, and coma.

Cerebrovascular disease is a major cause of morbidity and death. Patients with a history of stroke, transient ischemic attacks (TIAs), or asymptomatic extracranial vascular obstructions frequently present to the operating room for unrelated procedures. This chapter discusses a general approach to these patients as well as patients with other common neurologic disorders. Chapter 21 discusses anesthetic management of patients undergoing carotid artery surgery.

Nonvascular neurologic diseases and psychiatric disorders are less frequently encountered in surgical patients and are often overlooked. Fortunately, unless increased intracranial pressure (ICP) is present, special anesthetic techniques are not usually required. Nonetheless, the anesthesiologist must have a basic understanding of the major neurologic and psychiatric disorders and their drug therapy; failure to recognize potentially adverse anesthetic interactions may result in avoidable perioperative morbidity.

CEREBROVASCULAR DISEASE

Preoperative Considerations

The incidence of significant cerebrovascular disease in surgical patients is unknown but probably increases with age. Patients with known cerebrovascular disease typically have a history of **TIAs** or **stroke.** Asymptomatic cervical bruits occur in up to 4% of patients over age 40 but do not necessarily indicate significant carotid artery obstruction. Fewer than 10% of patients with completely asymptomatic bruits have hemodynamically significant carotid artery lesions. Moreover, the absence of a bruit does not exclude significant carotid obstruction.

The risk of postoperative stroke increases with patient age and varies with the type of surgery. The overall risk of stroke following nonneurologic surgery is low, but it is higher in patients undergoing cardiovascular surgery. Rates of stroke after general anesthesia and surgery range from 0.08 to 0.4%. Even in patients with known cerebrovascular disease, the risk is only 0.4–3.3%. An asymptomatic cervical bruit does not appear to increase the risk of stroke following surgery but may increase the likelihood of coexisting coronary artery disease (see Chapter 20). Patients undergoing open heart procedures for valvular disease are at highest risk for postoperative stroke (incidence of about 4%), as are patients undergoing operations on the thoracic aorta. The mortality rate following postoperative stroke may be as high as 26%. Strokes following open heart surgery are usually due to emboli of air, fibrin, or calcium debris. The pathophysiology of postoperative strokes following noncardiac surgery is less clear but may involve severe sustained hypotension or hypertension. Hypotension with severe hypoperfusion can result in intracerebral thrombosis and infarction, while hypertension can result in hemorrhage into a carotid plaque or intracerebral hemorrhage (hemorrhagic stroke); sustained hypertension can also disrupt the blood-brain barrier and promote cerebral edema (see Chapter 25). The period of time after which a patient may be safely anesthetized following a stroke has not been determined. Abnormalities in regional blood flow and metabolic rate usually

resolve after 2 weeks while alterations in CO_2 responsiveness and blood brain barrier may require more than four weeks. Most clinicians postpone elective procedures a minimum of 6–26 weeks following a completed stroke.

Patients with TIAs have a history of transient (< 24 hours) impairment and by definition have no residual neurologic impairment (see Chapter 21). These attacks are thought to result from emboli of fibrin-platelet aggregates or atheromatous debris from plaques in extracranial vessels. Unilateral visual impairment, numbness or weakness of an extremity, or aphasia is suggestive of carotid disease, while bilateral visual impairment, dizziness, ataxia, dysarthria, bilateral weakness, or amnesia is suggestive of vertebral-basilar disease. Patients with TIAs have a 30–40% chance of developing a thrombotic stroke within 5 years; most (50%) occur within the first year. Patients with TIAs should not undergo any elective surgical procedure without an adequate medical evaluation that generally includes at least noninvasive (Doppler) flow and imaging studies. The presence of an ulcerative plaque of greater than 60% occlusion is generally an indication for carotid endarterectomy (see Chapter 21).

PREOPERATIVE MANAGEMENT

Preoperative assessment requires careful neurologic and cardiovascular evaluations. The type of stroke, the presence of neurologic deficits, and the extent of residual impairment should be determined. **Thrombotic strokes** are most common and usually occur in patients with generalized atherosclerosis. Most patients are elderly and have comorbid conditions such as hypertension, hyperlipidemia, and diabetes. Coexisting coronary artery disease and renal impairment are common. **Embolic strokes** are most often associated with mitral valve disease or endocarditis or follow valve replacement. **Hemorrhagic strokes** are typically due to accelerated hypertension, rupture of a cerebral aneurysm, or an arteriovenous malformation. Many patients, following nonhemorrhagic strokes or TIAs, are placed on long-term warfarin or antiplatelet therapy. The risk of stopping such therapy perioperatively for a few days appears small. Clotting studies and a bleeding time should be used to confirm reversal of their effect prior to operation. Once surgical hemostasis has been achieved (12–48 hours), anticoagulants or aspirin may be resumed postoperatively.

Regardless of the procedure or the type of anesthetic to be administered, hypertension, angina, congestive heart failure, and hyperglycemia should be under good control preoperatively. With the exception of diuretics and insulin, all patients should receive their usual medications up to the time of surgery. The management of diabetes is discussed in Chapter 36.

INTRAOPERATIVE MANAGEMENT

Although some clinicians feel that regional anesthesia may be safer than general anesthesia for these patients, supporting studies are lacking. No one general anesthesia technique is clearly superior to another. Blood pressure should be maintained at or slightly higher than normal levels because of a rightward shift in cerebral autoregulation (Figure 27–1) (see Chapter 25). Vasopressors should not be relied upon to maintain blood pressure, as their overuse can precipitate myocardial ischemia (see Chapter 20). Vasodilators or adrenergic blockade may be necessary during periods of intense stimulation and during emergence. Use of a neuromuscular blocking agent (also called muscle relaxant) facilitates anesthetic management by providing optimal surgical conditions yet allowing appropriate adjustments in anesthetic depth. Wide swings in blood pressure are undesirable and may contribute to postoperative cardiac and cerebral complications.

The use of a paretic or paralyzed extremity for monitoring neuromuscular blockade can result in overdosage. Resistance to neuromuscular blockade—as assessed by train-of-four monitoring—may be observed in paretic extremities; neuromuscular blockade should therefore be monitored on the nonparetic side. Succinylcholine should be avoided in patients with a history of recent stroke as well as in those with extensive muscle wasting because of the risks of hyperkalemia.

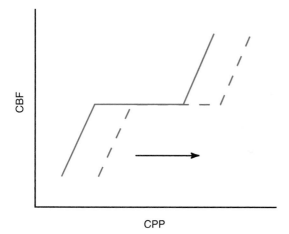

Figure 27–1. Rightward shift in cerebral blood flow (CBF) seen in patients with chronic hypertension. CPP = cerebral perfusion pressure.

Table 27–1. Classification of seizures.

Partial (focal)
    Simple
    Complex
    Partial evolving into generalized
Generalized
    Absence (petit mal)
    Myoclonic
    Clonic
    Tonic
    Tonic-clonic (grand mal)
    Atonic
    Unclassified

■ SEIZURE DISORDERS

Preoperative Considerations

Seizures represent abnormal synchronized electrical activity in the brain. They may be a manifestation of an underlying central nervous system disease, a systemic disorder, or may be idiopathic. Mechanisms are thought to include: (1) loss of inhibitory γ-aminobutyric acid (GABA) activity, (2) enhanced release of excitatory amino acids (glutamate), and (3) enhanced neuronal firing due to abnormal voltage-mediated calcium currents. Up to 2% of the population may experience a seizure in their lifetime. Epilepsy is a disorder characterized by recurrent paroxysmal seizure activity. Healthy individuals who experience an isolated nonrecurrent seizure are not considered to have epilepsy.

Seizure activity may be localized to a specific area in the brain or may be generalized. Moreover, initially localized (focal) seizures can subsequently spread, becoming generalized. A simple classification scheme is presented in Table 27–1. **Partial seizures** (also called **focal**) are clinically manifested by motor, sensory, autonomic, or psychic symptoms depending on the cortical area affected. Focal seizures associated with impairment in consciousness are termed "complex partial" (psychomotor or temporal lobe) seizures. **Generalized seizures** characteristically produce bilaterally symmetric electrical activity without local onset. They result in abnormal motor activity, loss of consciousness, or both. Generalized activity resulting in isolated and transient lapses in consciousness are called **absence (petit mal) seizures.** Other generalized seizures are usually classified according to the type of motor activity. **Tonic-clonic (grand mal) seizures** are most common and are characterized by a loss of consciousness followed by clonic and then tonic motor activity.

PREOPERATIVE MANAGEMENT

Preoperative evaluation of patients with a seizure disorder should focus on determining the cause and type of seizure activity and with what drugs the patient is being treated. Seizures in adults are most commonly due to structural brain lesions (head trauma, tumor, degeneration, or stroke) or metabolic abnormalities (uremia, hepatic failure, hypoglycemia, hypocalcemia, or drug toxicity or withdrawal). Idiopathic seizures occur most often in children but may persist into adulthood. Anesthetic evaluation should focus primarily on the underlying disorder and secondarily on the seizures. Management of patients with a mass lesion or increased ICP is discussed in Chapter 26.

Characterization of the type of seizure is important in detecting such activity perioperatively. Seizures—particularly grand mal seizures—are serious complicating factors in surgical patients and should be treated aggressively to prevent musculoskeletal injury, hypoventilation, hypoxemia, and aspiration of gastrointestinal content. Even partial seizures can progress to grand mal seizures. If a seizure occurs, maintaining an open airway and adequate oxygenation take first priority. Intravenous thiopental (50–100 mg), phenytoin (500–1000 mg slowly), or diazepam (5–10 mg) can be used to terminate the seizure.

Most patients with seizure disorders have been receiving antiepileptic drugs ([AEDs] anticonvulsants) preoperatively (Table 27–2). Drug therapy should be reviewed for efficacy and toxicity. Phenytoin, carbamazepine, and valproate are used for generalized tonic-clonic seizures. Phenytoin and valproate are often used for partial seizures. Adverse side effects and signs of toxicity should be excluded clinically and by laboratory investigations. Carbamazepine, ethosuximide, felbamate, and valprolate may cause bone marrow depression and hepatotoxicity. At toxic levels, most agents cause ataxia, dizziness, confusion, and sedation. Blood levels of AEDs are usually readily available from the hospital laboratory and should be checked in patients with signs of toxicity and those who give a history of recent seizures. AEDs should ideally be continued throughout the perioperative period to maintain therapeutic levels. Fortunately, most agents have a relatively long half-life, so that a delayed or even a missed dose is often not critical.

INTRAOPERATIVE MANAGEMENT

In selecting anesthetic agents, drugs with possible epileptogenic potential should be avoided. Ketamine and methohexital (in small doses) theoretically can precipitate seizure activity and should be avoided. Theoretically, large doses of atracurium or cisatracurium or meperidine may be contraindicated because of the reported epileptogenic potential of their metabolites, laudanosine and normeperidine, respectively. Hepatic microsomal enzyme induction should be expected from chronic AED therapy. Enzyme induction may increase dose requirement and frequency for intravenous anesthetics and nondepolarizing neuromuscular blocking agents and may increase the potential for hepatotoxicity from halothane. The use of enflurane in patients with a seizure disorder is questionable. Enflurane in high concentrations (> 2.5%) and in association with concomitant hypocapnia can precipitate electroencephalographic spike-and-wave patterns resembling seizures even in normal individuals.

Table 27–2. Commonly used anticonvulsants and their dose.

Drug	Daily Dose[1] (mg)
Carbamazepine	800–1600
Felbamate	2400–3600
Gabapentin	900–3600
Lamotrigine	300–500
Phenytoin	300–400
Tiagabine	32–56
Topiramate	200–400
Valproate	1000–3000

[1]Usual total daily dose for adults. (Reprinted with permission from: Samuels MA, Ann Intern Med 1998;129:878–885.)

■ DEGENERATIVE & DEMYELINATING DISEASES

PARKINSON'S DISEASE

Preoperative Considerations

Parkinson's disease typically afflicts patients 50–70 years of age. Also known as **paralysis agitans,** this slowly progressive disease is characterized by cogwheel rigidity, a resting (pill-rolling) tremor, a fixed facial expression, and festination gait. Increasing problems with rigidity and tremor eventually result in physical incapacitation, but intellectual function is usually preserved early in the disease. The disease appears to be related to progressive loss of dopamine in the nigrostriaum with an associated increase in activity of the GABA nuclei in the basal ganglia. The increase in GABA output from the basal ganglia inhibits thalamic and brainstem nuclei. Thalamic inhibition suppresses the motor system in the cortex leading to akinesia, rigidity, and tremor.

Treatment is directed at controlling the symptoms. Anticholinergics may be used for mild disease to control the resting tremor; these agents include amantadine and selegiline. Levodopa (a precursor of dopamine) is the most effective therapy and is used for moderate to severe symptoms (akinesia and postural imbalance). Levodopa is used because dopamine does not cross the blood-brain barrier. Side effects include nausea, vomiting, dyskinesia, cardiac irritability, and orthostatic hypotension. The latter may be due to catecholamine depletion (chronic negative feedback inhibition) and volume depletion perhaps secondary to a natriuretic effect. Preparations combining levodopa with a dopa decarboxylase inhibitor (carbidopa; Sinemet) increase central delivery and allow the use of smaller doses. Bromocriptine (Parlodel) or pergolide (Permax), both dopamine agonists, may also be used with benefit in some patients.

Anesthetic Considerations

Medication for Parkinson's disease should be continued perioperatively, including the morning of surgery, because the half-life of levodopa is short. Abrupt withdrawal of levodopa can cause worsening of muscle rigidity and may interfere with ventilation. Phenothiazines, butyrophenones (droperidol), and metoclopramide can exacerbate symptoms as a consequence of their antidopaminergic activity and should be avoided. Anticholinergics (atropine) or antihistamines (diphenhydramine) may be used for acute exacerbation of symptoms. Diphenhydramine is especially valuable for premedication and intraoperative sedation in patients 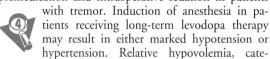 with tremor. Induction of anesthesia in patients receiving long-term levodopa therapy may result in either marked hypotension or hypertension. Relative hypovolemia, catecholamine depletion, autonomic instability, and sensitization to catecholamines are probably contributory. Arterial blood pressure should be monitored carefully. Significant hypotension should be treated with small doses of a direct-acting vasopressor such as phenylephrine. Cardiac irritability readily produces arrhythmias, so halothane, ketamine, and local anesthetic solutions containing epinephrine should be used cautiously if at all. Although the response to neuromuscular blocking agents is generally normal, a rare occurrence of hyperkalemia following succinylcholine has been reported. Adequacy of ventilation and airway reflexes should be carefully assessed prior to extubation of patients with moderate to severe disease.

ALZHEIMER'S DISEASE

Preoperative Considerations

The prevalence of Alzheimer's disease (AD) increases with age to as high as 20% in patients over 80. The disease is characterized by a slow decline in intellectual function (**dementia**). Loss of recent memory, depression, and emotional lability are common early—but often subtle—manifestations. Late in the course of the disease, severe extrapyramidal signs, apraxias, and aphasia are often present. Although some degree of brain atrophy is normal with advancing age, patients with AD usually show marked cortical atrophy with ventricular enlargement; the pathologic hallmarks of AD include neurofibrillary tangles, neuritic plaques, and neuronal thread protein.

In the absence of an effective cure, treatment is aimed at preventing further deterioration, and if not possible, slowing the rate of deterioration and treating symptoms. The cholinesterase inhibitors include tacrine, donepezil, and rivastigmine.

Anesthetic Considerations

Anesthetic management of patients with moderate to severe disease is often complicated by disorientation and uncooperativeness. Such patients require repeated reassurance and explanation. Consent must be obtained from the next of kin or a legal guardian if the patient is incapacitated. Because the use of centrally acting drugs must be minimized, premedication is usually not given. Regional anesthesia should be attempted only if the patient is cooperative. Inhalational agents may be preferable for general anesthesia because of their rapid elimination. Centrally acting anticholinergics, such as atropine and scopolamine, could theoretically contribute to postoperative confusion. Glycopyrrolate, which does not cross the blood-brain barrier, may be the preferred agent when an anticholinergic is required.

MULTIPLE SCLEROSIS

Preoperative Considerations

Multiple sclerosis is characterized by reversible demyelination at random and multiple sites in the brain and spinal cord; chronic inflammation, however, eventually produces scarring (gliosis). The disease may be an autoimmune disorder that is initiated by a viral infection. It primarily affects patients between 20 and 40 years of age with a 2:1 female predominance and typically follows an unpredictable course of frequent attacks and remissions. With time, remissions become less complete, and the disease is progressive and incapacitating; almost

50% of patients will require help with walking within 15 years of diagnosis. Clinical manifestations depend on the sites affected but frequently include sensory disturbances (paresthesias), visual problems (optic neuritis and diplopia), and motor weakness. Symptoms develop over the course of days and remit over weeks to months. Early diagnosis of exacerbations can often be confirmed by cerebrospinal fluid analysis and magnetic resonance imaging. Remyelination is limited and often fails to occur. Moreover, axonal loss can develop. Changes in neurologic function appear to be related to changes in axonal conduction. Conduction can occur across demyelinated axons but appears to be affected by multiple factors, especially temperature. Increases in body temperature cause exacerbation of symptoms, presumably by decreasing nerve conduction.

Treatment of multiple sclerosis may be primarily symptomatic or may attempt to arrest the disease process. Diazepam, dantrolene, or baclofen is used to control spasticity; bethanechol is useful for urinary retention. Painful dysesthesia may respond to carbamazepine, phenytoin, or antidepressants (see Chapter 18). ACTH (adrenocorticotropic hormone) or glucocorticoids may lessen the severity and duration of acute attacks. Interferon β-1b, interferon β-1a, and glatiramer acetate reduce the frequency of relapse by up to 30%. Immunosuppression with azathioprine or cyclophosphamide may also be attempted to halt disease progression.

Anesthetic Considerations

The effect of stress, anesthesia, and surgery on the course of the disease is controversial. A detrimental effect has been suggested but not substantiated. Overall, the effect of anesthesia is unpredictable. Elective surgery should be avoided during relapse regardless of the anesthetic technique employed. The preoperative consent record should document counseling of the patient to the effect that the stress of surgery and anesthesia might worsen the symptoms. Spinal anesthesia has been reported to cause exacerbation of the disease. Epidural and other regional techniques appear to have no adverse effect, especially in obstetrics. No specific interactions with general anesthetics are generally recognized. Patients with advanced disease may have a labile cardiovascular system due to autonomic dysfunction. In the setting of paresis or paralysis, succinylcholine should be avoided because of hyperkalemia. Regardless of the anesthetic technique employed, increases in body temperatures should be avoided. Demyelinated fibers are extremely sensitive to increases in temperature; an increase of as little as 0.5 °C may completely block conduction.

AMYOTROPHIC LATERAL SCLEROSIS

Amyotrophic lateral sclerosis (ALS) is the most common progressive disease of motor neurons. It is a rapidly progressive disorder of both upper and lower motor neurons. Clinically, patients present in the fifth or sixth decade of life with muscular weakness, atrophy, fasciculation, and spasticity. The disease may initially be asymmetric but over the course of 2–3 years becomes generalized, involving all skeletal and bulbar muscles. Progressive respiratory muscle weakness makes the patient susceptible to aspiration and eventually leads to death from ventilatory failure. Although the heart is unaffected, autonomic dysfunction can be seen. There is no specific treatment for ALS.

The primary emphasis in management is judicious respiratory care. As with other patients with lower motor neuron disease, succinylcholine is contraindicated because of the risk of hyperkalemia. Nondepolarizing neuromuscular blocking agents should be used sparingly, because patients often display enhanced sensitivity. Adequacy of ventilation should be carefully assessed both intraoperatively and postoperatively; an awake extubation is desirable. Difficulty in weaning patients off mechanical ventilation postoperatively is not uncommon in patients with moderate to advanced disease.

GUILLAIN-BARRÉ SYNDROME

Also known as **acute demyelinating polyneuropathy,** this disorder is characterized by a sudden onset of ascending motor paralysis, areflexia, and variable paresthesias. Bulbar involvement, including respiratory muscle paralysis, is a frequent complication. Pathologically, the disease appears to be an immunologic reaction against the myelin sheath of peripheral nerves, especially lower motor neurons. In most instances, the syndrome appears to follow viral respiratory or gastrointestinal infections; the disorder can also present as a paraneoplastic syndrome associated with Hodgkin's disease, or as a complication of human immunodeficiency virus (HIV) infection. Some patients respond to plasmapheresis. The prognosis is good, with most patients recovering completely.

In addition to the respiratory complications, anesthetic management is complicated by lability of the autonomic nervous system. Exaggerated hypotensive and hypertensive responses during anesthesia may be seen. As with other lower motor neuron disorders, succinylcholine should not be used because of the risk of hyperkalemia. The use of regional anesthesia in these patients remains controversial.

AUTONOMIC DYSFUNCTION

Preoperative Considerations

Autonomic dysfunction, or dysautonomia, may be due to generalized or segmental disorders of the central or peripheral nervous system. Symptoms can be generalized, segmental, or focal. These disorders may be congenital, familial, or acquired. Common manifestations include impotence; bladder and gastrointestinal dysfunction; abnormal regulation of body fluids; decreased sweating, lacrimation and salivation; and orthostatic hypotension. The latter is often the most serious manifestation of the dysfunction.

Acquired autonomic dysfunction can be isolated (pure autonomic failure), part of a more generalized degenerative process (Shy-Drager syndrome, Parkinson's disease, olivopontocerebellar atrophy), part of a segmental neurologic process (multiple sclerosis, syringomyelia, reflex sympathetic dystrophy, or spinal cord injury), or a manifestation of disorders affecting peripheral nerves (Guillain-Barré syndrome, diabetes, chronic alcoholism, amyloidosis, or porphyria). Treatment includes increasing salt intake, sleeping in a reverse Trendelenburg position (to minimize nocturnal diuresis and supine hypertension), and various drug therapies. The latter may include a mineralocorticoid (fludrocortisone–Florinef), prostaglandin inhibitor (ibuprofen), β-adrenergic blocker, sympathomimetic, or a dopamine antagonist (metoclopramide). The vasopressin analog desmopressin (DDAVP) or the somatostatin analog octreotide (Sandostatin) may also be tried.

Congenital or familial dysautonomia occurs most frequently in Ashkenazi Jewish children and is usually referred to as Riley-Day syndrome. Autonomic dysfunction is prominent and is associated with generalized diminished sensation and emotional lability. Moreover, patients are predisposed to dysautonomic crises triggered by stress and characterized by marked hypertension, tachycardia, abdominal pain, diaphoresis, and vomiting. Intravenous diazepam is effective in resolving such episodes. Hereditary dysautonomia associated with a deficiency of dopamine β-hydroxylase is described. Administration of α-dihydroxyphenylserine (α-DOPS) improves symptoms in these patients.

Anesthetic Considerations

The major risk in patients with autonomic dysfunction is severe hypotension, compromising cerebral and coronary blood flow. Marked hypertension can be equally deleterious. Most patients are chronically hypovolemic. The vasodilatory effects of spinal and epidural anesthesia are poorly tolerated. Similarly, the vasodilatory and cardiac depressant effects of most general anesthetic agents combined with positive airway pressure can be equally deleterious. Continuous intra-arterial blood pressure monitoring is desirable. Hypotension should be treated with fluids and direct-acting vasopressors. The latter are preferable to indirect-acting agents. Enhanced sensitivity to vasopressors due to denervation sensitivity may be observed. Blood loss also is usually poorly tolerated; central venous or pulmonary artery catheterization is invaluable when significant fluid shifts are expected. Body temperature should be monitored closely. Patients with anhidrosis are especially susceptible to hyperpyrexia.

SYRINGOMYELIA

Syringomyelia results in progressive cavitation of the spinal cord. In many cases, obstruction of cerebrospinal fluid outflow from the fourth ventricle appears to be contributory. Many patients have craniovertebral abnormalities, especially the **Arnold-Chiari malformation.** Increased pressure in the central canal of the spinal cord produces enlargement or diverticulation to the point of cavitation. Syringomyelia typically affects the cervical spine, producing sensory and motor deficits in the upper extremities and, frequently, thoracic scoliosis. Extension upward into the medulla (**syringobulbia**) leads to cranial nerve deficits. Ventricular-peritoneal shunting and other decompressive procedures have variable success in arresting the disease.

Anesthetic evaluation should focus on defining existing neurologic deficits as well as any pulmonary impairment due to scoliosis. Pulmonary function testing and arterial blood gas analysis may be useful. Autonomic instability should be expected in patients with extensive lesions. Succinylcholine should be avoided when muscle wasting is present because of the risk of hyperkalemia. Adequacy of ventilation and reversal of nondepolarizing neuromuscular blocking agents should be achieved prior to extubation.

■ SPINAL CORD INJURY

Preoperative Considerations

Most spinal cord injuries are traumatic and often result in partial or complete transection. The majority of injuries are due to fracture and dislocation of the vertebral column. The mechanism is usually either compression and flexion at the thoracic spine or extension at the cervical spine. Clinical manifestations depend on the level of the transection. Injuries above C3–5 (diaphragmatic innervation) require patients to receive ventilatory support to stay alive. Transections above T1 result in quadriplegia, while those above L4 result in paraplegia. The most common sites of transection are C5–6 and T12–L1. Acute spinal cord transection produces loss of sensation, flaccid paralysis, and loss of spinal reflexes below the level of injury. These findings characterize a period of **spinal shock** that typically lasts 1–3 weeks.

Over the course of the next few weeks, spinal reflexes gradually return, together with muscle spasms and signs of sympathetic overactivity. Compression in the low thoracic or lumbar spine results in **cauda equina (conus medullaris) syndrome.** The latter usually consists of incomplete injury to nerve roots rather than the spinal cord.

Overactivity of the sympathetic nervous system is common with transections at T5 or above, but is unusual with injuries below T10. Interruption of normal descending inhibitory impulses in the cord results in **autonomic hyperreflexia.** Cutaneous or visceral stimulation below the level of injury can induce intense autonomic reflexes: sympathetic discharge produces hypertension and vasoconstriction below the transection and a baroreceptor-mediated reflex bradycardia and vasodilation above the transection. Cardiac dysrhythmias are not unusual.

Emergent surgical management is undertaken whenever there is potentially reversible compression of the spinal cord due to dislocation of a vertebral body or bony fragment. Operative treatment is also indicated for spinal instability to prevent further injury. Patients can also present to the operating room as a result of delayed complications or unrelated disorders.

Anesthetic Considerations

A. ACUTE TRANSECTION:

Anesthetic management depends on the age of the injury. In the early care of acute injuries, the emphasis should be on preventing further spinal cord damage during patient movement, airway manipulation, and positioning. High-dose corticosteroid therapy (methylprednisolone: 30 mg/kg over first hour followed by 5.4 mg/kg/hour for 23 hours) is used for the first 24 hours following injury to improve neurologic outcome. The head should be maintained in neutral position using in-line stabilization with the help of an assistant or should remain in traction during intubation. Awake fiberoptic intubation after topical anesthesia may be safest. Patients with high transections often have impaired airway reflexes and are further predisposed to hypoxemia by a decrease in functional residual capacity. Hypotension and bradycardia are often present prior to induction. Direct arte-

rial pressure monitoring is indicated. Central venous and pulmonary artery pressure monitoring also facilitate management. An intravenous fluid bolus and the use of ketamine for anesthesia may help prevent further decreases in blood pressure; vasopressors may also be required. Succinylcholine can be used safely in the first 24 hours but should not be used thereafter because of the risk of hyperkalemia. The latter can occur within the first week following injury and is due to excessive release of potassium secondary to the proliferation of acetylcholine receptors outside the neuromuscular synaptic cleft.

B. CHRONIC TRANSECTION:

Anesthetic management of patients with nonacute transections is complicated by the possibility of autonomic hyperreflexia in addition to the risk of hyperkalemia. Autonomic hyperreflexia should be expected in patients with lesions above T6 and can be precipitated by surgical manipulations. Regional anesthesia and deep general anesthesia are effective in preventing hyperreflexia. Many clinicians, however, are reluctant to administer spinal and epidural anesthesia in these patients because of the difficulties encountered with determining the anesthetic level, exaggerated hypotension, and technical problems resulting from deformities. Severe hypertension can result in pulmonary edema, myocardial ischemia, or cerebral hemorrhage and should be treated aggressively. Direct arterial vasodilators and α-adrenergic blocking agents should be readily available. Although the risk of succinylcholine-induced hyperkalemia is reported to decrease 6 months after the injury, the use of nondepolarizing neuromuscular blocking agents are preferred. Administration of a small dose of a nondepolarizing neuromuscular blocking agent does not reliably prevent hyperkalemia. Body temperature should be monitored carefully, especially in patients with transections above T1, because chronic vasodilation and loss of normal reflex cutaneous vasoconstriction predispose to hypothermia.

Many patients eventually develop progressive renal insufficiency due to recurrent calculi and amyloid deposition. Drugs that are primarily renally excreted should be avoided in these patients (see Chapter 31).

■ PSYCHIATRIC DISORDERS

DEPRESSION

Depression is a mood disorder characterized by sadness and pessimism. Its cause is multifactorial, but pharmacologic treatment is based on the presumption that its manifestations are due to a brain deficiency of dopamine, norepinephrine, and serotonin, or altered receptor activities. Up to 50% of patients with major depression hypersecrete cortisol and have abnormal circadian secretion. Current pharmacologic therapy utilizes three classes of drugs that increase brain levels of these neurotransmitters, namely, tricyclic antidepressants, monoamine oxidase (MAO) inhibitors, and atypical antidepressants. The mechanisms of action of these drugs result in some potentially serious anesthetic interactions. Electroconvulsive therapy (ECT) is being increasingly used for refractory and severe cases and prophylactically once the patient returns to baseline. The use of general anesthesia for ECT is largely responsible for its safety and widespread acceptance.

Tricyclic Antidepressants

These agents may be used for the treatment of depression and chronic pain syndromes (see Chapter 18) (Table 27–3). All tricyclic antidepressants work at nerve synapses by blocking neuronal reuptake of catecholamines, serotonin, or both (see Table 18–7). Desipramine (Norpramin) and nortriptyline (Pamelor) are commonly used because they are less sedating and tend to have fewer side effects. Other agents are generally more sedating and include amitriptyline (Elavil), imipramine (Tofranil), protriptyline (Vivactil), amoxapine (Asendin), and doxepin (Sinequan). Clomipramine (Anafranil) is used in the treatment of obsessive-compulsive disorders. Most tricyclics also have significant anticholinergic (antimuscarinic) actions: dry mouth, blurred vision, prolonged gastric emptying, and urinary retention. Quinidine-like cardiac effects include tachycardia, T-wave flattening or inversion, and prolongation of the PR, QRS, and QT intervals. Amitriptyline has the most marked anticholinergic effects, while doxepin has the least cardiac effects.

St. John's wart is being used with increased frequency as an over-the-counter therapy for depression. Because it induces hepatic enzymes, blood levels of other drugs may decrease, with sometimes serious complications. During the preoperative evaluation, the use of all over-the-counter medications should be reviewed.

These drugs are generally continued perioperatively. Increased anesthetic requirements, presumably from enhanced brain catecholamine activity, have been reported with these agents. Potentiation of centrally acting anticholinergic agents (atropine and scopolamine) may increase the likelihood of postoperative confusion and delirium. The most important interaction during anesthesia is an exaggerated response to both indirect-acting vasopressors and sympathetic stimulation. Pancuronium, ketamine, meperidine, and epinephrine-containing local anesthetic solutions should be avoided (especially during halothane anesthesia). Because tricyclics lower the seizure threshold, the use of enflurane may also be questionable. Chronic therapy with tricyclic antidepressants is reported to deplete cardiac catecholamines, theoretically potentiating the cardiac depressant effects of anesthetics. If hypotension occurs, small doses of a direct-acting vasopressor should be used instead of an indirect-acting agent. Amitriptyline's anticholinergic action may occasionally contribute to postoperative delirium.

Monoamine Oxidase Inhibitors

These agents may be more effective for patients with depression accompanied by panic attacks and prominent anxiety. **MAO inhibitors** block the oxidative deamination of naturally occurring amines. At least two MAO isoenzymes (types A and B) with differential substrate selectivities have been identified. MAO A is selective for serotonin, dopamine, and norepinephrine, while MAO B is selective for tyramine and phenylethylamine. Currently available agents that are effective in treating depression are nonselective MAO inhibitors. They include phenelzine (Nardil), isocarboxazid (Marplan), and tranylcypromine (Parnate). Selective MAO-B inhibitors (see above) are not effective in the treatment of depression. Nonselective agents also appear to interfere with many enzymes other than monoamine oxidase. Side effects include orthostatic hypotension, agitation, tremor, seizures, muscle spasms, urinary retention, paresthesias, and jaundice. Their hypotensive effect may be related to the accumulation of false neurotransmitters (octopamine). The most serious sequela is a hypertensive crisis that occurs following ingestion of tyramine-containing foods (cheeses and red wines).

The practice of discontinuing MAO inhibitors at least 2 weeks prior to elective surgery is no longer recommended. With the exception of tranylcypromine, these agents produce irreversible enzyme inhibition; the 2-week delay allows sufficient regeneration of new enzyme. Studies suggest that patients may be safely anesthetized, at least for electroconvulsive therapy, without this waiting period. Phenelzine can decrease plasma cholinesterase activity and prolong the duration of succinylcholine. Opioids should generally be used with caution in patients receiving MAO inhibitors, since rare but serious reactions to opioids have been reported. Most serious reactions are associated with meperidine, resulting in hyperthermia, seizures, and coma. As with tricyclic antidepressants, exaggerated responses to vasopressors and sympathetic stimulation should be expected. If a vasopressor is necessary, a direct-acting agent in small doses should be employed. Drugs that enhance sympathetic

Table 27–3. Classification of antidepressants.

Class	Mechanism of Action	Generic Name (US Trade Name)
Selected newer antidepressants Selective serotonin reuptake inhibitors	Inhibit reuptake of 5-HT at presynaptic nerve membrane	Fluoxetine (Prozac) Fluvoxamine (Luvox) Paroxetine (Paxil) Sertraline (Zoloft) Citalopram (Celexa)
Serotonin and noradrenaline reuptake inhibitors	Potent inhibitors of 5-HT and NEPI uptake	Venlafaxine (Effexor) Mirtazapine (Remeron)
NEPI reuptake inhibitor	Selectively inhibit NEPI reuptake	Viloxazine[1] Reboxetine[2]
Reversible inhibitors of monoamine oxidase A	Selective, reversible inhibitors of monoamine oxidase A, increases NEPI, 5-HT, and dopamine	Moclobemide[2] Brofaromine[2]
5-HT$_2$ receptor antagonists	Mixed serotonin effects	Nefazodone (Serzone) Ritanserin[2]
5-HT$_{1a}$ receptor agonists	Partial agonist of serotonin 5-HT$_{1a}$	Gepirone[2] ipaspirone,[2] tandospirone,[2] felsinoxan[2]
GABAmimetics	GABA$_A$ and GABA$_B$ receptor agonists	Fengamine[2]
Dopamine reuptake inhibitor	Increases activity of NEPI and dopamine only; no affect on serotonin	Buproprion (Wellbutrin, Zyban)
Herbal remedies	Unclear	Hypericum (also known as St. John's wart)

Selected older antidepressants
  Mixed serotonin and NEPI reuptake inhibitors
    First-generation tricyclic anti-depressants
	Potentiate serotonin and NEPI activity; potency and selectivity differ by agent	Amitriptyline (Elavil, Endep)[3]
		Clomipramine (Anafranil)
		Doxepin (Adapin, Sinequan)[3]
		Imipramine (Tofranil)[3]
		Trimipramine (Surmontil)

Second-generation tricyclic antidepressants Tetracyclic antidepressant		Desipramine (Norpramin)[3] Nortriptyline (Pamelor)[3] Maprotiline (Ludiomil)[3]
Triazolopyridine	Mixed serotonin effects	Trazodone (Desyrel)
Monoamine oxidase inhibitors	Nonselective inhibitor of monoamine oxidase A and B	Phenelzine (Nardil) Tranylcypromine (Parnate)

HT = hydroxy-tryptophan; NEPI = norepinephrine; GABA = gamma-aminobutyric acid.

[1]Brand-name drugs are produced by the following manufacturers: Adapin, Fisons Pharmaceuticals, Rochester, New York; Anafranil and Tofranil, Novartis, East Hanover, New Jersey; Celexa, Forest Pharmaceuticals, Inc., St. Louis, Missouri; Desyrel and Serzone, Bristol-Myers Squibb, Princeton, New Jersey; Effexor and Surmontil, Wyeth-Ayerst, Philadelphia, Pennsylvania; Elavil, Zeneca Pharmaceuticals, Wilmington, Delaware; Endep, Hoffman-LaRoche, Nutley, New Jersey; Luvox, Solvay Pharmaceuticals, Inc., Marietta, Georgia; Nardil, Parke-Davis, Morris Plains, New Jersey; Norpramine, Aventis Pharmaceuticals, Parsippany, New Jersey; Pamelor and Ludiomil, Novartis, East Hanover, New Jersey; Paxil and Parnate, SmithKline Beecham Pharmaceuticals, Philadelphia, Pennsylvania; Prozac, Eli Lilly and Co., Indianapolis, Indiana; Remeron, Organon, Inc., West Orange, New Jersey; Wellbutrin and Zyban, Glaxo Wellcome, Research Triangle Park, North Carolina; Zoloft and Sinequan, Pfizer, New York, New York.

[2]Not available in the United States.

[3]Generic form available.

(Modified with permission from Williams JW et al. Ann Intern Med 2000;132:743.)

activity such as ketamine, pancuronium, and epinephrine (in local anesthetic solutions) should be avoided.

Atypical Antidepressants

Most atypical antidepressants are primarily selective serotonin reuptake inhibitors (SSRIs). These include fluoxetine (Prozac), sertraline (Zoloft), and paroxetine (Paxil), which some clinicians consider first-line agents of choice for depression. These agents have little or no anticholinergic activity and do not affect cardiac conduction. Their principal side effects are headache, agitation, and insomnia. Other atypical agents include bupropion (Wellbutrin), venlafaxine (Effexor), trazodone (Desyrel), nefazodone (Serzone), fluvoxamine (Luvox), and maprotiline (Ludiomil). The last is not commonly used because of a relatively high incidence of seizures. Bupropion may primarily inhibit dopamine reuptake. Anesthetic interactions with atypical antidepressants are not well documented.

MANIA

Mania is a mood disorder characterized by elation, hyperactivity, and flight of ideas. Manic episodes may alternate with depression in patients with a bipolar disorder. Mania is thought to be related to excessive norepinephrine activity in the brain. Lithium is the drug of choice for treating acute manic episodes, preventing their recurrence as well as suppressing episodes of depression. Concomitant administration of an antipsychotic (haloperidol) or a benzodiazepine (lorazepam) is usually necessary during acute mania. Alternative treatments include valproic acid, carbamazepine, as well as ECT.

Lithium's mechanism of action is poorly understood. It has a narrow therapeutic range, with a desirable blood concentration between 0.8 and 1.0 mEq/L. Side effects include reversible T-wave changes, mild leukocytosis, and, on rare occasions, hypothyroidism or a vasopressin-resistant diabetes insipidus-like syndrome. Toxic blood concentrations produce confusion, sedation, muscle weakness, tremor, and slurred speech. Still higher concentrations result in widening of the QRS complex, atrioventricular block, hypotension, and seizures.

Although lithium is reported to decrease minimum alveolar concentration and prolong the duration of some neuromuscular blocking agents, clinically these effects appear to be minor. Nonetheless, neuromuscular function should be closely monitored when neuromuscular blocking agents are used. The greatest concern is the possibility of perioperative toxicity. Blood levels should be checked perioperatively. Sodium depletion decreases renal excretion of lithium and can lead to lithium toxicity. Fluid restriction and overdiuresis should be avoided.

SCHIZOPHRENIA

Patients with schizophrenia display disordered thinking, withdrawal, paranoid delusions, and auditory hallucinations. This disorder is thought to be related to an excess of dopaminergic activity in the brain. Antipsychotic drugs remain the only effective treatment for controlling this disease.

The most commonly used antipsychotics include phenothiazines, thioxanthenes, oxoindoles, dibenzoxazepines, and butyrophenones. Commonly used agents include haloperidol (Haldol), chlorpromazine (Thorazine), risperidone (Risperdal), molindone (Moban), clozapine (Clozaril), fluphenazine (Prolixin), trifluoperazine (Stelazine), thiothixene (Navane), perphenazine (Trilafon), and droperidol (Inapsine). All these agents have similar properties with minor variations. Clozapine may be effective in patients refractory to other drugs. Their antipsychotic effect appears to be due to dopamine antagonist activity. Most are sedating and mildly anxiolytic. With the exception of thioridazine (Mellaril), all are potent antiemetics (see Chapter 8). Mild α-adrenergic blockade and anticholinergic activity are also observed. Side effects include orthostatic hypotension, acute dystonic reactions, and parkinsonism-like manifestations. Risperidone and clozapine have little extrapyramidal activity, but the latter has a significant incidence of granulocytopenia. T-wave flattening, ST segment depression, and prolongation of the PR and QT intervals may be seen, especially in patients taking thioridazine.

Generally, patients whose disease is controlled by antipsychotics present few problems. Continuing antipsychotic medication perioperatively is desirable. Reduced anesthetic requirements may be observed in some patients. α-Adrenergic blockade is usually well compensated. Enflurane and possibly ketamine should probably be avoided, since antipsychotics decrease the seizure threshold.

NEUROLEPTIC MALIGNANT SYNDROME

This syndrome is a rare complication of antipsychotic therapy that may occur hours or weeks after administration. Metoclopramide can also precipitate the disorder. The mechanism is related to dopamine blockade in the basal ganglia and hypothalamus and impairment of thermoregulation. In its most severe form, the presentation is similar to that of malignant hyperthermia. Muscle rigidity, hyperthermia, rhabdomyolysis, autonomic instability, and altered consciousness are seen. Creatine kinase levels are often high. The mortality rate approaches 20–30%, with deaths occurring primarily as a result of renal failure or dysrhythmias. Treatment with dantrolene appears to be effective; bromocriptine, a dopamine agonist, may also be effective. Although muscle biopsy is often normal, patients with a history of **neuroleptic malignant syndrome** should be treated in the same way as those susceptible to malignant hyperthermia (see Chapter 44).

SUBSTANCE ABUSE

Behavioral disorders from abuse of psychotropic (mind-altering) substances may involve a socially acceptable drug (alcohol), a medically prescribed drug (diazepam), or an illegal substance (cocaine). Environmental, social, and perhaps genetic factors lead to this type of behavior. A "need" for the substance develops ranging in intensity from a simple desire to a compulsion that consumes the patient's life. Characteristically with chronic abuse, patients develop tolerance to the drug and varying degrees of psychological and physical dependence. Physical dependence is most often seen with opioids, barbiturates, alcohol, and benzodiazepines. Life-threatening complications primarily due to sympathetic overactivity can develop during abstention. Barbiturate withdrawal is potentially the most lethal and dangerous of the withdrawal syndromes.

Knowledge of a patient's substance abuse preoperatively may prevent adverse drug interactions, predict tolerance to anesthetic agents, and facilitate the recognition of drug withdrawal. The history of substance abuse may be volunteered by the patient (usually only on direct questioning) or deliberately hidden. A high index of suspicion is often required. Sociopathic tendencies are difficult to detect during a short interview. The presence of numerous punctate scars with difficult venous access strongly suggests intravenous drug abuse. Such injecting drug users have a relatively high incidence of skin infections, thrombophlebitis, malnutrition, endocarditis, hepatitis B and C, and HIV infection.

Anesthetic requirements for substance abusers vary depending on whether the drug exposure is acute or chronic (see Table 27–3). Elective procedures should be postponed for acutely intoxicated patients and those with signs of withdrawal. When surgery is deemed necessary in patients with physical dependence, perioperative doses of the abused substance should be provided or specific agents given to prevent withdrawal. In the case of opioid dependence, any opioid can be used, while for alcohol a benzodiazepine is usually substituted. Tolerance to most anesthetic agents is often seen but is not always predictable. Regional anesthetics should be considered whenever possible. For general anesthesia, a technique primarily relying on a volatile inhalational agent may be preferable so that anesthetic depth can be readily adjusted according to individual

Table 27–4. Effect of acute and chronic substance abuse on anesthetic requirements.

Substance	Acute	Chronic
Opioids	↓	↑
Barbiturates	↓	↑
Alcohol	↓	↑
Marijuana	↓	0
Benzodiazepines	↓	↑
Amphetamines	↑[1]	↓
Cocaine	↑[1]	0
Phencyclidine	↓	?

[1]Associated with marked sympathetic stimulation.
↓ = decreases; ↑ = increases; 0 = no effect; ? = unknown.

need. Opioids with mixed agonist-antagonist activity should be avoided in opioid-dependent patients because such agents can precipitate acute withdrawal. Clonidine is a useful adjuvant in treatment of postoperative withdrawal syndromes.

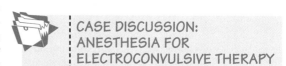

**CASE DISCUSSION:
ANESTHESIA FOR
ELECTROCONVULSIVE THERAPY**

A 64-year-old man with depression refractory to drug therapy is scheduled for electroconvulsive therapy (ECT).

How is ECT administered?

The electroconvulsive shock is applied to one or both cerebral hemispheres to induce a seizure. Variables include stimulus pattern, amplitude, and duration. The goal is to produce a therapeutic generalized seizure 30–60 seconds in duration. Electrical stimuli are usually administered until a therapeutic seizure is induced. A good therapeutic effect is generally not achieved until a total of 400–700 seizure seconds have been induced. Since only one treatment is given per day, patients are usually scheduled for a series of treatments, usually two or three a week. Progressive memory loss often occurs with an increasing number of treatments, especially when electrodes are applied bilaterally.

Why is anesthesia necessary?

When the efficacy of ECT was discovered, enthusiasm was tempered in the medical community because relaxants were not used to control the violent seizures caused by the procedure, thus engendering a relatively high incidence of musculoskeletal injuries. Moreover, when muscle relaxants were used alone, patients sometimes recalled being paralyzed and awake just prior to the shock. The routine use of general anesthesia to ensure amnesia and muscle paralysis to prevent injuries has renewed interest in ECT. The current mortality rate for ECT is estimated to be one death per 10,000 treatments. While some psychiatrists administer the anesthetic, the presence of an anesthesiologist is optimal for airway management and cardiovascular monitoring.

What are the physiologic effects of ECT-induced seizures?

Seizure activity is characteristically associated with an initial parasympathetic discharge followed by a more sustained sympathetic discharge. The initial phase is characterized by bradycardia and increased secretions. Marked bradycardia (< 30 beats/min) and even transient asystole (up to 6 seconds) are occasionally seen. The hypertension and tachycardia that follow are typically sustained for several minutes. Transient autonomic imbalance can produce arrhythmias and T-wave abnormalities on the electrocardiogram. Cerebral blood flow, ICP, intragastric pressure, and intraocular pressure all transiently increase.

Are there any contraindications to ECT?

Contraindications are a recent myocardial infarction (usually < 3 months), a recent stroke (usually < 1 month), an intracranial mass, or increased ICP from any cause. More relative contraindications include angina, poorly controlled heart failure, significant pulmonary disease, bone fractures, severe osteoporosis, pregnancy, glaucoma, and retinal detachment.

What are the important considerations in selecting anesthetic agents?

Amnesia is required only for the brief period (1–5 minutes) from when the muscle relaxant is given to when a therapeutic seizure has been successfully induced. The seizure itself usually results in a brief period of anterograde amnesia, somnolence, and often confusion. Consequently, only a short-acting induction agent is necessary. Moreover, since most induction agents (barbiturates, etomidate, benzodiazepines, and propofol) have anticonvulsant properties, small doses must be used. Seizure threshold is increased and seizure duration is decreased by all these agents.

Following adequate preoxygenation, methohexital, 0.5–1 mg/kg, is most commonly employed. Propofol, 1–1.5 mg/kg, may be used but higher doses reduce seizure duration. Benzodiazepines raise the seizure threshold and decrease duration. Ketamine increases seizure duration but is generally not used because it also increases the incidence of delayed awakening, nausea, and ataxia. Use of etomidate also prolongs recovery. Short-acting opioids such as alfentanil are not given alone because they do not consistently produce amnesia. However, alfentanil (10–25 mg/kg) can be a useful adjunct when very small doses of methohexital (10–20 mg) are required in patients with a high seizure threshold. In very small doses, methohexital may actually enhance seizure activity. Increases in seizure threshold are often observed with each subsequent ECT.

Muscle paralysis is required from the time of electrical stimulation till the end of the seizure. A short-acting agent such as succinylcholine (0.5–1 mg/kg) is most often selected. Controlled mask ventilation using a self-inflating bag device or an anesthesia circle system is required until spontaneous respirations resume.

Can seizure duration be increased without increasing the electrical stimulus?

Hyperventilation can increase seizure duration and is routinely employed in some centers. Intravenous caffeine, 125–250 mg (given slowly), has also been reported to increase seizure duration.

What monitors should be used during ECT?

Monitoring should be similar to that appropriate with the use of any other general anesthetic. Seizure activity is sometimes monitored by an unprocessed electroencephalogram. Seizure activity can also be monitored in an isolated limb: a tourniquet is inflated around one arm prior to injection of succinylcholine, preventing entry of the muscle relaxant and allowing observation of convulsive motor activity in that arm.

How can the adverse hemodynamic effects of the seizure be controlled in patients with limited cardiovascular reserve?

Exaggerated parasympathetic effects should be treated with atropine. In fact, premedication with glycopyrrolate is desirable in all patients to prevent both the profuse secretions associated with seizures and to attenuate the bradycardia. Nitroglycerin, nifedipine, and α- and β-adrenergic blockade have all been employed successfully to control sympathetic manifestations. High doses of β-*adrenergic blockers (esmolol 200 mg), however, are reported to decrease seizure duration.*

What if the patient has a pacemaker?

Patients with pacemakers may safely undergo electroconvulsive treatments, but a magnet should be readily available to convert the pacemaker to a fixed mode if necessary.

SUGGESTED READING

Atlee JL: *Complications in Anesthesia.* WB Saunders and Company, 1999.

Cucchiara RF, Black S, Michenfelder JD: *Clinical Neuroanesthesia.* Churchill Livingstone, 2nd ed. 1998.

Gilman AG et al (editors): *Goodman and Gilman's The Pharmacological Basis of Therapeutics,* 9th ed. McGraw-Hill, New York, 1996.

Newfield P, Cottrell JE: *Handbook of Neuroanesthesia,* 3rd ed. Lippincott Williams & Wilkins, 1999.

Schubert A: *Clinical Neuroanesthesia.* Butterworth-Heinemann, 1997.

Management of Patients With Fluid & Electrolyte Disturbances

28

KEY CONCEPTS

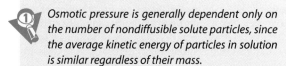 Osmotic pressure is generally dependent only on the number of nondiffusible solute particles, since the average kinetic energy of particles in solution is similar regardless of their mass.

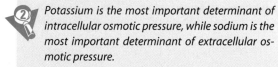 Potassium is the most important determinant of intracellular osmotic pressure, while sodium is the most important determinant of extracellular osmotic pressure.

③ Fluid exchange between the intracellular and interstitial spaces is governed by the osmotic forces created by differences in nondiffusible solute concentrations.

④ Serious manifestations of hyponatremia are generally associated with plasma sodium concentrations less than 120 mEq/L.

⑤ Very rapid correction of hyponatremia has been associated with demyelinating lesions in the pons (central pontine myelinolysis), resulting in serious permanent neurologic sequelae.

⑥ The major hazard of increases in extracellular volume is impaired gas exchange due to pulmonary interstitial edema, alveolar edema, or large collections of pleural or ascitic fluid.

⑦ Intravenous replacement of potassium chloride should usually be reserved for patients with or at

risk for serious cardiac manifestations or muscle weakness. Intravenous replacement should generally not exceed 240 mEq/d.

⑧ Because of its lethal potential, hyperkalemia exceeding 6 mEq/L should always be treated.

⑨ Symptomatic hypercalcemia requires rapid treatment. The most effective initial treatment is rehydration followed by a brisk diuresis (urinary output 200–300 mL/hour) with administration of intravenous saline infusion and a loop diuretic to accelerate calcium excretion.

⑩ Symptomatic hypocalcemia is a medical emergency and should be treated immediately with intravenous calcium chloride (3–5 mL of a 10% solution) or calcium gluconate (10–20 mL of a 10% solution).

⑪ Some patients with severe hypophosphatemia may require mechanical ventilation postoperatively.

⑫ Marked hypermagnesemia can lead to respiratory arrest.

⑬ Isolated hypomagnesemia should be corrected prior to elective procedures because of its potential for causing cardiac arrhythmias.

Fluid and electrolyte disturbances are extremely common in the perioperative period. Large amounts of intravenous fluids are frequently required to correct fluid deficits and compensate for blood loss during surgery. Anesthesiologists must therefore have a clear under-standing of normal water and electrolyte physiology. Major disturbances in fluid and electrolyte balance can rapidly alter cardiovascular, neurologic, and neuromuscular functions. This chapter examines the body's fluid compartments and common water and electrolyte derangements, their treatment, and anesthetic implications. Acid-base disorders and intravenous fluid therapy are discussed in subsequent chapters.

NOMENCLATURE OF SOLUTIONS

The system of international units (SI) has still not gained universal acceptance in clinical practice, and many older expressions of concentration remain in common use. Thus, for example, the quantity of a solute in a solution may be expressed in grams, moles, or equivalents. To complicate matters further, the concentration of a solution may be expressed either as quantity of solute per volume of solution or quantity of solute per weight of solvent.

MOLARITY, MOLALITY, & EQUIVALENCY

One **mole** of a substance represents 6.02×10^{23} molecules. The weight of this quantity in grams is commonly referred to as **gram-molecular weight. Molarity** is the standard SI unit of concentration that expresses the number of moles of solute per *liter* of solution. **Molality** is an alternative term that expresses moles of solute per *kilogram* of solvent. **Equivalency** is also commonly used for substances that ionize: the number of **equivalents** of an ion in solution is the number of moles multiplied by its charge (valence). Thus, a 1-molar solution of $MgCl_2$ yields 2 equivalents of magnesium per liter and 2 equivalents of chloride per liter.

OSMOLARITY, OSMOLALITY, & TONICITY

Osmosis is the net movement of water across a semipermeable membrane as a result of a difference in nondiffusible solute concentrations between the two sides. **Osmotic pressure** is the pressure that must be applied

to the side with more solute to prevent a net movement of water across the membrane to dilute the solute. Since

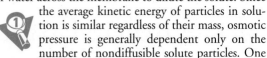

the average kinetic energy of particles in solution is similar regardless of their mass, osmotic pressure is generally dependent only on the number of nondiffusible solute particles. One **osmole** equals 1 mole of nondissociable substances. For substances that ionize, however, each mole results in *n* osmoles, where *n* is the number of ionic species produced. Thus, 1 mole of a highly ionized substance such as NaCl dissolved in solution should produce 2 osmoles; in reality ionic interaction between the cation and anion reduces the effective activity of each such that NaCl behaves as if it is only 75% ionized. A difference of 1 milliosmole per liter between two solutions results in an osmotic pressure of 19.3 mm Hg. The **osmolarity** of a solution is equal to the number of osmoles per *liter* of solution, while its **osmolality** equals the number of osmoles per *kilogram* of solvent. **Tonicity** is a term that is often used interchangeably with osmolarity and osmolality. More correctly, tonicity refers to the effect a solution has on cell volume. An isotonic solution has no effect on cell volume, while hypotonic and hypertonic solutions increase and decrease cell volume, respectively.

FLUID COMPARTMENTS

The average adult male is approximately 60% water by weight; females are 50%. This water is distributed between two major fluid compartments separated by cell membranes: intracellular fluid (ICF) and extracellular fluid (ECF). The latter can be further subdivided into intravascular and interstitial compartments. The interstitium includes all fluid that is both outside cells and outside the vascular endothelium. The relative contributions of each compartment to total body water (TBW) and body weight are set forth in Table 28–1.

Table 28–1. Body fluid compartments (based on average 70-kg male).

Compartment	Fluid as Percent Body Weight (%)	Total Body Water (%)	Fluid Volume (L)
Intracellular	40	67	28
Extracellular			
Interstitial	15	25	10.5
Intravascular	5	8	3.5
Total	60	100	42

Table 28–2. The composition of fluid compartments.

			Extracellular	
	Gram-molecular Weight	**Intracellular (mEq/L)**	*Intravascular (mEq/L)*	*Interstitial (mEq/L)*
Sodium	23.0	10	145	142
Potassium	39.1	140	4	4
Calcium	40.1	< 1	3	3
Magnesium	24.3	50	2	2
Chloride	35.5	4	105	110
Bicarbonate	61.0	10	24	28
Phosphorus	31.0*	75	2	2
Protein (g/dL)		16	7	2

*PO_4^{3-} is 95 g.

The volume of fluid (water) within a compartment is determined by its solute composition and concentrations (Table 28–2). Differences in solute concentrations are largely due to the characteristics of the physical barriers that separate compartments (see below). The osmotic forces created by "trapped" solutes govern the distribution of water between compartments and ultimately each compartment's volume.

INTRACELLULAR FLUID

The outer membrane of cells plays an important role in regulating intracellular volume and composition. A membrane-bound ATP-dependent pump exchanges Na^+ for K^+ in a 3:2 ratio. Because cell membranes are relatively impermeable to sodium and to a lesser extent potassium ions, potassium is concentrated intracellularly while sodium is concentrated extracellularly. As a result, potassium is the most important determinant of intracellular osmotic pressure, while sodium is the most important determinant of extracellular osmotic pressure.

The impermeability of cell membranes to most proteins results in a high intracellular protein concentration. Because proteins act as nondiffusible solutes (anions), the unequal exchange ratio of 3 Na^+ for 2 K^+ by the cell membrane pump is critical in preventing relative intracellular hyperosmolality. Interference with Na^+-K^+ ATPase activity, as occurs during ischemia or hypoxia, results in progressive swelling of cells.

EXTRACELLULAR FLUID

The principal function of extracellular fluid is to provide a medium for cell nutrients and electrolytes and for cellular waste products. Maintenance of a normal extracellular volume—especially the circulating component (intravascular volume)—is critical. For the reasons described above, sodium is quantitatively the most important extracellular cation and the major determinant of extracellular osmotic pressure and volume. Changes in extracellular fluid volume are therefore related to changes in total body sodium content. The latter is a function of sodium intake, renal sodium excretion, and extrarenal sodium losses (see below).

Interstitial Fluid

Very little interstitial fluid is normally in the form of free fluid. Most interstitial water is in chemical association with extracellular proteoglycans, forming a gel. Interstitial fluid pressure is generally thought to be negative (about −5 mm Hg). As interstitial fluid volume increases, interstitial pressure also rises and eventually becomes positive. When the latter occurs, the free fluid in the gel increases rapidly and appears clinically as edema.

Because only small quantities of plasma proteins can normally cross capillary clefts, the protein content of interstitial fluid is relatively low (2 g/dL). Protein entering the interstitial space is returned to the vascular system via the lymphatic system.

Intravascular Fluid

Intravascular fluid, commonly referred to as plasma, is restricted to the intravascular space by the vascular endothelium. Most electrolytes (small ions) freely pass between plasma and the interstitium, resulting in nearly identical electrolyte composition. However, the tight intercellular junctions between adjacent endothelial cells impede the passage of plasma proteins outside the intravascular compartment. As a result, plasma proteins (mainly albumin) are the only osmotically active solutes in fluid not normally exchanged between plasma and interstitial fluid.

Increases in extracellular volume are normally proportionately reflected in intravascular and interstitial volume. When interstitial pressure becomes positive, continued increases in ECF result in expansion of only the interstitial fluid compartment (Figure 28–1). In this way, the interstitial compartment acts as an overflow reservoir for the intravascular compartment. This can be seen clinically in the form of tissue edema.

EXCHANGE BETWEEN FLUID COMPARTMENTS

Diffusion is the random movement of molecules due to their kinetic energy and is responsible for the majority of fluid and solute exchange between compartments. The rate of diffusion of a substance across a membrane depends on (1) the permeability of that substance through that membrane, (2) the concentration diference for that substance between the two sides, (3) the pressure difference between either side because pressure imparts greater kinetic energy, and (4) the electrical potential across the membrane for charged substances.

Diffusion Through Cell Membranes

Diffusion between interstitial fluid and intracellular fluid may take place by one of several mechanisms: (1) directly through the lipid bilayer of the cell membrane, (2) through protein channels within the membrane, or (3) by reversible binding to a carrier protein that can traverse the membrane (facilitated diffusion). Oxygen, CO_2, water, and lipid-soluble molecules penetrate the cell membrane directly. Cations such as Na^+, K^+, and Ca^{2+} penetrate the membrane poorly because of the cell transmembrane voltage potential (which is positive to the outside) created by the Na^+-K^+ pump. Therefore, these cations can diffuse only through specific protein channels. Passage through these channels is dependent on membrane voltage and the binding of ligands (such as acetylcholine) to the membrane receptors. Glucose and amino acids diffuse with the help of membrane-bound carrier proteins.

 Fluid exchange between the intracellular and interstitial spaces is governed by the osmotic forces created by differences in nondiffusible solute concentrations. Relative changes in osmolality between the intracellular and interstitial compartments result in a net water movement from the hypo-osmolar to the hyperosmolar compartment.

Diffusion Through Capillary Endothelium

Capillary walls are typically 0.5 μm thick, consisting of a single layer of endothelial cells with their basement membrane. Intercellular clefts, 6–7 nm wide, separate each cell from its neighbors. Oxygen, CO_2, water, and lipid-soluble substances can penetrate directly through both sides of the endothelial cell membrane. Only low-molecular-weight water-soluble substances such as sodium, chloride, potassium, and glucose readily cross intercellular clefts. High-molecular-weight substances such as plasma proteins penetrate the endothelial clefts poorly (except in the liver and the lungs, where the clefts are larger).

Fluid exchange across capillaries differs from that across cell membranes in that it is governed by significant differences in hydrostatic pressures in addition to osmotic forces (Figure 28–2). These forces are operative on both arterial and venous ends of capillaries. As a result, there is a tendency for fluid to move out of capillaries at the arterial end and back into capillaries at the venous end. Moreover, the magnitude of these forces differs between the various tissue beds. Arterial capillary pressure is determined by precapillary sphincter tone. Thus capillaries that require a high pressure such as glomeruli have low precapillary sphincter tone while the normally low pressure capillaries of muscle have high precapillary sphincter tone. Normally, all but 10% of the fluid filtered is reabsorbed back into capillaries. That which is not reabsorbed (about 2 mL/min) enters interstitial fluid and is then returned by lymphatic flow to the intravascular compartment.

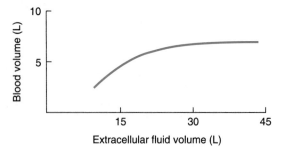

Figure 28–1. The relationship between blood volume and extracellular fluid volume. (Modified and reproduced, with permission, from Guyton AC: *Textbook of Medical Physiology,* 7th ed. WB Saunders and Company, 1986).

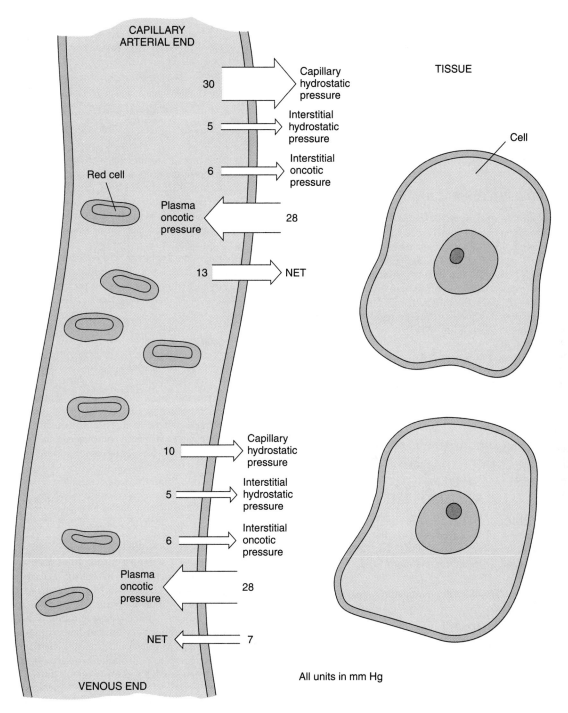

Figure 28–2. Capillary fluid exchange.

■ DISORDERS OF WATER BALANCE

The human body at birth is approximately 75% water by weight. By 1 month this value decreases to 65%, and by adulthood to 60% for males and 50% for females. The higher fat content in females decreases water content. For the same reason, obesity and advanced age further decrease water content.

NORMAL WATER BALANCE

The normal adult daily water intake averages 2500 mL, which includes approximately 300 mL as a by-product of the metabolism of energy substrates. Daily water loss necessarily averages 2500 mL and can roughly be accounted for by 1500 mL in urine, 400 mL in respiratory tract evaporation, 400 mL in skin evaporation, 100 mL in sweat, and 100 mL in feces. The evaporative losses are very important in thermoregulation because they normally account for 20–25% of heat loss (see Chapter 6).

Both ICF and ECF osmolalities are closely regulated in such a way as to maintain a normal water content in tissues. Changes in water content and cell volume can induce serious impairment of function especially in the brain (see below).

RELATIONSHIP BETWEEN PLASMA SODIUM CONCENTRATION, EXTRACELLULAR OSMOLALITY, & INTRACELLULAR OSMOLALITY

The osmolality of ECF is equal to the sum of the concentrations of all dissolved solutes. Because Na^+ together with its anions account for nearly 90% of these solutes, the following approximation is valid:

Plasma osmolality = $2 \times$ Plasma sodium concentration

Moreover, because ICF and ECF are in osmotic equilibrium, plasma sodium concentration $[Na^+]_{plasma}$ generally reflects total body osmolality:

$$[Na]_{plasma} \text{ Total body osmolality} = \frac{\text{Extracellular solutes} + \text{intracellular solutes}}{\text{TBW}}$$

Since sodium and potassium are the major intra- and extracellular solutes, respectively:

$$\text{Total body osmolality} = \frac{(Na^+_{extracellular} \times 2) + (K^+_{intracellular solutes} \times 2)}{\text{TBW}}$$

Combining the two approximations:

$$[Na^+]_{plasma} \approx \frac{Na^+_{extracellular} + K^+_{intracellular}}{\text{TBW}}$$

Using these principles, the effect of isotonic, hypotonic, and hypertonic fluid loads on compartmental water content and plasma osmolality can be calculated (Table 28–3). The potential importance of intracellular potassium concentration is readily apparent from this equation. Thus significant potassium losses may contribute to hyponatremia.

In pathologic states, glucose and—to a much lesser extent—urea can contribute significantly to extracellular osmolality. A more accurate approximation of plasma osmolality is therefore given by the following equation:

Plasma osmolality (mosm/kg) =

$$[Na^+] \times 2 + \frac{BUN}{2.8} + \frac{glucose}{18}$$

where $[Na^+]$ is expressed as mEq/L and blood urea nitrogen (BUN) and glucose as mg/dL. Urea is an ineffective osmole because it readily permeates cell membranes and is therefore frequently omitted from this calculation:

Effective plasma osmolality = $[Na^+] \times 2 + \frac{glucose}{18}$

Plasma osmolality normally varies between 280 and 290 mOsm/L. Plasma sodium concentration decreases approximately 1 mEq/L for every 62 mg/dL increase in glucose concentration. A discrepancy between the measured and calculated osmolality is referred to as an **osmolal gap.** Significant osmolal gaps indicate a high concentration of an abnormal osmotically active molecule in plasma such as ethanol, mannitol, methanol, ethylene glycol, or isopropyl alcohol. Osmolal gaps may also be seen in patients with chronic renal failure (attributed to retention of small solutes), patients with ketoacidosis (as a result of a high concentration of ketone bodies), and those receiving large amounts of glycine (as during transurethral resection of the prostate). Lastly, osmolal gaps may also be present in patients with marked hyperlipidemia or hyperproteinemia. In such instances, the protein or lipid part of plasma con-

Table 28–3. Effect of different fluid loads on extracellular and intracellular water contents.[1]

A. Normal

Total body solute	$= 280 \text{ mOsm/kg} \times 42 \text{ kg} = 11{,}760 \text{ mOsm}$
Intracellular solute	$= 280 \text{ mOsm/kg} \times 25 \text{ kg} = 7000 \text{ mOsm}$
Extracellular solute	$= 280 \text{ mOsm/kg} \times 17 \text{ kg} = 4760 \text{ mOsm}$

Extracellular sodium concentration $= 280 \div 2 = 140 \text{ mEq/L}$

	Intracellular	Extracellular
Osmolality	280	280
Volume (L)	25	17
Net water gain	0	0

B. Isotonic load: 2 L of Isotonic saline (NaCl)

Total body solute	$= 280 \text{ mOsm/kg} \times 44 \text{ kg} = 12{,}320 \text{ mOsm}$
Intracellular solute	$= 280 \text{ mOsm/kg} \times 25 \text{ kg} = 7000 \text{ mOsm}$
Extracellular solute	$= 280 \text{ mOsm/kg} \times 19 \text{ kg} = 5320 \text{ mOsm}$

	Intracellular	Extracellular
Osmolality	280	280
Volume (L)	25	19
Net water gain	0	2

Net effect: Fluid remains in extracellular compartment.

C. Free water (hypotonic) load: 2 L water

New body water	$= 42 + 2 = 44 \text{ kg}$
New body osmolality	$= 11{,}760 \text{ mOsm} \div 44 \text{ kg} = 267 \text{ mOsm/kg}$
New intracellular volume	$= 7000 \text{ mOsm} \div 267 \text{ mOsm/kg} = 26.2 \text{ kg}$
New extracellular sodium concentration	$= 267 \div 2 = 133 \text{ mEq/L}$

	Intracellular	Extracellular
Osmolality	267.0	267.0
Volume (L)	26.2	17.8
Net water gain	+1.2	+0.8

Net effect: Fluid distributes between both compartments.

D. Hypertonic load: 600 mEq NaCl (no water)

Total body solute	$= 11{,}760 + 600 = 12{,}360 \text{ mOsm/kg}$
New body osmolality	$= 12{,}360 \text{ mOsm/kg} \div 42 \text{ kg} = 294 \text{ mOsm}$
New extracellular solute	$= 600 + 4760 = 5360 \text{ mOsm}$
New extracellular volume	$= 5360 \text{ mOsm} \div 294 \text{ mOsm/kg} = 18.2 \text{ kg}$
New intracellular volume	$= 42 - 18.2 = 23.8 \text{ kg}$
New extracellular sodium concentration	$= 294 \div 2 = 147 \text{ mEq/L}$

	Intracellular	Extracellular
Osmolality	294.0	294.0
Volume (L)	23.8	18.2
Net water gain	−1.2	+1.2

Net effect: An intracellular to extracellular movement of water.

[1]Based on a 70-kg adult male.

tributes significantly to plasma volume; although plasma [Na$^+$] is decreased, [Na$^+$] in the water phase of plasma (true plasma osmolality) remains normal. The water phase of plasma is normally only 93% of its volume; the remaining 7% consists of plasma lipids and proteins.

CONTROL OF PLASMA OSMOLALITY

Plasma osmolality is closely regulated by osmoreceptors in the hypothalamus. These specialized neurons control the secretion of antidiuretic hormone (ADH) and the thirst mechanism. Plasma osmolality is therefore maintained within relatively narrow limits by varying both water intake and water excretion.

Secretion of Antidiuretic Hormone

Specialized neurons in the supraoptic and paraventricular nuclei of the hypothalamus are very sensitive to changes in extracellular osmolality. When ECF osmolality increases, these cells shrink and release ADH (arginine vasopressin, also called AVP) from the posterior pituitary. ADH markedly increases water reabsorption in renal collecting tubules (see Chapter 31), which tends to reduce plasma osmolality to normal again. Conversely, a decrease in extracellular osmolality causes osmoreceptors to swell and suppresses the release of ADH. Decreased ADH secretion allows a water diuresis, which tends to increase osmolality to normal. Peak diuresis occurs once circulating ADH is metabolized (90–120 minutes). With complete suppression of ADH secretion, the kidneys can excrete up to 10–20 L of water per day (see below).

Nonosmotic Release of Antidiuretic Hormone

The carotid baroreceptors and possibly atrial stretch receptors can also stimulate ADH release following a 5–10% decrease in blood volume (see below). Other nonosmotic stimuli include pain, emotional stress, and hypoxia.

Thirst

Osmoreceptors in the lateral preoptic area of the hypothalamus are also very sensitive to changes in extracellular osmolality. Activation of these neurons by increases in ECF osmolality induces thirst and causes the individual to drink water. Conversely, hypo-osmolality suppresses thirst.

Thirst is the major defense mechanism against hyperosmolality and hypernatremia, because it is the only mechanism that increases water intake. Unfortunately, the thirst mechanism is only operative in conscious individuals who are capable of drinking.

HYPEROSMOLALITY & HYPERNATREMIA

Hyperosmolality occurs whenever total body solute content increases relative to TBW and is usually but not always associated with hypernatremia ([Na$^+$] > 145 mEq/L). Hyperosmolality without hypernatremia may be seen during marked hyperglycemia or following the accumulation of abnormal osmotically active substances in plasma (see above). In the latter two instances, plasma sodium concentration may actually decrease as water is drawn from the intracellular to the extracellular compartment. For every 100 mg/dL increase in plasma glucose concentration, plasma sodium decreases approximately 1.6 mEq/L.

Hypernatremia is nearly always the result of either a loss of water in excess of sodium (hypotonic fluid loss) or the retention of large quantities of sodium. Even when renal concentrating ability is impaired, thirst is normally highly effective in preventing hypernatremia. Hypernatremia is therefore most commonly seen in debilitated patients who are unable to drink, the very aged, the very young, and patients with altered consciousness. Patients with hypernatremia may have a low, normal, or high total body sodium content (Table 28–4).

Hypernatremia & Low Total Body Sodium Content

These patients have lost both sodium and water, but the water loss is in excess of the sodium loss. Hypotonic

Table 28–4. Major causes of hypernatremia.

Impaired thirst
  Coma
  Essential hypernatremia
Solute diuresis
  Osmotic diuresis: diabetic ketoacidosis, nonketotic hyperosmolar coma, mannitol administration
Excessive water losses
  Renal
    Pituitary diabetes insipidus
    Nephrogenic diabetes insipidus
  Extrarenal
    Sweating
Combined disorders
  Coma plus hypertonic nasogastric feeding

---

losses can be renal (osmotic diuresis) or extrarenal (diarrhea or sweat). In either case, patients usually manifest signs of hypovolemia (see Chapter 29). Urinary sodium concentration is generally greater than 20 mEq/L with renal losses, and less than 10 mEq/L with extrarenal losses.

Hypernatremia & Normal Total Body Sodium Content

This group of patients generally manifests signs of water loss without overt hypovolemia unless the water loss is massive. Total body sodium content is generally normal. Nearly pure water losses can occur via the skin, respiratory tract, or kidneys. Occasionally transient hypernatremia is observed with movement of water into cells following exercise, seizures, or rhabdomyolysis. The most common cause of hypernatremia with a normal total body sodium content is **diabetes insipidus** (in conscious individuals). Diabetes insipidus is characterized by marked impairment in renal concentrating ability that is due either to decreased ADH secretion (central diabetes insipidus) or failure of the renal tubules to respond normally to circulating ADH (nephrogenic diabetes insipidus). Rarely, "essential hypernatremia" may be encountered in patients with central nervous system disorders. These patients appear to have reset osmoreceptors that function at a higher baseline osmolality.

A. CENTRAL DIABETES INSIPIDUS:

Lesions in or around the hypothalamus and the pituitary stalk frequently produce diabetes insipidus. Diabetes insipidus frequently develops with brain death. Transient diabetes insipidus is also commonly seen following neurosurgical procedures and head trauma (see Chapter 26). The diagnosis is suggested by a history of polydipsia, polyuria (often > 6 L/d), and the absence of hyperglycemia. In the perioperative setting, the diagnosis of diabetes insipidus is suggested by marked polyuria without glycosuria and a urinary osmolality lower than plasma osmolality. The absence of thirst in unconscious individuals leads to marked water losses and can rapidly produce hypovolemia. The diagnosis of central diabetes insipidus is confirmed by an increase in urinary osmolality following the administration of exogenous ADH. Aqueous vasopressin (5 U SC q4h) is the treatment of choice for acute central diabetes insipidus. Vasopressin in oil (0.3 mL IM qd) is longerlasting but is more likely to cause water intoxication. Desmopressin (DDAVP), a synthetic analogue of ADH with a 12- to 24-hour duration of action, is available as an intranasal preparation (5–10 mg qd or bid) that can be used both in the ambulatory and perioperative settings.

B. NEPHROGENIC DIABETES INSIPIDUS:

Nephrogenic diabetes insipidus can be congenital but is more commonly secondary to other disorders. These include chronic renal disease, certain electrolyte disorders (hypokalemia and hypercalcemia), and a variety of other disorders (sickle cell disease, hyperproteinemias). Nephrogenic diabetes insipidus can also be secondary to the side effects of some drugs (amphotericin B, lithium, demeclocycline, ifosfamide, mannitol). ADH secretion in all the above patients is normal, but the kidneys fail to respond to ADH. Urinary concentrating ability is therefore impaired. The mechanism may be either a decreased response to circulating ADH or interference with the renal countercurrent mechanism (see Chapter 31). The diagnosis is confirmed by failure of the kidneys to produce a hypertonic urine following the administration of exogenous ADH. Treatment is generally directed at the underlying illness and ensuring an adequate fluid intake. Volume depletion by a thiazide diuretic can paradoxically decrease urinary output by reducing water delivery to collecting tubules. Sodium and protein restriction can similarly reduce urinary output.

Hypernatremia & Increased Total Body Sodium Content

This condition most commonly results from the administration of large quantities of hypertonic saline solutions (3% NaCl or 7.5% $NaHCO_3$). Patients with primary hyperaldosteronism and Cushing's syndrome may also have small elevations in serum sodium concentration along with signs of increased sodium retention.

Clinical Manifestations of Hypernatremia

Neurologic manifestations predominate in patients with hypernatremia and are generally thought to result from cellular dehydration. Restlessness, lethargy, and hyperreflexia can progress to seizures, coma, and ultimately death. Symptoms correlate more closely with the rate of movement of water out of brain cells than with the absolute level of hypernatremia. Rapid decreases in brain volume can rupture cerebral veins and result in focal intracerebral or subarachnoid hemorrhage. Seizures and serious neurologic damage are common, especially in children with acute hypernatremia when plasma $[Na^+]$ exceeds 158 mEq/L. Chronic hypernatremia is generally better tolerated than the acute form. After 24–48 hours, intracellular osmolality begins to rise as a result of increases in intracellular inositol and amino acid (glutamine and taurine) concentrations. As intracellular solute concentration increases, neuronal water content slowly returns to normal.

Treatment of Hypernatremia

The treatment of hypernatremia is aimed at restoring plasma osmolality to normal as well as correcting the underlying problem. Water deficits should generally be corrected over 48 hours with a hypotonic solution such as 5% dextrose in water (see below). Abnormalities in extracellular volume must also be corrected (Figure 28–3). Hypernatremic patients with decreased total body sodium should be given isotonic fluids to restore plasma volume to normal *prior* to treatment with a hypotonic solution. Hypernatremic patients with increased total body sodium should be treated with a loop diuretic along with intravenous 5% dextrose in water. The treatment of diabetes insipidus is discussed above.

Rapid correction of hypernatremia can result in seizures, brain edema, permanent neurologic damage, and even death. Serial serum osmolalities should be obtained during treatment. In general, plasma sodium concentration should not be decreased faster than 0.5 mEq/L/hour.

EXAMPLE:

A 70-kg man is found to have a plasma $[Na^+]$ of 160 mEq/L. What is his water deficit?

If one assumes that the hypernatremia is from water loss only, then total body osmoles are unchanged. Thus, assuming he had a normal $[Na^+]$ of 140 mEq/L and a TBW content that is 60% of body weight:

$$\text{Normal TBW} \times 140 = \text{present TBW} \times [Na^+]_{plasma},$$
$$\text{or } (70 \times 0.6) \times 140 = \text{present TBW} \times 160$$

Solving the equation:

$$\text{Present TBW} = 36.7 \text{ L}$$
$$\text{Water deficit} = \text{normal TBW} - \text{present TBW},$$
$$\text{or } (70 \times 0.6) - 36.7 = 5.3 \text{ L}$$

To replace this deficit over 48 hours, one would give 5% dextrose in water intravenously, 5300 mL over 48 hours, or 110 mL/hour.

Note that this method ignores any coexisting isotonic fluid deficits, which if present should be replaced with an isotonic solution.

Anesthetic Considerations

Hypernatremia increases the minimum alveolar concentration for inhalational anesthetics in animal studies, but its clinical significance is more closely related to the associated fluid deficits. Hypovolemia accentuates any vasodilation or cardiac depression from anesthetic agents and predisposes to hypotension and hypoperfusion of tissues. Decreases in the volume of distribution for drugs necessitate dose reductions for most intravenous agents, while decreases in cardiac output enhance the uptake of inhalational anesthetics.

Elective surgery should be postponed in patients with significant hypernatremia (> 150 mEq/L) until the cause is established and fluid deficits are corrected. Both water and isotonic fluid deficits should be completely corrected prior to surgery.

HYPO-OSMOLALITY & HYPONATREMIA

Hypo-osmolality is nearly always associated with hyponatremia ($[Na^+]$ < 135 mEq/L). Table 28–5 lists rare instances in which hyponatremia does not necessarily

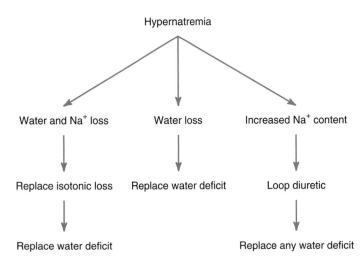

Figure 28–3. Algorithm for treatment of hypernatremia.

Table 28–5. Causes of pseudohyponatremia.

Hyponatremia with a normal plasma osmolality
 Asymptomatic
  Marked hyperlipidemia
  Marked hyperproteinemia
 Symptomatic
  Marked glycine absorption during transurethral surgery
Hyponatremia with an elevated plasma osmolality
 Hyperglycemia
 Administration of mannitol

Adapted from Rose RD: *Clinical Physiology of Acid-Base and Electrolyte Disorders,* 3rd ed. McGraw-Hill, 1989.

reflect hypo-osmolality (pseudohyponatremia). Routine measurement of plasma osmolality in hyponatremic patients rapidly excludes pseudohyponatremia.

Hyponatremia invariably reflects water retention from either an absolute increase in TBW or a loss of sodium in excess of water. The kidneys' normal capacity to produce dilute urine with an osmolality as low as 40 mOsm/kg (specific gravity 1.001) allows them to excrete over 10 L of free water per day if necessary. Because of this tremendous reserve, hyponatremia is nearly always the result of a defect in urinary diluting capacity (urinary osmolality > 100 mOsm/kg or specific gravity > 1.003). Rare instances of hyponatremia without an abnormality in renal diluting capacity (urinary osmolality < 100 mOsm/kg) are generally attributed to primary polydipsia or "reset" osmoreceptors; the latter two conditions can be differentiated by water restriction.

Clinically, hyponatremia is best classified according to total body sodium content (Table 28–6). Hyponatremia associated with transurethral resection of the prostate is discussed in Chapter 33.

Hyponatremia & Low Total Body Sodium

Progressive losses of both sodium and water eventually lead to extracellular volume depletion. As the intravascular volume deficit reaches 5–10%, nonosmotic ADH secretion is activated (see above). With further volume depletion, the stimuli for nonosmotic ADH release overcome any hyponatremia-induced suppression of ADH. Preservation of circulatory volume takes place at the expense of plasma osmolality.

Fluid losses resulting in hyponatremia may be renal or extrarenal in origin. Renal losses are most commonly related to thiazide diuretics and result in a urinary [Na$^+$] greater than 20 mEq/L. Extrarenal losses are typically gastrointestinal and usually produce a urine [Na$^+$] of less than 10 mEq/L. A major exception to the latter

is hyponatremia due to vomiting, which can result in a urinary [Na$^+$] greater than 20 mEq/L. In those instances, bicarbonaturia from the associated metabolic alkalosis (see Chapter 30) obligates concomitant excretion of Na$^+$ with HCO$_3^-$ to maintain electrical neutrality in the urine; urinary chloride concentration, however, is usually less than 10 mEq/L.

Hyponatremia & Increased Total Body Sodium

Edematous disorders are characterized by an increase in both total body sodium and TBW. When the increase in water exceeds that in sodium, hyponatremia occurs. Edematous disorders include congestive heart failure, cirrhosis, renal failure, and nephrotic syndrome. Hyponatremia in these settings results from progressive impairment of renal free water excretion and generally parallels underlying disease severity. Pathophysiologic mechanisms include nonosmotic ADH release and decreased delivery of fluid to the distal diluting segment in nephrons (see Chapter 31). The "effective" circulating blood volume is reduced (see below).

Hyponatremia With Normal Total Body Sodium

Hyponatremia in the absence of edema or hypovolemia may be seen with glucocorticoid insufficiency, hypothyroidism, drug therapy (chlorpropamide and cyclophosphamide), and the syndrome of inappropriate

Table 28–6. Classification of hyponatremia.

Decreased total sodium content
 Renal
  Diuretics
  Mineralocorticoid deficiency
  Salt-losing nephropathies
  Osmotic diuresis (glucose, mannitol)
  Renal tubular acidosis
 Extrarenal
  Vomiting
  Diarrhea
  "Third-spacing"
Normal total sodium content
 Syndrome of inappropriate antidiuretic hormone
 Glucocorticoid deficiency
 Hypothyroidism
 Drug-induced
Increased total sodium content
 Congestive heart failure
 Cirrhosis
 Nephrotic syndrome

antidiuretic hormone secretion (SIADH). The hyponatremia associated with adrenal hypofunction may be due to cosecretion of ADH with corticotropin releasing factor (CRF). Patients with AIDS often exhibit hyponatremia which may due to adrenal infection by cytomegalovirus or mycobacteria. Diagnosis of SIADH requires exclusion of other causes of hyponatremia and the absence of hypovolemia, edema, and adrenal, renal, or thyroid disease. A variety of malignant tumors, pulmonary diseases, and central nervous system disorders are commonly associated with SIADH. In most such instances, plasma ADH concentration is not elevated but is inadequately suppressed relative to the degree of hypo-osmolality in plasma; urine osmolality is usually > 100 mOsm/kg and urine sodium concentration is > 40 mEq/L.

Clinical Manifestations of Hyponatremia

Symptoms of hyponatremia are primarily neurologic and result from an increase in intracellular water. Their severity is generally related to the rapidity with which extracellular hypo-osmolality develops. Patients with mild to moderate hyponatremia ([Na$^+$] > 125 mEq/L) are frequently asymptomatic. Early symptoms are typically nonspecific and may include anorexia, nausea, and weakness. Progressive cerebral edema, however, results in lethargy, confusion, seizures, coma, and finally death. Serious manifestations are generally associated with plasma sodium concentrations less than 120 mEq/L. Compared with men, premenopausal women appear to be at greater risk of neurologic impairment and damage from hyponatremia.

Patients with slowly developing or chronic hyponatremia are generally less symptomatic. A gradual compensatory loss of intracellular solutes (primarily Na$^+$, K$^+$, and amino acids) appears to restore cell volume to normal. Neurologic symptoms in patients with chronic hyponatremia may be related more closely to changes in cell membrane potential (due to a low extracellular [Na$^+$]) than to changes in cell volume.

Treatment of Hyponatremia

As with hypernatremia, the treatment of hyponatremia (Figure 28–4) is directed at correcting both the underlying disorder as well as the plasma [Na$^+$]. Isotonic saline (see Chapter 29) is generally the treatment of choice for hyponatremic patients with decreased total body sodium content. Once the extracellular fluid deficit is corrected, spontaneous water diuresis returns plasma [Na$^+$] to normal. Conversely, water restriction is the primary treatment for hyponatremic patients with normal or increased total body sodium. More specific

treatments such as hormonal replacement in patients with adrenal or thyroid hypofunction and measures aimed at improving cardiac output in patients with heart failure (see Chapter 20) may also be indicated. Demeclocycline, a drug that antagonizes ADH activity at the renal tubules, has proved to be a useful adjunct to water restriction in the treatment of patients with SIADH.

Acute symptomatic hyponatremia requires prompt treatment. In such instances, correction of plasma [Na$^+$] to > 125 mEq/L is usually sufficient to alleviate symptoms. The amount of NaCl necessary to raise plasma [Na$^+$] to the desired value, the **Na$^+$ deficit,** can be estimated by the following formula:

$$\text{Na}^+ \text{ deficit} = \text{TBW} \times (\text{desired } [\text{Na}^+] - \text{present } [\text{Na}^+])$$

 Very rapid correction of hyponatremia has been associated with demyelinating lesions in the pons (**central pontine myelinolysis**), resulting in serious permanent neurologic sequelae. The rapidity with which hyponatremia is corrected should be tailored to the severity of symptoms. The following correction rates have been suggested: for mild symptoms, 0.5 mEq/L/hour or less; for moderate symptoms, 1 mEq/L/hour or less; and for severe symptoms, 1.5 mEq/L/hour or less.

EXAMPLE:

An 80-kg woman is lethargic and is found to have a plasma [Na$^+$] of 118 mEq/L. How much NaCl must be given to raise her plasma [Na$^+$] to 130 mEq/L?

$$\text{Na}^+ \text{ deficit} = \text{TBW} \times (130 - 118)$$

TBW is approximately 50% of body weight in females:

$$\text{Na}^+ \text{ deficit} = 80 \times 0.5 \times (130 - 118) = 480 \text{ mEq}$$

Since normal (isotonic) saline contains 154 mEq/L, the patient should receive 480 mEq ÷ 154 mEq/L, or 3.12 L of normal saline. For a correction rate of 0.5 mEq/L/hour, this amount of saline should be given over 24 hours (130 mL/hour).

Note that this calculation does not take into account any coexisting isotonic fluid deficits, which, if present, should also be replaced.

More rapid correction of hyponatremia can be achieved by giving a loop diuretic to induce water diuresis while replacing urinary sodium losses with isotonic saline. Even more rapid corrections can be achieved with intravenous hypertonic saline (3% NaCl). Hypertonic saline may be indicated in markedly symptomatic patients with a plasma [Na$^+$] less than 110

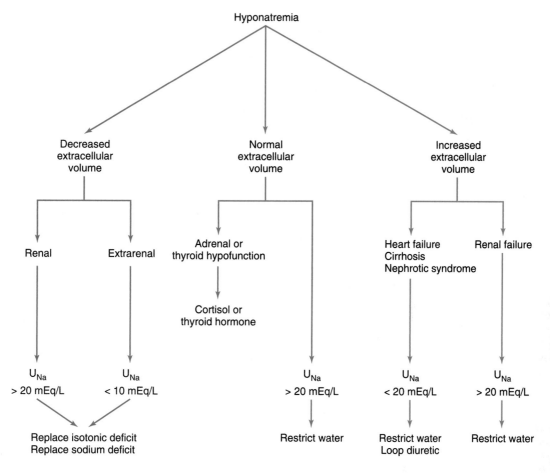

Figure 28–4. Algorithm for treatment of hyponatremia.

mEq/L. Three percent NaCl should be given cautiously since it can precipitate pulmonary edema, hypokalemia, hyperchloremic metabolic acidosis, and transient hypotension; bleeding has been associated with prolongation of the prothrombin time and activated partial thromboplastin time.

Anesthetic Considerations

Hyponatremia is often a manifestation of a serious underlying disorder and requires careful evaluation preoperatively. Plasma sodium concentrations above 130 mEq/L are generally considered safe for patients undergoing general anesthesia. Plasma $[Na^+]$ should be corrected above 130 mEq/L for all elective procedures, even in the absence of symptoms. Lower concentrations may result in significant cerebral edema that can be

manifested intraoperatively as a decrease in minimum alveolar concentration or postoperatively as agitation, confusion, or somnolence. Patients undergoing transurethral resection of the prostate can absorb significant amounts of water from irrigation fluids (as much as 20 mL/min) and are at high risk for rapid development of profound acute water intoxication (see Chapter 33).

■ DISORDERS OF SODIUM BALANCE

Extracellular fluid volume is directly proportionate to total body sodium content. Variations in ECF volume result from changes in total body sodium content. A positive sodium balance increases ECF volume, while a negative sodium balance decreases ECF volume. It is important to reemphasize that *extracellular (plasma) sodium concentration is more indicative of water balance than total body sodium content.*

NORMAL SODIUM BALANCE

Net sodium balance is equal to total sodium intake (adults average 170 mEq/d) minus both renal sodium excretion and extrarenal sodium losses. (One gram of sodium yields 43 mEq of sodium ions, whereas 1 g of sodium chloride yields 17 mEq of sodium ions.) The kidneys' ability to vary urinary sodium excretion from less than 1 mEq/L to more than 100 mEq/L allows them to play a critical role in sodium balance (see Chapter 31).

REGULATION OF SODIUM BALANCE & EXTRACELLULAR FLUID VOLUME

Because of the relationship between ECF volume and total body sodium content, regulation of one is intimately tied to the other. This regulation is achieved via sensors (see below) that detect changes in the most important component of ECF, namely, the "effective" intravascular volume. The latter correlates more closely with the rate of perfusion in renal capillaries than with measurable intravascular fluid (plasma) volume. Indeed, with edematous disorders (heart failure, cirrhosis, and renal failure), "effective" intravascular volume can be independent of the measurable plasma volume, ECF volume, and even cardiac output.

Extracellular fluid volume and total body sodium content are ultimately controlled by appropriate adjustments in renal sodium excretion. In the absence of renal disease, diuretic therapy, and selective renal ischemia, urinary sodium concentration reflects "effective" intravascular volume. A low urine sodium concentration (< 10 mEq/L) is therefore generally indicative of a low "effective" intravascular fluid volume and reflects secondary retention of sodium by the kidneys.

Control Mechanisms

The multiple mechanisms involved in regulating ECF volume and sodium balance normally complement one another but can function completely independently of one another. In addition to altering renal sodium excretion, some mechanisms also produce more rapid compensatory hemodynamic responses when "effective" intravascular volume is reduced (see Chapter 19).

A. SENSORS OF VOLUME:

The principal volume receptors in the body are really baroreceptors. Since blood pressure is the product of cardiac output and systemic vascular resistance (see Chapter 19), significant changes in intravascular volume (preload) not only affect cardiac output but also transiently affect arterial blood pressure. Thus, the baroreceptors at the carotid sinus and afferent renal arterioles (juxtaglomerular apparatus) indirectly function as sensors of intravascular volume. Changes in blood pressure at the carotid sinus modulate sympathetic nervous system activity and nonosmotic ADH secretion, while changes at the afferent renal arterioles modulate the renin-angiotensin-aldosterone system. Stretch receptors in both atria are also known to sense changes in intravascular volume; the degree of atrial distention modulates the release of atrial natriuretic hormone and ADH.

B. EFFECTORS OF VOLUME CHANGE:

Regardless of the mechanism, effectors of volume change ultimately alter urinary sodium excretion. Decreases in "effective" intravascular volume decrease urinary sodium excretion, while increases in the "effective" intravascular volume increase urinary sodium excretion. These mechanisms include the following:

1. Renin-angiotensin-aldosterone—Renin secretion increases the formation of angiotensin II. The latter increases the secretion of aldosterone and has some direct effect in enhancing sodium reabsorption in the proximal renal tubules. Angiotensin II is also a potent direct vasoconstrictor and potentiates the actions of norepinephrine. Aldosterone secretion enhances sodium reabsorption in the distal nephron (see Chapter 31) and is a major determinant of urinary sodium excretion.

2. Atrial natriuretic peptide (ANP)—This peptide is normally released from both right and left atrial cells following atrial distention. Atrial natriuretic peptide appears to have two major actions: arterial vasodilation and increased urinary sodium and water excretion in the renal collecting tubules. ANP-mediated afferent arteriolar dilation and efferent arteriolar constriction can also increase GFR. Other reported effects include the inhibition of both renin and aldosterone secretion and antagonism of ADH.

3. Pressure natriuresis—Even small elevations of blood pressure can result in a relatively large increase in urinary sodium excretion. Pressure diuresis appears to be independent of any known humorally or neurally mediated mechanism.

4. Sympathetic nervous system activity—Enhanced sympathetic activity increases sodium reabsorption in the proximal renal tubules, resulting in sodium retention, and mediates renal vasoconstriction, which reduces renal blood flow (see Chapter 31). Conversely, stimulation of left atrial stretch receptors results in decreases in renal sympathetic tone and increases renal blood flow (cardiorenal reflex) and, potentially, glomerular filtration.

5. Glomerular filtration rate and plasma sodium concentration—The amount of sodium filtered in the kidneys is directly proportionate to the product of the GFR and plasma sodium concentration. Since GFR is generally directly proportionate to intravascular volume, intravascular volume expansion can increase sodium excretion. Conversely, intravascular volume depletion decreases sodium excretion.

6. Tubuloglomerular balance—Despite wide variations in the amount of sodium filtered in nephrons, sodium reabsorption in the proximal renal tubules is normally controlled within narrow limits. Factors considered to be responsible for tubuloglomerular balance include the rate of renal tubular flow and changes in peritubular capillary hydrostatic and oncotic pressures. Altered sodium reabsorption in the proximal tubules can have a marked effect on renal sodium excretion.

7. Antidiuretic hormone—Although ADH secretion has little effect on sodium excretion, nonosmotic secretion of this hormone (see above) can play an important part in maintaining extracellular volume with moderate to severe decreases in the "effective" intravascular volume.

Extracellular Osmoregulation Versus Volume Regulation

Osmoregulation protects the normal ratio of solutes to water, whereas extracellular volume regulation preserves absolute solute and water content. Differences between the two mechanisms are highlighted in Table 28–7. As noted previously, volume regulation generally takes precedence over osmoregulation.

Anesthetic Implications

Problems related to altered sodium balance result from its manifestations as well as the underlying disorder. Disorders of sodium balance present either as hypovolemia (sodium deficit) or hypervolemia (sodium excess). Both disturbances require correction prior to elective surgical procedures. Cardiac, liver, and renal function should also be carefully evaluated in the presence of sodium excess (generally manifested as tissue edema).

Hypovolemic patients are sensitive to the vasodilating and negative inotropic effects of the volatile anesthetics, barbiturates, and agents associated with histamine release (morphine, meperidine, curare, atracurium). Dosage requirements for other drugs must also be reduced to compensate for decreases in their volume of distribution. Hypovolemic patients are especially sensitive to sympathetic blockade from spinal or epidural anesthesia. If an anesthetic must be administered prior to complete correction of the hypovolemia, ketamine may be the induction agent of choice for general anesthesia; etomidate may be a suitable alternative.

Table 28–7. Osmoregulation versus volume regulation.

	Volume Regulation	**Osmoregulation**
Purpose	Control extracellular volume	Control extracellular osmolality
Mechanism	Vary renal Na$^+$ excretion	Vary water intake Vary renal water excretion
Sensors	Afferent renal arterioles Carotid baroreceptors Atrial stretch receptors	Hypothalamic osmoreceptors
Effectors	Renin-angiotensin-aldosterone Sympathetic nervous system Tubuloglomerular balance Renal pressure natriuresis Atrial natriuresis peptide Antidiuretic hormone	Thirst Antidiuretic hormone

Adapted from Rose RD: *Clinical Physiology of Acid-Base and Electrolyte Disorders,* 3rd ed. McGraw-Hill, 1989.

Hypervolemia should generally be corrected pre-operatively with diuretics. Abnormalities in cardiac, renal, and hepatic function should also be corrected whenever possible. The major hazard of increases in extracellular volume is impaired gas exchange due to pulmonary interstitial edema, alveolar edema, or large collections of pleural or ascitic fluid.

DISORDERS OF POTASSIUM BALANCE

Potassium plays a major role in the electrophysiology of cell membranes (see Chapter 19) as well as carbohydrate and protein synthesis (see below). The resting cell membrane potential is normally dependent on the ratio of intracellular to extracellular potassium concentrations. Intracellular potassium concentration is estimated to be 140 mEq/L, while extracellular potassium concentration is normally about 4 mEq/L. Although the regulation of intracellular $[K^+]$ is poorly understood, extracellular $[K^+]$ generally reflects the balance between potassium intake and excretion.

Under some conditions (see below), a redistribution of K^+ between the ECF and ICF compartments can result in marked changes in extracellular $[K^+]$ without a change in total body potassium content.

NORMAL POTASSIUM BALANCE

Dietary potassium intake averages 80 mEq/d in adults (range, 40–140 mEq/d). About 70 mEq of that amount is normally excreted in urine while the remaining 10 mEq is lost through the gastrointestinal tract.

Renal excretion of potassium can vary from as little as 5 mEq/L to over 100 mEq/L. Nearly all the potassium filtered in glomeruli is normally reabsorbed in the proximal tubule and the loop of Henle. The potassium excreted in urine is the result of distal tubular secretion. Potassium secretion in the distal tubules is coupled to aldosterone-mediated reabsorption of sodium (see Chapter 31).

REGULATION OF EXTRACELLULAR POTASSIUM CONCENTRATION

Extracellular potassium concentration is closely regulated by cell membrane Na^+-K^+-ATPase activity as well as plasma $[K^+]$. The former regulates the distribution of potassium between cells and ECF, while the latter is the major determinant of urinary potassium excretion.

INTERCOMPARTMENTAL SHIFTS OF POTASSIUM

Intercompartmental shifts of potassium are known to occur following changes in extracellular pH (see Chapter 30), circulating insulin levels, circulating catecholamine activity, plasma osmolality, and possibly hypothermia. Insulin and catecholamines are known to directly affect Na^+-K^+-ATPase activity and decrease plasma $[K^+]$. Exercise can also transiently increase plasma $[K^+]$ as a result of the release of K^+ by muscle cells; the increase in plasma $[K^+]$ (0.3–2 mEq/L) is proportionate to the intensity and duration of muscle activity. Intercompartmental potassium shifts are also thought to be responsible for changes in plasma $[K^+]$ in syndromes of periodic paralysis (see Chapter 37).

Changes in extracellular hydrogen ion concentration (pH) directly affect extracellular $[K^+]$ because the ICF may buffer up to 60% of an acid load (see Chapter 30). During acidosis, extracellular hydrogen ions enter cells, displacing intracellular potassium ions; the movement of potassium ions out of cells maintains electrical balance but increases extracellular and plasma $[K^+]$. Conversely, during alkalosis, extracellular potassium ions move into cells to balance the movement of hydrogen ions out of cells; as a result, plasma $[K^+]$ decreases. Although the relationship can be quite variable, a useful rule of thumb is that plasma potassium concentration changes approximately 0.6 mEq/L per 0.1 unit change in arterial pH (range 0.2–1.2 mEq/L per 0.1 unit).

Changes in circulating insulin levels can directly alter plasma $[K^+]$ independent of glucose transport. Insulin enhances the activity of membrane-bound Na^+-K^+-ATPase, increasing cellular uptake of potassium in the liver and in skeletal muscle. In fact, insulin secretion may play an important role in the basal control of plasma potassium concentration and facilitates the handling of increased potassium loads.

Sympathetic stimulation also increases intracellular uptake of potassium by enhancing Na^+-K^+-ATPase activity. This effect is mediated through activation of β_2-adrenergic receptors. In contrast α-adrenergic activity may impair the intracellular movement of K^+. Plasma $[K^+]$ often decreases following the administration of β_2-adrenergic agonists as a result of uptake of potassium by muscle and the liver. Moreover, β-adrenergic blockade can impair the handling of a potassium load in some patients.

Acute increases in plasma osmolality (hypernatremia, hyperglycemia, or mannitol administration) are reported to increase plasma $[K^+]$ (about 0.6 mEq/L per 10 mOsm/L). In such instances, the movement of water out of cells (down its osmotic gradient) is accompanied by movement of K^+ out of cells. The latter may be the result of "solvent drag" or the increase in intracellular [K⁺] that follows cellular dehydration.

Hypothermia has been reported to lower plasma [K⁺] as a result of cellular uptake. Rewarming reverses this shift and may result in transient hyperkalemia if potassium was given during the hypothermia.

Urinary Excretion of Potassium

Urinary potassium excretion generally parallels its extracellular concentration. Potassium is secreted by tubular cells in the distal nephron (see Chapter 31). Extracellular [K⁺] is a major determinant of aldosterone secretion from the adrenal gland. Hyperkalemia stimulates aldosterone secretion, while hypokalemia suppresses aldosterone secretion. Renal tubular flow in the distal nephron may also be an important determinant of potassium secretion because high tubular flow rates (as during osmotic diuresis) increase potassium secretion by keeping the capillary to renal tubular gradient for potassium secretion high. Conversely, slow tubular flow rates increase [K⁺] in tubular fluid and decrease the gradient for K⁺ secretion.

Table 28–8. Major causes of hypokalemia.

Excess renal loss
Mineralocorticoid
Bartter's syndrome
Diuresis
Chronic metabolic alkalosis
Antibiotics
Carbenicillin
Gentamicin
Amphotericin B
Renal tubular acidosis
Distal, gradient-limited
Proximal
Liddle's syndrome
Ureterosigmoidostomy
Gastrointestinal losses
Vomiting
Diarrhea, particularly secretory diarrheas
ECF → ICF shifts
Acute alkalosis
Hypokalemic periodic paralysis
Barium ingestion
Insulin therapy
Vitamin B₁₂ therapy
Thyrotoxicosis (rarely)
Inadequate intake

HYPOKALEMIA

Hypokalemia is defined as plasma [K⁺] less than 3.5 mEq/L and can occur as a result of (1) an intercompartmental shift of K⁺ (see above), (2) increased potassium loss, or (3) an inadequate potassium intake (Table 28–8). Plasma potassium concentration typically correlates poorly with the total potassium deficit. A decrease in plasma [K⁺] from 4 mEq/L to 3 mEq/L usually represents a 100- to 200-mEq deficit, while a plasma [K⁺] below 3 mEq/L can represent a deficit anywhere between 200 mEq and 400 mEq.

Hypokalemia Due to the Intracellular Movement of Potassium

Hypokalemia due to the intracellular movement of potassium occurs with alkalosis, insulin therapy, β₂-adrenergic agonists, hypothermia, and during attacks of hypokalemic periodic paralysis (see above). Hypokalemia may also be seen following transfusion of frozen red cells; these cells lose potassium in the preservation process and take up potassium following reinfusion. Cellular K⁺ uptake by red blood cells (and platelets) also accounts for the hypokalemia seen in patients recently treated with folate or vitamin B₁₂ for megaloblastic anemia.

Hypokalemia Due to Increased Potassium Losses

Increased potassium losses are nearly always either renal or gastrointestinal. Renal wasting of potassium is most commonly the result of a diuresis or enhanced mineralocorticoid activity. Other renal causes include hypomagnesemia (see below), renal tubular acidosis (see Chapter 30), ketoacidosis, salt-wasting nephropathies, and some drug therapies (carbenicillin and amphotericin B). Increased gastrointestinal loss of potassium is most commonly due to vomiting, nasogastric suctioning, or diarrhea. Other gastrointestinal causes include losses from fistulae, laxative abuse, villous adenomas, and pancreatic tumors secreting vasoactive intestinal peptide.

Chronic increased sweat formation occasionally causes hypokalemia, especially when potassium intake is limited. Dialysis with a low-potassium-containing dialysate solution can also cause hypokalemia. Uremic patients may actually have a total body potassium deficit (primarily intracellular) despite a normal or even high plasma concentration; the absence of hypokalemia in these instances is probably due to an intercompartmental shift from the acidosis. Dialysis in these patients unmasks the total body potassium deficit and often results in hypokalemia.

Table 28–9. Effects of hypokalemia.

Cardiovascular
  Electrocardiographic changes/dysrhythmias
  Myocardial dysfunction
Neuromuscular
  Skeletal muscle weakness
  Tetany
  Rhabdomyolysis
  Ileus
Renal
  Polyuria (nephrogenic DI)
  Increased ammonia production
  Increased bicarbonate reabsorption
Hormonal
  Decreased insulin secretion
  Decreased aldosterone secretion
Metabolic
  Negative nitrogen balance
  Encephalopathy in patients with liver disease

Adapted from Schrier RW, ed: *Renal and Electrolyte Disorders,* 3rd ed. Little, Brown and Company, 1986.

A urinary [K$^+$] less than 20 mEq/L is generally indicative of increased extrarenal losses, while concentrations greater than 20 mEq/L suggest renal wasting of K$^+$.

Hypokalemia Due to Decreased Potassium Intake

Because of the kidney's ability to decrease urinary potassium excretion to as low as 5–20 mEq/L, marked reductions in potassium intake are required to produce hypokalemia. Low potassium intakes, however, often accentuate the effects of increased potassium losses.

Clinical Manifestations of Hypokalemia

Hypokalemia can produce widespread organ dysfunction (Table 28–9). Most patients are asymptomatic until plasma [K$^+$] falls below 3 mEq/L. Cardiovascular effects are most prominent and include an abnormal electrocardiogram (ECG), arrhythmias, decreased cardiac contractility, and a labile arterial blood pressure due to autonomic dysfunction. Chronic hypokalemia has also been reported to cause myocardial fibrosis. ECG manifestations are primarily due to delayed ventricular repolarization and include T-wave flattening and inversion, an increasingly prominent U wave, ST-segment depression, increased P-wave amplitude, and prolongation of the P–R interval (Figure 28–5). Increased myocardial cell automaticity and delayed repolarization promote both atrial and ventricular dysrhythmias.

Neuromuscular effects of hypokalemia include skeletal muscle weakness (especially the quadriceps), ileus, muscle cramping, tetany, and, rarely, rhabdomyolysis. Hypokalemia induced by diuretics is often associated with metabolic alkalosis; as the kidneys absorb sodium to compensate for intravascular volume depletion and in the presence of diuretic-induced hypochloremia, bicarbonate is absorbed. The end result is hypokalemia and hypochloremic metabolic alkalosis. Renal dysfunction is seen due to impaired concentrating ability (resistance to ADH, resulting in polyuria)

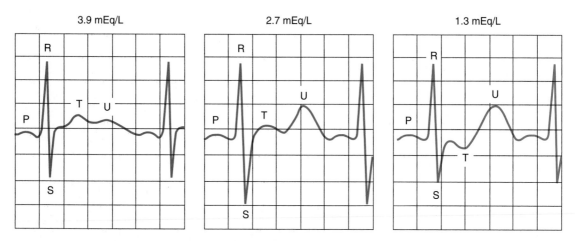

Figure 28–5. Electrocardiographic effects of hypokalemia. Note progressive flattening of the T wave, an increasingly prominent U wave, increased amplitude of the P wave, prolongation of the P–R interval, and ST-segment depression.

and increased production of ammonia resulting in impairment of urinary acidification. Increased ammonia production represents intracellular acidosis; hydrogen ions move intracellularly to compensate for intracellular potassium losses. The resulting metabolic alkalosis, together with increased ammonia production, can precipitate encephalopathy in patients with advanced liver disease. Chronic hypokalemia has been associated with renal fibrosis (tubulointerstitial nephropathy).

Treatment of Hypokalemia

The treatment of hypokalemia depends on the presence and severity of any associated organ dysfunction. Significant ECG changes such as ST-segment changes or dysrhythmias mandate continuous ECG monitoring, especially during intravenous K^+ replacement. Digoxin therapy—as well as the hypokalemia itself—sensitizes the heart to changes in potassium ion concentration. Muscle strength should also be periodically assessed in patients with weakness.

Oral replacement with potassium chloride solutions is generally safest (60–80 mEq/d). Replacement of the potassium deficit usually requires several days. Intravenous replacement should usually be reserved for patients with or at risk for serious cardiac manifestations or muscle weakness. The goal of intravenous therapy is to remove the patient from immediate danger and not necessarily to correct the entire potassium deficit. Peripheral intravenous replacement should not exceed 8 mEq/hour because of the irritative effect of potassium on peripheral veins. Dextrose-containing solutions should generally be avoided, because the resulting hyperglycemia and secondary insulin secretion may actually lower plasma $[K^+]$ even further. Faster intravenous replacement (10–20 mEq/hour) requires a central venous catheter and close monitoring of the ECG. Higher replacement rates may be safest through a femoral catheter, because very high localized K^+ concentrations may occur within the heart with standard central venous catheters. Intravenous replacement should generally not exceed 240 mEq/d.

Potassium chloride is the preferred potassium salt when a metabolic alkalosis is also present because it also corrects the chloride deficit discussed above. Potassium bicarbonate or equivalent (K^+ acetate or K^+ citrate) is preferable for patients with metabolic acidosis. Potassium phosphate is a suitable alternative with concomitant hypophosphatemia (diabetic ketoacidosis).

Anesthetic Considerations

Hypokalemia is a common preoperative finding. This decision to proceed with elective surgery is often arbi-

trarily based on lower limits somewhere between 3 and 3.5 mEq/L. The decision, however, should be based also on the rate at which the hypokalemia developed as well as the presence or absence of secondary organ dysfunction. In general, chronic mild hypokalemia (3–3.5 mEq/L) without ECG changes does not appear to substantially increase anesthetic risk. The latter may not apply to patients receiving digoxin, who may be at increased risk of developing digoxin toxicity from the hypokalemia; plasma $[K^+]$ values above 4 mEq/L are desirable in such patients.

The intraoperative management of hypokalemia requires vigilant ECG monitoring. Intravenous potassium should be given if atrial or ventricular dysrhythmias develop. Glucose-free intravenous solutions should be used and hyperventilation avoided to prevent further decreases in plasma $[K^+]$. Increased sensitivity to neuromuscular blocking agents (also called muscle relaxants) may be seen in some patients. Dosages of neuromuscular blocking agents should therefore be reduced 25–50%, and a nerve stimulator should be used to follow the degree of paralysis and the adequacy of reversal.

HYPERKALEMIA

Hyperkalemia exists when plasma $[K^+]$ exceeds 5.5 mEq/L. Hyperkalemia rarely occurs in normal individuals because of the kidney's tremendous capacity to excrete potassium. When potassium intake is increased slowly, the kidneys can excrete as much as 500 mEq of K^+ per day. The sympathetic system and insulin secretion also appear to play important roles in preventing acute increases in plasma $[K^+]$ following potassium loads.

Hyperkalemia can result from (1) an intercompartmental shift of potassium ions, (2) decreased urinary excretion of potassium, or, rarely, (3) an increased potassium intake (Table 28–10). Measurements of plasma potassium concentration can be spuriously elevated if red cells hemolyze in a blood specimen (most commonly due to prolonged application of a tourniquet while obtaining a venous sample). In vitro release of potassium from white cells in a blood specimen can also falsely indicate increased levels in the measured plasma $[K^+]$ when the leukocyte count exceeds $70,000 \times 10^9$/L. A similar release of potassium from platelets occurs when the platelet count exceeds $1,000,000 \times 10^9$/L.

Hyperkalemia Due to Extracellular Movement of Potassium

Movement of K^+ out of cells can be seen with succinylcholine administration, acidosis, cell lysis following chemotherapy, hemolysis, rhabdomyolysis, massive tissue trauma, hyperosmolality, digitalis overdoses, arginine hydrochloride administration, β_2-adrenergic

Table 28–10. Causes of hyperkalemia.

Pseudohyperkalemia
  Red cell hemolysis
  Marked leukocytosis/thrombocytosis
Intercompartmental shifts
  Acidosis
  Hypertonicity
  Rhabdomyolysis
  Severe exercise
  Periodic paralysis
  Succinylcholine
Decreased renal potassium excretion
  Renal failure
  Decreased mineralocorticoid activity
    Acquired immunodeficiency syndrome
    Competitive potassium-sparing diuretics
      Spironolactone
    ACE inhibitors
    Cyclosporine
    Nonsteroidal anti-inflammatory drugs
Increased potassium intake
  Salt substitutes

ACE = angiotensin-converting enzyme.

blockade, and during episodes of hyperkalemic periodic paralysis. The average increase in plasma [K^+] of 0.5 mEq/L following succinylcholine can be exaggerated following large burns or severe muscle trauma and in patients with spinal cord injuries (see Chapter 9). β_2-Adrenergic blockade accentuates the increase in plasma [K^+] that occurs following exercise. Digitalis inhibits Na^+-K^+ ATPase in cell membranes; digitalis overdose has been reported to cause hyperkalemia in some patients. Arginine hydrochloride, which is used to treat metabolic alkalosis, can cause hyperkalemia as the cationic arginine ions enter cells and potassium ions move out to maintain electroneutrality.

Hyperkalemia Due to Decreased Renal Excretion of Potassium

Decreased renal excretion of potassium can result from (1) marked reductions in glomerular filtration, (2) decreased aldosterone activity, or (3) a defect in potassium secretion in the distal nephron.

Glomerular filtration rates less than 5 mL/min are nearly always associated with hyperkalemia. Patients with lesser degrees of renal impairment can also readily develop hyperkalemia when faced with increased potassium loads (dietary, catabolic, or iatrogenic). Uremia may also impair Na^+-K^+-ATPase activity.

Hypokalemia due to decreased aldosterone activity can result from a primary defect in adrenal hormone

synthesis or a defect in the renin-aldosterone system. Patients with primary adrenal insufficiency (Addison's disease) and those with isolated 21-hydroxylase adrenal enzyme deficiency have marked impairment of aldosterone synthesis. Patients with the syndrome of isolated hypoaldosteronism (also called hyporeninemic hypoaldosteronism, or type IV renal tubular acidosis) are usually diabetics with some degree of renal impairment; they appear to have an impaired ability to increase aldosterone secretion in response to hyperkalemia. Although usually asymptomatic, these patients develop hyperkalemia when they increase their potassium intake or when given potassium-sparing diuretics. They also often have varying degrees of Na^+ wasting and a hyperchloremic metabolic acidosis. Similar findings have been reported in some patients with AIDS who may have relative adrenal insufficiency (due to cytomegalovirus infection).

Drugs interfering with the renin-aldosterone system have the potential to cause hyperkalemia, especially in the presence of any degree of renal impairment. Nonsteroidal anti-inflammatory drugs (NSAIDs) inhibit prostaglandin-mediated renin release. Angiotensin-converting enzyme (ACE) inhibitors interfere with angiotensin II-mediated release of aldosterone. Large doses of heparin can interfere with aldosterone secretion. The potassium-sparing diuretic spironolactone directly antagonizes aldosterone activity at the kidneys.

Decreased renal excretion of potassium can also occur as a result of an intrinsic or acquired defect in the distal nephron's ability to secrete potassium. Such defects may occur even in the presence of normal renal function and are characteristically unresponsive to mineralocorticoid therapy. The kidneys of patients with pseudohypoaldosteronism display an intrinsic resistance to aldosterone. Acquired defects have been associated with systemic lupus erythematosus, sickle cell anemia, obstructive uropathies, and cyclosporine nephropathy in transplanted kidneys.

Hyperkalemia Due to Increased Potassium Intake

Increased potassium loads rarely cause hyperkalemia in normal individuals unless large amounts are given rapidly and intravenously. Hyperkalemia, however, may be seen when potassium intake is increased in patients receiving β-blockers or those with renal impairment or insulin deficiency. Unrecognized sources of potassium include potassium penicillin, sodium substitutes (primarily potassium salts), and transfusion of stored whole blood. The plasma [K^+] in a unit of whole blood can increase to 30 mEq/L after 21 days of storage. The risk of hyperkalemia from multiple transfusions is reduced (but not eliminated) by minimizing the volume of plasma given through the use of packed red blood cell transfusions (see Chapter 29).

Clinical Manifestations of Hyperkalemia

The most important effects of hyperkalemia are on skeletal and cardiac muscle. Skeletal muscle weakness is generally not seen until plasma $[K^+]$ is greater than 8 mEq/L. The weakness is due to sustained spontaneous depolarization and inactivation of Na^+ channels of muscle membrane (similar to succinylcholine), eventually resulting in ascending paralysis. Cardiac manifestations (Figure 28–6) are primarily due to delayed depolarization and consistently present when plasma $[K^+]$ is greater than 7 mEq/L. ECG changes characteristically progress (in order) from symmetrically peaked T waves (often with a shortened QT interval) → widening of the QRS complex → prolongation of the P–R interval → loss of the P wave → loss of R-wave amplitude → ST-segment depression (occasionally elevation) → an ECG that resembles a sine wave—before progression to ventricular fibrillation and asystole. Contractility appears to be relatively well preserved. Hypocalcemia, hyponatremia, and acidosis accentuate the cardiac effects of hyperkalemia.

Treatment of Hyperkalemia

Because of its lethal potential, hyperkalemia exceeding 6 mEq/L should always be treated. Treatment is directed at reversing cardiac

manifestations, and skeletal muscle weakness, and restoring of plasma $[K^+]$ to normal. The number of treatment modalities employed (see below) depends on the severity of manifestations as well as the cause of hyperkalemia. Hyperkalemia associated with hypoaldosteronism can be treated with mineralocorticoid replacement. Drugs contributing to hyperkalemia should be discontinued and sources of increased potassium intake reduced or stopped.

Calcium (5–10 mL of 10% calcium gluconate or 3–5 mL of 10% calcium chloride) partially antagonizes the cardiac effects of hyperkalemia and is useful in patients with marked hyperkalemia. Its effects are rapid but unfortunately short-lived. Care must be exercised in patients taking digoxin, since calcium potentiates digoxin toxicity.

When metabolic acidosis is present, intravenous sodium bicarbonate (usually 45 mEq) will promote cellular uptake of potassium and can decrease plasma $[K^+]$ within 15 minutes. β-Agonists promote cellular uptake of potassium and may be useful in acute hyperkalemia associated with massive transfusions (see Chapter 29); low doses of epinephrine (0.5–2 mg/min) often rapidly decrease plasma $[K^+]$ and provide inotropic support in this setting. An intravenous infusion of glucose and insulin (30–50 g of glucose per 10 units of insulin) is also effective in promoting cellular uptake of potassium and lowering plasma $[K^+]$, but often takes up to 1 hour for peak effect.

For patients with some renal function, furosemide is a useful adjunct in increasing urinary excretion of

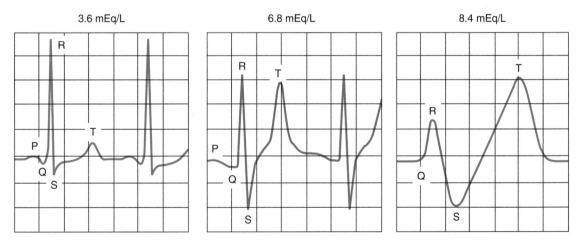

Figure 28–6. Electrocardiographic effects of hyperkalemia. Electrocardiographic changes characteristically progress from symmetrically peaked T waves, often with a shortened QT interval, to widening of the QRS complex, prolongation of the P–R interval, loss of the P wave, loss of R-wave amplitude, and ST-segment depression (occasionally elevation)—to an ECG that resembles a sine wave—before final progression into ventricular fibrillation or asystole.

potassium. In the absence of renal function, elimination of excess potassium can only be accomplished with nonabsorbable cation exchange resins such as oral or rectal sodium polystyrene sulfonate (Kayexalate). Each gram of resin binds up to 1 mEq of K^+ and releases 1.5 mEq of Na^+; the oral dose is 20 g in 100 mL of 20% sorbitol.

Dialysis is indicated in symptomatic patients with severe or refractory hyperkalemia. Hemodialysis is faster and more effective than peritoneal dialysis in decreasing plasma $[K^+]$. Maximal potassium removal with hemodialysis approaches 50 mEq/hour, compared with 10–15 mEq/hour for peritoneal dialysis.

Anesthetic Considerations

Elective surgery should not be undertaken in patients with hyperkalemia. Anesthetic management of hyperkalemic surgical patients is directed at both lowering the plasma potassium concentration and preventing any further increases. The ECG should be carefully monitored. Succinylcholine is contraindicated, as is the use of any potassium-containing intravenous solutions such as lactated Ringer's injection. The avoidance of metabolic or respiratory acidosis is critical to prevent further increases in plasma $[K^+]$. Ventilation should be controlled under general anesthesia; mild hyperventilation may even be desirable. Lastly, neuromuscular function should be monitored closely, since hyperkalemia can accentuate the effects of neuromuscular blocking agents.

◾ DISORDERS OF CALCIUM BALANCE

Although 98% of total body calcium is in bone, maintenance of a normal extracellular calcium concentration is critical to homeostasis. Calcium ions are involved in nearly all essential biologic functions, including muscle contraction, the release of neurotransmitters and hormones, blood coagulation, and bone metabolism. It is not surprising that abnormalities in calcium balance can result in profound physiologic derangements.

NORMAL CALCIUM BALANCE

Calcium intake in adults averages 600–800 mg/d. Intestinal absorption of calcium occurs primarily in the proximal small bowel but is quite variable. Calcium is also secreted into the intestinal tract; moreover, this secretion appears to be constant and independent of absorption. Up to 80% of the daily calcium intake is normally lost in feces.

The kidneys are responsible for calcium excretion. Renal calcium excretion averages 100 mg/d but can be varied from as low as 50 mg/d to more than 300 mg/d. Normally, 98% of the filterable calcium is reabsorbed. Calcium reabsorption parallels that of sodium in the proximal renal tubules and the ascending loop of Henle. In the distal tubules, however, calcium reabsorption is dependent on parathyroid hormone secretion, while sodium reabsorption is dependent on aldosterone secretion. Increased parathyroid hormone levels enhance distal calcium reabsorption and decrease urinary calcium excretion.

Plasma Calcium Concentration

The normal plasma calcium concentration is 8.5–10.5 mg/dL (2.1–2.6 mmol/L). Approximately, 50% is in the free ionized form, 40% is protein-bound (mainly to albumin), and 10% is complexed with anions such as citrate and amino acids. It is the free ionized calcium concentration ($[Ca^{2+}]$) that is physiologically most important. Plasma $[Ca^{2+}]$ is normally 4.75–5.3 mg/dL (2.38–2.66 mEq/L or 1.19–1.33 mmol/L). Changes in plasma albumin concentration affect total but not ionized calcium concentrations: for each increase or decrease of 1 g/dL in albumin, the total plasma calcium concentration increases or decreases approximately 0.8–1.0 mg/dL, respectively.

Changes in plasma pH directly affect the degree of protein binding and thus ionized calcium concentration. Ionized calcium increases approximately 0.16 mg/dL for each decrease of 0.1 unit in plasma pH and decreases by the same amount for each 0.1 unit increase in pH.

Regulation of Extracellular Ionized Calcium Concentration

Calcium normally enters extracellular fluid by either absorption from the intestinal tract or resorption of bone; only 0.5–1% of calcium in bone is exchangeable with extracellular fluid. In contrast, calcium normally leaves the extracellular compartment by: (1) deposition into bone, (2) urinary excretion, (3) secretion into the intestinal tract, and (4) sweat formation. Extracellular $[Ca^{2+}]$ is closely regulated by three hormones: parathyroid hormone, vitamin D, and calcitonin. These hormones act primarily on bone, the distal renal tubules, and the small bowel.

PTH is the most important regulator of plasma $[Ca^{2+}]$. Decreases in plasma $[Ca^{2+}]$ stimulate PTH secretion, while increases in plasma $[Ca^{2+}]$ inhibit PTH secretion. The calcemic effect of parathyroid hormone is due to (1) mobilization of calcium from bone, (2) enhancement of calcium reabsorption in the distal renal tubules, and (3) an indirect increase in intestinal absorption of calcium via acceleration of 1,25-dihydroxycholecalciferol synthesis in the kidneys (see below).

Vitamin D exists in several forms in the body, but 1,25-dihydroxycholecalciferol has the most important biologic activity. It is the product of the metabolic conversion of (primarily endogenous) cholecalciferol, first by the liver to 25-cholecalciferol and then by the kidneys to 1,25-dihydroxycholecalciferol. The latter transformation is enhanced by secretion of parathyroid hormone as well as hypophosphatemia. Vitamin D augments intestinal absorption of calcium, facilitates the action of parathyroid hormone on bone, and appears to augment renal reabsorption of calcium in the distal tubules.

Calcitonin is a polypeptide hormone that is secreted by parafollicular cells in the thyroid gland. Its secretion is stimulated by hypercalcemia and inhibited by hypocalcemia. Calcitonin inhibits bone reabsorption and increases urinary calcium excretion.

HYPERCALCEMIA

Hypercalcemia can occur as a result of a variety of disorders (Table 28–11). In primary hyperparathyroidism, parathyroid hormone secretion is increased and independent of $[Ca^{2+}]$. In contrast, in secondary hyperparathyroidism (chronic renal failure or malabsorption), the elevated parathyroid hormone levels are in response to chronic hypocalcemia (see Chapter 32). Prolonged secondary hyperparathyroidism, however, can occasionally result in autonomous secretion of

Table 28–11. Causes of hypercalcemia.

Hyperparathyroidism
Malignancy
Excessive vitamin D intake
Paget's disease of bone
Granulomatous disorders (sarcoidosis, tuberculosis)
Chronic immobilization
Milk-alkali syndrome
Adrenal insufficiency
Drug-induced
    Thiazide diuretics
    Lithium

PTH, resulting in a normal or elevated $[Ca^{2+}]$ (tertiary hyperparathyroidism).

Patients with cancer can present with hypercalcemia whether or not bone metastases are present. Direct bony destruction or secretion of humoral mediators of hypercalcemia (PTH-like substances, cytokines, or prostaglandins) is probably responsible in most patients. Hypercalcemia due to increased turnover of calcium from bone can also be encountered in patients with benign conditions such as Paget's disease and chronic immobilization. Increased gastrointestinal absorption of calcium can lead to hypercalcemia in patients with the milk-alkali syndrome (marked increase in calcium intake), hypervitaminosis D, or granulomatous diseases (enhanced sensitivity to vitamin D). The mechanisms responsible for other causes of hypercalcemia are poorly understood.

Clinical Manifestations of Hypercalcemia

Hypercalcemia often produces anorexia, nausea, vomiting, weakness, and polyuria. Ataxia, irritability, lethargy, or confusion can rapidly progress to coma. Hypertension is often present initially before hypovolemia supervenes. ECG signs include a shortened ST segment and a shortened QT interval. Hypercalcemia increases cardiac sensitivity to digitalis. Pancreatitis, peptic ulcer disease, and renal failure can also complicate hypercalcemia.

Treatment of Hypercalcemia

 Symptomatic hypercalcemia requires rapid treatment. The most effective initial treatment is rehydration followed by a brisk diuresis (urinary output 200–300 mL/hour) with administration of intravenous saline infusion and a loop diuretic to accelerate calcium excretion. Premature diuretic therapy prior to rehydration may aggravate the hypercalcemia by additional volume depletion. Renal loss of potassium and magnesium usually occurs during diuresis, and laboratory monitoring and intravenous replacement should be performed as necessary. Although hydration and diuresis may remove the potential risk of cardiovascular and neurologic complications of hypercalcemia, the serum calcium usually remains elevated above normal. Additional therapy with a bisphosphonate or calcitonin may be required to further lower the serum calcium. Severe hypercalcemia (> 15 mg/dL) usually requires additional therapy after saline hydration and lasix calciuresis. Biphosphonates (pamidronate 60–90 mg intravenously) or calcitonin (2–8 U/kg subcutaneously) are preferred agents. Pamidronate has become the agent of choice in this setting because of its prolonged duration of action, but it likely should be avoided in the setting of renal insufficiency (serum creatinine > 2.5 mg/dL). Dialysis may be necessary in the presence of renal or cardiac failure. Additional treatment depends on the underlying cause of the hypercalcemia and may include glucocorticoids in the setting of vitamin D–induced hypercalcemia such as granulomatous disease states. The use of older agents such as plicamycin (mithramycin) or phosphates is seldom used today because of their potential adverse effects.

It is necessary to look for the underlying etiology and direct appropriate treatment toward the cause of the hypercalcemia once the initial threat of hypercalcemia has been removed. Approximately 90% of all hypercalcemia is due to either malignancy or hyperparathyroidism. The best laboratory test for discriminating between these two main categories of hypercalcemia is the double-antibody parathyroid hormone (PTH) assay. The serum PTH concentration will usually be suppressed in malignancy states and elevated in hyperparathyroidism.

Anesthetic Considerations

Hypercalcemia is a medical emergency and should be corrected, if possible, prior to administration of any anesthetic. Ionized calcium levels should be monitored closely. If surgery must be performed, saline diuresis should be continued intraoperatively with great care to avoid hypovolemia; central venous or pulmonary artery pressure monitoring may be advisable for patients with decreased cardiac reserve. Serial measurements of $[K^+]$ and $[Mg^{2+}]$ are helpful in detecting iatrogenic hypokalemia and hypomagnesemia. Responses to anesthetic agents are not predictable. Ventilation should be controlled under general anesthesia. Acidosis should be avoided so as not to raise plasma $[Ca^{2+}]$ any further.

HYPOCALCEMIA

Hypocalcemia should be diagnosed only on the basis of the plasma ionized calcium concentration. When direct measurements of plasma $[Ca^{2+}]$ are not available, the total calcium concentration must be corrected for decreases in plasma albumin concentration (see above). The causes of hypocalcemia are listed in Table 28–12.

Hypocalcemia due to hypoparathyroidism is a relatively common cause of symptomatic hypocalcemia. Hypoparathyroidism may be surgical, idiopathic, part of multiple endocrine defects (most often with adrenal insufficiency), or associated with hypomagnesemia. Magnesium deficiency is postulated to impair the secretion of PTH and antagonize its effects on bone. Hypocalcemia during sepsis is also thought to be due to suppression of parathyroid hormone release. Hyper-

Table 28–12. Causes of hypocalcemia.

Hypoparathyroidism
Pseudohypoparathyroidism
Vitamin D deficiency
  Nutritional
  Malabsorption
    Postsurgical (gastrectomy, short bowel)
    Inflammatory bowel disease
  Altered vitamin D metabolism
Hyperphosphatemia
Precipitation of calcium
  Pancreatitis
  Rhabdomyolysis
  Fat embolism
Chelation of calcium
  Multiple rapid red blood transfusions or rapid infusion of large amounts of albumin

phosphatemia (see below) is also a relatively common cause of hypocalcemia, especially in patients with chronic renal failure. Hypocalcemia due to vitamin D deficiency may be the result of a markedly reduced intake (nutritional), vitamin D malabsorption, or abnormal vitamin D metabolism.

Chelation of calcium ions with the citrate ions in blood preservatives is an important cause of perioperative hypocalcemia; similar transient decreases in $[Ca^{2+}]$ are also theoretically possible following rapid infusions of large volumes of albumin. Hypocalcemia following acute pancreatitis is thought to be due to precipitation of calcium with fats (soaps) following the release of lipolytic enzymes and fat necrosis; hypocalcemia following fat embolism may have a similar basis. Precipitation of calcium (in injured muscle) may also be seen following rhabdomyolysis.

Less common causes of hypocalcemia include calcitonin-secreting medullary carcinomas of the thyroid, osteoblastic metastatic disease (breast and prostate cancer), and pseudohypoparathyroidism (familial unresponsiveness to parathyroid hormone). Transient hypocalcemia may also be seen following heparin, protamine, or glucagon administration and massive blood transfusion (from citrate).

Clinical Manifestations of Hypocalcemia

Manifestations include paresthesias, confusion, laryngeal stridor (laryngospasm), carpopedal spasm (Trousseau's sign), masseter spasm (Chvostek's sign), and seizures. Biliary colic and bronchospasm have also been described. Cardiac irritability can lead to dysrhythmias. Decreased cardiac contractility may result in heart failure, hypotension, or both. Decreased responsiveness to digitalis and β-adrenergic agonists have also been reported. ECG signs include prolongation of the QT interval. The severity of ECG manifestations does not necessarily correlate with the degree of hypocalcemia.

Treatment of Hypocalcemia

 Symptomatic hypocalcemia is a medical emergency and should be treated immediately with intravenous calcium chloride (3–5 mL of a 10% solution) or calcium gluconate (10–20 mL of a 10% solution). (Ten milliliters of 10% $CaCl_2$ contains 272 mg of Ca^{2+}, whereas 10 mL of 10% calcium gluconate contains only 93 mg of Ca^{2+}). To avoid precipitation, intravenous calcium should not be given with bicarbonate- or phosphate-containing solutions. Serial ionized calcium measurements are mandatory. Repeat boluses or a continuous infusion (Ca^{2+} 1–2 mg/kg/hour) may be necessary. Plasma magnesium concentration should be checked to exclude hypomagnesemia. In chronic hypocalcemia, oral calcium ($CaCO_3$) and vitamin D replacement are usually necessary. Treatment for hyperphosphatemia is discussed below.

Anesthetic Considerations

Hypocalcemia should be corrected preoperatively. Serial ionized calcium levels should be monitored intraoperatively in patients with a history of hypocalcemia. Alkalosis should be avoided to prevent further decreases in $[Ca^{2+}]$. Intravenous calcium may be necessary following rapid transfusions of citrated blood products or large volumes of albumin solutions (see Chapter 29). Potentiation of the negative inotropic effects of barbiturates and volatile anesthetics should be expected. Responses to neuromuscular blocking agents are inconsistent and require close monitoring with a nerve stimulator.

■ DISORDERS OF PHOSPHORUS BALANCE

Phosphorus is an important intracellular constituent. Its presence is required for the synthesis of (1) the phospholipids and phosphoproteins in cell membranes and intracellular organelles, (2) the phosphonucleotides involved in protein synthesis and reproduction, and (3) ATP used for the storage of energy. Only 0.1% of total body phosphorus is in extracellular fluid; 85% is in bone and 15% is intracellular.

NORMAL PHOSPHORUS BALANCE

Phosphorus intake averages 800–1500 mg/d in adults. About 80% of that amount is normally absorbed in the proximal small bowel. Vitamin D increases intestinal absorption of phosphorus. The kidneys are the major route for phosphorus excretion and are responsible for regulating total body phosphorus content. Urinary excretion of phosphorus depends on both intake and plasma concentration. Parathyroid hormone secretion can augment urinary phosphorus excretion by inhibiting its proximal tubular reabsorption. The latter effect may be offset by PTH-induced release of phosphate from bone.

Plasma Phosphorus Concentration

Plasma phosphorus exists in both organic and inorganic forms. Organic phosphorus is mainly in the form of phospholipids. Of the inorganic phosphorus fraction, 80% is filterable in the kidneys, while 20% is protein-bound. The majority of inorganic phosphorus is in the form of $H_2PO_4^-$ and HPO_4^{2-} in a 1:4 ratio. By convention, plasma phosphorus is measured as milligrams of elemental phosphorus. Normal plasma phosphorus concentration is 2.5–4.5 mg/dL (0.8–1.45 mmol/L) in adults and up to 6 mg/dL in children. Plasma phosphorus concentration is usually measured during fasting, because a recent carbohydrate intake transiently decreases the plasma phosphorus concentration. Hypophosphatemia increases vitamin D production, while hyperphosphatemia depresses it. The latter plays an important role in the genesis of secondary hyperparathyroidism in patients with chronic renal failure (see Chapter 32).

HYPERPHOSPHATEMIA

Hyperphosphatemia may be seen with increased phosphorus intakes (abuse of phosphate laxatives or excessive potassium phosphate administration), decreased phosphorus excretion (renal insufficiency), or massive cell lysis (following chemotherapy for lymphoma or leukemia).

Clinical Manifestations of Hyperphosphatemia

Although hyperphosphatemia itself does not appear to be directly responsible for any functional disturbances, its secondary effect on plasma $[Ca^{2+}]$ can be important. Marked hyperphosphatemia is thought to lower plasma $[Ca^{2+}]$ by precipitation and deposition of calcium phosphate in bone and soft tissues.

Treatment of Hyperphosphatemia

Hyperphosphatemia is generally treated with phosphate-binding antacids such as aluminum hydroxide or aluminum carbonate.

Anesthetic Considerations

While specific interactions between hyperphosphatemia and anesthesia are generally not described, renal function should be carefully evaluated (see Chapter 32). Secondary hypocalcemia should also be excluded.

HYPOPHOSPHATEMIA

Hypophosphatemia is usually the result of either a negative phosphorus balance or cellular uptake of extracellular phosphorus (an intercompartmental shift). Intercompartmental shifts of phosphorus can occur during alkalosis and following carbohydrate ingestion or insulin administration. Large doses of aluminum- or magnesium-containing antacids, severe burns, inadequate phosphorus supplementation during hyperalimentation, diabetic ketoacidosis, alcohol withdrawal, and prolonged respiratory alkalosis can all produce a negative phosphorus balance and lead to severe hypophosphatemia (< 0.3 mmol/dL or < 1.0 mg/dL). In contrast to respiratory alkalosis, metabolic alkalosis rarely leads to severe hypophosphatemia.

Clinical Manifestations of Hypophosphatemia

Mild to moderate hypophosphatemia (1.5–2.5 mg/dL) is generally asymptomatic. In contrast, severe hypophosphatemia (< 1.0 mg/dL) is often associated with widespread organ dysfunction. Cardiomyopathy, impaired oxygen delivery (decreased 2,3-diphosphoglycerate levels), hemolysis, impaired leukocyte function, platelet dysfunction, encephalopathy, skeletal myopathy, respiratory failure, rhabdomyolysis, skeletal demineralization, metabolic acidosis, and hepatic dysfunction have all been associated with severe hypophosphatemia.

Treatment of Hypophosphatemia

Oral phosphorus replacement is generally preferable to parenteral replacement because of the risk of hypocalcemia and metastatic calcification. Potassium or sodium phosphate (2–5 mg of elemental phosphorus per kilogram, or 10–45 mmol slowly over 6–12 hours) is generally used for intravenous correction of severe symptomatic hypophosphatemia.

Anesthetic Considerations

Anesthetic management of patients with hypophosphatemia requires familiarity with its complications (see above). Hyperglycemia and respiratory alkalosis should be avoided to prevent further decreases in plasma phosphorus concentration. Neuromuscular function must be monitored carefully when neuromuscular blocking agents are given. Some patients with severe hypophosphatemia may require mechanical ventilation postoperatively.

■ DISORDERS OF MAGNESIUM BALANCE

Magnesium is an important intracellular cation that functions as a cofactor in many enzyme pathways. Only 1–2% of total body magnesium stores are in the ECF compartment; 67% is contained in bone while the remaining 31% is intracellular.

NORMAL MAGNESIUM BALANCE

Magnesium intake averages 20–30 mEq/d (240–370 mg/d) in adults. Of that amount, only 30–40% is absorbed, mainly in the distal small bowel. Renal excretion is the primary route for elimination, averaging 6–12 mEq/d. Magnesium reabsorption by the kidneys is very efficient. Twenty-five percent of filtered magnesium is reabsorbed in the proximal tubule while 50–60% is reabsorbed in the thick ascending limb of the loop of Henle. Factors known to increase magnesium reabsorption in the kidneys include hypomagnesemia, parathyroid hormone, hypocalcemia, ECF depletion, and metabolic alkalosis. Factors known to increase renal excretion include hypermagnesemia, acute volume expansion, hyperaldosteronism, hypercalcemia, ketoacidosis, diuretics, phosphate depletion, and alcohol ingestion.

Plasma Magnesium Concentration

Plasma [Mg^{2+}] is closely regulated between 1.7 and 2.1 mEq/L (0.7–1 mmol/L or 1.7–2.4 mg/dL). Although the exact mechanisms involved remain unclear, they involve interaction of the gastrointestinal tract (absorption), bone (storage), and the kidneys (excretion). Approximately 50–60% of plasma magnesium is unbound and diffusible.

HYPERMAGNESEMIA

Increases in plasma $[Mg^{2+}]$ are nearly always due to excessive intake (magnesium-containing antacids or laxatives), renal impairment (GFR < 30 mL/min), or both. Iatrogenic hypermagnesemia can also occur during magnesium sulfate therapy for gestational hypertension in the mother as well as the fetus. Less common causes include adrenal insufficiency, hypothyroidism, rhabdomyolysis, and lithium administration.

Clinical Manifestations of Hypermagnesemia

Symptomatic hypermagnesemia typically presents with neurologic, neuromuscular, or cardiac manifestations. Hyporeflexia, sedation, and skeletal muscle weakness are characteristic features. Hypermagnesemia appears to impair the release of acetylcholine and decreases motor end-plate sensitivity to acetylcholine in muscle. Vasodilation, bradycardia, and myocardial depression can lead to hypotension at levels > 10 mmol/dL (> 24 mg/dL). ECG signs are inconsistent but often include prolongation of the P–R interval and widening of the QRS complex. Marked hypermagnesemia can lead to respiratory arrest.

Treatment of Hypermagnesemia

All sources of magnesium intake (most often antacids) should be stopped. Intravenous calcium (1 g calcium gluconate) can temporarily antagonize most of the effects of hypermagnesemia. A loop diuretic along with an infusion of 1/2-normal saline in 5% dextrose enhances urinary magnesium excretion. Diuresis with normal saline is generally not recommended to lessen the likelihood of iatrogenic hypocalcemia, because the latter potentiates the effects of hypermagnesemia. Dialysis may be necessary in patients with marked renal impairment.

Anesthetic Considerations

Hypermagnesemia requires close monitoring of the ECG, blood pressure, and neuromuscular function. Potentiation of the vasodilating and negative inotropic properties of anesthetics should be expected. Dosages of neuromuscular blocking agents should be reduced by 25–50%. A urinary catheter is required when diuretic and saline infusions are used to enhance magnesium excretion (see above). Serial measurements of $[Ca^{2+}]$ and $[Mg^{2+}]$ may be useful.

HYPOMAGNESEMIA

Hypomagnesemia is a common and frequently overlooked problem, especially in critically ill patients. Associated deficiencies of other intracellular components such as potassium and phosphorus are common. Deficiencies of magnesium are generally the result of inadequate intake, reduced gastrointestinal absorption, or increased renal excretion (Table 28–13). β-Adrenergic agonists may cause transient hypomagnesemia as the ion is taken up by adipose tissues. Drugs that cause renal wasting of magnesium include ethanol, theophylline, diuretics, cisplatin, aminoglycosides, cyclosporine, amphotericin B, pentamidine, and granulocyte colony stimulating factor.

Clinical Manifestations of Hypomagnesemia

Most patients with hypomagnesemia are asymptomatic, but anorexia, weakness, fasciculation, paresthesias, confusion, ataxia, and seizures may be encountered. Hypomagnesemia is frequently associated with both hypocalcemia (impaired parathyroid hormone secretion) and hypokalemia (due to renal K^+ wasting). Cardiac manifestations include electrical irritability and potentiation of digoxin toxicity; both factors are aggravated by hypokalemia. Hypomagnesemia is associated with an increased incidence of atrial fibrillation. Prolongation of

Table 28–13. Causes of hypomagnesemia.

Inadequate intake
Nutritional
Reduced gastrointestinal absorption
Malabsorption syndromes
Small bowel or biliary fistulas
Prolonged nasogastric suctioning
Severe diarrhea
Increased renal losses
Diuresis
Diabetic ketoacidosis
Hyperparathyroidism
Hyperaldosteronism
Hypophosphatemia
Drugs
Postobstructive diuresis
Multifactorial
Chronic alcoholism
Protein-calorie malnutrition
Hyperthyroidism
Pancreatitis
Burns

the P–R and QT intervals may also be present and usually reflects concomitant hypocalcemia.

Treatment of Hypomagnesemia

Asymptomatic hypomagnesemia can be treated orally (magnesium sulfate heptahydrate or magnesium oxide) or intramuscularly (magnesium sulfate). Serious manifestations such as seizures should be treated with intravenous magnesium sulfate, 1–2 g (8–16 mEq or 4–8 mmol) given slowly over 15–60 minutes.

Anesthetic Considerations

Although no specific anesthetic interactions are described, coexistent electrolyte disturbances such as hypokalemia, hypophosphatemia, and hypocalcemia are often present and should be corrected prior to surgery (see above). Isolated hypomagnesemia should also be corrected prior to elective procedures because of its potential for causing cardiac arrhythmias. Moreover, magnesium appears to have intrinsic antiarrhythmic properties and possibly cerebral protective effects (see Chapter 25), such that it is increasingly being administered prior to coming off cardiopulmonary bypass.

CASE DISCUSSION: ELECTROLYTE ABNORMALITIES FOLLOWING URINARY DIVERSION

A 70-year-old man with carcinoma of the bladder presents for radical cystectomy and ileal loop urinary diversion. He weighs 70 kg and has a 20-year history of hypertension. Preoperative laboratory measurements revealed normal plasma electrolyte concentrations and a blood urea nitrogen (BUN) of 20 mg/dL with a serum creatinine of 1.5 mg/dL. The operation lasts 4 hours and is performed under uncomplicated general anesthesia. The estimated blood loss is 900 mL. Fluid replacement consists of 3500 mL of lactated Ringer's injection and 750 mL of 5% albumin.

One hour after admission to the recovery room, the patient is awake, his blood pressure is 130/70 mm Hg, and he appears to be breathing well (18 breaths/min, $FiO_2 = 0.4$). Urinary output has been only 20 mL in the last hour. Laboratory measurements are as follows: Hb, 10.4 g/dL; plasma Na^+, 133 mEq/L; K^+, 3.8 mEq/L; Cl^-, 104 mEq/L; total CO_2, 20 mmol/L; PaO_2, 156 mm Hg; arterial blood pH, 7.29; $PaCO_2$, 38 mm Hg; and calculated HCO_3^-, 18 mEq/L.

What is the most likely explanation for the hyponatremia?

Multiple factors tend to promote hyponatremia postoperatively, including nonosmotic ADH secretion (surgical stress, hypovolemia, and pain), large evaporative and functional fluid losses (tissue sequestration), and the administration of hypotonic intravenous fluids. Hyponatremia is especially common postoperatively in patients who have received relatively large amounts of lactated Ringer's injection (130 mEq/L); the postoperative plasma $[Na^+]$ generally approaches 130 mEq/L in such patients. (Fluid replacement in this patient was appropriate considering basic maintenance requirements, blood loss, and the additional fluid losses usually associated with this type of surgery; see Chapter 29.)

Why is the patient hyperchloremic and acidotic (normal arterial blood pH is 7.35–7.45)?

Operations for supravesical urinary diversion utilize a segment of bowel (ileum, ileocecal segment, jejunum, or sigmoid colon) that is made to function as a conduit or reservoir. The simplest and most common procedure utilizes an isolated loop of ileum as a conduit: the proximal end is anastomosed to the ureters, and the distal end is brought through the skin, forming a stoma.

Whenever urine comes in contact with bowel mucosa, the potential for significant fluid and electrolyte exchange exists. The ileum actively absorbs chloride in exchange for bicarbonate and sodium in exchange for potassium or hydrogen ions. When chloride absorption exceeds sodium absorption, plasma chloride concentration increases while plasma bicarbonate concentration decreases—a hyperchloremic metabolic acidosis is established. In addition, the colon absorbs NH_4^+ directly from urine; the latter may also be produced by urea-splitting bacteria. Hypokalemia results if significant amounts of Na^+ are exchanged for K^+. Potassium losses through the conduit are increased by high urinary sodium concentrations. Moreover, a potassium deficit may be present— even in the absence of hypokalemia—because movement of K^+ out of cells (secondary to the acidosis) can prevent an appreciable decrease in extracellular plasma $[K^+]$.

Are there any factors that tend to increase the likelihood of hyperchloremic metabolic acidosis following urinary diversion?

The longer the urine is in contact with bowel, the greater the chance that hyperchloremia and acidosis will occur. Mechanical problems such as poor emptying or redundancy of a conduit—along with hypovolemia—thus predispose to hyperchloremic metabolic acidosis. Preexisting renal impairment also appears to be a major risk factor and probably represents an inability to compensate for the excessive bicarbonate losses.

What treatment, if any, is required for this patient?

The ileal loop should be irrigated with saline—through the indwelling catheter or stent—to exclude partial obstruction and ensure free drainage of urine. Hypovolemia should be considered and treated based on central venous pressure measurements or the response to a fluid challenge (see Chapter 29). A mild to moderate systemic acidosis (arterial pH > 7.25) is generally well tolerated by most patients. Moreover, hyperchloremic metabolic acidosis following ileal conduits is often transient and usually due to urinary stasis. Persistent or more severe acidosis requires treatment with sodium bicarbonate. Potassium replacement may also be required if hypokalemia is present.

Are electrolyte abnormalities seen with other types of urinary diversion?

Procedures employing bowel as a conduit (ileal or colonic) are less likely to result in a hyper-chloremic metabolic acidosis than those where bowel functions as a reservoir. The incidence of hyperchloremic metabolic acidosis approaches 80% following ureterosigmoidostomies. In contrast, newer techniques for continent reservoirs such as the Kock pouch and Indiana pouch appear to be associated with a very low incidence of electrolyte abnormalities postoperatively.

SUGGESTED READING

Boldt J: Volume replacement in the surgical patient—does the type of fluid make a difference? Br J Anaesth 2000;84:783.

Kokko JP, Tannen RL: *Fluids and Electrolytes.* 3rd ed. Saunders, 1996.

Paradis OC: *Fluids and Electrolytes.* 2nd ed. Lippincott, 1999.

Vincent JL: Strategies in body fluid replacement. Minerva Anestesiol 2000;66:278.

Webb AR: The appropriate role of colloids in managing fluid imbalance: a critical review of recent meta-analytic findings. Crit Care (Lond) 2000;4(Suppl 2):S26–32.

Fluid Management & Transfusion

KEY CONCEPTS

 While the intravascular half-life of a crystalloid solution is 20–30 minutes, most colloid solutions have intravascular half-lives between 3 and 6 hours.

 Patients with a normal hematocrit should generally be transfused only after losses greater than 10–20% of their blood volume. The exact point is based on the patient's medical condition and the surgical procedure.

 The most severe transfusion reactions are due to ABO incompatibility; naturally acquired antibodies can react against the absent (foreign) antigens, activate complement, and result in intravascular hemolysis.

 In anesthetized patients, an acute hemolytic reaction is manifested by a rise in temperature, unexplained tachycardia, hypotension, hemoglobinuria, and diffuse oozing in the surgical field.

 Transfusion of leukocyte-containing blood products appears to be immunosuppressive.

 The current rate of transmission of the HIV virus by transfusion is estimated to be 1:200,000 transfusions.

 Immunocompromised and immunosuppressed patients (eg, premature infants and organ transplant recipients) are particularly susceptible to severe cytomegalovirus (CMV) infections through transfusions. Such patients should only receive CMV-negative units.

 The most common cause of bleeding following massive blood transfusion is dilutional thrombocytopenia.

 Clinically significant hypocalcemia, causing cardiac depression, does not occur in most normal patients unless the transfusion rate exceeds 1 U every 5 minutes.

 The most consistent abnormality after massive blood transfusion is postoperative metabolic alkalosis.

All patients except those undergoing the most minor surgical procedures require venous access and intravenous fluid therapy. Some require transfusion of blood or blood components. Maintenance of a normal intravascular volume is highly desirable in the perioperative period. The anesthesiologist should be able to assess intravascular volume accurately and to replace any fluid or electrolyte deficits and ongoing losses. Errors in fluid replacement or transfusion may result in considerable morbidity or even death.

■ EVALUATION OF INTRAVASCULAR VOLUME

Clinical evaluation of intravascular volume must generally be relied upon, because measurements of fluid compartment volumes are not readily available. Intravascular volume can be assessed using physical or laboratory examinations or with the aid of sophisticated hemodynamic monitoring techniques. Regardless of the method employed, serial evaluations are necessary to confirm initial impressions and guide fluid therapy. Moreover, modalities should complement one another, because all parameters are indirect, nonspecific measures of volume; reliance on any one parameter may be erroneous and, therefore, hazardous.

PHYSICAL EXAMINATION

Physical examination is most reliable preoperatively. Invaluable clues to hypovolemia (Table 29–1) include: skin turgor, the hydration of mucous membranes, palpation of a peripheral pulse, the resting heart rate and blood pressure and their (orthostatic) changes from the supine to sitting or standing positions, and urinary flow rate. Unfortunately, many drugs used during anesthesia, as well as the physiologic effects of surgical stress, alter these signs and render them unreliable in the immediate postoperative period. Intraoperatively, the fullness of a peripheral pulse (radial or dorsalis pedis), urinary flow rate, and indirect signs, such as the response of blood pressure to positive pressure ventilation and the vasodilating or negative inotropic effects of anesthetics are most often used.

Pitting edema—presacral in the bedridden patient or pretibial in the ambulatory patient—and increased urinary flow are signs of hypervolemia in patients with normal cardiac, hepatic, and renal function. Late signs of hypervolemia include tachycardia, pulmonary crackles, wheezing, cyanosis, and pink, frothy respiratory secretions.

LABORATORY EVALUATION

Several laboratory measurements may be used as surrogates of intravascular volume and adequacy of tissue perfusion. These include serial hematocrits, arterial blood pH, urinary specific gravity or osmolality, urinary sodium or chloride concentration, serum sodium, and the serum creatinine to blood urea nitrogen (BUN) ratio. These measurements are only indirect indices of intravascular volume and often cannot be relied upon intraoperatively because they are affected by many other variables and results are often delayed. Laboratory signs of dehydration include a rising hematocrit, a progressive metabolic acidosis, a urinary specific gravity greater than 1.010, a urinary sodium less than 10 mEq/L, a urinary osmolality greater than 450 mOsm/kg, hypernatremia, and a BUN to creatinine ratio greater than 10:1. Evidence of volume overload is not consistently present with these measurements; only radiographic signs of increased pulmonary vascular and interstitial markings (Kerly "B" lines) or diffuse alveolar infiltrates are reliable.

HEMODYNAMIC MEASUREMENTS

Hemodynamic monitoring is discussed in Chapter 6. Central venous pressure monitoring is indicated in patients with normal cardiac and pulmonary function when volume status is difficult to assess by other means or when rapid or major alterations are expected. Central venous pressure readings must be interpreted in light of the clinical setting. Low values (< 5 mm Hg) may be normal unless associated with other signs of hy-

Table 29–1. Signs of fluid loss (hypovolemia).

Sign	Fluid Loss (Expressed as Percentage of Body Weight)		
	5%	10%	15%
Mucous membranes	Dry	Very dry	Parched
Sensorium	Normal	Lethargic	Obtunded
Orthostatic changes	None	Present	Marked
In heart rate			> 15 bpm ↑
In blood pressure			> 10 mm Hg ↓
Urinary flow rate	Mildly decreased	Decreased	Markedly decreased
Pulse rate	Normal or increased	Increased > 100 bpm	Markedly increased > 120 bpm
Blood pressure	Normal	Mildly decreased with respiratory variation	Decreased

bpm = beats per minute.

povolemia. Moreover, the response to a fluid bolus (250 mL) is equally as important: a small elevation (1–2 mm Hg) may indicate the need for more fluid, whereas a large increase (> 5 mm Hg) suggests the need for a slower rate of administration and a reevaluation of volume status. Central venous pressure readings greater than 12 mm Hg are elevated and imply hypervolemia in the absence of right ventricular dysfunction, increased intrathoracic pressure, or restrictive pericardial disease.

Pulmonary artery pressure monitoring is necessary if central venous pressures do not correlate with the clinical assessment or if the patient has primary or secondary right ventricular dysfunction; the latter is usually due to pulmonary or left ventricular disease, respectively. Pulmonary artery occlusion pressure (PAOP) readings of less than 8 mm Hg indicate hypovolemia in the presence of confirmatory clinical signs; however, values less than 15 mm Hg may be associated with relative hypovolemia in patients with poor ventricular compliance. PAOP measurements greater than 18 mm Hg are elevated and generally imply left ventricular volume overload. The presence of mitral valve disease (especially stenosis), severe aortic stenosis, or a left atrial myxoma or thrombus alters the normal relationship between PAOP and left ventricular end-diastolic volume (see Chapters 6, 19, 20, and 21). Increased thoracic and pulmonary airway pressures also introduce errors; consequently, all pressure measurements should always be obtained at end-expiration and interpreted in the context of the clinical setting.

Newer techniques of measuring ventricular volumes with transesophageal echocardiography or by radioisotopes are more accurate but are not as widely available.

■ INTRAVENOUS FLUIDS

Intravenous fluid therapy may consist of infusions of crystalloids, colloids, or a combination of both. Crystalloid solutions are aqueous solutions of low-molecular-weight ions (salts) with or without glucose, whereas colloid solutions also contain high-molecular-weight substances such as proteins or large glucose polymers. Colloid solutions maintain plasma colloid oncotic pressure (see Chapter 28) and for the most part remain intravascular, whereas crystalloid solutions rapidly equilibrate with and distribute throughout the entire extracellular fluid space.

Controversy exists regarding the use of colloid versus crystalloid fluids for surgical patients. Proponents of colloids justifiably argue that by maintaining plasma oncotic pressure, colloids are more effective in restoring normal intravascular volume and cardiac output. Crystalloid proponents, on the other hand, maintain that the crystalloid solutions are equally as effective when given in sufficient amounts. Concerns that colloids may enhance the formation of pulmonary edema fluid in patients with increased pulmonary capillary permeability appear to be unfounded, because pulmonary interstitial oncotic pressure parallels that of plasma (see Chapter 22). Several generalizations can be made:

(1) Crystalloids, when given in sufficient amounts, can be just as effective as colloids in restoring intravascular volume.

(2) Replacing an intravascular volume deficit with crystalloids generally requires three to four times the volume needed when using colloids.

(3) Most surgical patients have an extracellular fluid deficit that exceeds the intravascular deficit.

(4) Severe intravascular fluid deficits can be more rapidly corrected using colloid solutions.

(5) The rapid administration of large amounts of crystalloids (> 4–5 L) is more frequently associated with significant tissue edema.

Some evidence suggests—but does not prove—that marked tissue edema can impair oxygen transport, tissue healing, and return of bowel function following major surgery.

CRYSTALLOID SOLUTIONS

A wide variety of solutions are available (Table 29–2). Solutions are chosen according to the type of fluid loss being replaced. Losses primarily due to water loss are replaced with hypotonic solutions, also called **maintenance-type solutions.** Losses that involve both water and electrolyte deficits are replaced with isotonic electrolyte solutions, also called **replacement-type solutions.** Glucose is provided in some solutions to maintain tonicity or to prevent ketosis and hypoglycemia due to fasting. Children are prone to developing hypoglycemia (< 50 mg/dL) following 4- to 8-hour fasts (see Chapter 44). Women may be more likely to develop hypoglycemia following extended fasts (> 24 hours) as compared to men.

Since most intraoperative fluid losses are isotonic, replacement-type solutions are generally used. The most commonly used fluid is lactated Ringer's solution. Although it is slightly hypotonic, providing approximately 100 mL of free water per liter and tending to lower serum sodium to 130 mEq/L, lactated Ringer's generally has the least effect on extracellular fluid composition and appears to be the most physiologic solution when large volumes are necessary. The lactate in this solution is converted by the liver into bicarbonate.

Table 29–2. Composition of crystalloid solutions.

Solution	Toxicity (mOsm/L)	Na$^+$ (mEq/L)	Cl$^-$ (mEq/L)	K$^+$ (mEq/L)	Ca^{2+} (mEq/L)	Mg^{2+} (mEq/L)	Glucose (g/L)	Lactate (mEq/L)	HCO$_3^-$ (mEq/L)	Acetate (mEq/L)	Gluconate (mEq/L)
5% dextrose in water (D$_5$W)	Hypo (253)						50				
Normal saline (NS)	Iso (308)	154	154								
D$_5$¼NS	Iso (355)	38.5	38.5				50				
D$_5$⅓NS	Hyper (432)	77	77				50				
D$_5$NS	Hyper (586)	154	154				50				
Lactated Ringer's injection (LR)	Iso (273)	130	109	4	3			28			
D$_5$LR	Hyper (525)	130	109	4	3		50	28			
½NS	Hypo (154)	77	77								
3% S	Hyper (1026)	513	513								
5% S	Hyper (1710)	855	855								
7.5% NaHCO$_3$	Hyper (1786)	893							893		
Plasmalyte	Iso (294)	140	98	5		3				27	23

When given in large volumes, normal saline produces a dilutional hyperchloremic acidosis because of its high sodium and chloride content (154 mEq/L): plasma bicarbonate concentration decreases as chloride concentration increases (see Chapters 28 and 30). Normal saline is the preferred solution for hypochloremic metabolic alkalosis and for diluting packed red blood cells prior to transfusion. Five percent dextrose in water (D$_5$W) is used for replacement of pure water deficits and as a maintenance fluid for patients on sodium restriction. Hypertonic 3% saline is employed in therapy of severe symptomatic hyponatremia (see Chapter 28). Three to 7.5% saline solutions have been advocated for the resuscitation of patients in hypovolemic shock (see Chapter 41). These solutions must be administered slowly (preferably through a central venous catheter) because they readily cause hemolysis.

COLLOID SOLUTIONS

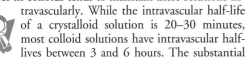

The osmotic activity of the high-molecular-weight substances in colloids tends to maintain these solutions intravascularly. While the intravascular half-life of a crystalloid solution is 20–30 minutes, most colloid solutions have intravascular half-lives between 3 and 6 hours. The substantial cost and occasional complications associated with colloids tend to limit their use. Generally accepted indications for colloids include (1) fluid resuscitation in patients with severe intravascular fluid deficits (eg, hemorrhagic shock) prior to the arrival of blood for transfusion, and (2) fluid resuscitation in the presence of severe hypoalbuminemia or conditions associated with large protein losses such as burns.

Many clinicians also use colloid solutions in conjunction with crystalloids when fluid replacement needs exceed 3–4 L prior to transfusion. It should be noted that these solutions are prepared in normal saline (Cl⁻ 145–154 mEq/L) and can also cause hyperchloremic metabolic acidosis (above).

Several colloid solutions are generally available. All are derived from either plasma proteins or synthetic glucose polymers and are supplied in isotonic electrolyte solutions.

Blood-derived colloids include albumin (5% and 25% solutions) and plasma protein fraction (5%). Both are heated to 60 °C for at least 10 hours to minimize the risk of transmitting hepatitis and other virally transmitted diseases. Plasma protein fraction contains alpha and beta globulins in addition to albumin and has occasionally resulted in hypotensive reactions. These reactions are allergic in nature and may involve activators of prekallikrein.

Synthetic colloids include dextrose starches and gelatins. Gelatins are associated with histamine-mediated allergic reactions and are not available in the United States. Dextran is available as dextran 70 (Macrodex) and dextran 40 (Rheomacrodex), which have average molecular weights of 70,000 and 40,000, respectively. Although dextran 70 is a better volume expander than dextran 40, the latter also improves blood flow through the microcirculation, presumably by decreasing blood viscosity. Antiplatelet effects are also described for dextrans. Infusions exceeding 20 mL/kg/d can interfere with blood typing, may prolong bleeding time (dextran 40), and have been associated with renal failure. Dextrans can also be antigenic, and both mild and severe anaphylactoid and anaphylactic reactions are described. Dextran 1 (Promit) may be administered prior to dextran 40 or dextran 70 to prevent severe anaphylactic reactions; it acts as a hapten and binds any circulating dextran antibodies.

Hetastarch (hydroxyethyl starch) is available as a 6% solution with an average molecular weight of 450,000. Small molecules are eliminated by the kidneys, while large molecules must be first broken down by amylase. Hetastarch is highly effective as a plasma expander and less expensive than albumin. Moreover, hetastarch is nonantigenic, and anaphylactoid reactions are rare. Coagulation studies and bleeding times are generally not significantly affected following infusions of up to 0.5–1.0 L. Whether or not kidney transplant patients do worse following hetastarch infusions is controversial. Pentastarch, a lower molecular weight starch solution, is less likely to cause adverse effects and may replace hetastarch.

■ PERIOPERATIVE FLUID THERAPY

Perioperative fluid therapy includes replacement of preexisting fluid deficits, of normal losses (maintenance requirements), and of surgical wound losses including blood loss.

NORMAL MAINTENANCE REQUIREMENTS

In the absence of oral intake, fluid and electrolyte deficits can rapidly develop as a result of continued urine formation, gastrointestinal secretions, sweating, and insensible losses from the skin and respiratory tract. Normal maintenance requirements can be estimated from Table 29–3. Solutions such as D$_5$¼NS and D$_5$½NS are most commonly used because these losses are normally hypotonic (more water loss than sodium loss).

Table 29–3. Estimating maintenance fluid requirements.

Weight	Rate
For the first 10 kg	4 mL/kg/h
For the next 10–20 kg	Add 2 mL/kg/h
For each kg above 20 kg	Add 1 mL/kg/h

Example: What are the maintenance fluid requirements for a 25-kg child?
Answer: 40 + 20 + 5 = 65 mL/h

PREEXISTING DEFICITS

Patients presenting for surgery after an overnight fast without any fluid intake will have a preexisting deficit proportionate to the duration of the fast. The deficit can be estimated by multiplying the normal maintenance rate by the length of the fast. For the average 70-kg person fasting for 8 hours, this amounts to (40 + 20 + 50) mL/hour × 8 hours, or 880 mL. (In reality, this deficit will be somewhat less as a result of renal conservation.)

Abnormal fluid losses frequently contribute to preoperative deficits. Preoperative bleeding, vomiting, diuresis, or diarrhea is often contributory. Occult losses (really redistribution; see below) due to fluid sequestration by traumatized or infected tissues or ascites can also be substantial. Increased insensible losses due to hyperventilation, fever, and sweating are often overlooked.

Ideally, all deficits should be replaced preoperatively in all patients. The fluids used should be similar in composition to the fluids lost (Table 29–4).

SURGICAL FLUID LOSSES

Blood Loss

One of the most important tasks of the anesthesiologist is to continually monitor and estimate blood loss. While estimates are complicated by occult bleeding into the wound or under the surgical drapes, accuracy is important to guide fluid therapy and transfusions.

The most commonly used method for estimating blood loss is measurement of blood in the surgical suction container and visually estimating the blood on surgical sponges and laparotomy pads ("laps"). A fully soaked sponge (4 × 4) is said to hold 10 mL of blood, whereas a soaked "lap" holds 100–150 mL. More accurate estimates are obtained if sponges and "laps" are weighed before and after use (particularly during pediatric procedures). Use of irrigating solutions complicates estimates, but their use should be noted and some attempt made to compensate for them. Serial hematocrits or hemoglobin concentrations reflect the ratio of blood cells to plasma, not necessarily blood loss; moreover, rapid fluid shifts and intravenous replacement affect measurements. Hematocrits may be useful during long procedures or when estimates are difficult.

Other Fluid Losses

Many surgical procedures are associated with obligatory losses of fluids other than blood. Such losses are due mainly to evaporation and internal redistribution of body fluids. Evaporative losses are most apparent with large wounds and directly proportionate to the surface area exposed and the duration of the surgical procedure.

Internal redistribution of fluids—often called "third spacing"—can cause massive fluid shifts and severe in-

Table 29–4. Electrolyte content of body fluids.

Fluid	Na⁺ (mEq/L)	K⁺ (mEq/L)	Cl⁻ (mEq/L)	HCO₃⁻ (mEq/L)
Sweat	30–50	5	45–55	
Saliva	2–40	10–30	6–30	30
Gastric juice				
High acidity	10–30	5–40	80–150	
Low acidity	70–140	5–40	55–95	5–25
Pancreatic secretions	115–180	5	55–95	60–110
Biliary secretions	130–160	5	90–120	30–40
Ileal fluid	40–135	5–30	20–90	20–30
Diarrheal stool	20–160	10–40	30–120	30–50

travascular depletion. Traumatized, inflamed, or infected tissue (as occurs with burns, extensive injuries, surgical dissections, or peritonitis) can sequester large amounts of fluid in its interstitial space and can translocate fluid across serosal surfaces (ascites) or into bowel lumen. The result is an obligatory increase in a nonfunctional component of the extracellular compartment, as this fluid does not readily equilibrate with the rest of the compartments. This fluid shift cannot be prevented by fluid restriction and is at the expense of both the functional extracellular and the intracellular fluid compartments. Cellular dysfunction as a result of hypoxia can produce an increase of the intracellular fluid volume, also at the expense of the functional extracellular compartment (see Chapter 28). Lastly, significant losses of lymphatic fluid may occur during extensive retroperitoneal dissections.

INTRAOPERATIVE FLUID REPLACEMENT

Intraoperative fluid therapy should include supplying basic fluid requirements and replacing residual preoperative deficits as well as intraoperative losses (blood, fluid redistribution, and evaporation). Selection of the type of intravenous solution depends upon the surgical procedure and the expected blood loss. For procedures involving minimal blood loss and fluid shifts, maintenance solutions can be used. For all other procedures, lactated Ringer's solution or fluid is generally used even for maintenance requirements.

Replacing Blood Loss

Ideally, blood loss should be replaced with crystalloid or colloid solutions to maintain intravascular volume (normovolemia) until the danger of anemia outweighs the risks of transfusion. At that point, further blood loss is replaced with transfusions of red blood cells to maintain hemoglobin concentration (or hematocrit) at that level. For most patients, that point corresponds to a hemoglobin between 7 and 8 g/dL (or a hematocrit of 21–24%).

Below a hemoglobin concentration of 7 g/dL, the resting cardiac output has to increase greatly to maintain a normal oxygen delivery (see Chapter 22). A level of 10 g/dL is generally used for elderly patients and those with significant cardiac or pulmonary disease. Higher limits may be used if continuing rapid blood loss is expected.

In practice, most clinicians give lactated Ringer's solution in approximately three to four times the volume of the blood lost, or colloid in a 1:1 ratio, until the transfusion point is reached. At that time, blood is replaced unit for unit as it is lost, with reconstituted packed red blood cells.

Table 29–5. Average blood volumes.

Age	Blood Volume
Neonates	
Premature	95 mL/kg
Full-term	85 mL/kg
Infants	80 mL/kg
Adults	
Men	75 mL/kg
Women	65 mL/kg

The transfusion point can be determined preoperatively from the hematocrit and by estimating blood volume (Table 29–5). Patients with a normal hematocrit should generally be transfused only after losses greater than 10–20% of their blood volume. The exact point is based on the patient's medical condition and the surgical procedure. The amount of blood loss necessary for the hematocrit to fall to 30% can be calculated as follows:

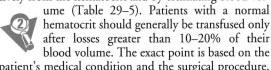

(1) Estimate blood volume from Table 29–5.

(2) Estimate the red blood cell volume (RBCV) at the preoperative hematocrit ($RBCV_{preop}$).

(3) Estimate red cell volume at a hematocrit of 30% ($RBCV_{30\%}$), assuming normal blood volume is maintained.

(4) Calculate the red cell volume lost when the hematocrit is 30%; $RBCV_{lost} = RBCV_{preop} - RBCV_{30\%}$.

(5) Allowable blood loss = $RBCV_{lost} \times 3$.

EXAMPLE:

An 85-kg woman has a preoperative hematocrit of 35%. How much blood loss will decrease her hematocrit to 30%?

Estimated blood volume = 65 mL/kg × 85 kg = 5525 mL.

$RBCV_{35\%}$ = 5525 × 35% = 1934 mL.
$RBCV_{30\%}$ = 5525 × 30% = 1658 mL.
Red cell loss at 30% = 1934 - 1658 = 276 mL.
Allowable blood loss = 3 × 276 mL = 828 mL.

Therefore, transfusion should only be considered when this patient's blood loss exceeds 800 mL. Increasingly, transfusions are not recommended until the hematocrit decreases to 24% (hemoglobin < 8.0 g/dL), but one must take into account the rate of blood loss and comorbid conditions, ie, cardiac disease in which case transfusion might be indicated if only 800 mL of blood is lost.

Other useful guidelines commonly used are as follows: (1) one unit of red blood cells will increase hemoglobin 1 g/dL and the hematocrit 2–3% (in adults);

Table 29–6. Redistribution and evaporative surgical fluid losses.

Degree of Tissue Trauma	Additional Fluid Requirement
Minimal (eg, hemiorrhaphy)	0–2 mL/kg
Moderate (eg, cholecystectomy)	2–4 mL/kg
Severe (eg, bowel resection)	4–8 mL/kg

and (2) a 10-mL/kg transfusion of red blood cells will increase hemoglobin concentration by 3 g/dL and the hematocrit by 10%.

Replacing Redistributive & Evaporative Losses

Since these losses are primarily related to wound size and the extent of surgical dissections and manipulations, procedures can be classified according to the degree of tissue trauma. These additional fluid losses can be replaced according to Table 29–6, based on whether tissue trauma is minimal, moderate, or severe. These values are only guidelines, and actual needs vary considerably from patient to patient.

■ TRANSFUSION

BLOOD GROUPS

Human red cell membranes are estimated to contain at least 300 different antigenic determinants. At least 20 separate blood group antigen systems are known; the expression of each is under genetic control from a separate chromosomal locus. Fortunately, only the ABO and the Rh systems are important in the majority of blood transfusions. Individuals often produce antibodies (alloantibodies) to the alleles they lack within each system. Such antibodies are responsible for the most serious reactions to transfusions. Antibodies may occur "naturally" or in response to sensitization from a previous transfusion or pregnancy.

The ABO System

Simplistically, the chromosomal locus for this system produces three alleles: A, B, and O. Each represents an enzyme that modifies a cell surface glycoprotein, producing a different antigen. (Actually, the O enzyme is functionally silent and there are two variants of A: A_1 and A_2.) Almost all individuals not having A or B "nat-

urally" produce antibodies (mainly IgM) against those antigens (Table 29–7) within the first year of life. The H antigen is functionally related to the ABO system but is produced by a different chromosomal locus. Absence of the H antigen (hh genotype, also called the Bombay phenotype) prevents expression of the A or B genes; these very rare individuals will have anti-A and anti-B antibodies regardless of their ABO genotype.

The Rh System

The genetics of the Rh gene is complicated, probably involving three chromosomal loci with a total of six alleles. For simplicity, only the presence or absence of the most common and most immunogenic allele, the D antigen, is considered. Approximately 80–85% of Caucasians have the D antigen. Individuals lacking this allele are called Rh-negative and usually develop antibodies against the D antigen only after exposure to a previous (Rh-positive) transfusion or pregnancy (an Rh-negative mother delivering an Rh-positive baby).

Other Systems

Other systems include the Lewis, P, Ii, MNS, Kidd, Kell, Duffy, Lutheran, Xg, Sid, Cartright, YK, and Chido Rodgers antigens. Fortunately, with a few exceptions, alloantibodies against these systems rarely cause serious hemolytic reactions.

COMPATIBILITY TESTING

The purpose of such testing is to predict and to prevent antigen-antibody reactions as a result of red blood cell transfusions. Donor and recipient blood are typed and checked for the presence of adverse antibodies.

ABO-Rh Testing

 The most severe transfusion reactions are due to ABO incompatibility; naturally acquired antibodies can react against the transfused (foreign) antigens, activate complement, and result in in-

Table 29–7. ABO blood grouping.

Type	Naturally Occurring Antibodies in Serum	Incidence*
A	Anti-B	45%
B	Anti-A	8%
AB	—	4%
O	Anti-A, anti-B	43%

*Rates are based on persons of western European ancestry.

travascular hemolysis. The patient's red cells are tested with serum known to have antibodies against A and against B to determine blood type. Because of the almost universal prevalence of natural ABO antibodies, confirmation of blood type is then made by testing the patient's serum against red cells with known antigen type.

The patient's red cells are also tested with anti-D antibodies to determine Rh. If the subject is Rh-negative, the presence of anti-D antibody is checked by mixing her or his serum against Rh-positive red cells. The probability of developing anti-D antibodies after a single exposure to the Rh antigen is 50–70%.

Crossmatching

A crossmatch mimics the transfusion: donor cells are mixed with recipient serum. Crossmatching serves three functions: (1) it confirms ABO and Rh typing (in less than 5 minutes), (2) it detects antibodies to the other blood group systems, and (3) it detects antibodies in low titers or those that do not agglutinate easily. The latter two require at least 45 minutes.

Antibody Screen

The purpose of this test is to detect in the serum the presence of the antibodies that are most commonly associated with non-ABO hemolytic reactions. The test (also known as the indirect Coombs test) requires 45 minutes and involves mixing the subject's serum with red cells of known antigenic composition; if specific antibodies are present, they will coat the red cell membrane, and addition of an anti-globulin antibody results in red cell agglutination. Screens are routinely done on all donor blood and may be done for a potential recipient instead of a crossmatch (below).

Type & Crossmatch Versus Type & Screen

The incidence of a serious hemolytic reaction after transfusion of an ABO- and Rh-compatible transfusion with a negative screen but without a crossmatch is less than 1%. Crossmatching, however, assures optimal safety and detects the presence of less common antibodies not usually tested for in a screen. Crossmatches are now performed only for elective surgical procedures where the probability of transfusion is high. Because of the time involved, (45 minutes) if two previous type and screen procedures have been documented, some centers have begun computer crossmatching—no actual crossmatch is performed.

Maximum Surgical Blood Ordering Schedule

Most hospitals compile a list of their most commonly performed operations and the maximum number of units that can be crossmatched preoperatively. Such practices prevent needless, excessive crossmatching of blood. Lists are usually based on each institution's own experience. A crossmatch-to-transfusion ratio less than 2.5:1 is considered acceptable. Only a type and screen is performed if the incidence of transfusion for a procedure is less than 10%. If transfusion is required, a crossmatch is performed. Allowances are typically made for anemic patients and those with coagulation disorders.

EMERGENCY TRANSFUSIONS

When a patient is exsanguinating, the need to transfuse arises prior to completion of a crossmatch, screen, or even blood typing. If the patient's blood type is known, an abbreviated crossmatch, requiring less than 5 minutes, will confirm ABO compatibility. If the recipient's blood type is not known with certainty and transfusion must be started before determination, type O Rh-negative (universal donor) blood may be used.

BLOOD BANK PRACTICES

Donors are screened to exclude medical conditions that might adversely affect the recipient. The hematocrit is determined, and if it is normal the blood is typed, screened for antibodies, and tested for hepatitis B, hepatitis C, syphilis, and HIV-1 and HIV-2. Most centers are doing nuclei acid testing for viral RNA to detect hepatitis B and C viruses and HIV. This is an extremely sensitive test and should narrow even further the window of positive virus but negative test. Most blood banks also test for the human T cell lymphotropic viruses I and II (HTLV-I and HTLV-II; see below).

Once blood is collected, a preservative-anticoagulant solution is added. The most commonly used solution is CPDA-1, which contains citrate as an anticoagulant (by binding calcium), phosphate as a buffer, dextrose as a red cell energy source, and adenine as a precursor for ATP synthesis. CPDA-1 preserved blood can be stored for 35 days, after which the viability of the red cells rapidly decreases. Alternatively, use of either AS-1 (Adsol) or AS-3 (Nutrice) extends the shelf-life to 6 weeks.

All units collected are separated into their component parts, namely, red blood cells, platelets, and plasma. When centrifuged, one unit of whole blood yields 250 mL of packed red blood cells (hematocrit 70%); following the addition of more saline preservative, the volume of a unit of packed red cells often reaches 350 mL. Red cells are normally stored at 1–6 °C. Red cells may be frozen in a hypertonic glycerol solution for up to 10 years. The latter technique is usually reserved for storage of blood with rare phenotypes.

The supernatant is centrifuged to yield platelets and plasma. The unit of platelets obtained generally contains 50–70 mL of plasma and can be stored at 20–24 °C for 5 days. The remaining plasma supernatant is further processed and frozen to yield fresh frozen plasma; rapid freezing helps prevent inactivation of labile coagulation factors (V and VIII). Slow thawing of fresh frozen plasma yields a gelatinous precipitate (cryoprecipitate) that contains high concentrations of Factor VIII and fibrinogen. Once separated, this cryoprecipitate can be refrozen for storage. One unit of blood yields 200 mL of plasma, which is frozen for storage; once thawed, it must be transfused within 24 hours.

Platelets may alternatively be obtained by automated plateletpheresis, which yields the equivalent of up to six regular units from a single patient.

INTRAOPERATIVE TRANSFUSION PRACTICES

Packed Red Blood Cells

Blood transfusions should be given as packed red blood cells, since doing so allows optimal utilization of blood bank resources. Packed red blood cells are ideal for patients requiring red cells but not volume replacement (eg, anemic patients in compensated congestive heart failure). Surgical patients require volume as well as red blood cells; a crystalloid can be infused simultaneously through second intravenous line for volume replacement.

Prior to transfusion, each unit should be carefully checked against the blood bank slip and the recipient's identity bracelet. The transfusion tubing should contain a 170-mm filter to trap any clots or debris; use of smaller filters (20–40 mm) is probably not necessary except for prevention of febrile transfusion reactions in sensitized patients (see below). Blood for intraoperative transfusion should be warmed to 37 °C during infusion, especially if more than 2–3 units are going to be transfused; failure to do so can result in profound hypothermia. The additive effects of hypothermia and the typically low levels of 2,3-diphosphoglycerate in stored blood can cause a marked leftward shift of the hemoglobin-oxygen dissociation curve (see Chapter 22) and, at least theoretically, promote tissue hypoxia. Blood warmers should be able to maintain blood temperature > 30 °C even at flow rates up to 150 mL/min.

Fresh Frozen Plasma

Fresh frozen plasma (FFP) contains all plasma proteins, including all clotting factors. Transfusions of FFP are indicated in the treatment of isolated factor deficiencies, the reversal of warfarin therapy, and the correction of coagulopathy associated with liver disease. Each unit of FFP generally increases the level of each clotting factor by 2–3% in adults. The initial therapeutic dose is usually 10–15 mL/kg. The goal is to achieve 30% of the normal coagulation factor concentration.

Fresh frozen plasma may also be used in patients who have received massive blood transfusions (see below) and continue to bleed following platelet transfusions. Patients with antithrombin III deficiency or thrombotic thrombocytopenic purpura also benefit from FFP transfusions.

Each unit of FFP carries the same infectious risk as a unit of whole blood. In addition, occasional patients may become sensitized to plasma proteins. ABO-compatible units should generally be given but are not mandatory. As with red cells, FFP should generally be warmed to 37 °C prior to transfusion.

Platelets

Platelet transfusions should be given to patients with thrombocytopenia or dysfunctional platelets in the presence of bleeding. Prophylactic platelet transfusions are also indicated in patients with platelet counts below $10,000–20,000 \times 10^9/L$ because of an increased risk of spontaneous hemorrhage.

Platelet counts less than $50,000 \times 10^9/L$ are associated with increased blood loss during surgery. Thrombocytopenic patients about to undergo surgery or invasive procedures should receive prophylactic platelet transfusions preoperatively: the platelet count should be increased to approximately $100,000 \times 10^9/L$. Vaginal delivery and minor surgical procedures may be performed in patients with lower platelet counts but with normal platelet function and counts greater than $50,000 \times 10^9/L$.

Each single unit of platelets may be expected to increase the count by $5,000-10,000 \times 10^9/L$. Plateletpheresis units contain the equivalent of six regular, single donor units (above). Lesser increases can be expected in patients with a history of prior platelet transfusions. Platelet dysfunction can also increase surgical bleeding even when the platelet count is normal and can be diagnosed preoperatively with a bleeding time. Platelet transfusions may also be indicated in patients with dysfunctional platelets and increased surgical bleeding.

ABO-compatible platelet transfusions are desirable but not necessary. Transfused platelets generally survive only 1–7 days following transfusion. ABO compatibility may increase platelet survival. Rh sensitization can occur in Rh-negative recipients owing to the presence of a few red cells in Rh-positive platelet units. Moreover, anti-A or anti-B antibodies in the 70 mL of plasma in each platelet unit can cause a hemolytic reaction against the recipient's red cells when a large number of ABO-incompatible platelet units are given. Administration of Rh immunoglobulin to Rh-negative individuals can protect against Rh sensitization following Rh-positive platelet transfusions. Patients who develop antibodies against HLA antigens (present on lymphocytes in platelet concentrates) or specific platelet antigens require HLA-compatible or single-donor units. Use of plateletpheresis transfusions may decrease the likelihood of sensitization.

Granulocyte Transfusions

Granulocyte transfusions, prepared by leukapheresis, may be indicated in neutropenic patients with bacterial infections not responding to antibiotics. Transfused granulocytes have a very short circulatory life span, so that daily transfusion of $10–30 \times 10^9$ granulocytes are usually required. Irradiation of these units decreases the incidence of graft-versus-host reactions, pulmonary endothelial damage, and other problems associated with transfusion of leukocytes (see below), but may adversely affect granulocyte function. The availability of filgrastim (granulocyte colony-stimulating factor, or G-CSF) and sargramostim (granulocyte-macrophage colony-stimulating factor, or GM-CSF) have greatly reduced the use of granulocyte transfusions.

■ COMPLICATIONS OF BLOOD TRANSFUSION

IMMUNE COMPLICATIONS

Immune complications following blood transfusions are primarily due to sensitization of the recipient to donor red cells, white cells, platelets, or plasma proteins. Less commonly, the transfused cells or serum may mount an immune response against the recipient.

1. Hemolytic Reactions

Hemolytic reactions usually involve specific destruction of the transfused red blood cells by the recipient's antibodies. Less commonly, hemolysis of a recipient's red blood cells occurs as a result of the transfusion of red cell antibodies. Incompatible units of platelet concentrates, FFP, clotting factor concentrates, or cryoprecipitate may contain small amounts of plasma with anti-A or anti-B (or both) alloantibodies. Transfusions of large volumes of such units can lead to intravascular hemolysis. Hemolytic reactions are commonly classified as either acute (intravascular) or delayed (extravascular).

Acute Hemolytic Reactions

Acute intravascular hemolysis is usually due to ABO blood incompatibility and is reported with the frequency of approximately 1:6000 transfusions. The most common cause is misidentification of a patient, blood specimen, or transfusion unit. These reaction are often severe. The risk of a fatal hemolytic reaction is about 1 in 100,000 transfusions. In awake patients, symptoms include chills, fever, nausea, and chest and flank pain. In anesthetized patients, the reaction is manifested by a rise in temperature, unexplained tachycardia, hypotension, hemoglobinuria, and diffuse oozing in the surgical field. Disseminated intravascular coagulation, shock, and renal shutdown can develop rapidly. The severity of a reaction often depends on how much incompatible blood has been given. If the volume of the incompatible blood given is less than 5% of total blood volume, the reaction is usually not severe.

Management of hemolytic reactions can be summarized as follows:

(1) Once a hemolytic reaction is suspected, the transfusion should be stopped immediately.

(2) The unit should be rechecked against the blood slip and the patient's identity bracelet.

(3) Blood should be drawn to identify hemoglobin in plasma, to repeat compatibility testing, and to obtain coagulation studies and a platelet count.

(4) A urinary catheter should be inserted, and the urine should be checked for hemoglobin.

(5) Osmotic diuresis should be initiated with mannitol and intravenous fluids.

(6) Low-dose dopamine may help preserve renal blood flow and support blood pressure.

(7) In the presence of rapid blood loss, platelets and FFP are indicated.

Delayed Hemolytic Reactions

This type of hemolytic reaction—also called extravascular hemolysis—is generally mild and is caused by antibodies to non-D antigens of the Rh system or to foreign alleles in other systems such as the Kell, Duffy, or Kidd antigens. Following an ABO and Rh D-compatible transfusion, patients have a 1–1.6% chance of forming antibodies directed against foreign antigens in these other systems. By the time significant amounts of these antibodies have formed (weeks to months), the transfused red cells have been cleared from the circulation. Moreover, the titer of these antibodies subsequently decreases and may become undetectable. Reexposure to the same foreign antigen during a subsequent red cell transfusion, however, triggers an anamnestic antibody response against the foreign antigen. The hemolytic reaction is therefore typically delayed 2–21 days after transfusion, and symptoms are generally mild, consisting of malaise, jaundice, and fever. The patient's hematocrit typically fails to rise in spite of the transfusion and the absence of bleeding. The serum unconjugated bilirubin increases as a result of hemoglobin breakdown.

Diagnosis of delayed antibody-mediated hemolytic reactions may be facilitated by the antiglobulin (Coombs) test. The direct Coombs test detects the presence of antibodies on the membrane of red cells. In this setting, however, this test cannot distinguish between recipient antibodies coated on donor red cells versus donor antibodies coated on recipient red cells. The latter requires a more detailed reexamination of pretransfusion specimens from both the patient and the donor.

The treatment of delayed hemolytic reactions is primarily supportive. The frequency of delayed hemolytic transfusion reactions is estimated to be approximately 1:2500–1500 transfusions. Pregnancy (exposure to fetal red cells) can also be responsible for the formation of alloantibodies to red cells.

2. Nonhemolytic Immune Reactions

Nonhemolytic immune reactions are due to sensitization of the recipient to the donor's white cells, platelets, or plasma proteins.

Febrile Reactions

White cell or platelet sensitization is typically manifested as a febrile reaction. Such reactions are relatively common (1–3% of transfusion episodes) and are characterized by an increase in temperature without evidence of hemolysis. Patients with a history of febrile reactions should receive white cell-poor red cell transfusions only. Red cell transfusions can be made leukocyte-poor by washing, centrifugation, filtration, or freeze-thaw techniques. Use of a 20- to 40-mm filter will trap most of the white cell and platelet contaminants.

Urticarial Reactions

Urticarial reactions are usually characterized by erythema, hives, and itching without fever. They are relatively common (1% of transfusions) and are thought to be due to sensitization of the patient to transfused plasma proteins. The use of packed red blood cells instead of whole blood lessens the likelihood of urticaria-type reactions. Urticarial reactions can be treated with antihistaminic drugs (H_1 and perhaps H_2 blockers).

Anaphylactic Reactions

Anaphylactic reactions are rare (approximately 1 in 150,000 transfusions). These severe reactions may occur after only a few milliliters of blood have been given, typically in IgA-deficient patients with anti-IgA antibodies who receive IgA-containing blood transfusions. The prevalence of IgA deficiency is estimated to be 1:600–800 in the general population. Such reactions call for treatment with epinephrine, fluids, corticosteroids, and H_1 and H_2 blockers. Patients with IgA deficiency should receive thoroughly washed packed red cells, deglycerolized frozen red cells, or IgA-free blood units.

Noncardiogenic Pulmonary Edema

An acute lung injury syndrome (*T*ransfusion-*R*elated *A*cute *L*ung *I*njury [TRALI]) is a rare complication of blood transfusion (< 1:10,000). It is thought to be due to transfusion of antileukocytic or anti-HLA antibodies that interact with and cause the patient's white cells to aggregate in the pulmonary circulation. Damage to the alveolar/capillary membrane triggers the syndrome. Alternatively, transfused white cells can interact with leukoagglutinins in the patient. Initial treatment of TRALI is similar to that for acute respiratory distress syndrome (ARDS) (see Chapter 50), but it typically resolves within 12 to 48 hours with supportive therapy.

Graft-Versus-Host Disease

This type of reaction may be seen in immune-compromised patients. Cellular blood products contain lymphocytes capable of mounting an immune response against the compromised (recipient) host. Use of special leukocyte filters alone does not reliably prevent graft-versus-host disease; irradiation (1500–3000 cGy) of red cell, granulocyte, and platelet transfusions effectively inactivates lymphocytes without altering the efficacy of such transfusions.

Posttransfusion Purpura

Profound thrombocytopenia can rarely occur following blood transfusions and is due to the development of platelet alloantibodies. For unknown reasons, these antibodies also destroy the patient's own platelets. The platelet count typically drops precipitously 1 week after transfusion. Plasmapheresis is generally recommended.

Immune Suppression

 Transfusion of leukocyte-containing blood products appears to be immunosuppressive. This is most clearly evident in renal transplant recipients, in whom preoperative blood transfusions appear to improve graft survival. Some studies suggest that recurrence of malignant growths may be more likely in patients who receive blood transfusion during surgery. Available evidence also suggests that transfusion of allogenic leukocytes can activate latent viruses in the recipient. Lastly, blood transfusion may increase the incidence of serious infections following surgery or trauma.

INFECTIOUS COMPLICATIONS

Viral Infections

A. HEPATITIS:

Until routine testing for hepatitis viruses was implemented, the incidence of hepatitis following blood transfusion was 7–10%. At least 90% of these cases were due to the hepatitis C virus. The incidence of **posttransfusion hepatitis** is presently less than 1% (between 1:150 and 1:5000 transfusions); 75% of these cases are anicteric, and at least 50% develop chronic liver disease. Moreover, of this latter group, at least 10–20% develop cirrhosis.

B. ACQUIRED IMMUNODEFICIENCY SYNDROME (AIDS):

The virus responsible for this disease, human immunodeficiency virus type 1 (HIV-1), is transmissible by blood transfusion. All blood is tested for the presence of anti-HIV-1 and 2 antibodies. Unfortunately, because of an estimated 6- to 8-week period required to develop the antibody after donor infection, infectious units can go undetected. The current rate of transmission of the HIV virus by transfusion is estimated to be 1:200,000 transfusions. Blood is also routinely tested for immunodeficiency virus type 2 (HIV-2) although this virus has not yet been implicated as a cause for transfusion-related AIDS.

C. OTHER VIRAL INFECTIONS:

Cytomegalovirus (CMV) and Epstein-Barr virus usually cause asymptomatic or mild systemic illness. Unfortunately, some individuals become asymptomatic infectious carriers; the white cells in blood units from such donors are capable of transmitting either virus. Immunocompromised and immunosuppressed patients (eg, premature infants and organ transplant recipients) are particularly susceptible to severe CMV infections through transfusions. Ideally, such patients should only receive CMV-negative units. Human T cell lymphotropic viruses I and II (HTLV-1 and HTLV-2) are leukemia and lymphoma viruses, respectively, that have been reported to be transmitted by blood transfusion; the for-

mer has also been associated with myelopathy. Parvovirus transmission has been reported following transfusion of coagulation factor concentrates and can result in transient aplastic crises in immunocompromised hosts. The use of special leukocyte filters appears to reduce but not eliminate the incidence of these complications.

Parasitic Infections

Parasitic diseases reported to be transmitted by transfusion include malaria, toxoplasmosis, and Chagas' disease. Fortunately, such cases are very rare.

Bacterial Infections

Both gram-positive (*Staphylococcus*) and gram-negative (*Yersinia* and *Citrobacter*) bacteria can rarely contaminate blood transfusions and transmit disease. To avoid the possibility of significant bacterial contamination, blood products should be administered over a period shorter than 4 hours. Specific bacterial diseases transmitted by blood transfusions from donors include syphilis, brucellosis, salmonellosis, yersiniosis, and various rickettsioses.

MASSIVE BLOOD TRANSFUSION

Massive transfusion is generally defined as the need to transfuse one to two times the patient's blood volume. For most adult patients, that is the equivalent of 10–20 units.

Coagulopathy

The most common cause of bleeding following massive blood transfusion is dilutional thrombocytopenia. Clinically significant dilution of the coagulation factors is unusual in previously normal patients. Coagulation studies and platelet counts, if readily available, ideally should guide platelet and FFP transfusion. Viscoelastic analysis of whole blood clotting (thromboelastography and Sonoclot analysis) may also be useful.

Citrate Toxicity

Calcium binding by the **citrate preservative** can theoretically become significant following transfusion of large volumes of blood or blood products. Clinically significant hypocalcemia, causing cardiac depression, does not occur in most normal patients unless the transfusion rate exceeds 1 U every 5 minutes. Because citrate metabolism is primarily hepatic, patients with hepatic disease or dysfunction (and possibly hypothermic patients) may require calcium infusion during massive transfusion (see Chapter 28).

Hypothermia

Massive blood transfusion is an absolute indication for warming all blood products and intravenous fluids to normal body temperature. Ventricular dysrhythmias progressing to fibrillation often occur at temperatures close to 30 °C. Hypothermia can hamper cardiac resuscitation. The use of rapid infusion devices with very efficient heat transfer has remarkably decreased the incidence of transfusion related hypothermia.

Acid-Base Balance

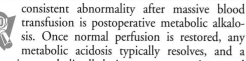 Although stored blood is acidic due to the citric acid anticoagulant and accumulation of red cell metabolites (carbon dioxide and lactic acid), significant metabolic acidosis due to transfusion is not common. The most consistent abnormality after massive blood transfusion is postoperative metabolic alkalosis. Once normal perfusion is restored, any metabolic acidosis typically resolves, and a progressive metabolic alkalosis supervenes as citrate and lactate contained in transfusions and resuscitation fluids are converted to bicarbonate by the liver.

Serum Potassium Concentration

The extracellular concentration of potassium in stored blood steadily increases with time. The amount of extracellular potassium transfused with each unit is typically less than 4 mEq per unit. Hyperkalemia can develop regardless of the age of the blood when transfusion rates exceed 100 mL/min. The treatment of hyperkalemia is discussed in Chapter 28. Hypokalemia is commonly encountered postoperatively, especially in association with metabolic alkalosis (see Chapters 28 and 30).

■ ALTERNATIVE STRATEGIES FOR MANAGEMENT OF BLOOD LOSS DURING SURGERY

AUTOLOGOUS TRANSFUSIONS

Patients undergoing elective surgical procedures with a high probability for transfusion can donate their own blood for use during that surgery. Collection is usually started 4–5 weeks prior to the procedure. The patient is allowed to donate a unit as long as the hematocrit is at least 34% or hemoglobin at least 11 g/dL. A minimum of 72 hours is required between donations to make certain

that plasma volume returns to normal. With iron supplementation and recombinant erythropoietin therapy (400 U weekly), at least three or four units can usually be collected prior to the operation. Some studies suggest that autologous blood transfusions do not adversely affect survival in patients undergoing operations for cancer. Although autologous transfusions likely reduce the risk of infection and transfusion reactions, they are not completely free of hazard. Risks include those of immunological reactions due to clerical errors in collection and labeling, contamination, and improper storage. Allergic reactions can occur due to allergens (eg, ethylene oxide) that dissolve into the blood from collection and storage equipment. Preoperative autologous blood collection is being used with decreasing frequency.

BLOOD SALVAGE & REINFUSION

This technique is used widely during cardiac and major reconstructive vascular and orthopedic surgery (see Chapter 21). The shed blood is aspirated intraoperatively together with an anticoagulant (heparin) into a reservoir. After a sufficient amount of blood is collected, the red blood cells are concentrated and washed to remove debris and anticoagulant and then reinfused into the patient. The concentrates obtained usually have hematocrits of 50–60%. To be used effectively, this technique requires blood losses greater than 1000–1500 mL. Contraindications include septic contamination of the wound and perhaps a malignant tumor, though concerns about the possibility of reinfusing malignant cells via this technique may be not justified. Newer, simpler systems allow reinfusion of shed blood without centrifugation.

NORMOVOLEMIC HEMODILUTION

Acute normovolemic hemodilution relies on the premise that if the concentration of red blood cells is decreased, total red cell loss is reduced when large amounts of blood are shed; moreover, cardiac output remains normal because intravascular volume is maintained. Blood is typically removed just prior to surgery from a large bore intravenous catheter and is replaced with crystalloid and colloids such that the patient remains normovolemic but has a hematocrit of 21–25%. The removed blood is stored in a CPD bag at room temperature (up to 6 hours) to preserve platelet function; the blood is given back to the patient after the blood loss or sooner if necessary.

DONOR-DIRECTED TRANSFUSIONS

Patients can request donated blood from family members or friends known to be ABO-compatible. Most blood banks discourage this practice and generally require donation at least 3 days prior to surgery to process the donated blood and confirm compatibility. Studies comparing the safety of donor-directed units to that of random donor units have found either no difference, or that blood bank units are safer.

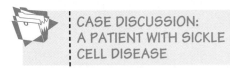

CASE DISCUSSION: A PATIENT WITH SICKLE CELL DISEASE

A 24-year-old black woman with a history of a hereditary sickle cell anemia presents with abdominal pain and is scheduled for cholecystectomy. The patient thinks she may have sickle cell anemia.

What is sickle cell anemia?

Sickle cell anemia *is a hereditary hemolytic anemia resulting from the formation of an abnormal hemoglobin (Hb S). Hb S differs structurally from the normal adult hemoglobin (Hb A) only in the substitution of valine for glutamic acid at the sixth position of the beta chain (see Chapter 22). Functionally, sickle hemoglobin has less affinity for oxygen (P_{50} = 31 mm Hg) as well as decreased solubility. Upon deoxygenation, Hb S readily polymerizes and precipitates inside red blood cells, causing them to sickle. Patients produce variable amounts (2–20%) of fetal hemoglobin (Hb F). It is likely that cells with large amounts of Hb F are somewhat protected from sickling. The continuous formation and destruction of irreversibly sickled cells leads to anemia. Hematocrits are typically 18–30% due to extravascular hemolysis. Red cell survival is reduced to 10–15 days, compared with up to 120 days in normal individuals.*

What is the difference between sickle cell anemia and sickle cell trait?

*When the genetic defect for adult hemoglobin is on both the maternally and paternally derived chromosomes (No. 11), the patient is homozygous for Hb S and has sickle cell anemia (Hb SS). When only one chromosome has the sickle gene, the patient is heterozygous and has sickle cell trait (Hb AS). Patients with sickle trait produce variable amounts of Hb A (55–60%) and Hb S (35–40%). Unlike those with Hb SS, they are generally not anemic, are asymptomatic, and have a normal life span. Sickling occurs only under extreme hypoxemia or in low-flow states. Sickling is especially apt to occur in the renal medulla; indeed, many patients with sickle trait have impaired renal concen-*trating ability. Some patients with Hb AS have been reported to have renal medullary, splenic, and pulmonary infarcts.*

What is the prevalence of sickle cell gene in black Americans?

Sickle cell anemia is primarily a disease of blacks of Central African ancestry. Approximately 0.2–0.5% of black Americans are homozygous for the sickle gene, while approximately 8–10% are heterozygous. Sickle cell anemia is less commonly found in patients of Mediterranean ancestry.

What is the pathophysiology?

Conditions favoring the formation of deoxyhemoglobin— eg, hypoxemia, acidosis, intracellular hypertonicity or dehydration, increased 2,3-DPG levels, or increased temperature—can precipitate sickling in patients with Hb SS. Hypothermia may also be detrimental because of the associated vasoconstriction (see below). Intracellular polymerization of Hb S distorts red cells, makes them less pliable and "more sticky," and increases blood viscosity. Sickling may initially be reversible but eventually becomes irreversible in some cells. Formation of red cell aggregates in capillaries can obstruct the microcirculation in tissues. A vicious cycle is established in which circulatory stasis leads to localized hypoxia, which, in turn, causes more sickling.

What symptoms do patients with sickle cell anemia usually present?

Patients with Hb SS generally first develop symptoms in infancy, when levels of fetal hemoglobin (Hb F) decline appreciably. The disease is characterized both by acute episodic crises and by chronic and progressive features (Table 29–8). Children display retarded growth and have recurrent infections. Recurrent splenic infarction leads to splenic atrophy and functional asplenism by adolescence. Patients usually die from recurrent infections or renal failure. Crises are often precipitated by infection, cold weather, dehydration, or other forms of stress. Crises may be divided into three types:

(1) Vaso-occlusive crises: *Depending on the vessels involved, these acute episodes can result in micro- or macroinfarctions. Most painful crises are thought to be due to microinfarcts in the various tissues. Clinically, they present as acute abdominal, chest, back, or joint pain. Differentiation between surgical and nonsurgical causes of abdominal pain is difficult. Most patients form pig-*

Table 29–8. Manifestations of sickle cell anemia.

Neurologic
  Stroke
  Subarachnoid hemorrhage
  Coma
  Seizures
Ocular
  Vitreous hemorrhage
  Retinal infarcts
  Proliferative retinopathy
  Retinal detachment
Pulmonary
  Increased intrapulmonary shunting
  Pleuritis
  Recurrent pulmonary infections
  Pulmonary infarcts
Cardiovascular
  Congestive heart failure
  Cor pulmonale
  Pericarditis
  Myocardial infarction
Gastrointestinal
  Cholelithiasis (pigmented stones)
  Cholecystitis
  Hepatic infarcts
  Hepatic abscesses
  Hepatic fibrosis
Hematologic
  Anemia
  Aplastic anemia
  Recurrent infections
  Splenic infarcts
  Splenic sequestration
  Functional asplenia
Genitourinary
  Hematuria
  Renal papillary necrosis
  Impaired renal concentrating ability (isosthenuria)
  Nephrotic syndrome
  Renal insufficiency
  Renal failure
  Priapism
Skeletal
  Synovitis
  Arthritis
  Aseptic necrosis of femoral head
  Small bone infarcts in hand and feet (dactylitis)
  Biconcave ("fishmouth") vertebrae
  Osteomyelitis
Skin
  Chronic ulcers

---

mented gallstones by adulthood, and many present with acute cholecystitis. Vaso-occlusive phenomena in larger vessels can produce thromboses resulting in splenic, cerebral, pulmonary, hepatic, renal, and, less commonly, myocardial infarctions.

(2) Aplastic crisis: *Profound anemia (Hb 2–3 g/dL) can rapidly occur when red cell production in the bone marrow is exhausted or suppressed. Infections and folate deficiency may play a major role. Some patients also develop leukopenia.*

(3) Splenic sequestration crisis: *Sudden pooling of blood in the spleen can occur in infants and young children and can cause life-threatening hypotension. The mechanism is thought to be partial or complete occlusion of venous drainage from the spleen.*

How is sickle cell anemia diagnosed?

Red blood cells from patients with sickle cell anemia readily sickle following addition of an oxygen-consuming reagent (metabisulfite) or a hypertonic ionic solution (solubility test). Confirmation requires hemoglobin electrophoresis.

What would be the best way to prepare patients with sickle cell anemia for surgery?

Optimal preoperative preparation is desirable for all patients undergoing surgery. Patients should be well-hydrated, infections should be controlled, and the hemoglobin concentration should be at an acceptable level. Preoperative transfusion therapy must be individualized to the patient and to the surgical procedure. Most authors advocate partial exchange transfusions before major surgical procedures. Unlike simple transfusions, exchange transfusions decrease blood viscosity. They also increase oxygen-carrying capacity and decrease the likelihood of sickling. The goal of such transfusions is generally to achieve a hematocrit of 35–40% with 40–50% normal hemoglobin (Hb A_1). Although the benefits of exchange transfusions for patients undergoing anesthesia have yet to be demonstrated, exchange transfusions clearly help patients experiencing a crisis.

Are there any special intraoperative considerations?

Conditions that might promote hemoglobin desaturation or low-flow states should be avoided. Every effort must be made to avoid hypothermia and hyperthermia, acidosis, and even mild degrees of hypoxemia, hypotension, or hypovolemia.

Generous hydration and a relatively high (> 50%) inspired oxygen tension are desirable. The major compensatory mechanism in these patients is an increased cardiac output, which should be maintained intraoperatively. Central venous pressure monitoring or pulmonary artery pressure with mixed venous oxygen saturation monitoring may be useful in some patients. Mild alkalosis may help avoid sickling, but even moderate degrees of respiratory alkalosis may have an adverse effect on cerebral blood flow. Many clinicians will also avoid the use of tourniquets. Studies are not available to support or reject the use of any one regional or general anesthetic technique.

Are there any special postoperative considerations?

The same principles applied intraoperatively hold for the postoperative period. Most perioperative deaths occur in the postoperative period. Hypoxemia and pulmonary complications appear to be major risk factors. Supplemental oxygen, optimal pain control, pulmonary physiotherapy, and early ambulation are desirable to avoid such complications.

What is the significance of sickle cell anemia and thalassemia in the same patient?

The combination of Hb S and thalassemia, most commonly sickle β-thalassemia, has a variable and unpredictable effect on disease severity. In general, the combination tends to be milder in black patients than in those of Mediterranean ancestry.

What is the pathophysiology of thalassemia?

Thalassemia is a hereditary defect in the production of one or more of the normal subunits of hemoglobin. Patients with thalassemia may be able to produce normal Hb A but have reduced amounts of alpha or beta chain production. The severity of this defect depends on the subunit affected and the degree with which hemoglobin production is affected. Symptoms may be absent or severe. Patients with α-thalassemia produce reduced amounts of α-subunit, while patients with β-thalassemia produce reduced amounts of the β-subunit. The formation of hemoglobins with abnormal subunit composition can alter the red cell membrane and lead to variable degrees of hemolysis as well as ineffective hematopoiesis. The latter can result in hypertrophy of the bone marrow and often an abnormal skeleton. Maxillary hypertrophy may make endotracheal intubation diffi-

cult. Thalassemias are most common in patients of Southeast Asian, African, Mediterranean, and Indian ancestry.

What is hemoglobin C disease?

Substitution of lysine for glutamic acid at position 6 on the β-subunit results in hemoglobin C (Hb C). Approximately 0.05% of black Americans carry the gene for Hb C. Patients homozygous for Hb C generally have only a mild hemolytic anemia and splenomegaly. They rarely develop significant complications. The tendency for Hb C to crystallize in hypertonic environments is probably responsible for the hemolysis and characteristically produces target cells on the peripheral blood smear.

What is the significance of the genotype Hb SC?

Nearly 0.1% of black Americans are simultaneously heterozygous for both Hb S and Hb C (Hb SC). These patients generally have a mild to moderate hemolytic anemia. Some patients occasionally have painful crises, splenic infarcts, and hepatic dysfunction. Eye manifestations similar to those associated with Hb SS disease are especially prominent. Females with Hb SC have a high rate of complications during the third trimester of pregnancy and delivery.

What is hemoglobin E?

Hemoglobin E is the result of a single substitution on the β chain and is the second most common hemoglobin variant worldwide. It is most often encountered in patients from Southeast Asia. Although oxygen-binding affinity is normal, the substitution impairs production of β chains (similar to β-thalassemia). Homozygous patients have marked microcytosis and prominent target cells, but are not usually anemic and lack any other manifestations.

What is the hematologic significance of glucose-6-phosphate dehydrogenase deficiency?

Red blood cells are normally well protected against oxidizing agents. The sulfhydryl groups on hemoglobin are protected by reduced glutathione. The latter is regenerated by NADPH (reduced nicotinamide adenine dinucleotide phosphate), which itself is regenerated by glucose metabolism in the hexose monophosphate shunt. Glucose-6-phosphate dehydrogenase (G6PD) is a critical enzyme in this pathway. A defect in this pathway results in an inadequate amount of reduced glutathione, which can potentially result in the ox-

Table 29–9. Drugs to avoid in patients with G6PD deficiency.

Drugs that may cause hemolysis
Sulfonamides
Antimalarial drugs
Nitrofurantoin
Nalidixic acid
Probenecid
Aminosalicylic acid
Phenacetin
Acetanilid
Ascorbic acid (in large doses)
Vitamin K
Methylene blue
Quinine[1]
Quinidine[2]
Chloramphenicol
Penicillamine
Dimercaprol
Other drugs
Prilocaine
Nitroprusside

G6PD = glucose-6-phosphate dehydrogenase.
[1]May be safe in patients with A⁻ variant.
[2]Should be avoided because of their potential to cause methemoglobinemia.

idation and precipitation of hemoglobin in red cells (seen as Heinz bodies) and hemolysis.

Abnormalities in G6PD are relatively common. Over 400 variants are described. Depending on the functional significance of the enzyme abnormality, clinical manifestations can be quite variable. Up to 15% of black American males have the common clinically significant A⁻ variant. A second variant is common in individuals of eastern Mediterranean ancestry, and a third in individuals of Chinese ancestry. Because the locus for the enzyme is on the X chromosome, abnormalities are X-linked traits, with males being primarily affected. As red blood cells age, G6PD activity normally decreases. Consequently, aging red cells are most susceptible to oxidation. This decay is markedly accelerated in patients with the Mediterranean variant but only moderately so in patients with the A⁻ variant. Most patients are typically not anemic but can develop hemolysis following oxidant stresses such as viral and bacterial infections or ingestions of some drugs (Table 29–9). Hemolysis can also be precipitated by metabolic acidosis. Hemolytic episodes can present with hemoglobinuria and hypotension. They are generally self-limited because only the older population of cells is destroyed. Mediterranean variants may be associated with some degree of chronic hemolytic anemia, and some patients are exquisitely sensitive to fava beans.

Treatment is primarily preventive. Measures aimed at preserving renal function (see above) are indicated in patients who develop hemoglobinuria.

SUGGESTED READING

Lake CL, Moore RA: *Blood: Hemotasis, Transfusion, and Alternatives in the Perioperative Period.* Raven, 1995.

Mollison PL, Engelfriet CP, Contreras M: *Blood Transfusion in Clinical Medicine,* 10th ed. Blackwell Science, 1997.

Pestana C: *Fluids and Electrolytes in the Surgical Patient,* 5th ed, Lippincott Williams & Wilkins, 2000.

Practice Guidelines for blood component therapy: a report by the American Society of Anesthesiologists Task Force on Blood Component Therapy. Park Ridge, IL: American Society of Anesthesiologists. Anesthesiology 1996;84:732.

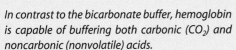

Nearly all biochemical reactions in the body are dependent on maintenance of a physiologic hydrogen ion concentration. The latter is closely regulated because changes in hydrogen ion concentration produce widespread organ dysfunction.

This regulation—often referred to as acid-base balance—is of prime importance to anesthesiologists. Changes in ventilation and perfusion are common during anesthesia and can rapidly alter acid-base balance. A thorough understanding of acid-base disturbances, their physiologic effects, and treatment is thus essential for proper anesthetic management.

This chapter examines acid-base physiology, common disturbances, and their anesthetic implications.

Clinical measurements of blood gases and their interpretation are also discussed.

■ DEFINITIONS

ACID-BASE CHEMISTRY

Hydrogen Ion Concentration & pH

In any aqueous solution, water molecules reversibly dissociate into hydrogen and hydroxide ions:

$$H_2O \leftrightarrow H^+ + OH^-$$

This process is described by the dissociation constant, K_W:

$$K_W = [H^+] + [HO] = 10^{-14}$$

The concentration of water is omitted from the denominator of this expression because it does not vary appreciably and is already included in the constant. Therefore, if one is given $[H^+]$ or $[OH^-]$, the concentration of the other ion can be readily calculated.

Example: If $[H^+] = 10^{-8}$ nEq/L, then $[OH^-] = 10^{-14} \div 10^{-8} = 10^{-6}$ nEq/L.

Arterial $[H^+]$ is normally 40 nEq/L, or 40×10^{-9} mol/L. Hydrogen ion concentration is more commonly expressed as pH, because dealing with numbers of this order of magnitude is awkward. The pH of a solution is defined as the negative logarithm (base 10) of $[H^+]$ (Figure 30–1). Normal arterial pH is therefore $-\log (40 \times 10^{-9}) = 7.40$. Hydrogen ion concentrations between 16 and 160 nEq/L (pH 6.8–7.8) are compatible with life.

Like most dissociation constants, K_W is affected by changes in temperature. Thus the electroneutrality point for water occurs at a pH of 7.0 at 25 °C but at about a pH of 6.8 at 37 °C; temperature-related

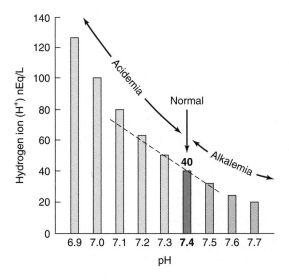

Figure 30–1. The relationship between pH and $[H^+]$. Note that between a pH of 7.10 and 7.50, the relationship between pH and $[H^+]$ is nearly linear. (Reproduced with permission from Narins RG, Emmett M: Simple and mixed acid-base disorders: a practical approach. *Medicine* 1980;49:161.)

changes may be important during hypothermia (see Chapter 21).

Equally important may be other factors that affect the dissociation of water into H^+ and OH^-, such as the strong ion difference (SID), the PCO_2, and the total weak acid concentration. (The latter two will be discussed below.) The SID is the net charge balance of all strong ions present (Na^+, K^+, Ca^{++}, Mg^{++}) minus Cl^- and other strong anions. Infusion of concentrated Na^+ lactate, for example, in a small volume could decrease the plasma H^+ concentration and raise the pH, but this does not happen because the lactate is metabolized to bicarbonate and to H_2O and CO_2. The pH increases because the infused Na^+ increases the SID and decreases the dissociation of water.

Acids & Bases

An acid is usually defined as a chemical species that can act as a proton (H^+) donor, while a base is a species that can act as a proton acceptor (Brönsted-Lowry definitions). The acidity of an aqueous solution therefore reflects its $[H^+]$. A strong acid is a substance that readily and almost irreversibly gives up an H^+ and increases $[H^+]$, while a strong base avidly binds H^+ and decreases $[H^+]$. In contrast, weak acids reversibly donate H^+, while weak bases reversibly bind H^+; both tend to have less of an effect on $[H^+]$. Most biologic compounds are either weak acids or weak bases.

For a solution containing the weak acid HA, where

$$HA \leftrightarrow H^+ + A^-$$

a dissociation constant, K, can be defined as follows:

$$K = \frac{[H^+][A^-]}{[HA]}, \text{ or } [H^+] = \frac{K[HA]}{[A^-]}$$

The negative logarithmic form of the latter equation is called the Henderson-Hasselbalch equation:

$$pH = pK + \log \left(\frac{[A^-]}{[HA]} \right)$$

From this equation, it is apparent that the pH of this solution is related to the ratio of the dissociated anion to the undissociated acid.

Conjugate Pairs & Buffers

When the weak acid HA is in solution, HA can act as an acid by donating an H^+, while A^- can act as a base by taking up H⁺. A⁻ is therefore often referred to as the conjugate base of HA. A similar concept can be applied for weak bases. Consider the weak base B, where

$$B + H^+ \leftrightarrow BH^+$$

BH⁺ is therefore the conjugate acid of B.

A buffer is a solution that contains a weak acid and its conjugate base or a weak base and its conjugate acid (conjugate pairs). Buffers minimize any change in [H⁺] by readily accepting or giving up hydrogen ions. From the Henderson-Hasselbalch equation, it is readily apparent that buffers are most efficient in minimizing changes in the [H⁺] of a solution (ie, [A⁻] = [HA]) when pH = pK. Moreover, the conjugate pair must be present in significant quantities in solution to act as an effective buffer.

CLINICAL DISORDERS

A clear understanding of acid-base disorders and compensatory physiologic responses requires precise terminology (Table 30–1). The suffix "-osis" is used here to denote any pathologic process that alters arterial pH. Thus, any disorder that tends to lower pH is an **acidosis**, while one tending to increase pH is termed an **alkalosis**. If the disorder primarily affects [HCO₃⁻], it is termed metabolic. If the disorder primarily affects PaCO₂, it is termed respiratory. Secondary compensatory responses (see below) should be referred to as just that and not as an "-osis." One might therefore refer to a metabolic acidosis with respiratory compensation.

When only one pathologic process occurs by itself, the acid-base disorder is considered to be **simple.** The presence of two or more primary processes comprises a **mixed** acid-base disorder.

The suffix "-emia" is used to denote the net effect of all primary processes and compensatory physiologic responses (see below) on arterial blood pH. Since arterial blood pH is normally 7.35–7.45 in adults, the term

Table 30–1. Defining acid-based disorders.

Disorder	Primary Change	Compensatory Response
Respiratory		
Acidosis	↑ PaCO₂	↑ HCO₃⁻
Alkalosis	↓ PaCO₂	↓ HCO₃⁻
Metabolic		
Acidosis	↓ HCO₃⁻	↓ PaCO₂
Alkalosis	↑ HCO₃⁻	↑ PaCO₂

"acidemia" signifies a pH < 7.35 while alkalemia signifies a pH > 7.45.

■ COMPENSATORY MECHANISMS

Physiologic responses to changes in [H⁺] are characterized by three phases: (1) immediate chemical buffering, (2) respiratory compensation (whenever possible), and (3) a slower but more effective renal compensatory response that may nearly normalize arterial pH even if the pathologic process is still present.

BODY BUFFERS

Physiologically important buffers in humans include bicarbonate (H₂CO₃/HCO₃⁻), hemoglobin (HbH/Hb⁻), other intracellular proteins (PrH/Pr⁻), phosphates (H₂PO₄⁻/HPO₄²⁻), and ammonia (NH₃/NH₄⁺). The effectiveness of these buffers in the various fluid compartments is related to their concentration (see Chapter 28). Bicarbonate is the most important buffer in the extracellular fluid compartment. Hemoglobin, though restricted inside red blood cells, also functions as an important buffer in blood. Other proteins probably play a major role in buffering the intracellular fluid compartment. Phosphate and ammonium ions are important urinary buffers.

Buffering of the extracellular compartment can also be accomplished by the exchange of extracellular H⁺ for Na⁺ and Ca²⁺ ions from bone and by the exchange of extracellular H⁺ for intracellular K⁺ (see Chapter 28). Acid loads can also demineralize bone and release alkaline compounds (CaCO₃ and CaHPO₄). Alkaline loads (NaHCO₃) increase the deposition of carbonate in bone.

Buffering by plasma bicarbonate is almost immediate while that due to interstitial bicarbonate requires 15–20 minutes. In contrast, buffering by intracellular proteins and bone is slower (2–4 hours). Up to 50–60% of acid loads may ultimately be buffered by bone and intracellular buffers.

The Bicarbonate Buffer

Although in the strictest sense, the bicarbonate buffer consists of H₂CO₃ and HCO₃⁻, CO₂ tension (PaCO₂) may be substituted for H₂CO₃, because:

$$H_2O + CO_2 \leftrightarrow H_2CO_3 \leftrightarrow H^+ + HCO_3^-$$

This hydration of CO₂ is catalyzed by carbonic anhydrase. If adjustments are made in the dissociation constant for the bicarbonate buffer and if the solubility coefficient for CO_2 (0.03 mEq/L) is taken into consideration, the Henderson-Hasselbalch equation for bicarbonate can be written as follows:

$$pH = pK' + \left(\frac{[HCO_3^-]}{0.03\ PaCO_2} \right)$$

where $pK' = 6.1$.

Note that its pK' is not close to the normal arterial pH of 7.40, which means that bicarbonate would not be expected to be an efficient extracellular buffer (see above). The bicarbonate system is, however, important for two reasons: (1) bicarbonate (HCO_3^-) is present in relatively high concentrations in extracellular fluid, and (2) more importantly—$PaCO_2$ and plasma $[HCO_3^-]$ are closely regulated by the lungs and the kidneys, respectively. The ability of these two organs to alter the $[HCO_3^-]/PaCO_2$ ratio allows them to exert important influences on arterial pH.

A simplified and more practical derivation of the Henderson-Hasselbalch equation for the bicarbonate buffer is as follows:

$$[H^+] = 24 \times \frac{PaCO_2}{[HCO_3^-]}$$

This equation is very useful clinically because pH can be readily converted to $[H^+]$ (Table 30–2). Note that below 7.40, $[H^+]$ increases 1.25 nEq/L for each 0.01 decrease in pH; above 7.40, $[H^+]$ decreases 0.8 nEq/L for each 0.01 increase in pH.

Example: If arterial pH = 7.28 and $PaCO_2$ = 24 mm Hg, what should the plasma $[HCO_3^-]$ be?

$$[H+] = 40 + [(40 - 28) \times 1.25] = 55\ nEq/L$$

Therefore,

$$55 = 24 \times \frac{24}{[HCO_3^-]}, \text{ and } [HCO_3^-] =$$

$$\frac{(24 \times 24)}{55} = 10.5\ mEq/L$$

 It should be emphasized that the bicarbonate buffer is effective against metabolic but *not* respiratory acid-base disturbances. If 3 mEq/L

Table 30–2. The relationship between pH and $[H^+]$.

pH	$[H^+]$ nEq/L
6.80	158
6.90	126
7.00	100
7.10	79
7.20	63
7.30	50
7.40	40
7.50	32
7.60	25
7.70	20

of a strong nonvolatile acid such as HCl is added to extracellular fluid, the following takes place:

$$3\ mEq/L\ of\ H^+ + 24\ mEq/L\ of\ HCO_3^- \rightarrow H_2CO^3 + H_2O +$$

$$3\ mEq/L\ of\ CO_2 + 21\ mEq/L\ of\ HCO_3^-$$

Note that HCO_3^- reacts with H^+ to produce CO_2. Moreover, the CO_2 generated is normally eliminated by the lungs such that $PaCO_2$ does not change. Consequently, $[H^+] = 24 \times 40 \div 21 = 45.7$ nEq/L and pH = 7.34. Furthermore, the decrease in $[HCO_3^-]$ reflects the amount of nonvolatile acid added.

In contrast, an increase in CO_2 tension (volatile acid) has a minimal effect on $[HCO_3^-]$. If, for example, $PaCO_2$ increases from 40 to 80 mm Hg, the dissolved CO_2 only increases from 1.2 mEq/L to 2.2 mEq/L. Moreover, the equilibrium constant for the hydration of CO_2 is such that an increase of this magnitude minimally drives the reaction to the left:

$$H_2O + CO_2 \leftrightarrow H_2CO_3 \leftrightarrow H^+ + HCO_3^-$$

If the valid assumption is made that $[HCO_3^-]$ does not appreciably change, then

$$[H^+] = \frac{24 \times 80}{24} = 80\ nEq/L\ and\ pH = 7.10$$

[H⁺] therefore increases by 40 nEq/L, and since HCO₃⁻ is produced in a 1:1 ratio with H⁺, [HCO₃⁻] also increases by 40 nEq/L. Thus, extracellular [HCO₃⁻] increases negligibly, from 24 mEq/L to 24.000040 mEq/L. Therefore, the bicarbonate buffer is not effective against increases in PaCO₂, and changes in [HCO₃⁻] do not reflect the severity of a respiratory acidosis.

Hemoglobin as a Buffer

Hemoglobin is rich in histidine, which is an effective buffer from pH 5.7 to 7.7 (pKa 6.8). Hemoglobin is the most important noncarbonic buffer in extracellular fluid. Simplistically, hemoglobin may be thought of as existing in red blood cells in equilibrium as a weak acid

(HHb) and a potassium salt (KHb). In contrast to the bicarbonate buffer, hemoglobin is capable of buffering both carbonic (CO₂) and noncarbonic (nonvolatile) acids:

$$H^+ + KHb \leftrightarrow HHb + K^+ \text{ and } H_2CO_3 + KHb \leftrightarrow HHb + HCO_3^-$$

PULMONARY COMPENSATION

Changes in alveolar ventilation responsible for pulmonary compensation of PaCO₂ are mediated by chemoreceptors within the brain stem (see Chapter 22). These receptors respond to changes in cerebrospinal spinal fluid pH. Minute ventilation increases 1–4 L/min for every 1 mm Hg increase in PaCO₂. In fact, the lungs are responsible for eliminating the approximately 15 mEq of carbon dioxide produced every day as a by-product of carbohydrate and fat metabolism. Pulmonary compensatory responses are also important in defending against marked changes in pH during metabolic disturbances.

Pulmonary Compensation During Metabolic Acidosis

Decreases in arterial blood pH stimulate medullary respiratory centers. The resulting increase in alveolar ventilation lowers PaCO₂ and tends to restore arterial pH towards normal. The pulmonary response to lower PaCO₂ occurs rapidly but may not reach a predictably steady state until 12–24 hours; pH is never completely restored to normal. PaCO₂ normally decreases 1–1.5 mm Hg below 40 mm Hg for every 1 mEq/L decrease in plasma [HCO₃⁻].

Pulmonary Compensation During Metabolic Alkalosis

Increases in arterial blood pH depress respiratory centers. The resulting alveolar hypoventilation tends to elevate PaCO₂ and restore arterial pH toward normal. The pulmonary response to metabolic alkalosis is generally less predictable than that to metabolic acidosis. Hypoxemia, as a result of progressive hypoventilation, eventually activates oxygen-sensitive chemoreceptors (see Chapter 22); the latter stimulates ventilation and limits the compensatory pulmonary response. Consequently, PaCO₂ usually does not rise above 55 mm Hg in response

to metabolic alkalosis. As a general rule, PaCO₂ can be expected to increase 0.25–1 mm Hg for each 1 mEq/L increase in [HCO₃⁻].

RENAL COMPENSATION

The kidneys' ability to control the amount of HCO₃⁻ reabsorbed from filtered tubular fluid, form new HCO₃⁻, and eliminate H⁺ in the form of titratable acids and ammonium ions (see Chapter 31) allows them to exert a major influence on pH during both metabolic and respiratory acid-base disturbances. In fact, the kidneys are responsible for eliminating the approximately 1 mEq/kg/d of sulfuric acid, phosphoric acid, and incompletely oxidized organic acids that are normally produced by the metabolism of dietary and endogenous proteins, nucleoproteins, and organic phosphates (from phosphoproteins and phospholipids). Metabolism of nucleoproteins also produces uric acid. Incomplete combustion of fatty acids and glucose produce keto acids and lactic acid. Endogenous alkali are produced during the metabolism of some anionic amino acids (glutamate and aspartate) and other organic compounds (citrate, acetate and lactate), but the quantity is insufficient to offset the endogenous acid production.

Renal Compensation During Acidosis

The renal response to acidemia is 3-fold: (1) increased reabsorption of the filtered HCO₃⁻, (2) increased excretion of titratable acids, and (3) increased ammonia production.

Although these mechanisms are probably activated immediately, their effects are generally not appreciable for 12–24 hours and may not be maximal for up to 5 days.

A. INCREASED REABSORPTION OF HCO₃⁻:

Bicarbonate reabsorption is shown in Figure 30–2. CO₂ within renal tubular cells combines with water in the presence of carbonic anhydrase. The carbonic acid (H₂CO₃) formed rapidly dissociates into H⁺ and HCO₃⁻. Bicarbonate ion then enters the bloodstream while the H⁺ is secreted into the renal tubule, where it reacts with filtered HCO₃⁻ to form H₂CO₃. Carbonic anhydrase associated with the luminal brush border cat-

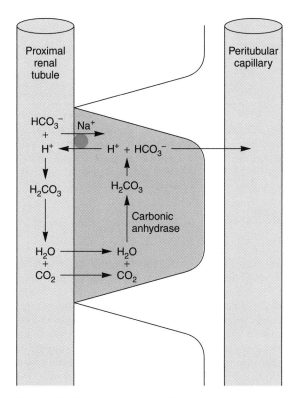

Figure 30–2. Reclamation of filtered HCO_3^- by the proximal renal tubules.

alyzes the dissociation of H_2CO_3 into CO_2 and H_2O. The CO_2 thus formed can diffuse back into the renal tubular cell to replace the CO_2 originally consumed. The proximal tubules normally reabsorb 80–90% of the filtered bicarbonate load along with sodium, while the distal tubules are responsible for the remaining 10–20%. Unlike the proximal H^+ pump, the H^+ pump in the distal tubule is not necessarily linked to sodium reabsorption, and is capable of generating steep H^+ gradients between tubular fluid and tubular cells. Urinary pH can decrease as low as 4.4 (compared with a pH of 7.40 in plasma).

B. Increased Excretion of Titratable Acids:

After all the HCO_3^- in tubular fluid is reclaimed, the H^+ secreted into the tubular lumen can combine with HPO_4^{2-} to form $H_2PO_4^-$ (Figure 30–3); the latter is not readily reabsorbed because of its charge and is eliminated in urine. The net result is that H^+ is excreted from the body as $H_2PO_4^-$, and the HCO_3^- that is generated in the process can enter the bloodstream. With a pK of 6.8, the $H_2PO_4^-/HPO_4^{2-}$ pair is normally an ideal urinary buffer. When urinary pH approaches 4.4,

however, all the phosphate reaching the distal tubule is in the $H_2PO_4^-$ form; HPO_4^{2-} ions are no longer available for eliminating H^+.

C. Increased Formation of Ammonia:

After complete reabsorption of HCO_3^- and consumption of the phosphate buffer, NH_3/NH_4^+ pair becomes the most important urinary buffer (Figure 30–4). Deamination of glutamine within the mitochondria of proximal tubular cells is the principal source of NH_3 production in the kidneys. Acidemia markedly increases renal NH_3 production. The ammonia formed is then able to passively cross the cell's luminal membrane, enter tubular fluid, and react with H^+ to form NH_4^+. Unlike NH_3, NH_4^+ does not readily penetrate the luminal membrane and is therefore trapped within the tubules. Thus, excretion of NH_4^+ in urine effectively eliminates H^+.

Renal Compensation During Alkalosis

The tremendous amount of HCO_3^- normally filtered and subsequently reabsorbed allows the kidneys to

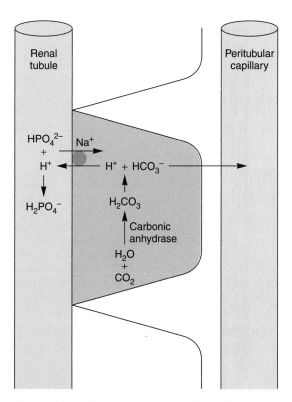

Figure 30–3. Formation of a titratable acid in urine.

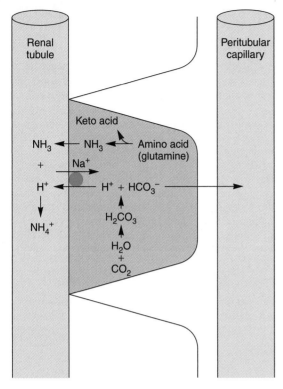

Figure 30–4. Formation of ammonia in urine.

rapidly excrete large amounts of bicarbonate if necessary (see Chapter 28). As a result, the kidneys are highly effective in protecting against metabolic alkalosis. Metabolic alkalosis therefore generally occurs only in association with concomitant sodium deficiency or mineralocorticoid excess. Sodium depletion decreases extracellular fluid volume and enhances Na$^+$ reabsorption in the proximal tubule (see Chapter 28). To maintain neutrality, the Na$^+$ ion is brought across with a Cl$^-$ ion. As Cl$^-$ ions decrease in number (< 10 mEq/L of urine), HCO$_3^-$ must be reabsorbed. In addition, increased H$^+$ secretion in exchange for augmented Na$^+$ reabsorption favors continued HCO$_3^-$ formation even in the face of metabolic alkalosis. Similarly, increased mineralocorticoid activity augments aldosterone-mediated Na$^+$ reabsorption in exchange for H$^+$ secretion in the distal tubules (see Chapter 28). The resulting increase in HCO$_3^-$ formation can initiate or propagate metabolic alkalosis. Metabolic alkalosis is commonly associated with increased mineralocorticoid activity even in the absence of sodium and chloride depletion (see Chapters 28 and 36).

Base Excess

Base excess is the amount of acid or base that must be added to return blood pH to 7.40 and PaCO$_2$ to 40 mm Hg at full O$_2$ saturation and 37 °C. Moreover, it adjusts for noncarbonic (hemoglobin) buffering in the blood. Simplistically, base excess represents the metabolic component of an acid-base disturbance. A positive value indicates metabolic alkalosis, while a negative value reveals metabolic acidosis. Base excess is usually derived graphically or electronically from a nomogram originally developed by Siggaard-Andersen and requires measurement of hemoglobin concentration (Figure 30–5).

ACIDOSIS

PHYSIOLOGIC EFFECTS OF ACIDEMIA

The overall effects of acidemia represent the balance between its direct effects and sympathoadrenal activation. With worsening acidosis (pH < 7.20), direct depressant effects predominate. Direct myocardial and smooth muscle depression reduces cardiac contractility and peripheral vascular resistance, resulting in progressive hypotension (see Chapter 19). Severe acidosis can lead to tissue hypoxia despite a rightward shift in hemoglobin affinity for oxygen (see Chapter 22). Both cardiac and vascular smooth muscle become less responsive to endogenous and exogenous catecholamines, and the threshold for ventricular fibrillation is decreased. Progressive hyperkalemia as a result of the movement of K$^+$ out of cells in exchange for extracellular H$^+$ (see Chapter 28) is also potentially lethal. Plasma [K$^+$] increases approximately 0.6 mEq/L for each 0.10 decrease in pH.

Central nervous system depression is more prominent with respiratory acidosis than with metabolic acidosis. This effect, often termed **CO$_2$ narcosis,** may be the result of intracranial hypertension secondary to increased cerebral blood flow, and severe intracellular acidosis. Unlike CO$_2$, H$^+$ ions do not readily penetrate the blood brain barrier (see Chapter 25).

RESPIRATORY ACIDOSIS

Respiratory acidosis is defined as a primary increase in PaCO$_2$ This increase drives the reaction H$_2$O + CO$_2$ ↔ H$_2$CO$_3$ ↔ H$^+$ + HCO$_3^-$ to the right, leading to an increase in [H$^+$] and a fall in arterial pH. For the reasons described above, [HCO$_3^-$] is minimally affected.

PaCO$_2$ represents the balance between CO$_2$ production and CO$_2$ elimination (see Chapter 22):

$$PaCO_2 = \frac{CO_2 \text{ production}}{\text{Alveolar ventilation}}$$

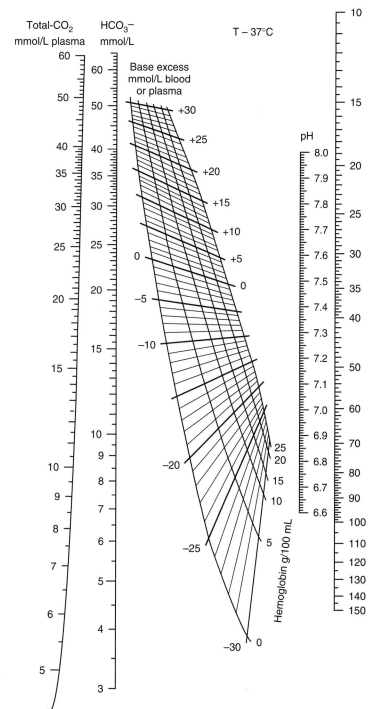

Figure 30–5. The Siggaard-Andersen nomogram for calculating base excess.

Carbon dioxide production is a by-product of fat and carbohydrate metabolism. Muscle activity, body temperature, and thyroid hormone activity can all have major influences on CO_2 production. Because CO_2 production does not appreciably vary under most circumstances, respiratory acidosis is usually the result of alveolar hypoventilation (Table 30–3). In patients with a limited capacity to increase alveolar ventilation, however, increased CO_2 production can precipitate respiratory acidosis.

Table 30–3. Causes of respiratory acidosis.

Alveolar hypoventilation
Central nervous system depression
  Drug-induced
  Sleep disorders
  Obesity hypoventilation (Pickwickian) syndrome
  Cerebral ischemia
  Cerebral trauma
Neuromuscular disorders
  Myopathies
  Neuropathies
Chest wall abnormalities
  Flail chest
  Kyphoscoliosis
Pleural abnormalities
  Pneumothorax
  Pleural effusion
Airway obstruction
  Upper airway
    Foreign body
    Tumor
    Laryngospasm
    Sleep disorders
  Lower airway
    Severe asthma
    Chronic obstructive pulmonary disease
    Tumor
Parenchymal lung disease
  Pulmonary edema
    Cardiogenic
    Noncardiogenic
  Pulmonary emboli
  Pneumonia
  Aspiration
  Interstitial lung disease
Ventilator malfunction
Increased CO_2 production
Large carbohydrate loads
Malignant hyperthermia
Intensive shivering
Prolonged seizure activity
Thyroid storm
Extensive thermal injury (burns)

Acute Respiratory Acidosis

The compensatory response to acute (6–12 hours) elevations in $PaCO_2$ is limited. Buffering is primarily provided by hemoglobin and the exchange of extracellular H^+ for Na^+ and K^+ from bone and the intracellular fluid compartment (see above). The renal response to retain more bicarbonate is very limited acutely. As a result, plasma $[HCO_3^-]$ increases only about 1 mEq/L for each 10 mm Hg increase in $PaCO_2$ above 40 mm Hg.

Chronic Respiratory Acidosis

"Full" renal compensation characterizes chronic respiratory acidosis. Renal compensation is appreciable only after 12–24 hours and may not peak until 3–5 days. During that time, the sustained increase in $PaCO_2$ has been present long enough to permit maximal renal compensation. During chronic respiratory acidosis, plasma $[HCO_3^-]$ increases approximately 4 mEq/L for each 10 mm Hg increase in $PaCO_2$ above 40 mm Hg.

Treatment of Respiratory Acidosis

The treatment of respiratory acidosis is to reverse the imbalance between CO_2 production and alveolar ventilation. In most instances, this is accomplished by increasing alveolar ventilation. Measures aimed at reducing CO_2 production (eg, dantrolene, muscle paralysis, antithyroid medication, or reduced carbohydrate intake) are useful only in specific instances (malignant hyperthermia, tetanus, thyroid storm, and total parenteral nutrition, respectively). Temporizing measures aimed at improving alveolar ventilation include bronchodilation, reversal of narcosis, administration of a respiratory stimulant (doxapram), or improving lung compliance (diuresis). Moderate to severe acidosis (pH < 7.20), CO_2 narcosis, and impending respiratory muscle fatigue are indications for mechanical ventilation (see Chapter 50). An increased inspired oxygen concentration is also usually necessary, since coexistent hypoxemia is common. Intravenous $NaHCO_3$ is rarely necessary unless pH is < 7.10 and HCO_3^- is < 15 mEq/L. Sodium bicarbonate therapy will transiently increase $PaCO_2$:

$$H^+ + HCO_3^- \leftrightarrow CO_2 + H_2O$$

Buffers that do not produce CO_2, such as carbicarb or tromethamine (THAM) have been proposed as alternatives but are not of proven benefit (below). Carbicarb is a mixture of 0.3 M sodium bicarbonate and 0.3 M sodium carbonate; buffering by this mixture mainly produces sodium bicarbonate instead of CO_2.

Tromethamine has the added advantage of lacking sodium and may be a more effective intracellular buffer.

Patients with a baseline chronic respiratory acidosis require special consideration (see Chapter 23). When such patients develop acute ventilatory failure, the goal of therapy should be to return $PaCO_2$ to the patient's "normal" baseline. Normalizing the patient's $PaCO_2$ to 40 mm Hg will result in respiratory alkalosis (see below). Oxygen therapy must also be carefully controlled, because the respiratory drive in these patients may become dependent on hypoxemia not $PaCO_2$ or may increase physiologic dead space (see Chapters 22 and 23); "normalization" of $PaCO_2$ or relative hyperoxia can precipitate severe hypoventilation.

METABOLIC ACIDOSIS

Metabolic acidosis is defined as a primary decrease in $[HCO_3^-]$. Pathologic processes can initiate metabolic acidosis by one of three mechanisms: (1) consumption of HCO_3^- by a strong nonvolatile acid, (2) renal or gastrointestinal wasting of bicarbonate, or (3) rapid dilution of the extracellular fluid compartment with a bicarbonate-free fluid.

A fall in plasma $[HCO_3^-]$ without a proportionate reduction in $PaCO_2$ decreases arterial pH. The pulmonary compensatory response in a simple metabolic acidosis (see above) characteristically does not reduce $PaCO_2$ to a level that completely normalizes pH but can produce marked hyperventilation (**Kussmaul's respiration**).

Table 30–4 lists disorders that can cause metabolic acidosis. Note that differential diagnosis of metabolic acidosis may be facilitated by calculation of the anion gap.

The Anion Gap

The anion gap in plasma is most commonly defined as the difference between the major measured cations and the major measured anions:

Anion Gap = Major plasma cations − Major plasma anions

or

$$\text{Anion Gap} = [Na^+] - ([Cl^-] + [HCO_3^-])$$

Some physicians include plasma K^+ in the calculation. Using normal values,

Anion Gap = 140 − (104 + 24) = 12 mEq/L
(normal range = 7 − 14 mEq/L)

Table 30–4. Causes of metabolic acidosis.

Increased anion gap
  Increased production of endogenous nonvolatile acids
    Renal failure
    Ketoacidosis
      Diabetic
      Starvation
    Lactic acidosis
    Mixed
      Nonketotic hyperosmolar coma
      Alcoholic
    Inborn errors of metabolism
  Ingestion of toxin
    Salicylate
    Methanol
    Ethylene glycol
    Paraldehyde
    Toluene
    Sulfur
  Rhabdomyolysis
Normal anion gap (hyperchloremic)
  Increased gastrointestinal losses of HCO_3^-
    Diarrhea
    Anion exchange resins (cholestyramine)
    Ingestion of $CaCl_2$, $MgCl_2$
    Fistulae (pancreatic, biliary, or small bowel)
    Ureterosigmoidostomy or obstructed ileal loop
  Increased renal losses of HCO_3^-
    Renal tubular acidosis
    Carbonic anhydrase inhibitors
    Hypoaldosteronism
  Dilutional
    Large amount of bicarbonate-free fluids
  Total parenteral nutrition
  Increased intake of chloride-containing acids
    Ammonium chloride
    Lysine hydrochloride
    Arginine hydrochloride

In reality, an anion gap cannot exist because electroneutrality must be maintained in the body; the sum of all anions must equal the sum of all cations. Therefore,

Anion Gap = Unmeasured anions − Unmeasured cations

"Unmeasured cations" include K^+, Ca^{2+}, and Mg^{2+}, while "unmeasured anions" include all organic anions (including plasma proteins), sulfates, and phosphates. Plasma albumin normally accounts for the largest fraction of the anion gap (about 11 mEq/L). The anion gap decreases by 2.5 mEq/L for every 1 g/dL reduction in plasma albumin concentration. Any process that increases "unmeasured anions" or decreases "unmeasured cations" will increase the anion gap. Conversely, any process that decreases "unmeasured anions" or increases "unmeasured cations" will decrease the anion gap.

Mild elevations of plasma anion gap up to 20 mEq/L may not be helpful diagnostically during acidosis, but values > 30 mEq/L usually indicate the presence of a high anion gap acidosis (below). Metabolic alkalosis can also produce a high anion gap because of extracellular volume depletion, an increased charge on albumin, and a compensatory increase in lactate production. A low plasma anion gap may be encountered with hypoalbuminemia, bromide or lithium intoxication, and multiple myeloma.

High Anion Gap Metabolic Acidosis

Metabolic acidosis with a high anion gap is characterized by an increase in relatively strong nonvolatile acids. These acids dissociate into H^+ and their respective anions; the H^+ consumes HCO_3^- to produce CO_2, while their anions (conjugate bases) accumulate and take the place of HCO_3^- in extracellular fluid (hence the anion gap increases). Nonvolatile acids can be endogenously produced or ingested.

A. Failure to Excrete Endogenous Nonvolatile Acids:

Endogenously produced organic acids are normally eliminated by the kidneys in urine (above). Glomerular filtration rates below 20 mL/min (renal failure) typically result in progressive metabolic acidosis from the accumulation of these acids.

B. Increased Endogenous Nonvolatile Acid Production:

Severe tissue hypoxia following hypoxemia, hypoperfusion (ischemia), or inability to utilize oxygen (cyanide poisoning) can result in **lactic acidosis.** Lactic acid is the end product of the anaerobic metabolism of glucose (glycolysis) and can rapidly accumulate under these conditions. Decreased utilization of lactate by the liver, and to a lesser extent the kidneys, is less commonly responsible for lactic acidosis; causes include hypoperfusion, alcoholism, and liver disease. Lactate levels can be readily measured and are normally 0.3 to 1.3 mEq/L. Acidosis resulting from D-lactic acid, which is not recognized by α-lactate dehydrogenase (and not measured by routine assays), may be encountered in patients with short bowel syndromes; this latter compound is formed by colonic bacteria from dietary glucose and starch and is absorbed systemically.

An absolute or relative lack of insulin can result in hyperglycemia and progressive ketoacidosis from accumulation of β-hydroxybutyric and acetoacetic acids. Ketoacidosis may also be seen following starvation and alcoholic binges. The pathophysiology of the acidosis often associated with severe alcoholic intoxication and nonketotic hyperosmolar coma is complex and may represent a build-up of lactic, keto, or other unknown acids.

Some inborn errors of metabolism, such as maple syrup urine disease, methylmalonic aciduria, propionic acidemia, and isovaleric acidemia, produce a high anion gap metabolic acidosis as a result of accumulation of abnormal amino acids.

C. Ingestion of Exogenous Nonvolatile Acids:

Ingestion of large amounts of salicylates frequently results in metabolic acidosis. Salicylic acid as well as other acid intermediates rapidly accumulate and produce a high anion gap acidosis. Because salicylates also produce direct respiratory stimulation, most adults develop mixed metabolic acidosis with superimposed respiratory alkalosis. Ingestion of methanol (methyl alcohol) frequently produces acidosis and visual disturbances (retinitis). Symptoms are typically delayed until the slow oxidation of methanol by alcohol dehydrogenase produces formic acid, which is highly toxic to the retina. The high anion gap represents the accumulation of many organic acids, including acetic acid. The toxicity of ethylene glycol is also the result of the action of alcohol dehydrogenase to produce glycolic acid. Glycolic acid, the principal cause of the acidosis, is further metabolized to form oxalic acid, which can be deposited in the renal tubules and result in renal failure.

Normal Anion Gap Metabolic Acidosis

Metabolic acidosis associated with a normal anion gap is typically characterized by hyperchloremia. Plasma $[Cl^-]$ increases to take the place of the HCO_3^- ions lost. Hyperchloremic metabolic acidosis most commonly results from abnormal gastrointestinal or renal losses of HCO_3^-.

Calculation of the anion gap in urine can be helpful in diagnosing a normal anion gap acidosis.

$$\text{Urine anion gap} = ([Na^+] + [K^+]) - [Cl^-]$$

The urine anion gap is normally positive or close to zero. The principle unmeasured urinary cation is normally NH_4^+ which should increase (along with Cl^-) during a metabolic acidosis; the latter results in a negative urinary anion gap. Impairment of H^+ or NH_4^+ secretion, as occurs in renal failure or renal tubular acidosis (below), results in a positive urine anion gap in spite of systemic acidosis.

A. INCREASED GASTROINTESTINAL LOSS OF HCO_3^-:

Diarrhea is the most common cause of hyperchloremic metabolic acidosis. Diarrheal fluid contains 20–50 mEq/L of HCO_3^-. Small bowel, biliary, and pancreatic fluids are all rich in HCO_3^-. Loss of large volumes of these fluids can lead to a hyperchloremic metabolic acidosis. Patients with ureterosigmoidostomies and those with ileal loops that are too long or that become partially obstructed frequently develop hyperchloremic metabolic acidosis (see Chapter 28). The ingestion of chloride-containing anion exchange resins (cholestyramine) or large amounts of calcium or magnesium chloride can result in increased absorption of chloride and loss of bicarbonate ions. These nonabsorbable resins bind bicarbonate ions, while calcium and magnesium combine with bicarbonate to form insoluble salts within the intestines.

B. INCREASED RENAL LOSS OF HCO_3^-:

Renal wasting of HCO_3^- can occur as a result of failure to reabsorb filtered HCO_3^- or to secrete adequate amounts of H^+ in the form of titratable acid or ammonium ion. These defects are encountered in patients taking carbonic anhydrase inhibitors such as acetazolamide and those with renal tubular acidosis.

Renal tubular acidosis comprises a group of nonazotemic defects of H^+ secretion by the renal tubules, resulting in a urinary pH that is too high for the systemic acidemia. These defects may be a result of a primary renal defect or secondary to a systemic disorder. The site of the H^+-secreting defect may be in the distal (type 1) or proximal (type 2) renal tubule. Hyporeninemic hypoaldosteronism is commonly referred to as type 4 renal tubular acidosis (see Chapter 28). With distal renal tubular acidosis, the defect occurs at a site after most of the filtered HCO_3^- has been reclaimed. As a result, there is a failure to acidify the urine, so that net acid excretion is less than daily net acid production. This disorder is frequently associated with hypokalemia, demineralization of bone, nephrolithiasis, and nephrocalcinosis. Alkali ($NaHCO_3$) therapy with 1–3 mEq/kg/d is usually sufficient to reverse those side effects. With the less common proximal renal tubular acidosis, defective H^+ secretion in the proximal tubule results in massive wasting of HCO_3^-. Concomitant defects in tubular reabsorption of other substances such as glucose, amino acids, or phosphates are common. The hyperchloremic acidosis results in volume depletion and hypokalemia. Treatment involves giving alkali (as much as 10–25 mEq/kg/d) and potassium supplements.

C. OTHER CAUSES OF HYPERCHLOREMIC ACIDOSIS:

A dilutional hyperchloremic acidosis can occur when extracellular volume is rapidly expanded with a bicarbonate-free fluid such as normal saline. The plasma HCO_3^- decreases proportional to the amount of fluid infused as extracellular HCO_3^- is diluted. Amino acid infusions (parenteral hyperalimentation) contain organic cations in excess of organic anions and can produce hyperchloremic metabolic acidosis because chloride is commonly used as the anion for the cationic amino acids. Lastly, the administration of large quantities of chloride-containing acids such as ammonium chloride or arginine hydrochloride (usually given to treat a metabolic alkalosis) can cause hyperchloremic metabolic acidosis if too much is given.

Treatment of Metabolic Acidosis

Several general measures can be undertaken to control the severity of acidemia until the underlying processes are corrected. Any respiratory component of the acidemia should be corrected. Respiration should be controlled if necessary; a $PaCO_2$ in the low 30s may be desirable to partially return pH towards normal. If arterial blood pH remains below 7.20, alkali therapy, usually in the form of $NaHCO_3$ (usually a 7.5% solution), may be necessary. $PaCO_2$ may transiently rise as HCO_3^- is consumed by acids (emphasizing the need to control ventilation in severe acidemia). The amount of $NaHCO_3$ given is decided empirically as a fixed dose (1 mEq/kg) or is derived from the base excess and the calculated bicarbonate space (see below). In either case, serial blood gas measurements are mandatory to avoid complications (namely, overshoot alkalosis and sodium overload) and to guide further therapy. Raising arterial pH to > 7.25 is usually sufficient to overcome the adverse physiologic effects of the acidemia. Profound or refractory acidemia may necessitate acute hemodialysis with a bicarbonate dialysate.

The routine use of large amounts of $NaHCO_3$ in treating cardiac arrest and low flow states is no longer recommended (see Chapter 48). Paradoxical intracellular acidosis may occur, especially when CO_2 elimination is impaired, because the CO_2 formed readily enters cells but bicarbonate ion does not. Alternate buffers that do not produce CO_2 may be theoretically preferable, but are unproved clinically.

Specific therapy for diabetic ketoacidosis includes replacement of the existing fluid deficit (as a result of a hyperglycemic osmotic diuresis) first as well as insulin, potassium, phosphate, and magnesium. The treatment of lactic acidosis should be directed first at restoring adequate oxygenation and tissue perfusion. Alkalinization of the urine with $NaHCO_3$ to a pH greater than 7.0 increases elimination of salicylate following salicylate poisoning. Ethanol infusions (an IV loading dose of 8–10 mL/kg of a 10% ethanol in D5 solution over 30 minutes with the concomitant administration of a continuous infusion at 0.15 mL/kg/hour to achieve a blood ethanol level of 100–130 mg/dL) are indicated following methanol or ethylene glycol intoxication. Ethanol competes for alcohol dehydrogenase and slows down the formation of formic acid from methanol and glycolic and oxalic acids from ethylene glycol, respectively.

BICARBONATE SPACE:

The bicarbonate space is defined as the volume that HCO_3^- will distribute to when given intravenously. While this theoretically should equal the extracellular fluid space (approximately 25% of body weight), in reality it ranges anywhere between 25% and 60% of body weight depending on the severity and duration of the acidosis. This variation is at least partly related to the amount of intracellular and bone buffering that has taken place.

Example: Calculate the amount of $NaHCO_3$ necessary to correct a base deficit (BD) of –10 mEq/L for a 70-kg man with an estimated HCO_3^- space of 30%:

$$NaHCO_3 = BD \times 30\% \times \text{body weight in L.}$$

$$NaHCO_3 = -10 \text{ mEq/L} \times 30\% \times 70 \text{ L} = 210 \text{ mEq}$$

In practice, only 50% of the calculated dose (105 mEq) is usually given, after which another blood gas is measured.

ANESTHETIC CONSIDERATIONS IN PATIENTS WITH ACIDOSIS

Acidemia can potentiate the depressant effects of most sedatives and anesthetic agents on the central nervous and circulatory systems. Since most opioids are weak bases, acidosis can increase the fraction of the drug in the nonionized form and facilitate penetration of the opioid into the brain. Increased sedation and depression of airway reflexes may predispose to pulmonary aspiration. The circulatory depressant effects of both volatile and intravenous anesthetics can also be exaggerated. Moreover, any agent that rapidly decreases sympathetic tone can potentially allow unopposed circulatory depression in the setting of acidosis. Halothane is more arrhythmogenic in the presence of acidosis. Succinylcholine should generally be avoided in acidotic patients with hyperkalemia to prevent further increases in plasma [K^+]. Lastly, respiratory—but not metabolic—acidosis augments nondepolarizing neuromuscular blockade and may prevent its antagonism by reversal agents.

■ ALKALOSIS

PHYSIOLOGIC EFFECTS OF ALKALOSIS

Alkalosis increases the affinity of hemoglobin for oxygen and shifts the oxygen dissociation curve to the left, making it more difficult for hemoglobin to give up oxygen to tissues (see Chapter 22). Movement of H^+ out of cells in exchange for the movement of extracellular K^+ into cells can produce hypokalemia (see Chapter 28). Alkalosis increases the number of anionic binding sites for Ca^{2+} on plasma proteins and can therefore decrease ionized plasma [Ca^{2+}], leading to circulatory depression and neuromuscular irritability (see Chapter 28). Respiratory alkalosis reduces cerebral blood flow (see Chapter 25), increases systemic vascular resistance, and may precipitate coronary vasospasm (see Chapter 19). In the lungs, respiratory alkalosis increases bronchial smooth muscle tone (bronchoconstriction) but decreases pulmonary vascular resistance (see Chapter 22).

RESPIRATORY ALKALOSIS

Respiratory alkalosis is defined as a primary decrease in $PaCO_2$. The mechanism is usually an inappropriate increase in alveolar ventilation relative to CO_2 production. Table 30–5 lists the most common causes of respiratory alkalosis. *Plasma* [HCO_3^-] usually decreases 2 mEq/L for each 10 mm Hg acute decrease in $PaCO_2$ below 40 mm Hg. The distinction between acute and chronic respiratory alkalosis is not always made, because the compensatory response to chronic respiratory alkalosis is quite variable: plasma [HCO_3^-] decreases 2–5 mEq/L for each 10 mm Hg decrease in $PaCO_2$ below 40 mm Hg.

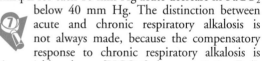

Treatment of Respiratory Alkalosis

Correction of the underlying process is the only treatment for respiratory alkalosis. For severe alkalemia (arterial pH > 7.60), intravenous hydrochloric acid, arginine chloride, or ammonium chloride may be indicated (see below).

METABOLIC ALKALOSIS

Metabolic alkalosis is defined as a primary increase in plasma [HCO_3^-]. Most cases of metabolic alkalosis can be divided into (1) those associated with NaCl deficiency and ECF depletion, often described as chloride-sensitive; and (2) those associated with enhanced mineralocorticoid activity, commonly referred to as chloride-resistant (Table 30–6).

Table 30–5. Causes of respiratory alkalosis.

Central stimulation
  Pain
  Anxiety
  Ischemia
  Stroke
  Tumor
  Infection
  Fever
  Drug-induced
    Salicylates
    Progesterone (pregnancy)
    Analeptics (doxapram)
Peripheral stimulation
  Hypoxemia
  High altitude
  Pulmonary disease
    Congestive heart failure
    Noncardiogenic pulmonary edema
    Asthma
    Pulmonary embolism
  Severe anemia
Unknown mechanism
  Sepsis
  Metabolic encephalopathies
Iatrogenic
  Ventilator-induced

25–100 mEq/L of H^+, 40–160 mEq/L of Na^+, about 15 mEq/L of K^+, and approximately 200 mEq/L of Cl^-. Vomiting or continuous loss of gastric fluid by gastric drainage (nasogastric suctioning) can result in marked metabolic alkalosis, extracellular volume depletion, and hypokalemia. Rapid normalization of $PaCO_2$ after plasma $[HCO_3^-]$ has risen in chronic respiratory acidosis results in metabolic alkalosis (posthypercapnic alkalosis; see above). Infants being fed formulas containing Na^+ without chloride readily develop metabolic alkalosis because of the increased H^+ (or K^+) secretion that must accompany sodium absorption.

Chloride-Resistant Metabolic Alkalosis

Increased mineralocorticoid activity commonly results in metabolic alkalosis even when it is not associated with extracellular volume depletion. Inappropriate (unregulated) increases in mineralocorticoid activity cause

Table 30–6. Causes of metabolic alkalosis.

Chloride-sensitive
  Gastrointestinal
    Vomiting
    Gastric drainage
    Chloride diarrhea
    Villous adenoma
  Renal
    Diuretics
    Posthypercapnic
    Low chloride intake
  Sweat
    Cystic fibrosis
Chloride-resistant
  Increased mineralocorticoid activity
    Primary hyperaldosteronism
    Edematous disorders (secondary hyperaldosteronism)
    Cushing's syndrome
    Licorice ingestion
    Bartter's syndrome
  Severe hypokalemia
Miscellaneous
  Massive blood transfusion
  Acetate-containing colloid solutions
  Alkaline administration with renal insufficiency
    Alkali therapy
    Combined antacid and cation exchange resin therapy
  Hypercalcemia
    Milk-alkali syndrome
    Bone metastases
  Sodium penicillins
  Glucose feeding after starvation

Chloride-Sensitive Metabolic Alkalosis

Extracellular fluid depletion causes the renal tubules to avidly reabsorb Na^+. Because not enough Cl^- is available to accompany all the Na^+ ions reabsorbed, increased H^+ secretion must take place to maintain electroneutrality. In effect, HCO_3^- ions that might otherwise have been excreted are reabsorbed, resulting in metabolic alkalosis. Physiologically, maintenance of extracellular fluid volume is therefore given priority over acid-base balance. Because secretion of K^+ ion can also maintain electroneutrality, potassium secretion is also enhanced. Moreover, hypokalemia augments H^+ secretion (and HCO_3^- reabsorption) and will also propagate metabolic alkalosis. Indeed, severe hypokalemia alone can cause alkalosis. Urinary chloride concentrations during a chloride-sensitive metabolic alkalosis are characteristically low (< 10 mEq/L).

Diuretic therapy is the most common cause of chloride-sensitive metabolic alkalosis. Diuretics such as furosemide, ethacrynic acid, and thiazides increase Na^+, Cl^-, and K^+ excretion, resulting in NaCl depletion, hypokalemia, and usually mild metabolic alkalosis. Loss of gastric fluid is also a common cause of chloride-sensitive metabolic alkalosis. Gastric secretions contain sodium retention and expansion of extracellular fluid volume. Increased H^+ and K^+ secretion takes place to balance enhanced mineralocorticoid-mediated sodium reabsorption, resulting in metabolic alkalosis and hypokalemia. Urinary chloride concentrations are typically greater than 20 mEq/L in such cases.

Other Causes of Metabolic Alkalosis

Metabolic alkalosis is rarely encountered in patients given even large doses of $NaHCO_3$ unless renal excretion of HCO_3^- is impaired. The administration of large amounts of blood products and some plasma protein-containing colloid solution frequently results in metabolic alkalosis. The citrate, lactate, and acetate contained in these fluids are converted by the liver into HCO_3^-. Patients receiving high doses of sodium penicillin (especially carbenicillin) can develop metabolic alkalosis. Because penicillins act as nonabsorbable anions in the renal tubules, increased H^+ (or K^+) secretion must accompany sodium absorption. For reasons that are not clear, hypercalcemia that results from nonparathyroid causes (milk-alkali syndrome and bone metastases) is also often associated with metabolic alkalosis. The pathophysiology of alkalosis following refeeding is also unknown.

Treatment of Metabolic Alkalosis

As with other acid-base disorders, correction of metabolic alkalosis is never complete until the underlying disorder is treated. When ventilation is controlled, any respiratory component contributing to alkalemia should be corrected by decreasing minute ventilation to normalize $PaCO_2$. The treatment of choice for chloride-sensitive metabolic alkalosis is intravenous saline (NaCl) administration and potassium (KCl) replacement. H_2 blocker therapy is useful when excessive loss of gastric fluid is a factor. Acetazolamide may also be useful in edematous patients. Alkalosis associated with primary increases in mineralocorticoid activity readily responds to aldosterone antagonists (spironolactone). When arterial blood pH is greater than 7.60, treatment with intravenous hydrochloric acid (0.1 mol/L), ammonium chloride (0.1 mol/L), arginine hydrochloride, or hemodialysis should be considered.

ANESTHETIC CONSIDERATIONS IN PATIENTS WITH ALKALEMIA

Respiratory alkalosis appears to prolong the duration of opioid-induced respiratory depression; this effect may result from increased protein binding of opioids. Cerebral ischemia can occur from marked reduction in cere-

 bral blood flow during respiratory alkalosis, especially during hypotension. The combination of alkalemia and hypokalemia can precipitate severe atrial and ventricular dysrhythmias. Potentiation of nondepolarizing neuromuscular blockade is reported with alkalemia but may be more directly related to concomitant hypokalemia.

■ DIAGNOSIS OF ACID-BASE DISORDERS

Interpretation of acid-base status from analysis of blood gases requires a systematic approach. A recommended approach follows (Figure 30–6):

(1) Look at arterial pH: Is acidemia or alkalemia present?

(2) Look at $PaCO_2$: Is the change in $PaCO_2$ consistent with a respiratory component?

(3) If the change in $PaCO_2$ does not explain the change in arterial pH, does the change in $[HCO_3^-]$ indicate a metabolic component?

(4) Make a tentative diagnosis (see Table 30–1).

(5) Compare the change in $[HCO_3^-]$ with the change in $PaCO_2$. Does a compensatory response exist (Table 30–7)? Because arterial pH is related to the ratio of $PaCO_2$ to $[HCO_3^-]$, both pulmonary and renal compensatory mechanisms are *always* such that $PaCO_2$ and $[HCO_3^-]$ change in

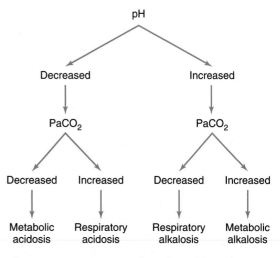

Figure 30–6. Diagnosis of simple acid-base disorders.

Table 30–7. Normal compensatory responses in acid-base disturbances.

Disturbance	Response	Expected Change
Respiratory acidosis		
Acute	↑ [HCO$_3^-$]	1 mEq/L/10 mm Hg increase in PaCO$_2$
Chronic	↑ [HCO$_3^-$]	4 mEq/L/10 mm Hg increase in PaCO$_2$
Respiratory alkalosis		
Acute	↓ [HCO$_3^-$]	2 mEq/L/10 mm Hg decrease in PaCO$_2^-$
Chronic	↓ [HCO$_3^-$]	4 mEq/L/10 mm Hg decrease in PaCO$_2$
Metabolic acidosis	↓ PaCO$_2$	1.2 × the decrease in [HCO$_3^-$]
Metabolic alkalosis	↑ PaCO$_2$	0.7 × the increase in [HCO$_3^-$]

the same direction. A change in opposite directions implies a mixed acid-base disorder.

(6) If the compensatory response is more or less than expected, by definition a mixed acid-base disorder exists.

(7) Calculate the plasma anion gap in the case of metabolic acidosis.

(8) Measure urinary chloride concentration in the case of metabolic alkalosis.

An alternate rapid but perhaps less precise approach is to correlate changes in pH with changes in CO_2 or HCO_3. For a respiratory disturbance, every 10 mm Hg change in CO_2 should change arterial pH by approximately 0.08 units in the opposite direction. During metabolic disturbances, every 6 mEq change in HCO_3 also changes arterial pH by 0.1 in the same direction. If the change in pH exceeds or is less than predicated, a mixed acid-base disorder is likely to be present.

MEASUREMENT OF BLOOD GAS TENSIONS & pH

Values obtained by routine blood gas measurement include oxygen and carbon dioxide tensions (PO_2 and PCO_2), pH, [HCO$_3^-$], base excess, hemoglobin, and the percentage oxygen saturation of hemoglobin. As a rule, only PO_2, PCO_2, pH are measured. Hemoglobin and percent oxygen saturation are measured with a cooximeter. [HCO$_3^-$] is derived using the Henderson-Hasselbalch equation and base excess from the Siggaard-Andersen nomogram.

Sample Source & Collection

Arterial blood samples are most commonly utilized clinically, though capillary or venous blood can be used if the limitations of such samples are recognized. Oxygen tension in venous blood (normally 40 mm Hg) reflects tissue extraction, not pulmonary function. Venous PCO_2 is usually 4–6 mm Hg higher than $PaCO_2$. Consequently, venous blood pH is usually 0.05 unit lower than arterial blood pH. Despite these limitations, venous blood is often useful in determining acid-base status. Capillary blood represents a mixture of arterial and venous blood, and the values obtained reflect this fact. Samples are usually collected in heparin-coated syringes and should be analyzed as soon as possible. Air bubbles should be eliminated, and the sample should be capped and placed on ice to prevent significant uptake of gas from blood cells or loss of gases to the atmosphere. Although heparin is highly acidic, excessive amounts of heparin in the sample syringe usually lower pH only minimally but decrease PCO_2 in direct proportion to the percent dilution, and have a variable effect on PO_2.

Temperature Correction

 Changes in temperature directly affect measurements of PCO_2, PO_2, and, indirectly, pH (above). Decreases in temperature lower the partial pressure of a gas in solution—even though the total gas content does not change—because gas solubility is inversely proportionate to temperature. Both PCO_2 and PO_2 therefore decrease during hypothermia, but pH increases because temperature does not appreciably alter [HCO$_3^-$]: $PaCO_2$ decreases, but [HCO$_3^-$] is unchanged. Since blood gas tensions and pH are always measured at 37 °C, controversy exists over whether to correct the measured values to the patient's actual temperature. "Normal" values at temperatures other than 37 °C are not known. Many clinicians use the measurements at 37 °C directly, regardless of the patient's actual temperature (see Chapter 21).

pH MEASUREMENT

When a metal is placed in solution with its salt, the tendency of the metal to ionize into the solution leaves the metal with a negative charge. If two different metals (electrodes) and their salts are separated by a porous partition (allowing transfer of charge), the tendency for one metal to go into solution more than the other results in an electromotive force between the two electrodes. For pH measurements, a silver/silver chloride electrode and a mercury/mercurous chloride (calomel) electrode are most commonly used. The silver electrode is in contact with the test solution through pH-sensitive glass. The calomel electrode interfaces with the test solution through a potassium chloride solution and a porous plug. The electromotive force developed between the two electrodes is proportionate to $[H^+]$.

CARBON DIOXIDE MEASUREMENT

Modification of the pH electrode system allows measurement of PCO_2. In this system (the Severinghaus electrode), the two electrodes are separated by sodium bicarbonate and potassium chloride solution. The test sample is in contact with the bicarbonate solution through a thin Teflon membrane that allows CO_2 to equilibrate between the test sample and the bicarbonate solution. As a result, the pH of the bicarbonate solution reflects the PCO_2 of the test solution.

OXYGEN MEASUREMENT

PO_2 is most commonly measured polarographically using the Clark electrode. In this system, platinum communicates with a silver/silver chloride electrode through an electrolyte solution (NaCl and KCl). The test sample is separated from the electrolyte solution by a membrane allowing oxygen to diffuse freely. When a negative voltage is applied to the platinum electrode, the electrical current that flows between the two electrodes is directly related to PO_2. In the process, molecules of oxygen take up electrons from the cathode and react with water to form hydroxide ions.

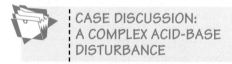

CASE DISCUSSION:
A COMPLEX ACID-BASE
DISTURBANCE

A 1-month-old male infant with an anorectal malformation undergoes anoplasty. Postoperatively, he is found to be in congestive heart failure resulting from coarctation of the aorta. He is noted to have tachypnea, decreased urinary output, poor peripheral perfusion, hepatomegaly, and cardiomegaly. Following endotracheal intubation, the infant is placed on a ventilator (pressure support ventilation, fraction of inspired oxygen [FiO_2] = 1.0). Initial arterial blood gas, hemoglobin, and electrolyte measurements are as follows:

$PaCO_2 = 11$ mm Hg
pH = 7.47
$PaO_2 = 209$ mm Hg
Calculated [HCO_3^-] = 7.7 mEq/L
Base deficit = −14.6 mEq/L

Hb = 9.5 g/dL
$[Na^+] = 135$ mEq/L
$[Cl^-] = 95$ mEq/L
$[K^+] = 5.5$ mEq/L
[Total CO_2] = 8 mEq/L

Note that the [total CO_2] normally measured with electrolytes includes both plasma [HCO_3^-] and dissolved CO_2 in plasma.

What is the acid-base disturbance?

Using the approach described above, the patient clearly has an alkalosis (pH > 7.45), which is at least partly respiratory in origin ($PaCO_2$ < 40 mm Hg). Since $PaCO_2$ has decreased by nearly 30 mm Hg, we would expect [HCO_3^-] to be 18 mEq/L:

$$(40 - 10) \times \frac{2\ mEq/L}{10} = 6\ mEq/L\ below\ 24\ mEq/L$$

In fact, the patient's [HCO_3^-] is nearly 10 mEq/L less than that! The patient therefore also has a mixed acid-base disturbance: primary respiratory alkalosis and primary metabolic acidosis. Note that the difference between the patient's [HCO_3^-] and the [HCO_3^-] expected for a pure respiratory alkalosis roughly corresponds to the base excess.

What are likely causes of these disturbances?

The respiratory alkalosis is probably the result of congestive heart failure, while the metabolic acidosis results from lactic acidosis secondary to poor perfusion. The latter is suggested by the calculated plasma anion gap:

$$Anion\ gap = 135 - (95 + 8) = 32\ mEq/L$$

The lactate level was in fact measured and found to be elevated at 14.4 mEq/L. It is probable that fluid overload precipitated the congestive heart failure.

What treatment is indicated?

Treatment should be directed at the primary process, ie, the congestive heart failure. The patient was treated with digoxin and furosemide. The hemoglobin concentration is low for this infant's age (normal, 14–16 g/L), so transfusion following diuresis is also probably indicated.

Following diuresis, the patient's tachypnea has improved, but perfusion still appears to be poor. Repeat laboratory measurements are as follows (FiO_2 = 0.5):

$PaCO_2 = 23$ mm Hg

$pH = 7.52$

$PaO_2 = 136$ mm Hg

Calculated $[HCO_3^-] = 18$ mEq/L

Base deficit $= -3.0$ mEq/L

$Hb = 10.3$ g/dL

$[Na^+] = 137$ mEq/L

$[Cl^-] = 92$ mEq/L

$[K^+] = 3.9$ mEq/L

$[Total\ CO_2] = 18.5$ mEq/L

What is the acid-base disturbance?

Respiratory alkalosis is still present, while the base deficit appears to have improved. Note that hemoglobin concentration has increased slightly, but [K+] has decreased as a result of the diuresis. With the new PaCO2, the expected [HCO3−] should be 20.6 mEq/L:

$$(40-23)\times\frac{2\ \text{mEq/L}}{10} = 3.4\ \text{mEq/L below 24 mEq/L}$$

Therefore, the patient still has metabolic acidosis because the [HCO3−] is 2 mEq/L less. Note again that this difference is close to the given base deficit and the anion gap is still high:

$$\text{Anion gap} = 137 - (92 + 18) = 27$$

The repeat lactate measurement is now 13.2 mEq/L.

The high anion gap and lactate level explain why the patient is still not doing well and indicate that a new process is masking the severity of the metabolic acidosis (which is essentially unchanged).

Given the clinical course, it is likely that the patient now has a triple acid-base disorder: respiratory alkalosis, metabolic acidosis, and now metabolic alkalosis. The latter probably resulted from hypovolemia secondary to excessive diuresis

(chloride-sensitive metabolic alkalosis). Note also that the metabolic alkalosis is nearly equal in magnitude to the metabolic acidosis.

The patient was subsequently given packed red blood cells in saline, and within 24 hours all three disorders began to improve:

$PaCO_2 = 35$ mm Hg

$pH = 7.51$

$PaO_2 = 124$ mm Hg

Calculated $[HCO_3^-] = 26.8$ mEq/L

Base excess $= +5.0$ mEq/L

$Hb = 15$ g/dL

$[Na^+] = 136$ mEq/L

$[Cl^-] = 91$ mEq/L

$[K^+] = 3.2$ mEq/L

$[Total\ CO_2] = 27$ mEq/L

Lactate $= 2.7$ mEq/L

Outcome

The respiratory alkalosis and the metabolic acidosis have now resolved, and the metabolic alkalosis is now most prominent.

Intravenous KCl replacement and a small amount of saline were judiciously given, followed by complete resolution of metabolic alkalosis. The patient subsequently underwent surgical correction of the coarctation.

SUGGESTED READING

Kraut JA, Madias NE: Approach to patients with acid-base disorders. Respiratory Care 2001; 46:392.

Longenecker JC: *High-yield Acid-base.* Williams & Wilkins, 1998.

Pestana C: *Fluids and Electrolytes in the Surgical Patient,* 5th ed. Lippincott Williams & Wilkins, 2000.

Rose BD: *Clinical Physiology of Acid-Base and Electrolyte Disorders,* 4th ed. McGraw-Hill, 1994.

Thompson WST, Adams JF, Cowan RA: *Clinical acid-base balance.* Oxford University Press, 1997.

Renal Physiology & Anesthesia

31

KEY CONCEPTS

 The combined blood flow through both kidneys normally accounts for 20–25% of total cardiac output.

 Autoregulation of renal blood flow normally occurs between mean arterial blood pressures of 80 and 180 mm Hg.

 Renal synthesis of vasodilating prostaglandins (PGD₂, PGE₂, and PGI₂) is an important protective mechanism during periods of systemic hypotension and renal ischemia.

 Dopamine dilates afferent and efferent arterioles via D₁-receptor activation. Low-dose dopamine infusion can at least partially reverse norepinephrine-induced renal vasoconstriction.

 Reversible decreases in renal blood flow, glomerular filtration rate, urinary flow, and sodium excretion occur during both regional and general anesthesia. These effects can be at least partially overcome by maintenance of an adequate intravascular volume and a normal blood pressure.

 The endocrine response to surgery and anesthesia is probably at least partly responsible for the transient postoperative fluid retention that is seen in many patients.

 Methoxyflurane has been associated with polyuric renal failure. Its nephrotoxicity is dose-related and is the result of release of fluoride ions from its metabolic degradation.

 High plasma fluoride concentrations following prolonged enflurane anesthesia may also occur in obese patients and those receiving isoniazid therapy,

 Compound A, breakdown product of sevoflurane that is formed at low flows, can cause renal damage in laboratory animals. Clinical studies have not detected significant renal injury in humans during sevoflurane anesthesia.

 Certain surgical procedures can significantly alter renal physiology. The pneumoperitoneum produced during laparoscopy produces an abdominal compartment syndrome–like state. The increase in intra-abdominal pressure typically produces oliguria (or anuria). Other surgical procedures that can significantly compromise renal function include cardiopulmonary bypass, cross-clamping of the aorta, and dissection near the renal arteries.

The kidneys play a vital role in regulating the volume and composition of body fluids, eliminating toxins, and elaborating hormones such as renin, erythropoietin, and the active form of vitamin D. Surgery and anesthesia can have important effects on renal function. Failure to take these effects into consideration could result in serious errors in patient management. Fluid overload, hypovolemia, and postoperative renal failure are major causes of postoperative morbidity and mortality.

Diuretics are an important class of drugs that are frequently employed in the perioperative period. Preoperative diuretic therapy is common in patients with hypertension and with cardiac, hepatic, and renal disease. Diuretics are also used intraoperatively, particularly during neurosurgical, cardiac, major vascular, ophthalmic, and urologic procedures. Familiarity with the various types of diuretics, their mechanisms of action, side effects, and potential anesthetic interactions is therefore essential.

■ THE NEPHRON

Each kidney is made up of approximately 1 million functional units called nephrons. Anatomically, a nephron consists of a tortuous tubule with at least six specialized segments. At its proximal end (**Bowman's capsule**), an ultrafiltrate of blood is formed, and as this fluid passes through the nephron, its volume and composition are modified by both the reabsorption and the secretion of solutes. The final product is eliminated as urine.

The six major anatomic and functional divisions of the nephron include the glomerular capillaries, the proximal convoluted tubule, the loop of Henle, the distal renal tubule, the collecting tubule, and the juxtaglomerular apparatus (Figure 31–1 and Table 31–1).

The Glomerular Capillaries

The **glomerulus** is composed of tufts of capillaries that jut into Bowman's capsule, providing a large surface area for the filtration of blood. Blood flow is provided by a single **afferent arteriole** and is drained by a single **efferent arteriole** (see below). Endothelial cells in glomeruli are separated from the epithelial cells of Bowman's capsule only by their fused basement membranes. The endothelial cells are perforated with relatively large fenestrae (70–100 nm), but the epithelial cells interdigitate tightly with one another, leaving relatively small filtration slits (about 25 nm). The two cell types with their basement membranes provide an effective filtration barrier for cells and large molecular weight substances. This barrier appears to have multiple anionic sites that give it a net negative charge, which favors the filtration of cations but somewhat hinders filtration of anions. A third cell type, **mesangial cells,** are located between the basement membrane and epithelial cells near adjacent capillaries. Mesangial cells are thought to play a significant role in regulation of glomerular filtration. They contain contractile proteins that respond to vasoactive substance such as angiotensin II, secrete various substances, and take up immune complexes.

Glomerular filtration pressure (about 60 mm Hg) is normally about 60% of mean arterial pressure and is opposed by both plasma oncotic pressure (about 25 mm Hg) and renal interstitial pressure (about 10 mm Hg). Both afferent and efferent arteriolar tones are important determinants of filtration pressure: Filtration

Table 31–1. Functional divisions of a nephron.[1]

Segment	Function
Glomerulus	Ultrafiltration of blood
Proximal tubule	Reabsorption Sodium[2] chloride Water Bicarbonate Glucose, protein, amino acids Potassium, magnesium, calcium Phosphates,[3] uric acid, urea Secretion Organic anions Organic cations Ammonia production
Loop of Henle	Reabsorption Sodium, chloride Water Potassium, calcium, magnesium Countercurrent multiplier
Distal tubule	Reabsorption Sodium[4] chloride Water Potassium Calcium[5] Bicarbonate Secretion Hydrogen ion[4] Potassium[4] Calcium
Collecting tubule	Reabsorption Sodium[4,7] chloride Water[6,7] Potassium Bicarbonate Secretion Potassium[4] Hydrogen ion[4] Ammonia production
Juxtaglomerular apparatus	Secretion of renin

[1]Adapted from Rose BD: *Clinical Physiology of Acid-Base and Electrolyte Disorders,* 3rd ed. McGraw-Hill, 1989.
[2]Partially augmented by angiotensin II.
[3]Inhibited by parathyroid hormone.
[4]At least partly aldosterone-mediated.
[5]Augmented by parathyroid hormone.
[6]Antidiuretic hormone-mediated.
[7]Inhibited by atrial natriuretic peptide.

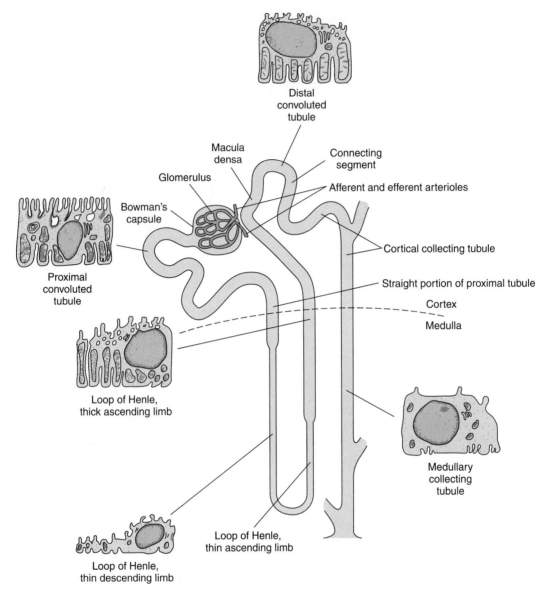

Figure 31–1. Major anatomic divisions of the nephron. (Modified and reproduced, with permission, from Ganong WF: *Review of Medical Physiology,* 20th ed. McGraw-Hill, 2001.)

pressure is directly proportionate to efferent arteriolar tone, but inversely proportionate to afferent arteriolar tone. Approximately 20% of plasma is normally filtered as blood passes through the glomerulus.

The Proximal Tubule

Sixty-five to 75 percent of the ultrafiltrate formed in Bowman's capsule is normally reabsorbed isotonically (proportionate amounts of water and sodium) in the proximal renal tubules (Figure 31–2). To be reabsorbed, most substances must first traverse the tubular (apical) side of the cell membrane, and then cross the basolateral cell membrane into the renal interstitium before entering peritubular capillaries. The major function of the proximal tubule is Na^+ reabsorption. Sodium is actively transported out of proximal tubular cells at their capillary side by membrane-bound Na^+-K^+

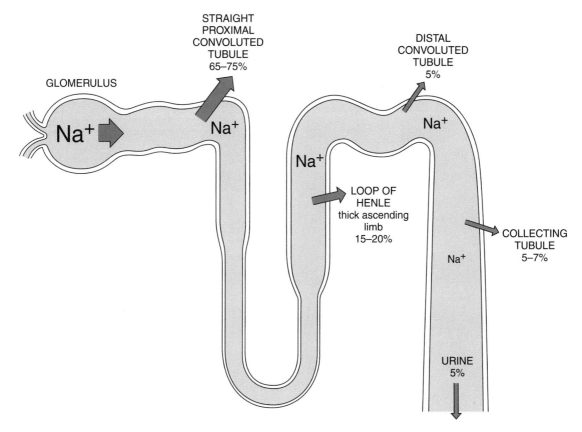

Figure 31–2. Sodium reabsorption in the nephron. Numbers represent the percentage of the filtered sodium reabsorbed at each site. (Modified and reproduced, with permission, from Cogan MG: *Fluid and Electrolytes: Physiology and Pathophysiology.* Appleton & Lange, 1991.)

adenosine triphosphatase (ATPase) (Figure 31–3). The resulting low intracellular concentration of Na^+ allows passive movement of Na^+ down its gradient from tubular fluid into epithelial cells. Angiotensin II and norepinephrine enhance Na^+ reabsorption in the early proximal tubule. In contrast, dopamine decreases the proximal reabsorption of sodium via D_1-receptor activation.

Sodium reabsorption is coupled with the reabsorption of other solutes and the secretion of H^+ (Figure 31–3). Specific carrier proteins use the low concentration of Na^+ inside cells to transport phosphate, glucose, and amino acids. The net loss of intracellular positive charges, the result of Na^+-K^+ ATPase activity (exchanging $3Na^+$ for $2K^+$), favors the absorption of other cations (K^+, Ca^{2+}, and Mg^{2+}). Thus, the Na^+-K^+ ATPase at the basolateral side of the renal cells provides the energy for the reabsorption of most solutes. Sodium reabsorption at the luminal membrane is also coupled with

countertransport (secretion) of H^+. The latter mechanism is responsible for reabsorption of 90% of the filtered bicarbonate ions (see Figure 30–2). Unlike other solutes, chloride can traverse the tight junctions between adjacent tubular epithelial cells. As a result, chloride reabsorption is generally passive and follows its concentration gradient. Active chloride reabsorption may also take place as a result of a K^+-Cl^- cotransporter that extrudes both ions at the capillary side of the cell membrane (Figure 31–3). Water moves passively out the proximal tubule along osmotic gradients. Specialized water channels, composed of a membrane protein called aquaporin-1, in the apical membranes of epithelial cells facilitate water movement.

The proximal tubules are capable of secreting organic cations and anions. Organic cations such as creatinine, cimetidine, and quinidine may share the same pump mechanism and thus can interfere with the excretion of one another. Organic anions such as urate, keto

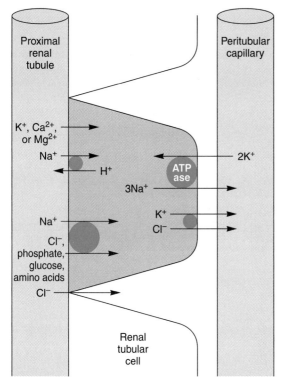

Figure 31–3. Reabsorption of solutes in proximal tubules. Note that Na⁺-K⁺ ATPase supplies the energy for reabsorption of most solutes by maintaining a low intracellular concentration of sodium.

acids, penicillins, cephalosporins, diuretics, salicylates, and most x-ray dyes also appear to share common secretory mechanisms. Both pumps probably play a major role in the elimination of many circulating toxins. Low molecular weight proteins, which are filtered by glomeruli, are normally reabsorbed by proximal tubular cells but are metabolized intracellularly.

The Loop of Henle

The loop of Henle consists of descending and ascending portions. The thin descending segment is a continuation of the proximal tubule and descends from the renal cortex into the renal medulla. In the medulla, the descending portion acutely turns back upon itself and rises back up toward the cortex as the ascending portion. The ascending portion consists of a functionally distinct, thin ascending limb, a medullary thick ascending limb, and a cortical thick ascending limb (Figure 31–1). Cortical nephrons (30–40%) have relatively short loops of Henle, while those near the medulla (jux-

tamedullary nephrons, 10%) loop deeply into the medulla. Cortical nephrons with short loops lack a thin ascending limb. Cortical nephrons outnumber juxtamedullary nephrons approximately 7:1. The loop of Henle is responsible for maintaining a hypertonic medullary interstitium and indirectly provides the collecting tubules with the ability to concentrate urine.

Only 25–35% of the ultrafiltrate formed in Bowman's capsule normally reaches the loop of Henle. This part of the nephron usually reabsorbs 15–20% of the filtered sodium load. With the notable exception of the ascending thick segments, solute and water reabsorption in the loop of Henle is passive and follows concentration and osmotic gradients, respectively. In the ascending thick segment, however, Na⁺ and Cl⁻ are reabsorbed in excess of water; moreover, Na⁺ reabsorption in this part of the nephron is directly coupled to both K⁺ and Cl⁻ reabsorption (Figure 31–4), and [Cl⁻] in tubular fluid appears to be the rate-limiting factor.

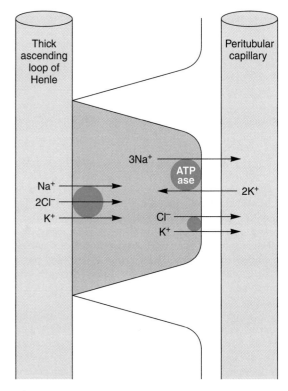

Figure 31–4. Sodium and chloride reabsorption in the thick ascending loop of Henle. All four sites on the luminal carrier protein must be occupied for transport to occur. The rate-limiting factor appears to be chloride concentration in tubular fluid.

Active Na^+ reabsorption still results from Na^+-K^+ ATPase activity on the capillary side of epithelial cells.

Unlike the descending limb and the thin ascending limb, the thick parts of the ascending limb are impermeable to water. As a result, tubular fluid flowing out of the loop of Henle is hypotonic (100–200 mOsm/L) and the interstitium surrounding the loop of Henle is therefore hypertonic. A countercurrent multiplier mechanism is established such that both the tubular fluid and medullary interstitium become increasingly hypertonic with increasing depth into the medulla (Figure 31–5). Urea also reaches high concentrations in the medulla and contributes substantially to its hypertonicity. The countercurrent mechanism includes the loop of Henle, the cortical and medullary collecting tubules, and their respective capillaries (**vasa recta**).

The thick ascending loop of Henle is also an important site for calcium and magnesium reabsorption. Parathyroid hormone may augment calcium reabsorption at this site.

The Distal Tubule

The distal tubule receives hypotonic fluid from the loop of Henle and is normally responsible for only minor modifications of tubular fluid. In contrast to more proximal portions, the distal nephron has very tight junctions between tubular cells and is relatively impermeable to water and sodium. It can therefore maintain the gradients generated by the loop of Henle. Sodium reabsorption in the distal tubule normally accounts for only about 5% of the filtered sodium load. As in other parts of the nephron, the energy is derived from Na^+-K^+ ATPase activity on the capillary side, but on the luminal side Na^+ is reabsorbed by a Na^+-Cl^- carrier. Sodium reabsorption in this segment is directly proportionate to Na^+ delivery. The distal tubule is the major site of parathyroid hormone– and vitamin D–mediated calcium reabsorption.

The late distal tubule is referred to as the **connecting segment.** Although it is also involved in hormone-

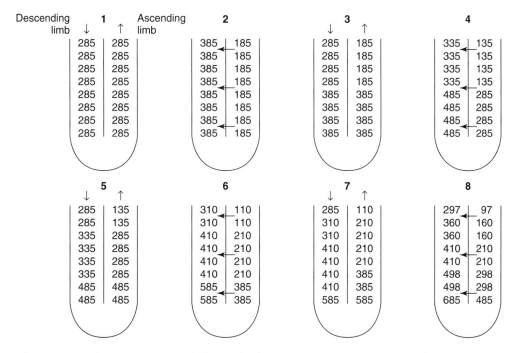

Figure 31–5. The countercurrent multiplier mechanism. This mechanism is dependent on differential permeability and transport characteristics between the descending and ascending limbs. The descending limb and the thin ascending limb are permeable to water, Na^+, Cl^-, and urea. The thick ascending limb is impermeable to water and urea, actively reabsorbs Na^+ and Cl^-, and therefore can generate an osmotic gradient. This figure depicts from "time zero" a progressive 200 mOsm/kg gradient between the descending and ascending limbs. Note that as urine flows, the gradient remains unchanged but the osmolality progressively increases at the bottom of the loop. (Adapted from Pitts RF: *Physiology of the Kidney and Body Fluids,* 3rd ed. Year Book, 1974.)

mediated calcium reabsorption, unlike more proximal portions, it participates in aldosterone-mediated Na+ reabsorption.

The Collecting Tubule

This tubule can be divided into cortical and medullary portions. Together, they normally account for the reabsorption of 5–7% of the filtered sodium load.

A. CORTICAL COLLECTING TUBULE:

This part of the nephron consists of two cell types: (1) principal cells (P cells), which primarily secrete potassium and participate in aldosterone-mediated Na+ reabsorption, and (2) intercalated cells (I cells), which are responsible for acid-base regulation. Because principal cells reabsorb Na+ via an electrogenic pump, either Cl− must be also be reabsorbed, or K+ must be secreted to maintain electroneutrality. Increases in intracellular [K+] favor K+ secretion. Aldosterone enhances Na+-K+ ATPase activity in this part of the nephron by increasing the number of open K+ and Na+ channels in the luminal membrane. Aldosterone also enhances the H+-secreting ATPase on the luminal border of intercalated cells (Figure 31–6). Intercalated cells additionally have a luminal K+-H+ ATPase pump, which reabsorbs K+ and secretes H+. Some intercalated cells are capable of secreting bicarbonate ion in response to large alkaline loads.

B. MEDULLARY COLLECTING TUBULE:

The medullary collecting tubule courses down from the cortex through the hypertonic medulla before joining collecting tubules from other nephrons to form a single ureter in each kidney. This part of the collecting tubule is the principal site of action for antidiuretic hormone (ADH), also called arginine vasopressin (AVP); this hormone activates adenylate cyclase via V_2 receptors. (V_1 receptors increase vascular resistance). ADH stimulates the expression of a water channel protein, aquaporin-2, in the cell membrane. The permeability of the luminal membrane to water is entirely dependent of the presence of ADH (see Chapter 28). Dehydration increases ADH secretion, rendering the luminal membrane permeable to water. As a result, water is osmotically drawn out of the tubular fluid passing through the medulla, and a concentrated urine (up to 1400 mOsm/L) is produced. Conversely, adequate hydration suppresses ADH secretion; the fluid in the collecting tubules therefore passes through the medulla unchanged and remains hypotonic (100–200 mOsm/L). The medullary collecting tubule also possesses principal and intercalated cells, but the latter predominate. Moreover, this part of the nephron is responsible for acidifying urine; the hydrogen ions secreted are ex-

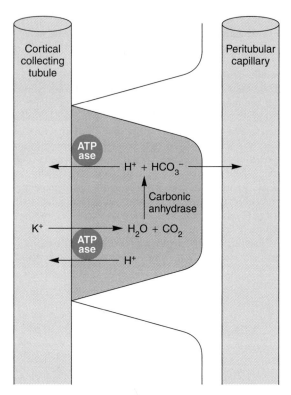

Figure 31–6. Secretion of hydrogen ions and reabsorption of bicarbonate and potassium in the cortical collecting tubule.

creted in the form of titratable acids (phosphates) and ammonium ions (see Chapter 30).

C. ROLE OF THE COLLECTING TUBULE IN MAINTAINING A HYPERTONIC MEDULLA:

Differential permeability for urea between the cortical and medullary collecting tubules accounts for up to half the hypertonicity of the renal medulla. Cortical collecting tubules are freely permeable to urea, whereas medullary collecting tubules are normally impermeable. In the presence of ADH, the innermost part of the medullary collecting tubules becomes even more permeable to urea. Thus, when ADH is secreted, water moves out of the collecting tubules and the urea becomes highly concentrated. Urea can then diffuse out deeply into the medullary interstitium, increasing its tonicity.

The Juxtaglomerular Apparatus

This small organ within each nephron consists of a specialized segment of the afferent arteriole, containing juxtaglomerular cells within its wall, and the end of the

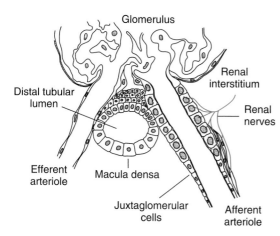

Figure 31–7. The juxtaglomerular apparatus. (Modified and reproduced, with permission, from Ganong WF: *Review of Medical Physiology*, 20th ed. McGraw-Hill, 2001.)

thick, ascending cortical segment of the loop of Henle, the **macula densa** (Figure 31–7). Juxtaglomerular cells contain the enzyme renin and are innervated by the sympathetic nervous system. Release of renin depends on β_1-adrenergic sympathetic stimulation, changes in afferent arteriolar wall pressure (see Chapter 28), and changes in chloride flow past the macula densa. Renin released into the bloodstream acts on angiotensinogen, a protein synthesized by the liver, to form angiotensin I. This inert decapeptide is then rapidly converted, primarily in the lungs, by angiotensin-converting enzyme (ACE) to form the octapeptide angiotensin II. Angiotensin II plays a major role in blood pressure regulation (see Chapter 19) and aldosterone secretion (see Chapter 28). Proximal renal tubular cells have converting enzyme as well as angiotensin II receptors. Moreover, intrarenal formation of angiotensin II enhances sodium reabsorption in proximal tubules. Some extrarenal production of renin and angiotensin II also takes place in vascular endothelium, the adrenal glands, and the brain.

■ THE RENAL CIRCULATION

Renal function is intimately related to renal blood flow. In fact, the kidneys are the only organs for which oxygen consumption is determined by blood flow; the reverse is true in other organs. The combined blood flow through both kidneys normally accounts for 20–25% of total cardiac output. In most persons, each kidney is supplied by a single renal artery arising from the aorta. The renal artery then divides at the renal pelvis into interlobar arteries, which in turn give rise to arcuate arteries at the junction between renal cortex and medulla (Figure 31–8). Arcuate arteries further divide into interlobular branches that eventually supply each nephron via a single afferent arteriole. Blood from each glomerulus is drained via a single efferent arteriole and then travels alongside adjacent renal tubules in a second (peritubular) system of capillaries. In contrast to the glomerular capillaries, which favor filtration, peritubular capillaries are primarily "reabsorptive." Venules draining the second capillary plexus finally return blood to the inferior vena cava via a single renal vein on each side.

RENAL BLOOD FLOW & GLOMERULAR FILTRATION

Clearance

The concept of clearance is frequently used in measurements of **renal blood flow** (RBF) and the **glomerular filtration rate** (GFR). The **renal clearance** of a substance is defined as the volume of blood that is completely cleared of that substance per unit of time (usually, per minute).

Renal Blood Flow

Renal plasma flow (RPF) is most commonly measured by *p*-aminohippurate (PAH) clearance. PAH at low plasma concentrations can be assumed to be completely cleared from plasma by filtration and secretion in one passage through the kidneys. Consequently—

$$RPF = \text{Clearance of PAH} = \left(\frac{[PAH]_{Urine}}{[PAH]_{Plasma}} \right) \times \text{Urine flow}$$

where $[PAH]_U$ = urinary concentration of PAH and $[PAH]_P$ = plasma PAH concentration.

If the hematocrit is known, then—

$$RBF = \frac{RPF}{(1 - \text{Hematocrit})}$$

Renal plasma flow and RBF are normally about 660 mL/min and 1200 mL/min, respectively.

Glomerular Filtration Rate

The GFR is normally about 20% of RPF. Clearance of inulin, a fructose polysaccharide that is completely fil-

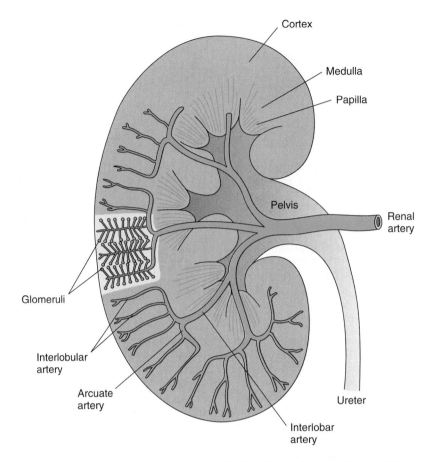

Figure 31–8. The renal circulation. (Modified and reproduced, with permission, from Leaf A, Cotran RS: *Renal Pathophysiology*. Oxford Univ Press, 1976.)

tered but is neither secreted nor reabsorbed, is a good measure of GFR. Normal values for GFR are about 120 ± 25 mL/min in men and 95 ± 20 mL/min in women. Although less accurate than measuring inulin clearance, creatinine clearance is a much more practical measurement of GFR (see Chapter 32). Creatinine clearance tends to overestimate GFR because some creatinine is normally secreted by renal tubules. Creatinine is a product of phosphocreatine breakdown in muscle. Creatinine clearance is calculated as follows:

Creatinine clearance =

$$\frac{([\text{Creatinine}]_U \times \text{Urinary flow rate})}{[\text{Creatinine}]_P}$$

where $[\text{creatinine}]_U$ = creatinine concentration in urine and $[\text{creatinine}]_P$ = creatinine concentration in plasma.

The ratio of GFR to RPF is called the **filtration fraction** (FF) and is normally 20%. GFR is dependent on the relative tones of both the afferent and efferent arterioles (see above). Afferent arteriolar dilatation or efferent arteriolar vasoconstriction can increase the FF and maintain GFR, even when RPF decreases. Afferent arteriolar tone appears to be responsible for maintaining GFR nearly constant over a wide range of blood pressures.

Control Mechanisms

Regulation of renal blood flow represents a complex interplay between intrinsic autoregulation, tubuloglomerular balance, and hormonal and neuronal influences.

A. Intrinsic Regulation:

 Autoregulation of RBF normally occurs between mean arterial blood pressures of 80 and 180 mm Hg. Blood flow is generally decreased at mean arterial pressures less than 70 mm Hg. Although the exact mechanism is not known, it is thought to be an intrinsic myogenic response of the afferent arterioles to changes in blood pressure. Within these limits, RBF (and GFR) can be kept relatively constant by afferent arteriolar vasoconstriction or vasodilation. Outside the autoregulation limits, RBF becomes pressure-dependent. Glomerular filtration generally ceases when mean systemic arterial pressure is less than 40–50 mm Hg.

B. TUBULOGLOMERULAR BALANCE AND FEEDBACK:

Changes in renal tubular flow rates affect GFR: Increases in tubular flow tend to reduce GFR, while decreases in flow tend to favor increases in GFR. Tubuloglomerular feedback probably plays an important role in maintaining GFR constant over a wide range of perfusion pressures. Although the mechanism is poorly understood, the macula densa appears to be responsible for tubuloglomerular feedback by inducing reflex changes in afferent arteriolar tone and possibly glomerular capillary permeability. Angiotensin II probably plays a permissive role in this mechanism. Local release of adenosine (which occurs in response to volume expansion) may inhibit renin release and dilate the afferent arteriole. The phenomenon of pressure natriuresis, or decreased sodium reabsorption in response to increases in blood pressure, likely reflects tubuloglomerular feedback.

C. HORMONAL REGULATION:

Increases in afferent arteriolar pressure stimulate renin release and formation of angiotensin II. Angiotensin II causes generalized arterial vasoconstriction and secondarily reduces RBF. Both afferent and efferent arterioles are constricted but because the efferent arteriole is smaller, its resistance becomes greater than that of the afferent arteriole; GFR therefore tends to be relatively preserved. Very high levels of angiotensin II constrict both arterioles and can markedly decrease GFR. Adrenal catecholamines (epinephrine and norepinephrine) directly and preferentially increase afferent arteriolar tone, but marked decreases in GFR are minimized indirectly through activation of renin release and angiotensin II formation. Relative preservation of GFR during increased aldosterone or catecholamine secretion appears to be at least partly mediated by angiotensin-induced prostaglandin synthesis and is blocked by inhibitors of prostaglandin synthesis (nonsteroidal anti-inflammatory drugs). Renal synthesis of vasodilating prostaglandins (PGD_2, PGE_2, and PGI_2) is an important protective mechanism during periods of systemic hypotension and renal ischemia.

Atrial natriuretic peptide (ANP) is released from atrial myocytes in response to distention. ANP is a direct smooth muscle dilator and antagonizes the vasoconstrictive action of norepinephrine and angiotensin II. It appears to preferentially dilate the afferent arteriole and may constrict the efferent arteriole, effectively increasing GFR (see Chapter 28). ANP also inhibits both the release of renin and angiotensin-induced secretion of aldosterone, and antagonizes the action of aldosterone in the distal and collecting tubules.

D. NEURONAL REGULATION:

Sympathetic outflow from the spinal cord at T_4–L_1 reaches the kidneys via the celiac and renal plexuses. Sympathetic nerves innervate the juxtaglomerular apparatus (β_1) as well as the renal vasculature (α_1). This innervation is probably responsible for stress-induced reductions in RBF (below). α_1-Adrenergic receptors enhance sodium reabsorption in proximal tubules while α_2 receptors decrease such reabsorption and promote water excretion. Dopamine dilates afferent and efferent arterioles via D_1-receptor activation. Low-dose dopamine infusion can at least partially reverse norepinephrine-induced renal vasoconstriction. Activation of D_2-receptors on presynaptic postganglionic sympathetic neurons can also vasodilate arterioles through inhibition of norepinephrine secretion (negative feedback). Dopamine, which is formed in the proximal tubules as well as released from nerve endings, reduces proximal reabsorption of Na^+. Some cholinergic vagal fibers are also present but their role is poorly understood.

Distribution of Renal Blood Flow

Approximately 80% of RBF normally goes to cortical nephrons, while only 10–15% goes to juxtamedullary nephrons. Redistribution of RBF away from cortical nephrons with short loops of Henle to larger juxtamedullary nephrons with long loops, is known to occur under certain conditions. Sympathetic stimulation, increased levels of catecholamines and angiotensin II, and heart failure can cause redistribution of RBF to the medulla. Although the significance of this redistribution remains controversial, it appears to be clinically associated with sodium retention.

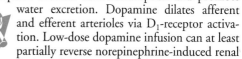

■ EFFECTS OF ANESTHESIA & SURGERY ON RENAL FUNCTION

Clinical studies attempting to define the effects of anesthetic agents on renal function are complicated by difficulties in differentiating between direct and indirect effects and often fail to control many important variables. These variables include the type of surgical procedure, fluid administration, and preexisting cardiac and renal function. Several conclusions, however, can be stated:

(1) Reversible decreases in RBF, GFR, urinary flow, and sodium excretion occur during both regional and general anesthesia.

(2) Changes are generally less marked during regional anesthesia.

(3) Most of these changes are indirect and are mediated by autonomic and hormonal influences.

(4) These effects can be at least partially overcome by maintenance of an adequate intravascular volume and a normal blood pressure.

(5) Only a few anesthetics (methoxyflurane and, theoretically, enflurane and sevoflurane) in high doses can cause specific renal toxicity.

INDIRECT EFFECTS

Cardiovascular Effects

Most inhalational and intravenous anesthetics cause some degree of cardiac depression or vasodilation and therefore are capable of decreasing arterial blood pressure. The sympathetic blockade associated with regional anesthesia (spinal or epidural) can similarly cause hypotension as a result of increased venous capacitance and arterial vasodilation. Decreases in blood pressure below the limits of autoregulation can therefore be expected to reduce RBF, GFR, urinary flow, and sodium excretion. Intravenous fluid administration often at least partially reverses the hypotension and ameliorates its effects on renal function.

Neural Effects

Sympathetic activation commonly occurs in the perioperative period as a result of light anesthesia, intense surgical stimulation, tissue trauma, or anesthetic-induced circulatory depression. Sympathetic overactivity increases renal vascular resistance and activates various hormonal systems. Both effects tend to reduce RBF, GFR, and urinary output.

Endocrine Effects

Endocrine changes during anesthesia generally reflect a stress response that may be induced by surgical stimulation, circulatory depression, hypoxia, or acidosis. Increases in catecholamines (epinephrine and norepinephrine), renin, angiotensin II, aldosterone, ADH, adrenocorticotropic hormone, and cortisol are com-

mon. Catecholamines, ADH, and angiotensin II all reduce RBF by inducing renal arterial constriction. Aldosterone enhances sodium reabsorption in the distal tubule and collecting tubule, resulting in sodium retention and expansion of the extracellular fluid compartment (see Chapter 28). Nonosmotic release of ADH also favors water retention and, if marked, may result in hyponatremia (see Chapter 28). The endocrine response to surgery and anesthesia is probably at least partly responsible for the transient postoperative fluid retention that is seen in many patients.

DIRECT ANESTHETIC EFFECTS

The direct effects of anesthetics on renal function are minor compared with the secondary effects described above.

Volatile Agents

Halothane, enflurane, and isoflurane have been reported to decrease renal vascular resistance. Studies of their effect on autoregulation have had conflicting results. In some animal studies, halothane appears to depress sodium reabsorption.

Methoxyflurane has been associated with a syndrome of polyuric renal failure. Its nephrotoxicity is dose-related and is the result of release of fluoride ions from its metabolic degradation. Plasma fluoride concentrations greater than 50 μmol/L have been associated with renal toxicity that is characterized by a defect in urinary concentrating ability. Methoxyflurane doses greater than 1 minimum alveolar concentration for 2 hours are associated with a high incidence of renal impairment. Fluoride production is negligible during halothane, desflurane, and isoflurane anesthesia but can become significant following the prolonged administration of enflurane and possibly sevoflurane. Since fluoride excretion is dependent on GFR, patients with preexisting renal impairment may be more susceptible to this syndrome.

High plasma fluoride concentrations following prolonged enflurane anesthesia may also occur in obese patients and those receiving isoniazid therapy, but an increased incidence of renal dysfunction has not been reported.

Compound A, breakdown product of sevoflurane that is formed at low flows, can cause renal damage in laboratory animals. Clinical studies have not detected significant renal injury in humans during sevoflurane anesthesia. Nonetheless, most authorities recommend fresh gas flow of at least 2 L/min with sevoflurane to prevent significant production of compound A.

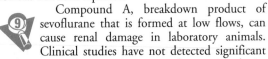

Intravenous Agents

Studies on opioids and barbiturates generally show minor effects when they are used alone. In the presence of nitrous oxide, these agents can produce effects similar to those observed with volatile agents. Ketamine is reported to minimally affect renal function and to preserve renal function during hemorrhagic hypovolemia. Agents with α-adrenergic blocking activity, such as droperidol, may prevent catecholamine-induced redistribution of RBF. Drugs with antidopaminergic activity—such as metoclopramide, phenothiazines, and droperidol—may impair the renal response to dopamine. Inhibition of prostaglandin synthesis by analgesics such as ketorolac prevents the renal production of vasodilatory prostaglandins in patients with high levels of angiotensin II and norepinephrine; attenuation of this protective response can decrease GFR and produce renal dysfunction in some patients. ACE inhibitors can similarly potentiate the detrimental effects of anesthetic agents on renal perfusion; these drugs block the protective effects of angiotensin II and may result in additional reductions in GFR during anesthesia.

Other Drugs

Many drugs and dyes that are used in the perioperative period can adversely affect renal function, especially in the setting of preexisting renal dysfunction. These include antibiotics (eg, aminoglycosides and amphotericin B), immunosuppressive agents (eg, cyclosporin and tacrolimus), and radiocontrast dyes. Mechanisms of injury include renal arterial vasospasm, direct cytotoxic properties, and renal microvascular or tubular obstruction.

Pretreatment with acetylcysteine (1200 mg orally in divided doses on the day before and on the day of the administration of the radiocontrast) has been shown to protect against radiocontrast dye–induced renal failure in patients with preexisting renal dysfunction. Acetylcysteine's protective action may be due to its free-radical scavenging or sulfhydryl donor (reducing) properties. Calcium channel agents (diltiazem) may protect against cyclosporine-induced nephrotoxicity. Although anecdotal experience suggests otherwise, clinical studies have not clearly demonstrated the renal protective effects of mannitol.

DIRECT SURGICAL EFFECTS

In addition to the physiologic changes associated with the neuroendocrine stress response to surgery, certain surgical procedures can significantly alter renal physiology. The pneumoperitoneum produced during laparoscopy produces an abdominal compartment syndrome–like state. The increase in intra-abdominal pressure typically produces oliguria (or anuria) that is generally proportional to the insufflation pressures. Mechanisms include central venous compression (renal vein and vena cava); renal parenchymal compression; decreased cardiac output; and increases in plasma levels of renin, aldosterone, and ADH. Other surgical procedures that can significantly compromise renal function include cardiopulmonary bypass (see Chapter 21), cross-clamping of the aorta (see Chapter 21), and dissection near the renal arteries (see Chapter 33). The potential effects of neurosurgical procedures on ADH physiology are discussed in Chapters 26 and 28.

◼ DIURETICS

Diuretics increase urinary output by decreasing the reabsorption of Na^+ and water. They are most commonly classified according to their mechanism of action. Unfortunately, many diuretics have more than one such mechanism, so the classification system is imperfect; only major mechanisms will be reviewed here.

The majority of diuretics exert their action on the luminal cell membrane from within the renal tubules. Because nearly all diuretics are highly protein-bound, relatively little of the free drug enters the tubules by filtration. Most diuretics must therefore be secreted by the proximal tubule (usually via the organic anion pump) to exert their action. Impaired delivery into the renal tubules accounts for resistance to diuretics in patients with impaired renal function.

OSMOTIC DIURETICS (MANNITOL)

Osmotically active diuretics are filtered at the glomerulus and undergo limited or no reabsorption in the proximal tubule. Their presence in the proximal tubule limits the passive water reabsorption that normally follows active sodium reabsorption. Although their major effect is to increase water excretion, in large doses, osmotically active diuretics also increase electrolyte (sodium and potassium) excretion. The same mechanism also impairs water and solute reabsorption in the loop of Henle.

Mannitol is the most commonly used osmotic diuretic. It is a six-carbon sugar that normally undergoes little or no reabsorption. In addition to its diuretic effect, mannitol appears to increase RBF. The latter can wash out some of the medullary hypertonicity and interfere with renal concentrating ability. Mannitol appears to activate the intrarenal synthesis of vasodilating prostaglandins. It also appears to be a free radical scavenger.

Uses

A. PROPHYLAXIS AGAINST ACUTE RENAL FAILURE IN HIGH-RISK PATIENTS:

This group of patients includes those with massive trauma, major hemolytic reactions, rhabdomyolysis, and severe jaundice as well as those undergoing cardiac or aortic operations. The efficacy of prophylaxis in these instances may be related to dilution of nephrotoxic substances within the renal tubules, prevention of sludging and obstruction within the tubules, maintenance of RBF, and perhaps reduction of cellular swelling and preservation of cellular architecture.

B. EVALUATION OF ACUTE OLIGURIA:

Mannitol in the presence of hypovolemia will augment urinary output. In contrast, it will have little effect in the presence of severe glomerular or tubular injury.

C. CONVERSION OF OLIGURIC RENAL FAILURE TO NONOLIGURIC RENAL FAILURE:

Although this indication is controversial, the lower mortality rate associated with nonoliguric renal failure still prompts many clinicians to use mannitol in that setting.

D. ACUTE REDUCTION OF INTRACRANIAL PRESSURE AND CEREBRAL EDEMA:

See Chapter 26.

E. ACUTE REDUCTION OF INTRAOCULAR PRESSURE IN THE PERIOPERATIVE PERIOD:

See Chapter 38.

Intravenous Dosage

Mannitol, 0.25–1 g/kg.

Side Effects

Mannitol solutions are hypertonic and acutely raise plasma and extracellular osmolality. A rapid intracellular to extracellular shift of water can transiently increase intravascular volume and precipitate cardiac decompensation and pulmonary edema in patients with limited cardiac reserve. Transient hyponatremia and reductions in hemoglobin concentration are also common and represent acute hemodilution resulting from rapid movement of water out of cells; a modest, transient increase in plasma potassium concentration may also be observed (see Chapter 28). It is also important to note that the initial hyponatremia does not represent hypo-

osmolality but reflects the presence of mannitol (see Chapter 28). If fluid and electrolyte losses are not replaced following diuresis, mannitol can result in hypovolemia, hypokalemia, and hypernatremia. The hypernatremia occurs because water is lost in excess of sodium.

LOOP DIURETICS

The loop diuretics include furosemide (Lasix), bumetanide (Bumex), ethacrynic acid (Edecrin), and torsemide (Demadex). All loop diuretics inhibit Na^+ and Cl^- reabsorption in the thick ascending limb. Sodium reabsorption at that site requires that all four sites on the Na^+-K^+-$2Cl^-$ luminal carrier protein be occupied. Loop diuretics compete with Cl^- for its binding site on the carrier protein (see Figure 31–4). With a maximal effect, they can lead to excretion of 15–20% of the filtered sodium load. Both urinary concentrating and urinary diluting capacities are impaired. The large amounts of Na^+ and Cl^- presented to the distal nephron overwhelm its limited reabsorptive capability. The resulting urine remains hypotonic. The reason for the latter is not clear but may relate to rapid urinary flow rates that prevent equilibration with the hypertonic renal medulla or interference with the action of ADH on the collecting tubules. A marked increase in diuresis may occur when loop diuretics are combined with thiazides, especially metolazone.

Some studies suggest that furosemide increases RBF and can reverse the redistribution of blood flow from the cortex to the medulla.

Loop diuretics increase urinary calcium and magnesium excretion. Ethacrynic acid is the only diuretic (other than mannitol and filtration diuretics) that is not a sulfonamide derivative, and it may for that reason be the diuretic of choice in patients allergic to sulfonamide drugs. Torsemide may have an antihypertensive action independent of its diuretic effect.

Uses

A. EDEMATOUS STATES (SODIUM OVERLOAD):

These disorders include heart failure, cirrhosis, the nephrotic syndrome, and renal insufficiency. When given intravenously, these agents can rapidly reverse cardiac and pulmonary manifestations.

B. HYPERTENSION:

Loop diuretics may be used as adjuncts to other hypotensive agents, particularly when thiazides (below) are ineffective.

C. EVALUATION OF ACUTE OLIGURIA:

The response to a small dose (10–20 mg) of furosemide may be useful in differentiating between oliguria resulting from hypovolemia and oliguria that results from re-distribution of RBF to juxtamedullary nephrons. Little or no response is seen with hypovolemia, whereas resumption of normal urinary output occurs with the latter.

D. CONVERSION OF OLIGURIC RENAL FAILURE TO NONOLIGURIC RENAL FAILURE:

Use of these drugs in this setting is as controversial as with mannitol. Moreover, mannitol may be more effective.

E. TREATMENT OF HYPERCALCEMIA:

See Chapter 28.

F. RAPID CORRECTION OF HYPONATREMIA:

See Chapter 28.

Intravenous Dosages

Furosemide, 20–100 mg; bumetanide, 0.5–1 mg; ethacrynic acid, 50–100 mg; torsemide 10–100 mg.

Side Effects

Increased delivery of Na^+ to the distal and collecting tubules increases K^+ and H^+ secretion at those sites and can result in hypokalemia and metabolic alkalosis. Marked Na^+ losses will also lead to hypovolemia and prerenal azotemia (see Chapter 48); secondary hyperaldosteronism often accentuates the hypokalemia and metabolic alkalosis. Hypercalciuria can result in stone formation and occasionally hypocalcemia. Hypomagnesemia may be seen in patients receiving long-term therapy. Hyperuricemia is thought to result from increased urate reabsorption and competitive inhibition of urate secretion in the proximal tubule. Reversible hearing loss has been reported with both furosemide and ethacrynic acid but may be more common with ethacrynic acid.

THIAZIDE-TYPE DIURETICS

This group of agents includes thiazides, chlorthalidone (Thalitone), quinethazone (Hydromox), metolazone (Zaroxolyn), and indapamide (Lozol). These diuretics act at the distal tubule, including the connecting segment. Inhibition of sodium reabsorption at this site impairs urinary diluting but not concentrating ability. The thiazide diuretics compete for the Cl^- site on the luminal Na^+-Cl^- carrier protein. When given alone, thiazide-type diuretics increase Na^+ excretion to only 3–5% of the filtered load because of enhanced compensatory Na^+ reabsorption in the collecting tubules. They also have some carbonic anhydrase inhibiting activity in the proximal tubule. The latter is normally masked by sodium reabsorption in the loop of Henle but is proba-

bly responsible for the often marked ("high ceiling") diuresis seen when thiazides are combined with loop diuretics. In contrast to their effects on sodium excretion, thiazide-type diuretics augment Ca^{2+} reabsorption in the distal tubule. Indapamide has some vasodilating properties and is the only thiazide-type diuretic with significant hepatic excretion.

Uses

A. HYPERTENSION:

Thiazides are often selected as first-line agents in the treatment of hypertension (see Chapter 20).

B. EDEMATOUS DISORDERS (SODIUM OVERLOAD):

These agents are exclusively used as oral agents for mild to moderate sodium overload.

C. HYPERCALCIURIA:

Thiazide diuretics are often used to decrease calcium excretion in patients with hypercalciuria who form renal stones.

D. NEPHROGENIC DIABETES INSIPIDUS:

The efficacy of these agents in this disorder reflects their ability to impair diluting capacity and increase urine osmolality (see Chapter 28).

Intravenous Dosages

These agents are only given orally.

Side Effects

Although thiazide-type diuretics deliver less sodium to the collecting tubules than do loop diuretics, the increase in sodium excretion is enough to enhance K^+ secretion and frequently results in hypokalemia. Enhanced H^+ secretion can also occur, enough to result in metabolic alkalosis. Impairment of renal diluting capacity may produce hyponatremia in some patients. Hyperuricemia, hyperglycemia, hypercalcemia, and hyperlipidemia may also be seen.

POTASSIUM-SPARING DIURETICS

These weak agents characteristically do not increase potassium excretion. Potassium-sparing diuretics inhibit Na^+ reabsorption in the collecting tubules and therefore can maximally excrete only 1–2% of the filtered Na^+ load. They are usually used in conjunction with more potent diuretics for their potassium-sparing effect.

1. Aldosterone Antagonists (Spironolactone)

Spironolactone (Aldactone) is a direct aldosterone receptor antagonist in collecting tubules. It acts to inhibit aldosterone-mediated Na^+ reabsorption and K^+ secretion. As a result, spironolactone is only effective in patients with hyperaldosteronism. This agent also has some antiandrogenic properties.

Uses

A. PRIMARY AND SECONDARY HYPERALDOSTERONISM:

Spironolactone is usually used as an adjuvant in the treatment of refractory edematous states associated with secondary hyperaldosteronism (see Chapter 28). It is especially effective in patients with advanced liver disease.

B. HIRSUTISM:

This less common indication relies on spironolactone's antiandrogenic properties.

Intravenous Dosage

Spironolactone is only given orally.

Side Effects

Spironolactone can result in hyperkalemia in patients with high potassium intake or renal insufficiency and in those receiving β-blockers or ACE inhibitors. Metabolic acidosis may also be seen. Other side effects include diarrhea, lethargy, ataxia, gynecomastia, and sexual dysfunction.

2. Noncompetitive Potassium-Sparing Diuretics

Triamterene (Dyrenium) and amiloride (Midamor) are not dependent on aldosterone activity in the collecting tubule. They inhibit Na^+ reabsorption and K^+ secretion by decreasing the number of open sodium channels in the luminal membrane of collecting tubules. Amiloride may also inhibit Na^+-K^+ ATPase activity in the collecting tubule.

Uses

A. HYPERTENSION:

These agents are often combined with thiazides to prevent hypokalemia.

B. CONGESTIVE HEART FAILURE:

They are often added to more potent (loop) diuretics in patients with marked potassium wasting.

Intravenous Dosages

These agents are only given orally.

Side Effects

Amiloride and triamterene can cause hyperkalemia and metabolic acidosis similar to spironolactone (see above). Both can also cause nausea, vomiting, and diarrhea. Amiloride is generally associated with fewer side effects, but paresthesias, depression, muscle weakness, and cramping may occasionally be seen. Triamterene on rare occasions has resulted in renal stones and is potentially nephrotoxic, especially when combined with nonsteroidal anti-inflammatory agents.

CARBONIC ANHYDRASE INHIBITORS

Carbonic anhydrase inhibitors such as acetazolamide (Diamox) interfere with Na^+ reabsorption and H^+ secretion in proximal tubules. They are weak diuretics because the former effect is limited by the reabsorptive capacities of more distal segments of nephrons. Nonetheless, these agents significantly interfere with H^+ secretion in the proximal tubule and impair HCO_3^- reabsorption (see Chapter 30).

Uses

A. CORRECTION OF METABOLIC ALKALOSIS IN EDEMATOUS PATIENTS:

Carbonic anhydrase inhibitors often potentiate the effects of other diuretics.

B. ALKALINIZATION OF URINE:

Alkalinization enhances urinary excretion of weakly acidic compounds such as uric acid.

C. REDUCTION OF INTRAOCULAR PRESSURE:

Inhibition of carbonic anhydrase in the ciliary processes reduces the formation of aqueous humor and, secondarily, intraocular pressure. This is a common indication during ophthalmic surgery.

Intravenous Dosage

Acetazolamide, 250–500 mg.

Side Effects

Carbonic anhydrase inhibitors generally produce only a mild hyperchloremic metabolic acidosis because of an apparently limited effect on the distal nephron. Large doses of acetazolamide have been reported to cause drowsiness, paresthesias, and confusion. Alkalinization of the urine can interfere with the excretion of amine drugs, such as quinidine.

OTHER "DIURETICS"

These agents may increase GFR by elevating cardiac output or arterial blood pressure. Drugs in this category are not primarily classified as diuretics because of their other major actions. These agents include methylxanthines (theophylline), cardiac glycosides (digitalis), inotropes, and saline infusions. Methylxanthines also appear to decrease sodium reabsorption in both the proximal and distal renal tubules. The renal effects of dopamine are discussed above.

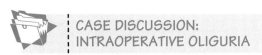

CASE DISCUSSION:
INTRAOPERATIVE OLIGURIA

A 58-year-old woman is undergoing radical hysterectomy under general anesthesia. She was in good health prior to the diagnosis of uterine carcinoma. An indwelling urinary catheter is placed following induction of general anesthesia. Total urinary output was 60 mL for the first 2 hours of surgery. After the third hour of surgery, only 5 mL of urine is noted in the drainage reservoir.

Should the anesthesiologist be concerned?

Decreases in urinary output during anesthesia are very common. Although decreases may be expected owing to the physiologic effects of surgery and anesthesia (above), a urinary output of less than 20 mL/hour in adults generally requires evaluation.

What issues should be addressed?

The following questions should be answered:

(1) Is there a problem with the urinary catheter and drainage system?

(2) Are hemodynamic parameters compatible with adequate renal function?

(3) Could the decrease in urinary output be directly related to surgical manipulations?

How can the urinary catheter and drainage system be evaluated intraoperatively?

Incorrect catheter placement is not uncommon and should be suspected if there has been total absence of urine flow since the time of catheter insertion. The catheter may be inadvertently placed and inflated in the urethra in men or the vagina in women. Catheter displacement, kinking, obstruction, or disconnection from the reservoir tubing

can all present with features similar to this case, with complete or near-complete cessation of urinary flow. The diagnosis of such mechanical problems requires retracing and inspecting the path of urine (often under the surgical drapes) from the catheter to the collection reservoir. Obstruction of the catheter can be confirmed by inability to irrigate the bladder with saline through the catheter.

What hemodynamic parameters should be evaluated?

Decreased urinary output during surgery is most commonly the result of hemodynamic changes. In most instances, a decrease in intravascular volume (hypovolemia), cardiac output, or mean arterial blood pressure is responsible. Redistribution of renal blood flow from the renal cortex to the medulla may also play a role.

Intravascular volume depletion can rapidly develop when intravenous fluid replacements do not match intraoperative blood loss, insensible fluid losses, and sequestration of fluid by traumatized tissues (third-spacing). Oliguria requires careful assessment of intravascular volume to exclude hypovolemia (see Chapter 29). An increase in urinary output following an intravenous fluid bolus is highly suggestive of hypovolemia. In contrast, oliguria in patients with a history of congestive heart failure may require inotropes, vasodilators, or diuretics. Central venous or pulmonary artery pressure monitoring is useful in patients with underlying cardiac, renal, or advanced hepatic disease, as well as in patients experiencing extensive blood loss (see Chapter 6).

When mean arterial blood pressure drops below the lower limit of renal autoregulation (80 mm Hg), urinary flow may become blood pressure-dependent. The latter may be especially true in patients with chronic systemic hypertension, in whom renal autoregulation occurs at higher mean arterial blood pressures. Reductions in anesthetic depth, intravenous fluid boluses, or the administration of a vasopressor may increase blood pressure and urinary output in such instances.

Occasionally, otherwise normal patients may exhibit decreased urinary output in spite of normal intravascular volume, cardiac output, and mean arterial blood pressure. A small dose of a loop diuretic (furosemide, 5–10 mg) usually restores normal urinary flow in such instances.

How can surgical manipulations influence urinary output?

In addition to the neuroendocrine response to surgery, mechanical factors related to the surgery itself can alter urinary output. This is especially true during pelvic surgery, when compression of the bladder by retractors, unintentional cystotomy, and ligation or severing of one or both ureters can dramatically affect urinary output. Retractor compression combined with a head-down (Trendelenburg) position commonly impedes emptying of the bladder. Excessive pressure on the bladder will often produce hematuria. When mechanical problems with the urinary catheter drainage system and hemodynamic factors are excluded (see above), a surgical explanation should be sought. The surgeon should be notified so that the position of retractors can be checked, the ureters identified, and their path retraced in the operative area. Intravenous methylene blue or indigo carmine—both dyes that are excreted in urine—are useful in identifying the site of an unintentional cystotomy or the end of a severed ureter. Note that the appearance of the dye in the urinary drainage reservoir does not exclude unilateral ligation of one ureter. Methylene blue and, to a much lesser extent, indigo carmine can transiently give falsely low pulse oximeter readings (see Chapter 6).

Outcome

After the integrity of the urinary catheter and drainage system was checked, 2 L of lactated Ringer's injection along with 250 mL of 5% albumin and 10 mg of furosemide were administered intravenously but failed to increase urinary output. Indigo carmine was given intravenously, and the proximal end of a severed left ureter was subsequently identified. A urologist was called, and the ureter was reanastomosed.

SUGGESTED READING

Better OS, Rubinstein I, Winaver JM, Knochel JP: Mannitol therapy revisited (1940–1997). Kidney Int 1997;52:886.

Colson P, Ryckwaert F, Coriat P: Renin angiotensin system antagonists and anesthesia. Anesth Analg 1999;89:1143.

Fawcett WJ, Haxby EJ, Male DA: Magnesium: Physiology and pharmacology. Br J Anaesth 1999;83:302.

Ganong WF: *Review of Medical Physiology,* 20th edition. McGraw-Hill, 2001.

Malhotra V: *Anesthesia for Renal and Genito-Urologic Surgery.* McGraw-Hill, 1996.

Anesthesia for Patients With Renal Disease

32

KEY CONCEPTS

 Creatinine clearance measurements are the most accurate method available for clinically assessing overall renal function.

 The accumulation of morphine and meperidine metabolites has been reported to prolong respiratory depression in some patients with renal failure.

 Succinylcholine can be used safely in the presence of renal failure if the serum potassium concentration is less than 5 mEq/L at the time of induction.

 The extracellular fluid overload from sodium retention—together with the increased demand imposed by anemia and hypertension—make patients with chronic renal failure especially prone to congestive heart failure and pulmonary edema.

 Delayed gastric emptying secondary to autonomic neuropathy can predispose patients with chronic renal failure to aspiration perioperatively.

 Controlled ventilation is safest for patients with renal failure. Spontaneous ventilation under anesthesia can result in respiratory acidosis that may exacerbate preexisting acidemia, leading to potentially severe circulatory depression and dangerous increases in serum potassium concentration.

 Procedures associated with a relatively high incidence of postoperative renal failure include cardiac and aortic reconstructive surgery.

 Intravascular volume depletion, sepsis, obstructive jaundice, crush injuries, recent contrast dye injections, and aminoglycoside, angiotensin-converting enzyme inhibitor, or nonsteroidal anti-inflammatory drug therapy are additional major risk factors for an acute deterioration in renal function.

 The consequences of excessive fluid overload—namely, pulmonary congestion or edema—are easier to treat than those of acute renal failure.

Diseases affecting the kidneys are often grouped into syndromes based on common clinical and laboratory findings: nephrotic syndrome, acute renal failure, chronic renal failure, nephritis, nephrolithiasis, and urinary tract obstruction and infection. The anesthetic care of patients with these syndromes is facilitated by grouping patients according to the status of their preoperative renal function rather than by syndrome. This chapter examines the basis for this approach and the anesthetic considerations applicable within each group. Renal physiology and the effects of anesthesia on renal function are discussed in Chapter 31.

■ EVALUATING RENAL FUNCTION

Accurate assessment of renal function relies heavily on laboratory determinations (Table 32–1). Renal impairment can be due to glomerular dysfunction, tubular dysfunction, or obstruction of the urinary tract. Because abnormalities of glomerular function cause the greatest derangements and are most readily detectable, the most useful laboratory tests are those related to the glomerular filtration rate (GFR; see Chapter 31).

Table 32–1. Grouping of patients according to glomerular function.

	Creatinine Clearance (mL/min)
Normal	100–120
Decreased renal reserve	60–100
Mild renal impairment	40–60
Moderate renal insufficiency	25–40
Renal failure	< 25
End-stage renal disease[1]	< 10

[1]This term applies to patients with chronic renal failure.

BLOOD UREA NITROGEN

The primary source of urea in the body is the liver. During protein catabolism, ammonia is produced from the deamination of amino acids. Hepatic conversion of ammonia to urea prevents the build-up of toxic ammonia levels:

$$2NH_3 + CO_2 \rightarrow H_2N - CO - NH_2 + H_2O$$

BUN is therefore directly related to protein catabolism and inversely related to glomerular filtration. As a result, BUN is not a reliable indicator of the GFR unless protein catabolism is normal and constant. Moreover, 40–50% of the filtrate is normally reabsorbed passively by the renal tubules; hypovolemia increases this fraction (below). Renal handling of urea is discussed in Chapter 31.

The normal BUN concentration is 10–20 mg/dL. Lower values can be seen with starvation or liver disease; elevations usually result from decreases in GFR or increases in protein catabolism. The latter may be due to a high catabolic state (trauma or sepsis), degradation of blood either in the gastrointestinal tract or in a large hematoma, or a high-protein diet. BUN concentrations greater than 50 mg/dL are generally associated with renal impairment.

SERUM CREATININE

Creatine is a product of muscle metabolism that is nonenzymatically converted to creatinine. Creatinine production in most persons is relatively constant and related to muscle mass, averaging 20–25 mg/kg in men and 15–20 mg/kg for women. Creatinine is then filtered (and to a minor extent secreted) but not reabsorbed in the kidneys (see Chapter 31). Serum creatinine concentration is therefore directly related to body muscle mass but inversely related to glomerular filtration (Figure 32–1). Because body muscle mass is usually fairly constant, serum creatinine measurements are generally reliable indices of GFR. The normal serum creatinine concentration is 0.8–1.3 mg/dL in men and 0.6–1 mg/dL in women. Note from Figure 32–1 that each doubling of the serum creatinine represents a 50% reduction in GFR. Large meat meals, cimetidine therapy, and increases in acetoacetate (as during ketoacidosis) can increase serum creatinine measurements without a change in GFR. Meat meals increase the creatinine load, while high acetoacetate concentrations interfere with the most common laboratory method for measuring creatinine. Cimetidine appears to inhibit creatinine secretion by the renal tubules.

GFR declines with increasing age in most persons (5% per decade after age 20), but because muscle mass also declines, the serum creatinine remains relatively normal; creatinine production may decrease to 10 mg/kg. Thus, in elderly patients, small increases in serum creatinine may represent large changes in GFR. Using age and lean body weight (in kg), GFR can be estimated by the following formula for men:

Creatinine clearance =

$$\frac{[(140 - age) \times lean\ body\ weight]}{(72 \times plasma\ creatinine)}$$

For women, this equation must be multiplied by 0.85 to compensate for a smaller muscle mass.

The serum creatinine concentration requires 48–72 hours to equilibrate at a new level following acute changes in GFR.

BLOOD UREA NITROGEN: CREATININE RATIO

Low renal tubular flow rates enhance urea reabsorption but do not affect creatinine handling. As a result, the

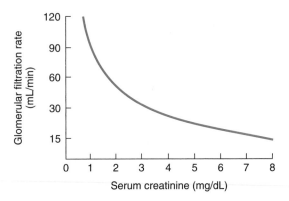

Figure 32–1. The relationship between the serum creatinine concentration and the glomerular filtration rate.

BUN to serum creatinine ratio increases above 10:1. Decreases in tubular flow can be caused by decreased renal perfusion or obstruction of the urinary tract. BUN:creatinine ratios greater than 15:1 are therefore seen in volume depletion and in edematous disorders associated with decreased tubular flow (eg, heart failure, cirrhosis, nephrotic syndrome) as well as in obstructive uropathies. Increases in protein catabolism can also increase this ratio (see above).

CREATININE CLEARANCE

 As discussed in Chapter 31, creatinine clearance measurements are the most accurate method available for clinically assessing overall renal function (really GFR). Although measurements are usually performed over 24 hours, 2-hour creatinine clearance determinations are reasonably accurate and easier to perform. Mild renal impairment generally results in creatinine clearances of 40–60 mL/min. Clearances between 25 and 40 mL/min produce moderate renal dysfunction and nearly always cause symptoms. Creatinine clearances less than 25 mL/min are indicative of overt renal failure.

Progressive renal disease enhances creatinine secretion in the proximal tubule. As a result, with declining renal function the creatinine clearance progressively overestimates the true GFR. Moreover, relative preservation of GFR may occur early in the course of progressive renal disease due to compensatory hyperfiltration in remaining nephrons and increases in glomerular filtration pressure. It is therefore important to look for other signs of deteriorating renal function such as hypertension, proteinuria, or other abnormalities in urine sediment.

URINALYSIS

Urinalysis continues to be the most common test routinely performed for evaluating renal function. Although its utility for that purpose is justifiably questionable, urinalysis can be helpful in identifying some disorders of renal tubular dysfunction as well as some nonrenal disturbances. A routine urinalysis typically includes pH, specific gravity, detection and quantification of glucose, protein, and bilirubin content, and microscopic examination of the urinary sediment. Urinary pH is helpful only when arterial pH is also known. A urinary pH greater than 7.0 in the presence of systemic acidosis is suggestive of renal tubular acidosis (see Chapter 30). Specific gravity is related to urinary osmolality; 1.010 usually corresponds to 290 momol/kg. A specific gravity greater than 1.018 after an overnight fast is indicative of adequate renal concentrating ability. A lower specific gravity in the presence of hyperosmolality in plasma is consistent with diabetes insipidus.

Glycosuria is the result either of a low tubular threshold for glucose (normally 180 mg/dL) or of hyperglycemia. Proteinuria detected by routine urinalysis should be evaluated by means of 24-hour urine collection. Urinary protein excretions greater than 150 mg/d are significant. Elevated levels of bilirubin in the urine are seen with biliary obstruction.

Microscopic analysis of the urinary sediment detects the presence of red or white blood cells, bacteria, casts, and crystals. Red cells may be indicative of bleeding due to tumor, stones, infection, coagulopathy, or trauma. White cells and bacteria are generally associated with infection. Disease processes at the level of the nephron produce tubular casts. Crystals may be indicative of abnormalities in oxalic acid, uric acid, or cystine metabolism.

■ ALTERED RENAL FUNCTION & THE EFFECTS OF ANESTHETIC AGENTS

Most drugs commonly employed during anesthesia are at least partly dependent on renal excretion for elimination. In the presence of renal impairment, dosage modifications may be required to prevent accumulation of the drug or active metabolites. Moreover, the systemic effects of azotemia can potentiate the pharmacologic actions of many of these agents. This latter observation may be the result of decreased protein binding of the drug, greater brain penetration due to some breach of the blood-brain barrier, or a synergistic effect with the toxins retained in renal failure.

INTRAVENOUS AGENTS

Barbiturates

Patients with renal disease often exhibit increased sensitivity to barbiturates during induction, even though pharmacokinetic profiles appear to be unchanged. The mechanism appears to be an increase in free circulating barbiturate as a result of decreased protein binding. Acidosis may also favor a more rapid entry of these agents into the brain by increasing the nonionized fraction of the drug (see Chapter 25).

Ketamine

Ketamine pharmacokinetics are minimally altered by renal disease. Some active hepatic metabolites are dependent on renal excretion and can potentially accumulate in renal failure. Ketamine's secondary hypertensive effect may be undesirable in hypertensive renal patients.

Propofol & Etomidate

The pharmacokinetics of both propofol and etomidate are not significantly affected by impaired renal function. Decreased protein binding of etomidate in patients with hypoalbuminemia may enhance its pharmacologic effects.

Benzodiazepines

These drugs undergo hepatic metabolism and conjugation prior to elimination in urine. Because most are highly protein-bound, increased sensitivity may be seen in patients with hypoalbuminemia. Diazepam should be used cautiously in the presence of renal impairment because of a potential for the accumulation of active metabolites.

Opioids

Most opioids currently in use in anesthetic management (morphine, meperidine, fentanyl, sufentanil, and alfentanil) are inactivated by the liver; some of these metabolites are then excreted in urine. With the exception of morphine and meperidine, significant accumulation of active metabolites generally does not occur with these agents. The accumulation of morphine (morphine-6-glucuronide) and meperidine metabolites has been reported to prolong respiratory depression in some patients with renal failure. Increased levels of normeperidine, a meperidine metabolite, have been associated with seizures. The pharmacokinetics of the most commonly used opioid agonist-antagonists (butorphanol, nalbuphine, and buprenorphine) are unaffected by renal failure.

Anticholinergic Agents

In doses used for premedication, atropine and glycopyrrolate can generally be used safely in patients with renal impairment. Because up to 50% of these drugs and their active metabolites are normally excreted in urine, however, the potential for accumulation exists following repeated doses. Scopolamine is less dependent on renal excretion, but its central nervous system effects can be enhanced by azotemia.

Phenothiazines, H₂ Blockers, & Related Agents

Most phenothiazines, such as promethazine, are metabolized to inactive compounds by the liver. Although pharmacokinetic profiles are not appreciably altered by renal impairment, potentiation of their central depressant effects by azotemia can also occur. Their antiemetic actions are particularly useful in the setting of preoperative nausea. Droperidol may be partly dependent on the kidneys for excretion. Although accumulation may be seen following large doses in patients with renal impairment, relatively small doses of droperidol (< 2.5 mg) are usually used clinically.

All H_2 receptor blockers are very dependent on renal excretion. Metoclopramide is partly excreted unchanged in urine and will also accumulate in renal failure. Although up to 50% of dolasetron is excreted in urine, no dosage adjustments are recommended for any of the 5-HT_3 blockers in patients with renal insufficiency.

INHALATIONAL AGENTS

Volatile Agents

Volatile anesthetic agents are nearly ideal for patients with renal dysfunction because of their lack of dependence on the kidneys for elimination, their ability to control blood pressure, and generally minimal direct effects on renal blood flow (see Chapter 31). Although patients with mild to moderate renal impairment do not exhibit altered uptake or distribution, accelerated induction and emergence may be seen in severely anemic patients (hemoglobin < 5 g/dL) with chronic renal failure; this observation may be explained by a decrease in the blood:gas partition coefficient or a decrease in minimum alveolar concentration (see Chapter 7). Because of its potential nephrotoxicity, methoxyflurane is the only volatile agent that should not be used (see Chapters 7 and 31). Enflurane and sevoflurane may also be considered undesirable for patients with renal disease undergoing long procedures because of a similar potential for fluoride accumulation.

Nitrous Oxide

Many clinicians omit or limit the use of nitrous oxide to 50% in patients with renal failure in an attempt to increase arterial oxygen content in the presence of anemia. This rationale may only be justified in severely anemic patients (hemoglobin < 7 g/dL), in whom even a small increase in the dissolved oxygen content may represent a significant percentage of the arterial to venous oxygen difference (see Chapter 22).

MUSCLE RELAXANTS

Succinylcholine

 Succinylcholine can be safely used in the presence of renal failure, provided the serum potassium concentration is known to be less than 5 mEq/L at the time of induction. When the serum potassium is higher or is in doubt, a nondepolarizing muscle relaxant should be used instead. Although decreased pseudocholinesterase levels have been reported in a few uremic patients following dialysis, significant prolongation of neuromuscular blockade is rarely seen.

Cisatracurium, Atracurium, & Mivacurium

Mivacurium is minimally dependent on the kidneys for elimination. Minor prolongation of effect may be observed due to reduced plasma pseudocholinesterase. Cisatracurium and atracurium are degraded in plasma by enzymatic ester hydrolysis and nonenzymatic Hofmann elimination. These agents may be the drugs of choice for muscle relaxation in patients with renal failure.

Vecuronium & Rocuronium

The elimination of vecuronium is primarily hepatic, but up to 20% of the drug is eliminated in urine. The effects of large doses of vecuronium (> 0.1 mg/kg) are only modestly prolonged in patients with renal insufficiency. Rocuronium primarily undergoes hepatic elimination, but prolongation by severe renal disease has been reported.

Curare

Elimination of curare is dependent on both renal and biliary excretion; 40–60% of a dose of curare is normally excreted in urine. Increasingly prolonged effects are observed following repeated doses in patients with significant renal impairment. Smaller doses and longer dosing intervals are therefore required for maintenance of optimal muscle relaxation.

Pancuronium, Pipecuronium, Alcuronium, & Doxacurium

All these agents are primarily dependent on renal excretion (60–90%). Although pancuronium is metabolized by the liver into less active intermediates, its elimination half-life is still primarily dependent on renal excretion (60–80%). Neuromuscular function should be closely monitored if these agents are used in patients with abnormal renal function.

Metocurine, Gallamine, & Decamethonium

All three agents are almost entirely dependent on renal excretion for elimination and should generally be avoided in patients with impaired renal function.

Reversal Agents

Renal excretion is the principal route of elimination for edrophonium, neostigmine, and pyridostigmine. The half-lives of these agents in patients with renal impairment are therefore prolonged at least as much as any of the above relaxants. Problems with inadequate reversal of neuromuscular blockade are usually related to other factors (see Chapter 9).

■ ANESTHESIA FOR PATIENTS WITH RENAL FAILURE

PREOPERATIVE CONSIDERATIONS

Acute Renal Failure

This syndrome is a rapid deterioration in renal function that results in retention of nitrogenous waste products (**azotemia**). These substances, many of which behave as toxins, are by-products of protein and amino acid metabolism. They include urea, guanidine compounds (including creatine and creatinine), urates, aliphatic amines, and various peptides and metabolites of aromatic amino acids. Impaired renal metabolism of circulating proteins and peptides may also contribute to widespread organ dysfunction.

Azotemia can be divided into prerenal, renal, and postrenal types depending on its causes (see Chapter 50). **Prerenal azotemia** results from an acute decrease in renal perfusion. **Renal azotemia** is usually due to intrinsic renal disease, renal ischemia, or nephrotoxins. **Postrenal azotemia** is the result of urinary tract obstruction or disruption. Both prerenal and postrenal azotemia are readily reversible in their initial stages but with time progress to renal azotemia. Most adult patients with renal failure develop oliguria. Nonoliguric patients (those with urinary outputs > 400 mL/d) continue to form urine that is qualitatively poor; these patients tend to have greater preservation of GFR. Although glomerular filtration and tubular function are impaired in both cases, abnormalities tend to be less severe in nonoliguric renal failure.

The course of acute renal failure varies widely, but the oliguria typically lasts for 2 weeks and is followed by a diuretic phase marked by a progressive increase in urinary output. This diuretic phase often results in very large urinary outputs and is usually absent in nonoliguric renal failure. Urinary function improves over the course of several weeks but may not return to normal for up to 1 year. A more complete discussion of acute renal failure is found in Chapter 50.

Chronic Renal Failure

This syndrome is characterized by a progressive and irreversible decline in renal function over the course of at

Table 32–2. Manifestations of uremia.

Neurologic
   Peripheral neuropathy
   Autonomic neuropathy
   Muscle twitching
   Encephalopathy
     Asterexis
     Myoclonus
     Lethargy
     Confusion
     Seizures
     Coma
Cardiovascular
   Fluid overload
   Congestive heart failure
   Hypertension
   Pericarditis
   Arrhythmia
   Conduction blocks
   Vascular calcification
   Accelerated atherosclerosis
Pulmonary
   Hyperventilation
   Interstitial edema
   Alveolar edema
   Pleural effusion
Gastrointestinal
   Anorexia
   Nausea and vomiting
   Delayed gastric emptying
   Hyperacidity
   Mucosal ulcerations
   Hemorrhage
   Adynamic ileus
Metabolic
   Metabolic acidosis
   Hyperkalemia
   Hyponatremia
   Hypermagnesemia
   Hyperphosphatemia
   Hypocalcemia
   Hyperuricemia
   Hypoalbuminemia
Hematologic
   Anemia
   Platelet dysfunction
   Leukocyte dysfunction
Endocrine
   Glucose intolerance
   Secondary hyperparathyroidism
   Hypertriglyceridemia
Skeletal
   Ostedystrophy
   Periarticular calcification
Skin
   Hyperpigmentation
   Ecchymosis
   Pruritus

least 3–6 months. The most common causes are hypertensive nephrosclerosis, diabetic nephropathy, chronic glomerulonephritis, and polycystic renal disease.

The full manifestations of this syndrome (Table 32–2)—often referred to as **uremia**—are seen only after the GFR decreases below 25 mL/min. Patients with clearances below 10 mL/min (often said to have end-stage renal disease) are dependent on dialysis for survival until they receive a successful transplant. Dialysis may take the form of intermittent hemodialysis employing an arteriovenous fistula or continuous peritoneal dialysis via an implanted catheter.

The generalized effects of uremia can usually be controlled by dialysis. Unfortunately, with time some uremic complications can become refractory. Moreover, some complications are directly related to the dialysis itself (Table 32–3). Hypotension, neutropenia, hypoxemia, and the disequilibrium syndrome are generally transient and resolve within hours after dialysis. Factors contributing to hypotension during dialysis include the vasodilating effects of acetate dialysate solutions, autonomic neuropathy, and rapid removal of fluid. The interaction of white cells with cellophane-derived dialysis membranes can result in neutropenia and leukocyte-mediated pulmonary dysfunction leading to hypox-

Table 32–3. Complications of dialysis.

Neurologic
   Disequilibrium syndrome
   Dementia
Cardiovascular
   Intravascular volume depletion
   Hypotension
   Arrhythmia
Pulmonary
   Hypoxemia
Gastrointestinal
   Ascites
Hematologic
   Anemia
   Transient neutropenia
   Residual anticoagulation
   Hypocomplementemia
Metabolic
   Hypokalemia
   Large protein losses
Skeletal
   Osteomalacia
   Arthropathy
   Myopathy
Infectious
   Peritonitis
   Transfusion-related hepatitis

emia. **Disequilibrium syndrome** is characterized by transient neurologic symptoms that appear to be related to a more rapid lowering of extracellular osmolality than intracellular osmolality.

Manifestations of Renal Failure

A. METABOLIC:

Multiple metabolic abnormalities, including hyperkalemia, hyperphosphatemia, hypocalcemia, hypermagnesemia, hyperuricemia, and hypoalbuminemia typically develop in patients with overt renal failure. Water and sodium retention can result in worsening hyponatremia and extracellular fluid overload, respectively. Failure to excrete nonvolatile acids produces a high anion gap metabolic acidosis (see Chapter 30). Hypernatremia and hypokalemia are uncommon complications.

Hyperkalemia is the most lethal of these abnormalities because of its effect on the heart (see Chapter 28). It is usually present in patients with creatinine clearances of less than 5 mL/min, but it can develop rapidly in patients with higher clearances when challenged with large potassium loads (trauma, hemolysis, infections, or potassium administration).

The hypermagnesemia is generally mild unless magnesium intake is increased (most commonly from magnesium-containing antacids). Hypocalcemia develops for unclear reasons. Proposed mechanisms include deposition of calcium into bone secondary to the hyperphosphatemia, resistance to parathyroid hormone, and decreased intestinal absorption secondary to decreased renal synthesis of 1,25-dihydroxycholecalciferol (see Chapter 28). Symptoms of hypocalcemia rarely develop unless patients are also made alkalotic.

Patients with renal failure also rapidly lose tissue proteins and readily develop hypoalbuminemia. Anorexia, protein restriction, and dialysis (especially peritoneal dialysis) are contributory.

B. HEMATOLOGIC:

Anemia is nearly always present when the creatinine clearance is below 30 mL/min. Hemoglobin concentrations are generally 6–8 g/dL. Decreased erythropoietin production, decreased red cell production, and decreased cell survival are thought to be responsible. Additional factors include gastrointestinal blood loss, hemodilution, and bone marrow suppression from recurrent infections. Even with transfusions, hemoglobin concentrations greater than 9 g/dL are often difficult to maintain. Erythropoietin administration appears to at least partially correct the anemia. Increased levels of 2,3-diphosphoglycerate develop in response to the decrease in oxygen-carrying capacity. 2,3-DPG facilitates the unloading of oxygen from hemoglobin (see Chapter 22). The metabolic acidosis (see above) also favors a rightward shift in the hemoglobin-oxygen dissociation curve. In the absence of symptomatic heart disease, most patients tolerate the anemia remarkably well.

Both platelet and white cell function are impaired in patients with renal failure. Clinically, this is manifested as a prolonged bleeding time and increased susceptibility to infections, respectively. Most patients have decreased platelet factor III activity, as well as decreased platelet adhesiveness and aggregation. Patients who have recently undergone hemodialysis may also have residual anticoagulant effects from heparin.

C. CARDIOVASCULAR:

Cardiac output has to increase in renal failure to maintain oxygen delivery in the face of a decrease in oxygen-carrying capacity. Sodium retention and abnormalities in the renin-angiotensin system result in systemic arterial hypertension. Left ventricular hypertrophy is a common finding in chronic renal failure. The extracellular fluid overload from sodium retention—together with the increased demand imposed by anemia and hypertension—make these patients especially prone to congestive heart failure and pulmonary edema. Increased permeability of the alveolar-capillary membrane may also be a predisposing factor (below). Conduction blocks are not uncommon and may be due to deposition of calcium in the conduction system. Arrhythmias are common and may be in part related to the metabolic abnormalities. **Uremic pericarditis** may develop in some patients; patients may be asymptomatic, may present with chest pain, or may develop cardiac tamponade. Patients with chronic renal failure also characteristically develop accelerated peripheral vascular and coronary artery disease.

Intravascular volume depletion may occur during the diuretic phase of acute renal failure if fluid replacement is inadequate. Hypovolemia also develops if too much fluid is removed during dialysis.

D. PULMONARY:

Without dialysis or bicarbonate therapy, patients may be dependent on an increase in minute ventilation to compensate for the metabolic acidosis (see Chapter 30). Pulmonary extravascular water is often increased in the form of interstitial edema, resulting in a widening of the alveolar to arterial oxygen gradient and predisposing to hypoxemia. Increased permeability of the alveolar-capillary membrane in some patients can result in pulmonary edema even with normal pulmonary capillary pressures; a characteristic picture resembling "butterfly wings" may be seen on the chest film.

E. ENDOCRINE:

Abnormal glucose tolerance is characteristic of renal failure and is thought to result from peripheral resistance to insulin; patients therefore often handle large glucose loads poorly. Secondary hyperparathyroidism in patients with chronic renal failure can produce metabolic bone disease, which may predispose to fractures. Abnormalities in lipid metabolism frequently lead to hypertriglyceridemia and probably contribute to accelerated atherosclerosis. Increases in the circulating levels of proteins and polypeptides normally degraded in the kidneys are often seen; these include parathyroid hormone, insulin, glucagon, growth hormone, luteinizing hormone, and prolactin.

F. Gastrointestinal:

Anorexia, nausea, vomiting, and adynamic ileus are commonly associated with azotemia. Hypersecretion of gastric acid increases the incidence of peptic ulceration and gastrointestinal hemorrhage, which occurs in 10–30% of patients. Delayed gastric emptying secondary to autonomic neuropathy can predispose patients to aspiration perioperatively. Patients with chronic renal failure also have a high incidence of viral hepatitis (types B and C), often followed by residual hepatic dysfunction.

G. Neurologic:

Asterixis, lethargy, confusion, seizures, and coma are manifestations of **uremic encephalopathy.** Symptoms generally correlate with the degree of azotemia. Autonomic and peripheral neuropathies are common in patients with chronic renal failure. Peripheral neuropathies are typically sensory and involve the distal lower extremities.

Preoperative Evaluation

The generalized effects of azotemia mandate a thorough evaluation of patients in renal failure. Most patients with acute renal failure requiring surgery are critically ill. Their renal failure is frequently associated with a postoperative complication or trauma. Patients with acute renal failure also tend to have accelerated protein breakdown. Optimal perioperative management is dependent on preoperative dialysis. Hemodialysis is more effective than peritoneal dialysis and can be readily accomplished via a temporary internal jugular, subclavian or femoral dialysis catheter. The need for dialysis in nonoliguric patients should be assessed on an individual basis. Indications for dialysis are listed in Table 32–4.

Patients with chronic renal failure most commonly present to the operating room for creation or revision of an arteriovenous fistula under local or regional anesthesia. Regardless of the procedure or the anesthetic employed, complete evaluation is required to make certain that they are in optimal medical condition; all reversible manifestations (Table 32–2) of uremia should

be controlled. Preoperative dialysis on the day of surgery or on the previous day is usually necessary.

Physical and laboratory evaluation should focus on both cardiac and respiratory functions. Signs of fluid overload or hypovolemia should be sought (see Chapter 29). Intravascular volume depletion often results from overzealous dialysis. A comparison of the patient's current weight with previous predialysis and postdialysis weights may be helpful. Hemodynamic data, if available, and a chest film are invaluable in confirming clinical impressions. Arterial blood gas analysis is also useful in detecting hypoxemia and evaluating acid-base status. The electrocardiogram should be examined carefully for signs of hyperkalemia or hypocalcemia (see Chapter 28) as well as ischemia, conduction blocks, and ventricular hypertrophy. Echocardiography can be invaluable for evaluating cardiac function in patients undergoing major surgical procedures because it can evaluate the ventricular ejection fraction, as well as detect and quantitate hypertrophy, wall motion abnormalities, and pericardial fluid. A friction rub may not be audible on auscultation in patients with a pericardial effusion.

Preoperative red blood cell transfusions should generally be given only to severely anemic patients (hemoglobin < 6–7 g/dL) or when significant intraoperative blood loss is expected. A bleeding time and coagulation studies are advisable, especially if regional anesthesia is being considered. Serum electrolyte, BUN, and creatinine measurements can assess the adequacy of dialysis. Glucose measurements are helpful in evaluating the potential need for perioperative insulin therapy.

Preoperative drug therapy should be carefully reviewed for drugs with significant renal elimination (Table 32–5). Dosage adjustments and measurements of blood levels (when available) are necessary to prevent drug toxicity.

Premedication

Alert patients who are relatively stable can be given reduced doses of an opioid (see Table 8–6) or a benzodiazepine (see Table 8–3). Promethazine, 12.5–25 mg in-

Table 32–4. Indications for dialysis.

Fluid overload
Hyperkalemia
Severe acidosis
Metabolic encephalopathy
Pericarditis
Coagulopathy
Refractory gastrointestinal symptoms
Drug toxicity

Table 32–5. Drugs with a potential for significant accumulation in patients with renal impairment.

Muscle relaxants
  Metocurine
  Gallamine
  Decamethonium
  Pancuronium
  Pipecurium
  Doxacurium
  Alcuronium
Anticholinergics
  Atropine
  Glycopyrrolate
Metoclopramide
H₂ receptor antagonists
  Cimetidine
  Ranitidine
Digitalis
Diuretics
Calcium channel antagonists
  Nifedipine
  Diltiazem
β-Adrenergic blockers
  Propranolol
  Nadolol
  Pindolol
  Atenolol
Antihypertensives
  Clonidine
  Methyldopa
  Captopril
  Enalapril
  Lisinopril
  Hydalazine
  Nitroprusside (thiocyanate)
Antiarrhythmics
  Procainamide
  Disopyramide
  Bretylium
  Tocainide
  Encainide (genetically determined)
Bronchodilators
  Terbutaline
Psychiatric
  Lithium
Antibiotics
  Penicillins
  Cephalosporins
  Aminoglycosides
  Tetracycline
  Vancomycin
Anticonvulsants
  Carbamazepine
  Ethosuximide
  Primidone

---

tramuscularly, is a useful adjunct for additional sedation and for its antiemetic properties. Aspiration prophylaxis with an H₂ blocker may be indicated in patients with nausea, vomiting, or gastrointestinal bleeding (see Chapter 15). Metoclopramide, 10 mg orally or slowly intravenously, may also be useful in accelerating gastric emptying, preventing nausea, and decreasing the risk of aspiration. Preoperative medications—especially antihypertensive agents—should be continued until the time of surgery (see Chapter 20). The management of diabetic patients is discussed in Chapter 36.

INTRAOPERATIVE CONSIDERATIONS

Monitoring

The surgical procedure as well as the patient's general medical condition dictate monitoring requirements. Because of the danger of occlusion, blood pressure should not be measured by a cuff in an arm with an arteriovenous fistula. Intra-arterial, central venous, and pulmonary artery monitoring are often indicated, especially for patients undergoing procedures associated with major fluid shifts (see Chapter 6); intravascular volume is often difficult to assess based on clinical signs alone. Direct intra-arterial blood pressure monitoring may also be indicated in poorly controlled hypertensive patients regardless of the procedure. Aggressive invasive monitoring may be indicated especially in diabetic patients with advanced renal disease undergoing major surgery; this group of patients may have up to 10 times the perioperative morbidity of diabetics without renal disease. The latter probably reflects the high incidence of advanced cardiovascular complications in the first group.

Induction

Patients with nausea, vomiting, or gastrointestinal bleeding should undergo rapid-sequence induction with cricoid pressure (see Chapter 15). The dose of the induction agent should be reduced in debilitated or critically ill patients. Thiopental 2–3 mg/kg or propofol 1–2 mg/kg is often used. Etomidate, 0.2–0.4 mg/kg may be preferable in hemodynamically unstable patients. An opioid, β-blocker (esmolol), or lidocaine may be used to blunt the hypertensive response to intubation (see Chapter 20). Succinylcholine, 1.5 mg/kg, can be used for endotracheal intubation if the serum potassium is less than 5 mEq/L. Rocuronium (0.6 mg/kg), cisatracurium (0.15 mg/kg) atracurium (0.4 mg/kg) or mivacurium (0.15 mg/kg) should be used for intubating patients with hyperkalemia. Atracurium in this dosage generally causes little histamine release (see

Chapter 9). Vecuronium, 0.1 mg/kg, may be a suitable alternative, but some prolongation of its effects should be expected.

Maintenance

The ideal maintenance technique should be able to control hypertension with minimal effects on cardiac output, because an increase in cardiac output is the principal compensatory mechanism for anemia. Volatile anesthetics, nitrous oxide, propofol, fentanyl, sufentanil, alfentanil, remifentanil, hydromorphone, and morphine are generally regarded as satisfactory maintenance agents. Isoflurane and desflurane may be the preferred volatile agents because they have the least effect on cardiac output (see Chapter 7). Nitrous oxide should be used cautiously in patients with poor ventricular function and should probably not be used in patients with very low hemoglobin concentrations (< 7 g/dL) to allow the administration of 100% oxygen (see above). Meperidine may not be a good choice because of the accumulation of normeperidine (see above). Morphine may be used, but some prolongation of its effects should be expected.

Controlled ventilation is safest for patients with renal failure. Spontaneous ventilation under anesthesia can result in respiratory acidosis that may exacerbate preexisting acidemia, leading to potentially severe circulatory depression and dangerous increases in serum potassium concentration (see Chapter 30). Respiratory alkalosis may also be detrimental because it shifts the hemoglobin dissociation curve to the left (see Chapter 22), can exacerbate preexisting hypocalcemia (see Chapter 28), and may reduce cerebral blood flow (see Chapter 25).

Fluid Therapy

Superficial operations involving minimal tissue trauma require replacement of only insensible fluid losses with 5% dextrose in water. Procedures associated with major fluid losses or shifts require isotonic crystalloids, colloids, or both (see Chapter 29). Lactated Ringer's injection is best avoided in hyperkalemic patients when large volumes of fluid may be required, because it contains potassium (4 mEq/L); normal saline may be used instead. Glucose-free solutions should generally be used because of the glucose intolerance associated with uremia. Blood loss should generally be replaced with packed red blood cells. Blood transfusion either has no effect or may be beneficial for patients in renal failure who are renal transplant candidates; such transfusion may decrease the likelihood of rejection following renal transplantation in some patients.

■ ANESTHESIA FOR PATIENTS WITH MILD TO MODERATE RENAL IMPAIRMENT

PREOPERATIVE CONSIDERATIONS

The kidneys normally exhibit a large reserve in function. GFR, as determined by creatinine clearance, can decrease from 120 to 60 mL/min without any clinically perceptible change in renal function. Even patients with creatinine clearances of 40–60 mL/min usually are asymptomatic. These patients have only mild renal impairment but should still be thought of as having decreased renal reserve. The emphasis in the care of these patients is preserving remaining renal function.

When creatinine clearance reaches 25–40 mL/min, renal impairment is moderate, and patients can be said to have renal insufficiency: Significant azotemia is always present, and hypertension and anemia are common. Correct anesthetic management of this group of patients is as critical as management of those with frank renal failure. The latter is especially true during procedures associated with a relatively high incidence of postoperative renal failure, such as cardiac and aortic reconstructive surgery. Intravascular volume depletion, sepsis, obstructive jaundice, crush injuries, recent contrast dye injections, and aminoglycoside, angiotensin-converting enzyme inhibitor, or nonsteroidal anti-inflammatory drug therapy are additional major risk factors for an acute deterioration in renal function. Hypovolemia appears to be an especially important factor in the development of acute postoperative renal failure. The emphasis in management of these patients is on prevention, because the mortality rate of postoperative renal failure is as high as 50–60%. The increased perioperative risk associated with the combination of advanced renal disease and diabetes has already been alluded to above.

Prophylaxis against renal failure with solute diuresis appears to be effective and indicated in high-risk patients undergoing cardiac, major aortic reconstructive, and possibly other surgical procedures. Mannitol (0.5 g/kg) is generally employed and should be started prior to or at the time of induction (see Chapter 31). Intravenous fluids should be given concomitantly to prevent intravascular volume depletion. Intravenous infusions of low-dose dopamine may also be beneficial by increasing renal blood flow via activation of vasodilatory dopaminergic receptors in the renal vasculature. A loop diuretic may also be necessary to maintain an adequate urinary output and prevent fluid overload. The value of prophylaxis with acetylcysteine prior to the administration of radiocontrast dyes is discussed in Chapter 31.

INTRAOPERATIVE CONSIDERATIONS

Monitoring

Standard monitors are used for procedures involving minimal fluid losses. For operations associated with significant blood or fluid losses, monitoring hourly urinary output and intravascular volume is critical (see Chapter 29). Although an adequate urinary output does not ensure preservation of renal function, urinary outputs greater than 0.5 mL/kg/hour are generally desirable. Intra-arterial pressure monitoring is also desirable if rapid changes in blood pressure may be encountered, such as in poorly controlled hypertensive patients and in those undergoing procedures associated with abrupt changes in cardiac preload or afterload.

Induction

Selection of an induction agent is not as critical as ensuring an adequate intravascular volume prior to induction. Induction of anesthesia in patients with renal insufficiency frequently results in hypotension when hypovolemia is present. Unless a vasopressor is given, the hypotension typically resolves only following intubation or surgical stimulation. Renal perfusion, which may already be compromised by the hypovolemia, deteriorates further, first as a result of hypotension and then from sympathetically or pharmacologically mediated renal vasoconstriction. If sustained, the decrease in renal perfusion could contribute to postoperative renal impairment. Preoperative hydration usually prevents this sequence of events.

Maintenance

All maintenance agents are acceptable with the possible exception of methoxyflurane and sevoflurane. Although enflurane can be used safely for short procedures, it is best avoided in patients with renal insufficiency because of the availability of other satisfactory agents. Deterioration in renal function during this period may result from any adverse hemodynamic effects of surgery (hemorrhage) or anesthesia (cardiac depression or hypotension), indirect hormonal effects (sympathoadrenal activation or antidiuretic hormone secretion), or positive pressure ventilation (impeded venous return; see Chapter 31). These effects are almost completely reversible when sufficient intravenous fluids are given to maintain a normal or slightly expanded intravascular volume. The administration of predominantly α-adrenergic vasopressors (phenylephrine, methoxamine, and norepinephrine) may also be detrimental. Once mean arterial blood pressure, cardiac output, and intravascular volume are adequate, a low-dose dopamine infusion (2–5 µg/kg/min) can be used in patients with marginal urinary output in an attempt to preserve renal blood flow and renal function. "Renal dose dopamine" has also been shown to, at least partially, reverse renal arterial vasoconstriction during infusions of α-adrenergic vasopressors (norepinephrine).

Fluid Therapy

As discussed above, judicious fluid administration is critical in managing patients with decreased renal reserve or renal insufficiency. Concern over fluid overload is justified, but problems are rarely encountered in patients with normal urinary outputs if rational guidelines and appropriate monitors are employed (see Chapter 29). Indeed, the consequences of excessive fluid overload—namely, pulmonary congestion or edema—are easier to treat than those of acute renal failure.

CASE DISCUSSION: A PATIENT WITH UNCONTROLLED HYPERTENSION

A 59-year-old man with a recent onset of hypertension is scheduled for reconstruction of a stenotic left renal artery. His preoperative blood pressure is 180/110 mm Hg.

What is the cause of this man's hypertension?

Renovascular hypertension is one of few surgically correctable forms of hypertension. Others include coarctation of the aorta, pheochromocytoma, Cushing's disease, and primary hyperaldosteronism.

Most studies suggest that renovascular hypertension accounts for 2–5% of all cases of hypertension. It characteristically presents either as a relatively sudden onset of hypertension in persons younger than 35 years or older than 55 years. Renal artery stenosis can also be responsible for the development of accelerated or malignant hypertension in previously hypertensive persons of any age.

What is the pathophysiology of the hypertension?

Unilateral or bilateral stenosis of the renal artery decreases the perfusion pressure to the kidneys distal to the obstruction. Activation of the juxtaglomerular apparatus and release of renin in-

creases circulating levels of angiotensin II and aldosterone, resulting in peripheral vascular constriction and sodium retention, respectively (see Chapter 31). The resulting systemic arterial hypertension is often marked.

In nearly two-thirds of patients, the stenosis results from an atheromatous plaque in proximal renal artery. These patients are typically men over the age of 55 years. In the remaining third, the stenosis is more distal and due to malformations of the arterial wall, commonly referred to as fibromuscular hyperplasia (or dysplasia). This latter lesion most commonly presents in women below the age of 35 years. Bilateral renal artery stenosis is present in 30–50% of patients with renovascular hypertension. Less common causes of stenosis include dissecting aneurysms, emboli, polyarteritis nodosa, radiation, trauma, extrinsic compression from retroperitoneal fibrosis or tumors, and hypoplasia of the renal arteries.

What clinical manifestations other than hypertension may be present?

Signs of secondary hyperaldosteronism can be prominent. These include sodium retention in the form of edema, a metabolic alkalosis, and hypokalemia. The latter can cause muscle weakness, polyuria, and even tetany.

How is the diagnosis made?

The diagnosis is suggested by the clinical presentation previously described. A midabdominal bruit may also be present, but the diagnosis requires laboratory and radiographic confirmation. The captopril test is a good screening test; it relies on the observation that administration of an angiotensin-converting enzyme (ACE) inhibitor to these patients decreases renal perfusion as assessed by an isotope scan. If the test is positive, digital subtraction angiography is used to demonstrate the stenosis. If the latter is not available, a rapid-sequence intravenous pyelogram can suggest the diagnosis when appearance of the dye is delayed on the affected side. Renal arteriography is often used to confirm the anatomic defect preoperatively.

Which patients are most likely to benefit from surgery?

The functional significance of the lesion is evaluated by selective catheterization of both renal veins and measurement of plasma renin activity in blood from each kidney. Plasma renin activity is typically elevated on the stenotic side. Patients with renal artery stenosis with a plasma renin ac-

tivity ratio on the two sides greater than 1.5:1 have a greater than 90% cure rate following surgery. Administration of an ACE inhibitor greatly magnifies the difference in renal vein plasma renin activity between the two sides. If the stenosis is bilateral, the split plasma renin activity ratios may be less than 1.5:1, yet the patient may still benefit from surgery.

Should this patient undergo the procedure given his present blood pressure?

The current emphasis in the treatment of renovascular stenosis is surgical because of the propensity for progressive loss of renal function with medical treatment alone. Nonetheless, optimal medical therapy is important in preparing these patients for surgery. When compared with well-controlled patients, those with poorly controlled hypertension have a high incidence of problems intraoperatively: marked hypertension, hypotension, myocardial ischemia, and arrhythmias (see Chapter 20). Ideally, arterial blood pressure should be well controlled—preferably in the normal range—prior to surgery. Metabolic disturbances such as hypokalemia should be corrected. Patients should be evaluated for preexisting renal dysfunction (see Chapter 31). Those patients older than 50 years should also be evaluated for the presence and severity of coexisting atherosclerotic disease, especially of the coronary arteries (see Chapter 20).

What antihypertensive agents are most useful for controlling blood pressure perioperatively in these patients?

The most useful agents in renovascular hypertension are those that decrease renin-angiotensin system activity, namely ACE inhibitors, β-blockers, and centrally acting agents that decrease sympathetic activity. Many ACE inhibitors are available; but only enalaprilat is available as an intravenous preparation (see Chapter 20). Side effects include transient hypotension, hyperkalemia, neutropenia, angioedema, urticaria, and rashes. ACE inhibitors can cause acute renal failure in patients with bilateral renal artery stenosis. Their role in perioperative blood pressure management is restricted to the preoperative period.

In contrast, β-adrenergic blocking drugs can be readily used intraoperatively and postoperatively for blood pressure control. They are especially effective because secretion of renin is partly mediated by β_1-adrenergic receptors. Although parenteral selective β_1-blocking agents such as metoprolol and esmolol would be expected to be *most effective, nonselective agents such as pro- pranolol appear equally effective. Esmolol may be the agent of choice because of its short half-life and titratability.*

Direct vasodilators such as nitroprusside and nitroglycerin are also invaluable in controlling in- traoperative hypertension. Fenoldopam offers the additional benefit increasing renal blood flow and may have renal protective properties. The role of saralasin, an angiotensin II receptor antagonist, is limited because of its partial agonist activity.

What are important intraoperative consider- ations for the anesthesiologist?

Revascularization of a kidney is a major proce- dure, with the potential for major blood loss, fluid shifts, and hemodynamic changes. One of several procedures may be performed, including transaor- tic renal endarterectomy, aortorenal bypass (using a saphenous vein, synthetic graft, or segment of the hypogastric artery), a splenic to (left) renal artery bypass, a hepatic or gastroduodenal to (right) renal artery bypass, or excision of the stenotic segment with reanastomosis of the renal artery to the aorta. Rarely, nephrectomy may be performed. Regardless of the procedure, an exten- sive retroperitoneal dissection usually necessitates relatively large volumes of intravenous fluid re- placement. Large-bore intravenous access is mandatory because of the potential for extensive blood loss. Heparinization contributes to in- creased blood loss. Depending on the surgical technique, aortic cross-clamping, with its associ- ated hemodynamic consequences, often compli- cates anesthetic management (see Chapter 21). Direct intra-arterial and central venous pressure monitoring are mandatory. Pulmonary artery pressure monitoring is indicated for patients with poor ventricular function (see Chapter 6). The choice of anesthetic technique is generally deter- mined by the patient's cardiovascular function.

Urinary output should be followed carefully. Measures to protect the affected as well as the nor- mal kidney against ischemic injury are necessary. Generous hydration together with solute diuresis with mannitol are generally advisable (see Chap- ter 31). Topical cooling of the affected kidney dur- ing the anastomosis may also be employed.

What are the important postoperative con- siderations?

Although in most patients hypertension is ulti- mately cured or significantly improved, arterial blood pressure is often quite labile in the early postoperative period. Close hemodynamic moni- toring should be continued well into the postoper- ative period. Reported operative mortality rates range from 1% to 6%, and most deaths are associ- ated with myocardial infarction. The latter proba- bly reflects the relatively high prevalence of coro- nary artery disease in older patients with renovascular hypertension.

SUGGESTED READING

Better OS, Rubinstein I, Winaver JM, Knochel JP: Mannitol ther- apy revisited (1940–1997). Kid Int 1997;52:886.

Colson P, Ryckwaert F, Coriat P: Renin angiotensin system antag- onists and anesthesia. Anesth Analg 1999;89:1143.

Fawcett WJ, Haxby EJ, Male DA: Magnesium: Physiology and pharmacology. Br J Anaesth 1999;83:302.

Gravenstein D: Transurethral resection of the prostate (TURP) syndrome: A review of the pathophysiology and manage- ment. Anesth Analg 1997;84:438.

Schrier RW (editor): *Renal and Electrolyte Disorders,* 5th ed. Lip- pencott Williams & Wilkins, 1997.

Stoelting RK, Dierdorf SE: *Anesthesia and Co-existing Disease,* 3rd ed. Churchill Livingstone, 1993.

Thapa S, Brull SJ: Succinylcholine-induced hyperkalemia in pa- tients with renal failure: An old question revisited. Anesth Analg 2000;91:237.

Anesthesia for Genitourinary Surgery

33

KEY CONCEPTS

 The lithotomy position is the most commonly used position for patients undergoing urologic and gynecologic procedures. Failure to properly position patients can result in iatrogenic injuries.

 The lithotomy position is associated with major physiologic alterations. Functional residual capacity decreases, predisposing patients to atelectasis and hypoxia. Elevation of the legs increases venous return acutely. Mean blood pressure often increases but cardiac output does not change significantly. Conversely, rapid lowering of the legs acutely decreases venous return and can result in hypotension. Blood pressure measurements should always be taken immediately after the legs are lowered.

 Because of the short duration (15–20 minutes) and the outpatient setting of most cystoscopies, general anesthesia is usually used.

 Both epidural and spinal blocks can provide satisfactory anesthesia. A sensory level to T10 provides excellent anesthesia for nearly all cystoscopic procedures.

 Manifestations of the TURP (transurethral resection of the prostate) syndrome are primarily those of circulatory fluid overload, water intoxication, and occasionally, toxicity from the solute in the irrigating fluid.

 Absorption of irrigation fluid appears to be dependent on the duration of the resection as well as the height (pressure) of the irrigation fluid.

 When compared with general anesthesia, regional anesthesia appears to reduce the incidence of postoperative venous thrombosis; it is also less likely to mask symptoms and signs of the TURP syndrome or bladder perforation.

 Patients with a history of cardiac arrhythmias and those with a pacemaker or automatic internal cardiac defibrillator (AICD) may be at risk for developing arrhythmias induced by shock waves during extracorporeal shock wave lithotripsy (ESWL). Shock waves can damage the internal components of pacemaker and AICD devices.

 Patients who are undergoing retroperitoneal lymph node dissection and who are receiving bleomycin preoperatively are at increased risk for developing postoperative pulmonary insufficiency. These patients appear to be especially sensitive to oxygen toxicity and fluid overload, and are at increased risk for developing acute respiratory distress syndrome postoperatively. Excessive intravenous fluid administration may also be contributory.

 The serum potassium concentration should be below 5.5 mEq/L and existing coagulopathies should be corrected in patients undergoing renal transplantation. Hyperkalemia has been reported after release of the vascular clamp following completion of the arterial anastomosis, especially in small and pediatric patients. Release of potassium contained in the preservative solution has been implicated in those cases.

Urologic procedures account for 10–20% of most anesthetic practices. Patients undergoing genitourinary procedures may be of any age, but most are elderly and many have coexisting medical illnesses, especially renal dysfunction. Anesthetic management of patients with renal impairment is discussed in Chapter 32, and the effects of anesthesia on renal function are discussed in Chapter 31. This chapter reviews the anesthetic management of common urologic procedures. Use of the lithotomy position, the transurethral approach, and extracorporeal shock waves (lithotripsy) complicates many of these procedures. Moreover, advances in surgical technique allow more patients to undergo radical procedures for urologic cancer, urinary diversion with bladder reconstruction, and renal transplantation.

CYSTOSCOPY

Preoperative Considerations

Cystoscopy is the most commonly performed urologic procedure. Indications for cystoscopy include hematuria, recurrent urinary infections, and urinary obstruction. Bladder biopsies, extraction or laser lithotripsy of renal stones, and placement or manipulation of ureteral catheters (stents) can also be performed through the cystoscope.

Anesthetic management varies with the age and gender of the patient and the purpose of the procedure. General anesthesia is necessary for children. Topical anesthesia in the form of viscous lidocaine with or without sedation is used for diagnostic studies in most women, because of a short urethra. Operative cystoscopies involving biopsies, cauterization, or manipulation of ureteral catheters require regional or general anesthesia. Most males prefer regional or general anesthesia even for diagnostic studies.

Intraoperative Considerations

A. LITHOTOMY POSITION:

 Next to the supine position, this is the most commonly used position for patients undergoing urologic and gynecologic procedures. Failure to properly position patients can result in iatrogenic injuries. Two persons are required to safely move the patient's legs simultaneously up or down. Straps around the ankles or special holders support the legs in position (Figure 33–1). The leg supports should be padded, and the legs should hang freely. Caution should be exercised to prevent the fingers from being caught between the mid and lower sections of the operating room table when the lower section is lowered and raised. Injury to the common peroneal nerve, resulting in loss of dorsiflexion of the

foot, may result if the lateral thigh rests on the strap support. If the legs are allowed to rest on medially placed strap supports, compression of the saphenous nerve can result in numbness along the medial calf. Excessive flexion of the thigh against the groin can injure the obturator and, less commonly, the femoral nerves. Extreme flexion at the thigh can also stretch the sciatic nerve. It should be noted that the most common nerve injury associated with lithotomy position is to the brachial plexus (see Chapter 47). A compartment syndrome of the lower extremities with rhabdomyolysis has been reported with prolonged lithotomy position.

 The lithotomy position is associated with major physiologic alterations. Functional residual capacity decreases, predisposing patients to atelectasis and hypoxia. This effect is accentuated by the head-down (Trendelenburg) position (> 30°). Elevation of the legs increases venous return acutely and may exacerbate congestive heart failure. Mean blood pressure often increases but cardiac output does not change significantly. Conversely, rapid lowering of the legs acutely decreases venous return and can result in hypotension. Vasodilation from either general or regional anesthesia accentuates the hypotension. For this reason, blood pressure measurements should always be taken immediately after the legs are lowered.

The Trendelenburg may also be used with lithotomy position.

B. CHOICE OF ANESTHESIA:

 1. General anesthesia—Because of the short duration (15–20 minutes) and the outpatient setting of most cystoscopies, general anesthesia is usually used. Most patients are apprehensive about the procedure and prefer to be asleep. Any anesthetic technique suitable for outpatients may be used (see Chapter 46). Oxygen saturation should be closely monitored when obese or elderly patients or those with marginal pulmonary reserve are placed in the lithotomy or Trendelenburg position. A laryngeal mask airway (LMA) is often used.

 2. Regional anesthesia—Both epidural and spinal blocks can provide satisfactory anesthesia. However, satisfactory sensory blockade may require 15–20 minutes for epidural anesthesia compared with 5 minutes for spinal anesthesia. Consequently, most clinicians prefer spinal anesthesia, especially for procedures lasting more than 30 minutes with elderly and high-risk patients. Some clinicians feel that the sensory level following injection of a hyperbaric anesthetic solution should be well established ("fixed") before the patient is moved into the lithotomy position; however, studies fail to demonstrate that im-

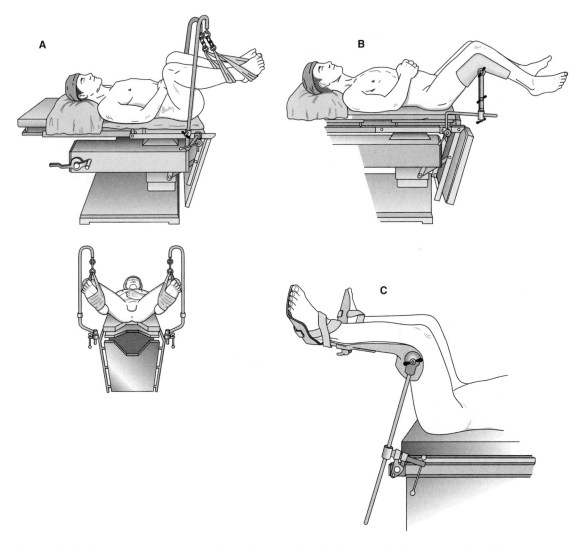

Figure 33–1. The lithotomy position. ***A:*** Strap stirrups. ***B:*** Bier-Hoff stirrups. ***C:*** Allen stirrups. (Modified and reproduced with permission, from Martin JT: *Positioning in Anesthesia.* WB Saunders and Company, 1988.)

mediate elevation of the legs following intrathecal injection increases the level of anesthesia or increases the likelihood of severe hypotension. A sensory level to T10 provides excellent anesthesia for nearly all cystoscopic procedures. Regional anesthesia, however, does not abolish the **obturator reflex** (external rotation and adduction of the thigh secondary to stimulation of the obturator nerve by electrocautery current through the lateral bladder wall). The reflex (muscle contraction) is reliably blocked only by muscle paralysis during general anesthesia.

TRANSURETHRAL RESECTION OF THE PROSTATE

Preoperative Considerations

Benign prostatic hypertrophy frequently leads to symptomatic bladder outlet obstruction in men older than 60 years. Because conservative treatment is often unsuccessful, most patients eventually ask for surgical relief. One of four operations may be selected to remove the hypertrophied and hyperplastic prostatic tissue: suprapubic (transvesical) prostatectomy, perineal prostatectomy, retropubic prostatectomy, or **transurethral resection of the prostate (TURP)**. With the possible exception of the suprapubic approach, morbidity and mortality rates are generally comparable. Nonetheless, the transurethral approach is nearly always selected for patients with prostate glands weighing less than 40–50 g. An alternative approach is chosen if the prostate is over 80 g. Patients with advanced prostatic carcinoma may also present for transurethral resections to relieve symptomatic urinary obstruction. Regardless of its cause, long-standing obstruction can lead to impaired renal function.

Patients undergoing TURP should be carefully evaluated for coexistent cardiac and pulmonary disease as well as renal dysfunction (see Chapters 20, 23, and 32). These patients have a relatively high (30–60%) prevalence of both cardiovascular and pulmonary disorders. The procedure is reported to carry a 0.2–6% mortality rate. Common causes of death include myocardial infarction, pulmonary edema, and renal failure.

Although a type and screen (see Chapter 29) is adequate for most patients, blood should be available and crossmatched for anemic patients as well as patients with large glands (> 40 g). Prostatic bleeding can be difficult to control through the cystoscope.

Intraoperative Considerations

The procedure is performed by passing a loop through a special cystoscope (resectoscope). Using continuous irrigation and direct visualization, prostatic tissue is resected by applying a cutting current to the loop. Because of the characteristics of the prostate and the large amounts of irrigation fluid often used, TURP can be associated with a number of serious complications (Table 33–1).

A. TURP SYNDROME: Transurethral prostatic resection often opens the extensive network of venous sinuses in the prostate and potentially allows systemic absorption of the irrigating fluid. The absorption of large amounts of fluid (2 L or more) results in a constellation of symptoms and signs commonly referred to as the TURP syndrome (Table 33–2). This syndrome presents intraoperatively or postoperatively as headache, restlessness, confusion, cyanosis, dyspnea, arrhythmias, hypotension, or seizures. Moreover, it can be rapidly fatal. The manifestations are primarily those of circulatory fluid overload, water intoxication, and occasionally, toxicity from the solute in the irrigating fluid.

Electrolyte solutions cannot be used for irrigation during TURP because they disperse the electrocautery current. Water provides excellent visibility because its hypotonicity lyses red blood cells, but significant absorption can readily result in acute water intoxication. Water irrigation is generally restricted to transurethral resection of bladder tumors only. For TURP, slightly hypotonic nonelectrolyte irrigating solutions such as glycine 1.5% (230 mOsm/L) or a mixture of sorbitol 2.7% and mannitol 0.54% (195 mOsm/L) are most commonly used. Less commonly used solutions include sorbitol 3.3%, mannitol 3%, dextrose 2.5–4%, and urea 1%. Because all these fluids are still hypotonic, significant absorption of water can nevertheless occur. Solute absorption can also occur because the irrigation fluid is under pressure. High irrigation pressures (bottle height) increases fluid absorption.

Absorption of irrigation fluid appears to be dependent on the duration of the resection as well as the height (pressure) of the irrigation fluid. Most resections last 45–60 minutes, and on the average 20 mL/min of the irrigating fluid is absorbed. Pulmonary congestion or florid pulmonary edema can readily result from the absorption of large amounts of irrigation fluid, especially in patients with limited cardiac reserve. The hypotonicity of these fluids also results in acute hyponatremia and hypo-osmolality, which can lead to serious neurologic manifestations (see Chapter 28). Symptoms of hyponatremia usually do not develop until the serum sodium concentration decreases below 120 mEq/L. Marked hypotonicity in

Table 33–1. Major complications associated with TURP.

Hemorrhage
TURP syndrome
Bladder perforation
Hypothermia
Septicemia
Disseminated intravascular coagulation

33–2. Manifestations of the TURP syndrome.

Hyponatremia
Hypo-osmolality
Fluid overload
Congestive heart failure
Pulmonary edema
Hypotension
Hemolysis
Solute toxicity
Hyperglycinemia (glycine)
Hyperammonemia (glycine)
Hyperglycemia (sorbitol)
Intravascular volume expansion (mannitol)

plasma ([Na⁺] < 100 mEq/L) may also result in acute intravascular hemolysis (see Chapter 29).

Toxicity may also arise from absorption of the solutes in these fluids. Marked **hyperglycinemia** has been reported with glycine solutions and is thought to contribute to circulatory depression and central nervous system toxicity. Plasma glycine concentrations in excess of 1000 mg/L have been recorded (normal is 13–17 mg/L). Glycine is known to be an inhibitory neurotransmitter in the central nervous system and has also been implicated in rare instances of transient blindness following TURP. Hyperammonemia, presumably from the degradation of glycine, has also been documented in a few patients with marked central nervous system toxicity following TURP. Blood ammonia levels in some patients exceeded 500 μmol/L (normal: 5–50 μmol/L). The use of large amounts of sorbitol or dextrose irrigating solutions can lead to hyperglycemia, which can be marked in diabetic patients. Absorption of mannitol solutions causes intravascular volume expansion and exacerbates fluid overload.

Treatment of TURP syndrome depends on early recognition and should be based on the severity of symptoms. The absorbed water must be eliminated, and hypoxemia and hypoperfusion must be avoided. Most patients can be managed with fluid restriction and a loop diuretic. Symptomatic hyponatremia resulting in seizures or coma should be treated with hypertonic saline (see Chapter 28). Seizure activity can be terminated with small doses of midazolam (2–4 mg), diazepam (3–5 mg), or thiopental (50–100 mg). Phenytoin, 10–20 mg/kg intravenously (no faster than 50 mg/min), should also be considered to provide more sustained anticonvulsant activity. Endotracheal intubation is generally advisable to prevent aspiration until the patient's mental status normalizes. The amount and rate of hypertonic saline solution (3% or 5%) to correct the hyponatremia to a safe level should be based on the patient's serum sodium concentration (see Chapter 28). Hypertonic saline solution should not be given at a rate faster than 100 mL/hour so as not to exacerbate circulatory fluid overload.

B. Hypothermia:

Large volumes of irrigating fluids at room temperature can be a major source of heat loss in patients. Irrigating solutions should be warmed to body temperature prior to use to prevent hypothermia. Postoperative shivering associated with hypothermia is especially undesirable, since it can dislodge clots and promote postoperative bleeding.

C. Bladder Perforation:

The incidence of **bladder perforation** during TURP is estimated to be approximately 1%. Perforation may re- sult from the resectoscope going through the bladder wall or from overdistention of the bladder with irrigation fluid. Most bladder perforations are extraperitoneal and are signaled by poor return of the irrigating fluid. Awake patients will typically complain of nausea, diaphoresis, and retropubic or lower abdominal pain. Large extraperitoneal and most intraperitoneal perforations are usually even more obvious, presenting as sudden unexplained hypotension (or hypertension) with generalized abdominal pain (in awake patients). Regardless of the anesthetic technique employed, perforation should be suspected in settings of sudden hypotension or hypertension, especially with bradycardia (vagally mediated).

D. Coagulopathy:

Disseminated intravascular coagulation (DIC) has on rare occasions been reported following TURP and is thought to result from the release of thromboplastins from the prostate into the circulation during surgery. Up to 6% of patients may have evidence of subclinical DIC. A dilutional thrombocytopenia can also develop during surgery as part of the TURP syndrome from absorption of irrigation fluids. Rarely, patients with metastatic carcinoma of the prostate develop a coagulopathy from primary fibrinolysis; the tumor is thought to secrete a fibrinolytic enzyme in such instances. The diagnosis of coagulopathy may be suspected from diffuse uncontrollable bleeding but must be confirmed by laboratory tests (see Case Discussion, Chapter 34). Primary fibrinolysis should be treated with ε-aminocaproic acid (Amicar) 5 g followed by 1 g/hour intravenously. The treatment of DIC in this setting may require heparin in addition to replacement of clotting factors and platelets. Consultation with a hematologist is advisable.

E. Septicemia:

The prostate is often colonized with bacteria and may harbor chronic infection. Extensive surgical manipulation of the gland together with the opening of venous sinuses can allow entry of organisms into the bloodstream. Bacteremia following transurethral surgery is not uncommon and can lead to septicemia or septic shock (see Chapter 50). Prophylactic antibiotic therapy (most commonly gentamicin or cephazolin) prior to TURP may decrease the likelihood of bacteremic and septic episodes.

F. Choice of Anesthesia:

Either spinal or epidural anesthesia with a T10 sensory level provides excellent anesthesia and good operating conditions for TURP. When compared with general anesthesia, regional anesthesia appears to reduce the incidence of postoperative venous thrombosis; it is also less likely to mask symptoms and signs of the TURP syndrome or bladder perforation. Clinical studies have failed to show any differences in blood loss, postoperative cognitive function, and mortality between regional and general anesthesia. The possibility of vertebral metastasis must be considered in patients with carcinoma, especially those with back pain. Metastatic disease to the lumbar spine is a contraindication to regional anesthesia. Acute hyponatremia from the TURP syndrome may delay or prevent emergence from general anesthesia.

G. MONITORING:

Evaluation of mental status in the awake patient is the best monitor for detection of early signs of the TURP syndrome and bladder perforation. A decrease in arterial oxygen saturation may be an early sign of fluid overload. Some studies have reported perioperative ischemic electrocardiographic changes in up to 18% of patients. Temperature monitoring should be used during long resections to detect hypothermia. Blood loss is especially difficult to assess because of the use of irrigating solutions, so clinical signs of hypovolemia must be relied upon (see Chapter 29). Blood loss averages about 3–5 mL/min of resection (usually 200–300 mL total) but rarely can be life-threatening. Transient, postoperative decreases in hematocrit may simply reflect hemodilution from absorption of irrigation fluid. About 2.5% of patients require intraoperative transfusion; factors associated with transfusion include duration of longer than 90 minutes and resection of greater than 45 g of prostate tissue.

EXTRACORPOREAL SHOCK WAVE LITHOTRIPSY

Extracorporeal shock wave lithotripsy is employed for disintegration of calculi in the kidneys or the upper two-thirds of the ureters (above the iliac crest). One of several techniques may be used to focus high-energy shock waves at the renal calculus. With high-energy units (Dornier HM3), the patient is placed in a hydraulic chair, immersed in a heated water bath, and positioned with the aid of two image intensifiers such that the stone is in the second focus of an elliptical reflector, while the source of the shock waves is in the first focus (Figure 33–2). Lower energy units (eg, Siemens Lithostar) require only a small amount of mineral oil on the skin to acoustically couple the patient to the energy source. The latter is enclosed in a water-filled casing and comes in contact with the patient via a plastic membrane.

Shock waves may be generated by discharging an underwater capacitor beneath the patient in the first focus of the elliptical reflector. Lower energy units gen-

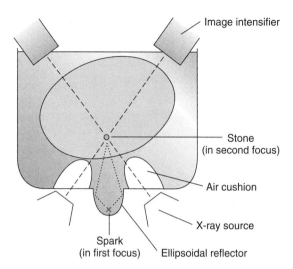

Figure 33–2. Schematic representation of a lithotripsy unit.

erate shock waves electromagnetically or from piezoelectric crystals. Because tissue has the same acoustic density as water, the waves travel through the body without damaging tissue. However, the change in acoustic impedance at the tissue-stone interface creates shear and tear forces on the stone. The stone is fragmented enough by the waves to allow its passage down the urinary tract. Ureteral stents are often placed cystoscopically prior to the procedure to facilitate the passage of large particles of stone. Tissue destruction can occur if the waves are focused at air-tissue interfaces such as in the lung and intestine. Inability to position the patient so that lung and intestine are away from the wave focus is a contraindication to the procedure. Other contraindications include urinary obstruction below the stone, untreated infection, a bleeding diathesis, and pregnancy. The presence of a nearby aortic aneurysm or orthopedic prosthetic device is considered a relative contraindication in some centers. Ecchymosis, bruising or blistering of the skin over the treatment site is not uncommon. Rarely, a large perinephric hematoma can develop and may be responsible for a significant decrease in hematocrit postoperatively.

Preoperative Considerations

Patients with a history of cardiac arrhythmias and those with a pacemaker or automatic internal cardiac defibrillator (AICD) may be at risk for developing arrhythmias induced by shock waves during ESWL. Shock waves can damage the internal components of pacemaker and AICD devices. The manufacturer should be contacted as to the best method for managing the device (eg, reprogramming or applying a magnet). Synchronization of the shock waves to the R wave from the electrocardiogram (ECG) decreases the incidence of arrhythmias during ESWL. The shock waves are usually timed to be 20 ms after the R wave to correspond to the ventricular refractory period (see Chapter 19). Studies suggest that asynchronous delivery of shocks can be safe in patients without heart disease.

Intraoperative Considerations

A. EFFECTS OF IMMERSION:

Immersion into a heated water bath (36–37 °C) initially results in vasodilation that can transiently lead to hypotension. Arterial blood pressure, however, subsequently rises as venous blood is redistributed centrally from the hydrostatic pressure of water on the legs and abdomen. Systemic vascular resistance (SVR) rises and cardiac output often decreases. The sudden increase in venous return and SVR can precipitate congestive heart failure in patients with marginal cardiac reserve. Moreover, the increase in intrathoracic blood volume significantly reduces functional residual capacity (30–60%) and predisposes some patients to hypoxemia.

B. CHOICE OF ANESTHESIA:

Pain during lithotripsy is from dissipation of a small amount of energy as shock waves enter the body through the skin. The pain is therefore localized to the skin and proportionate to the intensity of the shock waves. Lithotripsy with units employing a water bath (Dornier HM3) requires 1000–2400 relatively high-intensity shock waves (18–22 kV) that most patients do not tolerate without either regional or general anesthesia. In contrast, lithotripsy with units that are coupled directly to the skin utilizes 2000–3000 lower-intensity shock waves (10–18 kV) that usually require only light sedation.

C. REGIONAL ANESTHESIA:

Continuous epidural anesthesia is commonly used for ESWL using a water bath. A T6 sensory level assures adequate anesthesia, as renal innervation is derived from T10 to L2. Supplementation of the block with fentanyl, 50–100 mg epidurally, is often useful. As little air as possible should be used with the loss of resistance technique during insertion (see Chapter 16); large amounts of air in the epidural space can dissipate shock waves and theoretically may promote injury to neural tissue. Foam tape should not be used to secure the epidural catheter as this type of tape has been shown to dissipate the energy of the shocks when it is in their path. Light sedation is also generally desirable for most patients. Supplemental oxygen by face mask or nasal cannula is also useful in avoiding hypoxemia. Spinal anesthesia can also be used satisfactorily, but because of the potential for an increased incidence of post-dural puncture headache in a seated patient and less control over the sensory level with spinal anesthesia, epidural anesthesia is usually preferred. Regional anesthesia greatly facilitates positioning and monitoring. Prior intravascular volume expansion with 1000–1500 mL of lactated Ringer's injection may help prevent severe postural hypotension following the onset of neuraxial anesthesia, positioning in the hydraulic chair, and immersion in the warm bath.

A major disadvantage of regional anesthesia is the inability to control diaphragmatic movement. Excessive diaphragmatic excursion during spontaneous ventilation can move the stone in and out of the wave focus and may prolong the procedure. This problem can be partially solved by asking the patient to breathe in a more rapid but shallow respiratory pattern. Bradycardia from high sympathetic blockade also prolongs the procedure when shock waves are coupled to the ECG.

D. GENERAL ANESTHESIA:

General endotracheal anesthesia allows control of diaphragmatic excursion and is preferred by many patients. The procedure is complicated by the inherent risks associated with placing a supine anesthetized patient in a chair, elevating and then lowering the chair into a water bath to shoulder depth, and then reversing the sequence at the end. A light general anesthetic technique in conjunction with a muscle relaxant is preferable. The muscle relaxant ensures patient immobility and control of diaphragmatic movement. High-frequency jet ventilation during ESWL may be used to reduce diaphragmatic excursions to a minimum, but studies have failed to substantiate a decrease in the number of shocks required or in radiation exposure from fluoroscopy. As with regional anesthesia, intravenous fluid loading with 1000 mL of lactated Ringer's injection is generally advisable prior to moving patients upright into the hydraulic chair to prevent postural hypotension.

E. MONITORED ANESTHESIA CARE:

Intravenous sedation is usually adequate for low-energy lithotripsy. Low-dose propofol infusions together with midazolam and opioid supplementation are commonly used.

F. MONITORING:

Electrocardiograph pads should be attached securely with water-proof dressing prior to immersion. Even with R wave-triggered shocks, supraventricular arrhythmias can still occur and may require treatment.

Changes in functional residual capacity with immersion, mandate close monitoring of oxygen saturation, especially in patients at high risk for developing hypoxemia (see Chapter 22). The temperature of the bath and the patient should be monitored to prevent hypothermia or hyperthermia.

G. FLUID MANAGEMENT:

Intravenous fluid therapy is typically generous. Following the initial intravenous fluid bolus (above), an additional 1000–2000 mL of lactated Ringer's injection is usually given with a small dose of furosemide (10–20 mg) to maintain brisk urinary flow and flush stone debris and blood clots. Patients with poor cardiac reserve require more conservative fluid therapy.

NONCANCER SURGERY ON THE UPPER URETER AND KIDNEY

Open procedures for kidney stones in the upper ureter and renal pelvis, and nephrectomies for nonmalignant disease are often carried out in the "**kidney rest position**," also more accurately described as the **lateral flexed position.** With the patient in a full lateral position, the dependent leg is flexed and the other leg is extended. An axillary roll is placed underneath the dependent upper chest to prevent injury to the brachial plexus. The operating table is then extended to achieve maximal separation between the iliac crest and the costal margin on the operative side, and the kidney rest (a bar in the groove where the table bends) is elevated to raise the nondependent iliac crest higher and increase surgical exposure.

The lateral flexed position is associated with significant adverse respiratory and circulatory effects. Functional residual capacity is reduced in the dependent lung but may increase in the nondependent lung. In the anesthetized patient receiving controlled ventilation, ventilation/perfusion mismatching occurs because the dependent lung receives greater blood flow than the nondependent lung, whereas the nondependent lung receives greater ventilation, predisposing the patient to atelectasis in the dependent lung and hypoxemia. The arterial to end-tidal gradient for carbon dioxide progressively increases during general anesthesia in this position, indicating that dead space ventilation also increases in the nondependent lung. Moreover, elevation of the kidney rest can significantly decrease venous return to heart in some patients by compressing the inferior vena cava. Venous pooling in the legs decreases venous return and aggravates any anesthesia-induced vasodilation.

Because of the potential for large blood loss and limited access to major vascular structures in the lateral flexed position, a large-bore intravenous catheter is advisable. Inadvertent entry into the pleural space can produce a pneumothorax. Diagnosis requires a high index of suspicion. The pneumothorax may be subclinical intraoperatively but can be diagnosed postoperatively with a chest radiograph.

RADICAL SURGERY FOR UROLOGIC MALIGNANCIES

Demographic changes resulting in an increasingly elderly population together with improved survival rates for patients with urologic cancer following radical surgical resections have resulted in an increase in the number of procedures performed for prostatic, bladder, testicular, and renal cancer. Curative and palliative surgery plays an important role in treatment of these malignancies.

Many of these procedures are carried out in a **hyperextended supine position** to facilitate exposure of the pelvis during pelvic lymph node dissection, retropubic prostatectomy, or cystectomy (Figure 33–3). The patient is positioned supine with the iliac crest over the break in the operating table, and the table is extended such that distance between the iliac crest and the costal margin increases maximally. Care must be taken not to put excessive strain on the patient's back. The operating room table is also tilted head-down to make the operative field horizontal. The frog-leg position is a variation of this position where the knees are also flexed and the hips are abducted and externally rotated. For thoracoabdominal surgery, the patient is placed in hyperextended supine position close to the edge of the table on the operative side; the leg on the nonoperative is flexed 30-degrees while the knee is flexed 90-degrees, and the leg on the operative side remains straight (Figure 33–4). The shoulder on the ipsilateral side is elevated 30 degrees with a roll to allow that arm to come across the chest into an adjustable arm rest ("airplane"), while the other arm is extended on an arm board. Although the adverse effects of the hyperextended supine position have not been studied, its physiologic consequences appear to be similar to the Trendelenburg position. The potential for neurologic injuries and back injury exists because of the complex nature of the position. Careful positioning and generous padding of the arms and legs are therefore warranted. Positioning the pelvis above the heart may predispose patients to venous air embolism; however, this appears to be a rare complication.

1. Prostate Cancer

Preoperative Considerations

Adenocarcinoma of the prostate is the most common cancer in men. It is the second most common cause of

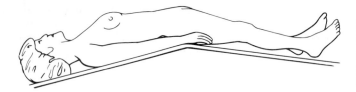

Figure 33–3. The hyperextended position. (Modified and reproduced, with permission, from Skinner DG, Lieskovsky G: *Diagnosis and Management of Genitourinary Cancer.* WB Saunders and Company, 1988.)

cancer deaths in men older than 55 years. The incidence of prostate cancer increases with age and is estimated to be 75% in patients over 75. Because of the tumor's wide spectrum of clinical behavior, management varies widely from surveillance to aggressive surgical therapy. Important variables include the grade and stage of the malignancy, patient age, and the presence of other medical illnesses. Transrectal ultrasound is used to evaluate tumor size and presence or absence of extracapsular extension. Clinical staging is also based on the Gleason score of the biopsy, computed tomography (CT) scan or magnetic resonance imaging (MRI), and bone scan.

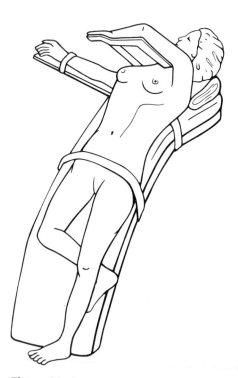

Figure 33–4. The thoracoabdominal incision. (Modified and reproduced, with permission, from Skinner DG, Lieskovsky G: *Diagnosis and Management of Genitourinary Cancer.* WB Saunders and Company, 1988.)

Intraoperative Considerations

Patients with prostate cancer may present to the operating room for a staging pelvic lymph node dissection, radical prostatectomy, salvage prostatectomy (following failure of radiation therapy), or bilateral orchiectomy for hormonal therapy.

A. PELVIC LYMPH NODE DISSECTION:

Although many urologists feel that the combination of the preoperative prostate-specific antigen (PSA) level together with the Gleason score of the biopsy provides sufficient information in the majority of patients to avoid the need for a staging lymph node dissection, laparoscopic pelvic lymph node dissection (LPLND) may be used in some centers to stage prostate cancer. LPLND differs from most other laparoscopic procedures in several aspects: (1) the use of steep Trendelenburg position and rotation from side to side for surgical exposure, (2) the potential for greater carbon dioxide absorption from the retroperitoneum, and (3) the potential for hypothermia from the copious fluid used to irrigate clots from the pelvic fossa. The procedure is carried out under general endotracheal anesthesia because of the length of the procedure, steep Trendelenburg position, necessity for abdominal distention, and desirability of being able to increase the patient's minute ventilation. Most clinicians avoid nitrous oxide to prevent bowel distention and expansion of residual intra-abdominal gas.

B. RADICAL RETROPUBIC PROSTATECTOMY:

Radical retropubic prostatectomy is usually performed together with a pelvic lymph node dissection through a lower, midline, abdominal position. It may be curative for localized prostatic cancer or occasionally used as a salvage procedure after failure of radiation. The prostate is removed en bloc with the seminal vesicles, ejaculatory ducts, and part of the bladder neck. A "nerve-sparing" technique may be used to help preserve sexual function. Following the prostatectomy, the remaining bladder neck is anastomosed directly to the urethra over an indwelling urinary catheter. The surgeon may ask for intravenous administration of indigo carmine for visualization of the ureters. This dye can be associated with hypertension or hypotension.

Radical retropubic prostatectomy is often associated with significant operative blood loss. Direct arterial pressure monitoring is generally advisable and allows controlled hypotension (see Chapter 13). Some authors also advocate routine use of central venous pressure monitoring. Blood loss appears to vary considerably from center to center; values less than 500 mL are not uncommon, but some institutions report average blood losses in excess of 1500 mL. Factors that may affect blood loss include positioning, pelvic anatomy, and size of the prostate; early ligation of the dorsal vein complex of the penis and temporary clamping of the hypogastric artery appear to reduce blood loss. Blood loss is similar in patients receiving general anesthesia and those having regional anesthesia; operative morbidity and mortality also appears to be similar. Neuraxial anesthesia requires a T6 sensory level but awake patients typically do not tolerate regional anesthesia without heavy sedation because of the hyperextended supine position. Moreover, the combination of prolonged Trendelenburg together with administration of large amounts of intravenous fluids can produce edema of the upper airway.

Clinical studies have found no differences in pain relief or recovery between patients receiving epidural opioids and intravenous patient-controlled analgesia. Ketorolac can be used as an analgesic adjuvant and has been reported to decrease opioid requirements, improve analgesia, and promote earlier return of bowel function without increasing transfusion requirements. Extensive surgical dissection around the pelvic veins increases the risk of thromboembolic complications. Although epidural anesthesia appears to reduce the incidence of postoperative deep venous thrombosis following prostatectomy, this beneficial effect may be negated by the routine use of warfarin or low molecular weight heparin prophylaxis postoperatively. Moreover, postoperative anticoagulation increases the risk of epidural hematoma. Prophylactic mini-dose unfractionated heparin has been reported to increase operative loss and transfusion requirements, while sequential pneumatic (leg) compression devices appear to delay but not reduce deep venous thrombosis. Other postoperative complications include hemorrhage; injuries to the obturator nerve, ureter, and rectum; as well as urinary incontinence and impotence.

C. Radical Perineal Prostatectomy:

Anesthetic management is complicated by the extreme (exaggerated) lithotomy position. Careful positioning can help reduce the likelihood of musculoskeletal or neurologic injuries. Patients typically require general endotracheal anesthesia because of this position, which is uncomfortable and interferes with diaphragmatic excursion. The procedure can be associated with considerable blood loss (> 2 L). Two large-bore intravenous

catheters and direct arterial pressure monitoring are generally indicated.

D. Bilateral Orchiectomy:

Bilateral orchiectomy is usually performed for local control of metastatic adenocarcinoma of the prostate. The procedure is relatively short (20–45 minutes) and performed through a single midline scrotal incision. Although bilateral orchiectomy can be performed under local anesthesia, most patients and many clinicians prefer general anesthesia, which is usually administered with an LMA.

2. Bladder Cancer

Preoperative Considerations

The bladder cancer incidence occurs at an average age of 65 years with a 3:1 male to female ratio. Transitional cell carcinoma of the bladder is the second most common malignancy of the genitourinary tract. The association of cigarette smoking with bladder carcinoma results in coexistent coronary artery and chronic obstructive pulmonary disease in many of these patients. Moreover, underlying renal impairment may be age-related or secondary to urinary tract obstruction. Staging includes cystoscopy and CT or MRI scans. Intravesical chemotherapy is used for superficial tumors, while transurethral resection is carried out for low-grade noninvasive bladder tumors. Some patients may receive preoperative radiation to shrink the tumor before radical cystectomy. Urinary diversion is usually performed immediately following the cystectomy.

Intraoperative Considerations

A. Radical Cystectomy:

Radical cystectomy is a major operation that is often associated with significant blood loss. It is usually performed through a midline incision that extends from the pubis to xiphoid process. All anterior pelvic organs including the bladder, prostate, and seminal vesicles are removed in males, while the uterus, cervix, ovaries, and part of the anterior vaginal vault may also be taken in females. Pelvic node dissection and urinary diversion are also carried out.

These procedures typically require 4–6 hours and frequently necessitate blood transfusion. General endotracheal anesthesia with a muscle relaxant provides optimal operating conditions. Controlled hypotensive anesthesia may reduce intraoperative blood loss and transfusion requirements. Many surgeons also feel controlled hypotension improves surgical visualization. Supplementation of general anesthesia with spinal or continuous epidural anesthesia can facilitate the induced hypotension, decreases general anesthetic requirements, and can provide a highly effective postoperative analgesia. A major drawback in the use of neuraxial anesthesia is the hyperperistalsis that produces a very small contracted bowel, which complicates construction of a urinary reservoir.

Close monitoring of blood pressure, intravascular volume, and blood loss is essential. Direct intra-arterial pressure monitoring is indicated in all patients, while central venous pressure monitoring is advisable in patients with limited cardiac reserve, while pulmonary artery pressure monitoring is indicated for those with a history of ventricular dysfunction. Urinary output should be monitored continuously and correlated with the progress of the operation, as the urinary path is interrupted at an early point during most of these procedures. An upper body forced-air warming blanket is essential in preventing hypothermia.

B. URINARY DIVERSION:

Urinary diversion is usually performed immediately following radical cystectomy. Many procedures are currently used, but all entail implanting the ureters into a segment of bowel. The selected bowel segment is either left in situ, such as in ureterosigmoidostomy or divided with its mesenteric blood supply intact and attached to a cutaneous stoma or urethra. Moreover, the isolated bowel can function either as a conduit (eg, ileal conduit) or be reconstructed to form a continent reservoir. Conduits may be formed from ileum, jejunum, or colon. Continent urinary diversions include ureterosigmoidostomy, and small bowel (Kock, Camey), and large bowel (Indiana).

Major anesthetic goals include keeping the patient well hydrated and maintaining a brisk urinary output once the ureters are opened. Central venous pressure monitoring is often employed to guide intravenous fluid administration. Neuraxial anesthesia often produces unopposed parasympathetic activity due to sympathetic blockade that results in a very contracted, hyperactive bowel that makes construction of a continent ileal reservoir technically difficult. Papaverine (100–150 mg as a slow intravenous infusion over 2–3 hours), large dose of an anticholinergic (glycopyrrolate, 1 mg), or glucagon (1 mg) may alleviate this problem.

Prolonged contact of urine with bowel mucosa (slow urine flow) may produce significant metabolic disturbances. Hyponatremia, hypochloremia, hyperkalemia, and metabolic acidosis can occur following jejunal conduits. In contrast, colonic and ileal conduits may be associated with hyperchloremic metabolic acidosis. The use of temporary ureteral stents and maintenance of high urinary flow help alleviate this problem in the early postoperative period.

3. Testicular Cancer

Preoperative Considerations

Testicular tumors are classified either as seminomas or nonseminomas. The initial treatment for all tumors is radical (inguinal) orchiectomy. Subsequent management depends on tumor histology. Nonseminomas include embryonal teratoma, choriocarcinoma, and mixed tumors. Retroperitoneal lymph node dissection (RPLND) plays a major role in the treatment of patients with nonseminomatous germ cell tumors. Low-stage disease is managed with RPLND or in some instances surveillance. High-stage disease is usually treated with chemotherapy followed by RPLND.

In contrast to nonseminomas, seminomas are very radiosensitive tumors that are primarily treated with retroperitoneal radiotherapy. Chemotherapy is used for patients who relapse after radiation. Patients with large bulky seminomas or those with increased α-fetoprotein levels (usually associated with nonseminomas) are treated primarily with chemotherapy. Chemotherapeutic agents commonly include cisplatin, vincristine, vinblastine, cyclophosphamide, dactinomycin, bleomycin, and etoposide. RPLND is usually undertaken for patients with residual tumor after chemotherapy.

Patients undergoing RPLND for testicular cancer are typically young (15–35 years old) but are at increased risk for morbidity from the residual effects of preoperative chemotherapy. In addition to bone marrow suppression, specific organ toxicity may be encountered such as renal impairment following cisplatin, pulmonary fibrosis following bleomycin, and neuropathy following vincristine.

Intraoperative Considerations

A. RADICAL ORCHIECTOMY:

Inguinal orchiectomy can be carried out with regional or general anesthesia; most patients prefer the latter. Anesthetic management may be complicated by reflex bradycardia from traction on the spermatic cord.

B. RETROPERITONEAL LYMPH NODE DISSECTION:

The retroperitoneum is usually accessed through a large thoracoabdominal incision that extends from the posterior axillary line over the eighth to tenth ribs to a paramedian line halfway between the xiphoid and the umbilicus (Figure 33–4). Alternatively, some surgeons use a transabdominal approach through a midline incision from the xiphoid to the pubis. All lymphatic tissue between the ureters from the renal vessels to the iliac bifurcation is removed. With the standard RPLND, all sympathetic fibers are disrupted resulting in loss of normal ejaculation and infertility; a modified technique that may preserve fertility limits the dissection below the inferior mesenteric artery to include lymphatic tissue only on the ipsilateral side of the tumor.

Patients receiving bleomycin preoperatively are at increased risk for developing postoperative pulmonary insufficiency. These patients appear to be especially sensitive to oxygen toxicity and fluid overload, and are at increased risk for developing acute respiratory distress syndrome postoperatively. Excessive intravenous fluid administration may also be contributory. Anesthetic management should generally include use of the lowest inspired concentration of oxygen compatible with acceptable oxygen saturation (> 90%). Positive end-expiratory pressure (5–10 cm H$_2$O) may be helpful in optimizing oxygenation. An air-oxygen mixture is generally used because prolonged nitrous oxide administration can produce bone marrow suppression.

Evaporative and redistributive fluid losses ("third spacing") can be considerable as a result of the large wound and the extensive surgical dissection. Fluid replacement should be sufficient to maintain an adequate urinary output (> 0.5 mL/kg/hour); the combined use of both colloid and crystalloid solutions in a ratio of 1:2 or 1:3 may be more effective in preserving urinary output than crystalloid alone. Mannitol (0.25–0.5 g/kg) is usually given prior to dissection near the renal arteries to prevent ischemic renal injury from surgically induced renal vasospasm. Retraction of the inferior vena cava during surgery often results in transient arterial hypotension.

The postoperative pain associated with thoracoabdominal incisions is severe and typically associated with considerable splinting. Aggressive postoperative analgesia is necessary to avoid atelectasis. Continuous epidural analgesia, interpleural analgesia, and intercostal nerve blocks can facilitate management. Because ligation of intercostal arteries during left-sided dissections has resulted in paraplegia—albeit rarely, it may be prudent to document normal motor function postoperatively prior to institution of epidural anesthesia. The arteria radicularis magna (artery of Adamkiewicz), which is supplied by these vessels and is responsible for most of the arterial blood to the lower half of the spinal cord (see Chapters 16 and 21), arises on the left side in most persons. It should be noted that unilateral sympathectomy following modified RPLND usually results in the ipsilateral leg being warmer than the contralateral one.

4. Renal Cancer

Preoperative Considerations

Adenocarcinoma of the kidney (renal cell carcinoma or hypernephroma) is often termed the internist's tumor because of a frequent association with paraneoplastic syndromes, such as erythrocytosis, hypercalcemia, hypertension, and nonmetastatic hepatic dysfunction. The classic triad of hematuria, flank pain, and palpable mass occurs only in 10% patients. Unfortunately, the tumor often causes symptoms only after it has grown considerably in size. It has a peak incidence between the 5th and 6th decades of life with 2:1 male to female ratio. Surgical treatment is undertaken for carcinomas confined to the kidneys. In approximately 5–10% of patients, the tumor extends into the renal vein and inferior vena cava as a thrombus, which does not necessarily preclude surgery. Staging includes CT or MRI scans and an arteriogram. Preoperative arterial embolization may reduce operative blood loss.

Preoperative evaluation should focus on defining the degree of renal impairment as well as searching for the presence of associated systemic diseases. Preexisting renal impairment depends on both tumor size in the affected kidney as well as underlying systemic disorders such as hypertension and diabetes. Smoking is a well established risk factor for renal adenocarcinoma; not surprisingly, patients have a high incidence of underlying coronary artery and chronic obstructive lung disease. Although some patients present with erythrocytosis, the majority of patients are anemic. Preoperative blood transfusion may be advisable to increase hemoglobin concentration > 10 g/dL when a large tumor is to be resected.

Intraoperative Considerations

A. RADICAL NEPHRECTOMY:

The operation may be carried out via an anterior subcostal, flank, midline, or thoracoabdominal incision. Many centers prefer a thoracoabdominal approach for large tumors, especially when a tumor thrombus is present. The kidney, adrenal gland, and perinephric fat are removed en bloc with the surrounding (Gerota's) fascia. General endotracheal anesthesia is used. The operation has the potential for extensive blood loss because these tumors are very vascular and often very large at presentation. Retraction of the inferior vena cava may be associated with transient arterial hypotension. Direct arterial pressure monitoring is indicated in most patients. Central venous cannulation is used for pressure monitoring as well as for rapid transfusion when necessary; pulmonary artery catheterization may be indicated for patients with impaired left ventricular function. Only brief periods of controlled hypotension should be used to reduced blood loss because of its potential to impair renal function. Reflex renal vasoconstriction in the nonaffected kidney can result in postoperative renal dysfunction. A mannitol infusion should be initiated prior to the surgical dissection.

B. RADICAL NEPHRECTOMY WITH EXCISION OF TUMOR THROMBUS:

Some medical centers routinely perform complicated resections of renal cancers with tumor thrombus extending into the inferior vena cava. A thoracoabdominal approach allows the use of cardioplumonary bypass when necessary. The thrombus may extend only into the inferior vena cava but below the liver (level I), up to the liver but below the diaphragm (level II), or above the diaphragm into the right atrium (level III). Surgery can significantly prolong life and improve the quality of life in selected patients, and in some patients, metastases may regress after resection of the primary tumor. A preoperative ventilation to perfusion scan can detect preexisting embolization of the thrombus.

The presence of a large thrombus (level II or III) greatly complicates anesthetic management. Invasive pressure monitoring and multiple large-bore intravenous catheters are necessary because transfusion requirements average 10–15 units of packed red blood cells and may exceed 50 units. Transfusion of platelets, fresh frozen plasma, and cryoprecipitate is usually required. Problems associated with massive blood transfusion should be expected (see Chapter 29). Central venous or pulmonary cannulation should be performed cautiously to prevent dislodgement and embolization of the tumor thrombus. A high central venous pressure is typical and reflects the degree of venous obstruction by the thrombus. The presence of a level III thrombus contraindicates flotation of a pulmonary artery catheter. A low-lying central venous catheter may be equally detrimental, especially on the right side. Intraoperative transesophageal echocardiography is useful in defining the extent of the thrombus and hemodynamic management.

Complete obstruction of the inferior vena cava increases blood loss because it markedly dilates venous collaterals from the lower body that traverse the abdominal wall, retroperitoneum, and the epidural space. Patients are also at significant risk for potentially catastrophic pulmonary embolization of the tumor. Tumor embolization may be heralded by sudden supraventricular arrhythmias, arterial desaturation, and/or profound systemic hypotension. Cardiopulmonary bypass is used when the tumor occupies more than 40% of the right atrium. Hypothermic circulatory arrest has been used in some centers (see Chapter 21). Heparinization and hypothermia greatly increase surgical blood loss.

RENAL TRANSPLANTATION

The success of renal transplantation, which is largely due to advances in immunosuppressive therapy, has greatly improved the quality of life for patients with end-stage renal disease. With modern immunosuppressive regimens, cadaveric transplants have achieved almost the same 3-year graft survival rates (80–90%) as living-related donor grafts. In addition, restrictions on candidates for renal transplantation have gradually decreased. Infection and cancer are the only remaining absolute contraindications. Advanced age (> 60 years) and severe cardiovascular disease are relative contraindications.

Preoperative Considerations

Preoperative optimization of the patient's medical condition with dialysis is mandatory (see Chapter 32). Current organ preservation techniques allow ample time (24–48 hours) for preoperative dialysis of cadaveric recipients. Living-related transplants are performed electively with the donor and recipient anesthetized simultaneously but in separate rooms. The recipient's serum potassium concentration should be below 5.5 mEq/L, and existing coagulopathies should be corrected.

Intraoperative Considerations

The transplant is carried out by placing the donor kidney retroperitoneally in the iliac fossa and anastomosing the renal vessels to the iliac vessels and the ureter to the bladder. Prior to temporary clamping of the iliac vessels, heparin is administered. Injection of a calcium channel blocker (verapamil) into the arterial circulation of the graft just prior to revascularization helps protect the kidney from reperfusion injury. Intravenous mannitol may also act as a radical free scavenger and helps establish an osmotic diuresis after reperfusion. Nephrectomy is performed only in the presence of intractable hypertension or chronic infection. Immunosuppression is started on the day of surgery with combinations of corticosteroids, cyclosporine (or tacrolimus), and azathioprine (or mycophenolate mofetil). Some centers avoid cyclosporine and tacrolimus in the first few days and use instead antithymocyte globulin, monoclonal antibodies directed against specific subsets of T lymphocytes (OKT3), or interleukin-2 receptor antibodies (daclizumab or basiliximab).

A. CHOICE OF ANESTHESIA:

Although both spinal and epidural anesthesia have been successfully employed, most transplants are done under general anesthesia. All general anesthetic agents, including methoxyflurane, enflurane, and sevoflurane have been employed without any apparent detrimental effect on graft function; nonetheless, these three agents are best avoided (see Chapter 32). Atracurium and rocuronium may be the muscle relaxants of choice, since they are not primarily dependent on renal excretion for elimination. Similarly, vecuronium may be used with only modest prolongation of its effects.

B. MONITORING:

Central venous pressure monitoring is very useful in ensuring adequate hydration but avoiding fluid overload. Normal saline or half-normal saline solutions are commonly used. A urinary catheter is placed preoperatively. A brisk urine flow following the arterial anastomosis generally indicates good graft function. The diuresis that follows may resemble nonoliguric renal failure (see Chapter 32). If the graft ischemic time was prolonged, an oliguric phase may precede the diuretic phase, in which case fluid therapy must be adjusted appropriately. The judicious use of furosemide or additional mannitol may be indicated in such cases. Hyperkalemia has been reported after release of the vascular clamp following completion of the arterial anastomosis, especially in small and pediatric patients. Release of potassium contained in the preservative solution has been implicated in those cases. Washout of the preservative solution with ice-cold lactated Ringer's solution just prior to the vascular anastomosis may help avoid this problem. Serum electrolyte concentrations should be monitored closely after completion of the anastomosis. Hyperkalemia may be suspected from peaking of the T wave on the ECG. Most patients can generally be extubated immediately after the procedure.

CASE DISCUSSION: HYPOTENSION IN THE RECOVERY ROOM

A 69-year-old man with a history of an inferior myocardial infarction was admitted to the recovery room following transurethral resection of the prostate (TURP) under general anesthesia. The procedure took 90 minutes and was reported as uncomplicated. On admission, the patient is extubated but still unresponsive, and vital signs are stable. Twenty minutes later, he is noted to be awake but restless. He begins to shiver intensely; his blood pressure decreases to 80/35 mm Hg; and his respirations increase to 40 breaths/min. The bedside monitor shows a sinus tachycardia of 140 beats/min and an oxygen saturation of 92%.

What is the differential diagnosis?

The differential diagnosis of hypotension following TURP should always include the following:

(1) Hemorrhage

(2) TURP syndrome

(3) Bladder perforation

(4) Myocardial infarction or ischemia

(5) Septicemia

(6) Disseminated intravascular coagulation (DIC).

Other possibilities (see Chapter 49) are less likely in this setting but should always be considered, especially when the patient fails to respond to appropriate measures (see below).

Based on the history, what is the most likely diagnosis?

A diagnosis cannot be made with reasonable certainty at this point, and the patient requires further evaluation. Nonetheless, the hypotension and shivering must be treated rapidly because of the history of coronary artery disease. The hypotension seriously compromises coronary perfusion, and the shivering markedly increases myocardial oxygen demand (see Chapter 20).

What diagnostic aids would be helpful?

A quick examination of the patient is extremely useful in narrowing down the possibilities. Hemorrhage from the prostate should be apparent from effluent of the continuous bladder irrigation system placed after the procedure. Relatively little blood in the urine makes it look red; brisk hemorrhage is often apparent as grossly bloody drainage. Occasionally, the drainage may be scant because of clots blocking the drainage catheter; irrigation of the catheter is indicated in such cases.

Clinical signs of peripheral perfusion are invaluable. Hypovolemic patients have decreased peripheral (radial) pulses, and their extremities are usually cool and may be cyanotic. Poor perfusion is consistent with hemorrhage, bladder perforation, DIC, and severe myocardial ischemia or infarction. A full bounding peripheral pulse with warm extremities is suggestive of, but not always present in, septicemia (see Chapter 50). Signs of fluid overload should be searched for, such as jugular venous distention, pulmonary crackles, and an S_3 gallop. Fluid overload is more consistent with TURP syndrome but may also be seen in myocardial infarction or ischemia.

The abdomen should be examined for signs of perforation. A rigid and tender or distended abdomen is very suggestive of perforation and should prompt immediate evaluation for laparotomy. When the abdomen is soft and nontender, perforation can reasonably be excluded.

Further evaluation requires laboratory measurements, an ECG, and a chest radiograph. Blood should be immediately obtained for arterial blood gas analysis and measurements of hematocrit, hemoglobin, electrolytes, glucose, a platelet count, and prothrombin and partial thromboplastin tests. If DIC is suggested by diffuse oozing, fibrinogen and fibrin split product measurements will confirm the diagnosis. A 12-lead ECG should be evaluated for signs of ischemia, electrolyte abnormalities (see Chapter 28), or an evolving myocardial infarction. A chest film should be obtained to search for evidence of pulmonary congestion, aspiration, pneumothorax, or cardiomegaly.

While laboratory measurements are being performed, what therapeutic and diagnostic measures should be undertaken?

Immediate measures aimed at avoiding hypoxemia and hypoperfusion should be instituted. Oxygen supplementation protects against hypoxemia and may increase oxygen delivery to tissues. If hypoventilation or respiratory distress is apparent, endotracheal intubation is indicated. Frequent blood pressure measurements should be obtained. If signs of fluid overload are absent, a diagnostic fluid challenge with 500 mL of crystalloid or 250 mL of colloid is helpful. A favorable response, as indicated by an increase in blood pressure and decrease in heart rate, is suggestive of hypovolemia and an indication for additional fluid boluses. Obvious bleeding in the setting of hypotension necessitates blood transfusion. Absence of a quick response should prompt further evaluation with invasive monitors. Administration of an inotrope, such as dopamine, is appropriate while the evaluation is being completed. Direct intra-arterial pressure measurement is invaluable in this setting. Central venous access should be established to measure central venous pressure and for possible placement of a pulmonary artery catheter. The latter is useful in patients with a history of congestive heart failure and when clinical signs are ambiguous. Cardiac output can then be measured by thermodilution, and pulmonary capillary wedge pressure measurements can be used to guide fluid or vasodilator therapy.

If signs of fluid overload are present, intravenous furosemide in addition to an inotrope is indicated. Further treatment with vasodilator therapy should only be initiated after full hemodynamic monitoring is established.

The patient's axillary temperature is 35.5 °C. Does the absence of obvious fever exclude sepsis?

No. Anesthesia is commonly associated with altered temperature regulation. Moreover, correlation between axillary and core temperatures is quite variable (see Chapter 6). A high index of suspicion is therefore required to diagnose sepsis. Leukocytosis is common following surgery and is not a reliable indicator of sepsis in this setting.

The mechanism of shivering in patients recovering from anesthesia is poorly understood. Although shivering is common in patients who become hypothermic during surgery (and presumably functions to raise body temperature back to normal), its relation to body temperature is inconsistent. Anesthetics probably alter the normal behavior of hypothalamic thermoregulatory centers in the brain. In contrast, infectious agents, circulating toxins, or immune reactions cause the release of cytokines (interleukin-1 and tumor necrosis factor) that stimulate the hypothalamus to synthesize prostaglandin (PG) E_2. The latter in turn activates neurons responsible for heat production, resulting in intense shivering.

How can the shivering be stopped?

Regardless of its cause, shivering has the undesirable effects of markedly increasing oxygen consumption (100–200%) and CO_2 production. Both cardiac output and minute ventilation must therefore increase. These effects are often poorly tolerated by patients with limited cardiac or pulmonary reserve. Although the ultimate therapeutic goal is to correct the underlying problem (such as hypothermia or sepsis), additional measures are indicated in this patient. Supplemental oxygen therapy (high FIO_2) helps prevent hypoxemia from the low mixed venous oxygen tension commonly associated with shivering; a low mixed venous oxygen tension tends to accentuate the effects of any intrapulmonary shunting (see Chapter 22). Unlike other opioid agonists, meperidine in small doses (20–50 mg intravenously) frequently terminates shivering regardless of the cause. Chlorpromazine, 10–25 mg, and butorphanol, 1–2 mg, may also be effective. These agents may have specific actions on temperature regulation centers in the hypothalamus. Shivering associated with sepsis and immune reactions can also be blocked by inhibitors of prostaglandin synthetase (aspirin, acetaminophen, and nonsteroidal anti-inflammatory agents) as well as glucocorticoids. Acetaminophen, which can be given rectally, is generally preferred perioperatively because it does not *affect platelet function. Rectal suppositories are, however, generally avoided following prostatic surgery to prevent bleeding from minor trauma to the gland during insertion.*

Outcome

Examination of the patient reveals warm extremities with a good pulse, even with the low blood pressure. The abdomen is soft and nontender. The irrigation fluid from the bladder was only slightly pink. A diagnosis of probable septicemia is made. Blood cultures are obtained and antibiotic therapy is initiated to cover gram-negative organisms and enterococci (the most common pathogens). The patient receives intravenous gentamicin, 80 mg, and ampicillin, 500 mg, and an intravenous dopamine infusion is started. The shivering ceases following administration of meperidine, 20 mg intravenously. The blood pressure increases to 110/60 mm Hg and the pulse slows to 110 beats/min following a 1000 mL intravenous fluid bolus and 5 mg/kg/min of dopamine. The serum sodium concentration was found to be 130 mEq/L. Four hours later, the dopamine was no longer needed, and the patient recovered uneventfully.

SUGGESTED READING

Battillo JA, Hendler MA: Effects of patient positioning during anesthesia. In Lebowitz RW: Anesthesia for urological surgery. Int Anesthesiol Clin 1993;31:67.

Better OS, Rubinstein I, Winaver JM, Knochel JP: Mannitol therapy revisited (1940–1997). Kid Int 1997;52:886.

Dobson PM, Caldicott LD, Gerrish SP, et al: Changes in hemodynamic variables during transurethral resection of the prostate: Comparison of general and spinal anaesthesia. Br J Anaesth 1994;72:267.

Eide TR: Anesthetic considerations for extracorporeal shock wave lithotripsy. In Lebowitz RW: Anesthesia for urological surgery. Int Anesthesiol Clin 1993;31:47.

Gravenstein D: Transurethral resection of the prostate (TURP) syndrome: A review of the pathophysiology and management. Anesth Analg 1997;84:438.

Liu S, Carpenter RL, Mulroy MF, et al: Intravenous versus epidural administration of hydromorphone: Effects on analgesia and recovery after radical retropubic prostatectomy. Anesthesiology 1995;82:682.

Malhotra V: *Anesthesia for Renal and Genito-Urologic Surgery.* McGraw-Hill, 1996.

Mathes DD: Bleomycin and hyperoxia exposure in the operating room. Anesth Analg 1995;81:624.

Mebust WK, Holtgrewe HL, Cockett ATK, et al: Transurethral prostatectomy—immediate and postoperative complications: A cooperative study of 13 participating institutions evaluating 3885 patients. J Urol 1989;141:243.

Monk TG, Goodnough LT, Brechner ME, et al: A prospective randomized comparison of three blood conservation strategies for radical prostatectomy. Anesthesiology 1999;91:24.

Richardson MG, Dooley JW: The effects of general versus epidural anesthesia for outpatient extracorporeal shock wave lithotripsy. Anesth Analg 1998;86:1214.

Shir Y, Frank SM, Brendler, et al: Postoperative morbidity is similar in patients anesthetized with epidural and general anesthesia for radical prostatectomy. Urology 1994;44:232.

Shir Y, Raja SN, Frank SM: The effect of epidural versus general anesthesia on postoperative pain and analgesic requirements in patients undergoing radical prostatectomy. Anesthesiology 1994;80:49.

Smith CE, Hunter JM: Anesthesia for renal transplantation: Relaxants and volatiles. Int Anesthesiol Clin 1995;33:69.

Warner MA, Martin JT, Schroeder DR, et al: Lower-extremity motor neuropathy associated with surgery performed on patients in a lithotomy position. Anesthesiology 1994;81:6.

Hepatic Physiology & Anesthesia

KEY CONCEPTS

 The hepatic artery supplies 45–50% of the liver's oxygen requirements while the portal vein supplies the remaining 50–55%.

 All coagulation factors—with the exception of factor VIII and von Willebrand factor—are produced by the liver. Vitamin K is a necessary cofactor in the synthesis of prothrombin (factor II) and factors VII, IX, and X.

 Liver tests that measure hepatic synthetic function include: serum albumin, prothrombin time (PT or international normalized ratio [INR]), cholesterol, and pseudocholinesterase.

 Albumin values less than 2.5 g/dL are generally indicative of chronic liver disease, acute stress, or severe malnutrition.

 The PT, which is normally 11–14 seconds (depending on the control), measures the activity of fibrinogen, prothrombin, and factors V, VII, and X.

 If an adequate intravascular volume is maintained, spinal and epidural anesthesia decrease hepatic blood flow primarily by lowering arterial blood pressure, while general anesthesia usually decreases it through reductions in blood pressure and cardiac output and sympathetic stimulation.

 Anesthetic interactions with bile formation and storage have not been reported. However, all opioids can potentially cause spasm of the sphincter of Oddi and increase biliary pressure (fentanyl > morphine > meperidine > butorphanol > nalbuphine).

 When the results of liver tests are elevated postoperatively, the usual cause is underlying liver disease or the surgical procedure itself.

 Epidemiologic studies have identified several risk factors that are associated with halothane-associated hepatitis, including middle age, obesity, female sex, and a repeat exposure to halothane (especially within 28 days).

The liver, which weighs approximately 1500–1600 g in adults, is the largest organ in the body. It is responsible for a seemingly endless number of complex and interrelated functions. Fortunately, because of the liver's large functional reserves, clinically significant hepatic dysfunction following anesthesia and surgery is uncommon. Such dysfunction is limited chiefly to patients with preexisting hepatic impairment and to those with rare idiosyncratic reactions to halogenated volatile anesthetics. This chapter reviews normal hepatic physiology, laboratory evaluation of hepatic function, and the effects of anesthesia on hepatic function. The anesthetic management of patients with liver disease is discussed in the following chapter.

FUNCTIONAL ANATOMY

The liver is separated by the **falciform ligament** into right and left anatomic lobes; the larger right lobe has two additional smaller lobes at its posterior-inferior surface, the **caudate** and **quadrate lobes.** In contrast, surgical anatomy divides the liver based on its blood supply. Thus the right and left surgical lobes are defined by the point of bifurcation of the **hepatic artery** and **portal vein (porta** hepatis); the falciform ligament therefore divides the left surgical lobe into medial and lateral segments. Surgical anatomy defines a total of eight segments.

The liver is made up of 50,000–100,000 discrete anatomic units called **lobules.** Each lobule is composed of plates of hepatocytes arranged cylindrically around a **centrilobular vein** (Figure 34–1). Four to five portal tracts surround each lobule. **Portal tracts** are composed of hepatic arterioles, portal venules, bile canaliculi, lymphatics, and nerves. In contrast to a lobule, **an acinus,** the functional unit of the liver, is defined by a portal tract in the middle and centrilobular veins at the periphery. Cells closest to the portal tract (zone 1) are well oxygenated, while those closest to centrilobular veins (zone 3) receive the least oxygen and are most susceptible to injury.

Blood from hepatic arterioles and portal venules commingles in the **sinusoidal channels,** which lie between the cellular plates and serve as capillaries. Two types of cells line the hepatic sinusoids: **endothelial cells** and **macrophages** (also called **Kupffer cells**). The **space of Disse** lies between the sinusoidal capillaries and the hepatocytes. Venous drainage from the central veins of **hepatic lobules** coalesces to form the **hepatic veins** (right, middle, and left), which empty into the inferior vena cava (Figure 34–2). The caudate lobe is usually drained by its own set of veins.

Bile canaliculi originate between hepatocytes within each plate and join to form **bile ducts.** An extensive system of lymphatic channels also forms within the plates and is in direct communication with the space of Disse.

The liver is supplied by sympathetic nerve fibers (T6–T11), parasympathetic fibers (right and left vagus), and as well by fibers from the right phrenic nerve. Some autonomic fibers synapse first in the celiac plexus while others reach the liver directly via splanchnic nerves and vagal branches before forming the hepatic plexus. The majority of sensory afferent fibers travel with sympathetic fibers.

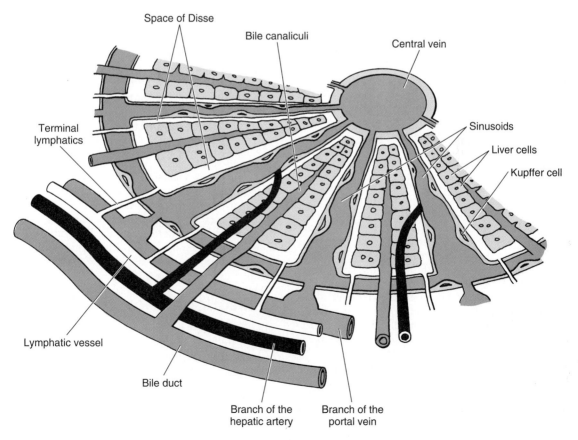

Figure 34–1. The hepatic lobule.

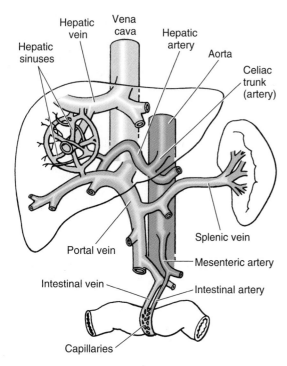

Figure 34–2. Hepatic blood flow. (Modified and reproduced, with permission, from Guyton AC: *Textbook of Medical Physiology,* 7th ed. WB Saunders and Company, 1986).

VASCULAR FUNCTIONS OF THE LIVER

Control of Hepatic Blood Flow

Normal **hepatic blood flow** is about 1500 mL/min in adults, of which 25–30% is derived from the hepatic artery and 70–75% from the portal vein (Figure 34–2). The hepatic artery supplies 45–50% of the liver's oxygen requirements while the portal vein supplies the remaining 50–55%. The pressure within the former is arterial, whereas that in the latter is normally less than 10 mm Hg. Portal vein oxygen saturation is normally 85%. The total blood flow from this dual supply represents 25–30% of total cardiac output. Hepatic arterial flow appears dependent on metabolic demand postprandially (autoregulation), while flow through the portal vein is dependent on blood flow to the gastrointestinal tract and the spleen. Although autoregulation of hepatic arterial flow may not be appreciable during fasting, a reciprocal though somewhat limited mechanism exists such that a decrease in either hepatic arterial or portal venous flow results in a compensatory increase in the other.

The hepatic artery has α_1-adrenergic vasoconstricting receptors as well as β_2-adrenergic, dopaminergic (D_1), and cholinergic vasodilator receptors. The portal vein has only α_1-adrenergic and dopaminergic (D_1) receptors. Sympathetic activation results in vasoconstriction of the hepatic artery and mesenteric vessels, decreasing hepatic blood flow. β-Adrenergic stimulation vasodilates the hepatic artery; β-blockers reduce blood flow and, therefore, decrease portal pressure.

Reservoir Function

Portal vein pressure is normally only about 7–10 mm Hg, but the low resistance of the hepatic sinusoids allows relatively large blood flows through the portal vein. Small changes in hepatic venous tone (and pressure) thus can result in large changes in hepatic blood volume, allowing the liver to act as a blood reservoir.

Normal hepatic blood volume is about 450 mL (almost 10% of total blood volume). A decrease in hepatic venous pressure, as occurs during hemorrhage, shifts blood from hepatic veins and sinusoids into the central venous circulation and augments circulating blood volume as much as 300 mL. In patients with congestive heart failure, the increase in central venous pressure is transmitted to the hepatic veins and causes blood to accumulate within the liver. As much as 1 L of blood can effectively be removed from the circulation in this way at the expense of causing hepatic congestion.

Blood-Cleansing Function

The Kupffer cells lining the sinusoids are part of the monocyte-macrophage (reticuloendothelial) system. Their functions include phagocytosis, processing of antigens, as well as the release of various proteins, enzymes, cytokines, and other chemical mediators. Their phagocytic activity is responsible for removing colonic bacteria and endotoxin entering the bloodstream from the portal circulation. Cellular debris, viruses, proteins, and particulate matter in the blood are also phagocytosed.

METABOLIC FUNCTIONS

The abundance of enzymatic pathways in the liver allow it to play a key role in the metabolism of carbohydrates, fats, proteins, and other substances (Figure 34–3).

Carbohydrate Metabolism

The final products of carbohydrate digestion are glucose, fructose, and galactose. With the exception of the large amount of fructose that is converted by the liver

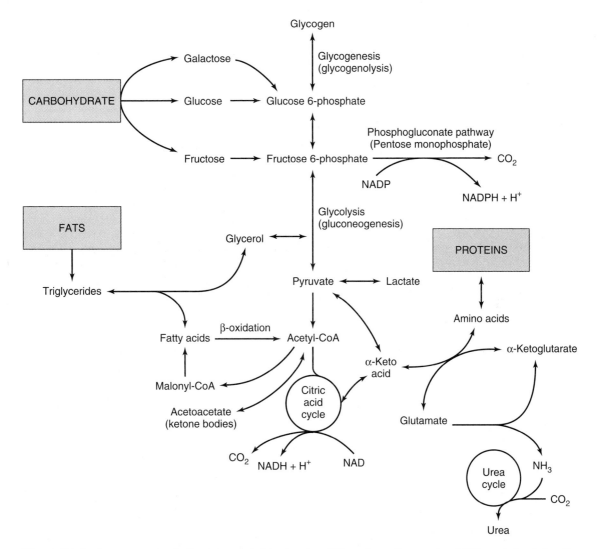

Figure 34–3. Important metabolic pathways in hepatocytes. Although small amounts of ATP are derived directly from some intermediary reactions, the overwhelming majority of ATP produced is the result of oxidative phosphorylation of the reduced forms of nicotinamide adenine dinucleotide (NADH) and nicotinamide adenine dinucleotide phosphate (NADPH).

to lactate, hepatic conversion of fructose and galactose into glucose makes glucose metabolism the final common pathway for most carbohydrates.

All cells utilize glucose to produce energy in the form of adenosine triphosphate (ATP) via glycolysis (anaerobically) or the citric acid cycle (aerobically). The liver (and adipose tissue) can also utilize the phosphogluconate pathway, and the latter not only provides energy but also produces an important cofactor in the synthesis of fatty acids. Most of the glucose absorbed

following a meal is normally stored as glycogen. When glycogen storage capacity is exceeded, excess glucose is converted into fat. Glycogen is a readily available source of glucose that does not contribute to intracellular osmolality. Only the liver and (to a lesser extent) muscle are able to store significant amounts of glycogen. Insulin enhances glycogen synthesis, while epinephrine and glucagon enhance glycogenolysis. Because hepatic glycogen stores are normally only about 70 g while glucose consumption averages 150 g/d, glycogen stores are depleted after 24 hours of fasting. After this period of fasting, de novo synthesis of glucose (gluconeogenesis) is necessary to provide an uninterrupted supply of glucose for other organs.

The liver and kidney are unique in their capacity to form glucose from lactate, pyruvate, amino acids (mainly alanine), and glycerol (derived from fat metabolism). Hepatic gluconeogenesis is very important in the maintenance of a normal blood glucose concentration. Glucocorticoids, catecholamines, glucagon, and thyroid hormone greatly enhance gluconeogenesis, while insulin inhibits it.

Fat Metabolism

When carbohydrate stores are saturated, the liver converts the excess ingested carbohydrates (and proteins) into fat. The fatty acids thus formed can be used immediately for fuel or stored in adipose tissue or the liver for later consumption. Nearly all cells utilize directly, as an energy source, fatty acids derived from ingested fats or those synthesized from intermediary metabolites of carbohydrates and protein. Only red blood cells and the renal medulla can utilize only glucose. Neurons normally utilize only glucose, but after a few days of starvation neurons can switch to break down products of fatty acids (ketone bodies) that have been made by the liver as an energy source.

In order to oxidize fatty acids, they are converted into acetylcoenzyme A (acetyl-CoA), which is then oxidized via the citric acid cycle to produce ATP. The liver is capable of high rates of fatty acid oxidation and can form acetoacetic acid (one of the ketone bodies) from excess acetyl-CoA. The acetoacetate released by hepatocytes serves as alternative circulating and readily available fuel (by reconversion into acetyl-CoA) for other cell types. Under some conditions (low insulin availability), glucagon increases ketone body production by the liver while insulin inhibits ketone body production.

Acetyl-CoA is also used by the liver for production of cholesterol and phospholipids, which are necessary in the synthesis of cellular membranes throughout the body. Hepatic synthesis of lipoproteins is also important in lipid transport by blood.

Protein Metabolism

The liver performs a critical role in protein metabolism. Without this function, death usually occurs within several days. The steps involved include (1) deamination of amino acids, (2) formation of urea (to eliminate the ammonia produced from deamination), (3) interconversions between nonessential amino acids, and (4) formation of plasma proteins.

Deamination is necessary for conversion of excess amino acids into carbohydrates and fats. The enzymatic processes (most commonly transamination) convert amino acids into their respective keto acids and produce ammonia as a by-product. The deamination of alanine plays a major role in hepatic gluconeogenesis. Although deamination also occurs to a minor extent in the kidneys (primarily glutamine; see Chapter 30), the liver is the principal site of deamination. With the exception of branched-chain amino acids (leucine, isoleucine, and valine), the liver normally deaminates most of the amino acids derived from dietary proteins. Branched-chain amino acids are primarily metabolized by skeletal muscle.

The ammonia formed from deamination (as well as that produced by colonic bacteria and absorbed through the gut) is highly toxic to tissues. Through a series of enzymatic steps, the liver combines two molecules of ammonia with CO_2 to form urea. The urea thus formed readily diffuses out of the liver and can then be excreted by the kidneys.

Hepatic transamination of the appropriate keto acid allows formation of nonessential amino acids and compensation for any dietary deficiency in these amino acids. Essential amino acids, by definition, cannot be readily synthesized through this mechanism and must be supplied exogenously.

Nearly all plasma proteins with the notable exception of immunoglobulins are formed by the liver. Quantitatively, the most important of these proteins are albumin, α_1-antitrypsin, and other proteases/elastases. Qualitatively, the coagulation factors are the most important proteins. Albumin is responsible for maintaining a normal plasma oncotic pressure and is the principal binding and transport protein for fatty acids and a large number of hormones and drugs. Consequently, changes in albumin concentration can affect the concentration of the pharmacologically active, unbound fraction of many drugs.

All coagulation factors—with the exception of factor VIII and von Willebrand factor—are produced by the liver. Vitamin K is a necessary cofactor in the synthesis of prothrombin (factor II) and factors VII, IX, and X. The liver also produces plasma cholinesterase (pseudocholinesterase), an enzyme that hydrolyzes esters, including some local anesthetics and succinylcholine. Other important proteins formed by the liver include protease inhibitors (antithrombin III, α_2-antiplasmin, and α_1-antitrypsin), transport proteins (transferrin, haptoglobin, and ceruloplasmin), complement, α_1-acid glycoprotein, C-reactive protein, and serum amyloid A.

Drug Metabolism

Many exogenous substances, including most drugs, undergo hepatic biotransformation. The end products of these reactions are generally either inactivated or more water-soluble substances that can be readily excreted in bile or urine. Hepatic biotransformations are often categorized as one of two types of reactions. **Phase I reactions** modify reactive chemical groups through mixed-function oxidases or the cytochrome P-450 enzyme systems, resulting in oxidation, reduction, deamination, sulfoxidation, dealkylation, or methylation. Barbiturates and benzodiazepines are inactivated by phase I reactions. **Phase II reactions,** which may or may not follow a phase I reaction, involve conjugation of the substance with glucuronide, sulfate, taurine, or glycine. The conjugated compound can then be readily eliminated in urine or bile.

Some enzyme systems, like those of **cytochrome P-450,** can be induced by a few drugs. Ethanol, barbiturates, ketamine, and perhaps benzodiazepines (eg, diazepam) are capable of enzyme induction, increasing production of the enzymes that metabolize those drugs. This can result in increased tolerance to the drugs' effects. Moreover, enzyme induction often promotes tolerance to other drugs that are metabolized by the same enzymes (**cross-tolerance**). Conversely, some agents, such as cimetidine and chloramphenicol, can prolong the effects of other drugs by inhibiting these enzymes.

Products of phase I reactions may in a few instances be more active than the parent compound or maybe cytotoxic. Such reactions are thought to be important in the toxicity of acetaminophen, isoniazid, and perhaps halothane (see below).

The metabolism of a few drugs—including lidocaine, morphine, verapamil, labetalol, and propranolol—is highly dependent on hepatic blood flow. These drugs have very high rates of hepatic extraction from the circulation. As a result, a decrease in their metabolic clearance usually reflects decreased hepatic blood flow rather than hepatocellular dysfunction.

Other Metabolic Functions

The liver plays a major role in hormone, vitamin, and mineral metabolism. Normal thyroid function is dependent on hepatic formation of the more active triiodothyronine (T_3) from thyroxine (T_4). Degradation of thyroid hormone is principally hepatic. The liver is also the major site of degradation for insulin, steroid hormones (estrogen, aldosterone, and cortisol), glucagon, and antidiuretic hormone. Hepatocytes are the principal storage sites for vitamins A, B_{12}, E, D, and K. Lastly, hepatic production of transferrin and haptoglobin is important because these proteins are involved in iron hemostasis, while ceruloplasmin is important in copper regulation.

BILE FORMATION & EXCRETION

Bile plays an important role in fat absorption and in the excretion of bilirubin, cholesterol, and many drugs. Hepatocytes continuously secrete bile salts, cholesterol, phospholipids, conjugated bilirubin, and other substances into bile canaliculi. Several mechanisms are responsible for bile formation: (1) osmotic filtration primarily due to secretion of bile salts into canaliculi (bile salt-dependent fraction), (2) Na^+-K^+ adenosine triphosphatase–mediated ion transport (bile salt-independent fraction), and (3) secretin-mediated sodium and bicarbonate transport by ductules.

Bile ducts from hepatic lobules join and eventually form the right and left hepatic ducts. These ducts, in turn, combine to form the hepatic duct, which together with the cystic duct from the gallbladder becomes the common bile duct (Figure 34–4). Biliary flow from the common bile duct into the duodenum is controlled by

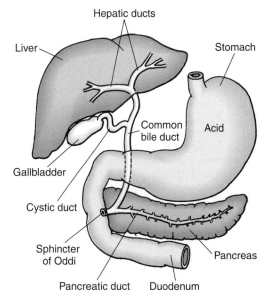

Figure 34–4. The biliary system. (Modified and reproduced, with permission, from Guyton AC: *Textbook of Medical Physiology,* 7th ed. WB Saunders and Company, 1986).

the sphincter of Oddi. The gallbladder serves as a reservoir for bile. Through active sodium transport and passive water reabsorption, the gallbladder concentrates biliary fluid between meals. Cholecystokinin, a hormone released by the intestinal mucosa in response to fat and protein, causes contraction of the gallbladder, relaxation of the sphincter of Oddi, and propulsion of bile into the small intestine.

Bile Acids & Fat Absorption

The bile acids formed by hepatocytes from cholesterol are essential for emulsifying the insoluble components of bile as well as facilitating the intestinal absorption of lipids. Bile acids also represent the major route of cholesterol elimination. Salts of the two principal acids formed, cholic acid and chenodeoxycholic acid, are usually conjugated with glycine and taurine before secretion into bile. Defects in the formation or secretion of bile salts interfere with the absorption of fats and fat-soluble vitamins (A, D, E, and K). Because of normally limited stores of vitamin K, a deficiency can develop in a few days. Vitamin K deficiency is manifested as a coagulopathy due to impaired formation of prothrombin and of factors VII, IX, and X.

Bilirubin Excretion

Bilirubin is primarily the end product of hemoglobin metabolism. It is formed from degradation of the heme ring in reticuloendothelial cells (macrophages). A much smaller amount is formed as a result of the breakdown of myoglobin and cytochrome enzymes. Heme oxygenase first breaks down hemoglobin into biliverdin, carbon monoxide, and iron; biliverdin reductase then converts the former into bilirubin. Bilirubin is then released into blood, where it readily binds albumin. Hepatic uptake of bilirubin from the circulation is passive, but binding to intracellular proteins traps the bilirubin inside hepatocytes. Inside the hepatocyte, bilirubin is conjugated (primarily with glucuronide) and actively excreted into bile canaliculi. A small fraction of the conjugated bilirubin is reabsorbed into the bloodstream. Half the bilirubin secreted into the intestine is converted by colonic bacteria into urobilinogen. A small amount of this substance is normally reabsorbed by the intestine, only to be excreted into bile again (enterohepatic recirculation). Urobilinogen is also renally excreted to a minor extent.

LIVER TESTS

Unfortunately, the most commonly performed liver tests are neither very sensitive nor very specific. Many tests such as serum transaminase measurements reflect hepatocellular integrity more than hepatic function. Tests that measure hepatic synthetic function include: serum albumin, prothrombin time (PT), cholesterol, and pseudocholinesterase. Moreover, because of the liver's large functional reserves, cirrhosis may be present with few or no laboratory abnormalities.

No one test reflects overall hepatic function. Each test generally reflects one aspect of hepatic function and must be interpreted in conjunction with the other tests along with clinical assessment of the patient.

Liver abnormalities can often be divided into either parenchymal disorders or obstructive disorders based on laboratory tests (Table 34–1). Obstructive disorders primarily affect biliary excretion of substances, while parenchymal disorders result in generalized hepatocellular dysfunction.

Serum Bilirubin

The normal total bilirubin concentration (conjugated and unconjugated) is less than 1.5 mg/dL (< 25 mmol/L) and reflects the balance between production and biliary excretion. Jaundice is usually clinically obvious when total bilirubin exceeds 3 mg/dL. A predominantly conjugated hyperbilirubinemia (> 50%) is associated with increased urinary urobilinogen and may reflect hepato-

Table 34–1. Abnormalities in liver tests.*

	Parenchymal (Hepatocellular) Dysfunction	Biliary Obstruction or Cholestasis
AST (SGOT)	↑ to ↑↑↑	↑
ALT (SGPT)	↑ to ↑↑↑	↑
Albumin	0 to ↓↓↓	0
Prothrombin time	0 to ↑↑↑	0 to ↑↑↑†
Bilirubin	0 to ↑↑↑	0 to ↑↑↑
Alkaline phosphatase	↑	↑ to ↑↑↑
5′-Nucleotidase	0 to ↑	↑ to ↑↑↑
γ-Glutamyl trans-peptidase	↑ to ↑↑↑	↑↑↑

AST = aspartate aminotransferase; SGOT = serum glutamic-oxaloacetic transaminase; ALT= alanine aminotransferase; SGPT= serum glutamic pyruvic-transferase.
*Adapted from Wilson JD et al (editors): *Harrison's Principles of Internal Medicine,* 12th ed. McGraw-Hill, 1991.
†Usually corrects with vitamin K.
↑ = increases, 0 = no change, ↓ = decreases.

cellular dysfunction, intrahepatic cholestasis, or extrahepatic biliary obstruction. Hyperbilirubinemia that is chiefly unconjugated may be seen with hemolysis or with congenital or acquired defects in bilirubin conjugation. In contrast to the conjugated form, unconjugated bilirubin is nontoxic to cells.

Serum Aminotransferases (Transaminases)

These enzymes are released into the circulation as a result of hepatocellular injury or death. Two aminotransferases are most commonly measured: serum aspartate aminotransferase (AST), also known as glutamic-oxaloacetic transaminase (SGOT); and serum alanine aminotransferase (ALT), also called glutamic pyruvic-transferase (SGPT). AST is present in many tissues, including the liver, heart, skeletal muscle, and kidneys. ALT is primarily located in the liver and is more specific for hepatic dysfunction. Normal AST and ALT levels are below 35–45 U/L. The circulating half-lives of these enzymes are about 18 and 36 hours, respectively. Mild elevations (< 300 U/L) can be seen with cholestasis or metastatic liver disease. Absolute levels correlate poorly with degree of hepatic injury in chronic conditions but are of great value in acute liver disease (drug overdose, ischemic injury, and fulminant hepatitis, for example).

Serum Alkaline Phosphatase

Alkaline phosphatase is produced by the liver, bone, small bowel, kidneys, and placenta and is excreted into bile. Normal serum alkaline phosphatase activity is generally 25–85 IU/L in most laboratories; children and adolescents have much higher levels reflecting active growth. Most of the circulating enzyme is normally derived from bone, but with biliary obstruction more hepatic alkaline phosphatase is synthesized and released into the circulation. The circulating half-life of the enzyme is about 7 days. Although mild elevations (up to twice normal) may be seen with hepatocellular injury or hepatic metastatic disease, higher levels are indicative of intrahepatic cholestasis or biliary obstruction.

Increased serum alkaline phosphatase levels may also be encountered with pregnancy (see Chapter 40) or bone disease (Paget's disease or bone metastases). Electrophoretic separation allows differentiation of hepatobiliary from other isoenzymes. It may be more practical to measure 5′-nucleotidase (5′-NT), leucine aminopeptidase (LAP), or serum γ-glutamyl transpeptidase to help exclude an extrahepatic source of alkaline phosphatase elevations. The combination of an elevated γ-glutamyl transpeptidase level together with an elevated alkaline phosphatase level strongly suggests hepatobiliary disease. In fact, elevated serum γ-glutamyl transpeptidase activity is the most sensitive indicator of hepatobiliary disease. Measurement of 5′-NT or LAP can alternately be used in nonpregnant patients; unlike γ-glutamyl transpeptidase, the latter two enzymes normally increase during late pregnancy.

Serum Albumin

The normal serum albumin concentration is 3.5–5.5 g/dL. Because its half-life is about 2–3 weeks, albumin concentration may initially be normal with acute liver disease. Albumin values less than 2.5 g/dL are generally indicative of chronic liver disease, acute stress, or severe malnutrition. Increased losses of albumin in the urine (nephrotic syndrome) or the gastrointestinal tract (protein-losing enteropathy) can also produce hypoalbuminemia.

Blood Ammonia

Significant elevations of blood ammonia levels usually reflect disruption of hepatic urea synthesis. Normal whole blood ammonia levels are 47–65 mmol/L (80–110 mg/dL). Marked elevations usually reflect severe hepatocellular damage. There is only a rough correlation between arterial ammonia levels and hepatic encephalopathy.

Prothrombin Time

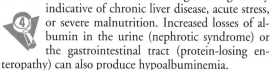

The PT, which is normally 11–14 seconds (depending on the control), measures the activity of fibrinogen, prothrombin, and factors V, VII, and X. The relatively short half-life of factor VII (4–6 hours) makes the PT useful in evaluating hepatic synthetic function of patients with acute or chronic liver disease. Prolongations of the PT greater than 3–4 seconds from the control are considered significant. This usually corresponds to an INR (International Normalized Ratio) greater than 1.5. Because only 20–30% of normal factor activity is required for normal coagulation, prolongation of the PT usually reflects severe liver disease unless vitamin K deficiency is present. Failure of the PT to correct following parenteral administration of vitamin K implies severe liver disease; correction normally requires 24 hours.

EFFECT OF ANESTHESIA ON HEPATIC FUNCTION

Hepatic Blood Flow

Hepatic blood flow usually decreases during regional and general anesthesia. Multiple factors are probably responsible, including both direct and indirect effects of anesthetic agents, the type of ventilation employed, and the type of surgery being performed.

All volatile anesthetic agents reduce portal hepatic blood flow. This decrease is greatest with halothane and least with isoflurane. Moreover, isoflurane appears to be the only volatile agent causing significant direct arterial vasodilation that can increase hepatic arterial blood flow. Nonetheless, even with isoflurane, total hepatic blood flow decreases because the decrease in portal blood flow usually offsets any increase in hepatic artery flow. All anesthetic agents indirectly reduce hepatic blood flow in proportion to any decrease in mean arterial blood pressure or cardiac output. Decreases in cardiac output reduce hepatic blood flow via reflex sympathetic activation, which vasoconstricts both the arterial and the venous splanchnic vasculature. If an adequate intravascular volume is maintained, spinal and epidural anesthesia therefore decrease hepatic blood flow primarily by lowering arterial blood pressure, while general anesthesia usually decreases it through reductions in blood pressure and cardiac output and sympathetic stimulation.

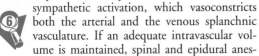

The hemodynamic effects of ventilation can also have a significant impact on hepatic blood flow. Controlled positive pressure ventilation with high mean airway pressures reduces venous return to the heart and decreases cardiac output; both mechanisms can compromise hepatic blood flow. The former increases hepatic venous pressure, while the latter can reduce blood pressure and increase sympathetic tone. Positive end-expiratory pressure (PEEP) further accentuates these effects. Spontaneous ventilation therefore may be more advantageous in maintaining hepatic blood flow. Hypoxemia decreases hepatic blood flow via sympathetic activation. Hypocapnia, hypercapnia, acidosis, and alkalosis have variable effects owing to the complex interaction between direct effects (increased flow with hypercapnia and acidosis but decreased flow with hypocapnia and alkalosis), secondary effects on the sympathetic system (activation with hypercapnia and acidosis), the ventilatory mode (spontaneous versus controlled ventilation), and the anesthetic agent used.

Surgical procedures near the liver can reduce hepatic blood flow up to 60%. Although the mechanisms are not clear, they most likely involve sympathetic activation, local reflexes, and direct compression of vessels in the portal and hepatic circulations.

β-Adrenergic blockers, α_1-adrenergic agonists, H_2-receptor blockers, and vasopressin reduce hepatic blood flow. Low-dose dopamine infusions may increase liver blood flow.

Metabolic Functions

The effects of the various anesthetic agents on hepatic intermediary metabolism (carbohydrate, fat, and protein) are poorly defined. An endocrine stress response secondary to fasting and surgical trauma is generally observed. This state is characterized by elevated circulating levels of catecholamines, glucagon, and cortisol. Mobilization of carbohydrate stores and proteins results in hyperglycemia and a negative nitrogen balance, respectively. The endocrine stress response may be at least partially blunted by regional anesthesia, deep general anesthesia, or pharmacologic blockade of the sympathetic system.

Drug Metabolism

Although halothane has been reported to directly inhibit the metabolism of several drugs (phenytoin, warfarin, and ketamine), it is probably the decreased hepatic blood flow associated with halothane and other anesthetics that is responsible for altered pharmacokinetics of other drugs (fentanyl, verapamil, and propranolol).

Biliary Function

 Anesthetic interactions with bile formation and storage have not been reported. However, all opioids can potentially cause spasm of the sphincter of Oddi and increase biliary pressure (fentanyl > morphine > meperidine > butorphanol > nalbuphine). The effects of alfentanil are similar to those of fentanyl but more short-lived. Intravenous opioid administration can therefore induce biliary colic or result in false-positive cholangiograms. Sphincter spasm may be less likely when the opioid is given slowly in small increments. Halothane and to a lesser extent enflurane may further blunt the increase in biliary pressure following opioid administration. Naloxone and glucagon (1–3 mg) are also reported to relieve opioid-induced spasm.

Liver Tests

Mild postoperative liver dysfunction in healthy persons is not uncommon if sensitive tests are employed. A combination of factors is probably responsible, including decreased blood flow that results from anesthesia, sympathetic stimulation, and the surgical procedure itself. Procedures in close proximity to the liver frequently result in modest elevations in lactate dehydrogenase and transaminase concentrations regardless of the anesthetic agent or technique employed.

When the results of liver function tests are elevated postoperatively, the usual cause is underlying liver disease or the surgical procedure itself. Persistent abnormalities in liver tests may be indicative of viral hepatitis (usually transfusion-related), sepsis, idiosyncratic drug reactions, or surgical complications. Postoperative jaundice can result from a variety of factors (Table 34–2), but the most common cause is overproduction of bilirubin because of resorption of a large hematoma or red cell breakdown following transfusion. Nonetheless, all other causes should be considered. Correct diagnosis requires a careful review of preoperative liver function as well as intraoperative and postoperative events such as transfusions, sustained hypotension or hypoxemia, and drug exposure.

HEPATIC DYSFUNCTION ASSOCIATED WITH HALOGENATED ANESTHETICS

Halothane, the first halogenated volatile anesthetic, was introduced in 1956, and shortly afterward the first cases of "halothane hepatitis" were reported. Since then, this disorder has been widely recognized, and cases associated with methoxyflurane, enflurane, and isoflurane have been described. Desflurane- and sevoflurane-related hepatitis have not been described.

Several mechanisms have been proposed for halothane-associated hepatitis, including the formation of hepatotoxic metabolic intermediates and immune hypersensitivity. Antibodies directed against hepatocyte components have been identified in some patients. A genetic susceptibility has been shown in rats and may also be operative in humans. Reductive metabolism under hypoxic conditions can produce hepatotoxic intermediates in some strains of laboratory animals. In contrast, oxidative metabolism, which produces trifluoroacetic acid, appears to be responsible in other models; trifluoroacetylation of tissue proteins can cause hepatotoxicity.

Halothane-associated hepatitis is a diagnosis of exclusion. Viral hepatitis—including that caused by hepatitis viruses (types A, B, and C), cytomegalovirus, Epstein-Barr virus, and herpes viruses—should be excluded. The severity of this syndrome can vary from an asymptomatic elevation in serum transaminases to fulminant hepatic necrosis. Although the incidence of a mild form of this syndrome has been reported as high as 20% in adults following a second exposure to halothane, the incidence of fatal hepatic necrosis is estimated to be approximately 1:35,000. Epidemiologic studies have identified several risk factors that are associated with this syndrome, including middle age, obesity, female sex, and a repeat exposure to halothane (especially within 28 days). Prepubertal children appear to be more resistant to this condition, with reported incidences of 1:200,000–1:80,000.

Hepatitis due to enflurane or isoflurane is very rare (estimated to be 1:500,000–1:300,000); indeed, the association between hepatitis and these two agents—especially isoflurane—is still questioned by many investigators.

**CASE DISCUSSION:
COAGULOPATHY IN A
PATIENT WITH LIVER DISEASE**

A 52-year-old man with a long history of alcohol abuse presents for a splenorenal shunt after three major episodes of upper gastrointestinal hemorrhage from esophageal varices. Coagulation studies reveal a prothrombin time of 17 seconds (control: 12 seconds) and a partial prothrombin time of 43 seconds (control: 29 seconds). The platelet count is 75,000/μL.

What factors can contribute to excessive bleeding during and following surgery?

Hemostasis following trauma or surgery is dependent on three major processes: (1) vascular spasm, (2) formation of a platelet plug (primary hemostasis), and (3) coagulation of blood (secondary hemostasis). The first two are nearly immediate (seconds), while the last is delayed (minutes). A defect in any of these processes can lead to a bleeding diathesis and increased blood loss.

Table 34–2. Causes of postoperative jaundice.

Prehepatic (increased bilirubin production)
  Large hematomas
  Transfusion
    Senescent red cell breakdown
    Delayed hemolytic reactions
Hepatic (hepatocellular dysfunction)
  Underlying liver disease
  Ischemic or hypoxemic injury
  Drug-induced
  Gilbert's syndrome
  Intrahepatic cholestasis
Posthepatic (biliary obstruction)
  Postoperative cholecystitis
  Postoperative pancreatitis
  Retained common bile duct stone

Outline the mechanisms involved in primary hemostasis.

Injury to blood vessels normally causes localized spasm as a result of the release of humoral factors (from platelets) as well as local myogenic reflexes. Sympathetic-mediated vasoconstriction is also probably operative in medium-sized vessels. Exposure of circulating platelets to the damaged endothelial surface causes them to undergo a series of changes that results in the formation of a platelet plug. If the break in a vessel is small, the plug itself can often completely stop bleeding. If the break is large, however, coagulation of blood is also necessary to stop the bleeding.

Formation of the platelet plug can be broken down into three stages: (1) adhesion, (2) release of platelet granules, and (3) aggregation. Following injury, circulating platelets adhere to subendothelial collagen via specific glycoprotein (GP) receptors on their membrane. This interaction is stabilized by a circulating GP called von Willebrand factor (vWF), which forms additional bridges between subendothelial collagen and platelets via GPIb. Collagen (as well as epinephrine and thrombin) activates platelet membrane-bound phospholipases A and C which, in turn, result in the formation of thromboxane A_2 (TXA$_2$) and degranulation, respectively. TXA$_2$ is a potent vasoconstrictor that promotes platelet aggregation. Platelet granules contain a large number of substances, including adenosine diphosphate (ADP), TXA$_2$, factor V, vWF, fibrinogen, and fibronectin. These factors attract and activate additional platelets. ADP alters a platelet membrane GPIIb/IIIa, which facilitates the binding of fibrinogen to activated platelets.

Describe the mechanisms involved in normal coagulation.

Coagulation, often referred to as secondary hemostasis, involves formation of a fibrin clot, which usually binds and strengthens a platelet plug. Fibrin can be formed via one of two mechanisms (pathways) that involve activation of soluble coagulation precursor proteins in blood (Table 34–3). Regardless of which pathway is activated, the coagulation cascade ends in the conversion of fibrinogen to fibrin. The extrinsic pathway of the coagulation cascade is triggered by the release of a tissue lipoprotein (thromboplastin) from the membranes of injured cells and is likely the more important pathway in humans. The intrinsic pathway (Figure 34–5) can be triggered by the interaction between subendothelial collagen with circulating Hageman factor (XII), high-molecular-

Table 34–3. Coagulation factors.

Factor	Approximate Half-Life (hrs)
I Fibrinogen	100
II Prothrombin	80
III Tissue thromboplastin	—
IV Calcium	—
V Proaccelerin	18
VII Proconvertin	6
VIII Antihemophilic factor	10
IX Christmas factor	24
X Stuart factor	50
XI Plasma thromboplastin antecedents	25
XII Hageman factor	60
XIII Fibrin-stabilizing factor	90

weight kininogen, and prekallikrein. The latter two substances are also involved in the formation of bradykinin.

Thrombin plays a central role in coagulation because it not only activates platelets (above) but also accelerates conversion of factors V, VIII, and XIII to their active forms. Conversion of prothrombin to thrombin is markedly accelerated by activated platelets. Thrombin then converts fibrinogen to soluble fibrin monomers that polymerize on the platelet plug. Cross-linking of fibrin polymers by factor XIII is necessary to form a strong, insoluble fibrin clot. Finally, retraction of the clot (which requires platelets) expresses fluid with the clot and helps pull the walls of the damaged blood vessel together.

What prevents coagulation of blood in normal tissues?

The coagulation process is limited to injured areas by localization of platelets to the injured area and maintenance of normal blood flow in uninjured areas. Normal endothelium produces prostacyclin (prostaglandin I_2 [PGI$_2$]), which is a potent vasodilator that inhibits platelet activation and helps confine the primary hemostatic process to the injured area. Normal blood flow is important in clearing activated coagulation factors, which are taken up by the monocyte-macrophage scavenger system (above). Multiple inhibitors of coagulation are normally present in plasma, in-

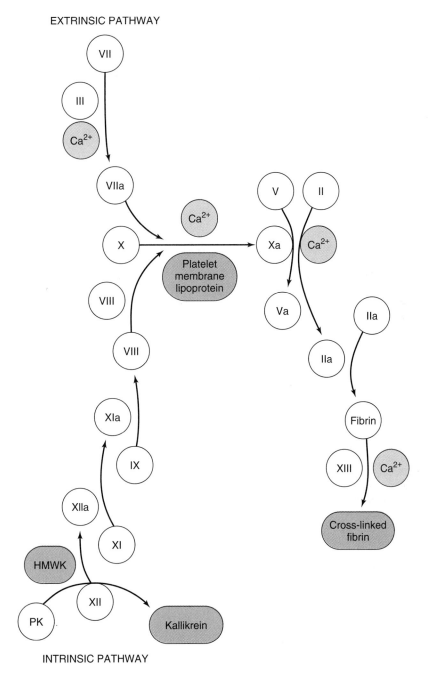

Figure 34–5. The intrinsic and extrinsic coagulation pathways.

cluding antithrombin III and proteins C and S, and tissue factor pathway inhibitor. Antithrombin III complexes with and inactivates circulating coagulation factors (with the notable exception of factor VII), while protein C specifically inactivates factors V and VIII. Heparin exerts its anticoagulant activity by augmenting the activity of antithrombin III. Protein S enhances the activity of protein C; deficiencies of these two proteins lead to hypercoagulability. Tissue factor pathway inhibitor antagonizes the action of activated factor VII.

What is the role of the fibrinolytic system in normal hemostasis?

The fibrinolytic system is normally activated simultaneously with the coagulation cascade and functions to maintain the fluidity of blood during coagulation. It is also responsible for clot lysis once tissue repair begins. When a clot is formed, a large amount of the protein plasminogen is incorporated. Plasminogen is then activated either by tissue plasminogen activator (tPA), which is usually released by endothelial cells in response to thrombin and fragments of Hageman factor. The resulting formation of plasmin degrades fibrin and fibrinogen as well as other coagulation factors. Urokinase (found in urine) and streptokinase (a product of bacteria) are also potent activators of plasminogen. The action of tPA is localized because: (1) it is absorbed into the fibrin clot, (2) tPA activates plasminogen more effectively on the clot, (3) free plasmin is rapidly neutralized by a circulating α_2-antiplasmin, and (4) circulating tPA is cleared by the liver. Plasmin degrades fibrin and fibrinogen into small fragments. These fibrin degradation products possess anticoagulant activity because they compete with fibrinogen for thrombin; they are normally cleared by the monocyte-macrophage system. The drugs ε-aminocaproic acid (EACA) and tranexamic acid inhibit the conversion of plasminogen to plasmin. Endothelium also normally secretes a plasminogen activator inhibitor (PAI-1) which antagonizes tPA.

What hemostatic defects are likely to be present in this patient?

Multifactorial coagulopathy often develops in patients with advanced liver disease. Three major causes are usually responsible: (1) vitamin K deficiency (impaired storage or absorption), (2) impaired hepatic synthesis of coagulation factors, and (3) splenic sequestration of platelets resulting from hypersplenism. To complicate matters further, patients with cirrhosis typically have multiple potential bleeding sites (esophageal varices, gas-

tritis, peptic ulcers, and hemorrhoids) and frequently require multiple blood transfusions. With severe liver disease, patients may also have decreased synthesis of coagulation inhibitors and fail to clear activated coagulation factors and fibrin split products (impaired Kupffer cell function); the coagulation defect resembles and becomes indistinguishable from disseminated intravascular coagulation (DIC).

What is DIC?

In DIC, the coagulation cascade is activated by the release of endogenous tissue thromboplastin or thromboplastin-like substances; or by direct activation of factor XII by endotoxin or foreign surfaces. Widespread deposition of fibrin in the microcirculation results in consumption of coagulation factors, secondary fibrinolysis, thrombocytopenia, and a microangiopathic hemolytic anemia. Diffuse bleeding and in some cases thromboembolic phenomena usually follow. Treatment is generally aimed at the underlying cause. Supportive measures include transfusion of coagulation factors and platelets. Heparin therapy is controversial but may benefit patients with thromboembolic phenomena.

What is primary fibrinolysis?

This bleeding disorder is due to uncontrolled fibrinolysis. Patients may have a deficiency of α_2-antiplasmin or impaired clearance of tPA. The latter may be common in patients with severe liver disease and during the anhepatic phase of liver transplantation (see Chapter 35). The disorder may occasionally be encountered in patients with carcinoma of the prostate (see Chapter 33). Diagnosis is often difficult but is suggested by a bleeding diathesis with a low fibrinogen level but relatively normal coagulation tests and platelet count (below). Treatment includes fresh frozen plasma or cryoprecipitate and possibly either EACA or tranexamic acid.

How are coagulation tests helpful in evaluating hemostasis?

The diagnosis of coagulation abnormalities can be facilitated by measurement of the activated partial thromboplastin time (aPTT), prothrombin time (PT), thrombin time (TT), and fibrinogen level (Table 34–4). The aPTT measures the intrinsic pathway (factors I, II, V, VIII, IX, X, XI, and XII). The whole blood clotting time and activated clotting time (ACT) also measure the intrinsic pathway (see Chapter 21). In contrast, the PT measures the extrinsic pathway (factors I, II, V, and

Table 34–4. Coagulation test abnormalities.

	PT	PTT	TT	Fibrinogen
Advanced liver disease	↑	↑	N or ↑	N or ↓
DIC	↑	↑	↑	↓
Vitamin K deficiency	↑↑	↑	N	N
Warfarin therapy	↑↑	↑	N	N
Heparin therapy	↑	↑↑	↑	N
Hemophilia				
Factor VIII deficiency	N	↑	N	N
Factor IX deficiency	N	↑	N	N
Factor VII deficiency	↑	N	N	N
Factor XIII deficiency	N	N	N	N

PT = prothrombin time; PTT = partial thromboplastin time; TT = thrombin time; N = normal; DIC = disseminated intravascular coagulation.

VII). The TT specifically measures conversion of fibrinogen to fibrin (factors I and II). The normal plasma fibrinogen level is 200–400 mg/dL (5.9–11.7 μmol/L). Since heparin therapy affects chiefly the intrinsic pathway, in low doses it usually prolongs the PTT only. In high doses, heparin also prolongs the PT. In contrast, warfarin primarily affects vitamin K–dependent factors (II, VII, IX, and X), so the PT is prolonged at usual doses and the PTT is prolonged only at high doses. In vivo plasmin activity can be evaluated by measuring circulating levels of peptides cleaved from fibrin and fibrinogen by plasmin, namely fibrin degradation products (FDP) and D-dimers. Patients with primary fibrinolysis usually have elevated FDPs but normal D-dimer levels.

What tests are most helpful in evaluating primary hemostasis?

The most commonly performed tests include a platelet count and a bleeding time. The bleeding time is generally not affected by the platelet count when the latter is greater than 100,000/μL. The normal platelet count is 150,000–450,000/μL. Patients with normally functioning platelets and platelet counts above 100,000/μL have normal primary hemostasis. When the platelet count is 50,000–100,000/μL, excessive bleeding generally occurs only with severe trauma or extensive surgery. In contrast, patients with platelet counts under 50,000/μL develop significant bleeding following even minor trauma. When the platelet count is under 20,000/μL, spontaneous bleeding is not unusual. Thrombocytopenia usually results from one of three mechanisms: (1) decreased platelet production, (2) splenic sequestration of platelets, or (3) increased platelet destruction. The last may fall under one of two categories of destruction: immune or nonimmune. Nonimmune destruction includes vasculitis or DIC.

A prolonged bleeding time with a normal platelet count implies a qualitative platelet defect. Although the bleeding time is somewhat dependent on the technique employed, values longer than 10 minutes are generally considered abnormal. Significant intraoperative and postoperative bleeding may be expected when the bleeding time exceeds 15 minutes. Specialized testing is required to diagnose specific platelet functional defects.

What are the most common causes of qualitative platelet defects?

The most common platelet defect is due to inhibition of TXA_2 production by aspirin and nonsteroidal anti-inflammatory drugs (NSAIDs). In contrast to aspirin, which irreversibly acetylates and inactivates cyclooxygenase for the life of the platelet (up to 7 days), enzyme inhibition by NSAIDs is reversible and generally lasts only 24 hours.

What is von Willebrand's disease?

The most common inherited bleeding disorder (1:800–1000 patients) is **von Willebrand's disease.** Patients with this disorder produce a defective vWF or low levels of a normal vWF (normal: 5–10 mg/L). Most patients are heterozygous and have relatively mild hemostatic defects that become apparent clinically when they are subjected to major surgery or trauma or following ingestion of aspirin or NSAIDs. In addition to helping link platelets, vWF serves as a carrier for coagulation factor VIII. As a result, patients typically have a prolonged bleeding time, decreased plasma vWF concentration, and decreased factor VIII activity. Acquired forms of von Willebrand's disease may be encountered in patients with some immune disorders and those with tumors that absorb vWF onto their surface. At least three forms of the disease are recognized, ranging in severity from mild to severe.

Treatment with desmopressin (DDAVP) can raise vWF levels in some patients with mild von Willebrand's disease (as well as normal individuals). The drug is usually administered at a dose of 0.3 μg/kg 30 minutes before surgery. Patients who do not respond to DDAVP should receive cryoprecipitate or factor VIII concentrates, both of which *are rich in vWF; prophylactic infusions are generally recommended before and after surgery twice a day for 2–4 days to guarantee surgical hemostasis. The risk of transmitting viral diseases is decreased with the use of purified and heat-treated factor VIII concentrates (see Chapter 29).*

What other hereditary hemostatic defects may be encountered in anesthetic practice?

The most common inherited defect in secondary hemostasis is **factor VIII deficiency** *(hemophilia A). This X-linked abnormality is estimated to affect 1:10,000 males. Disease severity is generally inversely related to factor VIII activity. Most symptomatic patients experience hemarthrosis, bleeding into deep tissues, and hematuria. Symptomatic patients generally have less than 5% of normal factor VIII activity. Classically, patients present with a prolonged aPTT but a normal PT and bleeding time. The diagnosis is confirmed by measuring factor VIII activity in blood. Affected patients generally do not experience increased bleeding during surgery when factor VIII levels are over 30%, but most clinicians recommend increasing factor VIII levels to more than 50% prior to surgery. Normal (fresh frozen) plasma, by definition, is considered to have 1 U of factor VIII activity per milliliter. In contrast, cryoprecipitate has 5–10 U/mL, while factor VIII concentrates have approximately 40 U/mL. Each unit of factor VIII transfused is estimated to raise factor VIII levels 2% per kilogram of body weight. Justifiable concern over transmission of viral disease has led to the development and increasing use of recombinant or monoclonal purified factor VIII. Twice-a-day transfusions are generally recommended following surgery because of the relatively short half-life of factor VIII (8–12 hours). Administration of DDAVP can raise factor VIII levels 2- to 3-fold in some patients. EACA or tranexamic acid may also be used as adjuncts.*

Hemophilia B (also known as Christmas disease) is the result of an X-linked hereditary deficiency of factor IX. The disease is very similar to hemophilia A but much less common (1:100,000 males). Measurement of factor IX levels establishes the diagnosis. Perioperative administration of fresh frozen plasma is generally recommended to maintain factor IX activity at more than 30% of normal. Recombinant or monoclonal purified factor IX should preferably be used when available.

Factor XIII deficiency is extremely rare but notable in that the aPTT, PT, TT, and bleeding times are normal. The diagnosis requires measurement of factor XIII levels. Since only 1% of normal factor XIII activity is generally required, patients are treated by a single transfusion of fresh frozen plasma.

Do normal laboratory values exclude a hemostatic defect?

A bleeding diathesis may exist even in the absence of gross abnormalities on routine laboratory tests. Some hemostatic defects are often not detected by routine testing but require additional specialized tests. A history of excessive bleeding after dental extractions, childbirth, minor surgery, minor trauma, or even during menstruation suggests a hemostatic defect. A family history of a bleeding diathesis may suggest an inherited coagulation defect but is often absent because the increased bleeding is often minor and goes unnoticed.

Hemostatic defects can often be differentiated by their clinical presentation. Bleeding in patients with primary hemostatic defects usually immediately follows minor trauma, is confined to superficial sites (skin or mucosal surfaces), and often can be controlled by local compression. Pinpoint small hemorrhage from capillaries in the dermis (petechiae) are typically present on examination. Bleeding into subcutaneous tissues (ecchymosis) from small arterioles or venules is also common in patients with platelet disorders. In contrast, bleeding that results from secondary hemostatic defects is usually delayed following injury, is typically deep (subcutaneous tissues, joints, body cavities, or muscles), and is often difficult to stop even with compression. Hemorrhages may be palpable as hematomas or may go unnoticed when located deeper (retroperitoneal). Coagulation may be impaired by systemic hypothermic or subnormal temperature of the site of bleeding even when coagulation test (PT, activated aPTT, bleeding time) results are normal and there is no history of hemostatic defects.

SUGGESTED READING

Kaplowitz N: Liver and Biliary Diseases, 2nd ed. Williams & Wilkins, 1996.

Park GR, Kang Y (editors): *Anesthesia and Intensive Care for Patients with Liver Disease.* Butterworth-Heinemann, 1995.

Stoelting RK, Dierdorf SF: *Handbook for Anesthesia and Co-existing Disease,* 2nd ed. Churchill Livingstone, 2002.

Anesthesia for Patients with Liver Disease

35

KEY CONCEPTS

 Elective surgery for the management of acute hepatitis should be postponed until the infection has resolved, as indicated by normalization of liver tests. Studies indicate increased perioperative morbidity (12%) and mortality (up to 10% with laparotomy) during acute viral hepatitis.

 Isoflurane is the volatile agent of choice because it has the least effect on hepatic blood flow. Factors known to reduce hepatic blood flow, such as hypotension, excessive sympathetic activation, and high mean airway pressures during controlled ventilation, should be avoided.

 In evaluating patients for chronic hepatitis, laboratory test results may show only a mild elevation in serum aminotransferase activity and often correlate poorly with disease severity.

In patients with cirrhosis, massive bleeding from gastroesophageal varices is a major cause of morbidity and mortality.

 Cirrhosis is typically characterized by a hyperdynamic circulatory state.

 Hypoxemia is frequently present and is due to right-to-left shunting (up to 40% of cardiac output).

 Factors known to precipitate hepatic encephalopathy in patients with cirrhosis include gastrointestinal bleeding, increased dietary protein intake, hypokalemic alkalosis (from vomiting or diuresis), infections, and worsening liver function.

 Intravenous colloid fluid replacement is often necessary to prevent profound hypotension and renal shutdown following the removal of large amounts of ascitic fluid.

 Anesthetic management for all hepatic surgeries can be complicated by large amounts of blood loss.

The prevalence of liver disease is increasing in the United States. Cirrhosis, the terminal pathology in a majority of liver diseases, appears to have a general incidence in some autopsy series as high as 5%. Cirrhosis is a major cause of death of men in their fourth and fifth decades, and mortality rates are increasing. Ten percent of the patients with liver disease undergo operative procedures during the final 2 years of their lives. The liver has remarkable functional reserve, and clinical manifestations of hepatic disease are often absent until extensive damage has occurred. Consequently, when these marginal patients with little reserve come to the operating room, effects from anesthetics and surgery (see Chapter 34) can precipitate further hepatic decompensation, leading to overt hepatic failure.

This chapter discusses the anesthetic management of patients with known liver disease. With some important exceptions, the anesthetic considerations tend to be similar in both acute and chronic liver disease. Although patients with cholelithiasis often have minimal hepatic impairment, the effects of anesthesia on the biliary system also require comment.

■ HEPATITIS

ACUTE HEPATITIS

Acute hepatitis is usually the result of viral infection, a drug reaction, or exposure to a hepatotoxin. The illness represents acute hepatocellular injury with variable amounts of cell necrosis. Clinical manifestations generally depend both on the severity of the inflammatory reaction and, more importantly, on the amount of necrosis. Mild inflammatory reactions may present as asymptomatic elevations in the serum transaminases, while massive hepatic necrosis presents as acute **fulminant hepatic failure.**

Viral Hepatitis

Viral hepatitis is most commonly due to hepatitis A, hepatitis B, or hepatitis C viruses (previously called blood-borne non-A, non-B). At least two other hepatitis viruses have also been recently identified: hepatitis D (delta virus) and hepatitis E (enteric non-A, non-B). Hepatitis types A and E are transmitted by the oral-fecal route, while types B and C are transmitted primarily percutaneously and by contact with body fluids. Hepatitis D is unique in that it may be transmitted by either route and requires the presence of hepatitis B virus in the host to be infective. Other viruses, including Epstein-Barr, herpes simplex, cytomegalovirus, and coxsackieviruses, may also cause hepatitis.

Patients with viral hepatitis often have a 1- to 2-week mild prodromal illness (fatigue, malaise, low-grade fever, or nausea and vomiting) that may or may not be followed by jaundice. The jaundice typically lasts 2–12 weeks, but complete recovery, as evidenced by serum transaminase measurements, usually takes 4 months. Because clinical manifestations overlap, serologic testing is necessary to determine the causative viral agent. The clinical course tends to be more complicated and prolonged with hepatitis B and C viruses. Less commonly, cholestasis (see below) is the major manifestation. Rarely, fulminant hepatic failure (massive hepatic necrosis) can develop.

The incidence of chronic active hepatitis (see below) is 3–10% following infection with hepatitis B virus and at least 50% following infection with hepatitis C virus. A small percentage of patients (mainly immunosuppressed patients and those on long-term hemodialysis regimens) become asymptomatic infectious carriers following infection with hepatitis B virus. Depending on the patient group studied, anywhere between 0.3% and 30% of patients remain infectious and have persistence of the B surface antigen (HBsAg) in their blood. Ap-proximately 0.5–1% of patients with hepatitis C infection become asymptomatic infectious carriers. Infectivity correlates with detection of hepatitis C viral RNA in peripheral blood. Most patients with chronic hepatitis C infection appear to have very low, intermittent, or absent circulating viral particles and are therefore not highly infective. However, infectious carriers pose a major health hazard to operating room personnel. In addition to "universal precautions" for avoiding direct contact with blood and secretions (gloves, mask, protective eyewear, and not recapping needles), immunization of health care personnel is highly effective against hepatitis B infection. A vaccine for hepatitis C is not available; moreover, unlike hepatitis B infection, hepatitis C infection does not appear to confer immunity to subsequent exposure. Postexposure prophylaxis with hyperimmune globulin is effective for hepatitis B but not for hepatitis C.

Drug-Induced Hepatitis

Drug-induced hepatitis (Table 35–1) can result from direct dose-dependent toxicity of a drug (or a metabolite), from an idiosyncratic drug reaction, or from a combination of the two causes. The clinical course often resembles viral hepatitis, making diagnosis difficult. Alcoholic hepatitis is probably the most commonly encountered type of drug-induced hepatitis, but the cause may not be obvious from the history. Chronic alcohol ingestion can also result in hepatomegaly from fatty infiltration of the liver, which reflects (1) impaired fatty acid oxidation, (2) increased uptake and esterification of fatty acids, and (3) diminished lipoprotein synthesis and secretion. Acetaminophen ingestion of 25 g or more usually results in fatal fulminant disease. A few drugs such as chlorpromazine and oral contraceptives characteristically cause cholestatic-type reactions (see below). Ingestion of potent hepatotoxins, such as carbon tetrachloride and certain species of mushrooms (*Amanita, Galerina*), are often associated with acute hepatic failure. Volatile anesthetics, most notably halothane, are associated with an idiosyncratic reaction hepatitis.

Preoperative Considerations

 Elective surgery should be postponed until the acute hepatitis has resolved, as indicated by normalization of liver tests. Studies indicate increased perioperative morbidity (12%) and mortality (up to 10% with laparotomy) during acute viral hepatitis. Although the risk with alcoholic hepatitis may not be as great, acute alcohol toxicity greatly complicates anesthetic management. Moreover, alcohol withdrawal during surgery may be associated with a

Table 35–1. Drugs and substances associated with hepatitis.

Toxic
Alcohol
Acetaminophen
Salicylates
Tetracyclines
Trichloroethylene
Vinyl chloride
Carbon tetrachloride
Yellow phosphorus
Poisonous mushrooms (*Amanita, Galerina*)
Idiosyncratic
Volatile anesthetics (halothane)
Phenytoin
Sulfonamides
Rifampin
Indomethacin
Toxic and idiosyncratic
Methyldopa
Isoniazid
Sodium valproate
Amiodarone
Primarily cholestatic
Chlorpromazine
Cyclosporine
Oral contraceptives
Anabolic steroids
Erythromycin estolate
Methimazole

---

mortality rate as high as 50%. Only truly emergent surgery should be considered in such instances. Patients with hepatitis are at risk for deterioration of hepatic function and the development of complications from hepatic failure, such as encephalopathy, coagulopathy, or hepatorenal syndrome (see below).

Laboratory evaluation should include blood urea nitrogen, serum electrolytes, creatinine, glucose, transaminases, bilirubin, alkaline phosphatase, and albumin as well as a prothrombin time (PT) and platelet count. Serum should be checked also for HBsAg whenever possible. A blood alcohol level is useful if the history or mental status is compatible with intoxication. Hypokalemia and metabolic alkalosis are not uncommon and are usually due to vomiting. Concomitant hypomagnesemia may be present in chronic alcoholics and predisposes to arrhythmias. The elevation in serum transaminases does not necessarily correlate with the amount of necrosis. The serum alanine aminotransferase (ALT) is generally higher than the serum aspartate aminotransferase (AST) except in alcoholic hepatitis, where the reverse occurs. Bilirubin and alkaline phosphatase are usually only moderately elevated, except with the cholestatic variant of hepatitis. The PT is the best indicator of hepatic synthetic function (see Chapter 34). Persistent prolongation greater than 3 seconds (INR > 1.5) following vitamin K administration is indicative of severe hepatic dysfunction. Hypoglycemia is not uncommon. Hypoalbuminemia is usually not present except in protracted cases, with severe malnutrition, or when chronic liver disease is present.

If a patient with acute hepatitis must undergo an emergent operation, the preanesthetic evaluation should focus on determining the cause and the degree of hepatic impairment. Information should be obtained regarding recent drug exposures, including alcohol intake, intravenous drug use, recent transfusions, and prior anesthetics. The presence of nausea or vomiting should be noted and dehydration and electrolyte abnormalities should be corrected. Mental status changes usually indicate severe hepatic impairment. Inappropriate behavior or obtundation in alcoholic patients may be signs of acute intoxication, while tremulousness and irritability usually reflect withdrawal. Hypertension and tachycardia are often also prominent with the latter. Vitamin K or fresh frozen plasma (FFP) may be necessary to correct a coagulopathy. Premedication is generally not given, in an effort to minimize drug exposure and not confound hepatic encephalopathy in patients with advanced liver disease. However, benzodiazepines and thiamine are indicated for alcoholic patients with acute withdrawal.

Intraoperative Considerations

The goal of intraoperative management is to preserve existing hepatic function and avoid factors that may be detrimental to the liver. Drug selection and dosage should be individualized. Some patients with viral hepatitis may exhibit increased central nervous system sensitivity to anesthetics, whereas alcoholic patients will often display cross-tolerance to both intravenous and volatile anesthetics. Alcoholic patients also require close cardiovascular monitoring, because the cardiac depressant effects of alcohol are additive to those of anesthetics; moreover, alcoholic cardiomyopathy develops in many alcoholic patients.

By definition, all anesthetics are central nervous system depressants, and for that reason the fewest number of agents should be used. Inhalational anesthetics are generally preferable to intravenous agents because most of the latter are dependent on the liver for metabolism or elimination. Standard induction doses of intravenous induction agents can generally be used because their action is terminated by redistribution rather than metabolism or excretion. A prolonged duration of action, however, may be encountered with large or repeated doses of intravenous agents, especially opioids.

Isoflurane is the volatile agent of choice because it has the least effect on hepatic blood flow (see Chapter 34). Factors known to reduce hepatic blood flow, such as hypotension, excessive sympathetic activation, and high mean airway pressures during controlled ventilation, should be avoided. Regional anesthesia may be employed in the absence of coagulopathy, provided hypotension is avoided.

CHRONIC HEPATITIS

Chronic hepatitis is defined as persistent hepatic inflammation for longer than 6 months, as evidenced by elevated serum aminotransferases. Patients can usually be classified as having one of three distinct syndromes based on a liver biopsy: chronic persistent hepatitis, chronic lobular hepatitis, or chronic active hepatitis. Those with chronic persistent hepatitis manifest chronic inflammation of portal tracts with preservation of normal cellular architecture on the biopsy; this type usually does not progress to cirrhosis. Clinically, these patients present with acute hepatitis (usually hepatitis B or C) that has a protracted course but eventually resolves. A recently described variant called chronic lobular hepatitis is characterized by acute hepatitis that resolves but is followed by recurrent exacerbations; foci of inflammation and necrosis are present in hepatic lobules. Like chronic persistent hepatitis, however, chronic lobular hepatitis usually does not progress to cirrhosis.

Patients with chronic active hepatitis have chronic hepatic inflammation with destruction of normal cellular architecture (piecemeal necrosis) on the biopsy. Evidence of cirrhosis is often present initially (20–50% of patients) or eventually develops. Although chronic active hepatitis appears to have many causes, it occurs most commonly as a sequela of hepatitis B or hepatitis C. Other postulated causes include drugs (methyldopa, oxyphenisatin, isoniazid, and nitrofurantoin) and autoimmune disorders. Both immunologic factors and a genetic predisposition appear to be responsible in most cases. Patients usually present with a history of fatigue and recurrent jaundice; extrahepatic manifestations, such as arthritis and serositis, are not uncommon. Manifestations of cirrhosis eventually predominate in patients with progressive disease. Laboratory test results may show only a mild elevation in serum aminotransferase activity and often correlate poorly with disease severity. Patients without chronic hepatitis B or C infection usually have a favorable response to immunosuppressants and are usually treated with long-term corticosteroid therapy with or without azathioprine.

Anesthetic Management

Patients with chronic persistent or chronic lobular hepatitis should be treated similarly to those with acute hepatitis (see above). In contrast, those with chronic active hepatitis should be assumed to have cirrhosis already and treated accordingly (see below). Patients with autoimmune chronic active hepatitis may also present problems related to other autoimmune manifestations (such as diabetes or thyroiditis) as well as long-term corticosteroid therapy (see Chapter 36).

■ CIRRHOSIS

Cirrhosis is a serious and progressive disease that eventually results in hepatic failure. The most common cause of cirrhosis in the United States is alcohol (Laennec's cirrhosis). Other causes include chronic active hepatitis (postnecrotic cirrhosis), chronic biliary inflammation or obstruction (biliary cirrhosis), chronic right-sided congestive heart failure (cardiac cirrhosis), hemochromatosis, Wilson's disease, and α_1-antitrypsin deficiency. Regardless of the cause, hepatocyte necrosis is followed by fibrosis and nodular regeneration. Distortion of the liver's normal cellular and vascular architecture obstructs portal venous flow and leads to **portal hypertension,** while impairment of the liver's normal synthetic and other diverse metabolic functions results in multisystem disease. Clinically, signs and symptoms often do not correlate with disease severity. Manifestations are typically absent initially, but jaundice and ascites eventually develop in most patients. Other signs include spider angiomas, palmar erythema, gynecomastia, and splenomegaly. Moreover, cirrhosis is generally associated with the development of three major complications: (1) variceal hemorrhage from portal hypertension, (2) intractable fluid retention in the form of ascites and the hepatorenal syndrome, and (3) hepatic encephalopathy or coma. Approximately 10% of patients also develop at least one episode of **spontaneous bacterial peritonitis,** and some may eventually develop hepatocellular carcinoma.

Few diseases can produce hepatic fibrosis without hepatocellular necrosis or nodular regeneration. They result mainly in portal hypertension and its associated complications (see below); hepatocellular function is often but not always preserved. These disorders include schistosomiasis, idiopathic portal fibrosis (Banti's syndrome), and congenital hepatic fibrosis. Obstruction of the hepatic veins or inferior vena cava (Budd-Chiari syndrome) can also cause portal hypertension. The latter may be the result of venous thrombosis (hypercoagulable state), a tumor thrombus (renal carcinoma), or occlusive disease of the sublobular hepatic veins.

Preoperative Considerations

The detrimental effects of anesthesia and surgery on hepatic blood flow are discussed in Chapter 34. Patients with cirrhosis are at increased risk for deterioration of liver function because of their limited functional reserves. Successful anesthetic management of these patients is dependent on recognizing the multisystem nature of cirrhosis and controlling or preventing its complications (Table 35–2).

Table 35–2. Manifestations of cirrhosis.

Gastrointestinal
Portal hypertension
Ascites
Esophageal varices
Hemorrhoids
Gastrointestinal bleeding
Circulatory
Hyperdynamic state (high cardiac output)
Systemic arteriovenous shunts
Pulmonary
Increased intrapulmonary shunting
Decreased functional residual capacity
Pleural effusions
Restrictive ventilatory defect
Respiratory alkalosis
Renal
Increased proximal reabsorption of sodium
Increased distal reabsorption of sodium
Impaired free water clearance
Decreased renal perfusion
Hepatorenal syndrome
Hematologic
Anemia
Coagulopathy
Hypersplenism
Thrombocytopenia
Leukopenia
Infectious
Spontaneous bacterial peritonitis
Metabolic
Hyponatremia
Hypokalemia
Hypomagnesemia
Hypoalbuminemia
Hypoglycemia
Neurologic
Encephalopathy

A. GASTROINTESTINAL MANIFESTATIONS:

Portal hypertension (> 10 mm Hg) leads to the development of extensive portal-systemic venous collateral channels. Four major collateral sites are generally recognized: gastroesophageal, hemorrhoidal, periumbilical, and retroperitoneal. Portal hypertension is often apparent preoperatively as evidenced by dilated abdominal wall veins (caput medusae). Massive bleeding from gastroesophageal varices is a major cause of morbidity and mortality in patients with cirrhosis. In addition to the effects of acute blood loss, the increased nitrogen load (from the breakdown of blood in the intestinal tract) can precipitate hepatic encephalopathy. Endoscopy is a valuable diagnostic and therapeutic tool. Identification of the site of bleeding is crucial because these patients may present with bleeding from a peptic ulcer or gastritis, which require different therapy.

The treatment of variceal bleeding is generally supportive (medical). Blood loss should be replaced with intravenous fluids and blood products (see Chapter 29). Nonsurgical treatment includes vasopressin (0.1–0.9 U/min intravenously), somatostatin (250 μg followed by 250 μg/hour), propranolol, balloon tamponade (with a Sengstaken-Blakemore tube), and endoscopic sclerosis of the varices. Vasopressin, somatostatin, and propranolol reduce the rate of blood loss. High doses of vasopressin can result in congestive heart failure or myocardial ischemia; concomitant infusion of intravenous nitroglycerin may lessen the likelihood of these complications as well as decrease the bleeding. Endoscopic sclerosis or ligation of the varices is usually effective in stopping the hemorrhage in 90% of bleeding episodes. Percutaneous transjugular intrahepatic portosystemic shunts (TIPS) can reduce portal hypertension and subsequent bleeding (however, it may increase the incidence of encephalopathy). When the bleeding fails to stop or it recurs, emergency surgery may be indicated. Surgical risk has been shown to correlate with the degree of hepatic impairment, based on clinical and laboratory findings (Child's classification; see Table 35–3). Shunting procedures are generally performed on low-risk patients, while ablative surgery, esophageal transection, and gastric devascularization are reserved for high-risk patients. Nonselective shunts (portacaval and proximal splenorenal) have generally been abandoned in favor of selective shunts (distal splenorenal). The latter decompress the varices but do not impair hepatic blood flow as much and are less likely to cause encephalopathy postoperatively (see below).

B. HEMATOLOGIC MANIFESTATIONS:

Anemia, thrombocytopenia, and, less commonly, leukopenia, may be present. The cause of the anemia is

Table 35–3. Child's classification for evaluating hepatic reserve.*

Risk Group	A	B	C
Bilirubin (mg/dL)	< 2.0	2.0–3.0	> 3.0
Serum albumin (g/dL)	> 3.5	3.0–3.5	< 3.0
Ascites	None	Controlled	Poorly controlled
Encephalopathy	Absent	Minimal	Coma
Nutrition	Excellent	Good	Poor
Mortality rate (%)	2–5	10	50

*Adapted from Child CG: *The Liver and Portal Hypertension.* WB Saunders and Company, 1964.

usually multifactorial and includes blood loss, increased red cell destruction, bone marrow suppression, and nutritional deficiencies. Congestive splenomegaly (from portal hypertension) is largely responsible for the thrombocytopenia and leukopenia. Coagulation factor deficiencies arise as a result of decreased hepatic synthesis. Enhanced fibrinolysis secondary to decreased clearance of activators of the fibrinolytic system may also contribute to the coagulopathy (see Chapter 34).

The need for preoperative blood transfusions should be balanced against the obligatory increase in nitrogen load. Protein breakdown from excessive blood transfusions can precipitate encephalopathy. However, coagulopathy should be corrected before surgery. Clotting factors should be replaced with appropriate blood products such as FFP and cryoprecipitate. Platelet transfusions should be considered immediately prior to surgery for counts less than 100,000/μL.

C. Circulatory Manifestations:

 Cirrhosis is typically characterized by a hyperdynamic circulatory state. Cardiac output is often increased, and generalized peripheral vasodilation is present. Arteriovenous shunting can occur in both the systemic and pulmonary circulations. The arteriovenous shunting together with the decrease in blood viscosity from anemia are at least partly responsible for the increased cardiac output. Patients with a superimposed alcoholic cardiomyopathy readily develop congestive heart failure.

D. Respiratory Manifestations:

Disturbances in pulmonary gas exchange as well as ventilatory mechanics are often present. Hyperventilation is common and results in a primary respiratory alkalosis. Hypoxemia is frequently present and is due to right-to-left shunting (up to 40% of cardiac output). Shunting is due to an increase in both pulmonary arteriovenous communications (absolute) and ventilation/perfusion mismatching (relative). Elevation of the diaphragm from ascites decreases lung volumes, especially functional residual capacity, and predisposes to atelectasis. Moreover, large amounts of ascites produce a restrictive ventilatory defect that increases the work of breathing.

Review of the chest film and arterial blood gas measurements is very useful preoperatively because atelectasis and hypoxemia are often not evident on clinical examination. Paracentesis should be considered for patients with massive ascites and pulmonary compromise but should be done with caution since removal of too much fluid can lead to circulatory collapse.

E. Renal Manifestations and Fluid Balance:

Derangements of fluid and electrolyte balance are manifested as ascites, edema, electrolyte disturbances, or the hepatorenal syndrome. Important mechanisms thought to be responsible for ascites include (1) portal hypertension, which increases the hydrostatic pressure and favors transudation of fluid across the intestine; (2) hypoalbuminemia, which decreases plasma oncotic pressure and favors fluid transudation; (3) seepage of protein-rich lymphatic fluid from the serosal surface of the liver secondary to distortion and obstruction of lymphatic channels in the liver; and (4) avid renal sodium (and often water) retention (see below). Both "underfilling" and "overflow" theories have been proposed to explain the sodium retention. The "underfilling" theory states that although the measurable total extracellular fluid and plasma volumes are increased in cirrhotic patients with ascites, "effective plasma volume" is decreased: sodium retention is secondary to relative hypovolemia and secondary hyperaldosteronism. The apparent discrepancy between the measured and "effective" plasma volumes may be accounted for by an increase in splanchnic blood volume. In contrast, the "overflow" theory holds that the primary abnormality is sodium retention by the kidneys and that the ascites represents transudation secondary to an expanded plasma volume. Patients with ascites have elevated levels of circulating catecholamines, which are thought to be due to enhanced sympathetic outflow. In addition to increased renin and angiotensin II, patients demonstrate an insensitivity to circulating atrial natriuretic peptide.

Regardless of the mechanisms involved, patients with cirrhosis and ascites have decreased renal perfusion, altered intrarenal hemodynamics, enhanced proximal and distal sodium reabsorption, and often an impairment of free water clearance. Hyponatremia and hypokalemia are common. The former is dilutional, while the latter is due to excessive urinary potassium losses (from secondary hyperaldosteronism or diuretics). The most severe expression of these abnormalities is seen with development of the hepatorenal syndrome.

The **hepatorenal syndrome** is a functional renal defect in patients with cirrhosis that usually follows gastrointestinal bleeding, aggressive diuresis, sepsis, or major surgery. It is characterized by progressive oliguria with avid sodium retention, azotemia, intractable ascites, and a very high mortality rate. Treatment is supportive and often unsuccessful unless liver transplantation is undertaken.

Judicious perioperative fluid management in patients with advanced liver disease is critical. The importance of preserving renal function perioperatively cannot be overemphasized. Overzealous preoperative diuresis should be avoided, and acute intravascular fluid deficits should be corrected with colloid infusions. Diuresis of ascites and edema fluid should be accomplished over several days. Loop diuretics are administered only after measures such as bed rest, sodium restriction (< 2 g NaCl/d), and spironolactone therapy are deemed ineffective. Daily body weight measurements are useful in preventing intravascular volume depletion during diuresis. For patients with both ascites and peripheral edema, no more than 1 kg/d should be lost during diuresis; while for those with ascites alone, no more than 0.5 kg/d should be lost. Hyponatremia (serum $[Na^+]$ < 130 mEq/L) also requires water restriction (< 1.5 L/d), while potassium deficits should be replaced preoperatively. Prophylactic perioperative mannitol infusions may be effective in preventing renal failure, but this has not been conclusively demonstrated.

F. CENTRAL NERVOUS SYSTEM MANIFESTATIONS:

Hepatic encephalopathy is characterized by alterations in mental status with fluctuating neurologic signs (asterixis, hyperreflexia, or an inverted plantar reflex) and characteristic electroencephalographic changes (symmetric high-voltage, slow-wave activity). Some patients also have elevated intracranial pressure. The metabolic encephalopathy appears to be related to both the amount of hepatocellular damage present as well as the degree of shunting of portal blood away from the liver and directly into the systemic circulation. The accumulation of substances originating in the gastrointestinal tract but normally metabolized by the liver has been implicated. These proposed toxins include ammonia, methionine metabolites (mercaptans), short-chain fatty acids, and phenols. Other reported abnormalities include increased blood levels of aromatic amino acids, decreased blood levels of branched-chain amino acids, increased permeability of the blood-brain barrier, and abnormally high levels of γ-aminobutyric acid in the brain. Factors known to precipitate hepatic encephalopathy include gastrointestinal bleeding, increased dietary protein intake, hypokalemic alkalosis (from vomiting or diuresis), infections, and worsening liver function.

Encephalopathy should be aggressively treated preoperatively. Precipitating causes should be corrected. Oral lactulose 30–50 mL q8h or neomycin 500 mg q6h is useful in reducing intestinal ammonia absorption. Lactulose acts as an osmotic laxative and like neomycin likely inhibits ammonia production by intestinal bacteria. Avoidance of sedatives in patients with encephalopathy is recommended.

Intraoperative Considerations

Patients with postnecrotic cirrhosis due to hepatitis B or C who are carriers of the virus may be infectious. Extra caution is indicated in preventing contact with blood and body fluids from these patients.

A. DRUG RESPONSES:

The response to anesthetic agents is unpredictable in patients with cirrhosis. Changes in central nervous system sensitivity, volumes of distribution, protein binding, drug metabolism, and drug elimination are common. Many patients display enhanced central nervous system sensitivity to thiopental, while some with an alcoholic history may appear to exhibit tolerance. An increase in the volume of distribution for highly ionized drugs, such as neuromuscular blocking agents (also called muscle relaxants), is due to the expanded extracellular fluid compartment; an apparent resistance may be observed, requiring larger than normal loading doses. However, smaller than normal maintenance doses of neuromuscular blocking agents dependent on hepatic elimination (pancuronium, rocuronium, and vecuronium) are needed. There may be a prolonged duration of action for succinylcholine as a result of reduced levels of pseudocholinesterase, but it is rarely of clinical consequence.

B. ANESTHETIC TECHNIQUE:

Because portal venous blood flow is reduced in cirrhosis, the liver becomes very dependent on hepatic arterial perfusion. Preservation of hepatic arterial blood flow and avoidance of agents with potentially adverse effects on hepatic function are critical (see Chapter 34). Regional anesthesia may be used in patients without thrombocytopenia or coagulopathy, but more care than normal must be directed to avoid hypotension. A barbiturate induction followed by isoflurane in oxygen or an oxygen-nitrous oxide mixture is most commonly employed for general anesthesia (see above). The use of halothane is generally avoided so as not to confuse the diagnosis if liver tests deteriorate postoperatively. Opioid supplementation reduces the dose of the volatile agent required, but the half-lives of opioids are often significantly prolonged, leading to prolonged respiratory depression. Cisatracurium may be the neuromuscular blocking agent of choice owing to its unique nonhepatic metabolism.

Preoperative nausea, vomiting, upper gastrointestinal bleeding, and abdominal distention due to massive ascites require a well-planned, methodical anesthetic induction. Preoxygenation and a rapid-sequence induction with cricoid pressure are most often performed. For unstable patients and those with active bleeding, either an awake intubation or a rapid-sequence induction with cricoid pressure using ketamine (or etomidate) and succinylcholine are best advised.

C. MONITORING:

Close respiratory and cardiovascular monitoring is necessary for patients undergoing abdominal procedures. Five-lead electrocardiographic monitoring of patients receiving vasopressin infusions is necessary to detect myocardial ischemia from coronary vasoconstriction. Pulse oximetry should be supplemented with arterial blood gas measurements to evaluate acid-base status. Patients with large right-to-left intrapulmonary shunts may not tolerate the addition of nitrous oxide and may require positive end-expiratory pressure (PEEP) to treat ventilation/perfusion inequalities and subsequent hypoxemia.

Intra-arterial pressure monitoring is generally indicated for most patients. Rapid changes in blood pressure occur as a result of excessive bleeding, rapid intercompartmental fluid shifts, and surgical manipulations. Intravascular volume status is often difficult to assess without central venous or pulmonary artery pressure monitoring. Such monitoring may be critical in preventing the hepatorenal syndrome. Urinary output must be followed closely; mannitol or low-dose dopamine should be considered for persistently low urinary outputs in spite of adequate intravascular fluid replacement (see Chapter 31).

D. FLUID REPLACEMENT:

Preoperatively, most patients are on sodium restriction, but intraoperatively preservation of intravascular volume and urinary output takes priority. The use of predominantly colloid intravenous fluids may be preferable in order to avoid sodium overload and to increase oncotic pressure (see Chapter 28). Intravenous fluid replacement should take into account the excessive bleeding and fluid shifts that often occur in these patients during abdominal procedures. Venous engorgement from portal hypertension, lysis of adhesions from previous surgery, and coagulopathy lead to excessive bleeding during surgical procedures, while evacuation of as-

cites and prolonged surgical procedures result in large fluid shifts. Intravenous colloid fluid replacement is often necessary to prevent profound hypotension and renal shutdown following the removal of large amounts of ascitic fluid.

Because most patients are anemic preoperatively and coagulopathic, red cell transfusions perioperatively are common. Significant transfusions may result in citrate toxicity. Citrate, the anticoagulant in stored red blood cell preparations, is normally readily metabolized by the liver. Toxicity occurs in patients with cirrhosis because metabolism is impaired. Citrate binds with serum calcium leading to the sequelae of hypocalcemia. Intravenous calcium is often necessary to reverse the negative inotropic effects of a drop in the blood ionized calcium concentration.

■ HEPATOBILIARY DISEASE

Hepatobiliary disease is often characterized by cholestasis, the suppression or stoppage of bile flow. The most common cause of cholestasis is extrahepatic obstruction of the biliary tract (obstructive jaundice). The biliary obstruction may be due to a gallstone, stricture, or tumor in the common hepatic duct. Patients with complete or near-complete obstruction present with progressive jaundice, a dark urine with pale stools, or pruritus.

Obstructive jaundice must be differentiated from intrahepatic cholestasis. The latter is due to suppression or obstruction of bile flow at the level of the hepatocyte or bile canaliculus. Intrahepatic cholestasis most commonly results from viral hepatitis or an idiosyncratic drug reaction (most commonly reactions to phenothiazines or oral contraceptives). The treatment for extrahepatic obstruction is usually surgical, whereas that for intrahepatic cholestasis is medical. Although pruritus (due to retained bile salts) is a prominent feature of intrahepatic cholestasis, correct diagnosis may not be possible based on clinical or laboratory grounds. Both entities produce a predominantly conjugated (> 50%) hyperbilirubinemia and moderate to marked elevations of serum alkaline phosphatase (see Chapter 34). Imaging studies (ultrasound, cholangiograms, radioisotopic or computed tomographic [CT] scans) are necessary to confirm extrahepatic biliary obstruction.

Gallstone disease (cholelithiasis) limited to the gallbladder is often asymptomatic and may affect 10–20% of the general population. The diagnosis is usually made by abdominal ultrasound. Symptomatic individuals usually present with biliary colic secondary to obstruction of the cystic duct. The triad of sudden right upper quadrant tenderness, fever, and leukocytosis suggests cholecystitis. The diagnosis can be confirmed by failure of the gallbladder to visualize on a radioisotope scan. Passage of a gallstone through the common duct may also produce transient jaundice (above). Concomitant chills or high fever may indicate an ascending bacterial infection of the biliary system (cholangitis). Less commonly, the gallstone can obstruct the pancreatic duct and cause acute pancreatitis. Approximately 75% of episodes of acute cholecystitis resolve within 2–7 days following medical treatment. The remaining 25% have a course complicated by failure to resolve the episode, empyema, perforation, gangrene, hydrops, fistula formation, or gallstone ileus. Five to ten percent of patients with an acute attack have acalculous cholecystitis. The latter typically occurs following or in association with serious trauma, burns, prolonged labor, major surgery, or critical illness. The diagnosis is usually made by ultrasound or CT scan of the abdomen.

Preoperative Considerations

Patients most commonly present to the operating room for cholecystectomy, relief of extrahepatic biliary obstruction, or both. The most common procedure is cholecystectomy, which is usually performed laparoscopically. Most patients with acute cholecystitis are stabilized medically prior to cholecystectomy. Medical treatment includes nasogastric suction, intravenous fluids, antibiotics, and opioid analgesics. Those in whom the acute attack resolves may defer surgery for a later time, while those suffering serious complications may require emergency cholecystectomy. Acalculous cholecystitis usually occurs in critically ill patients, and is associated with a high risk of gangrene and perforation; emergency operation is usually indicated in these patients.

Patients with extrahepatic biliary obstruction from whatever cause readily develop vitamin K deficiency. Vitamin K should be given parenterally but requires 24 hours for a full response. Failure of the PT to correct prior to surgery may necessitate administration of FFP. High bilirubin levels may be associated with an increased risk of postoperative renal failure; generous preoperative hydration is advised. Long-standing extrahepatic obstruction (> 1 year) produces secondary biliary cirrhosis and portal hypertension (see above).

Intraoperative Considerations

Laparoscopic cholecystectomy accelerates the patient's recovery but the insufflation of carbon dioxide into the abdomen can complicate anesthetic management (see Case Discussion, Chapter 23). Because all opioids can cause spasm of the sphincter of Oddi to varying degrees, their use has been questioned when an intraoperative cholangiogram is contemplated. Opioid-induced sphincteric spasm may theoretically result in a falsely positive intraoperative cholangiogram and needless exploration of the common bile duct. Although this point may have been overemphasized in the past, some clinicians withhold opioids until after the cholangiogram. If opioid-induced sphincter spasm is suspected, naloxone or glucagon can be given.

In patients with biliary tract obstruction, a prolonged duration of action of drugs primarily dependent on biliary excretion should be anticipated. Agents dependent on renal elimination are preferable (see Chapter 32). Urinary output should be monitored with an indwelling catheter. Maintenance of perioperative diuresis is desirable (see above).

Patients with acalculous cholecystitis and those with severe cholangitis are critically ill and have a high perioperative mortality rate. Invasive hemodynamic monitoring optimizes their anesthetic care (see Chapter 6).

■ HEPATIC SURGERY

Common hepatic procedures include repair of lacerations, drainage of abscesses, and resections for tumors (primary or metastatic). Up to 80–85% of the liver can be resected in many patients. Liver transplantation is also performed in many centers. Anesthetic management for all these procedures can be complicated by large amounts of blood loss. Cirrhosis greatly complicates anesthetic management and increases perioperative mortality. Multiple large-bore intravenous catheters and fluid (blood) warmers are necessary; rapid infusion devices facilitate management when massive blood transfusion is anticipated. Direct arterial and central venous pressure monitoring are also advisable. Some clinicians avoid hypotensive anesthesia because of its potentially deleterious effects on remaining liver tissue, while others feel that it can reduce blood loss when used judiciously. Administration of antifibrinolytics such as aprotinin, ε-aminocaproic acid, or tranexamic acid may reduce operative blood loss (see Chapter 21). Hypoglycemia may occur following large liver resections. Drainage of an abscess or cyst may be complicated by peritoneal contamination. In the case of a hydatid cyst, spillage can cause anaphylaxis due to *Echinococcus* antigens.

Postoperative complications include bleeding, sepsis, and hepatic dysfunction. Postoperative mechanical ventilation may be necessary in patients undergoing extensive resections.

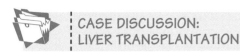

CASE DISCUSSION:
LIVER TRANSPLANTATION

A 23-year-old woman develops fulminant hepatic failure after ingesting wild mushrooms. She is not expected to survive without a liver transplant.

What are the indications for liver transplantation?

Orthotopic liver transplantation is usually performed in patients with end-stage liver disease who begin to experience life-threatening complications. Moreover, the complications become unresponsive to medical or nontransplant surgery. Transplantation is also carried out in patients with fulminant hepatic failure (from viral hepatitis or a hepatotoxin) when survival with medical management alone is judged unlikely.

In order of decreasing frequency, the most common indications for liver transplantation in children are biliary atresia, inborn errors of metabolism (usually α_1-antitrypsin deficiency, Wilson's disease, tyrosinemia, and Crigler-Najjar type I syndrome), and postnecrotic cirrhosis.

The most common indications in adults are postnecrotic (nonalcoholic) cirrhosis, primary biliary cirrhosis, and sclerosing cholangitis, and less commonly, primary malignant tumors in the liver. Considerable controversy exists over the justification for expenditure of scarce organs in transplanting patients with alcoholic cirrhosis, because of a general impression that a significant number of patients revert to habitual drinking afterward. Some studies, however, suggest the rate of recidivism is as low as 7% in patients who are able to abstain from alcohol for more than 6 months preoperatively.

What factors have contributed to the recent success of liver transplantation?

One-year survival rates for liver transplantations exceed 80–85% in some centers. Currently, 5-year survival rates are 50–60%. The success of this procedure owes much to the use of cyclosporine for immunosuppressant therapy. The drug selectively suppresses the activities of helper T cells (CD4 lymphocytes) by inhibiting production of interleukin-2 (IL-2) and other cytokines. IL-2 is required for the generation and proliferation of cytotoxic T cells responsible for graft rejection and for activating B cells responsible for T cell-dependent humoral responses. Cyclosporine is usually initially combined with corticosteroids and azathioprine. The use of anti-OKT-3, a monoclonal antibody directed against lymphocytes, has been extremely useful in treating steroid-resistant acute rejection. Tacrolimus (FK-506) has also proved effective in cyclosporine-resistant rejection and as an alternative to cyclosporine.

Additional factors may include greater understanding and experience with transplantation, the safe use of venovenous bypass, and the introduction of rapid infusion devices that allow transfusion of up to 2 L/min of warmed blood.

What major problems complicate anesthesia for liver transplantation?

These include the multisystem nature of cirrhosis. Often massive blood loss throughout the procedure, the hemodynamic consequences of clamping and unclamping the inferior vena cava and portal vein, the metabolic consequences of the anhepatic phase, and the risks of air embolism and hyperkalemia when circulation to the new liver is fully established.

Preoperative coagulation defects, thrombocytopenia, and previous abdominal surgery greatly increase blood loss. Extensive venous collaterals between the portal and systemic venous circulations also probably contribute to increased bleeding from the abdominal wall. Hypothermia, coagulopathies, hyperkalemia, citrate intoxication, and the potential transmission of infectious agents complicate massive blood transfusion (see Chapter 29). Typical transfusion requirements consist of 15–30 U of red blood cells, 15–30 U of FFP, 15–25 U of platelets, and 10–20 U of cryoprecipitate. Blood salvaging techniques can be extremely useful in reducing donor red cell transfusions. Aprotinin or ε-aminocaproic acid infusion may significantly reduce blood loss (see below and Chapter 21).

What is adequate venous access for these procedures?

Bleeding is a recurring problem during each phase of liver transplantation. Adequate venous access is paramount in anesthetic management. Several large-bore (14-gauge or larger) intravenous catheters should placed above the diaphragm. Specialized 8.5 F catheters can be placed in antecubital veins and used in conjunction with rapid infusion devices. Catheters should generally not be placed in the arm to be used for venovenous bypass. All transfusion lines should pass through a warming device that heats fluids to normal body temperature to prevent hypothermia; additional measures such as a forced-air surface warmer and humidification of respiratory gases are also necessary. Total blood replacement can range between 1 and 35 blood volumes.

What monitoring techniques are most useful during surgery?

All patients require direct intra-arterial pressure monitoring. A central venous or pulmonary artery catheter should be used to guide fluid replacement. The latter is preferred for most adult patients. Urinary output should be monitored carefully throughout surgery via an indwelling urinary catheter.

Laboratory measurements constitute an important part of intraoperative monitoring. Serial hematocrit measurements are mandatory to guide red blood cell replacement. Similarly, frequent measurements of arterial blood gases, serum electrolytes, serum ionized calcium, and serum glucose are necessary to detect and appropriately treat metabolic derangements. Coagulation can be monitored by measuring prothrombin time, activated partial thromboplastin time, and fibrinogen and by platelet counts, or by thromboelastography. The latter not only measures overall clotting and platelet function but can also detect fibrinolysis (below).

What anesthetic technique may be used for liver transplantation?

Premedication is usually administered unless the patient is in an advanced stage of hepatic encephalopathy. Intramuscular injections are avoided in patients with coagulopathy. Oral diazepam 5–10 mg or lorazepam 2–3 mg can be used for adults, while diazepam 0.1–0.2 mg/kg can be used orally for children. Most patients should be considered as having a "full stomach" often because of marked abdominal distention or recent upper gastrointestinal bleeding. General anesthesia is usually induced via a rapid-sequence induction with cricoid pressure. The semi-upright position during induction prevents rapid oxygen desaturation and facilitates ventilation until the abdomen is open. Thiopental, 4–5 mg/kg, ketamine, 1–2 mg/kg, or etomidate, 0.2–0.3 mg/kg, may be used. Succinylcholine, 1.5 mg/kg, is usually employed to facilitate rapid intubation. Hyperventilation may be beneficial in patients with severe encephalopathy because they may have increased intracranial pressure (see Chapter 25). Anesthesia is usually maintained with a volatile agent, usually isoflurane, and an intravenous opioid, usually fentanyl or sufentanil. The concentration of the volatile agent should be limited to less than 1 minimum alveolar concentration in patients with se-

vere encephalopathy (see Chapter 25). Nitrous oxide is usually avoided or used only until just prior to perfusion of the donor graft to prevent expansion of any intravascular air bubbles. Nitrous oxide can also cause marked distention of the bowel. The choice of a subsequent nondepolarizing neuromuscular blocking agent is generally at the discretion of the anesthesiologist. At the end of the procedure, many patients are routinely transferred to the intensive care unit intubated and mechanically ventilated.

Why are these operations so lengthy?

These procedures usually require an average of 8 hours of surgery (range 6–18 hours) that can be divided into three phases: a dissection phase, an anhepatic phase, and a revascularization phase.

(1) Dissection (preanhepatic) phase: Through a wide subcostal incision, the liver is dissected so that it remains attached only by the inferior vena cava, portal vein, hepatic artery, and common bile duct. Previous abdominal procedures greatly prolong the duration of and increase the blood loss associated with this phase.

(2) Anhepatic phase: Once the liver is freed, the inferior vena cava is clamped above and below the liver, as are the hepatic artery, portal vein, and common bile duct. The liver is then completely excised. Venovenous bypass (see below) may or may not be employed during this phase. The donor liver is then anastomosed to the supra- and infrahepatic inferior venae cavae and the portal vein.

(3) Revascularization and biliary reconstruction (neohepatic or postanhepatic) phase: Following completion of the venous anastomoses, venous clamps are removed and the circulation to the new liver is completed by anastomosing the hepatic artery. Lastly, the common bile duct of the donor liver is then usually connected to the recipient via a choledochocholedochostomy or Roux-en-Y choledochojejunostomy.

How are the circulatory effects of venous clamping managed?

When the inferior vena cava and portal vein are clamped, marked decreases in cardiac output and hypotension are typically encountered. Moreover, the increase in distal venous pressure can markedly increase bleeding and impair renal perfusion and often promotes edema and ischemia of intestines. Some patients (usually children) tolerate caval clamping because of extensive transdiaphragmatic collateral venous channels. For patients identified at increased risk with vena cava clamping, some surgeons use the technique of venovenous bypass in adults and in children weighing over 10 kg. This technique involves cannulating the inferior vena cava and the portal vein and diverting their blood flow (1–3 L/min) away from the liver and back to the heart, usually via an axillary vein. The pump and tubing are designed in such a way that heparinization of the patient is not necessary. Venovenous bypass can prevent severe hypotension, intestinal edema, ischemia, the build-up of acid metabolites, and postoperative renal dysfunction. Prophylactic measures such as mannitol or low-dose dopamine (2–3 µg/kg/min) prior to and during venous clamping may be beneficial in preserving renal function but are unproved. Temporary inotropic support (in addition to blood and fluid replacement) is often required transiently until effective venovenous bypass is established. Technical considerations have prevented the routine use of venovenous bypass for small children. The use of venovenous bypass is not without risk; it increases operative time; can be associated with air embolism, thromboembolic complications, and brachial plexus injuries; and may contribute to hypothermia.

What physiologic derangements are associated with the anhepatic phase?

When the liver is removed, the large citrate load from blood products is no longer metabolized and results in hypocalcemia and secondary myocardial depression (see Chapter 29). Periodic calcium chloride administration (200–500 mg) is necessary but should be guided by ionized calcium concentration measurements to avoid hypercalcemia. Electrocardiographic signs are unreliable for hypocalcemia but reliable for hyperkalemia (see Chapter 28). Progressive acidosis is also encountered because acid metabolites from the intestines (and lower body) are not cleared by the liver. Sodium bicarbonate therapy is therefore also necessary and should similarly be guided by arterial blood gas analysis. Excessive $NaHCO_3$ administration results in hypernatremia, hyperosmolality, and accentuation of the metabolic alkalosis that typically follows massive blood transfusions (see Chapter 29). Tromethamine should be considered when large amounts of alkali therapy is necessary (see Chapter 30). Although hypoglycemia can occur during the anhepatic phase, hyperglycemia is a more common occurrence. The large amounts of transfused blood products given usually provide a large glucose load. Glucose-containing intravenous solutions are therefore not used unless hypoglycemia is documented.

Pulmonary and systemic (paradoxic) air embolism can occur when the circulation is fully reestablished to the donor liver because air often enters hepatic sinusoids after harvesting. Systemic air embolism probably reflects the fact that many of these patients have extensive arteriovenous communications. Venous air embolism can be detected as a sudden increase in end-expired nitrogen concentration (see Chapter 26). The incidence of air embolism is decreased by infusing cold lactated Ringer's injection through the portal vein while the venous anastomoses are being constructed. In addition, after completion of the portal and suprahepatic caval anastomoses but before completion of the infrahepatic caval anastomosis, the portal vein clamp is released; blood from the portal vein then "flushes out" any air remaining in the liver, which can now escape through the incomplete infrahepatic caval anastomotic site. Marked hypotension is often encountered during this period and requires inotropic support as well as intravenous fluid replacement. After "flushing," venous clamps are reapplied until the infrahepatic caval anastomosis is completed. The anhepatic phase ends when the three venous clamps are removed and the donor liver is perfused. Thromboembolic phenomena are also described following reperfusion.

What problems may be anticipated during the revascularization phase?

Perfusion of the donor liver by the recipient's blood uniformly results in a transient increase in serum potassium concentration of usually 1–2 mEq/L and increased systemic acidosis. Acidosis accentuates the hyperkalemia (see Chapter 28). Reperfusion releases potassium from any remaining preservative solution (115–120 mEq/L of K^+) still within the liver as well as potassium released from tissues distal to venous clamps. Unclamping may also release a large acid load from ischemic tissue in the lower body (especially without venovenous bypass); prophylactic administration of $NaHCO_3$ is advocated by some.

When the circulation to the new liver is established, the sudden increase in blood volume, acidosis, and hyperkalemia can produce either tachyarrhythmias or, more commonly, bradyarrhythmias. In addition to $CaCl_2$ and $NaHCO_3$, inotropic support is also often required. Hyperfibrinolysis is commonly present and appears to be due to a marked increase in tissue plasminogen activator and decrease in plasminogen activator inhibitor during the anhepatic phase. Fibrinolysis can be detected by thromboelastography. ε-Aminocaproic acid or tranexamic acid inhibits the action of plasmin on fibrin, is indicated in those instances (if not used prophylactically).

What problems are encountered postoperatively?

Patients often have an uncomplicated postoperative course. Problems to be aware of include persistent hemorrhage, fluid overload, metabolic abnormalities (especially metabolic alkalosis and hypokalemia), respiratory failure, pleural effusions, paralysis of the right hemidiaphragm (secondary to injury of the right phrenic nerve), renal failure, systemic infections, and surgical complications such as bile leaks or stricture, or thrombosis of the hepatic or portal vessels. The last two complications may be suspected during Doppler ultrasound and are confirmed by angiography. Neurologic complications include seizures, intracranial hemorrhage, encephalopathy, and cyclosporine neurotoxicity. Renal dysfunction is often multifactorial in origin; contributory factors include periods of hypotension, impaired renal perfusion when the inferior vena cava is clamped (resulting in high pressures in the renal veins), and cyclosporine or antibiotic nephropathy. Measurement of cyclosporine levels may be helpful in avoiding toxicity.

Prophylactic antibiotics and antifungal agents are routinely given in many centers because of a high incidence of infections. Prophylactic ganci-clovir therapy may also be used in patients receiving anti-OKT3. Life-threatening infections include intra-abdominal, pulmonary, wound, urinary tract, and catheter-related infections. Pulmonary infections include those of common pathogens such as gram-negative bacteria as well as viruses (cytomegalovirus), fungi (Candida and Aspergillus), and parasites (Pneumocystis). Postoperative viral hepatitis may be due to cytomegalovirus, herpesvirus, Epstein-Barr virus, adenovirus (children), as well as hepatitis B and C viruses; de novo infection or viral reactivation may be responsible.

Rejection of the transplant is generally not a problem until 1–6 weeks after surgery. Graft function is usually monitored by the prothrombin time, serum bilirubin, aminotransferase activity, and lactate measurements. Diagnosis requires liver biopsy.

SUGGESTED READING

Benumof JL: *Anesthesia and Uncommon Diseases,* 4th ed. WB Saunders and Company, 1998.

Cecil RL, Goldman L, Bennett JC: *Cecil Textbook of Medicine,* 21st ed. WB Saunders and Company, 2000.

Sharpe MD, Gelb AW: *Anesthesia and Transplantation,* Butterworth-Heinemann, 1999.

Stoelting RK, Dierdorf SF: *Handbook for Anesthesia and Co-existing Disease,* 2nd ed. Churchill Livingstone, 2002.

Wu GY, Israel J: *Diseases of the Liver and Bile Ducts: A Practical Guide to Diagnosis and Treatment.* Humana Press, 1998.

Anesthesia for Patients with Endocrine Disease

36

KEY CONCEPTS

 Diabetic autonomic neuropathy, which may co-exist in diabetic patients with a history of hypertension, may limit the heart's ability to compensate for intravascular volume changes and may predispose patients to cardiovascular instability (eg, postinduction hypotension) and even sudden cardiac death.

 Diabetic patients should be routinely evaluated preoperatively for adequate temporomandibular joint and cervical spine mobility to help predict difficult intubations, which occur in approximately 30% of persons with type I diabetes.

 Hyperthyroid patients can be chronically hypovolemic and vasodilated and are prone to an exaggerated hypotensive response during induction of anesthesia.

 Hypothyroid patients are more susceptible to the hypotensive effect of anesthetic agents because of their diminished cardiac output, blunted baroreceptor reflexes, and decreased intravascular volume.

 Patients with Cushing's syndrome tend to be volume-overloaded and have hypokalemic metabolic alkalosis resulting from the mineralocorticoid activity of glucocorticoids.

 The key to the anesthetic management of patients with glucocorticoid deficiency is to ensure adequate steroid replacement therapy during the perioperative period.

 Anesthetic drugs or techniques that stimulate the sympathetic nervous system (eg, ephedrine, ketamine, hypoventilation), potentiate the dysrhythmic effects of catecholamines (eg, halothane), inhibit the parasympathetic nervous system (eg, pancuronium), or release histamine (eg, atracurium, morphine sulfate) may precipitate hypertension and are best avoided.

 Pay particular attention to the airway in obese patients because intubation is often difficult due to limited mobility of the temporomandibular and atlanto-occipital joints, a narrowed upper airway, and a shortened distance between the mandible and sternal fat pads.

 In patients with carcinoid syndrome, the key to anesthetic management is to avoid anesthetic techniques or agents that could cause the tumor to release vasoactive substances.

The underproduction or overproduction of hormones can have dramatic physiologic and pharmacologic consequences. Therefore, it is not surprising that endocrinopathies affect anesthetic management. This chapter briefly reviews the normal physiology and discusses the dysfunction of four endocrine organs: the pancreas, the thyroid, the parathyroids, and the adrenal gland. It also considers obesity and **carcinoid syndrome.**

■ THE PANCREAS

Physiology

Adults normally secrete approximately 50 units of insulin each day from the β cells of the islets of Langerhans in the pancreas. The rate of insulin secretion is primarily determined by the plasma glucose level. Insulin, the most important anabolic hormone, has multiple metabolic effects, including increased glucose and potassium entry into adipose and muscle cells; increased glycogen, protein, and fatty acid synthesis; and decreased glycogenolysis, gluconeogenesis, ketogenesis, lipolysis, and protein catabolism.

In general, insulin stimulates anabolism while its lack is associated with catabolism and a negative nitrogen balance (Table 36–1).

DIABETES MELLITUS

Clinical Manifestations

Diabetes mellitus is characterized by impairment of carbohydrate metabolism caused by a deficiency of insulin activity, which leads to hyperglycemia and glycosuria. The diagnosis is based on an elevated fasting plasma glucose (> 140 mg/dL) or blood glucose (126 mg/dL). Values are sometimes reported for blood glucose, which runs 12–15% lower than plasma glucose. Even when testing whole blood, newer glucose meters calculate and display plasma glucose. Diabetes has recently been reclassified to include four types (Table 36–2); type I (insulin-dependent) and type II (noninsulin-dependent) diabetes are the most common and well known. **Diabetic ketoacidosis** (DKA) is associated with type I diabetes mellitus, but there are individuals who present with DKA who phenotypically appear to have type II diabetes mellitus. Furthermore, individuals with an initial diagnosis of type II diabetes mellitus can later develop type I diabetes. Long-term complications of diabetes include hypertension, myocardial infarction, peripheral and cerebral vascular disease, peripheral and autonomic neuropathies, and renal failure. There are

Table 36–1. Endocrinologic effects of insulin.

Effects on liver
  Anabolic
    Promotes glycogenesis
    Increases synthesis of triglycerides, cholesterol, and VLDL
    Increases protein synthesis
    Promotes glycolysis
  Anticatabolic
    Inhibits glycogenolysis
    Inhibits ketogenesis
    Inhibits gluconeogenesis
Effects on muscle
  Promotes protein synthesis
    Increases amino acid transport
    Stimulates ribosomal protein synthesis
  Promotes glycogen synthesis
    Increases glucose transport
    Enhances activity of glycogen synthetase
    Inhibits activity of glycogen phosphorylase
Effects on fat
  Promotes triglyceride storage
    Induces lipoprotein lipase, making fatty acids available for absorption into fat cells
    Increases glucose transport into fat cells, thus increasing availability of α-glycerol phosphate for triglyceride synthesis
    Inhibits intracellular lipolysis

VLDL = very low-density lipoprotein.
Modified and reprinted, with permission from: Greenspan FS (editor): Basic & Clinical Endocrinology, 6th ed. McGraw-Hill, 2001.

three life-threatening acute complications: DKA, hyperosmolar nonketotic coma, and hypoglycemia.

Decreased insulin activity allows the catabolism of free fatty acids into ketone bodies (acetoacetate and β-hydroxybutyrate), some of which are weak acids (see Chapter 30). Accumulation of these organic acids results in an anion-gap metabolic acidosis—DKA. DKA can easily be distinguished from lactic acidosis, with which it can coexist; lactic acidosis is identified by elevated plasma lactate (> 6 mmol/L) and the absence of urine and plasma ketones. Alcoholic ketoacidosis can be differentiated by a history of recent heavy alcohol consumption (binge drinking) in a nondiabetic patient with a low or slightly elevated blood glucose level. Such patients may also have a disproportionate increase in β-hydroxybutyrate compared with acetoacetate.

Clinical manifestations of DKA include dyspnea (attempting to compensate for the metabolic acidosis), abdominal pain mimicking an acute abdomen, nausea and vomiting, and changes in sensorium. The treatment of DKA depends on correcting the hypovolemia,

Table 36–2. Diagnosis and classification of diabetes mellitus.

Diagnosis (based on blood glucose level)	
Fasting	126 mg/dL (7.0 mmol/L)
Glucose tolerance test	200 mg/dL (11.1 mmol/L)

Classification		
Type I		Absolute insulin deficiency secondary to immune-mediated or idiopathic
	II	Adult onset secondary to resistance/relative deficiency
	III	Specific types of diabetes mellitus secondary to genetic defects
	IV	Gestational

the hyperglycemia (which rarely exceeds 500 mg/dL), and total body potassium deficit, with a continuous infusion of insulin, potassium, and isotonic fluids.

The goal for decreasing blood glucose in ketoacidosis should be 75–100 mg/dL/hour or 10% an hour. Therapy can be begun with an intravenous infusion of 10 units per hour or 0.1 U/kg/hour of regular insulin, doubling the dose each hour until blood glucose begins to fall. These patients are often quite resistant to insulin therapy. As glucose moves intracellularly, so does potassium. Although this can quickly lead to a critical level of hypokalemia if not corrected, overaggressive replacement can cause an equally life-threatening hyperkalemia. Extreme swings in potassium represent the most common cause of death during treatment of ketoacidosis. Therefore, potassium, blood glucose, and serum ketones should be monitored at least hourly.

Several liters of normal saline (1–2 L the first hour, followed by 200–500 mL/hour) are typically required to correct the dehydration. Lactated Ringer's solution should be avoided since the liver eventually converts lactate to bicarbonate; in the face of potential poor tissue perfusion, volume expansion with normal saline is safest. When plasma glucose reaches 250 mg/dL, an infusion of D_5W is added to the insulin infusion to lessen the possibility of hypoglycemia and to provide a continuous source of glucose and insulin for eventual normalization of intracellular metabolism. These patients may require a nasogastric tube for gastric decompression and bladder catheterization to monitor urinary output.

Correction of severe acidosis (pH < 7.1) with bicarbonate is seldom necessary, as the acidosis corrects with volume expansion and with normalization of the hyperglycemia.

Ketoacidosis is not a feature of **hyperosmolar nonketotic coma** possibly because enough insulin is available to prevent ketone body formation. Instead, a hyperglycemic diuresis results in dehydration and hyperosmolality. Severe dehydration eventually leads to renal failure, lactic acidosis, and a predisposition to form intravascular thromboses. Hyperosmolality, frequently exceeding 360 mOsm/L, alters cerebral water balance, causing mental status changes and seizures. Severe hyperglycemia causes a factitious hyponatremia: each 100 mg/dL increase in plasma glucose lowers plasma sodium concentration by 1.6 mEq/L. Treatment includes fluid resuscitation, relatively small doses of insulin, and potassium supplementation.

Hypoglycemia in the diabetic patient is the result of an excess of insulin relative to carbohydrate intake. Furthermore, some diabetic patients are unable to counter hypoglycemia by secreting glucagon or epinephrine (**counter-regulatory failure**). The dependence of the brain on glucose as an energy source makes it the organ most susceptible to episodes of hypoglycemia. If hypoglycemia is not treated, mental status changes can progress from faintness or confusion to convulsions and permanent coma. Systemic manifestations of hypoglycemia result from catecholamine discharge and include diaphoresis, tachycardia, and nervousness. Most of the signs and symptoms of hypoglycemia will be masked by general anesthesia. Although normal plasma glucose levels are ill-defined and depend on age and sex, hypoglycemia can generally be considered to be levels of less than 50 mg/dL. The treatment of hypoglycemia is the intravenous administration of 50% glucose (each mL of 50% glucose will raise the blood glucose of a 70-kg patient by approximately 2 mg/dL).

Anesthetic Considerations

A. Preoperative:

The perioperative morbidity of diabetic patients is related to preoperative end-organ damage. In particular, the pulmonary, cardiovascular, and renal systems demand close examination. A preoperative chest radiograph in a diabetic patient is more likely to uncover cardiac enlargement, pulmonary vascular congestion, or pleural effusion. Diabetics also have an increased incidence of ST-segment and T-wave–segment abnormalities on preoperative electrocardiograms (ECGs). Myocardial ischemia may be evident on an ECG despite a negative history (**silent myocardial infarction**). Diabetic patients with hypertension have a 50% likelihood of coexisting **diabetic autonomic neuropathy** (Table 36–3). Reflex dysfunction of the autonomic nervous system may be worsened by old age, diabetes of longer than 10 years, coronary artery disease, or β-adrenergic blockade. This autonomic neuropathy may limit the heart's ability to compensate for intravascular volume changes and may predispose patients to cardiovascular instability (eg, postinduction hypotension) and even sudden car-

Table 36–3. Clinical signs of diabetic autonomic neuropathy.

Hypertension
Painless myocardial ischemia
Orthostatic hypotension
Lack of heart rate variability*
Reduced heart rate response to atropine and propranolol
Resting tachycardia
Early satiety
Neurogenic bladder
Lack of sweating
Impotence

*Normal heart rate variability during voluntary deep breathing (6 breaths/min) is greater than 10 beats/min.

diac death. Furthermore, autonomic dysfunction contributes to delayed gastric emptying (gastroparesis). Premedication with a histamine antagonist or metoclopramide would be especially prudent in an obese diabetic patient with signs of cardiac autonomic dysfunction (see Chapter 15). It must be appreciated, however, that autonomic dysfunction can affect the gastrointestinal tract without any signs of cardiac involvement.

Renal dysfunction is manifested first by proteinuria and later by elevated serum creatinine. By these criteria, most type I diabetic patients have evidence of renal failure by age 30. Because of a high incidence of infections related to a compromised immune system, strict attention to aseptic technique must accompany the placement of all intravenous catheters and invasive monitors.

Chronic hyperglycemia can lead to glycosylation of tissue proteins and a **limited-mobility joint syndrome.** Diabetic patients should be routinely evaluated preoperatively for adequate temporomandibular joint and cervical spine mobility to help predict difficult intubations, which occur in approximately 30% of persons with type I diabetes.

B. Intraoperative:

The primary goal of intraoperative blood sugar management is to avoid hypoglycemia. While attempting to maintain euglycemia is imprudent, unacceptably loose blood sugar control (> 180 mg/dL) also carries risk. Hyperglycemia has been associated with hyperosmolarity, infection, and poor wound healing. More important, hyperglycemia may worsen neurologic outcome following an episode of cerebral ischemia. Unless hyperglycemia is treated aggressively in type I diabetic patients, metabolic control may be lost, particularly in the face of major surgery or sepsis. Tight control probably benefits patients undergoing cardiopulmonary bypass by improving cardiac contractility and weaning, and by

decreasing infectious and neurologic complications. Tight control of the pregnant diabetic patient has been shown to improve fetal outcome. Nonetheless, as noted earlier, the brain's dependence on glucose as an energy supply makes it essential that hypoglycemia be avoided.

There are several perioperative management regimens for diabetic patients. In the most common, the patient receives a fraction—usually half—of the total morning insulin dose in the form of intermediate-acting insulin (Table 36–4). To lessen the risk of hypoglycemia, insulin is administered *after* intravenous access has been established and the morning blood glucose level is checked. For example, a patient who normally takes 20 units of NPH (neutral protamine Hagedorn; intermediate-acting) insulin and 10 units of regular or Lispro (short-acting) insulin or insulin analog each morning and whose blood sugar is at least 150 mg/dL would receive 15 units (half the normal morning dose) of NPH subcutaneously or intramuscularly before surgery along with an infusion of 5% dextrose solution (1.5 mL/kg/hour). Absorption of subcutaneous or intramuscular insulin depends on tissue blood flow, however, and can be unpredictable during surgery. Dedication of a small-gauge intravenous line for the dextrose infusion prevents interference with other intraoperative fluids and drugs. Supplemental dextrose can be administered if the patient becomes hypoglycemic (< 100 mg/dL). On the other hand, intraoperative hyperglycemia (> 180 mg/dL) is treated with intravenous regular insulin according to a sliding scale. One unit of regular insulin given to an adult usually lowers plasma glucose by 25–30 mg/dL. It must be stressed that these doses are approximations and do not apply to patients in catabolic states (eg, sepsis, hyperthermia).

An alternative method is to administer short-acting insulin as a continuous infusion. The advantages of this

Table 36–4. Two common techniques for perioperative insulin management in diabetes mellitus.

	Bolus Administration	Continuous Infusion
Preoperative	D$_5$W (1.5 mL/kg/h) NPH insulin (half usual AM dose)	D$_5$W (1 mL/kg/h) Regular insulin: Units / h = $\dfrac{\text{Plasma glucose}}{150}$
Intraoperative	Regular insulin (as per sliding scale)	Same as preoperative
Postoperative	Same as intraoperative	Same as preoperative

NPH = neutral protamine Hagedorn.

technique include more precise and predictable control of insulin delivery than can be achieved with a subcutaneous or intramuscular injection of NPH insulin, particularly in conditions associated with poor skin and muscle perfusion. From 10 to 15 units of regular insulin can be added to 1 L of 5% dextrose solution and infused at a rate of 1.0–1.5 mL/kg/hour (1 U/hour/70 kg). Mixing the glucose and the insulin ensures that if the intravenous line malfunctions, the patient cannot receive insulin or glucose alone. Infusing the 5% dextrose (1 mL/kg/hour) and insulin (50 units of regular insulin in 250 mL of normal saline) through separate intravenous lines, however, provides greater flexibility. As blood sugar fluctuates, the regular insulin infusion can be adjusted according to the following formula:

$$\text{Units per hour} = \frac{\text{Plasma glucose (mg / dL)}}{150}$$

For example, if the plasma glucose rose to 300 mg/dL, the rate of regular insulin infusion would be 2 U/hour (10 mL/hour of the insulin solution described above), while the glucose infusion would remain unchanged. A general target for the intraoperative maintenance of blood glucose is 120–180 mg/dL. The tighter control afforded by a continuous intravenous technique may be preferable in type I diabetics. Adding 30 mEq of KCl to each liter of dextrose might be prudent, since insulin causes an intracellular potassium shift. The effect of insulin absorption by intravenous tubing can be minimized by flushing the line before beginning the infusion. Some anesthesiologists also suggest placing the insulin infusion in a glass bottle to minimize absorption by a plastic IV bag. Because individual insulin needs can vary dramatically, any formula should be used only as a guideline.

If the patient is taking an oral hypoglycemic agent preoperatively instead of insulin, the drug can be continued until the day of surgery. Because of the long duration of action of some of these drugs (that of chlorpropamide is 1 to 3 days), a glucose infusion is begun and blood sugars are monitored as though intermediate-acting insulin had been given. The effects of oral hypoglycemic drugs with a short duration of action can be prolonged in the presence of renal failure. Many of these patients may require some exogenous insulin during the intraoperative and postoperative periods. This is because the stress of anesthesia and surgery cause elevations in counter-regulatory hormones (eg, catecholamines, glucocorticoids, growth hormone). Each of these imbalances contributes to stress hyperglycemia, which increases insulin requirements. Nonetheless, some type II diabetics will tolerate minor, brief surgical procedures without any exogenous insulin.

The key to any management regimen is to monitor plasma glucose levels frequently and appreciate the variation between patients. Patients with diabetes vary in their ability to produce endogenous insulin. Patients with brittle type I diabetes may need to have their glucose measured every hour, while every 2 or 3 hours is sufficient for many patients with type II diabetes. Likewise, insulin requirements vary with the stress of the surgical procedure. Patients receiving insulin in the morning but not going to surgery until the afternoon are prone to hypoglycemia despite a dextrose infusion. Unless an arterial line is available, drawing multiple blood specimens and sending them to the laboratory is time-consuming, expensive, and traumatic to the patient's veins. Portable **spectrophotometers** are capable of determining the glucose concentration in a drop of blood obtained from a finger stick within a minute. These devices measure the color conversion of a glucose-oxidase-impregnated strip that has been exposed to the patient's blood for a specified period. Their accuracy depends on, to a large extent, the care with which the measurements are made. Monitoring urine sugar is not accurate enough for intraoperative management.

Diabetic patients who require NPH or protamine zinc insulin are at a much greater risk for allergic reactions to protamine sulfate—including anaphylactic shock and death. Unfortunately, surgeries that require the use of heparin and subsequent reversal with protamine (eg, coronary artery bypass grafting) are more common in diabetic patients. These patients should receive a small protamine test dose of 1–5 mg over 5–10 minutes prior to the full reversal dose.

C. POSTOPERATIVE:

Close monitoring of the diabetic's blood sugar must continue postoperatively. One reason for this is the individual variation in onset and duration of action of insulin preparations (Table 36–5). For example, the onset of action of regular insulin may be less than 1 hour, but its duration of action may exceed 6 hours. NPH insulin typically has an onset of action within 2 hours, but the action can last longer than 24 hours. Another reason for close monitoring is the progression of stress hyperglycemia in the recovery period. If large volumes of lactate-containing intravenous fluids have been administered intraoperatively, blood sugar will tend to rise 24–48 hours postoperatively as the liver converts the lactate to glucose. Diabetic outpatients may require admission to the hospital overnight if persistent nausea and vomiting from gastroparesis prevent oral intake.

Table 36–5. Summary of bioavailability characteristics of the insulins.*

	Insulin Type	Onset	Peak Action	Duration
Short-acting	Lispro	10–20 min	30–90 min	4–6 hrs
	Regular, Actrapid, Velosulin	15–30	1–3 hrs	5–7 hrs
	Semilente, Semitard	30–60 min	4–6 hrs	12–16 hrs
Intermediate-acting	Lente, Lentard, Monotard, NPH, Insulatard	2–4 hrs	8–10 hrs	18–24 hrs
Long-acting	Ultralente, Ultratard, PZI	4–5 hrs	8–14 hrs	25–36 hrs

NPH = neutral protamine Hagedorn; PZI = protamine zinc insulin
*There is considerable patient-to-patient variation.

■ THE THYROID

Physiology

Dietary iodine is absorbed by the gastrointestinal tract, converted to iodide ion, and actively transported into the thyroid gland. Once inside, iodide is oxidized back to iodine, which is bound to the amino acid **tyrosine.** The end result is two hormones—**triiodothyronine** (T_3) and **thyroxine** (T_4)—which are bound to proteins and stored within the thyroid. Although the gland releases more T_4 than T_3, the latter is more potent and less protein-bound. Most T_3 is formed peripherally from partial deiodination of T_4. An elaborate feedback mechanism controls thyroid hormone synthesis and involves the hypothalamus (thyrotropin-releasing hormone), the anterior pituitary (thyroid-stimulating hormone, or TSH), and autoregulation (thyroid iodine concentration).

Thyroid hormone increases carbohydrate and fat metabolism and is an important factor in determining growth and metabolic rate. An increase in metabolic rate is accompanied by a rise in oxygen consumption and CO_2 production, indirectly increasing minute ventilation. Heart rate and contractility are also increased, presumably from an alteration in adrenergic-receptor physiology, as opposed to an increase in catecholamine levels.

HYPERTHYROIDISM

Clinical Manifestations

Excess thyroid hormone levels can be caused by Graves' disease, toxic multinodular goiter, thyroiditis, thyroid-stimulating-hormone-secreting pituitary tumors, functioning thyroid adenomas, or overdosage of thyroid replacement hormone. Clinical manifestations of excess thyroid hormones include weight loss, heat intolerance, muscle weakness, diarrhea, hyperactive reflexes, and nervousness. A fine tremor, exophthalmos, or goiter may be noted, particularly when the cause is Graves' disease. Cardiac signs range from sinus tachycardia to atrial fibrillation and congestive heart failure. The diagnosis of hyperthyroidism is confirmed by abnormal thyroid function tests, which may include an elevation in total (bound and unbound) serum thyroxine, serum triiodothyronine, and free (unbound) thyroxine.

Medical treatment of hyperthyroidism relies on drugs that inhibit hormone synthesis (eg, propylthiouracil, methimazole), prevent hormone release (eg, potassium, sodium iodide), or mask the signs of adrenergic overactivity (eg, propranolol). While β-adrenergic antagonists do not affect thyroid gland function, they do decrease the peripheral conversion of T_4 to T_3. Radioactive iodine destroys thyroid cell function but is not recommended for pregnant patients and may result in hypothyroidism. Subtotal thyroidectomy is now less commonly used as an alternative to medical therapy. Typically, it is reserved for patients with large toxic multinodular goiters or solitary toxic adenomas. Graves' disease is currently usually treated with thyroid drugs or radioiodine.

Anesthetic Considerations

A. PREOPERATIVE:

All elective surgical procedures, including subtotal thyroidectomy, should be postponed until the patient is rendered euthyroid with medical treatment. The days of a "thyroid steal" induction with covertly administered medications are past. Preoperative assessment should include normal thyroid function tests, and a resting heart rate less than 85 beats per minute has been recommended. Benzodiazepines are a good choice for preoperative sedation. Antithyroid medications and β-adrenergic antagonists are continued through the morning of surgery. If emergency surgery must proceed, the hyperdynamic circulation can be controlled by titration of an esmolol infusion.

B. INTRAOPERATIVE:

Cardiovascular function and body temperature should be closely monitored in patients with a history of hyperthyroidism. Patients' eyes should be well protected, since the exophthalmos of Graves' disease increases the risk of corneal abrasion or ulceration. The head of the operating table can be raised 15–20 degrees to aid venous drainage and decrease blood loss, although doing so increases the risk of venous air embolism. An armored endotracheal tube passed beyond the goiter will lessen the risk of kinking and airway obstruction.

Ketamine, pancuronium, indirect-acting adrenergic agonists, and other drugs that stimulate the sympathetic nervous system are avoided because of the possibility of exaggerated elevations in blood pressure and heart rate. Thiopental may be the induction agent of choice, since it possesses some antithyroid activity at high doses. Hyperthyroid patients can be chronically hypovolemic and vasodilated and are prone to an exaggerated hypotensive response during induction. Adequate anesthetic depth must be obtained, however, before laryngoscopy or surgical stimulation to avoid tachycardia, hypertension, and ventricular dysrhythmias.

Hyperthyroid patients display accelerated drug biotransformation and may theoretically be more susceptible to hepatic injury from halothane or kidney toxicity from enflurane. Neuromuscular blocking agents (also called muscle relaxants) should be administered cautiously, because thyrotoxicosis is associated with an increased incidence of myopathies and myasthenia gravis. Hyperthyroidism does not increase anesthetic requirements—ie, there is no change in minimum alveolar concentration.

C. POSTOPERATIVE:

The most serious threat to hyperthyroid patients in the postoperative period is **thyroid storm,** which is characterized by hyperpyrexia, tachycardia, altered consciousness (eg, agitation, delirium, coma), and hypotension. The onset is usually 6–24 hours after surgery but can occur intraoperatively, mimicking malignant hyperthermia. Unlike malignant hyperthermia, however, thyroid storm is not associated with muscle rigidity, elevated creatine kinase, or a marked degree of lactic and

respiratory acidosis. Treatment includes hydration and cooling, an esmolol infusion or intravenous propranolol (0.5-mg increments until the heart rate is < 100/min), propylthiouracil (250 mg every 6 hours orally or by nasogastric tube) followed by sodium iodide (1 g intravenously over 12 hours), and correction of any precipitating cause (eg, infection). Cortisol (100–200 mg every 8 hours) is recommended to prevent complications from coexisting adrenal gland suppression. Thyroid storm is a medical emergency that requires aggressive management and monitoring (see Case Discussion, Chapter 49).

Subtotal thyroidectomy is associated with several potential surgical complications. **Recurrent laryngeal nerve palsy** will result in hoarseness (unilateral) or aphonia and **stridor** (bilateral). Vocal cord function can be evaluated by laryngoscopy immediately following deep extubation. Failure of one or both cords to move may require intubation and exploration of the wound. **Hematoma formation** may cause airway compromise from collapse of the trachea in patients with tracheomalacia. Dissection into the compressible soft tissues of the neck may make intubation difficult. Immediate treatment includes opening the neck wound and evacuating the clot, then reassessing the need for reintubation. **Hypoparathyroidism** from unintentional removal of the parathyroid glands will cause acute hypocalcemia within 24–72 hours (see Clinical Manifestations under Hypoparathyroidism, below). Unintentional **pneumothorax** is a possible complication of neck exploration.

HYPOTHYROIDISM

Clinical Manifestations

Hypothyroidism can be caused by autoimmune disease (eg, Hashimoto's thyroiditis), thyroidectomy, radioactive iodine, antithyroid medications, iodine deficiency, or failure of the hypothalamic-pituitary axis (secondary hypothyroidism). Hypothyroidism during neonatal development results in cretinism, a condition marked by physical and mental retardation. Clinical manifestations in the adult are usually subtle and include weight gain, cold intolerance, muscle fatigue, lethargy, constipation, hypoactive reflexes, dull facial expression, and depression. Subclinical hypothyroidism commonly occurs in elderly patients with severe illnesses. Heart rate, myocardial contractility, stroke volume, and cardiac output decrease, and extremities are cool and mottled because of peripheral vasoconstriction. Pleural, abdominal, and pericardial effusions are common. The diagnosis of hypothyroidism may be confirmed by a low free T_4 level. Primary hypothyroidism is differentiated from secondary disease by an elevation in TSH. The treatment of hypothyroidism consists of oral replacement therapy with a thyroid hormone preparation, which takes several days to produce a physiologic effect and several weeks to evoke clear-cut clinical improvement.

Myxedema coma results from extreme hypothyroidism and is characterized by impaired mentation, hypoventilation, hypothermia, hyponatremia (from inappropriate antidiuretic hormone secretion), and congestive heart failure. It is more common in elderly patients and may be precipitated by infection, surgery, or trauma. Myxedema coma is a life-threatening disease that has been successfully treated with intravenous thyroid hormones. A loading dose of T_3 or T_4 (eg, 300–500 mg of levothyroxine sodium in patients without heart disease) is followed by a maintenance infusion (eg, 50 mg of levothyroxine per day). The ECG must be monitored during therapy to detect myocardial ischemia or dysrhythmias. Steroid replacement (eg, hydrocortisone, 100 mg intravenously every 8 hours) is routinely given in case of coexisting adrenal gland suppression. Some patients may require ventilatory support.

Anesthetic Considerations

A. PREOPERATIVE:

Patients with uncorrected severe hypothyroidism (T_4 < 1 mg/dL) or myxedema coma should not undergo elective surgery and should be treated with thyroid hormone prior to emergency surgery. While a euthyroid state is ideal, mild to moderate hypothyroidism does not appear to be an absolute contraindication to surgery. In fact, hypothyroid patients with symptomatic coronary artery disease may benefit from a delay in thyroid therapy until after coronary artery bypass surgery.

Hypothyroid patients usually do not require much preoperative sedation and may be prone to drug-induced respiratory depression. Consideration should be given to premedicating these patients with histamine H_2 antagonists and metoclopramide because of their slowed gastric-emptying times. Patients who have been rendered euthyroid may receive their usual dose of thyroid medication on the morning of surgery; it must be remembered, however, that most commonly used preparations have long half-lives (the t½ of T_4 is about 8 days).

B. INTRAOPERATIVE:

Hypothyroid patients are more susceptible to the hypotensive effect of anesthetic agents because of their diminished cardiac output, blunted baroreceptor reflexes, and decreased intravascular volume. For this reason, ketamine is often recommended for induction of anesthesia. The possi-

bility of coexistent primary adrenal insufficiency or congestive heart failure should be considered in cases of refractory hypotension. Decreased cardiac output may speed the rate of induction with an inhalational anesthetic, but hypothyroidism does not significantly decrease minimum alveolar concentration. Other potential problems include hypoglycemia, anemia, hyponatremia, difficulty during intubation because of a large tongue, and hypothermia from a low basal metabolic rate.

C. POSTOPERATIVE:

Recovery from general anesthesia may be delayed in hypothyroid patients by hypothermia, respiratory depression, or slowed drug biotransformation. These patients often require prolonged mechanical ventilation. Patients should remain intubated until awake and close to normothermic. Because hypothyroidism increases vulnerability to respiratory depression, a nonopioid such as ketorolac would be a good choice for postoperative pain relief.

■ THE PARATHYROID GLANDS

Physiology

Parathyroid hormone is the principal regulator of calcium homeostasis. It increases serum calcium by promoting bone resorption, limiting renal excretion, and indirectly enhancing gastrointestinal absorption by its effect on vitamin D metabolism. Parathyroid hormone decreases serum phosphate by increasing renal excretion. The effects of parathyroid hormone on calcium serum levels are countered in lower animals by calcitonin, a hormone excreted by parafollicular C-cells in the thyroid, but a physiologic calcium-lowering effect for calcitonin has not been demonstrated in humans (Table 36–6). Ninety-nine percent of total body calcium is in the skeleton. Of the calcium in the blood, 40% is bound to proteins and 60% is ionized or complexed to organic ions. Unbound ionized calcium is physiologically the more important of the two.

HYPERPARATHYROIDISM

Clinical Manifestations

Causes of **primary hyperparathyroidism** include adenoma, carcinoma, and hyperplasia of the parathyroid gland. **Secondary hyperparathyroidism** is an adaptive response to hypocalcemia produced by diseases such as renal failure or intestinal malabsorption syndromes. **Ec-**

Table 36–6. Actions of major calcium-regulating hormones.

	Bone	Kidney	Intestines
Parathyroid hormone	Increases resorption of calcium and phosphate	Increases reabsorption of calcium; decreases reabsorption of phosphate; increases conversion of $25OHD_3$ to $1,25 (OH)_2 D_3$; decreases reabsorption of bicarbonate	No direct effects
Calcitonin	Decreases resorption of calcium and phosphate	Decreases reabsorption of calcium and phosphate; questionable effect on vitamin D metabolism	No direct effects
Vitamin D	Maintains Ca^{2+} transport system	Decreases reabsorption of calcium	Increases absorption of calcium and phosphate

Reproduced with permission from: Greenspan FS (editor): Basic & Clinical Endocrinology, 6th ed. McGraw-Hill, 2001.

topic hyperparathyroidism is due to production of parathyroid hormone by rare tumors outside the parathyroid gland. Parathyroid hormone-related peptide may cause significant hypercalcemia when secreted by a carcinoma (eg, hepatoma, bronchogenic carcinoma) and is the most common cause of humoral hypercalcemia of malignancy.

Most of the clinical manifestations of hyperparathyroidism are due to hypercalcemia (Table 36–7). Causes of hypercalcemia (other than hyperparathyroidism) include bone metastases, vitamin D intoxication, milk-alkali syndrome, sarcoidosis, and prolonged immobilization (see Chapter 28). The treatment of hyperparathyroidism depends on the cause, but surgical removal of all four glands is usually required in the set-

Table 36–7. Effects of hyperparathyroidism.

Organ System	Clinical Manifestations
Cardiovascular	Hypertension, ventricular dysrhythmias, ECG changes (shortened QT interval)*
Renal	Impaired renal concentrating ability, hyperchloremic metabolic acidosis, polyuria, dehydration, polydipsia, renal stones, renal failure
Gastrointestinal	Ileus, nausea and vomiting, peptic ulcer disease, pancreatitis
Musculoskeletal	Muscle weakness, osteoporosis
Neurologic	Mental status change (eg, delirium, psychosis, coma)

ECG = electrocardiogram.
*The QT interval may be prolonged at serum calcium levels > 16 mg/dL.

ting of parathyroid hyperplasia. However, removal of a single adenoma cures many patients with sporadic primary hyperparathyroidism.

Anesthetic Considerations

Preoperative evaluation should include an assessment of volume status to avoid hypotension during induction. Hydration with normal saline and diuresis with furosemide usually decrease serum calcium to acceptable levels (< 14 mg/dL, 7 mEq/L, or 3.5 mmol/L). Rarely, more aggressive therapy with the intravenous bisphosphonates pamidronate (Aredia) or etridronate (Didronel) may be necessary. Plicamycin (Mithramycin), glucocorticoids, calcitonin, or dialysis may be necessary when intravenous bisphosphonates are not sufficient or are contraindicated. Hypoventilation should be avoided, since acidosis increases ionized calcium. Elevated calcium levels can cause cardiac dysrhythmias. The response to neuromuscular blocking agents may be altered in patients with preexisting muscle weakness caused by the effects of calcium at the neuromuscular junction. Osteoporosis worsened by hyperparathyroidism predisposes patients to vertebral compression during laryngoscopy and bone fractures during transport. The postoperative complications of parathyroidectomy are similar to those described above for subtotal thyroidectomy.

HYPOPARATHYROIDISM

Clinical Manifestations

Hypoparathyroidism is usually due to deficiency of parathyroid hormone following parathyroidectomy. Clinical manifestations of hypoparathyroidism are a result of hypocalcemia (Table 36–8), which is also caused by renal failure, hypomagnesemia, vitamin D defi-

Table 36–8. Effects of hypoparathyroidism.

Organ System	Clinical Manifestations
Cardiovascular	Hypotension, congestive heart failure, ECG changes (prolonged QT interval)
Musculoskeletal	Muscle cramps, weakness
Neurologic	Neuromuscular irritability (eg, laryngospasm, inspiratory stridor, tetany, seizures), perioral paresthesia, mental status changes (eg, dementia, depression, psychosis)

ECG = electrocardiogram.

ciency, and acute pancreatitis (see Chapter 28). Hypoalbuminemia decreases total serum calcium (a 1 g/dL drop in serum albumin causes a 0.8 mg/dL decrease in total serum calcium), but ionized calcium, the active entity, is unaltered. Neuromuscular irritability can be clinically confirmed by the presence of Chvostek's sign (painful twitching of the facial musculature following tapping over the facial nerve) or Trousseau's sign (carpopedal spasm following inflation of a tourniquet above systolic blood pressure for 3 minutes). These signs are also occasionally present in normal persons. Treatment of symptomatic hypocalcemia consists of intravenous administration of calcium chloride.

Anesthetic Considerations

Serum calcium should be normalized in any patient with cardiac manifestations of hypocalcemia. Anesthetics that depress the myocardium should be avoided in these patients. Alkalosis from hyperventilation or sodium bicarbonate therapy will further decrease ionized calcium. Although citrate-containing blood products do not usually lower serum calcium significantly, they should not be administered rapidly in patients with preexisting hypocalcemia. Other considerations include avoiding the use of 5% albumin solutions (which might bind and lower ionized calcium) and exploring the possibility of coagulopathy or a sensitivity to nondepolarizing neuromuscular blocking agents.

■ THE ADRENAL GLAND

Physiology

The adrenal gland is divided into two parts. The **adrenal cortex** secretes androgens, mineralocorticoids (eg, aldosterone), and glucocorticoids (eg, cortisol). The **adrenal medulla** secretes catecholamines (eg, epinephrine, norepinephrine, dopamine). The adrenal androgens have insignificant relevance for anesthetic management and will not be considered further.

Aldosterone is chiefly involved with fluid and electrolyte balance. Aldosterone secretion causes sodium to be reabsorbed in the distal renal tubule in exchange for potassium and hydrogen ions. The net effect is an expansion in extracellular fluid volume caused by fluid retention, a decrease in plasma potassium, and metabolic alkalosis. Aldosterone secretion is stimulated by the renin-angiotensin system (specifically, angiotensin II), pituitary ACTH (adrenocorticotropic hormone), and hyperkalemia. Hypovolemia, hypotension, congestive heart failure, and surgery result in an elevation of aldosterone concentrations.

Glucocorticoids are essential for life and have multiple physiologic effects. Metabolic actions include enhanced gluconeogenesis and inhibition of peripheral glucose utilization. These anti-insulin effects tend to raise blood glucose and worsen diabetic control. Glucocorticoids are required for vascular and bronchial smooth muscle to be responsive to catecholamines. Because these hormones are structurally related to aldosterone, they tend to promote sodium retention and potassium excretion (a mineralocorticoid effect). ACTH from the anterior pituitary is the principal regulator of glucocorticoid secretion. Secretion of ACTH and glucocorticoids exhibits a diurnal rhythm, is stimulated by stress, and is inhibited by circulating glucocorticoids. Endogenous production of cortisol, the most important glucocorticoid, averages 20 mg/day.

The structure, biosynthesis, physiologic effects, and metabolism of **catecholamines** are discussed in Chapter 12. Eighty percent of adrenal catecholamine secretion in humans is in the form of epinephrine. Catecholamine release is regulated mainly by cholinergic preganglionic fibers of the sympathetic nervous system that innervate the adrenal medulla. Stimuli include hypotension, hypothermia, hypoglycemia, hypercapnia, hypoxemia, pain, and fear.

MINERALOCORTICOID EXCESS

Clinical Manifestations

Intrinsic hypersecretion of aldosterone by the adrenal cortex (**primary aldosteronism** and patients with **Conn's syndrome**) can be due to a unilateral adenoma (aldosteronoma), bilateral hyperplasia, or carcinoma of the adrenal gland. Some diseases stimulate aldosterone secretion by affecting the renin-angiotensin system. For example, congestive heart failure, hepatic cirrhosis with ascites, nephrotic syndrome, and some forms of hypertension (eg, renal artery stenosis) can cause **secondary aldosteronism.** Although both primary and secondary aldosteronism are characterized by increased levels of aldosterone, only the latter is associated with increased renin activity. Clinical manifestations of mineralocorticoid excess include an elevation in blood pressure, hypervolemia, hypokalemia, muscle weakness, and metabolic alkalosis. Prolonged hypokalemia may lead to a renal concentrating defect and polyuria. Alkalosis will lower ionized calcium levels and can cause tetany. Serum sodium is often normal.

Anesthetic Considerations

Fluid and electrolyte disturbances can be corrected preoperatively with supplemental potassium and spironolactone. This aldosterone antagonist is a potassium-sparing diuretic with antihypertensive properties. Intravascular volume can be assessed preoperatively by testing for orthostatic hypotension or measuring cardiac filling pressures. Correction of plasma potassium, however, does not guarantee normal total body potassium.

MINERALOCORTICOID DEFICIENCY

Clinical Manifestations & Anesthetic Considerations

Atrophy or destruction of both adrenal glands results in a combined deficiency of mineralocorticoids and glucocorticoids (see Glucocorticoid Deficiency, below). Nonetheless, unilateral adrenalectomy, diabetes, or heparin therapy occasionally causes isolated hypoaldosteronism. These patients are hyperkalemic, acidotic, and usually hypotensive (the opposite of mineralocorticoid excess). Preoperative preparation includes treatment with an exogenously administered mineralocorticoid (eg, fludrocortisone).

GLUCOCORTICOID EXCESS

Clinical Manifestations

Glucocorticoid excess may be due to exogenous administration of steroid hormones, intrinsic hyperfunction of the adrenal cortex (eg, adrenocortical adenoma), ACTH production by a non-pituitary tumor (ectopic ACTH syndrome), or hypersecretion by a pituitary adenoma (Cushing's disease). Regardless of the cause, an excess of corticosteroids produces **Cushing's syndrome,** characterized by muscle wasting and weakness, osteoporosis, central obesity, abdominal striae,

glucose intolerance, hypertension, and mental status changes.

Anesthetic Considerations

Patients with Cushing's syndrome tend to be volume-overloaded and have hypokalemic metabolic alkalosis resulting from the mineralocorticoid activity of glucocorticoids. These abnormalities should be corrected preoperatively with supplemental potassium and spironolactone. Patients with osteoporosis are at risk for fracture during positioning, while preoperative weakness may indicate an increased sensitivity to neuromuscular blocking agents. If the cause of Cushing's syndrome is exogenous glucocorticoids, the patient's adrenal glands may not be able to respond to perioperative stresses, and supplemental steroids are indicated (see Glucocorticoid Deficiency, below). Likewise, patients undergoing adrenalectomy require intraoperative glucocorticoid replacement (intravenous hydrocortisone succinate, 100 mg every 8 hours). Other complications of adrenalectomy include significant blood loss during resection of a highly vascularized tumor and unintentional penetration of the pleura, causing pneumothorax.

GLUCOCORTICOID DEFICIENCY

Clinical Manifestations

Primary adrenal insufficiency (Addison's disease) is caused by destruction of the adrenal gland, which results in a combined mineralocorticoid and glucocorticoid deficiency. Clinical manifestations are due to aldosterone deficiency (hyponatremia, hypovolemia, hypotension, hyperkalemia, and metabolic acidosis) and cortisol deficiency (weakness, fatigue, hypoglycemia, hypotension, and weight loss). Etomidate suppresses adrenal function by inhibiting enzymes that are essential for the production of corticosteroid hormones (see Chapter 8); long-term etomidate therapy can lead to significant glucocorticoid deficiency.

Secondary adrenal insufficiency is a result of inadequate ACTH secretion by the pituitary. The most common cause of secondary adrenal insufficiency is iatrogenic, as a result of the administration of exogenous glucocorticoids. Because mineralocorticoid secretion is usually adequate in this disease, fluid and electrolyte disturbances are usually not present. Acute adrenal insufficiency (**addisonian crisis**), however, can be triggered in steroid-dependent patients who do not receive increased doses during periods of stress (eg, infection, trauma, surgery). The clinical features of this medical emergency include circulatory collapse, fever, hypoglycemia, and depressed mentation.

Anesthetic Considerations

 The key to the anesthetic management of patients with glucocorticoid deficiency is to ensure adequate steroid replacement therapy during the perioperative period. Because the risk of supplementation is probably quite low, all patients who have received potentially suppressive doses of steroids (eg, the daily equivalent of 5 mg of prednisone) by any route of administration (topical, inhalational, or oral) for a period of more than 2 weeks any time in the previous 12 months should be considered unable to respond appropriately to surgical stress.

What represents adequate steroid coverage is controversial. While adults normally secrete 20 mg of cortisol daily, this may increase to over 300 mg under conditions of maximal stress. Thus, one recommendation is to administer 100 mg of hydrocortisone phosphate every 8 hours beginning the evening before or on the morning of surgery. An alternative low-dose regimen (25 mg of hydrocortisone at the time of induction followed by an infusion of 100 mg during the subsequent 24 hours) achieves plasma cortisol levels equal to or higher than those reported in healthy patients undergoing similar elective surgery. This second regimen might be especially appropriate for diabetic patients, in whom glucocorticoid administration often interferes with control of blood glucose.

CATECHOLAMINE EXCESS

Clinical Manifestations

Pheochromocytoma is a catecholamine-secreting tumor that consists of cells originating from the embryonic neural crest (chromaffin tissue) and accounts for 0.1% of all cases of hypertension. While the tumor is usually benign and localized in a single adrenal gland, 10–15% are malignant, and another 10–15% are bilateral or extra-adrenal. The cardinal manifestations of pheochromocytoma are paroxysmal headache, hypertension, sweating, and palpitations. Unexpected intraoperative hypertension and tachycardia are occasionally the first indications of an undiagnosed pheochromocytoma. The pathophysiology, diagnosis, and treatment of these tumors require an understanding of catecholamine metabolism and of the pharmacology of adrenergic agonists and antagonists. The Case Discussion in Chapter 12 examines these aspects of pheochromocytoma management.

Anesthetic Considerations

Preoperative assessment should focus on the adequacy of adrenergic blockade and volume replacement. Specifically, resting arterial blood pressure, orthostatic blood pressure and heart rate changes, ventricular ectopy, and electrocardiographic evidence of ischemia should be evaluated.

A decrease in red cell mass and plasma volume contributes to the severe chronic hypovolemia seen in these patients. Although the hematocrit is usually elevated or normal, depending on the relative contribution of these two factors, it does not reliably reflect volume status. Preoperative α-adrenergic blockade with phenoxybenzamine helps correct the volume deficit, in addition to correcting hypertension and hyperglycemia. A drop in hematocrit should accompany the expansion of circulatory volume; this often unmasks an underlying anemia.

Potentially life-threatening variations in blood pressure—particularly during induction and manipulation of the tumor—indicate the need for direct arterial pressure monitoring. Large intraoperative fluid-volume shifts underscore the importance of good intravenous access and urinary output monitoring. Young patients with healthy hearts probably only need central venous pressure monitoring, although patients with evidence of catecholamine cardiomyopathy may benefit from the use of a pulmonary artery catheter.

Intubation should not be attempted until a deep level of anesthesia has been established. Intraoperative hypertension can be effectively treated with phentolamine, nitroprusside, or nicardipine. Nitroprusside is favored by some anesthesiologists because of a more rapid onset of action, a shorter duration of action, and increased familiarity with the drug. Phentolamine specifically blocks adrenergic receptors and prevents the effects of excessive circulating catecholamines. Nicardipine is being used more and more often preoperatively and intraoperatively. Anesthetic drugs or techniques that stimulate the sympathetic nervous system (eg, ephedrine, ketamine, hypoventilation), potentiate the dysrhythmic effects of catecholamines (eg, halothane), inhibit the parasympathetic nervous system (eg, pancuronium), or release histamine (eg, atracurium, morphine sulfate) may precipitate hypertension and are best avoided.

After tumor ligation and resection, the primary problem frequently becomes *hypotension* from hypovolemia, persistent adrenergic blockade, and prior tolerance to the high levels of endogenous catecholamines that have abruptly ended. Fluid resuscitation should include consideration of surgical bleeding and third-space fluid loss. Assessment of intravascular volume includes urinary output, central venous pressure, arterial blood pressure and, if available, pulmonary capillary occlusion pressure. Infusions of adrenergic agonists, such as phenylephrine or norepinephrine, may occasionally prove necessary. Postoperative *hypertension* may indicate the presence of occult tumors or volume overload.

■ OBESITY

Overweight and obesity are classified using the body mass index (BMI). Overweight is defined as a BMI of ≥ 30 kg/m². Extreme obesity (old term "morbid obesity") is defined as a BMI of ≥ 40 kg/m². Health risks increase with the degree of obesity and with increased abdominal distribution of weight. Men with a waist measurement of ≥ 40 inches and women with a waist measurement of ≥ 35 inches are at increased health risk. For a patient 1.8 meters tall and weighing 70 kg, the BMI would be as shown in the following formula:

$$BMI = \frac{\text{Weight (kg)}}{(\text{Height [meters]})^2} = \frac{70 \text{ kg}}{1.8^2} = \frac{70}{3.24} = 21.6 \text{ kg}/\text{m}^2$$

Clinical Manifestations

Obesity is associated with many diseases, including type II diabetes mellitus, hypertension, coronary artery disease, and cholelithiasis. Even in the absence of obvious coexisting disease, however, extreme obesity has profound physiologic consequences. Oxygen demand, CO_2 production, and alveolar ventilation are elevated because metabolic rate is proportional to body weight. Excessive adipose tissue over the thorax decreases chest wall compliance even though lung compliance may remain normal. Increased abdominal mass forces the diaphragm cephalad, yielding lung volumes suggestive of restrictive lung disease. Reductions in lung volumes are accentuated by the supine and Trendelenburg positions. In particular, functional residual capacity may fall below closing capacity. If this occurs, some alveoli will close during normal tidal volumes, causing a ventilation/perfusion mismatch.

While obese patients are often found to be hypoxic, only a few are hypercapnic, which should alert one to impending complications. Obesity-hypoventilation syndrome (**Pickwickian syndrome**) is a complication of extreme obesity characterized by hypercapnia, cyanosis-induced polycythemia, right-sided heart failure, and somnolence. These patients appear to have blunted respiratory drive and often suffer from loud snoring and upper-airway obstruction during sleep (**obstructive sleep apnea syndrome [OSAS]**). Patients often report dry mouths and short arousals, while bed partners frequently describe apnea pauses. OSAS has also been associated with increased perioperative complications including hypertension, hypoxia, dysrhyth-

mias, myocardial infarction, pulmonary edema, and stroke. Difficult airway management during induction and upper airway obstruction during recovery should be anticipated.

Patients are particularly vulnerable during the postoperative period if opioids or other sedatives have been given, and if they are placed supine, making the upper airway even more prone to obstruction. For patients with known or suspected OSAS, a trial of postoperative CPAP (continuous positive airway pressure) should be considered until such time as the anesthesiologist can be sure that the patient can protect his or her airway and maintain spontaneous ventilation without evidence of obstruction.

The heart is also exposed to an increased workload, since cardiac output and blood volume rise in order to perfuse additional fat stores. The elevation in cardiac output (0.1 L/min/kg of adipose tissue) is achieved through an increase in stroke volume—as opposed to heart rate—and frequently results in arterial hypertension and left ventricular hypertrophy. Elevations in pulmonary blood flow and pulmonary artery vasoconstriction from persistent hypoxia can lead to pulmonary hypertension and cor pulmonale.

Obesity is also associated with gastrointestinal pathophysiology, including hiatal hernia, gastroesophageal reflux, poor gastric emptying, and hyperacidic gastric fluid, and it has also been associated with an increased risk of gastric cancer. Fatty infiltration of the liver also occurs and may be associated with abnormal liver tests, but the extent of infiltration does not correlate well with the degree of liver test abnormality.

Anesthetic Considerations

A. PREOPERATIVE:

For the reasons outlined above, obese patients are at an increased risk for developing aspiration pneumonia. Routine pretreatment with H_2 antagonists and metoclopramide should be considered. Premedication with respiratory depressant drugs must be avoided in patients with evidence of preoperative hypoxia, hypercapnia, or obstructive sleep apnea. Intramuscular injections are often unreliable owing to the thickness of the overlying adipose tissue.

Preoperative evaluation of extremely obese patients undergoing major surgery should attempt to assess cardiopulmonary reserve with a chest radiograph, an ECG, arterial blood gases, and pulmonary function tests. Classic physical signs of cardiac failure (eg, sacral edema) may be difficult to identify. Blood pressures must be taken with the appropriate size cuff (see Figure 6–10). Intravenous and intra-arterial access sites should be checked in anticipation of technical difficulties. Obscured landmarks, difficult positioning, and extensive layers of adipose tissue may make regional anesthesia impossible with standard equipment and techniques.

The airway should receive particular attention, since these patients are often difficult to intubate as a result of limited mobility of the temporomandibular and atlanto-occipital joints, a narrowed upper airway, and a shortened distance between the mandible and sternal fat pads.

B. INTRAOPERATIVE:

Because of the risk of aspiration, obese patients are usually intubated for all but the shortest of general anesthetics. Furthermore, controlled ventilation with large tidal volumes often provides better oxygenation than do shallow, spontaneous respirations. If intubation appears likely to be difficult, keeping the patient awake and intubating with a fiberoptic bronchoscope is strongly recommended. Breath sounds may be difficult to appreciate; confirmation of tracheal intubation requires detection of end-tidal CO_2. Even controlled ventilation may require relatively high-inspired oxygen concentrations to prevent hypoxia, especially in the lithotomy, Trendelenburg, or prone position. Subdiaphragmatic abdominal laparotomy packs can cause further deterioration of pulmonary function and a reduction of arterial blood pressure by impairing venous return. The addition of positive end-expiratory pressure worsens pulmonary hypertension in some patients with extreme obesity.

Volatile anesthetics may be metabolized more extensively in obese patients. This is of particular concern with respect to the defluorination of halothane and enflurane. Increased metabolism and a predisposition to hypoxia may explain the increased incidence of halothane hepatitis in obese patients. Volatile anesthetics distribute so slowly to the lipid stores that increasing the fat reservoir has little clinical effect on wake-up time, even during long surgical procedures.

Theoretically, larger fat stores provide an increased volume of distribution for lipid-soluble drugs (eg, benzodiazepines, opioids). Thus, a larger loading dose would be required to produce the same plasma concentration. This is the rationale for basing some drug doses on actual body weight in obese patients. By the same reasoning, maintenance doses should be administered less frequently because clearance would be expected to be slower with a larger volume of distribution. In contrast, water-soluble drugs (eg, neuromuscular blocking agents) have a much more limited volume of distribution, which should not be influenced by fat stores. The dosing of these drugs should therefore be based on ideal body weight to avoid overdosing. In reality, however, clinical practice does not always validate these expectations.

The technical difficulties associated with regional anesthesia have been mentioned. Although dosage requirements for epidural and spinal anesthesia are difficult to predict, obese patients usually require 20–25% less local anesthetic because of epidural fat and distended epidural veins. A high level of blockade can easily result in respiratory compromise. Continuous epidural anesthesia has the advantage of providing pain relief and lessening respiratory complications in the postoperative period.

C. POSTOPERATIVE:

Respiratory failure is the major postoperative problem of extremely obese patients. The risk of postoperative hypoxia is increased by preoperative hypoxia and by surgery involving the thorax or upper abdomen (especially vertical incisions). Extubation should be delayed until the effects of neuromuscular blocking agents are completely reversed and the patient is fully awake. An obese patient should remain intubated until there is no doubt that an adequate airway and tidal volume will be maintained. This does *not* mean that all obese patients need to remain on ventilators overnight in an intensive care unit. If the patient is extubated in the operating room, supplemental oxygen should be provided during transportation to the recovery room. A 45-degree modified sitting position will unload the diaphragm and improve ventilation and oxygenation. The risk of hypoxia extends for several days into the postoperative period, and providing supplemental oxygen should be routinely considered. Other common postoperative complications in obese patients include wound infection, deep venous thrombosis, and pulmonary embolism.

CARCINOID SYNDROME

Carcinoid syndrome is the complex of signs and symptoms caused by the secretion of vasoactive substances (eg, serotonin, kallikrein, histamine) from enterochromaffin tumors (**carcinoid tumors**). Since most of these tumors are located in the gastrointestinal tract, their metabolic products are released into the portal circulation and destroyed by the liver before they can cause systemic effects. However, the products of nonintestinal tumors (eg, pulmonary, ovarian) or hepatic metastases bypass the portal circulation and, therefore, can cause a variety of clinical manifestations.

Clinical Manifestations

The most common manifestations of carcinoid syndrome are cutaneous flushing, bronchospasm, profuse diarrhea, dramatic swings in arterial blood pressure

Table 36–9. Principal mediators of carcinoid syndrome and their clinical manifestations.

Mediator	Clinical Manifestations
Serotonin	Vasoconstriction (coronary artery spasm, hypertension), increased intestinal tone, water and electrolyte imbalance (diarrhea) tryptophan deficiency (hypoproteinemia, pellagra)
Kallikrein	Vasodilation (hypotension, flushing), bronchoconstriction
Histamine	Vasodilation (hypotension, flushing), dysrhythmias, bronchoconstriction

(usually hypotension), and supraventricular dysrhythmias (Table 36–9). Carcinoid syndrome is associated with right-sided heart disease caused by valvular and myocardial plaque formation. Lung metabolism of serotonin evidently prevents involvement of the left side of the heart. The diagnosis of carcinoid syndrome is confirmed by detection of serotonin metabolites in the urine (5-hydroxyindoleacetic acid) or suggested by elevated plasma levels of chromogranin A. Treatment varies depending on tumor location but may include surgical resection, symptomatic relief, or specific serotonin and histamine antagonists. Somatostatin, an inhibitory peptide, reduces the release of vasoactive tumor products.

Anesthetic Considerations

The key to anesthetic management of these patients is to avoid anesthetic techniques or agents that could cause the tumor to release vasoactive substances. For example, hypotension, which can itself cause hormone release, should be treated with volume expansion. Catecholamine administration has been associated with kallikrein activation. Regional anesthesia may limit perioperative stress and the subsequent release of vasoactive agents. Clearly, histamine-releasing drugs (eg, morphine and atracurium) should be avoided. Surgical manipulation of the tumor can cause a massive release of hormones. Monitoring should include an arterial line and a central venous or pulmonary artery catheter because of the hemodynamic instability and intrinsic heart disease caused by carcinoid syndrome. Alterations in carbohydrate metabolism may lead to unsuspected hypoglycemia or hyperglycemia. Consultation with an endocrinologist may help clarify the role of antihistamine, antiserotonin drugs (eg, methysergide), octreotide (a long-acting somatostatin analog), or antikallikrein drugs (eg, corticosteroids) in specific patients.

CASE DISCUSSION: MULTIPLE ENDOCRINE NEOPLASIA

An isolated thyroid nodule is discovered during physical examination of a 36-year-old woman complaining of diarrhea and headaches. Work-up of the tumor reveals hypercalcemia and an elevated calcitonin level, which leads to the diagnosis of medullary cancer. During induction of general anesthesia for total thyroidectomy, the patient's blood pressure rises to 240/140 mm Hg and her heart rate approaches 140 beats/min, with frequent premature ventricular contractions. The surgery is canceled, an arterial line is placed, and the patient is treated with intravenous phentolamine, propranolol, lidocaine, and sodium nitroprusside.

What is the probable cause of this patient's hypertensive crisis during induction of general anesthesia?

Multiple endocrine neoplasia (MEN) is characterized by tumor formation in several endocrine organs. MEN type I consists of pancreatic (gastrinomas, insulinomas), pituitary (chromophobes), and parathyroid tumors. MEN type II consists of medullary thyroid carcinoma, pheochromocytoma, and hyperparathyroidism (type IIa) or multiple mucosal neuromas (type IIb or type III). The hypertensive episode in this case may be due to a previously undiagnosed pheochromocytoma. The pheochromocytoma in MEN often consists of small multiple tumors. These patients are typically young adults with strong family histories of MEN. If multiple surgeries are planned, pheochromocytoma resection will usually be scheduled first.

What is calcitonin, and why is it associated with medullary cancer?

Calcitonin is a polypeptide manufactured by the parafollicular cells (C cells) in the thyroid gland. It is secreted in response to increases in plasma ionic calcium and tends to lower calcium levels by affecting kidney and bone function. Therefore, it acts as an antagonist of parathyroid hormone (see Table 36–6).

Why is this patient hypercalcemic if calcitonin lowers serum calcium?

An excess or deficiency of calcitonin has minor effects in humans compared with the effects of parathyroid disorders. This patient's hypercal-

cemia may be due to coexisting primary hyper-parathyroidism (MEN type IIa).

Are headache and diarrhea consistent with the diagnosis of MEN?

The history of headaches suggests the possibility of pheochromocytoma, while diarrhea may be due to calcitonin or one of the other peptides often produced by medullary thyroid carcinoma (eg, ACTH [adrenocorticotropin hormone], somatostatin, β-endorphin).

What follow-up is required for this patient?

Because of the life-threatening hemodynamic changes associated with pheochromocytoma, this entity must be medically controlled before surgery can be considered (see Case Discussion, Chapter 12). Because MEN syndromes are hereditary, family members should be screened for early signs of pheochromocytoma, thyroid cancer, and hyper-parathyroidism.

SUGGESTED READING

Adams JP, Murphy PG: Obesity in anaesthesia and intensive care. Br J Anaesth 2000; 85:91.

Graham GW, Unger BP, Coursin DB: Perioperative management of selected endocrine disorders. Int Anesthesiol Clin 2000; 38:31.

Kirby RR: *Clinical Anesthesia Practice,* 2nd ed. Saunders, 2000.

Prys-Roberts C: Phaeochromocytoma—recent progress in its management. Br J Anaesth 2000; 85:44.

Stoelting RK, Dierdorf SF: *Handbook of Anesthesia and Co-existing Disease,* 2nd ed., Churchill Livingstone, 2002.

Wilson JD, Foster DW, Kronenberg HM, et al: *Williams Textbook of Endocrinology,* 9th ed. WB Saunders and Company, 1998.

Anesthesia for Patients with Neuromuscular Disease

37

KEY CONCEPTS

 The weakness associated with myasthenia gravis is thought to be due to autoimmune destruction or inactivation of postsynaptic acetylcholine receptors at the neuromuscular junction, leading to a reduced number of receptors and loss of folds on the postsynaptic membrane.

 Patients who have myasthenia gravis with respiratory muscle or bulbar involvement are at increased risk for pulmonary aspiration.

 Many patients with myasthenia gravis are exquisitely sensitive to nondepolarizing muscle relaxants.

 The following factors have been suggested as being predictive of the need for postoperative ventilation following thymectomy in patients who have myasthenia gravis with bulbar involvement: disease duration of more than 6 years, concomitant pulmonary disease, a peak inspiratory pressure of < –25 cm H_2O (ie, –20 cm H_2O), a vital capacity < 4 mL/kg, and a pyridostigmine dose > 750 mg/d.

 Patients with the myasthenic syndrome are very sensitive to both depolarizing and nondepolarizing muscle relaxants.

 Succinylcholine has been used safely in some patients with Duchenne's and Becker's muscular dystrophies but is best avoided because of unpredictable responses and the risks of inducing severe hyperkalemia or triggering malignant hyperthermia.

 Anesthetic management of patients with periodic paralysis is directed toward preventing attacks. Careful electrocardiographic monitoring is necessary to detect attacks and arrhythmias during anesthesia.

 In patients with periodic paralysis, the response to muscle relaxants is unpredictable. Increased sensitivity to nondepolarizing relaxants is especially apt to be encountered in those with hypokalemic periodic paralysis.

Although neuromuscular disorders are relatively uncommon, patients present to the operating room with some regularity at tertiary medical centers for diagnostic studies, for treatment of complications, or for surgical management of unrelated disorders. Diminished respiratory muscle strength and enhanced sensitivity to muscle relaxants (also called neuromuscular blocking agents) predispose these patients to postoperative ventilatory failure. A basic understanding of the major disorders and their potential interaction with anesthetic agents is necessary to avoid postoperative morbidity of this nature.

MYASTHENIA GRAVIS

Myasthenia gravis is characterized by weakness and easy fatigability of skeletal muscle. The incidence of myasthenia is about 1:10,000 and is highest in women during their third decade; in men, it typically presents in the sixth and seventh decades. The weakness is thought to be due to autoimmune destruction or inactivation of postsynaptic acetylcholine receptors at the neuromuscular junction, leading to a reduced number of receptors and loss of folds on the postsynaptic membrane. Antibodies against the acetylcholine receptor in neuromuscular junctions are found in over 90% of patients with generalized myasthenia gravis and up to 80% of patients with ocular myasthenia. Fifteen percent of myasthenics develop a thymoma, while 65% have thymic hyperphasia. Other autoimmune disorders (hypothyroidism, hyperthyroidism, rheumatoid arthritis) are also present in 10% of patients.

The course of the disease is marked by exacerbations and remissions. Remissions may be partial or complete. The weakness can be asymmetric, confined to one group of muscles, or generalized. Ocular muscles are most commonly affected, resulting in fluctuating ptosis and diplopia. With bulbar involvement, laryngeal and pharyngeal muscle weakness can result in dysarthria, difficulty in chewing and swallowing, problems clearing secretions, or pulmonary aspiration. Severe disease is usually also associated with proximal muscle weakness (primarily in the neck and shoulders) and involvement of respiratory muscles. Muscle strength characteristically improves with rest but deteriorates rapidly with exertion. Infection, stress, surgery, and pregnancy have unpredictable effects on the disease but often lead to exacerbations.

Treatment is with anticholinesterase drugs, immunosuppressants, glucocorticoids, plasmapheresis, intravenous immunoglobulin, and thymectomy. Anticholinesterase drugs are the most commonly used agents. These drugs increase the amount of acetylcholine at the neuromuscular junction through inhibition of end-plate acetylcholinesterase. Pyridostigmine is the most commonly used agent; when given orally, it has an effective duration of 2–4 hours. Excessive administration of an anticholinesterase may precipitate **cholinergic crisis,** which is characterized by increased weakness and excessive muscarinic effects, including salivation, diarrhea, miosis, and bradycardia. An **edrophonium test** may help differentiate a cholinergic from a myasthenic crisis. Increased weakness after up to 10 mg of intravenous edrophonium indicates cholinergic crisis, whereas increasing strength implies **myasthenic crisis.** If this test is equivocal or if the patient clearly has manifestations of cholinergic hyperactivity, then all cholinesterase drugs should be discontinued and the patient monitored closely (in most cases in an intensive care unit). Up to 85% of patients under the age of 55 show clinical improvement following thymectomy even in the absence of a tumor, but improvement may be delayed up to several years. Therapy with corticosteroids and immunosuppressants (ie, azathioprine, mycophe-

nolate mofetil, cyclosporine or cyclophosphamide) is also effective. Plasmapheresis or intravenous immunoglobulin may be used to treat impending or developed crisis (ie, severe dysphagia or respiratory failure) or to prepare moderately to severely affected patients for thymectomy.

Anesthetic Considerations

Patients with myasthenia may present for thymectomy or for unrelated surgical or obstetric procedures. In all cases, patients should be under the best possible medical control prior to operation. Patients scheduled for thymectomy often have deteriorating muscle strength, while those undergoing other elective procedures may be well controlled or in remission. Adjustments in anticholinesterase medication, immunosuppressants, or steroid therapy may be necessary. Management of anticholinesterase therapy in the perioperative period is controversial but should probably be individualized. Potential problems in continuing such therapy include altered patient requirements following surgery, increased vagal reflexes, and the possibility of disrupting bowel anastomoses secondary to hyperperistalsis. Moreover, because these agents also inhibit plasma cholinesterase, they can prolong the duration of ester-type local anesthetics and succinylcholine. Conversely, patients with advanced generalized disease may deteriorate significantly when anticholinesterase agents are withheld.

When in doubt, it is often best to withhold cholinesterase inhibitors in the immediate postoperative period and, if necessary, treat severe myasthenia manifestations with plasmapheresis or intravenous immunoglobulin. However, the majority of patients can withstand withdrawal of cholinesterase drugs for a few days without difficulty. These medications can be restarted when the patient resumes oral intake. When necessary, cholinesterase inhibitors can also be given parenterally at 1/30 the oral dose.

Preoperative evaluation should focus on the recent course of the disease, the muscle groups affected, drug therapy, and coexisting illnesses. Patients with respiratory muscle or bulbar involvement are at increased risk for pulmonary aspiration. Premedication with metoclopramide or an H_2 blocker may decrease this risk, but supporting studies are lacking in this group of patients. Because some patients with myasthenia are often very sensitive to respiratory depressants, premedication with opioids, benzodiazepines, and similar drugs is usually omitted.

With the exception of muscle relaxants, standard anesthetic agents may be used in patients with myasthenia gravis. Marked respiratory depression, however, may be encountered following even moderate doses of barbiturates or opioids. Propofol may be preferable because of its short duration of action. A volatile agent–based anesthetic is generally most satisfactory. Deep anesthesia with a volatile agent alone in patients with myasthenia may provide sufficient relaxation for endotracheal intubation as well as most surgical procedures. Some clinicians routinely try to avoid muscle relaxants. The response to succinylcholine is unpredictable. Patients may manifest a relative resistance, a prolonged effect, or an unusual response (phase II block; see Chapter 9). The dose of succinylcholine may be increased to 2 mg/kg to overcome any resistance, but a prolonged effect should be anticipated. Many patients are exquisitely sensitive to nondepolarizing muscle relaxants. Even a defasciculating dose in some patients can result in nearly complete paralysis. If a muscle relaxant is necessary, small doses of a relatively short-acting nondepolarizing agent (cisatracurium, mivacurium, or rapacuronium*) is preferred. Neuromuscular blockade should be monitored very closely with a nerve stimulator. Ventilatory function should be evaluated carefully prior to extubation. Patients with bulbar involvement may be at greatest risk for postoperative respiratory failure. Disease duration of more than 6 years, concomitant pulmonary disease, a peak inspiratory pressure of < −25 cm H_2O (ie, −20 cm H_2O), a vital capacity < 4 mL/kg, and a pyridostigmine dose > 750 mg/d have been suggested as predictive of the need for postoperative ventilation following thymectomy.

Women with myasthenia can experience increased weakness in the last trimester of pregnancy and the early postpartum period. Epidural anesthesia is generally preferable for these patients because it avoids potential problems with respiratory depression and muscle relaxants during general anesthesia. Excessively high levels of motor blockade, however, can also result in hypoventilation. Babies of myasthenic mothers may show transient myasthenia for 1–3 weeks, induced by transplacental transfer of acetylcholine receptor antibodies, sometimes necessitating controlled mechanical ventilation.

LAMBERT-EATON MYASTHENIC SYNDROME

The **Lambert-Eaton myasthenic syndrome (LEMS)**, is a paraneoplastic syndrome characterized by proximal

---

* At the time of publication, rapacuronium had been voluntarily withdrawn by the manufacturer. See Chapter 9 for details.

muscle weakness that typically begins in the lower extremities, but may spread to involve upper limb, bulbar, and respiratory muscles. Dry mouth, male impotence, and other manifestations of autonomic dysfunction are also very common. LEMS is usually associated with small cell carcinoma of the lung. It may also be seen with other occult malignancies or as an idiopathic autoimmune disease. The disorder results from presynaptic defect of neuromuscular transmission. Antibodies to voltage-gated calcium channels on the nerve terminal markedly reduce the quantal release of acetylcholine at the motor end-plate. Small cell carcinoma cells express identical voltage-gated calcium channels, serving as a trigger for the autoimmune response in patients with paraneoplastic LEMS.

In contrast to myasthenia gravis, muscle weakness improves with repeated effort and is improved less dramatically by anticholinesterase drugs. Guanidine hydrochloride and 3,4-diaminopyridine (DAP), which increases the release of acetylcholine, often produce significant improvement in LEMS. The use of guanidine is limited by hepatoxicity. DAP is only available on a compassionate-use basis in the United States, but is widely available in other countries. Many patients with LEMS improve with immunosuppression or plasmapheresis.

Patients with the **myasthenic syndrome** are very sensitive to both depolarizing and nondepolarizing muscle relaxants. The response to other drugs used in anesthesia is usually normal. Volatile agents alone are usually sufficient to provide muscle relaxation for both intubation and most surgical procedures. Muscle relaxants should be given only in small increments and with careful neuromuscular monitoring. The management of autonomic defects is discussed in Chapter 27.

MUSCULAR DYSTROPHIES

Preoperative Considerations

Muscular dystrophies are a group of hereditary disorders characterized by progressive weakness and degeneration of muscle. Sporadic cases are presumably due to mutations. **Duchenne's muscular dystrophy** is the most common and most severe form. Other major variants include Becker's, myotonic facioscapulohumeral, and limb-girdle dystrophies.

Duchenne's Muscular Dystrophy

An X-linked recessive disorder, Duchenne's muscular dystrophy affects males almost exclusively. It has an incidence of approximately 1–3 cases per 10,000 live male births and most commonly presents between 3 and 5 years of age. Affected individuals produce abnormal **dystrophin,** a protein found on the sarcolemma of muscle fibers. Patients characteristically develop symmetric proximal muscle weakness that is manifested as a gait disturbance. Fatty infiltration typically causes enlargement (pseudohypertrophy) of muscles, especially the calves. Progressive weakness and contractures eventually result in kyphoscoliosis. By age 12, most patients are confined to wheelchairs. Disease progression may be delayed by up to 2 to 3 years with glucocorticoid therapy in some patients. Intellectual impairment is common but generally nonprogressive. Plasma creatine kinase (CK) levels are 10 to 100 times normal even early in the disease and are thought to reflect an abnormal increase in the permeability of muscle cell membranes. Female carriers often also have high plasma CK levels, variable degrees of muscle weakness and, rarely, cardiac involvement. Plasma myoglobin concentration may also be elevated. The diagnosis is confirmed by muscle biopsy. Detection of deletions or duplications in the dystrophin gene may be detected by Southern blot analysis or polymerase chain reaction methods in 65% of patients with Duchenne's or Becker's muscular dystrophy.

Degeneration of the respiratory muscles interferes with an effective coughing mechanism and leads to retention of secretions and frequent pulmonary infections. The combination of marked kyphoscoliosis and muscle wasting produces a severe restrictive ventilatory defect. Pulmonary hypertension is common with disease progression. Degeneration of cardiac muscle is common, but results in dilated or hypertrophic cardiomyopathy in only 10% of patients. Mitral regurgitation secondary to papillary muscle dysfunction can also be documented in up to 25% of patients. Electrocardiographic (ECG) abnormalities include P–R interval prolongation, QRS and ST-segment abnormalities, and prominent R waves over the right precordium with deep Q waves over the left precordium. Atrial arrhythmias are common. Death is usually due to recurrent pulmonary infections, respiratory failure, or cardiac failure by the age of 15 to 25 years.

Becker's Muscular Dystrophy

This less common disorder (1:30,000 male births) is also an X-linked recessive muscular dystrophy. It is also thought to be due to a deletion or point mutation in the dystrophin gene, leading to a defect in dystrophin production. Manifestations are virtually identical to those of Duchenne's muscular dystrophy except that they usually present later in life (adolescence) and progress more slowly. Mental retardation is less common. Patients often reach the fourth or fifth decade, although they may survive into their 80s. Death is usually from respiratory complications. Cardiomyopathy may occur in some cases and may precede severe skeletal weakness.

Myotonic Dystrophy

Myotonic dystrophy (MD) is a multisystem disorder that is the most common cause of myotonia—slowing of relaxation after muscle contraction in response to electrical or percussive stimuli. The disease is transmitted in an autosomal dominant fashion and has an incidence of 1:8000. The most common form is localized to chromosome 19,locusq12.3; the gene codes for a serine/threonine protein kinase. An abnormally long trinucleotide repeat is thought to lead to the disease. MD manifests in the second to third decade of life; however, patients can present from infancy to late life. Myotonia is the principle manifestation early in the disease, but as the disease progresses, muscle weakness and atrophy become more prominent. This weakness and atrophy usually affect cranial muscles (orbicularis oculi and oris, masseter, and sternocleidomastoid) and result in the typical facial appearance. As opposed to most myopathies, distal muscles are more involved than proximal muscles. Plasma CK levels are normal or slightly elevated.

Multiple organ systems are involved in the disease as evidenced by presenile cataracts; premature frontal baldness; hypersomnolence with sleep apnea; and endocrine dysfunction leading to pancreatic, adrenal, thyroid, and gonadal insufficiency. Respiratory involvement leads to decreased vital capacity. Alveolar hypoventilation is caused by either pulmonary or central nervous system dysfunction. Chronic hypoxemia may lead to cor pulmonale. Gastrointestinal hypomotility can predispose patients to pulmonary aspiration. Uterine atony can prolong labor and increases the incidence of retained placenta. Cardiac manifestations, which are often present before other clinical symptoms appear, consist of atrial arrhythmias, varying degrees of heart block and, less frequently, depression of ventricular function.

The myotonia is usually described by patients as a "stiffness" that may ease with continued activity, the so-called "warm-up" phenomenon. Cold temperatures are often reported by patients to worsen stiffness, although electrophysiological studies have shown improvement in myotonic discharges with cooling. Antimyotonic treatment can be undertaken with membrane stabilizing medications. Phenytoin, quinine sulfate, and procainamide have all been used in this manner. Phenytoin does not appear to worsen cardiac conduction abnormalities, while quinine and procainamide may prolong the P–R interval. Mexiletine and tocainide should not be used in patients with MD. A cardiac pacemaker should be placed in patients with significant conduction defect, even if asymptomatic.

Facioscapulohumeral Dystrophy

This dystrophy is an autosomal dominant variant with an incidence of approximately 1–3:100,000, due to a DNA deletion on chromosome 4q35. It affects both males and females, although more females with the gene defect are asymptomatic. Patients usually present in the second or third decade of life with weakness that is confined chiefly to the muscles of the face and the shoulder girdle. Muscles in the lower extremities are less commonly affected, and respiratory muscles are usually spared. The disease is slowly progressive and has a variable course. Plasma CK levels are usually normal or only slightly elevated. Cardiac involvement is rare, but atrial paralysis has been reported in a few patients. The latter results in loss of all atrial electrical activity and an inability to atrially pace the heart; ventricular pacing is still possible. Longevity is minimally affected in most of these patients.

Limb-Girdle Dystrophy

Limb-girdle muscular dystrophy is a heterogeneous entity composed of several variants of neuromuscular diseases, which are further being defined by molecular genetics. Limb-girdle syndromes include severe childhood autosomal recessive muscular dystrophy (SCARMD, chromosome 13), autosomal recessive muscular dystrophy (chromosome 15), and other incompletely defined autosomal recessive syndromes such as Erb's (scapulohumeral type) and Leyden-Mobius (pelvifemoral type). Most patients present in childhood to the second or third decade of life with muscle weakness that may involve the shoulder girdle, the hip girdle, or both. The disease tends to be very slowly progressive. Plasma CK levels are usually elevated. Cardiac involvement, similar to that which occurs in Duchenne's muscular dystrophy, can present as frequent arrhythmias or congestive heart failure but is relatively uncommon. Respiratory complications, such as hypoventilation and recurrent respiratory infections, may occur early in the disease but is more common after long-standing disease (> 30 years).

Anesthetic Considerations

DUCHENNE'S AND BECKER'S MUSCULAR DYSTROPHIES:

The anesthetic management of these patients is complicated not only by muscle weakness but also by cardiac and pulmonary manifestations. An association with malignant hyperthermia has been suggested but is controversial. Preoperative premedication with sedatives or opioids is best avoided, because patients may be at increased

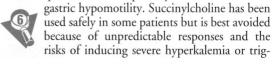 risk for aspiration from respiratory muscle weakness or gastric hypomotility. Succinylcholine has been used safely in some patients but is best avoided because of unpredictable responses and the risks of inducing severe hyperkalemia or triggering malignant hyperthermia. Although some patients exhibit a normal response to nondepolarizing muscle relaxants, others may be very sensitive. Marked respiratory and circulatory depression may be seen with volatile anesthetics in patients with advanced disease. Regional or local anesthesia may therefore be preferable in these patients. Respiratory complications are largely responsible for perioperative morbidity. Patients with vital capacities less than 30% of predicted appear to be at greatest risk and often require temporary postoperative mechanical ventilation.

MYOTONIC DYSTROPHY:

Patients with MD are at high risk for perioperative respiratory and cardiac complications. Surgery with general anesthesia should be avoided, therefore, when not absolutely necessary. Knowledge of the patients' diagnosis of MD is obviously vital to patient care; however, patients with the disease may not volunteer this information, and some patients may be simply presymptomatic and undiagnosed. The diagnosis of MD has been made in some patients only after prolonged apnea after general anesthesia. Most perioperative problems arise in MD patients with severe weakness and in those cases where surgeons and anesthesiologists are unaware of the diagnosis.

Patients with MD have altered responses to a number of anesthetic medicines. They are often very sensitive to even small doses of opioids, sedatives, and inhalational and intravenous (thiopental) agents, all of which may cause sudden and prolonged apnea. Premedication should therefore be avoided, if possible. Succinylcholine has been relatively contraindicated because it may precipitate intense myotonic contractions; trismus can prevent opening the mouth for intubation. Myotonic contraction of respiratory, chest wall, or laryngeal muscles can make ventilation difficult or impossible. Other drugs that act on the motor end-plate, such as decamethonium, neostigmine, and physostigmine, can aggravate myotonia. Regional anesthesia can be employed but does not always prevent myotonic contractions. Troublesome myotonia rarely occurs, but can be reduced by injecting procaine in the muscles or by giving quinine hydrochloride 300 to 600 mg intravenously.

The response to nondepolarizing neuromuscular blocking agents is reported to be normal; however, they do not consistently prevent or relieve myotonic contractions. As reversal of nondepolarizing neuromuscular blocking agents can induce myotonic contractions, the use of short-acting nondepolarizing agents (cisatracurium, mivacurium, rapacuronium*) is recommended. The postoperative shivering commonly associated with volatile agents, especially when associated with decreased body temperature, can induce myotonic contractions in the recovery room. Small doses of meperidine can often prevent such shivering and perhaps the myotonic contractions.

Induction of anesthesia without complications has been reported for a number of agents including thiopental, inhalational agents, and propofol (with or without ketamine). Neuromuscular blockade, if needed, should be performed with short-acting agents. Nitrous oxide and inhalational agents can be used as maintenance anesthesia. Reversal with anticholinesterases is to be avoided, if possible. There is no association of the type of anesthesia used and any postoperative complications.

The main postoperative complications are pulmonary: prolonged ventilatory failure, pneumonia, and atelectasis. Aggressive pulmonary hygiene with physical therapy, incentive spirometry, and careful postoperative monitoring are indicated. Aspiration prophylaxis is also probably indicated (see Chapter 15). Patients undergoing upper abdominal surgery or those with severe proximal weakness are more likely to experience this type of complication. Perioperative cardiac conduction abnormalities are less likely to occur but still warrant close cardiovascular monitoring.

As association between MD and malignant hyperthermia has been suggested but has not been firmly established. It does not seem, therefore, that patients with MD are at an increased risk for malignant hyperthermia. Interestingly, both disorders map to chromosome 19, albeit in different locations.

OTHER FORMS OF MUSCULAR DYSTROPHY:

Patients with facioscapulohumeral and limb-girdle muscular dystrophy generally have normal responses to anesthetic agents. Nonetheless, because of the great variability and overlap between the various forms of muscular dystrophy, nondepolarizing muscle relaxants should be used cautiously, and succinylcholine should probably be avoided.

MYOTONIAS

Myotonia Congenita & Paramyotonia Congenita

Myotonia congenita is a disorder manifested early in life with generalized myotonia. The disease is caused by mutations of a gene on chromosome 7q35 encoding a

chloride channel of the skeletal muscle fiber surface membrane. Both autosomal dominant (Thomsen's) and recessive (Becker's) forms exist. The disease is confined to skeletal muscle and produces no, minimal, or nonprogressive weakness. Many patients, in fact, have very well developed musculature due to near constant muscle contraction. Myotonia is usually more bothersome in patients with myotonia than in those with MD. Antimyotonic therapy includes phenytoin, mexiletine, quinine sulfate, or procainamide. Other medicines that have been used include tocainide, dantrolene, prednisone, acetazolamide, and taurine. There is no cardiac involvement in myotonia congenita, and a normal life span is expected.

Paramyotonia congenita is a very rare autosomal dominant disorder localized to chromosome 17q. Mutations in the α-subunit of the sodium channel are associated with the disease. Symptoms of paramyotonia congenita include transient stiffness (myotonia) and, occasionally, weakness after exposure to cold temperatures. The stiffness worsens with activity, in contrast to true myotonia, thus the term "paramyotonia." Serum potassium concentration may rise following an attack similar to hyperkalemic periodic paralysis (see below). Medicines that have been used to block the cold response include mexiletine and tocainide.

Anesthetic management of patients with myotonia congenita and paramyotonia is complicated by an abnormal response to succinylcholine, troublesome intraoperative myotonic contractions, and the need to avoid hypothermia. Neuromuscular blocking agents may paradoxically cause generalized muscle spasms, including trismus, leading to difficulty with intubation and ventilation.

Infiltration of muscles in the operative field with a dilute local anesthetic may alleviate refractory myotonic contraction. No patients with these types of myotonia have been reported with positive in vitro tests for malignant hyperthermia. Excised muscle in these patients does, however, display a prolonged myotonic contraction when exposed to a depolarizing neuromuscular blocking agent. Excessive muscle contraction during anesthesia, therefore, likely represents aggravation of myotonia and not malignant hyperthermia.

PERIODIC PARALYSIS

This group of disorders is characterized by sudden attacks of transient muscle weakness or paralysis. Symptoms usually begin in childhood. The attacks generally last a few hours and typically spare respiratory muscles. Secondary abnormalities in serum potassium concentration are common and are thought to reflect abnormal sodium and potassium transport across cell membranes. These entities are classified into primary genetic

---

* At the time of publication, rapacuronium had been voluntarily withdrawn by the manufacturer. See Chapter 9 for details.

channelopathies and secondary acquired forms. The genetic or inherited types are in two major categories. There is a dominantly inherited disorder in which there is a defect in voltage-gated, calcium channels. This entity is typically associated with low serum potassium levels during spells of weakness. A dominantly inherited defect in sodium channels, which also results in periodic paralysis, is typically associated with elevated serum potassium levels during episodes of weakness. Both defects result in inexcitable muscle membranes to both direct and indirect stimulation due to either decreased potassium conductance or increased sodium conductance, respectively. Both are associated with fluid and electrolyte shifts. Both disorders are inherited as autosomal dominant traits, but both have a number of allelic variants resulting in different presentations in different families. Paramyotonia with sensitivity to cold is one example of the sodium channelopathies.

The primary forms of these disorders have a number of clinical similarities. They are characterized by sporadic episodes of weakness. Muscle strength and serum potassium concentrations are usually normal between attacks. The disorder is characterized by worsening by hypothermia. The weakness lasts less than 1 hour, but can last 2 days, and frequent attacks can lead to progressive long-term weakness in some patients. Episodes can be increased by rest after vigorous exercise, but minimized by continued muscle exercise.

1. Voltage-Gated Calcium Channelopathy (Hypokalemic Periodic Paralysis)

The hypokalemic variant usually presents in childhood to early adulthood. As time progresses, there is usually an increased frequency of attacks, although they may subside in later life.

The hypokalemic variant is most common and may be inherited, occur sporadically, or be associated with hyperthyroidism. Up to 10% of hyperthyroid men of Latin or Asian descent have episodes of hypokalemic periodic paralysis. The episodes are characterized by weakness or paralysis of limb muscles that last 3–4 hours, but they may last for days. Episodes are most common in the early morning and can be precipitated by strenuous exertion or high carbohydrate meals. Mild exertion can actually prevent or delay paralysis. Interestingly, local anesthetics with antiphlogistics can precipitate an episode. During an attack, the potassium level is normal to moderately decreased, along with the phosphorus level. The kidneys retain sodium, potassium, chloride, and water, which are associated with increased intracellular fluid volume and decreased extracellular volume. This order may be associated with oliguria, obstipation, and diaphoresis. There may be ECG changes (see Chapter 28) consistent with a low potassium level. As noted, permanent muscle damage can develop as the attacks increase in frequency.

The diagnosis is usually made by a careful family history, the patient's history, and notation of changing potassium levels during an attack. There is no evidence of myotonia on electromyography. An acute attack is typically treated with 2–10 g of oral potassium without glucose, with mild physical activity being encouraged. Intravenous potassium is no longer recommended because it may lead to hyperkalemia. This disorder may be prevented by the administration of low-dose acetazolamide. Glucose solutions should be avoided, as uptake of glucose by cells, associated with changes in serum potassium, can exacerbate the hypokalemia and weakness.

A secondary form of this same disorder is associated with thyrotoxicosis. It resembles the primary form but is much more common in men than women, especially in persons of Asiatic descent and in young adults. Once the thyroid condition is treated, the episodes usually cease. The disorder can develop in anywhere from 10–25% of hyperthyroid Asian men. The metabolic sequelae and fluid and electrolyte shifts that are seen in the primary form are also seen in secondary hypokalemic periodic paralysis. Treatment involves the management of the hyperthyroidism, avoidance of high carbohydrate and low potassium meals, and potassium chloride for acute attacks.

Secondary hypokalemic paralysis can also develop if there are marked losses of potassium through the kidneys or through the gastrointestinal tract. It is associated with weakness, which is at times episodic. Potassium levels are much lower than in any other variant. There are many causes of this entity. Therapy of the primary disease with potassium replacement as well as treating acidosis or alkalosis is important in preventing attacks.

Persons who consume large amounts of barium salts, because they block potassium channels, can also develop hypokalemic period paralysis. This condition is treated by stopping the barium salts and administering oral potassium.

Sodium Channelopathy (Hyperkalemic Periodic Paralysis)

Patients with this type of periodic paralysis are prone to shorter (1–2 hours) but more frequent attacks. It is a primary hyperkalemic muscle membrane sodium channelopathy. Although it is dominant, there are multiple allelic mutations. The paralysis is triggered by abnormal inactivation of sodium channels by a mild increase in potassium. Sodium and water flow into the cells with prolonged depolarization. There is hemoconcentration associated with the elevation in serum potassium levels.

The clinical presentation is usually during childhood with early morning episodes, which increase in frequency over time. The episodes are more frequent and worse with rest after strenuous exercise. However, mild exercise prevents paralysis in the same muscles. The frequency of the attacks decrease later in life. Hypothermia, pregnancy, the administration of glucocorticoids, and potassium aggravate the condition. During an attack, the potassium levels usually increase to over 6 mEq/L but remain normal between attacks. Because of the shift of sodium and water into cells, it may also be associated with hyponatremia and hemoconcentration. Other electrolyte shifts have been noted. Hypothermia can induce weakness or make it worse.

Normokalemic periodic paralysis resembles hyperkalemic periodic paralysis and often has the same genotype. They differ in the lack of benefit from glucose, because the potassium level is normal during an episode. Even though potassium levels are normal, these patients also can develop persistent myopathy.

A high potassium level between episodes of weakness suggests a secondary form of the disorder. In these circumstances, the diagnosis is made based on a careful review of the family history, clinical documentation of an elevated potassium level between attacks, and electromyogram demonstrating myotonia associated with vigorous exercise followed by rest. In this circumstance, therapy is with frequent high-carbohydrate meals, maintenance of a low potassium diet if possible, and avoidance of strenuous activity and cold. Acetazolamide may help prevent attacks. Interestingly, paramyotonia congenita is an allelic variant of the sodium channel mutation.

There is a secondary hyperkalemic disorder seen in persons, men more often than women, with potassium levels over 7 mEq/L. Weakness persists between attacks. There are multiple medical causes, but common to all the hyperkalemic disorders is weakness with rest after exercise. Treatment is targeted toward the primary disease and restriction of potassium.

Anesthetic Considerations

Regardless of the type of periodic paralysis, anesthetic management of patients with the disorder is directed toward preventing attacks. Careful ECG monitoring is necessary to detect attacks and arrhythmias during anesthesia. Frequent intraoperative measurements of plasma potassium concentration is advisable whenever possible. Glucose-containing intravenous fluids should not be used in patients with hypokalemic paralysis, whereas such solutions may benefit patients with hyperkalemic and normokalemic paralysis (see above). Neuromuscular function should be

carefully monitored during general anesthesia. The response to muscle relaxants is unpredictable. Increased sensitivity to nondepolarizing relaxants is especially apt to be encountered in patients with hypokalemic periodic paralysis. Succinylcholine is contraindicated in hyperkalemic paralysis and perhaps other variants as well because of the risk of hyperkalemia. Because shivering and hypothermia may trigger attacks, maintenance of core temperature intraoperatively is important (see Chapter 6).

CASE DISCUSSION: ANESTHESIA FOR MUSCLE BIOPSY

A 16-year-old boy with progressive proximal muscle weakness is suspected of having a primary myopathy and is scheduled for biopsy of the quadriceps muscle.

What other potential abnormalities should concern the anesthesiologist?

The diagnosis of myopathy can be difficult and may include any one of several hereditary, inflammatory, endocrine, metabolic, or toxic disorders. A muscle biopsy may be necessary to supplement clinical, laboratory, nerve conduction, and electromyographic findings and help establish the diagnosis. Although the cause of the myopathy in this case is not yet clear, the clinician must always consider potential problems that can be associated with primary myopathies.

Respiratory muscle involvement should always be suspected in patients with muscle weakness. Pulmonary reserve can be assessed clinically by questions regarding dyspnea and activity level. Pulmonary function tests (see Chapter 22) are indicated if significant dyspnea on exertion is present. An increased risk of pulmonary aspiration is suggested by a history of dysphagia, regurgitation, recurrent pulmonary infections, or abdominal distention. Cardiac abnormalities may be manifested as arrhythmias, mitral valve prolapse, or cardiomyopathy. A 12-lead electrocardiogram is also helpful in excluding conduction abnormalities. A chest radiograph can evaluate inspiratory effort, the pulmonary parenchyma, and cardiac size; gastric distention secondary to smooth muscle or autonomic dysfunction may also be evident. Preoperative laboratory evaluation should have excluded a metabolic cause with measurement of serum sodium, potassium, magnesium, calcium, and phosphate concentrations. Similarly, thyroid, adrenal, and pituitary disorders should have been excluded. Plasma creatine kinase (CK) measurement may not be helpful, but very high levels (10 times normal) generally suggest a muscular dystrophy or polymyositis.

What anesthetic technique should be used?

The choice of anesthesia should be based on both patient and surgical requirements. Most muscle biopsies can be performed under local or regional anesthesia with supplemental intravenous sedation, using small doses of midazolam. Since most procedures are performed on an outpatient basis, spinal and epidural anesthesia are often avoided. A femoral nerve block (see Chapter 17) can provide excellent anesthesia for biopsy of the quadriceps muscle; a separate injection may be necessary for the lateral femoral cutaneous nerve to anesthetize also the anterolateral thigh. General anesthesia should be reserved for uncooperative patients or for times when local anesthesia proves to be inadequate. The anesthesiologist must therefore always be prepared with a plan for general anesthesia.

What agents may be safely used for general anesthesia?

The same principles discussed in the preceding chapter should be applied. Major goals include preventing pulmonary aspiration, avoiding excessive respiratory or circulatory depression, avoiding muscle relaxants if possible, and perhaps avoiding agents known to trigger malignant hyperthermia.

A normal response to a previous general anesthetic in the patient or a family member may be reassuring but does not guarantee the same response subsequently. General anesthesia may be induced and maintained with a combination of a barbiturate (thiopental or methohexital), benzodiazepine (midazolam), propofol, or opioid (alfentanil) and nitrous oxide. Patients at increased risk for aspiration should be intubated (see above). When a muscle relaxant is necessary, a short-acting nondepolarizing agent (cisatracurium or mivacurium) should be used. Succinylcholine should generally be avoided because of the unknown risk of an unusual response (myotonic contractions, prolonged duration, or phase II block), of inducing severe hyperkalemia, or of triggering malignant hyperthermia.

SUGGESTED READING

Booij LH, Vree TB: Skeletal muscle relaxants: Pharmacodynamics and pharmacokinetics in different patient groups. Clin Pract 2000; 54:526.

Mathieu J, Allard P, Gobeil G, et al: Anesthetic and surgical complications in 219 cases of myotonic dystrophy. Neurology 1997;49:1646.

Pourmand R: *Neuromuscular Diseases: Expert Clinician's Views.* Butterworth-Heineman, 2001.

Stoelting RK, Dierdorf SF: *Handbook for Anesthesia and Co-existing Disease.* 2nd ed. Churchill Livingstone, 2002.

Anesthesia for Ophthalmic Surgery 38

KEY CONCEPTS

 1 Any factor that increases intraocular pressure in a normal eye will tend to decrease intraocular volume in an open eye by causing drainage of aqueous or extrusion of vitreous through a surgical or traumatic wound. This loss of intraocular contents can permanently worsen vision.

 2 Succinylcholine increases intraocular pressure by 5–10 mm Hg for 5–10 minutes after administration, principally through prolonged contracture of the extraocular muscles.

 3 Traction on extraocular muscles or pressure on the eyeball can elicit a wide variety of cardiac dysrhythmias ranging from bradycardia and ventricular ectopy to sinus arrest or ventricular fibrillation.

 4 Complications involving the intraocular expansion of gas bubbles, such as intraocular hypertension and retinal detachment, can be avoided by discontinuing nitrous oxide at least 15 minutes prior to the injection of air or sulfur hexafluoride.

 5 Topically applied ophthalmic drugs are absorbed at a rate intermediate between absorption following intravenous and subcutaneous injection.

 6 Echothiophate is an irreversible cholinesterase inhibitor used in the treatment of glaucoma. It inhibits both acetylcholinesterase (true cholinesterase) and plasma cholinesterase (pseudocholinesterase). Because succinylcholine is metabolized by the latter enzyme, echothiophate will prolong succinylcholine's duration of action.

 7 The key to inducing anesthesia in a patient with an open eye injury is controlling intraocular pressure with a smooth induction. Specifically, coughing during intubation must be avoided by achieving a deep level of anesthesia and profound paralysis.

 8 The post-retrobulbar apnea syndrome is probably due to injection of local anesthetic into the optic nerve sheath, with spread into the cerebrospinal fluid.

 9 Regardless of the technique employed for intravenous sedation, ventilation and oxygenation must be continuously monitored (preferably by pulse oximetry), and equipment to provide positive pressure ventilation must be immediately available.

Eye surgery provides several unique challenges for the anesthesiologist, including regulation of intraocular pressure, prevention of the oculocardiac reflex, management of its consequences, control of intraocular gas expansion, and the need to deal with the possible systemic effects of ophthalmic drugs. An understanding of the mechanisms and management of these potential problems can favorably influence surgical outcome. This chapter also considers specific techniques of general and regional anesthesia in ophthalmic surgery.

INTRAOCULAR PRESSURE DYNAMICS

Physiology of Intraocular Pressure

The eye can be considered a hollow sphere with a rigid wall. If the contents of the sphere increase, the intraocular pressure (normal: 12–20 mm Hg) must rise. For example, glaucoma is caused by an obstruction to aqueous humor outflow. Similarly, intraocular pressure will rise if the volume of blood within the globe is increased. A rise in venous pressure will increase intraocular pressure by decreasing aqueous drainage and increasing choroidal blood volume. Extreme changes in arterial blood pressure and ventilation can also affect intraocular pressure (Table 38–1). Any anesthetic event that alters these parameters can affect intraocular pressure (eg, laryngoscopy, intubation, airway obstruction, coughing, Trendelenburg position).

Alternatively, decreasing the size of the globe without a proportional change in the volume of its contents will increase intraocular pressure. Pressure on the eye from a tightly fitted mask, improper prone positioning, or retrobulbar hemorrhage can lead to marked increases in pressure.

Intraocular pressure helps maintain the shape and therefore the optical properties of the eye. Temporary variations in pressure are usually well tolerated in normal eyes. In fact, blinking raises intraocular pressure by 5 mm Hg and squinting by 26 mm Hg. Even transient episodes of increased intraocular pressure in patients with low ophthalmic artery pressure (eg, deliberate hypotension, arteriosclerotic involvement of the retinal artery), however, may jeopardize retinal perfusion and cause retinal ischemia.

When the globe is open during certain surgical procedures (Table 38–2) or after traumatic perforation, in-

Table 38–1. The effect of cardiac and respiratory variables on intraocular pressure (IOP).

Variable	Effect on IOP
Central venous pressure	
Increase	↑↑↑
Decrease	↓↓↓
Arterial blood pressure	
Increase	↑
Decrease	↓
PaCO$_2$	
Increase (hypoventilation)	↑↑
Decrease (hyperventilation)	↓↓
PaO$_2$	
Increase	0
Decrease	↑

↓ = decrease (mild, moderate, marked).
↑ = increase (mild, moderate, marked).
0 = no effect.

Table 38–2. Open-eye surgical procedures.

Cataract extraction
Corneal laceration repair
Corneal transplant (penetrating keratoplasty)
Peripheral iridectomy
Removal of foreign body
Ruptured globe repair
Secondary intraocular lens implantation
Trabeculectomy (and other filtering procedures)
Vitrectomy (anterior and posterior)
Wound leak repair

traocular pressure approaches atmospheric pressure. Any factor that normally increases intraocular pressure will tend to decrease intraocular volume by causing drainage of aqueous or extrusion of vitreous through the wound. The latter is a serious complication that can permanently worsen vision.

Effect of Anesthetic Drugs on Intraocular Pressure

Most anesthetic drugs either lower or have no effect on intraocular pressure (Table 38–3). Inhalational anesthetics decrease intraocular pressure in proportion to the depth of anesthesia. The decrease has multiple causes: A drop in blood pressure reduces choroidal volume, relaxation of the extraocular muscles lowers wall tension, and pupillary constriction facilitates aqueous outflow. Intravenous anesthetics also decrease intraocular pressure. A possible exception is ketamine, which usually raises arterial blood pressure and does not relax extraocular muscles.

Topically administered anticholinergic drugs result in pupillary dilation (mydriasis), which may precipitate angle-closure glaucoma. Premedication doses of systemically administered atropine are not associated with intraocular hypertension, however, even in patients with glaucoma. The bulky quaternary ammonium structure of glycopyrrolate may provide an even greater margin of safety by preventing its passage into the central nervous system.

Succinylcholine increases intraocular pressure by 5–10 mm Hg for 5–10 minutes after administration, principally through prolonged contracture of the extraocular muscles. Unlike other skeletal muscle, extraocular muscles contain cells with multiple neuromuscular junctions. Repeated depolarization of these cells by succinylcholine causes the prolonged contracture. The resulting increase in intraocular pressure may have several effects. It will cause

Table 38–3. The effect of anesthetic agents on intraocular pressure (IOP).

Drug	Effect on IOP
Inhaled anesthetics	
Volatile agents	↓↓
Nitrous oxide	↓
Intravenous anesthetics	
Barbiturates	↓↓
Benzodiazepines	↓↓
Ketamine	?
Narcotics	↓
Muscle relaxants	
Depolarizers (succinylcholine)	↑↑
Nondepolarizers	0/↓

↓ = decrease (mild, moderate).
↑ = increase (mild, moderate).
0/↓ = no change or mild decrease.
? = conflicting reports.

spurious measurements of intraocular pressure during examinations under anesthesia in glaucoma patients, potentially leading to unnecessary surgery. Furthermore, a rise in intraocular pressure may cause extrusion of ocular contents through an open surgical or traumatic wound. A final effect of prolonged contracture of the extraocular muscles is shown as an abnormal **forced duction test** for 20 minutes. This maneuver evaluates the cause of extraocular muscle imbalance and may influence the type of strabismus surgery performed. Congestion of choroidal vessels may also contribute to the rise in intraocular pressure. Nondepolarizing muscle relaxants do not increase intraocular pressure.

THE OCULOCARDIAC REFLEX

 Traction on extraocular muscles or pressure on the eyeball can elicit a wide variety of cardiac dysrhythmias ranging from bradycardia and ventricular ectopy to sinus arrest or ventricular fibrillation. This reflex, originally described in 1908, consists of a trigeminal afferent (V_1) and a vagal efferent pathway. The oculocardiac reflex is most common in pediatric patients undergoing strabismus surgery. Nonetheless, it can be evoked in all age groups and during a variety of ocular procedures, including cataract extraction, enucleation, and retinal detachment repair. In awake patients, the oculocardiac reflex may be associated with somnolence and nausea.

Anticholinergic medication is often helpful in preventing the oculocardiac reflex. Intravenous atropine or

glycopyrrolate immediately prior to surgery is more effective than intramuscular premedication. It should be remembered that anticholinergic medications can be hazardous in elderly patients, who often have some degree of coronary artery disease. Retrobulbar blockade or deep inhalational anesthesia may also be of value, but these procedures impose risks of their own. Retrobulbar blockade can, in fact, elicit the oculocardiac reflex. The need for any routine prophylaxis is controversial.

Management of the oculocardiac reflex when it occurs consists of the following procedures: (1) immediate notification of the surgeon and temporary cessation of surgical stimulation until heart rate increases; (2) confirmation of adequate ventilation, oxygenation, and depth of anesthesia; (3) administration of intravenous atropine (10 μg/kg) if the conduction disturbance persists; and (4) in recalcitrant episodes, infiltration of the rectus muscles with local anesthetic. The reflex eventually fatigues itself (self-extinguishes) with repeated traction on the extraocular muscles.

INTRAOCULAR GAS EXPANSION

A gas bubble may be injected by the ophthalmologist into the posterior chamber during vitreous surgery. Intravitreal air injection will tend to flatten a detached retina and allow anatomically correct healing. The air bubble is absorbed within 5 days by gradual diffusion through adjacent tissue and into the bloodstream. If the patient is breathing nitrous oxide, the bubble will increase in size. This is because nitrous oxide is 35 times more soluble than nitrogen in blood (see Chapter 7). Thus, nitrous oxide tends to diffuse into an air bubble more rapidly than nitrogen (the major component of air) is absorbed by the bloodstream. If the bubble expands after the eye is closed, intraocular pressure will rise.

Sulfur hexafluoride (SF_6) is an inert gas that is less soluble in blood than is nitrogen—and much less soluble than nitrous oxide. Its longer duration of action (up to 10 days) compared with an air bubble can provide an advantage to the ophthalmologist. Bubble size doubles within 24 hours after injection because nitrogen from inhaled air enters the bubble more rapidly than the sulfur hexafluoride diffuses into the bloodstream. Even so, unless high volumes of pure sulfur hexafluoride are injected, the slow bubble expansion does not usually raise intraocular pressure. If the patient is breathing nitrous oxide, however, the bubble will rapidly increase in size and may lead to intraocular hypertension. A 70% inspired nitrous oxide concentration will almost triple the size of a 1-mL bubble and may double the pressure in a closed eye within 30 minutes. Subsequent discontinuation of nitrous oxide will lead to reabsorption of the bubble, which has become a mixture of nitrous oxide and sulfur hexafluoride. The consequent fall in intraocular pressure may precipitate another retinal detachment.

These complications involving the intraocular expansion of gas bubbles can be avoided by discontinuing nitrous oxide at least 15 minutes prior to the injection of air or sulfur hexafluoride. Obviously, the amount of time required to eliminate nitrous oxide from the blood will depend on several factors, including fresh gas flow rate and adequacy of alveolar ventilation. Depth of anesthesia should be maintained by substituting other anesthetic agents. Nitrous oxide should be avoided until the bubble is absorbed (5 days after air and 10 days after sulfur hexafluoride injection).

SYSTEMIC EFFECTS OF OPHTHALMIC DRUGS

Topically applied eye drops are absorbed by vessels in the conjunctival sac and the nasolacrimal duct mucosa (see Case Discussion, Chapter 11). One drop (typically 1/20 mL) of 10% **phenylephrine** contains 5 mg of drug. Compare this with the intravenous dose of phenylephrine (0.05–0.1 mg) used to treat an adult patient with hypotension. Topically applied drugs are absorbed at a rate intermediate between absorption following intravenous and subcutaneous injection (toxic subcutaneous

dose of phenylephrine is 10 mg). Children and the elderly are at particular risk for the toxic effects of topically applied medications and should receive at most a 2.5% phenylephrine solution (Table 38–4). Coincidentally, these patients are the ones most apt to require eye surgery.

Echothiophate is an irreversible cholinesterase inhibitor used in the treatment of glaucoma. Topical application leads to systemic absorption and a reduction in plasma cholinesterase activity. Because succinylcholine is metabolized by this enzyme, echothiophate will prolong succinylcholine's duration of action. Paralysis usually does not exceed 20 or 30 minutes, however, and postoperative apnea is unlikely (see Chapter 9). The inhibition of cholinesterase activity lasts for 3–7 weeks after discontinuation of echothiophate drops. Muscarinic side effects—such as bradycardia during induction—can be prevented with intravenous anticholinergic drugs (eg, atropine, glycopyrrolate).

Epinephrine eye drops can cause hypertension, tachycardia, and ventricular dysrhythmias; the dysrhythmogenic effects are potentiated by halothane. Direct instillation of epinephrine into the anterior chamber of the eye has not been associated with cardiovascular toxicity.

Timolol, a nonselective β-adrenergic antagonist, reduces intraocular pressure by decreasing aqueous humor production. Topically applied timolol eye drops, commonly used to treat glaucoma, have in rare cases been associated with atropine-resistant bradycar-

Table 38–4. Systemic effects of ophthalmic medications.

Drug	Mechanism of Action	Effect
Acetylcholine	Cholinergic agonist (miosis)	Bronchospasm, bradycardia, hypotension
Acetazolamide	Carbonic anhydrase inhibitor (decreases IOP)	Diuresis, hypokalemic metabolic acidosis
Atropine	Anticholinergic (mydriasis)	Central anticholinergic syndrome*
Cyclopentolate	Anticholinergic (mydriasis)	Disorientation, psychosis, convulsions
Echothiophate	Cholinesterase inhibitor (miosis, decreases IOP)	Prolongation of succinylcholine paralysis, bronchospasm
Epinephrine	Sympathetic agonist (mydriasis, decreases IOP)	Hypertension, bradycardia, tachycardia, headache
Phenylephrine	α-Adrenergic agonist (mydriasis, vasoconstriction)	Hypertension, tachycardia, dysrythmias
Scopolamine	Anticholinergic (mydriasis, vasoconstriction)	Central anticholinergic syndrome*
Timolol	β-Adrenergic blocking agent (decreases IOP)	Bradycardia, asthma, congestive heart failure

*See Chapter 11 Case Discussion.
IOP = intraocular pressure.

dia, hypotension, and bronchospasm during general anesthesia.

GENERAL ANESTHESIA FOR OPHTHALMIC SURGERY

The choice between general and local anesthesia should be made jointly by the patient, anesthesiologist, and surgeon. Some patients refuse even to discuss local anesthesia. This apprehension is often due to the fear of being awake during a surgical procedure or the recollection of pain during prior regional techniques. Although there is no conclusive evidence that one form of anesthesia is safer than the other, local anesthesia seems to be less stressful. General anesthesia is indicated in uncooperative patients, since even small head movements can prove disastrous during microsurgery. In other patients, local anesthesia is contraindicated for surgical reasons. In any event, a definitive decision must be made. **Local-general anesthesia**—a technique of deep sedation with questionable airway control—should be avoided because it imposes the combined risks of both local and general anesthesia.

PREMEDICATION

Patients undergoing eye surgery may be apprehensive, especially if they have undergone multiple procedures and there is a possibility of permanent blindness. Pediatric patients often have associated congenital disorders (eg, rubella syndrome, Goldenhar's syndrome, Down syndrome). Adult patients are usually elderly, with myriad systemic illnesses (eg, hypertension, diabetes mellitus, coronary artery disease). All of these factors must be considered when selecting premedication.

INDUCTION

The choice of induction technique for eye surgery usually depends more on the patient's other medical problems than on the patient's eye disease or the type of surgery contemplated. One exception is the patient with a ruptured globe. The key to inducing anesthesia in a patient with an open eye injury is controlling intraocular pressure with a smooth induction. Specifically, coughing during intubation must be avoided by achieving a deep level of anesthesia and profound paralysis. The intraocular pressure response to laryngoscopy and endotracheal intubation can be somewhat blunted by prior administration of intravenous lidocaine (1.5 mg/kg) or an opioid (eg, alfentanil 20 μg/kg). A nondepolarizing

muscle relaxant is used instead of succinylcholine because of the latter's influence on intraocular pressure. Most patients with open globe injuries have full stomachs and require a rapid-sequence induction technique (see Case Discussion, below).

MONITORING & MAINTENANCE

Eye surgery necessitates positioning the anesthesiologist away from the patient's airway, making pulse oximetry mandatory for all ophthalmologic procedures. Continuous monitoring for breathing-circuit disconnections or unintentional extubation is also crucial. The possibility of kinking and obstruction of the endotracheal tube can be minimized by using a reinforced or preformed right-angle endotracheal tube (see Figure 39–1). The possibility of dysrhythmias caused by the oculocardiac reflex increases the importance of constantly scrutinizing the electrocardiograph. In contrast to most pediatric surgery, infant body temperature often rises during ophthalmic surgery because of head-to-toe draping and insignificant body-surface exposure. End-tidal CO_2 analysis helps differentiate this from malignant hyperthermia.

The pain and stress evoked by eye surgery are considerably less than during a major intra-abdominal procedure. A lighter level of anesthesia would be satisfactory if the consequences of patient movement were not so catastrophic. The lack of cardiovascular stimulation inherent in most eye procedures combined with the need for adequate anesthetic depth can result in hypotension in elderly individuals. This problem is usually avoided by ensuring adequate intravenous hydration, administering small doses of ephedrine (2–5 mg), or establishing intraoperative paralysis with nondepolarizing muscle relaxants. The latter allows maintenance of a lighter level of anesthesia.

Emesis caused by vagal stimulation is a common postoperative problem, particularly following strabismus surgery. The Valsalva effect and the increase in central venous pressure that accompany vomiting can be detrimental to the surgical result and increase the risk of aspiration. Intraoperative administration of intravenous metoclopramide (10 mg in adults) or small doses of droperidol (20 μg/kg) may be beneficial. Because of its expense, ondansetron is usually reserved for patients with a history of postoperative nausea and vomiting.

EXTUBATION & EMERGENCE

Although modern suture materials and wound-closure techniques lessen the risk of postoperative wound dehiscence, a smooth emergence from general anesthesia is still desirable. Coughing on the endotracheal tube can be prevented by extubating the patient during a moderately deep level of anesthesia. As the end of the surgical procedure approaches, muscle relaxation is reversed and spontaneous respirations return. Anesthetic agents may be continued during suction of the airway. Nitrous oxide is then discontinued, and intravenous lidocaine (1.5 mg/kg) can be given to blunt cough reflexes temporarily. Extubation proceeds 1–2 minutes after the lidocaine and during spontaneous respiration of 100% oxygen. Proper airway control is crucial until the patient's cough and swallowing reflexes return. Obviously, this technique is not suitable in patients at increased risk for aspiration (see Case Discussion below).

Severe postoperative pain is unusual following eye surgery. Scleral buckling procedures, enucleation, and ruptured-globe repair are the most painful operations. Small doses of intravenous narcotics (eg, 15–25 mg of meperidine for an adult) are usually sufficient. Severe pain may signal intraocular hypertension, corneal abrasion, or other surgical complications.

■ REGIONAL ANESTHESIA FOR OPHTHALMIC SURGERY

Regional anesthesia for eye surgery has traditionally consisted of a **retrobulbar block,** a facial nerve block, and intravenous sedation. Although less invasive than general anesthesia with endotracheal intubation and less likely to be associated with postoperative nausea, local anesthesia is not without possible complications. In addition, the block may not provide adequate akinesia or analgesia of the eye, or the patient may be unable to lie perfectly still for the duration of the surgery. For these reasons, equipment and personnel required to treat the complications of local anesthesia and to induce general anesthesia must be readily available. At one time, the term **local-standby** described the anesthesiologist's role in these cases. This term has now been replaced by **monitored anesthesia care,** since the anesthesiologist should be continually monitoring the patient during surgery and not just standing by.

RETROBULBAR BLOCKADE

In this technique, local anesthetic is injected behind the eye into the cone formed by the extraocular muscles (Figure 38–1). A blunt-tipped 25-gauge needle penetrates the lower lid at the junction of the middle and lateral one-third of the orbit (usually 0.5 cm medial to the lateral canthus). The patient is instructed to stare supranasally as the needle is advanced 3.5 cm toward the apex of the muscle cone. After aspiration to preclude intravascular injection, 2–5 mL of local anesthetic are injected and the needle is removed. Choice of local anesthetic varies, but lidocaine and bupivacaine are most common. Hyaluronidase, a hydrolyzer of connective tissue polysaccharides, is frequently added to enhance the retrobulbar spread of the local anesthetic. A successful retrobulbar block is accompanied by anesthesia, akinesia, and abolishment of the oculocephalic reflex (ie, a blocked eye does not move during headturning).

Complications of retrobulbar injection of local anesthetics include retrobulbar hemorrhage, globe perforation (especially of eyes with an axial length greater than 26 mm), optic nerve atrophy, frank convulsions, oculocardiac reflex, acute neurogenic pulmonary edema, trigeminal nerve block, and respiratory arrest. Forceful injection of local anesthetic into the ophthalmic artery causes retrograde flow toward the brain and may result in an instantaneous seizure. The **post-retrobulbar apnea syndrome** is probably due to injection of local anesthetic into the optic nerve sheath, with spread into the cerebrospinal fluid. The central nervous system is exposed to high concentrations of local anesthetic, leading to apprehension and unconsciousness. Apnea occurs within 20 minutes and resolves within an hour. In the meantime, treatment is supportive, with positive pressure ventilation to prevent hypoxia, bradycardia, and cardiac arrest. Adequacy of ventilation must be constantly monitored in patients who have received retrobulbar anesthesia.

Retrobulbar injection is usually not performed in patients with bleeding disorders (because of the risk of retrobulbar hemorrhage), extreme myopia (the longer globe increases the risk of perforation), or an open eye injury (the pressure from injecting fluid behind the eye may cause extrusion of intraocular contents through the wound).

FACIAL NERVE BLOCK

A facial nerve block prevents squinting of the eyelids during surgery and allows placement of a lid speculum. There are several techniques of facial nerve block: van Lint, Atkinson, and O'Brien (Figure 38–2). The major complication of these blocks is subcutaneous hemorrhage. Another procedure, Nadbath's technique, blocks the facial nerve as it exits the stylomastoid foramen under the external auditory canal, in close proximity to the vagus and glossopharyngeal nerves. This block is not recommended because it has been associated with vocal cord paralysis, laryngospasm, dysphagia, and respiratory distress.

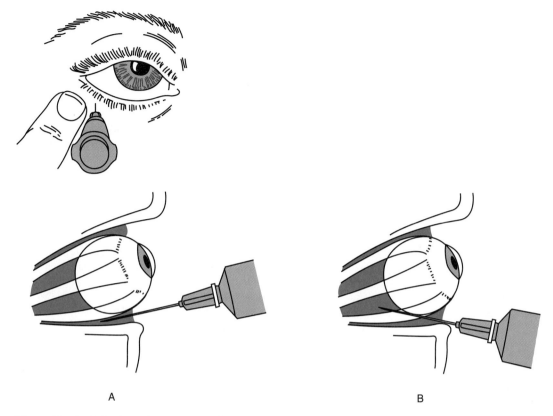

Figure 38–1. ***A:*** During administration of a retrobulbar block, the patient looks supranasally as a needle is advanced 1.5 cm along the inferotemporal wall of the orbit. ***B:*** The needle is then redirected upward and nasally toward the apex of the orbit and advanced until its tip penetrates the muscle cone.

LESS INVASIVE REGIONAL TECHNIQUES

Over the last several years, less traumatic regional techniques have evolved for anterior chamber (eg, cataract) and glaucoma surgeries. Alternatives include peribulbar anesthesia by injection of a small volume of local anesthetic (eg, 0.5 mL) into the superior quadrant of the subconjunctiva toward the sub-Tenon's space. This may be accomplished with a small 27-gauge needle or a blunt curved cannula, the latter avoiding any risk of globe perforation. A more recently described technique eliminates anesthetic injection altogether. After topical instillation of anesthetic drops (0.5% proximethacaine chlorhydrate) repeated at 5-minute intervals for 5 applications, an anesthetic gel (lidocaine chlorhydrate plus 2% methylcellulose) is applied with a cotton swab to the inferior and superior conjunctival sacs. These newer, less invasive techniques are not appropriate for posterior chamber surgery (eg, retinal detachment repair with a buckle) and work

best for surgeons with fast but gentle surgical technique.

INTRAVENOUS SEDATION

Several techniques of intravenous sedation are available for eye surgery. The particular drug used is less important than the dose. Deep sedation should be avoided because it increases the risk of apnea and unintentional patient movement during surgery. On the other hand, retrobulbar and facial nerve blocks can be quite uncomfortable. As a compromise, some anesthesiologists administer a small dose of a short-acting barbiturate (eg, 10–20 mg of methohexital or 25–75 mg of thiopental) to produce a brief state of unconsciousness during the regional block. Alternatively, a small bolus of alfentanil (375–500 µg) allows a brief period of intense analgesia. Other anesthesiologists, believing that the risks of respiratory arrest and aspiration are unac-

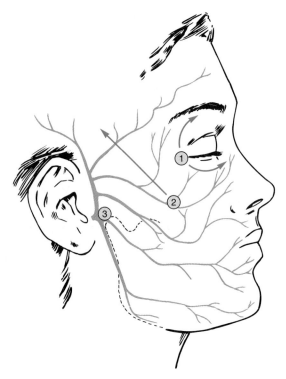

Figure 38–2. There are many techniques of facial nerve block, including (1) van Lint, (2) Atkinson, and (3) O'Brien.

ceptable, limit their doses to provide minimal relaxation and amnesia. Midazolam (1–3 mg) with or without fentanyl (12.5–25 μg) is a common regimen. Doses vary considerably between patients and should be administered in small increments. Regardless of the technique employed, ventilation and oxygenation must be continuously monitored (preferably by pulse oximetry), and equipment to provide positive pressure ventilation must be immediately available.

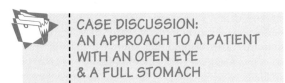

CASE DISCUSSION:
AN APPROACH TO A PATIENT
WITH AN OPEN EYE
& A FULL STOMACH

A 12-year-old boy arrives at the emergency room after being shot in the eye with a pellet gun. A brief examination by the ophthalmologist reveals intraocular contents presenting at the wound. The

boy is scheduled for emergency repair of the ruptured globe.

What should be stressed in the preoperative evaluation of this patient?

Aside from taking a routine history and performing a physical examination, one should establish as accurately as possible the time of last oral intake before or after the injury. The patient must be considered to have a full stomach if the injury occurred within 8 hours after the last meal, even if the patient did not eat for several hours after the injury: gastric emptying is delayed by the pain and anxiety that follow trauma.

What is the significance of a full stomach in a patient with an open globe injury?

Managing patients who have sustained penetrating eye injuries provides a challenge to anesthesiologists because of the need to develop an anesthetic plan that is consistent with at least two conflicting objectives. One obvious objective is to prevent further damage to the eye by avoiding increases in intraocular pressure. A second important objective is to prevent pulmonary aspiration in a patient with a full stomach.

Many of the common strategies used to achieve these objectives are in direct conflict with one another, however (Tables 38–5 and 38–6). For example, while regional anesthesia (eg, retrobulbar block) minimizes the risk of aspiration pneumonia, it is relatively contraindicated in patients with penetrating eye injuries because injecting local anesthetic behind the globe increases intraocular pressure and may lead to expulsion of

Table 38–5. Strategies to prevent increases in intraocular pressure (IOP).

- Avoid direct pressure on the globe
    Patch eye with Fox shield
    No retrobulbar or peribulbar injections
    Careful face mask technique
- Avoid increases in central venous pressure
    Prevent coughing during induction and intubation
    Ensure a deep level of anesthesia and relaxation prior to laryngoscopy*
    Avoid head-down positions
    Extubate deeply asleep*
- Avoid pharmacologic agents that increases IOP
    Succinylcholine
    Ketamine(?)

---

*These strategies are not recommended for patients with full stomachs.

Table 38–6. Strategies to prevent aspiration pneumonia.

- Regional anesthesia with minimal sedation*
- Premedication
  Metoclopramide
  Histamine H₂-receptor antagonists
  Antacids
- Evacuation of gastric contents
  Nasogastric tube*
- Rapid-sequence induction
  Cricoid pressure
  A rapid-acting induction agent
  Succinylcholine,* rocuronium, or rapacuronium
  Avoidance of positive pressure ventilation
  Intubation as soon as possible
- Extubation awake

---

*These strategies are not recommended for patients with penetrating eye injuries.

intraocular contents. Therefore, these patients require general anesthesia—despite the increased risk of aspiration pneumonia.

What preoperative preparation should be considered in this patient?

The goal of preoperative preparation is to minimize the risk of aspiration pneumonia by decreasing gastric volume and acidity (see Case Discussion, Chapter 15). Aspiration in patients with eye injuries is prevented by proper selection of pharmacologic agents and anesthetic techniques. Evacuation of gastric contents with a nasogastric tube may lead to coughing, retching, and other responses that can dramatically increase intraocular pressure.

Metoclopramide *increases lower esophageal sphincter tone, speeds gastric emptying, lowers gastric fluid volume, and exerts an antiemetic effect. It should be given intravenously (10–20 mg) as soon as possible and repeated every 2–4 hours until surgery.*

Ranitidine *(50 mg intravenously),* ***cimetidine*** *(300 mg intravenously), and* ***famotidine*** *(20 mg intravenously) are H₂-histamine–receptor antagonists that inhibit gastric acid secretion. Because they have no effect on the pH of gastric secretions present in the stomach prior to their administration, they have limited value in patients presenting for emergency surgery.*

Unlike H₂-receptor antagonists, antacids have an immediate effect. Unfortunately, they increase intragastric volume. Nonparticulate antacids (preparations of sodium citrate, potassium citrate, and citric acid) lose effectiveness within

30–60 minutes and should be given immediately prior to induction (15–30 mL orally).

Which induction agents are recommended in patients with penetrating eye injuries?

The ideal induction agent for patients with full stomachs would provide a rapid onset of action in order to minimize the risk of regurgitation. Ketamine, thiopental, propofol, and etomidate have essentially equally rapid onsets of action (ie, one-arm-to-brain circulation time).

Furthermore, the ideal induction agent would not increase the risk of ocular expulsion by raising intraocular pressure. (In fact, most intravenous induction agents lower intraocular pressure.) While investigations of the effects of ketamine on intraocular pressure have provided conflicting results, ketamine is not recommended in penetrating eye injuries owing to the high rate of blepharospasm and nystagmus.

Although etomidate may prove valuable in some patients with cardiac disease, it is associated with an incidence of myoclonus ranging from 10% to 60%. An episode of severe myoclonus may have contributed to complete retinal detachment and vitreous prolapse in one patient with an open globe injury and limited cardiovascular reserve.

Propofol and thiopental have a rapid onset of action and decrease intraocular pressure; however, neither prevents the hypertensive response to laryngoscopy and intubation. Similarly, neither prevents the increase in intraocular pressure that accompanies laryngoscopy and intubation. Prior administration of fentanyl (3–5 µg/kg), alfentanil (20 µg/kg), esmolol (0.5–1 mg/kg), or lidocaine (1.5 mg/kg) attenuates this response with varying degrees of success.

How does the choice of muscle relaxant differ in these patients from other patients at risk for aspiration?

The choice of muscle relaxant in patients with penetrating eye injuries has provided controversy for more than three decades. Succinylcholine definitely increases intraocular pressure. Although there is conflicting research, it is probably most prudent to conclude that this rise in pressure is not consistently and reliably prevented by pretreatment with a nondepolarizing agent or self-taming doses of succinylcholine, lidocaine, or diazepam. Contradictory findings by various investigators using different regimens are probably due to differences in doses and timing of the pretreatment drugs.

Some anesthesiologists argue that the relatively small and transient rise in intraocular pres-

sure caused by succinylcholine is insignificant when compared with changes caused by laryngoscopy and intubation. They claim that a slight rise in intraocular pressure is a small price to pay for two distinct advantages that succinylcholine offers: a rapid onset of action that decreases the risk of aspiration, and profound muscle relaxation that decreases the chance of a Valsalva response during intubation. Furthermore, these advocates of succinylcholine usually point to the lack of case reports documenting further eye injury when succinylcholine has been used.

Nondepolarizing muscle relaxants do not increase intraocular pressure. Until the release of rocuronium, however, nondepolarizing agents did not provide a rapid enough onset of action. Rapacuronium(1.5–2.5 mg/kg) had largely settled this debate because of its rapid onset of action, lack of effect on intraocular pressure, and short duration of action. However, the manufacturer of rapacuronium voluntarily withdrew it from the market due to several reports of serious bronchospasm, including a few unexplained fatalities. Regardless of the muscle relaxant chosen, intubation should not be attempted until a level of paralysis is achieved that will definitely prevent coughing on the endotracheal tube.

How do induction strategies vary in pediatric patients without an intravenous line?

A hysterical child with a penetrating eye injury and a full stomach provides an anesthetic challenge for which there is no perfect solution. Once again, the dilemma is due to the need to avoid increases in intraocular pressure yet minimize the risk of aspiration. For example, screaming and crying can lead to tremendous increases in intraocular pressure. Attempting to sedate children with rectal suppositories or intramuscular injections, however, often heightens their state of agitation and may worsen the eye injury. Similarly, although preoperative sedation may increase the risk of aspiration by obtunding airway reflexes, it is often necessary for establishing an intravenous line for a rapid-sequence induction. An ideal strategy would be to administer enough sedation painlessly to allow placement of an intravenous line yet maintain a level of consciousness adequate to protect airway reflexes. While this solution is currently hard to achieve, the introduction of new drugs and innovative delivery systems, such as opioid-containing lollipops, may provide some acceptable alternatives. In the meantime, the prudent strategy is to do everything possible to avoid aspiration—even at the cost of further eye damage.

Are there special considerations during extubation and emergence?

Patients at risk for aspiration during induction are also at risk during extubation and emergence. Therefore, extubation must be delayed until the patient is awake and has intact airway reflexes (eg, spontaneous swallowing and coughing on the endotracheal tube). Deep extubation risks vomiting and aspiration. Intraoperative administration of antiemetic medication and nasogastric-tube suctioning may decrease the incidence of emesis during emergence, but they do not guarantee an empty stomach.

SUGGESTED READING

Dell R, Williams B: Anaesthesia for strabismus surgery: A regional survey. Br J Anaesth 1999;82:761. This paper deals with the effect of succinylcholine on the forced duction test.

Gomez RS, Andrade LOF, Costa JRR: Brainstem anesthesia after peribulbar anesthesia. Can J Anaesth 1997;44:732. Peribulbar anesthesia may be safer than retrobulbar block, but serious complications can still occur.

Johnson RW: Anatomy for ophthalmic anaesthesia. Br J Anaesth 1995;75:80. A comprehensive review of the orbit and its contents.

McGoldrick KE (editor): *Anesthesia for Ophthalmic and Otolaryngologic Surgery.* WB Saunders and Company, 1992. The concluding chapters of this book provide a detailed discussion of all aspects of ophthalmic anesthesia.

Murphy DF: Anesthesia and intraocular pressure. Anesth Analg 1985;64:520. A comprehensive review article on the determinants of intraocular pressure.

Rosenfeld SI, Litinsky SM, Snyder DA, et al: Effectiveness of monitored anesthesia care in cataract surgery. Ophthalmology 1999;106:1256. The presence of anesthesia personnel during monitored anesthesia care for cataract surgery appeared warranted in this study.

Schein OD, Katz J, Bass EB, et al: The value of routine preoperative medical testing before cataract surgery. N Engl J Med 2000;342:168. A review of almost 20,000 cataract surgeries revealed no effect of routine preoperative medical testing on perioperative morbidity or mortality.

Smith GB: *Ophthalmic Anaesthesia: A Practical Handbook,* 2nd ed. Oxford University Press, 1996. An overview from the British perspective.

Anesthesia for Otorhinolaryngologic Surgery

39

KEY CONCEPTS

 The anesthetic goals for endoscopy include profound muscle paralysis in order to provide masseter muscle relaxation for introduction of the suspension laryngoscope and an immobile surgical field, adequate oxygenation and ventilation during surgical manipulation of the airway, and cardiovascular stability during periods of rapidly varying surgical stimulation.

 It is crucial to monitor chest wall motion constantly during endoscopy for proper tidal volumes and to allow sufficient time for exhalation in order to avoid air trapping and barotrauma.

 The greatest fear during laser airway surgery is an endotracheal tube fire. This can be avoided by using a technique of ventilation that does not involve a flammable tube or catheter (eg, intermittent apnea or jet ventilation through the laryngoscope side port).

 Techniques to minimize intraoperative blood loss during nasal and sinus surgery include supplementation with cocaine or an epinephrine-containing local anesthetic, maintaining a slightly head-up position, and providing a mild degree of controlled hypotension.

 If airway management has the potential for being complicated (ie, an obstructing lesion or distorted anatomy due to preoperative radiation therapy), avoid an intravenous induction in favor of awake direct or fiberoptic laryngoscopy (cooperative patient) or an inhalational induction, maintaining spontaneous ventilation (uncooper-

ative patient). In any case, the equipment and personnel required for an emergency tracheostomy must be immediately available.

 The surgeon may request the omission of neuromuscular blocking agents during neck dissection or parotidectomy to identify nerves (eg, spinal accessory, facial nerves) by direct stimulation and to preserve them.

 Bilateral neck dissection may result in postoperative hypertension and loss of hypoxic drive because of denervation of the carotid sinuses and bodies. Manipulation of the carotid sinus and stellate ganglion during radical neck dissection (right side more than the left) has been associated with wide swings in blood pressure, bradycardia, dysrhythmias, sinus arrest, and prolonged QT intervals.

 Providing anesthesia in patients undergoing craniofacial and orthognathic surgery is a challenge. If there are any forewarning signs of problems with mask ventilation or endotracheal intubation, the airway should be secured prior to induction.

 The patient should be left intubated after craniofacial or orthognathic surgery if there is a chance of postoperative edema involving structures that could obstruct the airway (eg, tongue).

 Nitrous oxide is either avoided during tympanoplasty or discontinued prior to graft placement because of the risk of graft dislodgment.

Never are cooperation and communication between surgeon and anesthesiologist more important than during head and neck surgery. Establishing, maintaining, and protecting an airway in the face of abnormal anatomy and simultaneous surgical intervention can test the skills and patience of any anesthesiologist. Clearly, a thorough understanding of airway anatomy (see Chapter 5) and an appreciation of common otorhinolaryngologic procedures will prove invaluable in handling these demanding anesthetic challenges.

ENDOSCOPY

Endoscopy includes laryngoscopy (diagnostic and operative), microlaryngoscopy (laryngoscopy aided by an operating microscope), esophagoscopy, and bronchoscopy (discussed in Chapter 24). Endoscopic procedures may be accompanied by laser surgery.

Preoperative Considerations

Patients presenting for endoscopic surgery are often being evaluated for hoarseness, stridor, or hemoptysis. Possible causes include foreign body aspiration, trauma to the aerodigestive tract, papillomatosis, tracheal stenosis, obstructing tumors, or vocal cord dysfunction. Thus, a meticulous preoperative physical examination and medical history, with particular attention to potential airway problems, must precede any decisions regarding the anesthetic plan. In some patients, flow-volume loops (see Case Discussion, Chapter 24) or special radiographic studies (eg, tomograms, computed tomography, or magnetic resonance imaging) may be available for review. Many patients will have undergone indirect laryngoscopy by the surgeon in clinic, and the importance of discussing the findings and plans with the surgeon preoperatively cannot be overemphasized.

The most important questions that must be answered are whether the patient will be easy to ventilate with a face mask and easy to intubate with direct laryngoscopy. If there is any reason to doubt either ability, the patient's airway should be secured prior to induction by using an alternative technique such as described in the Chapter 5 Case Discussion (eg, use of a fiberoptic bronchoscope, a tracheostomy under local anesthesia). It should be stressed that even securing an airway with tracheotomy does not necessarily prevent intraoperative airway obstruction due to surgical manipulation and techniques.

Sedative premedication is contraindicated in any patient with any significant degree of upper airway obstruction. Administering glycopyrrolate (0.2–0.3 mg IM) 1 hour before surgery may prove helpful by minimizing secretions, thereby facilitating airway visualization.

Intraoperative Management

 The anesthetic goals for endoscopy include profound muscle paralysis in order to provide masseter muscle relaxation for introduction of the suspension laryngoscope and an immobile surgical field, adequate oxygenation and ventilation during surgical manipulation of the airway, and cardiovascular stability during periods of rapidly varying surgical stimulation.

A. Muscle Relaxation:

Intraoperative muscle relaxation can be achieved by either a continuous infusion of succinylcholine or intermittent boluses of intermediate-duration nondepolarizing muscle relaxants (eg, rocuronium, vecuronium, atracurium). A disadvantage of a succinylcholine drip is the potential of developing a phase II block during unexpectedly long procedures (see Chapter 9). On the other hand, an intermediate-duration nondepolarizing block may prove difficult to reverse and may delay return of protective airway reflexes and extubation. These problems may be avoided by administering an intermittent bolus or continuous infusion of mivacurium or rapacuronium,* short-acting nondepolarizing muscle relaxants. It should be noted that although profound relaxation is needed until the very end of the surgery, rapid recovery is important since endoscopy is often an outpatient procedure.

B. Oxygenation and Ventilation:

Several methods have successfully been used to provide oxygenation and ventilation during endoscopy. Most commonly, the patient is intubated with a small-diameter (4.0–6.0 mm) endotracheal tube through which conventional positive pressure is administered. Standard endotracheal tubes of this size, however, are designed for pediatric patients. They therefore tend to be too short for the adult trachea, with a low-volume cuff that will exert high pressure against it. A 4.0-, 5.0-, or 6.0-mm microlaryngeal tracheal tube (MLT tube, Mallinckrodt Critical Care) is the same length as an adult tube, has a disproportionately large high-volume low-pressure cuff, and is stiffer and less prone to compression than a regular endotracheal tube. The advantages of intubation include protection against aspiration and the ability to administer inhalational anesthetics and to continuously monitor end-tidal CO_2.

In some cases (eg, those involving the posterior commissure), intubation with an endotracheal tube may interfere with the surgeon's visualization or perfor-

---

* At the time of publication, rapacuronium had been voluntarily withdrawn by the manufacturer. See Chapter 9 for details.

mance of the procedure. A simple alternative is **insufflation** of high flows of oxygen through a small catheter placed in the trachea. While oxygenation may be maintained for brief periods in patients with good lung function, ventilation is inadequate for longer procedures unless the patient is allowed to breathe spontaneously.

Another possibility is the **intermittent-apnea technique,** in which periods of ventilation with oxygen by face mask or endotracheal tube are alternated with periods of apnea, during which the surgery is performed. The duration of apnea, usually 2–3 minutes, is determined by how well the patient maintains oxygen saturation as measured by a pulse oximeter. Hypoventilation and pulmonary aspiration are risks of this technique.

A more sophisticated approach involves connecting a **manual jet ventilator** (see Figure 48–6) to a side port of the laryngoscope (Saunders jet injector). During inspiration (1–2 seconds), a high-pressure (30–50 psig) source of oxygen is directed through the glottic opening and entrains room air gas into the lungs (Venturi effect). Expiration (4–6 seconds duration) is passive. It is crucial to monitor chest wall motion constantly for proper tidal volumes and to allow sufficient time for exhalation in order to avoid air trapping and barotrauma. A variation of this technique is **high-frequency jet ventilation,** which utilizes a small cannula or tube in the trachea, through which gas is injected 80–300 times per minute (see Chapter 50). For example, the Carden tube is made of malleable copper with a Luer connector at the proximal end that attaches to the jet ventilator; its rounded distal end lies below the larynx. Both these techniques require an intravenous anesthetic. Capnography will tend to greatly underestimate the $PaCO_2$ during jet ventilation due to constant and sizable dilution of alveolar gases.

C. CARDIOVASCULAR STABILITY:

Blood pressure and heart rate often fluctuate strikingly during endoscopy procedures for two reasons. First, many of these patients have a long history of heavy tobacco and alcohol use that predisposes them to cardiovascular diseases. In addition, the procedure resembles a series of stress-filled laryngoscopies and intubations, separated by varying periods of minimal surgical stimulation. Attempting to maintain a patient at a constant level of anesthesia invariably results in alternating intervals of hypertension and hypotension. Providing a modest baseline level of anesthesia allows supplementation with short-acting anesthetics (eg, propofol, remifentanil) or sympathetic antagonists (eg, esmolol) as needed during periods of increased stimulation. Alternatively, regional nerve block of the glossopharyngeal nerve and superior laryngeal nerve would minimize in-

traoperative swings in blood pressure (see Chapter 5, Case Discussion). Invasive monitoring of arterial blood pressure should be considered in patients with a history of hypertension or coronary heart disease, even if the surgeon anticipates a short procedure.

Laser Precautions

Laser (*Light Amplification by Stimulated Emission of Radiation*) light differs from ordinary light in three ways: It is monochromatic (ie, it possesses one wavelength), coherent (it oscillates in the same phase), and collimated (it exists as a narrow, parallel beam). These characteristics offer the surgeon excellent precision and hemostasis with minimal postoperative edema or pain. Unfortunately, they also introduce some major hazards into the operating room.

The potential uses and side effects of a laser vary with its wavelength, which is determined by the medium in which the laser beam is generated. For example, a medium of CO_2 gas produces a long wavelength laser (the CO_2 laser has a 10,600-nm wavelength), while a medium of yttrium-aluminum-garnet (YAG) gem results in a shorter wavelength (the YAG laser has a 1060-nm wavelength). The longer the wavelength, the greater the absorption by water, and the less tissue is penetrated. Thus, the CO_2 laser's effects are much more localized and superficial than those of the YAG laser.

General precautions include evacuation of toxic fumes (laser plume) from tissue vaporization; these may have the potential to transmit microbacterial diseases. Depending on the wavelength of laser being used, all operating room personnel should wear some type of eye protection, and the patient's eyes should be taped shut.

 The greatest fear during laser airway surgery is an **endotracheal tube fire.** This can be avoided by using a technique of ventilation that does not involve a flammable tube or catheter (eg, intermittent apnea or jet ventilation through the laryngoscope side port). Some procedures, however, require an endotracheal tube because of the expected duration of the case, location of the lesion, or preexisting lung problems in the patient. In these cases, using an endotracheal tube that is *relatively* resistant to **laser ignition** may be warranted (Table 39–1). In an effort to protect endotracheal tubes from laser ignition, tubes can be wrapped with a variety of metallic tapes; however, they should be used with caution (Table 39–2).

It must be emphasized that no cuffed endotracheal tube or any currently available tube protection is completely laser-proof. Therefore, whenever laser airway surgery is being performed with an endotracheal tube in place, the following precautions should be observed:

Table 39–1. Advantages and disadvantages of various endotracheal tubes for laser airway surgery.

Type of Tube	Advantages	Disadvantages
Polyvinyl chloride	Inexpensive, nonreflective	Low melting point, highly combustible*
Red rubber	Puncture-resistant, maintains structure, nonreflective	Highly combustible*
Silicone rubber	Nonreflective	Combustible,* turns to toxic ash
Metal	Combustion-resistant,* kink-resistant	Thick-walled flammable cuff, transfers heat, reflects laser, cumbersome

*Combustibility depends on fraction of inspired oxygen and laser energy.

- Inspired oxygen concentration should be as low as possible (many patients tolerate an FiO_2 of 21%).
- Nitrous oxide supports combustion and should be replaced with air (nitrogen) or helium.
- The endotracheal tube cuff should be filled with saline dyed with methylene blue to dissipate heat and signal cuff rupture. A cuffed tube will minimize oxygen concentration in the pharynx. The addition of 2% lidocaine jelly (a 1:2 mixture with saline) into the cuff has been suggested as a method to seal small laser-induced cuff leaks, potentially preventing combustion.
- Laser intensity and duration should be limited as much as possible.
- Saline-soaked pledgets (completely saturated) should be placed in the airway to limit risk of ignition.

Table 39–2. Disadvantages of wrapping an endotracheal tube with metallic tape.

No cuff protection
Adds thickness to tube
Not an FDA-approved device
Protection varies with type of metal foil
Adhesive backing may ignite
May reflect laser onto non-targeted tissue
Rough edges may damage mucosal surfaces

- A source of water (eg, 60-mL syringe) should be immediately available in case of fire.

Since taking all these precautions limits, but does not eliminate, the risk of an airway fire, anesthesiologists must always be prepared for that eventuality (Table 39–3).

NASAL & SINUS SURGERY

Common nasal and sinus surgeries include polypectomy, endoscopic sinus surgery, maxillary sinusotomy (Caldwell-Luc procedure), rhinoplasty, and septoplasty.

Preoperative Considerations

Patients undergoing nasal or sinus surgery may have a considerable degree of preoperative nasal obstruction caused by polyps, a deviated septum, or mucosal congestion from infection. This may make face mask ventilation difficult, particularly if combined with other causes of difficult ventilation (eg, obesity, craniofacial deformities).

Nasal polyps are often associated with allergic disorders such as asthma. Patients who also have a history of allergic reactions to aspirin should not be given any nonsteroidal anti-inflammatory drugs (eg, ketorolac). Nasal polyps are a common feature of cystic fibrosis.

Because of the rich vascular supply of the nasal mucosa, the preoperative interview should concentrate on questions concerning drug use (eg, aspirin) and any history of bleeding problems.

Intraoperative Management

Many nasal procedures can be satisfactorily performed under local anesthesia with sedation. The anterior ethmoidal nerve and sphenopalatine nerves (see Figure 5–3) provide sensory innervation to the nasal septum and lateral walls. Both can be blocked by packing the nose with gauze or cotton-tipped applicators soaked with local anesthetic. The topical anesthetic should be allowed to remain in place at least 10 minutes before

Table 39–3. Airway-fire protocol.

1. Stop ventilation and remove endotracheal tube.
2. Turn off oxygen and disconnect circuit from machine.
3. Submerge tube in water.
4. Ventilate with face mask and reintubate.
5. Assess airway damage with bronchoscopy and blood gases.
6. Consider bronchial lavage and steroids.

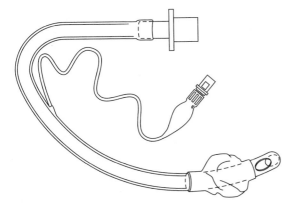

Figure 39–1. An oral RAE endotracheal tube has a preformed right-angle bend at the level of the teeth so that it exits the mouth away from the surgical field during ophthalmic or nasal surgery.

General anesthesia is often preferred for nasal surgery because of the discomfort and incomplete block that may accompany topical anesthesia. Special considerations during induction include using an oral airway during face mask ventilation to mitigate the effects of nasal obstruction, intubation with a reinforced or preformed right-angle endotracheal tube (eg, oral RAE tube, Mallinckrodt Critical Care; Figure 39–1), and tucking the patient's padded arms to the side. Because of the proximity of the surgical field, it is important to tape the patient's eyes closed to avoid a **corneal abrasion.** One exception to this is during endoscopic sinus surgery, when the surgeon may wish to periodically check for eye movement during dissection because of the close proximity of the sinuses and orbit (Figure 39–2). Similarly, muscle relaxation is strongly suggested because of the potential neurologic or ophthalmic complications that might arise if the patient moves during sinus instrumentation.

Techniques to minimize intraoperative blood loss include supplementation with cocaine or an epinephrine-containing local anesthetic, maintaining a slightly head-up position, and providing a mild degree of controlled hypotension. A posterior pharyngeal pack is often placed to limit the risk of aspiration of blood. Despite these precautions, the anesthesiologist must be prepared for significant blood loss, especially during the resection of vascular tumors (eg, juvenile nasopharyngeal angiofibroma).

Ideally, extubation should be smooth, with a minimum of coughing or straining, since these will increase

instrumentation is attempted. Supplementation with submucosal injections of local anesthetic is often required, particularly if scar tissue is present from prior surgery. Use of an epinephrine-containing solution or cocaine (usually a 4% or 10% solution) will shrink the nasal mucosa and potentially decrease intraoperative blood loss. Intranasal cocaine (maximum dose, 3 mg/kg) is rapidly absorbed (reaching peak levels in 30 minutes) and may cause detrimental cardiovascular effects (see Chapter 14).

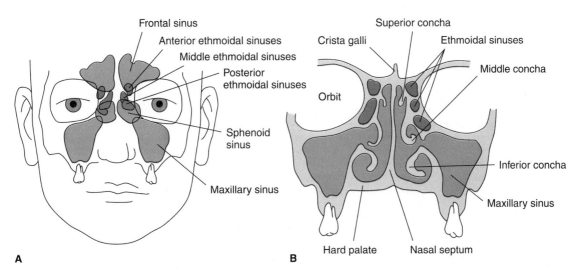

A   **B**

Figure 39–2. The proximity of the sinuses to the orbit (**A,** frontal view; **B,** coronal section) introduces the possibility of orbital fracture during endoscopic sinus surgery. (Reproduced and modified with permission from Snell RS, Katz J: *Clinical Anatomy for Anesthesiologists,* Appleton & Lange, 1988.)

venous pressure and tend to increase postoperative bleeding. Unfortunately, strategies that accomplish this goal also tend to increase the risk of aspiration (eg, deep extubation).

HEAD & NECK CANCER SURGERY

Surgery for cancer of the head and neck includes laryngectomy, glossectomy, pharyngectomy, parotidectomy, hemimandibulectomy, and radical neck dissection. An endoscopic examination often precedes these procedures, while the timing of a tracheostomy depends on the patient's preoperative airway compromise. Some procedures may include reconstructive surgery, such as the transplantation of a free microvascular muscle flap.

Preoperative Considerations

The typical patient presenting for head and neck cancer surgery is elderly and has a long history of heavy tobacco and alcohol use. Preexisting medical conditions that often need preoperative evaluation and optimization include chronic obstructive pulmonary disease, coronary artery disease, chronic alcoholism, aspiration pneumonia, and malnutrition.

Airway management may be complicated by an obstructing lesion or preoperative radiation therapy that has further distorted the patient's anatomy. As always, if there is serious doubt regarding potential airway problems, an intravenous induction should be avoided in favor of awake direct or fiberoptic laryngoscopy (cooperative patient) or an inhalational induction, maintaining spontaneous ventilation (uncooperative patient). In any case, the equipment and personnel required for an emergency tracheostomy must be *immediately* available. Elective tracheostomy under local anesthesia is a prudent option, particularly if indirect laryngoscopy shows the lesion to be susceptible to dislodgment during intubation.

Intraoperative Management

A. MONITORING:

Because of the substantial blood loss associated with many of these procedures and the prevalence of coexisting cardiopulmonary disease, these patients often require arterial cannulation for blood pressure, blood gas, and hematocrit monitoring. If a central venous line or pulmonary artery catheter is deemed necessary, antecubital or femoral veins provide the best access. Arterial lines and intravenous cannulas should not be placed in the arms if a radial forearm flap is planned. A minimum of two large-bore intravenous lines should be secured and a urinary catheter (preferably with temperature-monitoring capability) placed. Inspiratory gases should be heated and

humidified, and a forced-air warming blanket positioned over the lower extremities will help maintain normal body temperature. Intraoperative hypothermia and consequent vasoconstriction can be particularly detrimental for perfusion of a microvascular free flap.

B. TRACHEOSTOMY:

Intraoperative tracheostomy is often a part of head and neck cancer surgery. During ventilation with 100% oxygen, the endotracheal tube and hypopharynx should be thoroughly suctioned to limit the risk of aspiration of blood and secretions. After dissection down to the trachea, the endotracheal tube cuff is deflated to avoid perforation by the scalpel. When the tracheal wall is transected, the endotracheal tube is withdrawn so that its tip is just cephalad to the incision. Ventilation during this period is difficult because of the large leak through the trachea. A sterile wire-reinforced endotracheal tube or J-shaped laryngectomy tube is placed in the trachea, connected to a sterile breathing circuit, and sutured to the chest wall. As soon as correct positioning is confirmed by capnography and chest auscultation, the old endotracheal tube may be removed. An increase in peak inspiratory pressure immediately after tracheostomy usually signals a malpositioned tube, bronchospasm, or debris in the trachea.

C. MAINTENANCE OF ANESTHESIA:

 The surgeon may request the omission of muscle relaxants during neck dissection or parotidectomy to identify nerves (eg, spinal accessory, facial nerves) by direct stimulation and to preserve them. A mild hypotensive technique may be helpful in limiting blood loss. Cerebral perfusion pressure may be severely compromised, however, when the tumor involves the carotid artery (decreased cerebral arterial pressure) or jugular vein (increased cerebral venous pressure). Furthermore, a head-up tilt may increase the chance of venous air embolism. Following reanastomosis of a microvascular free flap, blood pressure should be maintained at the patient's baseline level. Vasoconstrictive agents (eg, phenylephrine) should be avoided because even though systemic blood pressure increases, flap perfusion decreases due to vasoconstriction of graft vessels. Likewise, vasodilators (eg, sodium nitroprusside) should be avoided due to decreased perfusion pressures.

D. TRANSFUSION:

Blood loss can be rapid and substantial. Transfusion decisions must balance the patient's medical problems with the possibility of an increased posttransfusion cancer recurrence rate as a result of immune suppression. Rheologic factors make a relatively low hematocrit (eg, 25–27%) desirable when microvascular free flaps are performed. Diuresis should be avoided during microvascular free-flap surgery to allow adequate graft perfusion in the postoperative period.

E. CARDIOVASCULAR INSTABILITY:

Manipulation of the carotid sinus and stellate ganglion during radical neck dissection (right side more than the left) has been associated with wide swings in blood pressure, bradycardia, dysrhythmias, sinus arrest, and prolonged QT intervals. Infiltration of the carotid sheath with local anesthetic will usually ameliorate this problem. Bilateral neck dissection may result in postoperative hypertension and loss of hypoxic drive because of denervation of the carotid sinuses and bodies.

CRANIOFACIAL RECONSTRUCTION & ORTHOGNATHIC SURGERY

Craniofacial reconstruction is often required to correct the effects of trauma (eg, LeFort fractures), congenital malformations (eg, hypertelorism), or radical cancer surgeries (eg, mandibulectomy). Orthognathic procedures (eg, LeFort osteotomies, mandibular osteotomies) for dental malocclusion share many of the same surgical and anesthetic techniques.

Preoperative Considerations

These patients often pose the greatest airway challenges to the anesthesiologist. Preoperative airway evaluation must be detailed and thorough. Particular attention should be focused on jaw opening, mask fit, neck mobility, micrognathia, retrognathia, maxillary protrusion (overbite), macroglossia, dental pathology, nasal patency, and the existence of any intraoral lesions or debris.

If there are any forewarning signs of problems with mask ventilation or endotracheal intubation, the airway should be secured prior to induction. This may involve fiberoptic nasal intubation, fiberoptic oral intubation, or tracheostomy. Nasal intubation with a preformed tube (nasal RAE) or a straight tube with a flexible angle connector (Figure 39–3) is usually preferred in dental and oral surgery. The endotracheal tube can then be directed cephalad and connected to breathing tubes coming over the patient's head. On the other hand, nasal intubation is specifically avoided in LeFort II and III fractures because of the possibility of a coexisting basilar skull fracture and cerebrospinal fluid rhinorrhea (Figure 39–4).

Intraoperative Management

Reconstructive and orthognathic surgeries can be associated with substantial blood loss. Strategies to mini-

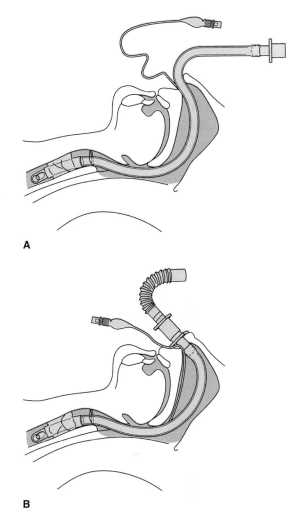

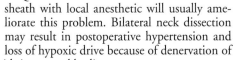

A

B

Figure 39–3. ***A:*** A nasal RAE endotracheal tube has a preformed right-angle bend at the level of the nose so that the tube is directed over the forehead; ***B:*** Alternatively, a regular straight endotracheal tube can be cut at the level of the nares and a flexible connector attached.

mize bleeding include a slight head-up position, controlled hypotension, and local infiltration with epinephrine solutions. Because the patient's arms are typically tucked at their sides, at least two intravenous lines should be established prior to surgery. This is especially important if one line is used for delivery of an intravenous anesthetic or hypotensive agent. An arterial line can be helpful during high-blood-loss cases, particularly since a surgeon leaning against the patient's arm may interfere with noninvasive blood pressure cuff readings.

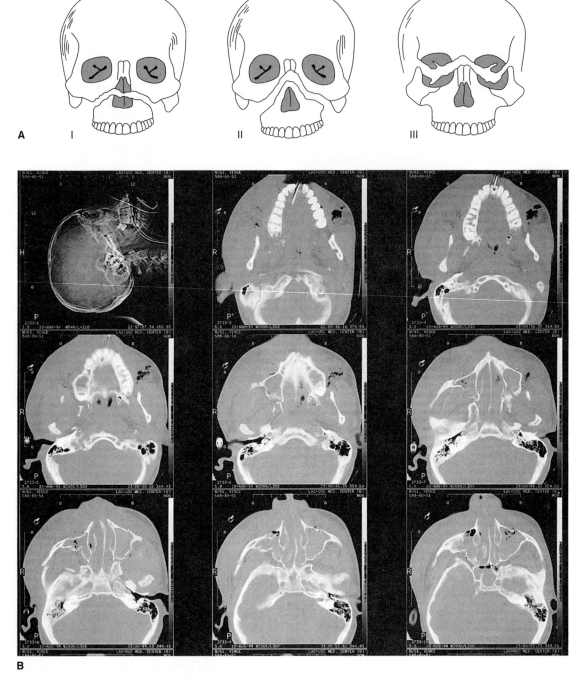

Figure 39–4. **A:** Diagrammatic representation of LeFort I, II, and III fractures. LeFort II and III may coexist with a basilar skull fracture, a contraindication to nasal intubation. **B:** CT scan demonstrating evidence of LeFort II fracture. There is no evidence of basilar skull fracture on these slices.

An oropharyngeal pack is often placed to minimize the amount of blood and other debris reaching the larynx and trachea.

Because of the proximity of the airway to the surgical field, the anesthesiologist's location is more remote than usual. This increases the likelihood of serious intraoperative airway problems such as endotracheal tube kinking, disconnection, or perforation by a surgical instrument. Airway monitoring of end-tidal CO_2, peak inspiratory pressures, and esophageal stethoscope breath sounds assume increased importance in such cases.

At the end of surgery, the oropharyngeal pack must be removed and the pharynx suctioned. While it is not unusual for there to be some bloody debris during initial suctioning, repeat efforts should be less productive. If there is a chance of postoperative edema involving structures that could potentially obstruct the airway (eg, tongue), the patient should be left intubated. Otherwise, extubation can be attempted once the patient is fully awake and there are no signs of continued bleeding. Patients with intermaxillary fixation (eg, maxillomandibular wiring) should have appropriate cutting tools at their bedside in case of vomiting or other airway emergencies.

EAR SURGERY

Frequently performed ear surgeries include stapedectomy (usually under local anesthesia), tympanoplasty, and mastoidectomy. Myringotomy with insertion of tympanostomy tubes is the most common pediatric surgical procedure and is discussed in Chapter 44.

Intraoperative Management

A. NITROUS OXIDE:

Because nitrous oxide is more soluble than nitrogen in blood, it diffuses into air-containing cavities more rapidly than nitrogen (the major component of air) can be absorbed by the bloodstream (see Chapter 7). Normally, changes in middle ear pressures caused by nitrous oxide are well tolerated as a result of passive venting through the eustachian tube. Patients with a history of chronic ear problems (eg, otitis media, sinusitis), however, often suffer from obstructed eustachian tubes and may rarely experience hearing loss or tympanic membrane rupture during nitrous oxide anesthesia.

During tympanoplasty, the middle ear is open to the atmosphere and there is no pressure build-up. Once the surgeon has placed a tympanic membrane graft, the middle ear becomes a closed space. If nitrous oxide is allowed to diffuse into this space, middle ear pressure will rise, and the graft may be displaced. Conversely, discontinuing nitrous oxide after graft placement will create a negative middle ear pressure that could also cause graft dislodgment. Therefore, nitrous oxide is either entirely avoided during tympanoplasty or discontinued prior to graft placement. Obviously, the exact amount of time required to wash out the nitrous oxide depends on many factors, including alveolar ventilation and fresh gas flows (see Chapter 7), but 15–30 minutes is usually recommended.

B. HEMOSTASIS:

As with any form of microsurgery, even small amounts of blood can obscure the operating field. Techniques to minimize blood loss during ear surgery include mild (15-degree) head elevation, infiltration or topical application of epinephrine (1:50,000–1:200,000), and controlled hypotension. The use of controlled hypotension in ear surgery is somewhat controversial because of its inherent risks and questionable necessity. Because coughing on an endotracheal tube during awakening (especially during head bandaging) will increase venous pressure and may cause bleeding, a deep extubation may prove helpful.

C. FACIAL NERVE IDENTIFICATION:

Preservation of the facial nerve is an important consideration during some types of ear surgery (eg, resection of a glomus tumor or acoustic neuroma). During these cases, intraoperative paralysis with muscle relaxants may confuse the interpretation of facial nerve stimulation and should be avoided.

D. POSTOPERATIVE NAUSEA AND VOMITING:

Because the inner ear is intimately involved with the sense of balance, it should not be surprising that ear surgery may cause postoperative dizziness (vertigo), nausea, and vomiting. Induction and maintenance with propofol has been shown to decrease postoperative nausea and vomiting in patients undergoing middle ear surgery. Routine prophylaxis with an antiemetic should be considered.

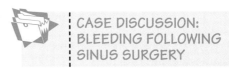

CASE DISCUSSION:
BLEEDING FOLLOWING
SINUS SURGERY

A 50-year-old man has a paroxysm of coughing in the recovery room while awakening following uneventful endoscopic sinus surgery. Immediately afterwards, his respirations appear labored with a loud inspiratory stridor.

What is the differential diagnosis of inspiratory stridor?

The acute onset of inspiratory stridor in a postoperative patient may be due to laryngospasm, laryngeal edema, foreign body aspiration, or vocal cord dysfunction. Laryngospasm, an involuntary spasm of the laryngeal musculature, may be triggered by blood or secretions stimulating the superior laryngeal nerve (see Chapter 5). Laryngeal edema may be caused by an allergic drug reaction, hereditary or iatrogenic angioedema, or a traumatic intubation. Vocal cord dysfunction could be due to residual muscle relaxant effect, hypocalcemic alkalotic tetany, intubation trauma, or paradoxical vocal cord motion (ie, hysterical stridor).

Another paroxysm of coughing is accompanied by hemoptysis. What would be your immediate management?

Bleeding after nose or throat surgery can be very serious. If the patient is not fully awake, he may continue to gag and cough on the secretions, increasing venous pressure and worsening the bleeding. Furthermore, he may aspirate blood and other secretions. Fortunately, because of its physiologic pH, aspiration of blood is not as serious as the aspiration of acidic gastric contents. Nonetheless, the airway should be immediately secured in the obtunded patient. This may be accomplished with an awake intubation or a rapid-sequence induction.

If the patient is awake and alert enough to cough and swallow and does not appear to be aspirating blood, the first priority should be to decrease the bleeding as quickly as possible. Immediate measures that should be considered include raising the head of the bed to decrease venous and arterial pressures at the site of bleeding and aggressively treating any degree of systolic hypertension with intravenous antihypertensive agents. Sedation should be avoided so that airway reflexes are not compromised.

Despite these measures the bleeding continues, and surgical intervention appears necessary. Describe your strategy for induction of anesthesia in this patient.

Before induction of general anesthesia in the bleeding patient, hypovolemia should be corrected with isotonic crystalloid or colloid. The degree of hypovolemia is difficult to assess because much of the blood may be swallowed but may be estimated by changes in vital signs, postural hypotension, and hematocrit. Cross-matched blood should be readily available, and a second large-bore intravenous line secured. It must be appreciated that from an anesthetic standpoint, this is an entirely different patient than the one who presented for surgery initially: he now has a full stomach, is hypovolemic, and may prove to be a more difficult intubation.

The preferred technique in this patient is a rapid-sequence induction with cricoid pressure. Drug choice (eg, ketamine, etomidate) and dosage should anticipate the possibility of hypotension from persistent hypovolemia. Personnel and equipment for an emergency tracheostomy should be readily available. An orogastric tube should be passed to decompress the stomach.

Which arteries supply blood to the nose?

The arterial supply of the nose is provided by the internal maxillary artery and the anterior ethmoid artery. These may need to be ligated in uncontrollable epistaxis.

Describe extubation.

Because this patient is still at risk for aspiration, extubation should not be attempted until the patient has fully awakened and regained airway reflexes. While it is desirable to limit coughing and "bucking" on the endotracheal tube during emergence, these are difficult to achieve in the awakening patient. Some authorities suggest the intravenous administration of lidocaine (1.5 mg/kg) during this period.

SUGGESTED READING

Banic A, Krejci V, Erni D, Wheatley AM, Sigurdsson G: Effects of sodium nitroprusside and phenylephrine on blood flow in free musculocutaneous flaps during general anesthesia. Anesthesiology 1999;90:147. Free flap survival can be greatly influenced by anesthetic management.

Bargainnier DR, Hasnain JU, Matjasko MJ: How do you manage the patient requiring subglottic laser surgery? Survey Anesth 1992;6:275.

Brooker CR, Hunsaker DH, Zimmerman AA: A new anesthetic system for microlaryngeal surgery. Otolaryngol Head Neck Surg 1998;118:55. This system combines a nonflammable tube and a subglottic jet ventilator with special safety features.

Fujii Y, Toyooka H, Tanaka H: Prophylactic antiemetic therapy with a combination of granisetron and dexamethasone in patients undergoing middle ear surgery. Br J Anaesth 1998; 81:754. The high incidence of nausea and vomiting following middle ear surgery requires combination antiemetic therapy.

Jensen NF: Glomus tumors of the head and neck: Anesthetic considerations. Anesth Analg 1994;78:112. An excellent review of the implications of surgery on this rare type of paraganglioma that can mimic pheochromocytoma and carcinoid syndrome.

Magnusson L, Lang FJW, Monnier P, Ravussin P: Anaesthesia for tracheal resection: Report of 17 cases. Can J Anaesth 1997;44:1282. This paper describes the use of high frequency jet ventilation for tracheal resection surgery.

McGoldrick KE (editor): *Anesthesia for Ophthalmic and Otolaryngologic Surgery.* WB Saunders and Company, 1992. The first 12 chapters of this book are devoted to anesthetic considerations in otolaryngologic surgery, including airway anatomy, management of difficult intubations, laser surgery, and emergency surgery.

Rampil IJ: Anesthetic considerations for laser surgery. Anesth Analg 1992;74:424. This article reviews the physics of laser light, clinical applications of laser hardware, laser hazards, and strategies to avoid endotracheal tube fires.

Sitzman BT, Rich GF, Rockwell JJ, et al: Local anesthetic administration for awake direct laryngoscopy: Are glossopharyngeal nerve blocks superior? Anesthesiology 1997;86:34. A 2-minute swish and gargle of 2% viscous lidocaine followed by a 10% lidocaine spray was found to provide better anesthesia for direct laryngoscopy than bilateral glossopharyngeal nerve blocks.

Sosis MB (editor): *Anesthesia for Otolaryngologic and Head and Neck Surgery.* Vol 11, No. 3 of *Anesth Clin N Am.* WB Saunders and Company, 1993.

Webster AC, Morley-Forster PK, Janzen V: Anesthesia for intranasal surgery: A comparison between tracheal intubation and the flexible reinforced laryngeal mask airway. Anesth Analg 1999;88:421. The authors demonstrate a lower incidence of laryngospasm, hemoglobin desaturation, and hoarseness following use of a laryngeal mask airway for intranasal surgery.

Anesthesia for Orthopedic Surgery | 40

KEY CONCEPTS

 Fat embolism syndrome classically presents within 72 hours following long-bone or pelvic fracture, with the triad of dyspnea, confusion, and petechiae.

 During general anesthesia, signs of fat embolism syndrome may include a decline in end-tidal carbon dioxide and arterial oxygen saturation, or a rise in pulmonary artery pressures.

 Flexion and extension lateral radiographs of the cervical spine should be obtained preoperatively in all patients with rheumatoid arthritis severe enough to require steroids or methotrexate. If atlantoaxial instability exceeds 5 mm, intubation should be performed with neck stabilization and an awake fiberoptic technique.

 Drugs that specifically inhibit COX-2 (eg, celecoxib, rofecoxib, parecoxib, valdecoxib) would be expected to have a lower risk of side effects than nonspecific nonsteroidal anti-inflammatory drugs (NSAIDs). Because of their greater cost, COX-2 agents are typically reserved for patients at increased risk for side effects (eg, prior history of gastrointestinal bleeding or reflux, coagulopathy, concurrent steroid use).

 Pulmonary artery monitoring in patients undergoing bilateral hip arthroplasties reliably signals embolization by a rise in pulmonary vascular resistance. If pulmonary artery pressures rise above normal (300 dynes × sec × cm^{-5}) during the first hip arthroplasty, the contralateral surgery should be postponed.

 Regional anesthesia decreases the incidence of deep venous thrombosis and pulmonary embolism following hip replacement surgery.

 Although most clinicians agree that full anticoagulation or fibrinolytic therapy (eg, urokinase) represents an unacceptable risk for epidural hematoma, the danger in patients receiving low-dose anticoagulation or patients with mild platelet dysfunction (eg, nonspecific NSAID) has not been adequately defined.

 Pneumatic tourniquets are often used in knee arthroscopic surgeries because they create a bloodless field, which greatly facilitates the procedure. However, tourniquets are associated with potential problems of their own, including hemodynamic changes, pain, metabolic alterations, arterial thromboembolus, and pulmonary embolism.

 During spinal surgery, with the patient in the prone position, extreme caution is necessary to avoid retinal ischemia from pressure on either globe or pressure necrosis of the nose, ears, forehead, female breasts, or male genitalia.

 Despite preservation of somatosensory evoked potentials (SSEPs) during spinal surgery, postoperative motor deficits are possible because SSEPs monitor dorsal column sensory function, not motor function.

 Successful reimplantation and transplantation surgery depends on good arterial blood flow following reanastomosis. The avoidance of hypothermia and hypovolemia becomes a critical responsibility of the anesthesiologist.

Orthopedic surgery challenges the anesthesiologist with its diversity. Orthopedic patients range from neonates with congenital anomalies to healthy young athletes to immobile geriatric patients with end-stage multiorgan failure. The degree of surgical trespass varies from finger surgery to hemipelvectomy. Blood loss may be limited by a tourniquet, or it may be uncontrollable despite all conventional strategies. Almost every conceivable patient position has been advocated at one time or another for some orthopedic procedure. Regional anesthetic techniques play a more important role in orthopedic surgery than in any other surgical subspecialty. Although this chapter addresses several concerns specific to orthopedic surgery, the successful orthopedic anesthesiologist must possess a wide range of anesthetic skills and knowledge.

■ HIP SURGERY

Common hip procedures encountered in adult patients include repair of hip fracture, total hip arthroplasty, and closed reduction of hip dislocation.

FRACTURE OF THE HIP

Preoperative Considerations

Most patients presenting for hip surgery are frail and elderly. This is particularly true of patients with hip fractures. Studies have reported mortality rates following hip fracture of 10% during the initial hospitalization and over 25% within 1 year. Many of these patients have concomitant diseases such as coronary artery disease, cerebral vascular disease, chronic obstructive pulmonary disease, or diabetes. Investigations of a new protective cup that rests over the greater trochanter have demonstrated a marked decrease of hip fractures in high-risk populations (eg, nursing home patients).

Patients presenting with hip fractures are frequently dehydrated because of inadequate oral intake. Depending on the site of the hip fracture, occult blood loss may be significant and further compromise intravascular volume. In general, intracapsular (subcapital, transcervical) fractures are associated with less blood loss than extracapsular (base of femoral neck, intertrochanteric, subtrochanteric) fractures (Figure 40–1).

Another characteristic of hip-fracture patients is preoperative hypoxia that is largely due to fat embolism. While some degree of fat embolism probably occurs in all cases of long-bone fracture, **fat embolism syndrome** is a less frequent but often fatal (10–20%) event. Fat embolism syndrome classically presents within 72 hours following

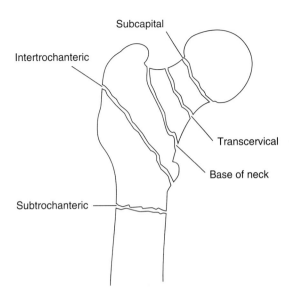

Figure 40–1. Blood loss from hip fracture depends on the location of the fracture (subtrochanteric, intertrochanteric > base of femoral neck > transcervical, subcapital) because the capsule contains blood loss by acting like a tourniquet.

long-bone or pelvic fracture, with the triad of dyspnea, confusion, and petechiae. Fat embolism syndrome can also be seen following cardiopulmonary resuscitation, parental feeding with lipid infusion, and liposuction. Two theories have been proposed for its pathogenesis. The most popular theory holds that fat globules are released by the disruption of fat cells in the fractured bone and enter the circulation through tears in medullary vessels. An alternative theory proposes that the fat globules are chylomicrons resulting from the aggregation of circulating free fatty acids caused by changes in fatty acid metabolism. Regardless of their source, the increased free fatty acid levels can have a toxic effect on the capillary-alveolar membrane leading to the release of vasoactive amines and prostaglandins and the development of acute respiratory distress syndrome (see Chapter 50). Neurologic manifestations (agitation, confusion, stupor, or coma) probably represent capillary damage to the cerebral circulation and cerebral edema and may be exacerbated by hypoxia.

The diagnosis of fat embolism syndrome is suggested by petechiae on the chest, upper extremities, axillae, and conjunctiva. Fat globules may be found in the retina, urine, or sputum. Coagulation abnormalities such as thrombocytopenia or prolonged clotting times are occasionally present. Serum lipase activity may be elevated, but bears no relationship to disease severity. Pulmonary involvement typically progresses from mild hypoxia and a normal chest radiograph to severe hypoxia and a chest film showing diffuse patchy pulmonary infiltrates. Most of the classic signs and symptoms of fat embolism syndrome occur 1 to 3 days after the precipitant event. Signs during general anesthesia may include a decline in end-tidal carbon dioxide and arterial oxygen saturation, or a rise in pulmonary artery pressures. Electrocardiography may show ischemic-appearing ST-segment changes and right-sided heart strain.

Treatment is 2-fold: prophylactic and supportive. Early stabilization of the fracture decreases the incidence of fat embolism syndrome. Supportive treatment consists of oxygen therapy with continuous positive airway pressure ventilation. Treatment with heparin or alcohol has generally been disappointing. High-dose corticosteroid therapy may be beneficial, especially in the presence of cerebral edema.

Intraoperative Management

The choice between regional (spinal or epidural) and general anesthesia has been extensively evaluated for hip-fracture surgery. Many studies have found a lower mortality in the early postoperative period following regional anesthesia, presumably because of a decrease in thromboembolic disease. After 2 months, however, the mortality rates for regional and general anesthesia have not been consistently different.

Several possible mechanisms may explain the reduction in thromboembolic complications following regional anesthesia. These include greater lower-extremity venous blood flow, decreased platelet reactivity, attenuated postoperative increase in factor VIII and von Willebrand factor, attenuated postoperative decrease in antithrombin III, and alterations in stress hormone release. Intravenous lidocaine has been shown to prevent thrombosis, enhance fibrinolysis, and decrease platelet aggregation.

A continuous epidural technique, with or without concomitant general anesthesia, provides the additional advantage of postoperative pain control. If a spinal anesthetic is planned, a hypobaric technique allows easier positioning because the patient does not have to lie on the fractured hip and can remain in the same position for the surgery.

TOTAL HIP ARTHROPLASTY

Preoperative Considerations

Most patients undergoing total hip replacement suffer from osteoarthritis or rheumatoid arthritis. **Osteoarthritis** is a degenerative disease affecting the articular surface of one or more joints (most commonly the hip and knee). The etiology of osteoarthritis appears to involve repetitive joint trauma (eg, morbid obesity). Because the spine is often involved, neck positioning during intubation should be as gentle as possible to avoid nerve root compression or nucleus pulposus protrusion.

Rheumatoid arthritis differs from osteoarthritis in three key aspects. First, rheumatoid arthritis is characterized by an immune-mediated joint destruction with chronic and progressive inflammation of synovial membranes, as opposed to articular wear and tear. Second, but very important to the anesthesiologist, is the systemic involvement that can accompany rheumatoid arthritis (Table 40–1). In addition, rheumatoid arthritis typically involves multiple joints, including the small joints of the hands, wrists, and feet, in a symmetric fashion. Inserting invasive catheters and even gaining intravenous access are a challenge in patients with severe deformities.

Debilitation and limited joint mobility prohibit assessment of exercise tolerance, potentially masking underlying coronary artery disease and pulmonary dysfunction. The cardiovascular status of patients unable to exercise, yet at risk for coronary artery disease (eg, a history of angina, diabetes, congestive heart failure, myocardial infarction) can be evaluated with dipyridamole thallium scanning, dipyridamole echocardiography, or dobutamine echocardiography.

Extreme cases of rheumatoid arthritis can involve almost all synovial membranes, including those in the cervical spine and temporomandibular joint. **Atlantoaxial subluxation,** which can be diagnosed radiologically, may lead to protrusion of the odontoid process into the foramen magnum during intubation, compromising ver-

Table 40–1. Systemic manifestations of rheumatoid arthritis.

Organ System	Abnormalities
Cardiovascular	Pericardial thickening and effusion, myocarditis, coronary arteritis, conduction defects, vasculitis, cardiac valve fibrosis (aortic regurgitation)
Pulmonary	Pleural effusion, pulmonary nodules, interstitial pulmonary fibrosis
Hematopoietic	Anemia, eosinophilia, platelet dysfunction (from aspirin therapy), thrombocytopenia
Endocrine	Adrenal insufficiency (from glucocorticoid therapy), impaired immune system
Dermatologic	Thin and atrophic skin from the disease and immunosuppressive drugs

tebral blood flow and compressing the spinal cord or brainstem (Figure 40–2). Flexion and extension lateral radiographs of the cervical spine should be obtained preoperatively in all patients with rheumatoid arthritis severe enough to require steroids or methotrexate. If atlantoaxial instability exceeds 5 mm, intubation should be performed with neck stabilization and an awake fiberoptic technique. Involvement of the temporomandibular joint can limit jaw mobility and range of motion to such a degree that successful intubation will require a nasal fiberoptic technique. Hoarseness or inspiratory stridor may signal a narrowing of the glottic opening caused by **cricoary-tenoid arthritis.** Despite the use of a smaller-diameter

endotracheal tube, this condition may lead to postextubation airway obstruction.

Patients with rheumatoid arthritis or osteoarthritis commonly receive nonsteroidal anti-inflammatory drugs (NSAIDs) for pain management. These drugs can have serious side effects such as life-threatening gastrointestinal bleeding, renal toxicity, and platelet dysfunction. The mechanism of action of NSAIDs has been related to their inhibition of the synthesis of prostaglandins by the cyclooxygenase (COX) enzyme, of which there are two isoforms (COX-1 and COX-2). It appears that the pain relief and anti-inflammatory properties are related to COX-2 inhibition, while most of the side effects are principally due to COX-1 inhibi-

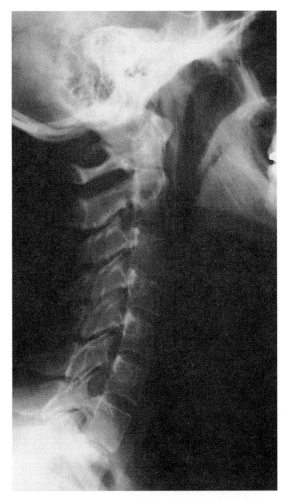 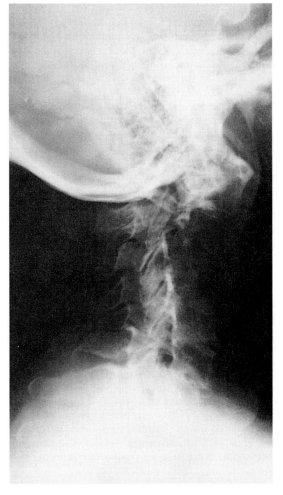

Figure 40–2. Because instability of the cervical spine may be asymptomatic, lateral radiographs are mandatory in patients with severe rheumatoid arthritis. Figure 40–2 (left) is a radiograph of a normal lateral cervical spine. Figure 40–2 (right) shows a lateral cervical spine of a patient with rheumatoid arthritis; note the severe C1–C2 instability.

tion (renal toxicity may be an exception). Thus, drugs that specifically inhibit COX-2 (eg, celecoxib, rofecoxib, parecoxib, valdecoxib) would be expected to have a lower risk of side effects than nonspecific NSAIDs. On the other hand, COX-2 inhibitors would not be expected to confer the benefits of long-term platelet inhibition (ie, prevention of myocardial infarction and stroke). Because of their greater cost, COX-2 agents are typically reserved for patients at increased risk for side effects (eg, prior history of gastrointestinal bleeding or reflux, coagulopathy, concurrent steroid use). Likewise, the perioperative period may be a rationale time to choose COX-2 drugs to decrease the risk of wound bleeding or epidural hematoma.

Intraoperative Management

Total hip replacement (THR) involves several surgical steps including placement and positioning of the patient in the lateral decubitus position (see Chapter 47), dislocation and removal of the femoral head, reaming of the acetabulum and insertion of a prosthetic acetabular cup (with or without cement), and reaming of the femur and insertion of a femoral component (femoral head and stem) into the femoral shaft (with or without cement). THR is also associated with three potentially life-threatening complications: bone cement implantation syndrome, perioperative hemorrhage, and thromboembolism.

Methylmethacrylate cement interdigitates within the interstices of cancellous bone and strongly binds the prosthetic device to the patient's bone. Mixing polymerized methylmethacrylate powder with liquid methylmethacrylate monomer causes polymerization and crosslinking of the polymer chains. This exothermic reaction leads to cement hardening and expansion against the prosthetic components. The resultant intramedullary hypertension (> 500 mm Hg) causes embolization of fat, bone marrow, cement, and air into the femoral venous channels. Residual methylmethacrylate monomer can produce vasodilation and a decrease in systemic vascular resistance. The release of tissue thromboplastin may trigger platelet aggregation, microthrombus formation in the lungs, and cardiovascular instability as a result of the circulation of vasoactive substances.

The clinical manifestations of this **bone cement implantation syndrome** include hypoxia (increased pulmonary shunt), hypotension, dysrhythmias (including heart block and sinus arrest), pulmonary hypertension (increased pulmonary vascular resistance), and decreased cardiac output. Thus, there are many reasons why invasive arterial monitoring is generally recommended for these procedures. Emboli most frequently occur during insertion of the femoral prosthesis. Strategies to minimize the effects of this complication include

increasing inspired oxygen concentration prior to cementing, maintaining euvolemia by monitoring central venous pressure, creating a vent hole in the distal femur to relieve intramedullary pressure, performing high-pressure lavage of the femoral shaft to remove debris (potential microemboli), or using an uncemented femoral component.

Bilateral hip arthroplasties can be safely performed during one anesthetic, assuming the absence of significant pulmonary embolization after insertion of the first femoral component. Pulmonary artery monitoring reliably signals embolization by a rise in pulmonary vascular resistance (PVR). This is usually indicated by a rise in pulmonary artery pressures ($\overline{PA}$) in the face of unchanged pulmonary artery occlusion pressure (PAOP) and falling cardiac output:

$$PVR = \frac{\overline{PA} - PAOP}{\text{Cardiac output}} \times 80$$

If pulmonary artery pressures rise above normal (300 dynes $\times$ sec $\times$ cm^{-5}) during the first hip arthroplasty, the contralateral surgery should be postponed.

Hip-replacement surgery, particularly revision of a prior hip arthroplasty, may be associated with significant perioperative blood loss. Blood loss depends on many factors, including the experience and skill of the surgeon, the surgical technique used, and the type of prosthesis chosen. **Controlled hypotension** (see Chapter 13 Case Discussion) can decrease intraoperative bleeding. Some studies have suggested that blood loss may be less during hip surgery using a regional technique (eg, spinal or epidural anesthesia) than with general anesthesia in spite of maintaining similar mean arterial blood pressures. The reasons for this dichotomy remain uncertain but may include differences in the resulting vasodilation of the venous and arterial vascular systems, leading to a redistribution of blood flow. By providing a dry bone surface, controlled hypotension also improves prosthetic cementing and shortens the duration of surgery. Because the majority of hip replacement patients require perioperative blood transfusions, preoperative autologous blood donation and intraoperative blood salvage should be considered (see Chapter 29). High-dose aprotinin, a proteinase inhibitor of fibrinolytic activity and the intrinsic coagulation pathway by decreasing activation of plasminogen, may reduce intraoperative blood loss in some patients. It is usually reserved for high-risk cases (eg, coagulopathies), however, because of its propensity to produce immunologic sensitization. Preoperative administration of recombinant human erythropoietin (Epoetin alfa: 600 IU/kg SQ weekly beginning 21 days before surgery and ending on the day of surgery) represents another alternative for decreasing the need for perioperative allogeneic blood transfusion. Erythropoietin increases red blood cell production by stimulating the division and differentiation of erythroid progenitors in the bone marrow. Maintaining normal body temperature during hip replacement surgery has been shown to reduce blood loss.

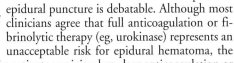

Venous thromboembolism is a significant cause of morbidity and mortality following hip-replacement surgery. For the reasons discussed earlier, regional anesthesia decreases the incidence of deep venous thrombosis and pulmonary embolism. Other strategies for minimizing the risk of perioperative thromboembolism include intermittent leg-compression devices and low-dose anticoagulant prophylaxis. Whether the latter contraindicates spinal or epidural puncture is debatable. Although most clinicians agree that full anticoagulation or fibrinolytic therapy (eg, urokinase) represents an unacceptable risk for epidural hematoma, the danger in patients receiving low-dose anticoagulation or patients with mild platelet dysfunction (eg, nonspecific NSAID) has not been adequately defined. A major concern is that a regional anesthetic could mask the hallmarks of an expanding hematoma and cord compression (eg, lower back pain and lower-extremity weakness), thus delaying diagnosis and treatment.

CLOSED REDUCTION
HIP DISLOCATION

There is a 3% incidence of hip dislocation following primary hip arthroplasty and a 20% incidence following total hip revision. Because less force is required to dislocate a prosthetic hip, patients with hip implants require special precautions during positioning for subsequent surgical procedures. Extremes of hip flexion (> 90 degrees), internal rotation (> 20 degrees), and adduction (> 20 degrees) increase the risk of dislocation and should be avoided. Hip dislocations are usually correctable with closed reduction. General anesthesia with a face mask is usually sufficient for this very brief procedure. Profound paralysis as provided by succinylcholine will facilitate the surgeon's manipulations by relaxing the hip musculature. Successful reduction may need to be confirmed radiologically prior to the patient's awakening.

■ KNEE SURGERY

The two most frequently performed knee surgeries are arthroscopy and total joint replacement.

KNEE ARTHROSCOPY
Preoperative Considerations

Arthroscopy has revolutionized surgery of many joints, including the knee, shoulder, ankle, and wrist. Joint arthroscopies are usually outpatient procedures. Although the typical patient undergoing knee arthroscopy is often thought of as being a healthy young athlete, knee arthroscopies are frequently performed in elderly patients with multiple medical problems.

Intraoperative Management

A bloodless field greatly facilitates arthroscopic surgery. Fortunately, knee surgery lends itself to the use of a pneumatic tourniquet. Tourniquets are associated with potential problems of their own, however, including hemodynamic changes, pain, metabolic alterations, arterial thromboembolus, and pulmonary embolism. Prolonged inflation (> 2 hours) routinely leads to transient muscle dysfunction and may be associated with permanent peripheral nerve injury. Tourniquet inflation has been associated with increases in body temperature in pediatric patients undergoing leg surgery.

Exsanguination of a lower extremity and tourniquet inflation cause a shift of blood volume into the central circulation. Although this is usually not clinically significant, bilateral Esmarch bandage exsanguination can cause a rise in central venous pressure and arterial blood pressure that may not be well tolerated in patients with left ventricular dysfunction.

Anyone who has had a tourniquet on the thigh inflated to 100 mm Hg above systolic blood pressure for more than a few minutes appreciates the potential for **tourniquet pain.** Although the mechanism and neural pathways for this severe aching and burning sensation defy precise explanation, unmyelinated, slow-conduction C fibers, which are relatively resistant to local anesthetic blockade, probably play a critical role. Tourniquet pain gradually becomes so severe that patients may require substantial supplemental analgesia, if not general anesthesia, despite a regional block that is adequate for surgical incision. Even during general anesthesia, tourniquet pain can be revealed as a gradually increasing mean arterial blood pressure beginning about ½ to 1 hour after cuff inflation. The likelihood of tourniquet pain and its accompanying hypertension may be influenced by many factors, including anesthetic technique (intravenous regional > epidural > spinal > general anesthesia), intensity and level of the block, choice of local anesthetic (hyperbaric spinal with tetracaine > isobaric bupivacaine), and supplementation of the block with opioids.

Cuff deflation invariably and immediately relieves the sensation of tourniquet pain and its hypertension.

In fact, cuff deflation can be accompanied by a significant fall in central venous pressure and arterial blood pressure. Heart rate usually increases and core temperature decreases. Washout of accumulated metabolic wastes in the ischemic extremity increases $PaCO_2$, $ETCO_2$, and serum lactate and potassium levels. These metabolic alterations can cause an increase in minute ventilation in the spontaneously breathing patient and, rarely, heart dysrhythmias. Ironically, cuff deflation and blood reoxygenation have been demonstrated to worsen ischemic tissue injury due to the formation of lipid peroxides. This reperfusion injury may be attenuated by propofol anesthetic techniques, which have been shown to limit superoxide generation.

Tourniquet-induced ischemia of a lower extremity may lead to the development of deep venous thrombosis. Transesophageal echocardiography has detected subclinical pulmonary embolism (miliary emboli) following tourniquet deflation in cases as minor as diagnostic knee arthroscopy. Rare episodes of massive pulmonary embolism during total knee arthroplasty have been reported during leg exsanguination, after tourniquet inflation, following tourniquet deflation, and even during cases in which no tourniquet was used. Tourniquets are generally contraindicated in patients with significant calcific arterial disease. They have been safely used in patients with sickle cell disease, although particular attention should be paid to maintaining oxygenation, normocarbia or hypocarbia, hydration, and normothermia.

Postoperative Pain Relief

Successful outpatient recovery depends on early ambulation, adequate pain relief, and minimal nausea and vomiting. Techniques that avoid large doses of systemic opioids have obvious appeal. Intra-articular bupivacaine (15–30 mL of 0.25–0.5% bupivacaine with 1:200,000 epinephrine) often provides satisfactory analgesia for a few hours postoperatively. The addition of 1–5 mg of morphine may prolong analgesia for several hours in some patients. The presumed mechanism of this somewhat controversial effect involves interactions with peripheral opioid receptors in the joint. Other pain-control strategies include systemic ketorolac, intra-articular corticosteroid injection (eg, 10 mg triamcinolone acetonide in 20 mL saline), a three-in-one (lateral femoral cutaneous, obturator, and femoral nerves) lumbar plexus block (see Chapter 17), or the placement during wound closure of a multi-orifice catheter connected to a portable pump.

TOTAL KNEE REPLACEMENT
Preoperative Considerations

Patients presenting for total knee replacement closely resemble those undergoing total hip replacement (eg, rheumatoid arthritis, osteoarthritis).

Intraoperative Management

The duration of total knee arthroplasty tends to be shorter than with hip replacement; patients remain in a supine position, and blood loss is limited by the use of a tourniquet. Cooperative patients usually tolerate a regional technique with intravenous sedation. An epidural catheter can prove helpful with the postoperative course, which can be more painful than that following hip replacement surgery.

Bone cement implantation syndrome following femoral prosthesis insertion is possible, but is less likely than during hip arthroplasty. Subsequent release of emboli into the systemic circulation may exaggerate any tendency for hypotension following tourniquet release. Like bilateral hip replacement, monitoring during bilateral knee replacement should include pulmonary artery and PAOP measurements.

■ SPINAL SURGERY

Spinal surgery is most often performed for symptomatic nerve root or cord compression secondary to degenerative disorders. Compression may occur from protrusion of an intervertebral disk or osteophyte (spondylosis) into the spinal canal or intervertebral foramen. Herniation of an intervertebral disk usually occurs at either the fifth-to-sixth cervical or the fourth-to-fifth lumbar levels in patients 30–50 years old. Spondylosis tends to affect the lower cervical spine more than lumbar spine and typically afflicts older patients. Surgery may also be undertaken to correct scoliosis (see Chapter 44), decompress the cord, stabilize the spine following spinal trauma, or resect a tumor, a vascular malformation, or an abscess. Spinal surgeries range in complexity from percutaneous diskectomy under local anesthesia to correction of severe rotational deformities with devices such as Harrington rods.

Preoperative Considerations

Preoperative evaluation should focus on any existing ventilatory impairment and the airway. Anatomic abnormalities and limited neck movement from disease, traction, or braces complicate airway management and necessitate special techniques. For example, securing the airway can be a major problem in patients with an unstable cervical spine. An awake, fiberoptic, nasal intubation should be considered in these patients (see Chapter 5). Preexisting neurologic deficits should be identified and documented. Most patients with degenerative diseases have considerable pain preoperatively and should be given an opioid-containing premedication. Conversely, premedication is best avoided in patients with difficult airways or ventilatory impairment.

Intraoperative Management

The prone position complicates the anesthetic management of spinal surgery (Tables 47–5 and 47–6). Use of the supine position with head traction for anterior cervical fusion introduces the possibility of injury to the trachea, esophagus, recurrent laryngeal nerve, sympathetic chain, carotid artery, or jugular vein. Recurrent laryngeal nerve injury has been diagnosed intraoperatively by electromyographic testing of vocal cord function using a special endotracheal tube with built-in electrode wires. A transthoracic approach to the anterior thoracic spine requires a double-lumen tube and one-lung anesthesia (see Chapter 24).

Following placement of any invasive monitoring lines, securing of the airway, and induction of general anesthesia in the supine position, the patient may be turned prone in a single movement. This usually requires four people, with the anesthesiologist supporting the head, neck, and shoulders. Care must be taken to maintain the neck in a neutral position. Once prone, the head usually remains face down on a cushioned holder or suspended with head traction. Extreme caution is necessary to avoid retinal ischemia from pressure on either globe or pressure necrosis of the nose, ears, forehead, female breasts, or male genitalia. The chest should rest on parallel foam rolls or special supports to facilitate ventilation. The shoulders should be abducted less than 90 degrees, with the elbows flexed or the arms tucked at the sides. Prone positioning limits access to peripheral intravenous lines and invasive monitors.

Turning the patient prone can create significant problems. Monitor disconnections are hard to avoid and are often complicated by hypotension from blunted postural sympathetic reflexes. Abdominal compression, especially in obese patients, may impede venous return and contribute to excessive intraoperative blood loss from engorgement of epidural veins. The use of specially designed frames that allow the abdomen to hang free may alleviate these problems.

An alternative technique for short lumbar procedures (eg, a single-level microdiscectomy) allows the patient to position themselves on the operative table in the prone position. A single shot of epidural anesthetic (eg, 25 mL of 0.75% bupivacaine with 5 mg morphine) is administered along with mild intravenous sedation. Obviously, this technique requires a cooperative patient and expeditious surgeon. A continuous epidural placed two or more segments above the planned incision can be used for surgery of moderate duration.

Spinal operations involving multiple levels, fusion, and instrumentation are also complicated by the poten-tial for large intraoperative blood loss. Invasive monitoring of arterial blood pressure and central venous pressure should be undertaken prior to positioning. In suitable candidates, controlled hypotension (see Case Discussion, Chapter 13) and wound infiltration with a weak epinephrine solution may decrease blood loss. Massive blood loss from aortic or vena caval injury can occur intraoperatively or postoperatively and is often initially occult.

Instrumentation of the spine (eg, derotational rods, pedicle screws) requires the ability to distinguish—intraoperatively—spinal cord injury from excessive distraction. Intraoperative wake-up techniques, using balanced anesthesia with a short-acting opioid and muscle relaxant allow testing of motor function at critical junctures (see Suggested Readings). If preservation of motor function below the level of the surgery appears jeopardized, spinal instrumentation is immediately removed. Monitoring somatosensory evoked potentials (SSEPs) avoids the problems associated with intraoperative awakening. Although volatile anesthetics interfere with SSEP monitoring, opioid techniques do so to a lesser degree. Unfortunately, SSEPs monitor dorsal column sensory function, not motor function. Thus, postoperative motor deficits are possible despite intraoperative preservation of SSEPs. Furthermore, potential attenuation or loss may signify peripheral nerve dysfunction instead of spinal cord ischemia. Monitors of motor tract function (eg, motor evoked potentials, spinal cord evoked potentials) are under development.

■ LIMB REIMPLANTATION & GRAFT TRANSPLANTATION SURGERY

Preoperative Considerations

The development of microsurgical techniques that allow reanastomosis of arteries and nerves has led to the potential of reattaching severed limbs and transplantation of autologous muscle grafts (free flaps). This tedious, meticulous surgery can require several hours of anesthesia. Patients presenting with a traumatic limb amputation are usually young and healthy, while those requiring graft transplantation have often been debilitated by a prolonged and complicated medical course.

Intraoperative Management

Successful reimplantation and transplantation surgery depends on good arterial blood flow following reanastomosis. The avoidance of hypothermia and hypovolemia becomes a critical responsibility of the anesthesiologist. These patients should be actively heated with forced-air warming blankets, intravenous fluid warmers, increased operating room temperature, and breathing-circuit humidifiers. Urinary output and, in longer cases associated with significant blood loss, central venous pressure should be monitored. Although blood volume must be aggressively maintained, a mild degree of anemia enhances blood flow by beneficially altering blood rheology. Dextran 40 improves microcirculatory blood flow by decreasing viscosity and inhibiting platelet function. Sympathectomy with continuous regional nerve blocks may improve regional blood flow by arterial dilatation and prevention of vasospasm. As with any long surgical procedure, patient positioning and pressure-point padding must be painstakingly done.

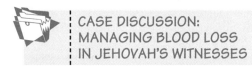

CASE DISCUSSION: MANAGING BLOOD LOSS IN JEHOVAH'S WITNESSES

A 58-year-old Jehovah's Witness presents for hemipelvectomy because of a malignant bone tumor (osteogenic sarcoma). The patient has received chemotherapy over the last 2 months with multiple drugs, including doxorubicin. The patient has no other medical problems and the preoperative hematocrit is 47%.

How does the care of Jehovah's Witnesses particularly challenge the anesthesiologist?

Jehovah's Witnesses, a fellowship of more than 1 million Americans, object to the administration of blood for any indication. This objection stems from their interpretation of the Bible ("to keep abstaining from . . . blood," Acts 15:28,29), not for medical reasons (eg, the fear of hepatitis). Physicians are obliged to honor the principle of bodily integrity, *which states that patients have final authority over what is done to them. Witnesses sign a waiver that relieves physicians of responsibility for any consequences of blood refusal.*

Which intravenous fluids will Witnesses accept?

Witnesses abstain from blood and blood products (eg, packed red blood cells, fresh frozen plasma, platelets) but not non-blood-containing solutions. They accept crystalloids, hetastarch, and dextran replacement solutions. Witnesses view albumin, erythropoietin (because of the use

of albumin), immune globulins, and hemophiliac preparations as a gray area that requires a personal decision by the believer.

Do they allow the use of autologous blood?

According to their religion, any blood that is removed from the body should be discarded ("You should pour it out upon the ground as water," Deuteronomy 12:24) and not stored. Thus, the usual practice of autologous preoperative collection and storage would not be allowed. Techniques of acute normovolemic hemodilution and intraoperative blood salvaging have been accepted by some Witnesses, however, as long as their blood maintains continuity with their circulatory systems at all times. For example, up to 4 units of blood could be drawn from the patient immediately before surgery and kept in anticoagulant-containing bags that maintain a constant link to the patient's body. The blood would be replaced by an acceptable colloid or crystalloid solution, and reinfused as needed during the surgery.

How would the inability to transfuse blood affect intraoperative monitoring decisions?

Hemipelvectomy involves radical resection that can lead to massive blood loss. This is particularly true for large tumors and if an internal approach, rather than the classic external hemipelvectomy, is planned. Invasive arterial blood pressure and central venous pressure monitors would probably be indicated in most patients undergoing this procedure. Techniques that minimize intraoperative blood loss (eg controlled hypotension, aprotinin) should be considered. In a Jehovah's Witness, the management of life-threatening anemia (Hb < 5 g/dL) may be improved by monitoring cardiac output, oxygen delivery, and oxygen consumption. Thus, a pulmonary artery catheter with continuous mixed venous oxygen saturation monitoring capability might prove useful. Continuous electrocardiograph ST-segment analysis may signal myocardial ischemia. Hypoventilation-induced decreases in cerebral blood flow can be prevented by continuous end-tidal carbon dioxide monitoring.

What physiologic effects result from severe anemia?

Assuming the maintenance of normovolemia and the absence of preexisting major end-organ dysfunction, most patients tolerate severe anemia surprisingly well. Decreased blood viscosity and vasodilation lower systemic vascular resistance and increase blood flow. Augmentation of stroke volume increases cardiac output, allowing arterial blood pressure and heart rate to remain relatively unchanged. Coronary and cerebral blood flows increase in the absence of coronary artery disease and carotid artery stenosis. A decrease in venous oxygen saturation reflects an increase in tissue oxygen extraction. Oozing from surgical wounds as a result of dilutional coagulopathy may accompany extreme degrees of anemia.

What are some of the anesthetic implications of preoperative doxorubicin therapy?

This anthracycline antibiotic has well-recognized cardiac side effects, ranging from transient dysrhythmias and electrocardiograph changes (eg, ST-segment and T-wave abnormalities) to irreversible cardiomyopathy and congestive heart failure. The risk of cardiomyopathy appears to increase with a cumulative dose greater than 550 mg/m^{-2}, prior radiotherapy, and concurrent cyclophosphamide treatment. Mild degrees of cardiomyopathy can be detected preoperatively with endomyocardial biopsy, echocardiography, or exercise radionuclide angiography. Doxorubicin's other important toxicity is myelosuppression (eg, thrombocytopenia, leukopenia, anemia).

Are there any special considerations regarding postoperative pain management in the Jehovah's Witness?

Witnesses generally refrain from any mind-altering drugs or medications, although opioids prescribed by a physician for severe pain are accepted by some believers. Insertion of an epidural catheter could provide pain relief with local anesthetics, with or without opioids.

SUGGESTED READING

Berman M, Grande CM (editors): *Pediatric Trauma Anesthesia.* Intl Anesthesiol Clin. Little Brown, 1994.

Capdevila X, Biboulet P, Bouregba M: Comparison of the three-in-one and fascia iliaca compartment blocks in adults: Clinical and radiographic analysis. Anesth Analg 1998;86:1039. These blocks can provide very effective anesthesia for lower limb surgery.

Capdevila X, Barthelet Y, Biboulet P, et al: Effects of perioperative analgesic technique on the surgical outcome and duration of rehabilitation after major knee surgery. Anesthesiology 1999; 91:8. Continuous femoral block shortened hospital stay compared with patient-controlled analgesia, and had fewer side effects than continuous epidural infusion.

Carson JL, Duff A, Berlin JA, et al: Perioperative blood transfusion and postoperative mortality. JAMA 1998;279:199. Preopera-

tive blood transfusion in patients with a hemoglobin of at least 8.0 g/dL did not affect mortality following hip fracture repair.

Conroy JM, Dorman BH: *Anesthesia for Orthopedic Surgery.* Raven Press, 1994. An up-to-date reference with extensive discussions of patient positioning, regional anesthesia, spinal cord monitoring, and pain considerations.

Ereth MH, Weber JG, Abel MD, et al: Cemented versus noncemented total hip arthroplasty–embolism, hemodynamics, and intrapulmonary shunting. Mayo Clin Proc 1992;67:1066. A prospective study using transesophageal echocardiography and pulmonary artery monitoring.

Hiippala ST, Strid LJ, Wennerstrand MI, et al: Traexamic acid radically decreases blood loss and transfusions associated with total knee arthroplasty. Anesth Analg 1997;84:839. The benefits of decreased blood loss must be weighed against the cost and risk of thromboembolic complications.

Karakaya D, Ustun E, Tur A, et al: Acute normovolemic hemodilution and nitroglycerin-induced hypotension: Comparative effects on tissue oxygenation and allogeneic blood transfusion requirement in total hip arthroplasty. J Clin Anesth 1999; 11:368. This study found that acute normovolemic hemodilution was more effective than deliberate hypotension with nitroglycerine for reducing allogeneic blood transfusions.

Kearon C, Hirsh J: Management of anticoagulation before and after elective surgery. N Engl J Med 1997;336:1506. Recommendations regarding the cessation of warfarin and institution of heparin in the perioperative period.

Koscielniak-Nielsen ZJ, Stens-Pedersen HL, Hesselbjerg L: Midazolam-flumazenil versus propofol anaesthesia for scoliosis surgery with wake-up tests. Acta Anaesthesiol Scand 1998;42: 111.

Lafont ND, Kalonji MK, Barre J, Guillaume C, Boogaerts JG: Clinical features and echocardiography of embolism during cemented hip arthroplasty. Can J Anaesth 1997;44:112.

Pietak S, Holmes J, Matthews R, Petrasek A, Porter B: Cardiovascular collapse after femoral prosthesis surgery for acute hip fracture. Can J Anaesth 1997;444:198. Two cases of fatal hemodynamic collapse coinciding with femoral reaming and placement of prosthesis.

Sharrock NE, Cazan MG, Hargett JL, et al: Changes in mortality after total hip and knee arthroplasty over a ten-year period. Anesth Analg 1995;80:242. A 3-fold decrease in perioperative mortality was documented in this study.

Schmied H, Schiferer A, Sessler DI: The effects of red-cell scavenging, hemodilution, and active warming on allogenic blood requirements in patients undergoing hip or knee arthroplasty. Anesth Analg 1998;86:387. All three techniques effectively cut transfusion requirements.

Skues MA, Welchew EA: Anaesthesia and rheumatoid arthritis. Anaesthesia 1993;48:989. A review of the anesthetic implications of rheumatoid arthritis emphasizing systemic manifestations, pharmacologic changes, and airway management.

Slappendel R, Weber EW, Dirksen R: Optimization of the dose of intrathecal morphine in total hip surgery: A dose finding study. Anesth Analg 1999;88:822. The optimal dose of intrathecal morphine for total hip replacement surgery was 0.1 mg.

Steele SM, Slaughter TF, Greenberg CS, Reves JG: Epidural anesthesia and analgesia: Implications for perioperative coagulability. Anesth Analg 1991;73:683. An editorial that reviews current evidence and opinion regarding epidural anesthesia in anticoagulated patients.

Stowell CP, Chandler H, Jove M, Guilfoyle M, Wacholtz MC: An open-label, randomized study to compare the safety and efficacy of perioperative Epoetin alfa with preoperative autologous blood donation in total joint arthroplasty. Orthopedics 1999;22:s105.

Sulek CA, Davies LK, Enneking FK: Cerebral microembolism diagnosed by transcranial Doppler during total knee arthroplasty: Correlation with transesophageal echocardiography. Anesthesiology 1999;91:672. Over 50% of the patients studied had evidence of cerebral fat emboli following tourniquet deflation, with a higher average number of emboli following bilateral versus unilateral knee arthroplasty.

Reuben SS, Connelly NR: Postarthroscopic meniscus repair analgesia with intraarticular ketorolac or morphine. Anesth Analg 1996;82:1036.

Wedel DJ (editor): *Orthopedic Anesthesia.* Churchill Livingstone, 1993. A well-referenced source that covers most areas of interest to the orthopedic anesthesiologist.

Weiss SJ, Cheung AT, Stecker MM, Garino JP, Hughes JE, Murphy FL: Fatal paradoxical cerebral embolization during bilateral knee arthroplasty. Anesthesiology 1996;84:721.

Wolfe MM, Lichtenstein DR, Singh G: Gastrointestinal toxicity of nonsteroidal antiinflammatory drugs. N Engl J Med 1999; 340:1888. A review article that discusses the risks, causes, and treatment of NSAID-related gastroduodenal disease.

Anesthesia for the Trauma Patient   **41**

KEY CONCEPTS

 The initial assessment of the trauma patient can be divided into primary and secondary surveys. The primary survey resembles the ABC sequence suggested for cardiopulmonary resuscitation: Airway, Breathing, and Circulation. Resuscitation and assessment proceed simultaneously. Trauma resuscitation includes two additional phases: control of hemorrhage and definitive repair of the injury. A more comprehensive secondary survey of the patient follows the primary survey.

 A cervical spine fracture must be assumed in trauma patients, even if there is no known injury above the level of the clavicle. The incidence of cervical spine trauma is approximately 2% whether or not the patient has a closed head injury.

 Neck hyperextension and excessive axial traction must be avoided, and manual immobilization of the head and neck by an assistant should be used to stabilize the cervical spine during laryngoscopy ("in-line stabilization").

 The mainstay of therapy of hemorrhagic shock is intravenous fluid resuscitation and transfusion.

 Rapid-infusion systems that use large-bore tubing and rapidly warm fluids are invaluable during massive transfusions. A convection forced-air warming blanket and heated humidifier will also help maintain body temperature. Hypothermia worsens acid-base disorders, coagulopathies

(platelet sequestration and red blood cell deformities), and myocardial function.

 Hypotension in patients with hypovolemic shock should be aggressively treated with intravenous fluids, not vasopressors unless there is profound hypotension that is unresponsive to fluid therapy, coexisting cardiogenic shock, or cardiac arrest.

 Commonly used induction agents for hypovolemic patients include ketamine and etomidate. Even drugs such as ketamine and nitrous oxide that indirectly stimulate cardiac function in normal patients can display cardiodepressant properties in shock patients who already have maximal sympathetic stimulation.

 The key to the safe anesthetic management of shock patients is to administer small incremental doses of whichever agents are selected.

 Any trauma victim with altered consciousness must be considered to have a brain injury. The level of consciousness is assessed by serial Glasgow Coma Scale evaluations.

 Brain injuries are often accompanied by increased intracranial pressure from cerebral hemorrhage or edema. Intracranial hypertension is controlled by a combination of fluid restriction (except in the presence of hypovolemic shock), diuretics (eg, mannitol, 0.5 g/kg), barbiturates, and deliberate hypocapnia ($PaCO_2$ of 26–30 mm Hg).

Trauma is the leading cause of death in Americans from the first to the thirty-fifth year of age. One-third of all hospital admissions in the United States are directly related to trauma. Fifty percent of trauma deaths occur immediately, with another 30% occurring within a few hours of injury (the "golden hour"). Because many trauma victims require immediate surgery, anesthesiologists can directly affect their survival. In fact, the role of the anesthesiologist is often that of primary resuscitator, while providing anesthesia becomes a secondary activity. It is important for the anesthesiologist to remember that these patients have an increased likelihood of being drug abusers, acutely intoxicated, and carriers of hepatitis or HIV. This chapter presents a framework for the initial assessment of the trauma victim and anesthetic considerations in the treatment of patients with injuries of the head and spine, chest, abdomen, and extremities. The Case Discussion at the end of the chapter discusses burn trauma.

■ INITIAL ASSESSMENT

The initial assessment of the trauma patient can be divided into primary and secondary surveys. The primary survey resembles the *ABC* sequence suggested for cardiopulmonary resuscitation: *A*irway, *B*reathing, and *C*irculation. If the function of any of these three systems is impaired, resuscitation must be initiated immediately. In critically ill patients, resuscitation and assessment proceed simultaneously by a team of trauma practitioners. The principles of cardiopulmonary resuscitation are presented in detail in Chapter 48. Trauma resuscitation includes two additional phases: control of hemorrhage and definitive repair of the injury. A more comprehensive secondary survey of the patient follows the primary survey.

PRIMARY SURVEY

Airway

A cervical spine fracture must be assumed in trauma patients, even if there is no known injury above the level of the clavicle. The incidence of cervical spine trauma is approximately 2% whether or not the patient has a closed head injury. To avoid neck hyperextension, the jaw-thrust maneuver is the preferred means of establishing an airway. Oral and nasal airways may help maintain airway patency. The possibility of cervical spine injury is commonly evaluated by examining all seven vertebrae in a cross-table lateral radiograph and a swimmer's view. Although these studies detect 80–90% of fractures, only a normal computed tomographic scan reliably rules out significant cervical spine trauma. Cervical spine injury is unlikely in alert patients without neck pain or tenderness.

While a simple jaw thrust may alleviate airway obstruction as a result of unconsciousness (see Figure 48–1), a major trauma patient is *always* considered to be at increased risk for aspiration, and the airway must be secured as soon as possible with an endotracheal tube or tracheostomy. Neck hyperextension and excessive axial traction must be avoided, and manual immobilization of the head and neck by an assistant should be used to stabilize the cervical spine during laryngoscopy ("in-line stabilization"). The assistant places his or her hands on either side of the head, holding down the occiput and preventing any head rotation. Studies have demonstrated neck movement, however, particularly C1 and C2, during mask ventilation and direct laryngoscopy despite attempts at stabilization (eg, sandbags, forehead tape, Philadelphia collar). For this reason, some clinicians prefer nasal intubation, blind or fiberoptic, in spontaneously breathing patients with suspected cervical spine injury, although this technique may be associated with a higher risk of pulmonary aspiration. Clearly, the expertise of the individual clinician may affect expediency and the risk of complications and should influence the choice of nasal or oral intubation. Most practitioners have greater familiarity with oral intubation, and this technique should be considered in patients who are apneic and require immediate intubation. Furthermore, nasal intubation should be avoided in patients with midface or basilar skull fractures. If an esophageal obturator airway has been placed in the field, it should not be removed until the trachea has been intubated because of the likelihood of regurgitation (see Chapter 48).

Laryngeal trauma makes a complicated situation worse. Open trauma may be associated with bleeding from major neck vessels, obstruction from hematoma or edema, subcutaneous emphysema, and cervical spine injuries. Closed trauma is less obvious but can present as neck crepitations, hematoma, dysphagia, hemoptysis, or poor phonation. An awake intubation with a small endotracheal tube (6.0 in adults) under direct laryngoscopy or fiberoptic bronchoscopy with topical anesthesia can be attempted if the larynx can be well-visualized. If facial or neck injuries preclude endotracheal intubation, tracheostomy under local anesthesia should be considered. Acute obstruction from upper airway trauma may require emergency cricothyrotomy, or percutaneous or surgical tracheostomy (see Case Discussion, Chapter 5).

Breathing

Most critically ill trauma patients require assisted—if not controlled—ventilation. Bag-valve devices (eg, a self-inflating bag with a nonrebreathing valve) usually provide adequate ventilation immediately after intubation and during periods of patient transport. A 100% oxygen concentration is delivered until oxygenation is assessed by arterial blood gases. If the patient arrives in the operating room already intubated, correct positioning of the endotracheal tube must be verified. Patients with suspected head trauma are hyperventilated to decrease intracranial pressure. Ventilation may be compromised by pneumothorax, flail chest, obstruction of the endotracheal tube, or direct pulmonary injury.

Circulation & Fluid Resuscitation

A. HEMORRHAGE:

The term **shock** denotes circulatory failure leading to inadequate vital organ perfusion and oxygen delivery. While there are many causes of shock (Table 41–1), in the trauma patient it is usually due to hypovolemia. Physiologic responses to hemorrhage range from tachycardia, poor capillary perfusion, and a decrease in pulse pressure to hypotension, tachypnea, and delirium (Table 41–2). Serum hematocrit and hemoglobin concentrations are often not accurate indicators of acute blood loss. Peripheral somatic nerve stimulation and massive tissue injury appear to exacerbate the reductions in cardiac output and stroke volume seen in hypovolemic shock. The hemodynamic lability of these patients demands invasive arterial blood pressure monitoring. In severe hypovolemia, the pulse waveform can almost disappear during the inspiratory phase of mechanical ventilation. The degree of hypotension on presentation to the emergency room and operating room correlates strongly with the mortality rate.

Obvious sites of hemorrhage should be identified and controlled with direct pressure on the wound. Occult bleeding in the thorax, abdomen, or extremities is more difficult to assess and manage. Pneumatic antishock garments can decrease bleeding in the abdomen and lower extremities, increase peripheral vascular resistance, and augment perfusion of the heart and brain. Bleeding wounds above the level of the suit (eg thorax or head) contraindicate the use of these garments because of the risk of increasing hemorrhage.

The mainstay of therapy of hemorrhagic shock is intravenous fluid resuscitation and transfusion. Multiple short (1.5–2 inches), large-bore (14–16 gauge, or 7–8.5F) catheters are placed in whichever veins are easily accessible. Patients with possible vena caval or hepatic injury should have intravenous access established in both caval

Table 41–1. Classification of shock by mechanism and common causes.

Hypovolemic shock
Loss of blood (hemorrhagic shock)
  External hemorrhage
    Trauma
    Gastrointestinal tract bleeding
  Internal hemorrhage
    Hematoma
    Hemothorax or hemoperitoneum
Loss of plasma
  Burns
  Exfoliative dermatitis
Loss of fluid and electrolytes
  External
    Vomiting
    Diarrhea
    Excessive sweating
    Hyperosmolar states (diabetic ketoacidosis, hyperosmolar nonketotic coma)
  Internal ("third-spacing")
    Pancreatitis
    Ascites
    Bowel obstruction
Cardiogenic shock
Dysrhythmia
  Tachyarrhythmia
  Bradyarrhythmia
Pump failure (secondary to myocardial infarction or other cardiomyopathy)
Acute valvular dysfunction (especially regurgitant lesions)
Rupture of ventricular septum or free ventricular wall
Obstructive shock
Tension pneumothorax
Pericardial disease (tamponade, constriction)
Disease of pulmonary vasculature (massive pulmonary emboli, pulmonary hypertension)
Cardiac tumor (atrial myxoma)
Left atrial mural thrombus
Obstructive valvular disease (aortic or mitral stenosis)
Distributive shock
Septic shock
Anaphylactic shock
Neurogenic shock
Vasodilator drugs
Acute adrenal insufficiency

Reproduced, with permission, from Ho MT, Saunders CE: *Current Emergency Diagnosis & Treatment,* 4th ed. Appleton & Lange, 1992.

systems in case cross-clamping becomes necessary during vascular repair. Although central lines may provide useful information regarding volume status, they may be time-consuming and introduce the possibility of life-threatening complications (eg, pneumothorax).

Table 41–2. Clinical classification of shock.*

	Pathophysiology	Clinical Manifestations
Mild (< 20% of blood volume lost)	Decreased peripheral perfusion only of organs able to withstand prolonged ischemia (skin, fat, muscle, and bone). Arterial pH normal.	Patient complains of feeling cold. Postural hypotension and tachycardia. Cool pale moist skin; collapsed neck veins; concentrated urine.
Moderate (20–40% of blood volume lost)	Decreased central perfusion of organs able to tolerate only brief ischemia (liver, gut, kidneys). Metabolic acidosis present.	Thirst. Supine hypotension and tachycardia (variable). Oliguria and anuria.
Severe (> 40% of blood volume lost)	Decreased perfusion of heart and brain. Severe metabolic acidosis. Respiratory acidosis possibly present.	Agitation, confusion, or obtundation. Supine hypotension and tachycardia invariably present. Rapid, deep respiration.

Modified and reprinted, with permission, from Ho MT, Saunders CE: *Current Emergency Diagnosis & Treatment,* 4th ed. Appleton & Lange, 1992.
*These clinical findings are most consistently observed in hemorrhagic shock but apply to other types of shock as well.

Peripheral lines are usually sufficient for initial resuscitation.

Massive hemorrhage depletes the intravascular fluid compartment. Fluid shifts intravascularly from the interstitial compartment to maintain cardiovascular integrity, and interstitial fluid also moves into cells. Anaerobic metabolism leads to adenosine triphosphate (ATP) depletion, dysfunction of the ATP-dependent Na^+-K^+ pump, and progressive cellular edema.

B. FLUID THERAPY:

The choice of initial fluid therapy is determined chiefly by availability. While fully cross-matched whole blood is ideal, typing and cross-matching take 45–60 minutes. Type-specific blood (preferably type and screen blood) may cause minor antibody reactions but is appropriate therapy as soon as it is available (5–10 minutes). Uncrossed O-negative packed red blood cells should be reserved for life-threatening blood loss that cannot be adequately replaced by other fluids (eg, exsanguination). Complications associated with massive blood transfusions are discussed in Chapter 29.

Crystalloid solutions are readily available and inexpensive. Resuscitation requires large quantities, however, because most crystalloid solution does not remain in the intravascular compartment. Lactated Ringer's injection is less likely to cause hyperchloremic acidosis than is normal saline, although calcium in the former makes it less compatible with blood transfusions. Dextrose-containing solutions may exacerbate ischemic brain damage and should be avoided in the absence of documented hypoglycemia. Even lactated Ringer's solution is slightly hypotonic and when administered in large volumes can aggravate cerebral edema. Hypertonic solutions such as 3% or 7.5% saline are effective for volume resuscitation and appear to be associated with less cerebral edema than lactated Ringer's solution or normal saline in the presence of brain injury. Although small volumes of hypertonic saline rapidly expand plasma volume, its use is limited by progressive hypernatremia (see Chapters 28 and 29). Transient vasodilation and hypotension may also be observed.

Colloid solutions are far more expensive than crystalloids, but they are more effective in rapidly restoring intravascular volume. Nonetheless, the interstitial fluid deficit associated with hypovolemic shock may be better treated with a crystalloid solution. Albumin is usually selected over dextran or hetastarch solutions because of the fear of inducing a coagulopathy (see Chapter 29).

Whichever fluid is chosen, it must be warmed prior to administration. Rapid-infusion systems that use large-bore tubing and rapidly warm fluids are invaluable during massive transfusions. A convection forced-air warming blanket and heated humidifier will also help maintain body temperature. Hypothermia worsens acid-base disorders, coagulopathies (platelet sequestration and red blood cell deformities), and myocardial function (see Table 6–7). It also shifts the oxygen-hemoglobin curve to the left and decreases the metabolism of lactate, citrate, and some anesthetic drugs. The amount of fluid administered is based on improvement of clinical signs, particularly blood pressure, pulse pressure, and heart rate. Central venous pressure and urinary output also provide indications of restoration of vital organ perfusion.

Inadequate organ perfusion interferes with aerobic metabolism, producing lactic acid and metabolic acidosis. Sodium bicarbonate, which dissociates into bicarbonate ion and CO_2, may temporarily worsen intracellular acidosis because cell membranes are relatively insoluble to bicarbonate compared with CO_2. Acid-base imbalances will eventually resolve with hydration and improved organ perfusion. Lactate will be metabolized in the liver to bicarbonate, and H^+ will be excreted by the kidneys.

Hypotension in patients with hypovolemic shock should be aggressively treated with intravenous fluids, *not* vasopressors unless there is profound hypotension that is unresponsive to fluid therapy, coexisting cardiogenic shock, or cardiac arrest. Some clinicians advocate a low-dose infusion of dopamine (3 μg/kg/min) in an attempt to increase renal blood flow.

Regional anesthesia is usually impractical in hemodynamically unstable patients with life-threatening injuries. If possible, hypovolemia should be corrected prior to induction of general anesthesia. In unstable patients, anesthesia may consist primarily of muscle relaxants (also called neuromuscular blocking agents), with general anesthetic agents titrated as tolerated (mean arterial pressure > 50–60 mm Hg) in an effort to provide at least amnesia. Commonly used induction agents for hypovolemic patients include ketamine and etomidate (see Chapter 8). Even drugs such as ketamine and nitrous oxide that indirectly stimulate cardiac function in normal patients can display cardiodepressant properties in shock patients who already have maximal sympathetic stimulation. Intermittent small doses of ketamine (25 mg every 15 minutes) are often well tolerated and may help reduce the incidence of recall, especially when used with low concentrations of a volatile agent (< 0.5 minimum alveolar concentration). Other adjuncts that may be useful in preventing recall include midazolam (intermittent 1 mg) or scopolamine (0.3 mg). Many clinicians avoid nitrous oxide entirely in these patients because of the possibility of a pneumothorax and because it limits inspired oxygen concentration. Obviously, drugs that tend to lower blood pressure (eg, tubocurarine) should be avoided in patients in hypovolemic shock. The rate of rise of alveolar concentration of inhalational anesthetics is greater in shock because of lower cardiac output and increased ventilation (see Chapter 7). Higher alveolar anesthetic partial pressures lead to higher arterial partial pressures and greater myocardial depression. Similarly, the effects of intravenous anesthetics are exaggerated since they are injected into a smaller intravascular volume. The key to the safe anesthetic management of shock patients is to administer small incremental doses of whichever agents are selected.

Shock that is refractory to aggressive fluid therapy may be due to uncontrolled hemorrhage that exceeds the rate of transfusion or to cardiogenic shock (eg, pericardial tamponade, myocardial contusion, myocardial infarction), neurogenic shock (eg, brainstem dysfunction, spinal cord transection), septic shock (a late complication), pulmonary failure (eg, pneumothorax, hemothorax), or severe acidosis or hypothermia.

SECONDARY SURVEY

In the secondary survey, the patient is evaluated from head to toe and the indicated studies (eg, radiographs, laboratory tests, invasive diagnostic procedures) are obtained. The neurologic examination includes evaluation of consciousness, pupillary signs, motor function, and sensory loss. Fixed dilated pupils do not necessarily imply irreversible brain damage. The patient should be undressed and examined for any hidden injuries. The chest is inspected for fractures and functional integrity (flail chest). Diminished breath sounds may reveal a **pneumothorax,** which is an indication for chest tube placement. Similarly, distant heart sounds, a narrow pulse pressure, and distended neck veins may signal **pericardial tamponade,** calling for pericardiocentesis. A normal examination does not definitely eliminate the possibility of these problems. Examination of the abdomen should consist of inspection, auscultation, and palpation. Peritoneal lavage may confirm intra-abdominal hemorrhage, but its sensitivity is less than 90%. The extremities are examined for fractures, dislocations, and peripheral pulses.

■ ANESTHETIC CONSIDERATIONS PERTAINING TO SPECIFIC ANATOMIC REGIONS

HEAD & SPINAL CORD TRAUMA

Any trauma victim with altered consciousness must be considered to have a brain injury (see Chapter 26 also). The level of consciousness is assessed by serial Glasgow Coma Scale evaluations (see Table 26–1). Other signs of brain damage include restlessness, convulsions, and cranial nerve dysfunction (eg, a nonreactive pupil). The classic Cushing triad (hypertension, bradycardia, and respiratory disturbances) is a late and unreliable sign that usually just precedes brain herniation. Hypotension is rarely due to head injury alone. Patients suspected of sustaining head trauma should not receive any premedication that will alter their mental status (eg, sedatives, analgesics) or neurologic examination (eg, anticholinergic-induced pupillary dilation).

Brain injuries are often accompanied by increased intracranial pressure from cerebral hemorrhage or edema. Intracranial hypertension is controlled by a combination of fluid restriction (except in the presence of hypovolemic shock), diuretics (eg, mannitol, 0.5 g/kg), barbiturates, and deliberate hypocapnia ($PaCO_2$ of 26–30 mm Hg). The latter two require endotracheal intubation, which also protects against aspiration caused by altered airway reflexes. Hypertension or tachycardia during intubation can be attenuated with intravenous lidocaine or fentanyl. Awake intubations cause a precipitous rise in intracranial pressure. Nasal passage of an endotracheal tube or nasogastric tube in patients with basal skull fractures risks cribriform plate perforation and cerebrospinal fluid infection. Slight elevation of the head will improve venous drainage and decrease intracranial pressure. Role of corticosteroids in head injury is controversial; most studies have shown either an adverse effect or no benefit. Anesthetic agents that increase intracranial pressure should be avoided (eg, ketamine). Hyperglycemia should also be avoided and treated with insulin if present. Mild hypothermia may prove beneficial in the head injury patient because of its proven value in preventing ischemia-induced injury.

Because autoregulation of cerebral blood flow is usually impaired in areas of brain injury, arterial hypertension can worsen cerebral edema and increase intracranial pressure. In addition, episodes of arterial hypotension will cause regional cerebral ischemia. In general, cerebral perfusion pressure (the difference between mean arterial pressure at the level of the brain and the larger of central venous pressure or intracranial pressure) should be maintained above 60 mm Hg. Deliberate hypocapnia can improve autoregulation.

Patients with severe head injuries are more prone to arterial hypoxemia from pulmonary shunting and ventilation/perfusion mismatching. These changes may be due to aspiration, atelectasis, or direct neural effects on the pulmonary vasculature. Intracranial hypertension may predispose patients to pulmonary edema because of an increase in sympathetic outflow.

The degree of physiological derangement following spinal cord injury is proportional to the level of the lesion. Great care must be taken to prevent further injury during transportation and intubation. Lesions of the cervical spine may involve the phrenic nerves (C3–C5) and cause apnea. Loss of intercostal function limits pulmonary reserve and the ability to cough. High thoracic injuries will eliminate sympathetic innervation of the heart (T1–T4), leading to bradycardia. Acute high spinal cord injury can cause **spinal shock,** a condition characterized by loss of sympathetic tone in the capacitance and resistance vessels below the level of the lesion,

resulting in hypotension, bradycardia, areflexia, and gastrointestinal atony. In fact, venous distention in the legs is a sign of spinal cord injury. Hypotension in these patients requires aggressive fluid therapy—tempered by the possibility of pulmonary edema after the acute phase has resolved. Succinylcholine is reportedly safe during the first 48 hours following the injury but is associated with life-threatening hyperkalemia afterward. Short-term high-dose corticosteroid therapy with methylprednisolone (30 mg/kg followed by 5.4 mg/kg/hour for 23 hours) improves the neurologic outcome of patients with spinal cord trauma. **Autonomic hyperreflexia** is associated with lesions above T5 but is not a problem during acute management.

CHEST TRAUMA

Trauma to the chest may severely compromise the function of the heart or lungs, leading to cardiogenic shock or hypoxia. A **simple pneumothorax** is an accumulation of air between the parietal and visceral pleura. The ipsilateral collapse of lung tissue results in a severe ventilation/perfusion abnormality and hypoxia. The overlying chest wall is hyperresonant to percussion, breath sounds are decreased or absent, and a chest film confirms lung collapse. Nitrous oxide will expand a pneumothorax and is contraindicated in these patients. Treatment includes placement of a chest tube in the fourth or fifth intercostal space, anterior to the midaxillary line. A persistent air leak following chest tube placement may indicate injury to a major bronchus.

A **tension pneumothorax** develops from air entering the pleural space through a one-way valve in the lung or chest wall. In either case, air is forced into the thorax with inspiration but cannot escape during expiration. As a result, the ipsilateral lung completely collapses and the mediastinum and trachea are shifted to the contralateral side. A simple pneumothorax may develop into a tension pneumothorax when positive pressure ventilation is instituted. Venous return and expansion of the contralateral lung are impaired. Clinical signs include ipsilateral absence of breath sounds and hyperresonance to percussion, contralateral tracheal shift, and distended neck veins. Insertion of a 14-gauge over-the-needle catheter (3–6 cm long) into the second intercostal space at the midclavicular line will convert a tension pneumothorax to an open pneumothorax. Definitive treatment includes chest tube placement as described above.

Multiple rib fractures may compromise the functional integrity of the thorax, resulting in **flail chest.** Hypoxia is often worsened in these patients by underlying pulmonary contusion or hemothorax. **Pul-**

monary **contusion** results in worsening respiratory failure over time. **Hemothorax** is differentiated from pneumothorax by dullness to percussion over silent lung fields. Massive hemoptysis may require isolation of the affected lung with a double-lumen tube (DLT) to prevent blood from entering the healthy lung. Use of a single-lumen endotracheal tube with a bronchial blocker may be safer whenever laryngoscopy is difficult or problems are encountered with the DLT. A large bronchial injury also requires lung separation and ventilation of the unaffected side only (see Chapter 24). High-frequency jet ventilation may alternately be used to ventilate at lower airway pressures and help minimize the bronchial air leak when the bronchial leak is bilateral or the lung separation is not possible. Air leakage from traumatized bronchi can track an open pulmonary vein causing pulmonary and systemic air embolism. The source of the leak must be quickly identified and controlled.

Cardiac tamponade is a life-threatening chest injury that must be recognized early. The presence of Beck's triad (neck vein distention, hypotension, and muffled heart tones), pulsus paradoxus (a > 10 mm Hg decline in blood pressure during spontaneous inspiration), and a high index of suspicion will help make the diagnosis. Pericardiocentesis provides temporary relief. This is performed by directing a 16-gauge over-the-needle catheter (at least 15 cm long) from the xiphochondral junction toward the tip of the left scapula at a 45-degree angle, under the guidance of transthoracic echocardiography or the electrocardiogram. Electrocardiographic changes during pericardiocentesis indicate over-advancement of the needle into the myocardium. Definitive treatment of pericardial tamponade requires thoracotomy. Anesthetic management of these patients should maximize cardiac inotropism, chronotropism, and preload. For these reasons, ketamine is a favored induction agent. Penetrating injuries to the heart or great vessels require immediate exploration without delay. Repeated manipulation of the heart often results in intermittent episodes of bradycardia and profound hypotension.

Myocardial contusion is usually diagnosed by electrocardiographic changes consistent with ischemia (ST-segment elevation), cardiac enzyme elevations (creatine kinase MB [muscle band] determinations or troponin levels) or an abnormal echocardiogram. Wall motion abnormalities may be observed with transthoracic echocardiography. Patients are at increased risk for dysrhythmias, such as heart block and ventricular fibrillation. Elective surgery should be postponed until all signs of heart injury resolve.

Other possible injuries following chest trauma include aortic transection or dissection, avulsion of the subclavian artery, aortic or mitral valve disruption, traumatic diaphragmatic herniation, and esophageal rupture. Aortic transection usually occurs just distal to the left subclavian artery following a severe deceleration injury; it classically presents as wide mediastinum on the chest radiograph and may be associated with a fracture of the first rib.

Acute respiratory distress syndrome (ARDS) is usually a delayed pulmonary complication of trauma that has multiple causes: sepsis, direct thoracic injury, aspiration, head injury, fat embolism, massive transfusion, and oxygen toxicity. Clearly, the trauma patient is often at risk for several of these factors. Even with advances in technology, the mortality rate of ARDS approaches 50%. In some cases, ARDS may present early in the operating room. Mechanical ventilators on anesthesia machines are often incapable of sustaining adequate gas flows in these patients who rapidly develop poor lung compliance; use of an intensive care unit ventilator capable of sustaining adequate gas flows at high airway pressure may be necessary.

ABDOMINAL TRAUMA

Intra-abdominal injury is often indicated by the presence of a penetrating wound to the abdomen or lower thorax, paralytic ileus, or peritoneal irritation (eg, muscle guarding, percussion tenderness). Large quantities of unclotted blood may be present in the abdomen (eg, hepatic or splenic injury), however, with minimal signs. The diagnosis may be confirmed by free air on an abdominal radiograph or a bloody aspirate from peritoneal lavage. Management of abdominal trauma usually includes an exploratory laparotomy. Profound hypotension may follow opening of the abdomen as the tamponading effect of extravasated blood (and bowel distention) is lost. Whenever time permits, preparations for immediate fluid and blood resuscitation with a rapid infusion device should be completed prior to the laparotomy. Nitrous oxide is avoided to prevent worsening of bowel distention. A nasogastric tube will help prevent gastric dilation but should be placed orally if a cribriform plate fracture is suspected. The potential for massive blood transfusion (see Chapter 29) should be anticipated, particularly when abdominal trauma is associated with vascular, hepatic, splenic, or renal injuries, pelvic fractures, or retroperitoneal hemorrhage. Transfusion-induced hyperkalemia is equally as lethal as exsanguination and must be treated aggressively (see Chapters 28 and 29).

Massive abdominal hemorrhage may require packing of bleeding areas and/or clamping of the abdominal aorta until bleeding sites are identified and the resuscitation can catch up with the blood loss. Prolonged aortic clamping leads to ischemic injury to the liver, kidneys, intestines, and in some instances a compartment syndrome of the lower extremities; the latter can produce rhabdomyolysis and acute renal failure. The use of a mannitol infusion and a loop diuretic (prior to aortic cross-clamping), along with resuscitation fluid may prevent renal failure in such instances but is controversial. Rapid resuscitation with fluids and blood products via a rapid transfusion device, together with control of the bleeding, shortens cross-clamp time and likely reduces the incidence of such complications.

Progressive bowel edema from injuries and fluid resuscitation may preclude abdominal closure at the end of the procedure. Tight abdominal closures markedly increase intra-abdominal pressure, resulting in an abdominal compartment syndrome that can produce renal and splanchnic ischemia. Oxygenation and ventilation are often severely compromised, even with complete muscle paralysis. Oliguria and renal shut down follow. In such cases, the abdomen should be left open (but sterilely covered—often with IV bag plastic) for 48–72 hours until the edema subsides and secondary closure can be undertaken.

EXTREMITY TRAUMA

Extremity injuries can be life-threatening because of associated vascular injuries and secondary infectious complications. Vascular injuries can lead to massive hemorrhage and threaten extremity viability. For example, a femoral fracture can be associated with 3 U of occult blood loss, and closed pelvic fractures can cause hypovolemic shock. Delay of treatment or indiscriminate positioning can worsen dislocations and further compromise neurovascular bundles. **Fat emboli** are associated with pelvic and long-bone fractures and may cause pulmonary insufficiency, dysrhythmias, skin petechiae, and mental deterioration within 1–3 days after the traumatic event (see Chapter 40). The laboratory diagnosis of fat embolism depends on elevation of serum lipase, fat in the urine, and thrombocytopenia.

Modern surgical techniques frequently allow the reimplantation of severed extremities and digits (see Chapter 40). If these are isolated injuries, a regional technique (eg, brachial plexus block) is often recommended to increase peripheral blood flow by interrupting sympathetic innervation. If general anesthesia is

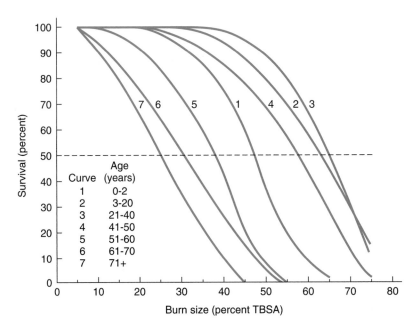

Figure 41–1. Sigmoid curves showing survival of humans as a function of total percentage of body surface burned and age. Survival curves are estimated by probit analysis for seven age categories. (Reproduced, with permission, from Merrell SW et al: Increased survival after major thermal injury. Am J Surg 1987;154:623.)

chosen, the patient should be kept warm, and emergence shivering must be avoided in order to maximize perfusion.

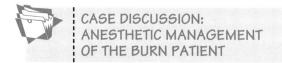

CASE DISCUSSION: ANESTHETIC MANAGEMENT OF THE BURN PATIENT

A 43-year-old man who suffered a major thermal burn 7 days previously is scheduled for excision and grafting under general anesthesia.

How are burn injuries classified?

Burn injuries are described according to the percentage of body surface area involved and the depth of the skin destroyed. Survival is influenced by the percentage surface area involved and the age of the patient (Figure 41–1). The **rule of nines** divides the body's surface area into areas of 9% or multiples of 9% (Figure 41–2). The surface area of one side of the patient's hand represents 1% of total body surface area.

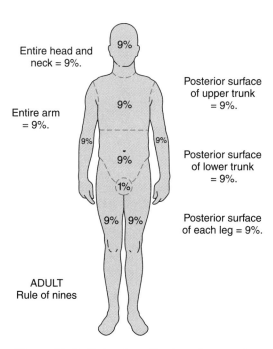

Figure 41–2. Estimation of body surface area in burns. (Modified and reproduced, with permission, from Tierney LM Jr et al: *Current Medical Diagnosis & Treatment 2002.* McGraw-Hill, 2002.)

First-degree burns are limited to the epithelium, while second-degree burns extend into the dermis, and third-degree burns destroy the entire skin thickness. It is ironic that since third-degree burns devastate nerve endings, they are not as painful as second-degree burns. A major thermal burn is considered to be a second-degree burn involving at least 25% of body surface area or a third-degree burn of at least 10% of body surface area. Electrical burns are typically more serious than superficial inspection would indicate because of underlying tissue damage. Pulmonary involvement, particularly with an underlying pneumonia, adds dramatically to the mortality rate.

How should one describe the pulmonary pathophysiology associated with major burn injuries?

Pulmonary function can be directly or indirectly affected. Direct inhalational injury is usually limited to upper airway edema that can lead to life-threatening airway obstruction. Nonetheless, lower airways can also be subjected to direct thermal insult (eg, steam) or can be injured by exposure to smoke and toxic products of combustion. Deactivation of surfactant can lead to atelectasis and pulmonary shunting. Indications of inhalational injury include stridor, hoarseness, facial burns, singed nasal hair or eyebrows, soot in sputum or in the oropharynx, respiratory distress, or a history of combustion in a closed space. Many patients with inhalational injury, however, do not demonstrate any signs until several hours postexposure.

Major burns can alter pulmonary function even in the absence of direct lung injury. For example, permeability can be increased throughout the entire microvascular system and may contribute to the development of pulmonary edema and acute respiratory distress syndrome. Circumferential burns of the thorax may decrease chest wall compliance and further increase peak inspiratory pressures.

Carbon monoxide inhalation shifts the oxygen-hemoglobin curve to the left (interfering with the unloading of oxygen at tissues) and decreases oxyhemoglobin saturation. PaO_2 and skin color may remain normal, but carboxyhemoglobin concentration will be increased (normal COHb < 1.5% in nonsmokers, < 10% in smokers). As opposed to laboratory cooximeters, pulse oximeters using two wavelengths cannot detect carboxyhemoglobin (see Chapter 6). Carbon monoxide's affinity for hemoglobin is 200 times greater than that of oxygen.

Administration of 100% oxygen will shorten the half-life of carboxyhemoglobin from 4 hours in room air to less than 1 hour. The use of hyperbaric oxygen is controversial, but it should be considered if available. Hydrogen cyanide released from synthetic materials will further limit oxygen availability and utilization (the normal blood cyanide level is < 0.2 μg/mL) and may provide another indication for hyperbaric oxygen therapy.

Metabolism is markedly increased during the healing phase of a burn injury. This hypermetabolic state is reflected by increased oxygen consumption and CO_2 production. Therefore, alveolar ventilation must be proportionately increased and supplemental oxygen supplied.

What cardiovascular effects are associated with major burn injuries?

Increases in permeability at the site of injury and throughout the microvasculature cause a tremendous shift of fluid from the plasma volume to the interstitial space. Despite red blood cell destruction, hematocrit may rise as a result of the contraction of intravascular volume. This decrease in intravascular volume is most pronounced during the first 24 hours and is typically replaced with crystalloid solutions (eg, lactated Ringer's injection, 2–4 mL/kg per percentage of body surface burned). Cardiac output declines as a result of the contraction of plasma volume and a circulating myocardial depressant factor. Perfusion of vital organs is monitored by measurement of urinary output through a Foley catheter. If volume replacement does not provide an adequate diuresis (1 mL/kg/hour), inotropic support with dopamine may be beneficial.

After 24–48 hours, capillary integrity returns to normal, and colloid solutions will remain intravascular. Interstitial fluid reabsorption, increased metabolic demands, and high levels of circulating catecholamines may lead to high-output failure. Blood pressure and heart rate are typically elevated.

What electrolyte derangements can be found in burn patients?

Hyperkalemia from tissue destruction may complicate management during the acute resuscitation phase. Later, renal wasting and gastric losses may result in hypokalemia. Topical antibiotic therapy may also cause electrolyte imbalances. Mafenide acetate inhibits carbonic anhydrase, causing hyperchloremic acidosis. Another topical medication, silver nitrate, decreases serum sodium, chloride, and potassium levels. Significant methemoglobinemia is a rare complication of topical silver nitrate therapy. Electrical burns are associated with such severe muscle cell damage that myoglobinuria can lead to renal failure.

Which monitors would be useful during this excision and grafting procedure?

Excision of dead tissue after a major burn injury is usually associated with significant blood loss. This is especially true if surgery is delayed more than a few days after the burn or if the burn is not limited to areas that can be isolated with tourniquets. In these situations, at least two large-bore intravenous lines, an arterial line, and often a central venous catheter or pulmonary artery catheter are indicated. A central triple-lumen catheter can be helpful in patients with difficult intravenous access. If possible, a noninvasive blood pressure unit should be used as a backup to the arterial line, which may malfunction if the patient is frequently repositioned.

Electrocardiograph skin electrodes will not stick to burned areas, and they interfere with chest wall excision. As an alternative, needle electrodes are often sutured in place. Patients with respiratory insufficiency should be monitored with pulse oximetry if a suitable probe location is available.

Heat loss through denuded skin is a serious problem in the burn patient and should be closely monitored. Hypothermia can be minimized by using warming blankets and heat lamps, increasing operating room temperature, humidification of inspired gases, and warming intravenous fluids.

Are there any special intubation considerations in these patients?

Burn victims with inhalational injury will often be intubated prior to surgery. Indications for early intubation include hypoxia not correctable with a face mask, upper airway edema that may progress to obstruction, or the presence of copious secretions. If in doubt, or if periods of questionable airway monitoring are anticipated (eg, during transport), intubate before edema develops and intubation becomes technically difficult. This is particularly important if the patient is being stabilized prior to transfer to another hospital. Impending airway obstruction or severe facial contractures call for an awake fiberoptic intubation. Precautions to prevent emesis and aspiration should be considered in the acute resuscitation phase, during episodes of sepsis, or if the patient is receiving large doses of narcotics. Tracheostomies have been associated with increased morbidity in burn patients because of pulmonary sepsis.

How does a burn injury affect the pharmacology of anesthetic drugs?

Succinylcholine is contraindicated in burn patients after the first 24 hours. Its administration has caused cardiac arrest because of dramatic increases in serum potassium levels. Prolonged muscle depolarization following succinylcholine appears to be related to an increase in postjunctional acetylcholine receptors. This response has even been documented in patients with less than a 10% body surface area burn. In contrast, burn patients require higher than normal doses of nondepolarizing muscle relaxants. This resistance is due to altered protein binding and an increased number of extrajunctional acetylcholine receptors, which bind nondepolarizing drug without causing a neuromuscular effect.

Volatile anesthetics will exacerbate myocardial depression but are useful after the acute phase. Because of the potential for serious dysrhythmias, halothane is best avoided if epinephrine-soaked bandages are being used to decrease blood loss.

SUGGESTED READING

Resources for Optimal Care of the Injured Patient: 1999 Committee on Trauma, American College of Surgeons, 1998.

Boffard KD, Brooks AJ: Pancreatic trauma—injuries to the pancreas and pancreatic duct. Eur J Surg 2000;166:4.

Brooks AJ, Rowlands BJ: Blunt abdominal injuries. Br Med Bull 1999;55:844.

Dabrowski GP, Steinberg SM, Ferrara JJ, Flint LM: A critical assessment of endpoints of shock resuscitation. Surg Clin N Am 2000;80:825.

Dykes EH: Paediatric trauma. Br J Anaesth 1999;83:130.

Ferrada R, Birolini D: New concepts in the management of patients with penetrating abdominal wounds. Sur Clin N Am 1999;79:1331.

Ho AM, Ling E: Systemic air embolism after lung trauma. Anesthesiology 1999;90:564.

Kao CC, Garner WL: Acute burns. Plastic Reconstruct Surg 2000;105:2482.

King BS, Gupta R, Narayan RK: The early assessment and intensive care unit management of patients with severe traumatic brain and spinal cord injuries. Surg Clin N Am 2000;80:855.

Parks RW, Chrysos E, Diamond T: Management of liver trauma. Br J Surg 1999;86:1121.

Peach SE, Trunkey D: Blunt injury of the thoracic aorta. Eur J Surg 1999;165:1110.

Rosenberg AD, Grande C, Bernstein RL: *Pain Management and Regional Anesthesia in Trauma.* WB Saunders and Company, 1999.

Strong RW: The management of blunt liver injuries. Australian N Zealand J Surg 1999;69:609.

Trunkey DD, Lewis FR: *Current Therapy of Trauma,* 4th edition. Mosby-Yearbook, 1999.

Maternal & Fetal Physiology & Anesthesia

42

KEY CONCEPTS

 The minimal alveolar concentration (MAC) progressively decreases during pregnancy—at term, by as much as 40%—for all general anesthetic agents; MAC returns to normal by the third day after delivery.

 Pregnant patients display enhanced sensitivity to local anesthetics during regional anesthesia; dose requirements may be reduced as much as 30%.

 Obstruction of the inferior vena cava by the enlarging uterus distends the epidural venous plexus and increases the risk of intravascular injection during epidural anesthesia.

 Up to 20% of women at term develop the supine hypotension syndrome, which is characterized by hypotension associated with pallor, sweating, or nausea and vomiting.

The reduction in gastric motility and the tone of the gastroesophageal sphincter as well as hypersecretion of gastric acid place the parturient at high risk for regurgitation and pulmonary aspiration.

 Ephedrine is considered the vasopressor of choice for treating hypotension during pregnancy because it has predominantly β-adrenergic activity.

 Transfer of a drug across the placenta is reflected by the ratio of its fetal umbilical vein to maternal venous concentrations (UV/MV), while its uptake by fetal tissues can be correlated with the ratio of its fetal umbilical artery to umbilical vein concentrations (UA/UV).

 Volatile inhalational anesthetics decrease blood pressure and, consequently, uteroplacental blood flow. Their effects are generally minor, however, in concentrations of less than 1 MAC.

 The greatest strain on the parturient's heart occurs immediately after delivery, when intense uterine contraction and involution suddenly relieve inferior vena caval obstruction and increase cardiac output as much as 80% above prelabor values.

 Because the maturation of the lungs occurs later in fetal development, extrauterine life is not possible until after 24–26 weeks of gestation, when pulmonary capillaries are formed and come to lie in close approximation to an immature alveolar epithelium.

Pregnancy produces profound physiologic changes that alter the usual responses to anesthesia. Moreover, anesthetic care of the pregnant patient is unique in that two patients are cared for simultaneously: the parturient and the fetus. Failure to take these facts into consideration can have disastrous consequences.

This chapter reviews the normal physiologic changes associated with pregnancy, labor, and delivery. Uteroplacental physiology and its response to common anesthetic agents are also discussed. Much of this knowledge forms the basis for current anesthetic practices for labor and delivery (see Chapter 43). Lastly, care of the neonate in the obstetric suite or the intensive care unit requires an understanding of the physiologic transition from fetal to neonatal life.

PHYSIOLOGIC CHANGES DURING PREGNANCY

Pregnancy affects virtually every organ system (Table 42–1). Many of these physiologic changes appear to be adaptive and useful to the mother in tolerating the stresses of pregnancy, labor, and delivery. Other changes lack obvious benefits but nonetheless require special consideration in caring for the parturient.

Central Nervous System Effects

 The minimal alveolar concentration (MAC) progressively decreases during pregnancy—at term, by as much as 40%—for all general anesthetic agents; MAC returns to normal by the third day after delivery. Changes in maternal hor-

Table 42–1. Average maximum physiologic changes associated with pregnancy.

Parameter	Change
Neurologic	
MAC	−40%
Respiratory	
Oxygen consumption	+20 to 50%
Minute ventilation	+50%
Tidal volume	+40%
Respiratory rate	+15%
PaO₂	+10%
PaCO₂	−15%
HCO₃	−15%
FRC	−20%
Cardiovascular	
Blood volume	+35%
Plasma volume	+45%
Cardiac output	+40%
Stroke volume	+30%
Heart rate	+15 to 30%
Peripheral resistance	−15%
Hematologic	
Hemoglobin	−20%
Platelets	−10 to 20%
Clotting factors	+50 to 250%
Renal	
GFR	+50%

MAC = minimum alveolar concentration; FRC = functional residual capacity; GFR = glomerular filtration rate.

monal and endogenous opiate levels have been implicated. Progesterone, which is sedating when given in pharmacologic doses, increases up to 20 times normal at term and is probably at least partly responsible for this observation. A surge in β-endorphin levels during labor and delivery also likely plays a major role.

 At term, pregnant patients also display enhanced sensitivity to local anesthetics during regional anesthesia; dose requirements may be reduced as much as 30%. This phenomenon appears to be hormonally mediated but may also be related to engorgement of the epidural venous plexus. Neural blockade occurs at lower concentrations of local anesthetics. Contrary to previous studies, more recent data suggests that pregnancy does not increase susceptibility to local anesthetic toxicity. Obstruction of the inferior vena cava by the enlarging uterus distends the epidural venous plexus and increases epidural blood volume. The latter has three major effects: (1) decreased spinal cerebrospinal fluid volume, (2) decreased potential volume of the epidural space, and (3) increased epidural (space) pressure. The first two effects enhance the cephalad spread of local anesthetic solutions during spinal and epidural anesthesia, respectively, while the last may predispose to a higher incidence of dural puncture with epidural anesthesia (see Chapter 16). Bearing down during labor further accentuates all these effects. Positive epidural pressures have been recorded in parturients and complicate identification of the epidural space without dural puncture. Engorgement of the epidural veins also increases the likelihood of placing an epidural catheter in a vein, resulting in an unintentional intravascular injection (see Chapter 16).

Respiratory Effects

Oxygen consumption and minute ventilation progressively increase during pregnancy. Both tidal volume and, to a lesser extent, respiratory rate increase. By term, oxygen consumption has increased about 20–40%, while minute ventilation has increased 40–50%. PaCO₂ decreases to 28–32 mm Hg; significant respiratory alkalosis is prevented by a compensatory decrease in plasma bicarbonate concentration. Hyperventilation may also increase PaO₂ slightly. Elevated levels of 2,3-diphosphoglycerate offset the effect of hyperventilation on hemoglobin's affinity for oxygen (see Chapter 22). The P-50 for hemoglobin increases from 27 to 30 mm Hg; the combination of the latter with an increase in cardiac output (see section on Cardiovascular Effects below) enhances oxygen delivery to tissues.

The maternal respiratory pattern changes as the uterus enlarges. In the third trimester, elevation of the diaphragm is compensated by an increase in the antero-posterior diameter of the chest; diaphragmatic motion, however, is not restricted. Thoracic breathing is favored over abdominal breathing. Both vital capacity and closing capacity are minimally affected but functional residual capacity (FRC) decreases up to 20% at term; FRC returns to normal within 48 hours of delivery. This decrease is principally due to a reduction in expiratory reserve volume as a result of larger than normal tidal volumes (see Chapter 22). Flow-volume loops are unaffected, and airway resistance may actually decrease. Physiologic dead space decreases but intrapulmonary shunting increases towards term. A chest film often shows prominent vascular markings due to increased pulmonary blood volume and an elevated diaphragm. Pulmonary vasodilatation prevents pulmonary pressures form rising.

The combination of a decreased FRC and increased oxygen consumption promotes rapid oxygen desaturation during periods of apnea (see Chapter 22). Preoxygenation prior to induction of general anesthesia is therefore mandatory to avoid hypoxemia in pregnant patients. Closing volume exceeds FRC in up to half of all pregnant women when they are supine at term. Under these conditions, atelectasis and hypoxemia readily occur. Parturients should not lie flat without supplemental oxygen. The decrease in FRC coupled with the increase in minute ventilation accelerates the uptake of all inhalational anesthetics. The reduction in dead space narrows the arterial end-tidal CO_2 gradient.

Capillary engorgement of the respiratory mucosa during pregnancy predisposes the upper airways to trauma, bleeding, and obstruction. Gentle laryngoscopy and the use of small endotracheal tubes (6–7 mm) should be employed during general anesthesia.

Cardiovascular Effects

Cardiac output and blood volume increase to meet accelerated maternal and fetal metabolic demands. An increase in plasma volume in excess of an increase in red cell mass produces dilutional anemia and reduces blood viscosity. Hemoglobin concentration, however, usually remains greater than 11 g/dL. Moreover, in terms of tissue oxygen delivery, the reduction in hemoglobin concentration is offset by the increase in cardiac output and the rightward shift of the hemoglobin dissociation curve (see section on Respiratory Effects). A decrease in systemic vascular resistance by the second trimester decreases both diastolic and, to a lesser degree, systolic blood pressure. The response to adrenergic agents and vasoconstrictors is blunted.

At term, maternal blood volume has increased by 1000–1500 mL in most women, allowing them to easily tolerate the blood loss associated with delivery; total blood volume reaches 90 mL/kg. Average blood loss during vaginal delivery is 400–500 mL, compared with 800–1000 mL for a cesarean section. Blood volume does not return to normal until 1–2 weeks after delivery.

The increase in cardiac output (40% at term) is due to increases in both heart rate (15–30%) as well as stroke volume (30%). Cardiac chambers enlarge and myocardial hypertrophy is often noted on echocardiography. Pulmonary artery, central venous, and pulmonary artery wedge pressures, however, remain unchanged. Most of these effects are observed in the first and, to a lesser extent, the second trimester. In the third trimester, cardiac output does not appreciably rise, except during labor. The greatest increases in cardiac output are seen during labor and immediately after delivery (see section on effect of labor on maternal physiology). Cardiac output often does not return to normal until 2 weeks after delivery.

Decreases in cardiac output can occur in the supine position after the 28th week of pregnancy. (Some authors suggest even earlier.) Such decreases have been shown to be secondary to impeded venous return to the heart as the enlarging uterus compresses the inferior vena cava. Up to 20% of women at term develop the **supine hypotension syndrome,** which is characterized by hypotension associated with pallor, sweating, or nausea and vomiting. The cause of this syndrome appears to be complete or near-complete occlusion of the inferior vena cava by the gravid uterus. Turning the patient on her side typically restores venous return from the lower body and corrects the hypotension in such instances. Trendelenburg position may exacerbate caval compression. The gravid uterus also compresses the aorta in most parturients when they are supine. This latter effect decreases blood flow to the lower extremities and, more importantly, to the uteroplacental circulation. Uterine contraction relieves caval compression but exacerbates aortic compression.

Aortocaval compression is an important but preventable cause of fetal distress. The combination of systemic hypotension (due to decreased venous return), increased uterine venous pressure, and uterine arterial hypoperfusion severely compromise uterine and placental blood flows. When combined with the hypotensive effects of regional or general anesthesia, **aortocaval compression** can readily produce fetal asphyxia. Parturients with a 28-week or longer gestation should not be placed supine without left uterine displacement. This maneuver is most readily accomplished by placing a wedge (> 15 degrees) under the right hip.

Chronic partial caval obstruction in the third trimester predisposes to venous stasis, phlebitis, and edema in the lower extremities. Moreover, compression of the inferior vena cava below the diaphragm distends and increases blood flow through collateral venous drainage, ie, the paravertebral venous plexus (including the epidural veins) and to a minor degree the abdominal wall.

Lastly, elevation of the diaphragm shifts the heart's position in the chest, resulting in the appearance of an enlarged heart on a plain chest film, and left axis deviation and T wave changes on the ECG. Physical examination often reveals a systolic ejection flow murmur (grade I or II) and exaggerated splitting of the first heart sound (S_1); a third heart sound (S_3) may be audible. A few patients develop small, asymptomatic pericardial effusions.

Renal Effects

Renal vasodilatation increases renal blood flow early during pregnancy but autoregulation is preserved. The kidneys often enlarge. Increased renin and aldosterone levels promote sodium retention. Renal plasma flow and the glomerular filtration rate increase as much as 50% during the first trimester; glomerular filtration declines toward normal in the third trimester. Serum creatinine and blood urea nitrogen may decrease to 0.5–0.6 mg/dL and 8–9 mg/dL, respectively. A decreased renal tubular threshold for glucose and amino acids is common and often results in mild glycosuria (1–10 g/d) or proteinuria (< 300 mg/d). Plasma osmolality decreases by 8–10 mOsm/kg.

Gastrointestinal Effects

Gastroesophageal reflux and esophagitis are common during pregnancy. Upward and anterior displacement of the stomach by the uterus promotes incompetence of the gastroesophageal sphincter. Elevated progesterone levels reduce the tone of the gastroesophageal sphincter, while placental gastrin secretion causes hypersecretion of gastric acid. These factors place the parturient at high risk for regurgitation and pulmonary aspiration. Intragastric pressure is unchanged. Data with regard to gastric emptying are conflicting; some studies suggest normal gastric emptying is preserved until the onset of labor, while others report delayed gastric emptying early in pregnancy. Nonetheless, nearly all parturients have a gastric pH under 2.5, and over 60% of them have gastric volumes greater than 25 mL. Both factors have been associated with an increased risk of severe aspiration pneumonitis. Narcotics and anticholinergics reduce lower esophageal sphincter pressure, may facilitate gastroesophageal reflux, and delay gastric emptying. These physiologic effects, together with recent food ingestion just prior to labor and the delayed gastric emptying associated with labor pains, predispose parturients to nausea and vomiting.

Hepatic Effects

Overall hepatic function and blood flow are unchanged; minor elevations in serum transaminases and lactic dehydrogenase levels may be observed in the third trimester. Elevations in serum alkaline phosphatase are due to its secretion by the placenta (see Chapter 34). A mild decrease in serum albumin is due to an expanded plasma volume; as a result, colloid oncotic pressure is reduced. A 25–30% decrease in serum pseudocholinesterase activity is also present at term but rarely produces significant prolongation of succinylcholine's action. The breakdown of mivacurium and ester-type local anesthetics is not appreciably altered. Pseudocholinesterase activity may not return to normal until up to 6 weeks postpartum. High progesterone levels appear to inhibit the release of cholecystokinin, resulting in incomplete emptying of the gallbladder. The latter, together with altered bile acid composition, can predispose to formation of cholesterol gallstones.

Hematologic Effects

Pregnancy is associated with a hypercoagulable state that may be beneficial in limiting blood loss at delivery. Fibrinogen and factors VII, VIII, IX, X, and XII concentrations all increase; only factor XI levels may decrease. Accelerated fibrinolysis can be observed late in the third trimester. In addition to the dilutional anemia (see section on cardiovascular effects), leukocytosis (up to $21,000/\mu L$) and a 10–20% decrease in platelet count may be encountered during the third trimester. Because of fetal utilization, iron and folate deficiency anemias readily develop if supplements of these nutrients are not taken. Cell-mediated immunity is markedly depressed and may increase susceptibility to viral infections.

Metabolic Effects

Complex metabolic and hormonal changes occur during pregnancy. Altered carbohydrate, fat, and protein metabolism favors fetal growth and development. These changes resemble starvation, because blood glucose and amino acid levels are low whereas free fatty acids, ketones, and triglyceride levels are high. Nonetheless, pregnancy is a diabetogenic state; insulin levels steadily rise during pregnancy. Secretion of human placental lactogen, also called human chorionic somatomammotropin, by the placenta is probably responsible for the relative insulin resistance associated with pregnancy. Pancreatic B cell hyperplasia occurs in response to an increased demand for insulin secretion.

Secretion of human chorionic gonadotropin and elevated levels of estrogens promote hypertrophy of the thyroid gland and increase thyroid-binding globulin; although T_4 and T_3 levels are elevated, free T_4, free T_3, and thyrotropin (thyroid-stimulating hormone) remain normal. Serum calcium levels decrease, but ionized calcium concentration remains normal.

Musculoskeletal Effects

Elevated levels of relaxin throughout pregnancy help prepare for delivery by softening the cervix, inhibiting uterine contractions, and relaxing the pubic symphysis and pelvic joints. Ligamentous laxity of the spine increases the risk of back injury. The latter may contribute to the relatively high incidence of back pain during pregnancy.

UTEROPLACENTAL CIRCULATION

A normal uteroplacental circulation (Figure 42–1) is critical in the development and maintenance of a healthy fetus. Uteroplacental insufficiency is an important cause of intrauterine fetal growth retardation and when severe can result in fetal demise. The integrity of this circulation is, in turn, dependent on both adequate uterine blood flow and normal placental function.

Uterine Blood Flow

At term, **uterine blood flow** represents about 10% of the cardiac output, or 600–700 mL/min (compared with 50 mL/min in the nonpregnant uterus). Eighty percent of uterine blood flow normally supplies the placenta, while the remainder goes to the myometrium. Pregnancy maximally dilates the uterine vasculature, so that autoregulation is absent, but it remains sensitive to α-adrenergic agonists. Uterine blood flow is not usually significantly affected by respiratory gas tensions, but extreme hypocapnia ($PaCO_2$ < 20 mm Hg) can reduce uterine blood flow and causes fetal hypoxemia and acidosis.

Blood flow is directly proportionate to the difference between uterine arterial and venous pressures but inversely proportionate to uterine vascular resistance. Although not under appreciable neural control, the uterine vasculature has an abundant supply of α-adrenergic and possibly some β-adrenergic receptors.

Three major factors decrease uterine blood flow during pregnancy: (1) systemic hypotension, (2) uterine vasoconstriction, and (3) uterine contractions. Common causes of hypotension during pregnancy include aortocaval compression, hypovolemia, and sympathetic blockade following regional anesthesia. Stress-induced release of endogenous catecholamines (sympathoadrenal activation) during labor causes uterine arterial vasoconstriction. Any drug with α-adrenergic activity (eg, phenylephrine) is also capable of decreasing uterine blood flow by vasoconstriction. Ephedrine, which has predominantly β-adrenergic activity, is therefore generally considered the vasopressor of choice for hypotension during pregnancy. Paradoxically, hypertensive disorders are often associated with decreased uterine blood flow due to generalized vasoconstriction. Uterine contractions decrease blood flow by elevating uterine venous pressure and, when intense, compressing arterial vessels as they traverse the myometrium. Hypertonic contractions during labor or during oxytocin infusions can critically compromise uterine blood flow.

Placental Function

The fetus is dependent on the placenta for respiratory gas exchange, nutrition, and waste elimination. The placenta is formed by both maternal and fetal tissues and derives a blood supply from each. The resulting exchange membrane has a functional area of about 1.8 m^2.

A. PHYSIOLOGIC ANATOMY:

The placenta (Figure 42–2) is composed of projections of fetal tissue (villi) that lie in maternal vascular spaces (intervillous spaces). As a result of this arrangement, the fetal capillaries within villi readily exchange substances with the maternal blood that bathes them. Maternal blood in the intervillous spaces is derived from spiral branches of the uterine artery and drains into the uterine veins. Fetal blood within villi is derived from umbilical cord via two umbilical arteries and returns to the fetus via a single umbilical vein.

B. PLACENTAL EXCHANGE:

Placental exchange can occur by one of five mechanisms:

1. Diffusion—Respiratory gases and small ions are transported by diffusion. Most drugs used in anesthesia have molecular weights well under 1000 and consequently can diffuse across the placenta.

2. Bulk flow—Water moves across by bulk flow.

3. Active transport—Amino acids, vitamins, and some ions (calcium and iron) utilize this mechanism.

4. Pinocytosis—Large molecules, such as immunoglobulins, are transported by pinocytosis.

5. Breaks—Breaks in the placental membrane and mixing of maternal and fetal blood are probably responsible for Rh sensitization (see Chapter 29).

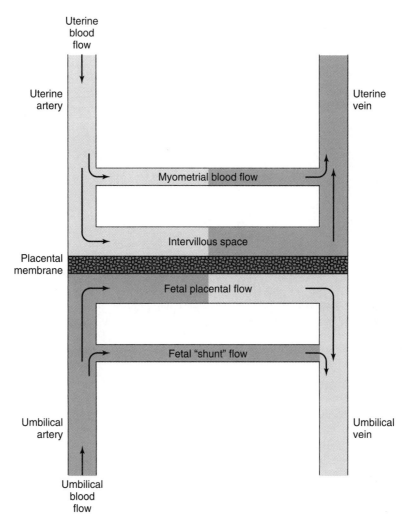

Figure 42–1. The uteroplacental circulation. (Modified and reproduced, with permission, from Schnider S, Levinson G: Anesthesia for Obstetrics, 2nd ed. Williams & Wilkins, 1987.)

Respiratory Gas Exchange

Of all the substances exchanged across the placenta, oxygen has the lowest storage to utilization ratio. At term, fetal oxygen consumption averages about 21 mL/min, yet fetal oxygen stores are normally estimated to be only 42 mL. Fortunately, because of multiple adaptive mechanisms, the normal fetus at term can survive 10 minutes or longer instead of the expected 2 minutes of total oxygen deprivation. Partial or complete oxygen deprivation can result from umbilical cord compression, umbilical cord prolapse, placental abruption, severe maternal hypoxemia, or hypotension.

Compensatory mechanisms include redistribution of fetal blood flow primarily to the brain, heart, placenta, and adrenal gland; decreased oxygen consumption; and anaerobic metabolism.

Transfer of oxygen across the placenta is dependent on the ratio of maternal uterine blood flow to fetal umbilical blood flow. Animal studies suggest that the reserve for oxygen transfer is small even during normal pregnancy. Well-oxygenated fetal blood from the placenta has a PaO_2 of only 40 mm Hg. To aid oxygen transfer, the fetal hemoglobin oxygen dissociation curve is shifted to the left such that fetal hemoglobin has greater affinity for oxygen than does maternal hemoglo-

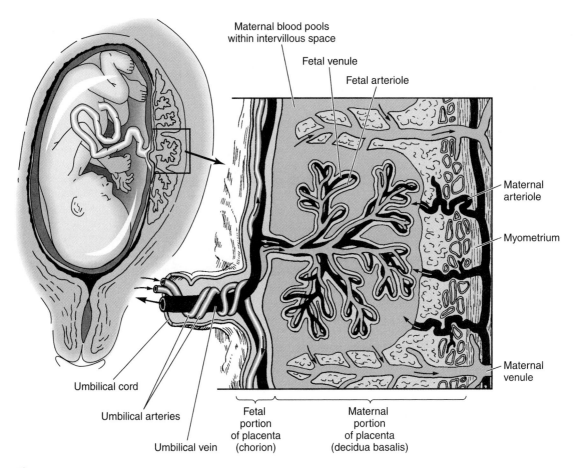

Figure 42–2. The placenta.

bin (whose curve is already shifted to the right; see section on respiratory effects). In addition, fetal hemoglobin concentration is usually 15 g/dL (compared with approximately 12 g/dL in the mother).

Carbon dioxide readily diffuses across the placenta. Maternal hyperventilation (see section on respiratory effects) increases the gradient for the transfer of carbon dioxide from the fetus into the maternal circulation. Fetal hemoglobin also appears to have less affinity for carbon dioxide than does maternal hemoglobin.

Placental Transfer of Anesthetic Agents

Transfer of a drug across the placenta is reflected by the ratio of its fetal umbilical vein to maternal venous concentrations (UV/MV), while its uptake by fetal tissues can be correlated with the ratio of its fetal umbilical artery to umbilical vein concentrations (UA/UV). Fetal effects of drugs administered to parturients depend on multiple factors including route of administration (intramuscular, intravenous, epidural, or intrathecal), dose, timing of administration (both relative to delivery as well as contractions), and maturity of the fetal organs (brain and liver). Thus, giving a drug hours before delivery or as a single intravenous bolus during a uterine contraction just prior to delivery (when uterine blood flow is maximally reduced) is least likely to produce high fetal levels. Effects on the fetus can be evaluated intrapartum by changes in fetal heart rate pattern or acid-base status, or postpartum by Apgar scores or neurobehavioral examinations (see Chapter 43). Fortunately, current anesthetic techniques for labor and delivery (see Chapter 43) generally have minimal fetal effects despite significant placental transfer of anesthetic agents and adjuncts.

All inhalational agents and most intravenous agents freely cross the placenta. Inhalational agents generally produce little fetal depression when they are given in limited doses (< 1 MAC) and delivery occurs within 10 minutes of induction. Thiopental, ketamine, propofol, and benzodiazepines readily cross the placenta and can be detected in the fetal circulation. Fortunately, when these agents, with the exception of benzodiazepines, are used in usual induction doses, drug distribution, metabolism, and possibly placental uptake may limit fetal effects. Although most opiates readily cross the placenta, their effects on neonates at delivery vary considerably. Newborns appear to be more sensitive to the respiratory depressant effect of morphine compared with that of other opioids. Although respiratory depression is significant with meperidine, peaking 1–3 hours after administration, it is still less than morphine; butorphanol and nalbuphine produce even less respiratory depression, but still may have significant neurobehavioral depressant effects. Although fentanyl readily crosses the placenta, it appears to have minimal neonatal effects unless large intravenous doses (> 1 μg/kg) are given immediately before delivery. Epidural or intrathecal fentanyl, sufentanil, and to a lesser extent morphine (see Chapter 43) generally produce minimal neonatal effects. Alfentanil causes neonatal depression similar to meperidine. The highly ionized property of muscle relaxants impedes placental transfer, resulting in minimal effects on the fetus.

Local anesthetics are weakly basic drugs that are principally bound to α_1-acid glycoprotein. Placental transfer depends on three factors: (1) pK_a (see Chapter 14), (2) maternal and fetal pH, and (3) degree of protein binding. Except in the case of chloroprocaine, fetal acidosis produces higher fetal to maternal drug ratios because binding of hydrogen ions to the nonionized form causes trapping of the local anesthetic in the fetal circulation. Highly protein-bound agents diffuse poorly across the placenta; thus, greater protein binding of bupivacaine and ropivacaine, compared with that of lidocaine, likely accounts for their lower fetal blood levels. Chloroprocaine has the least placental transfer because it is rapidly broken down by plasma cholinesterase in the maternal circulation.

Most commonly used anesthetic adjuncts also readily cross the placenta. Thus, maternally administered ephedrine, β-adrenergic blockers (such as labetalol and esmolol), vasodilators, phenothiazines, antihistamines (H_1 and H_2), and metoclopramide are transferred to the fetus. Atropine and scopolamine but not glycopyrrolate cross the placenta; the latter's quaternary ammonium (ionized) structure results in only limited transfer.

Effect of Anesthetic Agents on Uteroplacental Blood Flow

Intravenous anesthetic agents have variable effects on uteroplacental blood flow. Barbiturates and propofol are typically associated with small reductions in uterine blood flow due to mild to moderate, dose-dependent decreases in maternal blood pressure. A small induction dose, however, can produce greater reductions in blood flow as a result of sympathoadrenal activation (due to light anesthesia). Ketamine, in doses < 1.5 mg/kg, does not appreciably alter uteroplacental blood flow; its hypertensive effect typically counteracts any vasoconstriction. Compared with thiopental and propofol, midazolam may be more likely to produce transient systemic hypotension when used as an induction agent. Etomidate likely has minimal effects, but its actions on uteroplacental circulation are not well described.

Volatile inhalational anesthetics decrease blood pressure and, consequently, uteroplacental blood flow. In concentrations of less than 1 MAC, however, their effects are generally minor. Halothane and isoflurane may dilate the uterine arteries. Nitrous oxide has minimal effects.

High blood levels of local anesthetics—particularly lidocaine—cause uterine arterial vasoconstriction. Such levels are seen only with unintentional intravascular injections and occasionally following paracervical blocks (in which the injection site is in close proximity to the uterine arteries). Spinal and epidural anesthesia typically do not decrease uterine blood flow, provided arterial hypotension is avoided. Moreover, uterine blood flow during labor may actually improve in preeclamptic patients following epidural anesthesia; a reduction in circulating endogenous catecholamines likely decreases uterine vasoconstriction. The addition of dilute concentrations of epinephrine to local anesthetic solutions does not appreciably alter uterine blood flow. Intravascular uptake of the epinephrine from the epidural space may result in only minor systemic β-adrenergic effects.

THE PHYSIOLOGY OF NORMAL LABOR

Labor commences on the average 40 ± 2 weeks following the last menstrual period. The factors involved in the initiation of labor are as yet not entirely elucidated but likely involve overdistention of the uterus, enhanced myometrial sensitivity to oxytocin, and altered prostaglandin synthesis by fetal membranes and decidual tissues. Although circulating oxytocin levels often do not increase at the beginning of labor, the number of myometrial oxytocin receptors rapidly increases. Several prodromal events also usually precede true labor about 2–4 weeks prior to delivery: the fetal presenting part settles into the pelvis (lightening); patients develop uterine (Braxton Hicks) contractions that are characteristically irregular in frequency, duration, and intensity; and the cervix softens and thins out (cervical effacement). Approximately 1 week to 1 hour before true labor, the cervical mucous plug (which is often bloody) breaks free (bloody show).

True labor begins when the sporadic and haphazard Braxton Hicks contractions increase in strength (25–60 mm Hg), coordination, and frequency (15–20 min apart). Amniotic membranes may rupture spontaneously prior or subsequent to the onset of true labor. Following progressive cervical dilatation, the contractions propel first the fetus and then the placenta through the pelvis and perineum. By convention, labor is divided into three stages. The first stage is defined by the onset of true labor and ends with complete cervical dilatation. The second stage begins with full cervical dilatation, is characterized by fetal descent, and ends with complete delivery of the fetus. Finally, the third stage extends from the birth of the baby to the delivery of the placenta.

Based on the rate of cervical dilatation, the first stage is further divided into a slow **latent phase** followed by a faster **active phase** (Figure 42–3). The latent phase is characterized by progressive cervical effacement and minor dilatation (2–4 cm). The subsequent active phase is characterized by more frequent contractions (3–5 min apart) and progressive cervical dilatation up to 10 cm. The first stage usually lasts 8–12 hours in nulliparous patients and about 5–8 hours in multiparous patients.

Contractions during the second stage occur 1.5–2 minutes apart and last 1–1.5 minutes. Although contraction intensity does not appreciably change, the parturient, by bearing down, can greatly augment intrauterine pressure and facilitate expulsion of the fetus. The second stage usually lasts 15–120 minutes, while the third stage typically takes 15–30 minutes.

The course of labor is monitored by uterine activity, cervical dilatation, and fetal descent. Uterine activity refers to the frequency and magnitude of uterine contractions. The latter may be measured directly, with a catheter inserted through the cervix, or indirectly, with a tocodynamometer applied externally around the abdomen. Cervical dilatation and fetal descent are assessed by pelvic examination. Fetal station refers to the level of descent (in cm) of the presenting part relative to the ischial spines (eg, –1 or +1).

Effect of Labor on Maternal Physiology

During intense painful contractions, maternal minute ventilation may increase up to 300%. Oxygen consumption also increases another 60% above third-trimester values. With excessive hyperventilation, $PaCO_2$ falls below 20 mm Hg. Marked hypocapnia can cause periods of hypoventilation and transient maternal and fetal hypoxemia in between contractions. Excessive maternal hyperventilation also reduces uterine blood flow and promotes fetal acidosis.

Each contraction places an additional burden on the heart by displacing 300–500 mL of blood from the

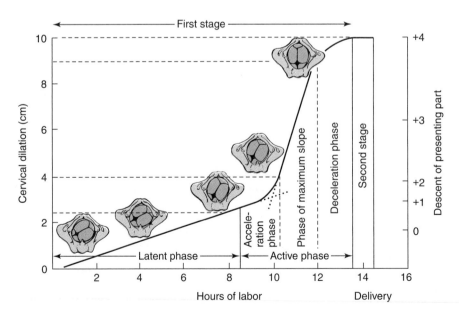

Figure 42–3. The course of normal labor. (Reproduced, with permission, from DeCherney AH, Pernoll ML, (editors): *Current Obstetric & Gynecologic Diagnosis & Treatment,* 9th ed. McGraw-Hill, 2001.)

uterus into the central circulation (analogous to an autotransfusion). Cardiac output rises 45% over third-trimester values. The greatest strain on the heart, however, occurs immediately after delivery, when intense uterine contraction and involution suddenly relieve inferior vena caval obstruction and increase cardiac output as much as 80% above prelabor values.

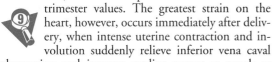

Effect of Anesthetic Agents on Uterine Activity and Labor

A. INHALATIONAL AGENTS:

Halothane, enflurane, isoflurane, sevoflurane, and desflurane depress uterine activity equally at equipotent doses; all cause dose-dependent uterine relaxation. Low doses (< 0.75 MAC) of these agents, however, do not interfere with oxytocin's effect on the uterus. Higher doses can result in uterine atony and increase blood loss at delivery. Nitrous oxide has minimal if any effects.

B. PARENTERAL AGENTS:

Opioids minimally decrease the progression of labor, while ketamine appears to have little effect.

C. REGIONAL ANESTHESIA:

The effects of regional anesthesia are complex, predominantly indirect, and somewhat controversial. Direct effects are only observed with toxic systemic levels of local anesthetics, producing tetanic contractions. Indirect effects relate to the duration of labor and the efficiency of maternal expulsive efforts. The traditional view is that regional anesthesia administered early in the course of labor may prolong it, whereas a regional block given once labor is well established has little effect. Studies suggest that epidural (or spinal) anesthesia up to a T10 sensory level has little effect on labor provided that: (1) the parturient is already in the active phase, (2) epinephrine-containing solutions are not used, and (3) hypotension and aortocaval compression are avoided. Moreover, decreases in uterine activity are said to be readily reversible with an oxytocin infusion. Some evidence suggests that intrathecal and epidural analgesia in some instances may shorten the first stage of labor.

In the past, controversy existed regarding whether regional anesthesia increased the incidence of low forceps deliveries. Regional analgesia/anesthesia removes the urge to bear down during the second stage (Ferguson reflex), potentially prolonging the second stage of delivery. With proper coaching, however, patients who are unable to feel contractions during the second stage can usually expel the fetus without the help of forceps if more time is allowed for the second stage. Use of dilute local anesthetic/opioid (see Chapter 43) can preserve motor function and may allow more effective pushing.

D. VASOPRESSORS:

Uterine muscle has both α- and β-receptors. α_1-Receptor stimulation causes uterine contraction, while β_2-receptor stimulation produces relaxation. α-Adrenergic agents such as methoxamine and phenylephrine, in addition to causing uterine arterial constriction, can produce tetanic uterine contractions in large doses. Small doses of phenylephrine (50 μg) may increase uterine blood flow in normal parturients by raising arterial blood pressure. In contrast, ephedrine has little effect on uterine contractions and is considered the vasopressor choice for obstetric patients. The use of epinephrine-containing local anesthetic solutions for epidural anesthesia can theoretically prolong the first stage of labor if absorption of epinephrine from the epidural space results in significant systemic β-adrenergic effects. Although somewhat controversial, prolongation of labor is generally not clinically observed with very dilute epinephrine-containing local anesthetics.

E. OXYTOCIN:

Oxytocin (Pitocin) is usually administered intravenously to induce or augment uterine contractions, or to maintain uterine tone postpartum. It has a half-life of 3–5 minutes. Induction doses for labor are 0.5–8 mU/min. Complications include fetal distress due to hyperstimulation, uterine tetany, and less commonly, maternal water intoxication. Rapid intravenous infusion can also cause transient systemic hypotension due to relaxation of vascular smooth muscle; reflex tachycardia may also be noted.

F. ERGOT ALKALOIDS:

Methylergonovine (Methergine) causes intense and prolonged uterine contractions. It is therefore only given after delivery (postpartum) to treat uterine atony. Moreover, because it also constricts vascular smooth muscle and can cause severe hypertension, the drug is usually only administered either as 0.2 mg intramuscularly or as a slow intravenous infusion.

G. MAGNESIUM:

Magnesium is used in obstetrics both to stop premature labor (tocolysis) and to prevent eclamptic seizures (see Chapter 43). It is usually administered as a 4 g intravenous loading dose (over 20 min) followed by a 2 g/hour infusion. Therapeutic serum levels are considered to be 6–8 mg/dL. Serious side effects include hypotension, heart block muscle weakness and sedation (see Chapter 28).

H. β_2-AGONISTS:

The β_2-adrenergic agonists, ritodrine and terbutaline, inhibit uterine contractions and are used to treat premature labor (see Chapter 43).

FETAL PHYSIOLOGY

The placenta, which receives nearly one-half of the fetal cardiac output, is responsible for respiratory gas exchange. As a result, the lungs receive little blood flow and the pulmonary and systemic circulations are parallel instead of in series, as in the adult (Figures 42–4 and 42–5). This arrangement is made possible by two cardiac shunts—the **foramen ovale** and the **ductus arteriosus:**

1. (1) Well-oxygenated blood from the placenta (approximately 80% oxygen saturation) mixes with venous blood returning from the lower body (25% oxygen saturation) and flows via the inferior vena cava into the right atrium.

2. Right atrial anatomy preferentially directs blood flow from the inferior vena cava (67% oxygen saturation) through the foramen ovale into the left atrium.

3. Left atrial blood is then pumped by the left ventricle to the upper body (mainly the brain and the heart).

4. Poorly oxygenated blood from the upper body returns via the superior vena cava to the right atrium.

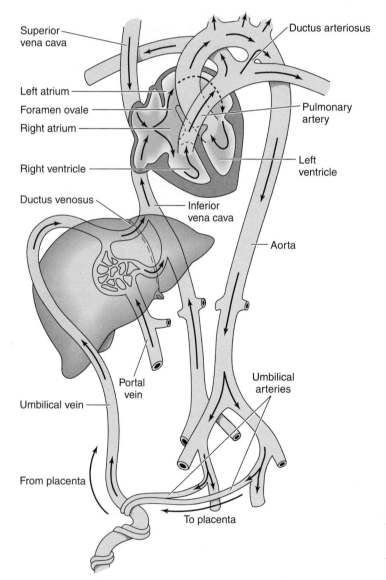

Figure 42–4. The fetal circulation before and after birth. (Reproduced, with permission, from Ganong WF: *Review of Medical Physiology,* 20th ed. McGraw-Hill, 2001.)

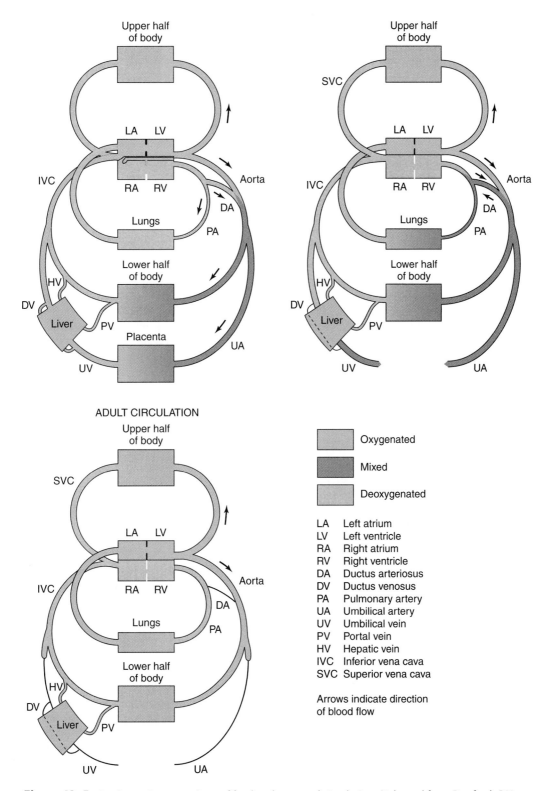

Figure 42–5. A schematic comparison of fetal and neonatal circulation. (Adapted from Danforth DN, Scott JR: *Obstetrics and Gynecology,* 5th ed. Lippincott, 1986.)

5. Right atrial anatomy preferentially directs flow from the superior vena cava into the right ventricle.

6. Right ventricular blood is pumped into the pulmonary artery.

7. Because of high pulmonary vascular resistance, 95% of the blood ejected from the right ventricle (60% oxygen saturation) is shunted across the ductus arteriosus, into the descending aorta, and back to the placenta and lower body.

The parallel circulation results in unequal ventricular flows; the right ventricle ejects two-thirds of the combined ventricular outputs, while the left ventricle ejects only one-third.

Up to one-half of the well-oxygenated blood in the umbilical vein can pass directly to the heart via the ductus venosus, bypassing the liver. The remainder of the blood flow from the placenta mixes with blood from the portal vein (via the portal sinus) and passes through the liver before reaching the heart. The latter may be important in allowing relatively rapid hepatic degradation of drugs (or toxins) that are absorbed from the maternal circulation.

In contrast to the fetal circulation, which is established very early during intrauterine life, maturation of the lungs lags behind. Extrauterine life is not possible until after 24–26 weeks of gestation, when pulmonary capillaries are formed and come to lie in close approximation to an immature alveolar epithelium. At 30 weeks, the cuboidal alveolar epithelium flattens out and begins to produce pulmonary surfactant. This substance provides alveolar stability and is necessary to maintain normal lung expansion after birth (see Chapter 22). Sufficient pulmonary surfactant is usually present after 34 weeks of gestation. Administration of glucocorticoids to the mother can accelerate fetal surfactant production.

PHYSIOLOGIC TRANSITION OF THE FETUS AT BIRTH

The most profound adaptive changes at birth involve the circulatory and respiratory systems. Failure to make this transition successfully results in fetal death or permanent neurologic damage.

At term, the fetal lungs are developed but contain about 90 mL of a plasma ultrafiltrate. During expulsion of the fetus at delivery, this fluid is normally squeezed from the lungs by the forces of the pelvic muscles and the vagina acting on the baby (the vaginal squeeze). Any remaining fluid is reabsorbed by the pulmonary capillaries and lymphatics. Catecholamine in the neonate during labor may augment release of surfactant from type II pneumocytes. Small (preterm) neonates

and neonates delivered via cesarean section do not benefit from the vaginal squeeze and thus typically have greater difficulty in maintaining respirations (transient tachypnea of the newborn). Respiratory efforts are normally initiated within 30 seconds after birth and become sustained within 90 seconds. Mild hypoxia and acidosis as well as sensory stimulation—cord clamping, pain, touch, and noise—help initiate and sustain respirations, while the outward recoil of the chest at delivery aids in filling the lungs with air.

Lung expansion increases both alveolar and arterial oxygen tensions and decreases pulmonary vascular resistance. The increase in oxygen tension is a potent stimulus for pulmonary arterial vasodilatation. The resultant increase in pulmonary blood flow and augmented flow to the left heart elevates left atrial pressure and functionally closes the foramen ovale. The increase in arterial oxygen tension also causes the ductus arteriosus to contract and functionally close. Other chemical mediators that may play a role in ductal closure include acetylcholine, bradykinin, and prostaglandins. The overall result is elimination of right-to-left shunting and establishment of the adult circulation (Figure 42–5). Anatomic closure of the ductus arteriosus does not usually occur until about 2–3 weeks, while closure of the foramen ovale takes months if at all.

Hypoxia or acidosis during the first few days of life can prevent or reverse these physiologic changes, resulting in persistence of (or return to) the fetal circulation. A vicious circle is established where the right-to-left shunting promotes hypoxemia and acidosis, which in turn promote more shunting (Figure 42–6). Right-to-left shunting may occur across the foramen ovale, the ductus arteriosus, or both. Unless this circle is broken, neonatal demise can occur rapidly.

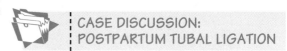

CASE DISCUSSION: POSTPARTUM TUBAL LIGATION

A 36-year-old woman is scheduled for bilateral tubal ligation 12 hours after delivery of a healthy baby.

Is this patient still at increased risk for pulmonary aspiration?

Controversy exists over when the increased risk for pulmonary aspiration diminishes following pregnancy. Certainly, many factors contributing to delayed gastric emptying are alleviated shortly after delivery: mechanical distortion of the stomach is relieved, labor pains cease, and the circulating progesterone level rapidly declines. In addition, a period of 8–12 hours of elective fasting is possible. Some studies suggest that the risk of pul-

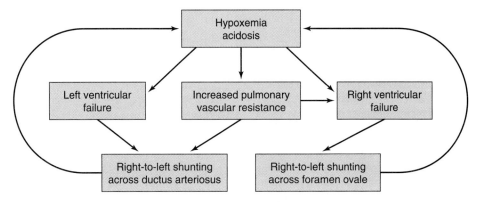

Figure 42–6. Pathophysiology of persistent fetal circulation. (Modified and reproduced, with permission, from Gregory GA: *Pediatric Anesthesia,* 2nd ed. Churchill Livingstone 1989.)

monary aspiration as judged by gastric volume and gastric fluid pH (see section on gastrointestinal effects) normalizes within 24 hours. Unfortunately, even these studies report up to a 30–60% incidence of either a gastric volume greater than 25 mL or a gastric fluid pH less than 2.5. Therefore, most clinicians still consider the postpartum patient at increased risk for pulmonary aspiration and take appropriate precautions (see Chapters 15 and 43). It is not known when the risk returns to that associated with elective surgical patients. Although some physiologic changes associated with pregnancy may require up to 6 weeks for resolution, the increased risk of pulmonary aspiration probably returns to "normal" well before that time.

Other than aspiration risk, what factors determine the "optimal" time for postpartum sterilization?

The decision when to perform postpartum tubal ligation (or laparoscopic fulguration) is complex and varies according to patient and obstetrician preferences as well as local practices. In addition, the decision may be based on whether the patient had a vaginal delivery or cesarean section and whether an anesthetic was administered for labor (epidural anesthesia) or delivery (epidural or general anesthesia).

Postpartum tubal ligation or fulguration may be: (1) performed immediately following delivery of the baby and repair of the uterus during a cesarean section, (2) delayed 8–48 hours following delivery to allow an elective fasting period, or (3) deferred until after the postpartum period (generally 6 weeks). Many obstetricians are reluctant to do immediate postpartum sterilizations because the patient may change her mind later, especially

if something untoward happens to the baby. Furthermore, they want to ensure that the patient is stable, especially after a complicated delivery. On the other hand, sterilization is technically much easier to perform in the immediate postpartum period because of the enlargement of the uterus and tubes. Postpartum sterilizations following natural vaginal delivery are generally performed within 48 hours of delivery, because bacterial colonization of the reproductive tract thereafter is thought to increase the risk of postoperative infection.

What factors determine selection of an anesthetic technique for postpartum sterilization?

When general or continuous epidural anesthesia is administered for a cesarean section, the same technique can easily be continued for immediate sterilization (provided that the patient is stable). When continuous epidural anesthesia was administered for labor and vaginal delivery, the epidural catheter may be left in place up to 48 hours for subsequent tubal ligation. The delay allows a period of elective fasting. A T4–5 sensory level with regional anesthesia is usually necessary to ensure a pain-free anesthetic experience. Lower sensory levels (as low as T10) may be adequate but sometimes fail to prevent pain during surgical traction on viscera.

When the patient has not had anesthesia for delivery, postpartum sterilization may be performed under either regional or general anesthesia. Because of the increased risk of pulmonary aspiration, regional anesthesia usually is preferred for bilateral tubal ligation via a minilaparotomy. Many clinicians prefer spinal over epidural anes-

thesia in this setting because of the risk of unintentional intravascular or intrathecal injections with the latter (see Chapter 16). Moreover, the risk of a precipitous decrease in blood pressure following spinal anesthesia may be significantly diminished following delivery (especially when preceded by an intravenous fluid bolus). In addition, the incidence of post-dural puncture headache is as low as 1% when a 25-gauge or smaller needle is used. Dosage requirements for regional anesthesia generally return to normal within 24–36 hours after delivery. Tetracaine, 7–10 mg, bupivacaine, 8–12 mg, or lidocaine, 60–90 mg, may be used for spinal anesthesia. For epidural anesthesia, 15–20 mL of lidocaine 1.5–2%, chloroprocaine 3%, or bupivacaine 0.5% are most commonly used.

In contrast, when laparoscopic tubal fulguration is planned, general endotracheal anesthesia is usually preferred. Insufflation of gas during laparoscopy impairs pulmonary gas exchange and predisposes the patient to nausea, vomiting, and possibly pulmonary aspiration. Endotracheal intubation generally ensures adequate ventilation and protects the airway.

What are important considerations for postpartum patients undergoing general anesthesia?

Preoperative concerns include a decreased blood hemoglobin concentration and the persistent increased risk of pulmonary aspiration. Anemia is nearly always present as a result of the physiologic effects of pregnancy combined with blood loss during and following delivery. Hemoglobin concentrations are usually greater than 9 g/dL, but levels as low as 7 g/dL are generally considered safe. Fortunately, sterilization procedures are rarely associated with significant blood loss.

The risk of pulmonary aspiration is diminished by a minimum of 8 hours of fasting, premedication with an H$_2$ histamine blocker (ranitidine), a clear antacid (sodium citrate), or metoclopramide

(see Chapters 15 and 43). In addition, induction of anesthesia should employ a rapid-sequence technique with cricoid pressure prior to endotracheal intubation, and the patient should be extubated only when she is awake. Decreased plasma cholinesterase levels persist after delivery (see section on hepatic effects) and generally prolong the effect of succinylcholine by only 3–5 minutes. The duration of vecuronium but not atracurium has also been reported to be prolonged in postpartum women. High concentrations of volatile agents should be avoided because of the at least theoretic risk of increasing uterine blood loss or inducing postpartum hemorrhage secondary to uterine relaxation. Intravenous opioids may be used to supplement inhalational agents. Intravenous drugs administered intraoperatively to mothers who are breast-feeding appear to have minimal if any effects on their neonates. Nonetheless, it may be prudent to avoid breast-feeding 12–24 hours following general anesthesia.

SUGGESTED READING

Birnbach DJ, Datta S, Gatt SP: *Textbook of Obstetric Anesthesia.* Churchill Livingstone, 2000.

Bucklin BA, Smith CV: Postpartum Tubal Ligation: Safety, Timing, and Other Implications for Anesthesia. Anesth Analg 1999;89:1269.

Chestnut DH: *Obstetric Anesthesia,* 2nd ed. Mosby, 1999.

Eisenach JC: Combined spinal-epidural analgesia in obstetrics. Anesthesiology 1999;91:299.

Holdcroft TT: *Principles and Practice of Obstetric Anaesthesia.* Blackwell, 2000.

Koren G, Pastuszak A, Ito S: Drugs in Pregnancy. N Engl J Med 1998;338:1128.

Norris MC: *Obstetric Anesthesia,* 2nd ed. Lippincott Williams & Wilkins, 1998.

Rosen MA: Management of anesthesia for the pregnant surgical patient. Anesthesiology 1999;91:1159.

Obstetric Anesthesia

43

KEY CONCEPTS

 Regardless of the time of last oral intake, all obstetric patients are considered to have a full stomach and to be at risk for pulmonary aspiration.

 Nearly all parenteral opioid analgesics and sedatives readily cross the placenta and can affect the fetus. Regional anesthetic techniques are preferred for management of labor pain.

 Using a local anesthetic-opioid mixture for lumbar epidural analgesia during labor significantly reduces drug requirements, compared with using either agent alone.

Optimal analgesia for labor requires neural blockade at the T10 to L1 in the first stage of labor and T10 to S4 for the second stage.

 Even when aspiration does not yield blood or cerebrospinal fluid, unintentional intravascular or intrathecal placement of an epidural needle or catheter is possible.

 Hypotension is the most common side effect of regional anesthetic techniques and must be treated aggressively with ephedrine and intravenous (IV) fluid boluses to prevent fetal compromise. IV fluid boluses prior to neural blockade may help reduce the severity of arterial hypotension following spinal or epidural anesthesia, but glucose-free intravenous fluid boluses are used to avoid mater-

nal hyperglycemia and hypersecretion of insulin by the fetus.

 Spinal or epidural anesthesia is preferred to general anesthesia for cesarean section because regional anesthesia is associated with lower maternal mortality.

Spinal anesthesia for cesarean section is easier to perform and results in more rapid and intense neural blockade than epidural anesthesia. Epidural anesthesia allows greater control over sensory level and results in a more gradual fall in arterial blood pressure.

 Systemic, local anesthetic toxicity during epidural anesthesia may be best avoided by slowly administering dilute solutions for labor pain and fractionating the total dose for cesarean section into 5-mL increments.

 In general anesthesia for cesarean section, if endotracheal intubation fails, the life of the mother takes priority over delivery of the fetus. In the absence of fetal distress, the patient should be awakened, and an awake intubation, regional or local (infiltration) anesthesia may be tried. In the presence of fetal distress, if spontaneous or positive ventilation with cricoid pressure is possible, delivery of the fetus may be attempted.

Obstetric anesthesia is a demanding but gratifying subspecialty of anesthesiology. The widespread acceptance and use of regional anesthesia for labor has made obstetric anesthesia a major part of most anesthetic practices. The American College of Obstetricians and Gynecologists and American Society of Anesthesiologists guidelines require that anesthesia service be readily available continuously and that cesarean section be started within 30 minutes of the recognition for its need. Moreover, high-risk patients, such as those undergoing a trial of vaginal birth after a previous cesarean delivery (VBAC), may require the immediate availability of anesthesia services.

Although most parturients are young and healthy, they nonetheless represent a high-risk group of patients for all the reasons discussed in the preceding chapter. Anesthesia is the sixth leading cause of obstetric death in the United States; overall maternal mortality between 1985 and 1990 was 1.7 deaths per 1,000,000 births, compared with an estimated 32 per 1,000,000 for patients receiving general anesthesia and 1.9 per 1,000,000 for regional anesthesia. Most deaths occurred during or after cesarean section. Moreover, the risk of an adverse outcome appears to be much greater with emergency cesarean sections than with elective ones. Pregnancy and childbirth are the most frequent conditions associated with malpractice claims against anesthesiologists. Indeed anesthesia for cesarean section carries almost twice the risk of a malpractice claim as any surgical procedure.

This chapter focuses on the practice of obstetric anesthesia; techniques for analgesia and anesthesia during labor, vaginal delivery, and cesarean section are presented. The chapter ends with a review of neonatal resuscitation. The suggested procedures are intended to serve only as guidelines consistent with our current understanding of maternal and fetal physiology.

GENERAL APPROACH TO THE OBSTETRIC PATIENT

All patients entering the obstetric suite potentially require anesthesia, whether planned or emergent. The anesthesiologist should therefore be aware of the presence and relevant history of all patients in the suite. Pertinent historic items include age, parity, duration of the pregnancy, and any complicating factors. Patients definitely requiring anesthetic care (for labor or cesarean section) should undergo a preanesthetic evaluation as early as possible (see Chapter 1).

All women in true labor should be managed with intravenous fluids (usually lactated Ringer's injection with dextrose) to prevent dehydration. An 18-gauge or larger intravenous catheter is employed in case rapid transfusion should become necessary. Blood should be sent for typing and screening. Regardless of the time of last oral intake, all patients are considered to have a full stomach and to be at risk for pulmonary aspiration. Because the duration of labor may be prolonged, guidelines often allow small amounts of clear liquid for uncomplicated labor. In contrast, patients at high risk for an operative delivery should take nothing by mouth. The minimum fasting period for elective cesarean section should be 6 hours. Prophylactic administration of a clear antacid (15–30 mL of 0.3-M sodium citrate PO) every 3 hours can help maintain gastric pH greater than 2.5 and may decrease the likelihood of severe aspiration pneumonitis. An H_2-blocking drug (ranitidine, 100–150 mg PO) or metoclopramide, 10 mg PO, should also be considered in patients expected to receive general or regional anesthesia. H_2-blockers reduce both gastric volume and pH but have no effect on the gastric contents already present. Metoclopramide accelerates gastric emptying, decreases gastric volume, and increases lower esophageal sphincter tone. All patients should ideally have a tocodynamometer and fetal heart rate monitor. The supine position should be avoided unless a left uterine displacement device (> 15-degree wedge) is placed under the right hip. Uterine contractions can be directly measured via a catheter in patients with ruptured membranes, especially those receiving oxytocin or those undergoing a trial of VBAC.

ANESTHESIA FOR LABOR & VAGINAL DELIVERY

PAIN PATHWAYS DURING LABOR

Pain during the first stage of labor results from uterine contractions and cervical dilatation. It is usually initially confined to the T11–T12 dermatomes during the latent phase but eventually involves the T10–L1 dermatomes as the labor enters the active phase. Much of labor pain arises from dilatation of the cervix and lower uterine segment, but contraction of the myometrium against the resistance of the cervix and perineum also plays a major role. The visceral afferent fibers responsible for labor pain travel with sympathetic nerve fibers first to the uterine and cervical plexuses, then through the hypogastric and aortic plexuses before entering the spinal cord with the T10–L1 nerve roots (see Chapter 18). The onset of perineal pain at the end of the first stage signals the beginning of fetal descent and the second stage of labor. Stretching and compression of pelvic and perineal structures intensifies the pain. Sensory innervation of the perineum is provided by the pudendal nerve (S2–4) so pain during the second stage of labor involves the T10–S4 dermatomes.

PSYCHOLOGIC & NONPHARMACOLOGIC TECHNIQUES

Psychologic and nonpharmacologic techniques are based on the premise that the pain of labor can be suppressed by reorganizing one's thoughts. Patient education and positive conditioning about the birthing process are central to such techniques. Pain during labor tends to be accentuated by fear of the unknown or previous unpleasant experiences. Techniques include those of Bradley, Dick-Read, Lamaze, Duola, and LeBoyer. The Lamaze technique, one of the most popular, coaches the parturient to take a deep breath at the beginning of each contraction followed by rapid shallow breathing for the duration of the contraction. The parturient also concentrates on an object in the room and attempts to focus her thoughts away from the pain. Less common nonpharmacologic techniques include hypnosis, transcutaneous electrical nerve stimulation, biofeedback, and acupuncture (see Chapter 18). The success of all these techniques varies considerably from patient to patient, but most patients require additional forms of pain relief.

PARENTERAL AGENTS

 Nearly all parenteral opioid analgesics and sedatives readily cross the placenta and can affect the fetus. Concern over fetal depression limits the use of these agents to the early stages of labor or to situations in which regional anesthetic techniques are not available. Central nervous system depression in the neonate may be manifested by a prolonged time to sustain respirations, respiratory acidosis, or an abnormal neurobehavioral examination. Moreover, loss of beat-to-beat variability in the fetal heart rate (seen with most central nervous system depressants) and decreased fetal movements complicate the evaluation of fetal well-being during labor. Long-term fetal heart variability is affected more than short-term variability. The degree and significance of these effects depend on the specific agent, the dose, the time elapsed between its administration and delivery, and fetal maturity. Premature neonates exhibit the greatest sensitivity. In addition to maternal respiratory depression, opioids can also induce maternal nausea and vomiting and delay gastric emptying. Some clinicians have advocated use of opioids via patient-controlled analgesia devices (see Chapter 18) early in labor because this technique appears to reduce total opioid requirements.

Meperidine, the most commonly used opioid, can be given in doses of 10–25 mg intravenously or 25–50 mg intramuscularly, usually up to a total of 100 mg. Maximal maternal and fetal respiratory depression are seen in 10–20 minutes following intravenous administration and in 1–3 hours following intramuscular administration. Consequently, meperidine is usually administered early in labor when delivery is not expected for at least 4 hours. Intravenous fentanyl 50–100 μg/hour has also been used for labor. Fentanyl in

25–100-μg doses has a 3–10-minute analgesic onset that lasts about 60 minutes. However, maternal respiratory depression outlasts the analgesia. Lower doses of fentanyl appear to be associated with little or no neonatal respiratory depression and are reported to have no effect on Apgar scores. Morphine is not used because in equianalgesic doses it appears to cause greater respiratory depression in the fetus than do meperidine and fentanyl. Agents with mixed agonist-antagonist activity (butorphanol 1–2 mg and nalbuphine 10–20 mg IV or IM) are effective and associated with little or no cumulative respiratory depression (ceiling effect), but excessive sedation with repeat doses can be problematic.

Promethazine (25–50 mg IM) and hydroxyzine (50–100 mg IM) can be useful alone or in combination with meperidine. Both drugs reduce anxiety, opioid requirements, and the incidence of nausea but do not add appreciably to neonatal depression. A significant disadvantage of hydroxyzine is pain at the injection site following intramuscular administration. Nonsteroidal anti-inflammatory agents, such as ketorolac, are not recommended because they suppress uterine contractions and promote closure of the fetal ductus arteriosus.

Benzodiazepines, especially longer acting agents such as diazepam, are not used during labor because of their potential to cause prolonged neonatal depression. The amnestic properties of benzodiazepines make them undesirable agents for parturients because they usually want to remember the experience of delivery.

Low-dose intravenous ketamine is a powerful analgesic. In doses of 10–15 mg intravenously, good analgesia can be obtained in 2–5 minutes without loss of consciousness. Unfortunately, fetal depression with low Apgar scores are associated with doses greater than 1 mg/kg. Large boluses of ketamine (> 1 mg/kg) can be associated with hypertonic uterine contractions. Low-dose ketamine is most useful just prior to delivery or as an adjuvant to regional anesthesia. Some clinicians avoid ketamine because of its potential to produce unpleasant psychotomimetic effects (see Chapter 8).

INHALATIONAL ANALGESIA

This once popular technique, which has been largely supplanted by regional techniques, involves giving subanesthetic doses of a volatile agent (isoflurane, enflurane, methoxyflurane, or halothane) or nitrous oxide during the late first stage and second stage of labor. The gas may be self-administered (via special apparatus) but is safest when given by an experienced anesthetist (via mask and anesthesia machine). Nitrous oxide analgesia for labor is a popular technique outside the United States. Ideally, the patient remains awake, free of pain, and cooperative, with intact laryngeal reflexes; the anesthetist must remain in constant communication with the parturient. Overdosage with loss of protective airway reflexes and vomiting can lead to pulmonary aspiration and is a major hazard. Confusion, excitement, or drowsiness is indicative of overdose and the need to reduce the concentration. When given alone in oxygen, these agents are carefully titrated, with concentration limits of 50% for nitrous oxide, 1% for enflurane and 0.7% for isoflurane. Supplementation with a pudendal nerve block or perineal infiltration of a local anesthetic is helpful during the second stage. Environmental contamination is also a problem without a scavenging apparatus.

PUDENDAL NERVE BLOCK

Pudendal nerve blocks are often combined with perineal infiltration of local anesthetic to provide perineal anesthesia during the second stage of labor when other forms of anesthesia are not employed or prove to be inadequate. A special needle (Koback) or guide (Iowa trumpet) is used to place the needle transvaginally underneath the ischial spine on each side (see Chapter 18); the needle is advanced 1–1.5 cm through the sacrospinous ligament, and 10 mL of 1% lidocaine or 2% chloroprocaine is injected following careful aspiration. The needle guide is used to limit the depth of injection and protect the fetus and vagina from the needle. Other potential complications include intravascular injection, retroperitoneal hematoma, and retropsoas or subgluteal abscess.

PARACERVICAL PLEXUS & SYMPATHETIC NERVE BLOCKS

Some obstetricians may perform paracervical plexus blocks when other regional anesthetic techniques are not available. Such blocks may be associated with a relatively high rate (up to 33%) of fetal bradycardia, especially with some local anesthetic agents like lidocaine. Moreover, the technique only provides pain relief for the first stage of labor. This block involves injecting local anesthetic (5 mL) submucosally in the vagina at the 3 o'clock and 9 o'clock positions on either side of the cervix. Visceral sensory fibers from the uterus, cervix, and upper vagina are blocked in these positions as they pass through the paracervical plexus (Frankenhäuser's ganglia). A Koback needle or Iowa trumpet guide is also used for this block, which is typically performed prior to 8 cm cervical dilation to prevent fetal injury. The injection depth is also limited to 3 mm, because the close proximity of the injection site to the uterine artery can result in uterine arterial vasoconstriction, uteroplacental insufficiency, and high fetal blood levels of the local anesthetic. Uterine activity can also increase after paracervical block. The use of chloropro-

caine is associated with less fetal depression than are amide local anesthetics but unfortunately provides only brief analgesia. Prilocaine and possibly bupivacaine may be associated with less risk of fetal bradycardia. Other complications include hematoma of the broad ligament, unintentional sciatic nerve block, and neuropathy secondary to sacral plexus injury.

Sensory fibers from the lower uterus and the cervix join the sympathetic chain between L2 and L3. Bilateral paravertebral sympathetic block beneath the spinous process of L2 can therefore provide good analgesia for the first stage of labor. However, lumbar sympathetic block (see Chapter 18) is rarely performed because it is technically difficult without fluoroscopy and has limited duration following a single injection on each side. To avoid radiation exposure, a loss of resistance technique is used to identify penetration of the psoas muscle fascia before local anesthetic is injected. Complications include hypotension, intravascular injection, and retroperitoneal hematoma. A transient increase in uterine contractions may be observed.

REGIONAL ANESTHETIC TECHNIQUES

Regional techniques employing the epidural or intrathecal route (see Chapter 16), alone or in combination, are currently the most popular methods of pain relief during labor and delivery. They can provide excellent pain relief, yet allow the mother to be awake and cooperative during labor. Although spinal opioids or local anesthetics alone can provide satisfactory analgesia, techniques that combine the two have proved to be the most satisfactory in most parturients. Moreover, the apparent synergy between the two types of agents decreases dose requirements and provides excellent analgesia with few maternal side effects and little or no neonatal depression.

1. Spinal Opioids Alone

Preservative-free opioids may be given intraspinally as a single injection or intermittently via an epidural or intrathecal catheter (Table 43–1). These techniques are

Table 43–1. Spinal opioid dosages for labor and delivery.

Agent	Intrathecal	Epidural
Morphine	0.5–1 mg	7.5–10 mg
Meperidine	10–20 mg	100 mg
Fentanyl	10–25 μg	50–150 μg
Sufentanil	3–10 μg	10–30 μg

most useful for high-risk patients who may not tolerate the functional sympathectomy associated with spinal or epidural anesthesia (see Chapter 16). This group includes patients with hypovolemia or significant cardiovascular disease such as aortic stenosis, tetralogy of Fallot, Eisenmenger's syndrome, or pulmonary hypertension. With the exception of meperidine, which has local anesthetic properties, spinal opioids alone do not produce motor blockade or maternal hypotension (sympathectomy). Thus, they do not impair the ability of the parturient to push the baby out. Disadvantages include less complete analgesia, lack of perineal relaxation, and such side effects as pruritus, nausea, vomiting, sedation, and respiratory depression (see Chapter 18). Side effects may improve with low doses of naloxone (0.1–0.2 mg/hour intravenously).

Intrathecal Opioids

Intrathecal morphine in doses of 0.5–1 mg may produce satisfactory and prolonged (6–8 hours) analgesia during the first stage of labor. Unfortunately, the onset of analgesia is slow (45–60 minutes), and these doses are associated with a relatively high incidence of side effects. Morphine is therefore rarely used alone. The combination of morphine, 0.25 mg, and fentanyl, 25 μg, (or sufentanil, 5–10 μg) may result in a more rapid onset of analgesia (5 min) but a shorter duration (4–5 hours). Intermittent boluses of 10–20 mg of meperidine, 5–10 μg of fentanyl, or 3–10 μg of sufentanil via an intrathecal catheter can also provide satisfactory analgesia for labor. Spinal meperidine has some weak local anesthetic properties and therefore can decrease blood pressure. Hypotension following intrathecal sufentanil for labor is likely related to the analgesia and decreased circulating catecholamine levels.

Epidural Opioids

Relatively high doses (≥ 7.5 mg) of morphine are required for satisfactory analgesia during labor; the analgesia is most effective for the early first stage of labor. The onset of analgesia may take 30–60 minutes but lasts up to 24 hours. Unfortunately, such doses are associated with an unacceptably high incidence of significant side effects. Epidural meperidine, 100 mg, provides consistently good but relatively brief analgesia (1–3 hours). Epidural fentanyl, 50–200 μg, or sufentanil, 10–50 μg, usually produces analgesia within 5–10 minutes with few side effects, but it has a short duration (1–2 hours). Although "single-shot" epidural opioids do not appear to cause significant neonatal depression, caution should be exercised following repeated administrations. Combinations of a lower dose of morphine, 2.5 mg, with fentanyl, 25–50 μg, (or

sufentanil, 10–20 μg) may result in a more rapid onset and prolongation of analgesia (4–5 hours) with fewer side effects.

2. Local Anesthetics Alone

Epidural anesthesia and spinal (intrathecal) anesthesia can be used safely for labor and delivery. Pain relief during the first stage requires a T10–L1 sensory level, while pain relief during the second stage requires blockade of T10–S4. Continuous lumbar epidural anesthesia is the most versatile and most commonly employed technique, because it can be used for pain relief for the first stage of labor as well as anesthesia for subsequent vaginal delivery or cesarean section, if necessary. "Single-shot" epidural, spinal, and caudal anesthesia may be appropriate when pain relief is initiated just prior to vaginal delivery (the second stage).

Absolute contraindications to regional anesthesia include infection over the injection site, coagulopathy, marked hypovolemia, true allergies to local anesthetics, and the patient's refusal or inability to cooperate for regional anesthesia. Preexisting neurologic disease, back disorders, and some forms of heart disease (see Chapter 20) are relative contraindications. The use of regional anesthesia in patients on minidose heparin is controversial. A previous VBAC is not considered a contraindication to regional anesthesia during labor. Concern that the anesthesia masks the pain associated with uterine rupture may not be justified, because dehiscence of a lower segment scar frequently does not cause pain even without epidural anesthesia; moreover, changes in uterine tone and contraction pattern may be more reliable signs.

Before performing any regional block, appropriate equipment and supplies for resuscitation should be checked and made immediately available. Minimum supplies include an oxygen supply, suction, a mask with a positive pressure device for ventilation, a functioning laryngoscope, endotracheal tubes (6 or 7 mm), oral or nasal airways, intravenous fluids, ephedrine, atropine, thiopental (or propofol), and succinylcholine. The capability for frequent monitoring of at least blood pressure and heart rate is mandatory. A pulse oximeter and capnograph should also be readily available.

Lumbar Epidural Anesthesia

Epidural anesthesia is typically administered only when labor is well established. It may be advantageous to place an epidural catheter early, when the patient is comfortable and can be positioned easily, but local anesthetics should generally only be administered when labor is progressing well and the patient becomes uncomfortable. Although exact criteria for initiation of epidural anesthesia tend to vary somewhat, commonly accepted criteria include no fetal distress; good regular contractions 3–4 minutes apart and lasting about 1 minute; adequate cervical dilatation, ie, 5–6 cm for nulliparous patients and 4–5 cm for multiparous patients; and engagement of the fetal head. Epidural anesthesia is often administered earlier to parturients who are receiving an oxytocin infusion once a good contraction pattern is achieved. Moreover, some evidence suggests that epidural analgesia can be started as early as after 3 cm cervical dilatation in nulliparous women without increasing the incidence of a cesarean delivery or need for oxytocin augmentation.

A. TECHNIQUE:

The technique of epidural anesthesia is described in Chapter 16. Parturients may be positioned on their sides or in the sitting position for the block. The sitting position is often more useful for identifying the midline in obese patients. When epidural anesthesia is being given for vaginal delivery (second stage), the sitting position helps ensure good sacral spread.

Because the epidural space pressure may be positive in some parturients, correct identification of the epidural space may be difficult, and unintentional dural puncture can readily occur; the incidence of wet taps in obstetric patients is 1–4%. Some clinicians advocate the midline approach, while others favor the paramedian approach. If air is used for detecting loss of resistance, the amount injected should be limited as much as possible; injection of excessive amounts air in the epidural space has been associated with patchy or unilateral analgesia. The average depth of the epidural space in obstetric patients is reported to be 5 cm from the skin. Placement of the epidural catheter at the L3–4 or L4–5 interspace is generally optimal for achieving a T10–S5 neural blockade. If unintentional dural puncture occurs, the anesthetist has two choices: (1) place the epidural catheter in the subarachnoid space for continuous spinal analgesia and anesthesia (see below), or (2) remove the needle and attempt placement at a higher spinal level.

B. CHOICE OF EPIDURAL CATHETER:

Many clinicians advocate use of a multi-holed catheter instead of a single-holed catheter for obstetric anesthesia. Use of a multi-holed catheter appears to be associated with fewer unilateral blocks, and greatly reduces the incidence of false-negative aspiration for intravascular catheter placement. Advancing a multi-holed catheter 7–8 cm into the epidural space appears to be optimal for obtaining adequate sensory levels. Shorter insertion depths (< 5 cm), especially in obese patients, may favor lodgment of the catheter out of the epidural space following flexion/extension movements of the spine. Spiral wire–reinforced catheters are very resistant to kinking. The spiral or spring tip, especially when used without a stylet, is associated with fewer, less intense paresthesias and may also be associated with a lower incidence of inadvertent intravascular insertion.

C. CHOICE OF LOCAL ANESTHETIC:

Anesthetic solutions in common use include lidocaine 1%, chloroprocaine 2%, bupivacaine 0.25%, and ropivacaine 0.2%. The effect of epinephrine-containing solutions on the course of labor is somewhat controversial. Many clinicians only use epinephrine-containing solutions for intravascular test doses because of concern that the solutions may slow the progression of labor or adversely affect the fetus; others use only very dilute concentrations of epinephrine such as 1:800,000 or 1:400,000. Studies comparing these various agents have failed to find any differences in neonatal Apgar scores, acid-base status, or neurobehavioral evaluations. In spite of its potential for cardiotoxicity, bupivacaine's long duration of action makes it a popular agent for labor. Ropivacaine may be preferable because of less motor blockade and its reduced potential for cardiotoxicity. Experience with levobupivacaine (the L enantiomer of bupivacaine), which has less cardiotoxicity, is limited. Chloroprocaine has almost immediate onset of action, but some clinicians have abandoned it because of controversy over its potential for neurotoxicity. Studies suggest that cases of chloroprocaine neurotoxicity were related to a relatively high concentration of sodium bisulfite used as an antioxidant in its solutions and a very low pH. New formulations of chloroprocaine contain ethylenediaminetetraacetic acid (EDTA) instead of bisulfite; unfortunately, the EDTA may increase the incidence of backache, especially when more than 20 mL of chloroprocaine is administered. The use of local anesthetic-opioid mixtures is discussed in the following section on local anesthetic and opioid mixtures.

D. EPIDURAL ACTIVATION FOR THE FIRST STAGE OF LABOR:

Epidural injection of local anesthetic may be done either before or after the catheter is placed. Activation through the needle can facilitate catheter placement. The following sequence is suggested for epidural activation:

1. Administer a 500- to 1000-mL intravenous bolus of lactated Ringer's injection. Rapid infusion of intravenous fluids can transiently decrease uterine activity. Glucose-free intravenous fluid boluses are used to avoid maternal hyperglycemia and hypersecretion of insulin by the fetus. When pla-

cental transfer of glucose ceases abruptly following delivery, persistent high circulating levels of insulin in the neonate can result in transient hypoglycemia.

2. Test for unintentional subarachnoid or intravascular placement of the needle or catheter with a 3- to 4-mL test dose of a local anesthetic with 1:200,000 epinephrine (controversial; see following section on preventing unintentional intravascular and intrathecal injections).

3. If after 5 minutes signs of intravascular or intrathecal injection are absent, give an additional 4–8 mL of local anesthetic to achieve a T10–L1 sensory level.

4. Monitor with frequent blood pressure measurements for 20–30 minutes or until the patient is stable. Pulse oximetry should also be used. Oxygen is administered via face mask if there are any significant drops in blood pressure or oxygen saturation readings.

5. Repeat steps 2 through 4 when pain recurs until the first stage of labor is completed; alternatively, a continuous epidural infusion technique may be employed using bupivacaine, 0.125–0.25%; ropivacaine, 0.1–0.2%; or lidocaine, 0.5–1.0% at an initial rate of 10 mL/hour, subsequently adjusted according to the patient's needs.

E. EPIDURAL ACTIVATION DURING THE SECOND STAGE OF LABOR:

Activation for the second stage of labor extends the block to include the S2–4 dermatomes. Whether a catheter is already in place or epidural anesthesia is just being initiated, the following steps should be undertaken:

1. Give a 1000- to 1500-mL intravenous bolus of lactated Ringer's injection.

2. If the patient does not already have a catheter in place, the epidural space is identified in the sitting position. If the patient already has an epidural catheter in place, she is placed in a semiupright or sitting position prior to injection.

3. Give a 3- or 4-mL test dose of local anesthetic with 1:200,000 epinephrine.

4. If after 5 minutes signs of an intravascular or intrathecal injection are absent, give 10–15 mL of additional local anesthetic at a rate not faster than 5 mL every 30 seconds.

5. Administer oxygen by face mask and lay the patient supine with left uterine displacement and monitor blood pressure every 1–2 minutes for the first 15 minutes, then every 5 minutes thereafter.

F. PREVENTION OF UNINTENTIONAL INTRAVASCULAR AND INTRATHECAL INJECTIONS:

Safe administration of epidural anesthesia is critically dependent on avoiding unintentional intrathecal or intravascular injections. Unintentional intravascular or intrathecal placement of an epidural needle or catheter is possible even when aspiration fails to yield blood or cerebrospinal fluid (CSF). The incidence of unintentional intravascular or intrathecal placement of an epidural catheter is 5–15% and 0.5–2.5%, respectively. Even a properly placed catheter can subsequently erode into an epidural vein or an intrathecal position. This possibility should be excluded each time local anesthetic is injected through an epidural catheter.

Test doses of lidocaine, 45–60 mg, bupivacaine, 7.5–10 mg, ropivacaine, 6–8 mg, or chloroprocaine, 100 mg, can be given to exclude unintentional intrathecal placement. Signs of sensory and motor blockade usually become apparent within 2–3 minutes and 3–5 minutes, respectively, if the injection is intrathecal.

Test dose techniques for unintentional intravascular injections may not be reliable in parturients. The best method for detecting intravascular injections is controversial in obstetric anesthesia. In patients not receiving β-adrenergic antagonists, the intravascular injection of a local anesthetic solution with 15–20 μg of epinephrine, consistently increases the heart rate by 20–30 beats/min within 30–60 seconds if the catheter (or epidural needle) is intravascular. This technique is not always reliable in parturients because they often have marked spontaneous baseline variations in heart rate with contractions. In fact, bradycardia has been reported in a parturient following intravenous injection of 15 μg of epinephrine. Moreover, in animal studies, 15 μg IV of epinephrine reduces uterine blood flow, and the dose has been associated with fetal distress in humans. Alternative methods of detecting unintentional intravascular catheter placement include eliciting tinnitus or perioral numbness following a 100-mg test dose of lidocaine, eliciting a chronotropic effect following injection of 5 μg of isoproterenol, or injecting 1 mL of air while monitoring the patient with a precordial Doppler. With the possible exception of the precordial Doppler, false-negative responses may be encountered with all methods; false-positives can also be observed. The use of dilute local anesthetic solutions and slow injection rates may also enhance detection of unintentional intravascular injections before catastrophic complications develop.

G. MANAGEMENT OF COMPLICATIONS:

1. Hypotension—Generally defined as a 20–30% decrease in blood pressure or a systolic pressure less than

100 mm Hg, hypotension is the most common side effect of regional anesthesia. It is primarily due to decreased sympathetic tone and is greatly accentuated by aortocaval compression and an upright or semiupright position. Treatment should be aggressive and consists of intravenous boluses of ephedrine (5–15 mg), supplemental oxygen, left uterine displacement, and an intravenous fluid bolus. Small intravenous doses of phenylephrine (25–50 µg) may also be used safely. Use of the head-down (Trendelenburg) position is controversial because of its potentially detrimental effects on pulmonary gas exchange.

2. Unintentional intravascular injections—Early recognition of intravascular injections, detected by the use of small incremental doses of local anesthetic, may prevent more serious local anesthetic toxicity, such as seizures or cardiovascular collapse. Intravascular injections of toxic doses of lidocaine or chloroprocaine usually present as seizures. Thiopental, 50–100 mg, will cease frank seizure activity. Small doses of propofol may also terminate seizures but experience with it is limited. Maintenance of a patent airway and adequate oxygenation are of paramount importance. Immediate endotracheal intubation with succinylcholine and cricoid pressure should be considered. Intravascular injections of bupivacaine can cause rapid and profound cardiovascular collapse as well as seizure activity. Cardiac resuscitation may be exceedingly difficult and is especially aggravated by acidosis and hypoxia. Bretylium and possibly amiodarone appear to be useful in reversing bupivacaine-induced decreases in the threshold for ventricular tachycardia.

3. Unintentional intrathecal injection—If dural puncture is recognized immediately after injection of local anesthetic, an attempt to aspirate the local anesthetic may be tried but is usually unsuccessful. The patient should be gently placed supine with left uterine displacement. Head elevation accentuates hypotension and should be avoided. The hypotension should be treated aggressively with ephedrine and intravenous fluids. A high spinal level can also result in diaphragmatic paralysis, which necessitates intubation and ventilation with 100% oxygen. Delayed onset of a very high and often patchy or unilateral block may be due to unrecognized subdural injection (see Chapter 16), which is managed similarly.

4. Post-dural puncture headache (PDPH)—Headache frequently follows unintentional dural puncture in parturients. It is due to decreased intracranial pressure with compensatory cerebral vasodilatation. Bed rest, hydration, oral analgesics, epidural saline injection (50–100 mL), and caffeine sodium benzoate (500 mg IV) may be effective in patients with mild headaches. Patients with moderate to severe headaches usually require an epidural blood patch (10–20 mL) (see Chapter 16). Prophylactic epidural blood patches are generally not recommended; delaying a blood patch for 48 hours may increase its efficacy.

Caudal Anesthesia

Lumbar epidural anesthesia is generally superior to caudal anesthesia because the former is technically easier to perform and requires less local anesthetic. Moreover, early paralysis of the pelvic muscles during caudal anesthesia may interfere with normal rotation of the fetal head. The principal advantage of caudal anesthesia is the rapidity of onset of perineal anesthesia when it is administered just prior to delivery. The technique for caudal anesthesia in pregnant patients differs only in that once the needle is positioned in the sacral canal—and prior to injection—rectal examination may be necessary to exclude accidental puncture of the fetus. Fifteen to 20 mL of local anesthetic is required for a T10–S5 nerve block, and a catheter may be left in place.

Spinal Anesthesia

Spinal anesthesia given just prior to delivery—also known as saddle block—provides profound anesthesia for vaginal delivery. A 500- to 1000-mL fluid bolus is given prior to the procedure, which is performed with the patient in the sitting position. Use of a 22-gauge or smaller, pencil-point spinal needle (Whitacre, Sprotte, or Gertie Marx) decreases the likelihood of PDPH. Hyperbaric tetracaine (3–4 mg), bupivacaine (6–7 mg), or lidocaine (20–40 mg) usually provides excellent perineal anesthesia. A T10 sensory level can be obtained with slightly larger amounts of local anesthetic. The intrathecal injection should be given slowly over 30 seconds and in between contractions to minimize excessive cephalad spread. Three minutes after injection, the patient is placed in the lithotomy position with left uterine displacement.

3. Local Anesthetic and Opioid Mixtures

Epidural Analgesia

The addition of opioids to local anesthetic solutions for epidural anesthesia has dramatically changed the practice of obstetric anesthesia. The synergy between epidural opioids and local anesthetic solutions appears to reflect separate sites of action, namely, opiate receptors and neuronal axons, respectively. When the two are combined, very low concentrations of both local anesthetic and opioid can be used. More importantly, the incidence of adverse side effects, such as hypotension and drug toxicity, is likely reduced. Chloroprocaine is not a suitable agent for continuous epidural infusion with opioids because studies suggest it interferes with their efficacy.

Once a 10-mL initial bolus is administered, the mixture is then most commonly given as continuous epidural infusion at a rate of 10–15 mL/hour. The initial bolus is usually 0.1–0.2% of ropivacaine or 0.0625–0.125% of bupivacaine combined with either 50–100 μg of fentanyl or 10–20 μg of sufentanil. Table 43–2 lists commonly used mixtures. These very dilute local anesthetic mixtures generally do not produce motor blockade and may allow some patients to ambulate ("walking epidural"). Moreover, they do not appear to have any adverse effects on the fetus. Patient-controlled epidural analgesia using very dilute mixtures has been advocated by some clinicians; patient satisfaction may be higher. Migration of the epidural catheter into a blood vessel during a continuous infusion may be heralded by loss of effective analgesia; a high index of suspicion is required because overt signs of systemic toxicity may be absent. Erosion of the catheter through the dura results in a slowly progressive motor blockade of the lower extremities and a rising sensory level.

Intrathecal Analgesia

Addition of small doses of local anesthetic agents to intrathecal opioid injection greatly potentiates their analgesia and can significantly reduce opioid requirements. Thus, many clinicians will inject 2.5 mg of preservative-free bupivacaine or 2–4 mg of ropivacaine with intrathecal opioids for analgesia in the first stage of labor (Table 43–2). Addition of 200 μg of epinephrine pro-

Table 43–2. Local anesthetic-opioid mixtures for labor and delivery.

Epidural
Bupivacaine 0.125% + fentanyl 1 μg/mL
Bupivacaine 0.0625% + fentanyl 2 μg/mL
Bupivacaine 0.125% + sufentanil 0.2 μg/mL
Bupivacaine 0.0625% + sufentanil 0.3 μg/mL
Bupivacaine 0.0625% + sufentanil 0.5 μg/mL
Ropivacaine 0.2% + fentanyl 1 μg/mL
Ropivacaine 0.1% + fentanyl 2 μg/mL
Ropivacaine 0.2% + sufentanil 0.2 μg/mL
Ropivacaine 0.1% + sufentanil 0.3 μg/mL
Ropivacaine 0.1% + sufentanil 0.5 μg/mL
Intrathecal
Bupivacaine 2.5 mg + fentanyl 10–25 μg
Bupivacaine 2.5 mg + sufentanil 3–10 μg
Ropivacaine 4 mg + fentanyl 10–25 μg
Ropivacaine 4 mg + sufentanil 3–10 μg

longs the analgesia with such mixtures but not for intrathecal opioids alone.

Continuous spinal anesthesia is a reasonable option following unintentional dural puncture while placing an epidural catheter. The catheter should be advanced no more than 2–2.5 cm into the lumbar subarachnoid space and left in place to provide analgesia for labor and vaginal delivery (or spinal anesthesia for cesarean section, if necessary). Intermittent injection of local anesthetic-opioid mixtures should be carefully titrated to produce the desired clinical response.

Combined Spinal & Epidural (CSE) Analgesia

Techniques using CSE analgesia and anesthesia (see Chapter 16) may especially benefit patients in early labor and those who receive anesthesia just prior to delivery. Intrathecal opioid and local anesthetic are injected and an epidural catheter is left in place. The intrathecal drugs provide almost immediate pain control and have minimal effects on the early progress of labor, while the epidural catheter provides a route for subsequent anesthesia for labor or operative delivery. Table 43–2 lists commonly used drug combinations for labor and delivery. Some studies suggest that CSE techniques may be associated with greater patient satisfaction than is epidural analgesia alone. A 24–27-gauge pencil-point spinal needle (Whitacre, Sprotte, or Gertie Marx) is used to minimize the incidence of PDPH.

The spinal and epidural needles may be placed at different interspaces, but most clinicians use the same interspace. Use of saline for identification for the epidural space (see Chapter 16) is best avoided because of potential confusion of saline for CSF. With the needle-through-needle technique, the epidural needle is placed in the epidural space and then a long spinal needle is then introduced through it and advanced further into the subarachnoid space. A distinct pop is felt as the needle penetrates the dura. The needle-beside-needle technique typically employs a specially designed epidural needle that has a channel for the spinal needle. After the intrathecal injection and withdrawal of the spinal needle, the epidural catheter is then threaded into position and the epidural needle is withdrawn. The risk of advancing the epidural catheter through the dural hole created by the spinal needle appears to be very small when a 25-gauge needle or smaller is used. The epidural catheter, however, should be aspirated carefully and local anesthetic should always be given slowly and in small increments to avoid unintentional intrathecal injections. Moreover, epidural drugs should be administered and titrated carefully because the dural hole appears to increase the flux of epidural drugs into CSF and enhance their effects.

Table 43–3. Indications for general anesthesia during vaginal delivery.

Fetal distress during the second stage
Tetanic uterine contractions
Breech extraction
Version and extraction
Manual removal of a retained placenta
Replacement of an inverted uterus
Psychiatric patients who become uncontrollable

GENERAL ANESTHESIA

Because of the increased risk of aspiration, general anesthesia for vaginal delivery is indicated only when emergency operation is necessary. Many indications for general anesthesia share the need for uterine relaxation. Intravenous nitroglycerin, 50–100 μg, has been shown to be effective in inducing uterine relaxation and may obviate the need for general anesthesia in these cases. Table 43–3 lists common indications for general anesthesia during vaginal delivery.

Suggested Technique for Vaginal Delivery

(1) Place a wedge under the right hip for left uterine displacement.

(2) Preoxygenate the patient for 3–5 minutes as monitors are applied. Defasciculation with curare or another nondepolarizing muscle relaxant is usually not necessary, because most pregnant patients do not fasciculate following succinylcholine. Moreover, fasciculations do not appear to promote regurgitation, because any increase in intragastric pressure is matched by a similar increase in the lower esophageal sphincter.

(3) Once all monitors are applied and the obstetrician is ready, proceed with a rapid-sequence induction while cricoid pressure is applied and intubate with a 6- to 7-mm endotracheal tube. Thiopental, 4 mg/kg, (or propofol, 2 mg/kg) and succinylcholine, 1.5 mg/kg, are most commonly used unless the patient is hypovolemic or hypotensive, in which case ketamine, 1 mg/kg, is used as the induction agent.

(4) After successful intubation, use 1–2 minimum alveolar concentration (MAC) of any potent volatile inhalational agent (see Chapter 7) in 100% oxygen while carefully monitoring blood pressure.

(5) If skeletal muscle relaxation is necessary, a short- to intermediate-acting, nondepolarizing muscle relaxant (atracurium, rapacuronium,* or rocuronium) is used.

(6) Once the fetus and placenta are delivered, the volatile agent is decreased to less than 0.5 MAC or discontinued; an oxytocin infusion is started (20–40 U/L of IV fluid); and a nitrous oxide-opioid technique can be used.

(7) An attempt to aspirate gastric contents may be made via an orogastric tube to decrease the likelihood of pulmonary aspiration on emergence.

(8) At the end of the procedure, the skeletal nondepolarizing muscle relaxant is reversed, the gastric tube (if placed) is removed, and the patient is extubated awake.

■ ANESTHESIA FOR CESAREAN SECTION

Common indications for cesarean section are listed in Table 43–4. The choice of anesthesia for cesarean section is determined by multiple factors, including the indication for operating, its urgency, patient and obstetrician preferences, and the skills of the anesthetist. Cesarean section rates vary between institutions and generally vary between 15–25%. Approximately 80% are performed under regional anesthesia in the United States, nearly evenly split between spinal and epidural anesthesia. Regional anesthesia has become the preferred technique because general anesthesia has been associated with higher maternal mortality (see the introduction). Deaths associated with general anesthesia are generally related to airway problems, such as inability to intubate, inability to ventilate, or aspiration pneumonitis, while deaths associated with regional anesthesia are generally related to excessively high neural blockade or local anesthetic toxicity.

Other advantages of regional anesthesia include (1) less neonatal exposure to potentially depressant drugs; (2) a decreased risk of maternal pulmonary aspiration; (3) an awake mother at the birth of her child, with the father also present if desired; and (4) the option of using spinal opioids for postoperative pain relief. The choice between spinal and epidural anesthesia is often based on physician preferences. Epidural anesthesia is preferred over spinal anesthesia by some clinicians because of the more

---

*At the time of publication, rapacuronium had been voluntarily withdrawn by the manufacturer. See Chapter 9 for details.

Table 43–4. Major indications for cesarean section.

Labor unsafe for mother and fetus
   Increased risk of uterine rupture
      Previous classic cesarean section
      Previous extensive myomectomy or uterine reconstruc-tion
   Increased risk of maternal hemorrhage
      Central or partial placenta previa
      Abruptio placentae
      Previous vaginal reconstruction
Dystocia
   Abnormal fetopelvic relations
      Fetopelvic disproportion
      Abnormal fetal presentation
         Transverse or oblique lie
         Breech presentation
   Dysfunctional uterine activity
Immediate or emergent delivery necessary
   Fetal distress
   Umbilical cord prolapse
   Maternal hemorrhage
   Amnionitis
   Genital herpes with ruptured membranes
   Impending maternal death

---

gradual decrease in blood pressure associated with epidural anesthesia. Continuous epidural anesthesia also allows better control over the sensory level. Conversely, spinal anesthesia is easier to perform, has a more rapid, predictable onset, may produce a more intense (complete) block, and does not have the potential for serious systemic drug toxicity (because of the smaller dose of local anesthetic employed). Regardless of the regional technique chosen, the ability to administer a general anesthetic at any time during the procedure is mandatory. Moreover, administration of a nonparticulate antacid 1 hour prior to surgery should also be considered.

General anesthesia offers (1) a very rapid and reliable onset, (2) control over the airway and ventilation, and (3) potentially less hypotension than regional anesthesia. General anesthesia also facilitates management in the event of severe hemorrhagic complications such as placenta accreta. Its principal disadvantages are the risk of pulmonary aspiration, the potential inability to intubate or ventilate the patient, and drug-induced fetal depression. Present anesthetic techniques, however, limit the dose of intravenous agents such that fetal depression is usually not clinically significant with general anesthesia when delivery occurs within 10 minutes of induction of anesthesia. Regardless of the type of anes-

thesia, neonates delivered more than 3 minutes after uterine incision have lower Apgar scores and acidotic blood gases.

REGIONAL ANESTHESIA

Cesarean section requires a T4 sensory level. Because of the associated high sympathetic blockade, all patients should receive a 1500- to 2000-mL bolus of lactated Ringer's injection prior to neural blockade. Crystalloid boluses do not consistently prevent hypotension but can be helpful in some patients. Smaller volumes (250–500 mL) of colloid solutions, such as hetastarch, are more effective. After injection of the anesthetic, the patient is placed supine with left uterine displacement; supplemental oxygen (40–50%) is given; blood pressure is measured every 1–2 minutes until it stabilizes. Intravenous ephedrine, 5–10 mg, should be used to maintain systolic blood pressure > 100 mm Hg. Small intravenous doses of phenylephrine, 25–50 µg, may also be used safely. Prophylactic administration of intramuscular ephedrine (25 mg) has been advocated by some clinicians for spinal anesthesia, as precipitous hypotension may be seen. Hypotension following epidural anesthesia typically has a slower onset. Slight Trendelenburg positioning facilitates achieving a T4 sensory level and may also help prevent severe hypotension. Extreme degrees of Trendelenburg may interfere with pulmonary gas exchange.

1. Spinal Anesthesia

The patient is usually placed in the lateral decubitus or sitting position, and a hyperbaric solution of tetracaine (7–10 mg), lidocaine (60–80 mg), or bupivacaine (10–15 mg) is injected. Epinephrine 0.1–0.2 mg can enhance the quality of the block and may prolong its duration (see Chapter 16). Use of 22-gauge or smaller, pencil-point spinal needle (Whitacre, Sprotte, or Gertie Marx) decreases the incidence of PDPH. Adding 10–25 µg of fentanyl or 5–10 µg of sufentanil, to the local anesthetic solution enhances the intensity of the block and prolongs its duration without adversely affecting neonatal outcome. Addition of preservative-free morphine, 0.2–0.3 mg, can prolong postoperative analgesia up to 24 hours but requires special monitoring for delayed postoperative respiratory depression. Regardless of the anesthetics agents used, considerable variability in the maximum sensory level should be expected (see Chapter 16).

Continuous spinal anesthesia is also a reasonable option following unintentional dural puncture while placing an epidural catheter for cesarean section. After the catheter is advanced 2–2.5 cm into the lumbar subarachnoid space and secured, it can then be used to inject anesthetic agents; moreover, it allows later supplementation of the anesthesia if necessary.

2. Epidural Anesthesia

Epidural anesthesia for cesarean section is generally most satisfactory when an epidural catheter is used. The catheter facilitates achieving an initial T4 sensory level, allows supplementation if necessary, and provides an excellent route for postoperative opioid administration. After a negative test dose, a total of 15–25 mL of local anesthetic is injected slowly in 5-mL increments. Lidocaine 2% (with or without 1:200,000 epinephrine), chloroprocaine 3%, bupivacaine 0.5%, or ropivacaine 0.5% is most commonly used. Addition of fentanyl, 50–100 μg, or sufentanil, 10–20 μg, greatly enhances the intensity of the block and prolongs its duration without adversely affecting neonatal outcome. Some practitioners also add sodium bicarbonate (7.5% or 8.4% solution) to local anesthetic solutions (1 mEq/10 mL of lidocaine and 0.05 mEq/10 mL of bupivacaine or ropivacaine) to increase the concentration of the nonionized free base and produce a faster onset and more rapid spread of epidural anesthesia. If pain develops as the sensory level recedes, additional local anesthetic is given in 5-mL increments to maintain a T4 sensory level. "Patchy" anesthesia prior to delivery of the baby can be treated with 10–20 mg IV of ketamine or 30% nitrous oxide. After delivery, intravenous opioid supplementation may also be used, provided excessive sedation and loss of consciousness are avoided. Pain that remains intolerable in spite of a seemingly adequate sensory level and that proves unresponsive to these measures necessitates general anesthesia with endotracheal intubation. Nausea can be treated intravenously with 0.625 mg of droperidol, 10 mg of metoclopramide, or 4 mg of ondansetron.

Epidural morphine, 5 mg, at the end of surgery provides good to excellent pain relief postoperatively for 6–24 hours. An increased incidence (3.5–30%) of recurrent herpes simplex labialis infection has been reported 2–5 days following epidural morphine in some studies. Postoperative analgesia can also be provided by continuous epidural infusions of fentanyl, 50–100 μg/hour, or sufentanil, 10–20 μg/hour, at a volume rate of approximately 10 mL/hour. Epidural butorphanol, 2 mg, can also provide effective postoperative pain relief, but marked somnolence is often a troublesome side effect.

3. CSE Anesthesia

The technique for CSE is described in the above section on combined spinal epidural analgesia. For ce-

sarean section, it combines the benefit of rapid, reliable, intense blockade of spinal anesthesia together with the flexibility of an epidural catheter. The catheter also allows supplementation of anesthesia and can be used for postoperative analgesia. As mentioned previously, epidurally administered drugs should be administered and titrated carefully because the dural hole created by the spinal needle increases the flux of epidural drugs into CSF and enhance their effects.

GENERAL ANESTHESIA

Pulmonary aspiration of gastric contents (incidence: 1:500–400 for obstetric patients versus 1:2000 for all patients) and failed endotracheal intubation (incidence: 1:300 versus 1:2000 for all patients) during general anesthesia are the major causes of maternal morbidity and mortality. Every effort should be made to ensure optimal conditions prior to the start of anesthesia and to follow measures aimed at preventing these complications.

All patients should possibly receive prophylaxis against severe nonparticulate aspiration pneumonia with 30 mL of 0.3-M sodium citrate 30–45 minutes prior to induction. Patients with additional risk factors predisposing them to aspiration should also receive ranitidine, 100–150 mg, and/or metoclopramide, 10 mg, 1–2 hours prior to induction; such factors include morbid obesity, symptoms of gastroesophageal reflux, a potentially difficult airway, or emergent surgical delivery without an elective fasting period. Premedication with oral omeprazole, 40 mg, at night and in the morning also appears to be highly effective in high-risk patients undergoing elective cesarean section. Although anticholinergics theoretically may reduce lower esophageal sphincter tone, premedication with a small dose of glycopyrrolate (0.1 mg) helps reduce airway secretions and should be considered in patients with a potentially difficult airway.

Anticipation of a difficult endotracheal intubation may help reduce the incidence of failed intubations. Examination of the neck, mandible, dentition, and oropharynx often helps predict which patients may be difficult. Useful predictors of a difficult intubation include Mallampati classification, short neck, receding mandible, and prominent maxillary incisors (see Chapter 5). The higher incidence of failed intubations in pregnant patients compared with nonpregnant surgical patients may be due to airway edema, a full dentition, or large breasts that can obstruct the laryngoscope handle in patients with short necks. Proper positioning of the head and neck may facilitate endotracheal intubation in obese patients: elevation of the shoulders, flexion of the cervical spine, and extension of the atlanto-occipital joint (Figure 43–1). A variety of laryngoscope

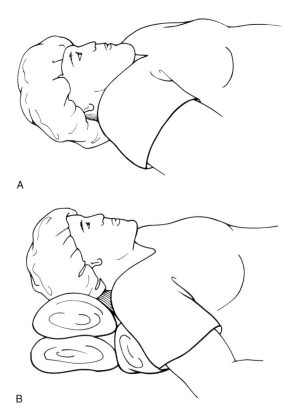

A

B

Figure 43–1. Optimal positioning for obese patients with a short neck. ***A:*** The normal supine position often prevents extension of the head and makes endotracheal intubation difficult. ***B:*** Elevation of the shoulder allows some neck flexion with more optimal extension of the head at the atlanto-occipital joint, facilitating intubation.

blades, a short laryngoscope handle, at least one extra styleted endotracheal tube (6 mm), Magill forceps (for nasal intubation), laryngeal mask airway (LMA), an intubating LMA (Fastrach), fiberoptic bronchoscope, the capability for transtracheal jet ventilation and possibly an esophageal-tracheal Combitube should be readily available (see Chapter 5). When a difficult airway is suspected, alternatives to the standard rapid-sequence induction, such as regional anesthesia or awake fiberoptic techniques, should be considered. Moreover, a clear plan should be formulated for a failed endotracheal intubation following induction of anesthesia (Figure 43–2). Note that the life of the mother takes priority over delivery of the fetus. In the absence of fetal distress, the patient should be awakened, and an awake intubation, regional or local (infiltration) anesthesia may be tried. In the

presence of fetal distress, if spontaneous or positive ventilation (by mask or LMA) with cricoid pressure is possible, delivery of the fetus may be attempted. In such instances, a potent volatile agent in oxygen is employed for anesthesia, but once the fetus is delivered, nitrous oxide can be added to reduce the concentration of the volatile agent; halothane or sevoflurane is usually selected because it may be least likely to depress ventilation. Inability to ventilate the patient at any time mandates immediate cricothyrotomy or tracheostomy.

Suggested Technique for Cesarean Section

(1) The patient is placed supine with a wedge under the right hip for left uterine displacement.

(2) Preoxygenation is accomplished with 100% oxygen for 3–5 minutes while monitors are applied. Defasciculation is generally not necessary (see section on suggested technique for vaginal delivery).

(3) The patient is prepared and draped for surgery.

(4) When the surgeons are ready, a rapid-sequence induction with cricoid pressure is performed using 4 mg/kg of thiopental (or 2 mg/kg of propofol) and 1.5 mg/kg of succinylcholine. Ketamine, 1 mg/kg, is used instead of thiopental in hypovolemic or asthmatic patients. Other agents, including methohexital, etomidate, and midazolam, offer little benefit in obstetric patients. In fact, midazolam may be more likely to produce maternal hypotension and neonatal depression.

(5) Surgery is begun only after proper placement of the endotracheal tube is confirmed by capnography. Excessive hyperventilation (PaCO$_2$, 25 mm Hg) should be avoided because it can reduce uterine blood flow and has been associated with fetal acidosis.

(6) Fifty percent nitrous oxide in oxygen with up to 0.75 MAC of a low concentration of a volatile agent (eg, 1% sevoflurane, 0.75% isoflurane, or 3% desflurane) is used for maintenance. The low dose of volatile agent helps ensure amnesia but is generally not enough to cause excessive uterine relaxation or prevent uterine contraction following oxytocin. A muscle relaxant of intermediate duration (atracurium, rapacuronium,* or rocuronium) is used for relaxation.

(7) After the neonate and placenta are delivered, 20–30 U of oxytocin is added to each liter of in-

---

* At the time of publication, rapacuronium had been voluntarily withdrawn by the manufacturer. See Chapter 9 for details.

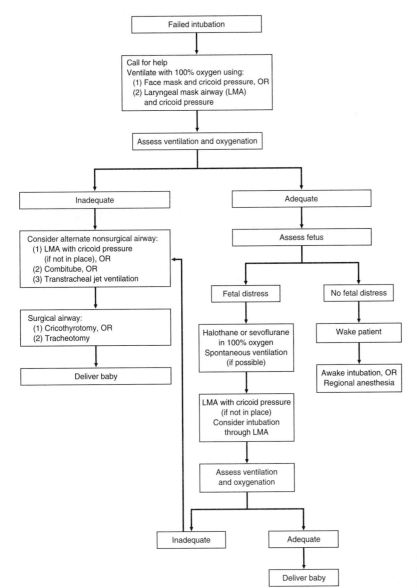

Figure 43–2. An algorithm for a difficult intubation in obstetric patients.

travenous fluid. The nitrous oxide concentration may be then increased to 70% and/or additional intravenous agents, such an opioid or benzodiazepine, can be given to ensure amnesia.

(8) If the uterus does not contract readily, an opioid should be given, and the halogenated agent is discontinued. Methylergonovine (Methergine), 0.2 mg intramuscularly, may also be given but can increase arterial blood pressure (see Chapter 42).

15-Methyl prostaglandin F2α (Hemabate), 0.25 mg IM, may also be used.

(9) An attempt to aspirate gastric contents may be made via an oral gastric tube to decrease the likelihood of pulmonary aspiration on emergence.

(10) At the end of surgery, muscle relaxants are completely reversed, the gastric tube (if placed) is removed, and the patient is extubated awake to reduce the risk of aspiration.

ANESTHESIA FOR EMERGENCY CESAREAN SECTION

Indications for emergency cesarean section include massive bleeding (placenta previa or accreta, abruptio placentae, or uterine rupture), umbilical cord prolapse, and severe fetal distress. The distinction must be made between a true emergency requiring immediate delivery (previous referred to as "crash") versus one where some delay is possible. Close communication with the obstetrician is necessary to determine whether fetus, mother, or both are in immediate jeopardy requiring general anesthesia or there is time to safely administer regional anesthesia. In the first instance, even if the patient has an epidural catheter in place, the delay in establishing adequate epidural anesthesia generally prohibits its use. Moreover, regional anesthesia is contraindicated in severely hypovolemic or hypotensive patients. Adequate preoxygenation may be achieved rapidly with four maximal breaths of 100% oxygen while monitors are being applied. Ketamine, 1 mg/kg, should be substituted for thiopental in hypotensive or hypovolemic patients.

Table 43–5 lists commonly accepted signs of fetal distress, an imprecise and poorly defined term. In most instances the diagnosis is primarily based on fetal heart rate monitoring (see below). Because worrisome fetal heart rate patterns have a relatively high incidence of false-positive results, careful interpretation of other parameters, such as fetal blood gas tensions or fetal pulse oximetry, may also be necessary. Moreover, continuation of fetal monitoring in the operating room may help avoid unnecessary induction of general anesthesia for fetal distress when additional time for use of regional anesthesia is possible. In selected instances where immediate delivery is not absolutely mandatory, epidural anesthesia with 3% chloroprocaine (or alkalinized 2% lidocaine) or spinal anesthesia may be appropriate.

■ ANESTHESIA FOR THE COMPLICATED PREGNANCY

UMBILICAL CORD PROLAPSE

Prolapse of the umbilical cord complicates 0.2–0.6% of deliveries. Umbilical cord compression following prolapse can rapidly lead to fetal asphyxia. Predisposing factors include excessive cord length, malpresentation, low birth weight, grand parity (> 5 pregnancies), multiple gestations, and artificial rupture of membranes. The diagnosis is suspected after sudden fetal bradycardia or profound decelerations and confirmed by physical ex-

Table 43–5. Signs of fetal distress.

Nonreassuring fetal heart rate pattern
Repetitive late decelerations
Loss of fetal beat-to-beat variability associated with late or deep decelerations
Sustained fetal heart rate < 80 beats/min
Fetal scalp pH < 7.20
Meconium-stained amniotic fluid
Oligohydramnios
Intrauterine growth restriction

amination. Treatment includes immediate steep Trendelenburg or knee-chest position and manual pushing of the presenting fetal part back up into the pelvis until immediate cesarean section under general anesthesia. If the fetus is not viable, vaginal delivery is allowed to continue.

DYSTOCIA AND ABNORMAL FETAL PRESENTATIONS & POSITIONS

Dystocia, or difficult labor, may be due to ineffective uterine contractions; abnormal lie, position, presentation, position; or cephalopelvic disproportion that is either due to a large fetus or small maternal pelvis. Abnormal fetal positions and presentations increase maternal and fetal morbidity and mortality. They also increase the likelihood that anesthesia will be required.

The fetus may lie longitudinally, transversely, or obliquely in the uterus. Fetal presentation refers to the body part that overlies the pelvic inlet. Spontaneous vaginal delivery can occur only with a longitudinal lie, in which either the head (vertex), or buttocks or legs (breech) descend first. The posture (attitude) of the fetus is normally flexion but may be extension. A vertex presentation with flexion together with rotation of the head into an occiput anterior position allows for optimal passage of the fetal skull through the pelvis.

Primary Dysfunctional Labor

Failure for labor to progress normally (see Chapter 42) may be due to inadequate or ineffective uterine contractions, which is referred to as primary dysfunctional labor. Although in most instances abnormal uterine contractility is responsible, anatomic abnormalities may also play a major role (see section on abnormal vertex presentations).

A **prolonged latent phase** is defined as exceeding 20 hours in a nulliparous parturient and 14 hours in a multiparous patient. The cervix usually remains at 4 cm or less but is completely effaced. The etiology is likely ineffective contractions without a dominant myometrial pacemaker. **Arrest of dilatation** is present when the cervix undergoes no further change after 2 hours in the active phase of labor. A **protracted active phase** refers to slower than normal cervical dilatation, defined as < 1.2 cm/hour in a nulliparous patient and < 1.5 cm/hour in a multiparous parturient. A **prolonged deceleration phase** occurs when cervical dilatation slows markedly after 8 cm. The cervix becomes very edematous and appears to lose effacement. A **prolonged second stage** (disorder of descent) is defined as the presenting descending less than 1 cm/hour and 2 cm/hour in nulliparous and multiparous parturients, respectively. Failure of the head to descend 1 cm in station after adequate pushing is referred to as **arrest of descent**.

Oxytocin (see Chapter 42) is generally the treatment of choice for uterine contractile abnormalities. The drug is given intravenously at 1–6 mU/min and increased in increments of 1–6 mU/min every 15–40 minutes, depending on the protocol. Use of amniotomy is controversial. Treatment is usually expectant management, as long as the fetus and mother are tolerating the prolonged labor. When a trial of oxytocin is unsuccessful or when malpresentation or cephalopelvic disproportion may also be present, operative vaginal delivery or cesarean section is indicated.

Breech Presentation

Breech presentations complicate 3–4% of deliveries and significantly increase both maternal and fetal morbidity and mortality rates. The most common cause is prematurity. Breech presentations increase neonatal mortality more than 5-fold. The incidence of cord prolapse is up to 10%. **External cephalic version** may be attempted after 36–38 weeks gestation and prior to the onset of labor; the procedure attempts to reverse the fetal lie and guide the head into the pelvis. Some obstetricians may also administer a tocolytic agent at the same time. In some centers, epidural anesthesia is used; the epidural catheter can then be used for analgesia after induction of labor. Although external version is successful in 75% of patients it can cause placental abruption and umbilical cord compression necessitating immediate cesarean section.

Because the shoulders or head can become trapped after vaginal delivery of the body, some obstetricians employ cesarean section for all breech presentations. The cesarean section rate for breech is 80–100%. Manual or forceps-assisted partial breech extraction is usually necessary with vaginal delivery. The need for breech extraction does not appear to be increased when epidural anesthesia is used for labor—if labor is well established prior to epidural activation. Moreover,

epidural anesthesia may lessen the likelihood of a trapped head, because the former relaxes perineum. Nonetheless, the fetal head can become trapped in the uterus even during cesarean section under regional anesthesia; rapid induction of general endotracheal anesthesia and administration of a volatile agent is necessary in such instances to relax the uterus. Alternatively, nitroglycerin 50–100 μg intravenously can be tried.

Abnormal Vertex Presentations

When the fetal occiput fails to spontaneously rotate anteriorly, a **persistent occiput posterior** presentation results in a more prolonged and painful labor. Manual or forceps rotation is usually necessary but increases the likelihood of maternal and fetal injuries. Regional anesthesia can be used to provide perineal analgesia and pelvic relaxation, allowing manual or forceps rotation followed by forceps delivery.

A **face presentation** occurs when the fetal head is hyperextended. Vaginal delivery of a face presentation is possible only if the chin is directed anteriorly (mentum anterior). **Persistent mentum posterior** requires cesarean section. **Brow presentation** is often associated with prolonged and dysfunctional labor. Vaginal delivery can occur only if the head extends into a face presentation or flexes into a normal vertex presentation. **Shoulder presentations** occur with an oblique lie or transverse lie. Vaginal delivery is usually impossible. It typically leads to dysfunctional labor and predisposes to cord prolapse when the membranes rupture. Delivery requires cesarean section. A **compound presentation** occurs when an extremity enters the pelvis along with either the head or the buttocks. Vaginal delivery is usually still possible as the extremity often withdraws as the labor progresses.

Impaction of a shoulder against the pubic symphysis, or **shoulder dystocia**, complicates 0.2–2% of deliveries and is one of major causes of birth injuries. The most important risk factor is fetal macrosomia. Shoulder dystocias are often difficult to predict. Several obstetric maneuvers can be used to relieve it, but a prolonged delay in the delivery could result in fetal asphyxia. Induction of general anesthesia may be necessary, if an epidural catheter is not already in place.

MULTIPLE GESTATIONS

Multiple gestations account for 1 birth in 90 and are commonly associated with two complications: breech presentation and prematurity. Anesthesia may be necessary for version, extraction, or cesarean section. The second baby (and any subsequent ones) is often more depressed and asphyxiated than the first. Regional anesthesia provides effective pain relief during labor, minimizes the need for central nervous system depressants, and may shorten the interval between the birth of the first and second baby. Some studies suggest that the acid-base status of the second twin is better when epidural anesthesia is used. Patients with multiple gestations, however, are more prone to develop hypotension from aortocaval compression, especially after regional anesthesia. Left lateral uterine displacement and intravenous fluid loading are mandatory prior to regional anesthesia. Either regional or general anesthesia may be used for cesarean section; regional anesthesia may be associated with less neonatal depression.

ANTEPARTUM HEMORRHAGE

Placenta Previa

The incidence of this complication is 0.5% of pregnancies. Placenta previa often occurs in patients who have had previous cesarean section or uterine myomectomy; other risk factors include multiparity, advanced maternal age, and a large placenta. The placenta may completely cover the internal cervical os (**central or complete placenta previa**), may partially cover the os (**partial placenta previa**), or may be close to the internal cervical os without extending beyond its edge (lowlying or **marginal placenta**). Placenta previa usually presents as painless vaginal bleeding. Although the bleeding often stops spontaneously, severe hemorrhage can occur at any time. When the gestation is less than 37 weeks in duration and the bleeding is mild to moderate, the patient is usually treated with bed rest and observation. After 37 weeks of gestation, delivery is usually accomplished via cesarean section. Patients with low-lying placenta may be allowed—although rarely—to deliver vaginally if the bleeding is mild.

All parturients with vaginal bleeding are assumed to have placenta previa until proved otherwise. An abdominal ultrasound examination can localize the placenta and establishes the diagnosis. If the patient is stable and fluid resuscitation has already taken place, regional anesthesia may be considered. Active bleeding or an unstable patient requires immediate cesarean section under general anesthesia. The patient should have two large-bore intravenous catheters in place; intravascular volume deficits must be vigorously replaced; and blood must be available for transfusion. A central venous line may be useful in monitoring and provides excellent access for rapid transfusion. The bleeding can continue after delivery because the placental implantation site in the lower uterine segment often does not contract well like the rest of the uterus.

A history of a previous placenta previa or cesarean section increases the risk of **placenta accreta**, **placenta increta**, and **placenta percreta** in subsequent pregnancies. In these conditions, the placenta becomes adherent to the surface, invades the muscle, or completely penetrates the myometrium, respectively. The placenta becomes difficult or impossible to separate from the uterus. Moreover, these conditions regularly produce life-threatening maternal hemorrhage. Hysterectomy following delivery of the fetus is usually required to control profuse bleeding following separation of the placenta. Coagulopathy is common and requires correction with blood components.

Abruptio Placentae

Premature separation of a normal placenta complicates approximately 1–2% of pregnancies; it is said to be the most common cause of intrapartum fetal death. Bleeding into the basal layers of the decidua causes placental separation. Expansion of the hematoma can progressively extend the separation. The blood occasionally may extend into the myometrium (Couvelaire uterus). Most abruptions are mild (grade I) but up to 25% are severe (grade III). Risk factors include hypertension, trauma, a short umbilical cord, multiparity, alcohol abuse, cocaine use, and an abnormal uterus. Patients usually experience painful vaginal bleeding with uterine contraction and tenderness. The diagnosis is made by excluding placenta previa on abdominal ultrasound. Mild to moderate abruptions may be managed with vaginal delivery if the fetus is over 37 weeks of gestational age, but immediate cesarean section is carried out after any signs of fetal distress. The choice between regional and general anesthesia must factor in the urgency for delivery, maternal hemodynamic stability, and any coagulopathy. The bleeding may remain concealed inside the uterus and cause underestimation of blood loss. Severe abruptio placentae can cause coagulopathy, especially following fetal demise. Fibrinogen levels are mildly reduced (150–250 mg/dL) with moderate abruptions but are typically less than 150 mg/dL with fetal demise. The coagulopathy is thought to be due to activation of circulating plasminogen (fibrinolysis) and the release of tissue thromboplastins that precipitate disseminated intravascular coagulation (DIC). Platelet count and factors V and VIII are low, and fibrin split products are elevated. Severe abruption is a life-threatening emergency that necessitates a crash emergency cesarean section under general anesthesia. Massive blood transfusion, including replacement of coagulation factors and platelets are necessary.

Uterine Rupture

Uterine rupture is relatively uncommon (1:1000–3000 deliveries) but can occur during labor as a result of (1) dehiscence of a scar from a previous (usually classic) cesarean section (VBAC), extensive myomectomy, or uterine reconstruction; (2) intrauterine manipulations or use of forceps (iatrogenic); or (3) spontaneous rupture following prolonged labor in patients with hypertonic contractions (especially with oxytocin infusions), fetopelvic disproportion, or a very large, thin, and weakened uterus. Uterine rupture can present either as frank hemorrhage or as hypotension with occult bleeding into the abdomen. Even when epidural anesthesia is employed for labor, uterine rupture is often heralded by the abrupt onset of continuous abdominal pain and hypotension. The use of dilute concentrations of local anesthetics for epidural anesthesia during labor may facilitate early recognition. Treatment requires volume resuscitation and immediate laparotomy under general anesthesia. Ligation of the internal iliac (hypogastric) arteries, with or without hysterectomy, may be necessary to control intraoperative bleeding.

PREMATURE RUPTURE OF MEMBRANES & CHORIOAMNIONITIS

Premature rupture of membranes (PROM) is present when leakage of amniotic fluid occurs before the onset of labor. The pH of amniotic fluid cause nitrazine paper to change color from blue to yellow. PROM complicates 10% of all pregnancies and up to 35% of premature deliveries. Predisposing factors include a short cervix, prior history of PROM or preterm delivery, infection, multiple gestations, polyhydramnios, and smoking. Spontaneous labor commences within 24 hours of ruptured membranes in 90% of patients. Management of PROM balances the risk of infection versus that of fetal prematurity. Delivery is usually indicated after 34 weeks gestation. Patients with a gestation less than 34 weeks gestation can be managed expectantly with prophylactic antibiotics and tocolytics for 5–7 days to allow some additional maturation of fetal organs. The longer the interval between rupture and the onset of labor, the higher the incidence of chorioamnionitis. PROM also predisposes to postpartum endometritis.

Chorioamnionitis represents infection of the chorionic and amnionic membranes, and may involve the placenta, uterus, umbilical cord, and fetus. It complicates up to 1–2% of pregnancies and is usually but not always associated with ruptured membranes. The contents of the amniotic cavity are normally sterile, but become vulnerable to ascending bacterial infection from the vagina when the cervix dilates or the membranes rupture. Intra-amniotic infections are less commonly caused by hematogenous spread of bacteria or retrograde seeding through the fallopian tubes. The princi-

pal maternal complications of chorioamnionitis are dysfunctional labor, often leading to cesarean section, intra-abdominal infection, septicemia, and postpartum hemorrhage. Fetal complications include premature labor, acidosis, hypoxia, and septicemia.

Diagnosis of chorioamnionitis requires a high index of suspicion. Clinical signs include fever (> 38 °C), maternal and fetal tachycardia, uterine tenderness, and foul smelling or purulent amniotic fluid. Blood leukocyte count is useful only if markedly elevated because it normally increases during labor (normal average 15,000/μL). C-reactive protein levels are usually elevated (> 2 mg/dL). Gram stain of amniotic fluid obtained by amniocentesis is helpful in ruling out infection.

The use of regional anesthesia in patients with chorioamnionitis is controversial because of the theoretical risk of promoting the development of meningitis or an epidural abscess. Available evidence suggests that this risk is very low and that concerns may be unjustified. Moreover, antepartum antibiotic therapy appears to reduce maternal and fetal morbidity. Nonetheless, concerns over hemodynamic stability following sympathectomy are justified, especially in patients with chills, high fever, tachypnea, mental status changes, or borderline hypotension. Therefore, in the absence of overt signs of septicemia, thrombocytopenia, or coagulopathy, most clinicians offer regional anesthesia to patients with chorioamnionitis following antibiotic therapy. When general anesthesia is being considered, the relative risks of failed intubation and aspiration must be weighed against those of a spinal infection following regional anesthesia.

PRETERM LABOR

Preterm labor by definition occurs between the 20th and 37th weeks of gestation and is the most common complication of the third trimester. Approximately 8% of liveborn infants in the United States are delivered before term. Important contributory maternal factors include extremes of age, inadequate prenatal care, unusual body habitus, increased physical activity, infections, and other medical illnesses or complications during pregnancy.

Because of their small size and incomplete development, preterm infants—especially those under 30 weeks of gestational age or weighing less than 1500 g—experience a greater number of complications than term infants. Premature rupture of membranes complicates a third of premature deliveries; the combination of premature rupture of membranes and premature labor increases the likelihood of umbilical cord compression resulting in fetal hypoxemia and asphyxia. Preterm infants with a breech presentation are especially prone to prolapse of the umbilical cord during labor. Moreover, inadequate pulmonary surfactant production frequently leads to the idiopathic respiratory distress syndrome (hyaline membrane disease) after delivery. Surfactant levels are generally adequate only after the 35th week of gestation. Lastly, a soft, poorly calcified cranium predisposes these neonates to intracranial hemorrhage during vaginal delivery.

When preterm labor occurs before 35 weeks of gestation, bed rest and tocolytic therapy are usually initiated. Treatment is successful in 75% of patients. Labor is inhibited until the lungs mature and sufficient pulmonary surfactant is produced, as judged by amniocentesis. The risk of respiratory distress syndrome is markedly reduced when amniotic fluid lecithin/sphingomyelin ratio is greater than 2. Glucocorticoid (betamethasone) may be given to induce production of pulmonary surfactant, which requires a minimum of 24–48 hours. Prophylactic antibiotics (penicillins) are given to patients until cultures for group B streptococcus are determined to be negative. The most commonly used tocolytics are β_2-adrenergic agonists (ritodrine or terbutaline) and magnesium (6 g intravenously over 30 minutes followed by 2–4 g/hour); intravenous alcohol is no longer used. Ritodrine (given intravenously as 100–350 µg/min) and terbutaline (given orally as 2.5–5 mg every 4–6 hours) also have some β_1-adrenergic receptor activity, which accounts for some of their side effects. Maternal side effects include tachycardia, arrhythmias, myocardial ischemia, mild hypotension, hyperglycemia, hypokalemia and, rarely, pulmonary edema. Other tocolytic agents include calcium channel blockers (nifedipine), prostaglandin synthetase inhibitors, oxytocin antagonists (atosiban) and possibly nitric oxide. Fetal ductal constriction can occur after 32 weeks gestation with nonsteroidal anti-inflammatory drugs, such as indomethacin, but it is usually transient and resolves after discontinuation of the drug; renal impairment in the fetus may also cause oligohydramnios.

When tocolytic therapy fails to stop labor, anesthesia often becomes necessary. The goal during vaginal delivery of a preterm fetus is a slow controlled delivery with minimal pushing by the mother. A large episiotomy and low forceps are often employed. Spinal or epidural anesthesia allows complete pelvic relaxation. Cesarean section is performed for fetal distress, breech presentation, intrauterine growth retardation, or failure of labor to progress. Regional or general anesthesia may be employed, but because preterm infants may be more sensitive to all central nervous system depressants, regional anesthesia may be preferable. Residual effects from β-adrenergic agonists may complicate general anesthesia. The half-life of ritodrine may be as long as 3 hours. Halothane, pancuronium, ketamine, and ephe-

drine should be used cautiously (if at all). Hypokalemia is usually due to an intracellular uptake of potassium and rarely requires treatment; however, it may increase sensitivity to muscle relaxants. Magnesium therapy potentiates muscle relaxants, may predispose to hypotension (secondary to vasodilatation). Residual effects from tocolytics interfere with uterine contraction following delivery. Lastly, preterm newborns are often depressed at delivery and frequently need resuscitation. Preparations for resuscitation should be completed prior to delivery.

PREGNANCY-INDUCED HYPERTENSION

The syndrome of **pregnancy-induced hypertension (PIH),** also called **preeclampsia** (or **toxemia**), refers to the triad of hypertension, proteinuria (> 500 mg/d), and edema (hand and face) occurring after the 20th week of gestation and resolving within 48 hours after delivery. PIH is usually defined as a systolic blood pressure greater than 140 mm Hg or diastolic pressure greater than 90 mm Hg; or, alternatively, as a consistent increase in systolic or diastolic pressure by 30 mm Hg and 15 mm Hg, respectively, above the patient's normal baseline. When seizures occur, the syndrome is termed **eclampsia**. In the United States, preeclampsia and eclampsia complicate approximately 7–10% and one in 10,000–15,000 pregnancies, respectively. Together, they cause or contribute to 20–40% of cases maternal deaths and 20% of perinatal deaths. Maternal deaths are usually due to stroke, pulmonary edema, and hepatic necrosis or rupture.

Pathophysiology & Manifestations

PIH affects chiefly primigravidas, but it can occur in multiparous women, especially those with vascular disorders. Some evidence suggests that it may have an immunogenetic basis. The pathophysiology of this multisystem disease remains obscure but appears to be related to abnormal prostaglandin metabolism and endothelial dysfunction that lead to vascular hyperreactivity. Patients with PIH have elevated levels of thromboxane A_2 (TXA_2) production and decreased prostacyclin (PGI_2) production. TXA_2 is a potent vasoconstrictor and promoter of platelet aggregation, while PGI_2 is a potent vasodilator and inhibitor of platelet aggregation. Endothelial dysfunction may reduce nitric oxide production and increase endothelin-1. The latter is also potent vasoconstrictor and activator of platelets. Abnormal regulation of oxygen-derived free radical and lipid peroxidation may also play an important role. Marked vascular reactivity and endothelial injury reduce placental perfusion and can lead to widespread systemic manifestations.

Other major manifestations of PIH include (1) generalized vasospasm, (2) reduced intravascular volume, (3) decreased glomerular filtration, and (4) generalized edema (Table 43–6). Severe PIH substantially increases both maternal and fetal morbidity and mortality and is defined by a blood pressure greater than 160/110 mm Hg, proteinuria in excess of 5 g/d, oliguria (< 500 mL/d), pulmonary edema, central nervous system manifestations (headache, visual disturbances, or seizures), hepatic tenderness, or the **HELLP syndrome** (*h*emolysis, *e*levated *l*iver enzymes, and a *l*ow *p*latelet count). Hepatic rupture may also occur in patients with the HELLP syndrome.

Patients with severe preeclampsia or eclampsia have widely differing hemodynamic profiles. Most patients have low-normal cardiac filling pressures with high systemic vascular resistance, but cardiac output may be low, normal, or high.

Table 43–6. Complications of pregnancy-induced hypertension.

Neurologic
 Headache
 Visual disturbances
 Hyperexcitability
 Seizures
 Intracranial hemorrhage
 Cerebral edema
Pulmonary
 Upper airway edema
 Pulmonary edema
Cardiovascular
 Decreased intravascular volume
 Increased arteriolar resistance
 Hypertension
 Heart failure
Hepatic
 Impaired function
 Elevated enzymes
 Hematoma
 Rupture
Renal
 Proteinuria
 Sodium retention
 Decreased glomerular filtration
 Renal failure
Hematologic
 Coagulopathy
  Thrombocytopenia
  Platelet dysfunction
  Prolonged partial thromboplastin time
 Microangiopathic hemolysis

Treatment

Treatment consists of bed rest, sedation, antihypertensive drugs (usually labetalol 5–10 mg IV, hydralazine 5 mg IV, or methyldopa 250-500 mg PO), and magnesium sulfate (4 g IV loading, followed by 1–3 g/hour) to treat hyperreflexia and prevent convulsions. Therapeutic magnesium levels are 4–6 mEq/L. Unlike labetalol, esmolol can have significant, potentially adverse fetal effects. Calcium channel blockers are generally not used because of their tocolytic action and potentiation of magnesium-induced circulatory depression.

Invasive arterial, central venous, and possibly pulmonary artery monitoring are probably indicated in patients with severe hypertension, pulmonary edema, or refractory oliguria; an intravenous vasodilator (nitroglycerin or nitroprusside) is often necessary. Definitive treatment is delivery of the fetus and placenta.

Anesthetic Management

Patients with mild PIH generally only require extra caution during anesthesia; standard anesthetic practices may be used. Spinal and epidural anesthesia are associated with similar decreases in arterial blood pressure in these patients. Patients with severe disease, however, are critically ill and require stabilization prior to administration of any anesthetic. Hypertension should be controlled and hypovolemia corrected before anesthesia. In the absence of coagulopathy, continuous epidural anesthesia is the anesthetic of choice for most patients with PIH during labor, vaginal delivery, and cesarean section. Moreover, continuous epidural anesthesia avoids the increased risk of a failed intubation due to severe edema of the upper airway.

A platelet count and coagulation profile should be checked prior to the institution of regional anesthesia in patients with severe PIH. Regional anesthesia is contraindicated if the platelet count is less than 100,000/μL. Although some patients have a qualitative platelet defect, the usefulness of a bleeding time is questionable. Continuous epidural anesthesia has been shown to decrease catecholamine secretion and improve uteroplacental perfusion in these patients, provided hypotension is avoided. Judicious colloid fluid boluses (250–500 mL) before epidural activation may be more effective than crystalloids in correcting the hypovolemia and preventing profound hypotension. A central venous line may be used to guide volume replacement; however, a pulmonary artery catheter should be used in severe cases (such as marked hypertension, refractory oliguria, hypoxemia, or frank pulmonary edema). Use of an epinephrine-containing test dose for epidural anesthesia is controversial because of its questionable reliability (see the above section on preventing unintentional intravascular injection) and the risk of exacerbating hypertension. Hypotension should be treated with small doses of vasopressors (ephedrine, 5 mg) because patients tend to be very sensitive to these agents.

Intra-arterial blood pressure monitoring is indicated in patients with severe hypertension during both general and regional anesthesia. Intravenous nitroprusside, trimethaphan, or nitroglycerin is usually necessary to control blood pressure during general anesthesia. Intravenous labetalol (5–10 mg increments) can also be effective in controlling the hypertensive response to intubation and does not appear to alter placental blood flow. Because magnesium potentiates muscle relaxants, doses of nondepolarizing muscle relaxants should be reduced in patients receiving magnesium therapy and guided by a peripheral nerve stimulator.

HEART DISEASE

The marked cardiovascular changes associated with pregnancy, labor, and delivery often cause pregnant patients with heart disease (2% of parturients) to decompensate during this period. Although most patients have rheumatic heart disease, an increasing number of parturients are presenting with congenital heart lesions. Anesthetic management is directed toward employing techniques that minimize the added stresses of labor and delivery. Specific management of the various lesions is discussed elsewhere. Most patients can be divided into one of two groups. Patients in the first group include those with mitral valve disease, aortic insufficiency, or congenital lesions with left-to-right shunting. These patients benefit from regional techniques, particularly continuous epidural anesthesia. The induced sympathectomy reduces both preload and afterload, relieves pulmonary congestion, and in some cases increases forward flow (cardiac output).

Patients in the second group include those with aortic stenosis, congenital lesions with right-to-left or bidirectional shunting, or primary pulmonary hypertension. Regional anesthesia is generally detrimental in this group. Reductions in venous return (preload) or afterload are usually poorly tolerated. These patients are better managed with intraspinal opioids alone, systemic medications, pudendal nerve blocks and, if necessary, general anesthesia.

AMNIOTIC FLUID EMBOLISM

Amniotic fluid embolism is a rare (1:20,000 deliveries) but potentially lethal complication (86% mortality rate in some series) that can occur during labor, delivery, cesarean section, or postpartum. The mortality exceeds 50% in the first hour. Entry of amniotic fluid into the maternal circulation can occur through any break in the uteroplacental membranes. Such breaks may occur during normal delivery or cesarean section or following placental abruption, placenta previa, or uterine rupture. In addition to desquamated fetal debris, amniotic fluid contains various prostaglandin and leukotrienes, which appear to play an important role in the genesis of this syndrome. The alternate term "anaphylactoid syndrome of pregnancy" has been suggested to emphasize the role of chemical mediators in this syndrome.

Patients typically present with sudden tachypnea, cyanosis, shock, and generalized bleeding. Three major pathophysiologic manifestations are responsible: (1) acute pulmonary embolism, (2) DIC, and (3) uterine atony. Seizures and pulmonary edema may develop; the latter has both cardiogenic and noncardiogenic components. Acute left ventricular dysfunction appears to be a common feature. Although the diagnosis can be firmly established only by demonstrating fetal elements in the maternal circulation (usually at autopsy or less commonly by aspirating amniotic fluid from a central venous catheter), amniotic fluid embolism should always be suggested by sudden respiratory distress and circulatory collapse. The presentation may initially mimic acute pulmonary thromboembolism, venous air embolism, overwhelming septicemia, or hepatic rupture or cerebral hemorrhage in a patient with toxemia.

Treatment consists of aggressive cardiopulmonary resuscitation, stabilization, and supportive care. When cardiac arrest occurs prior to delivery of the fetus, the efficacy of closed-chest compressions appears to be marginal at best. Aortocaval compression impairs resuscitation in the supine position, while chest compressions are less effective in a lateral tilt position. Moreover, expeditious delivery appears to improve maternal and fetal outcome; immediate (cesarean) delivery should therefore be carried out. Once the patient is resuscitated, stabilization with mechanical ventilation, fluids, and inotropes is best carried out with full invasive hemodynamic monitoring. Uterine atony is treated with oxytocin and methylergonovine, while significant coagulopathies are treated with platelets and coagulation factors based on laboratory findings.

POSTPARTUM HEMORRHAGE

This complication is usually considered present when the postpartum blood loss exceeds 500 mL. Up to 4% of parturients may experience postpartum hemorrhage, which is often associated with a prolonged third stage of labor, preeclampsia, multiple gestations, forceps delivery, and mediolateral episiotomy. Common causes include uterine atony, a retained placenta, obstetric lacerations, uterine inversion, and use of tocolytic agents prior to delivery. Atony is often associated with uterine overdistention (multiple gestation and polyhydramnios). Less commonly, a clotting defect may be responsible.

The anesthesiologist may be consulted to assist in venous access or fluid (and blood) resuscitation, as well as provide anesthesia for careful examination of the vagina, cervix, and uterus. Perineal lacerations can usually be repaired with local infiltration of anesthetic or pudendal nerve blocks. Residual anesthesia from prior institution of epidural or spinal anesthesia facilitates examination of the patient; however, supplementation with an opioid, nitrous oxide, or both may be required. Induction of spinal or epidural anesthesia in the face of hypovolemia is contraindicated. General anesthesia is usually required for bimanual massage of the uterus, manual extraction of a retained placenta, reversion of an inverted uterus, or repair of a major laceration. Uterine atony should be treated with oxytocin (20–30 U/L of intravenous fluid), methylergonovine (0.2 mg IM), and 15-methyl prostaglandin F2α (0.25 mg IM). Emergency laparotomy and hysterectomy may be necessary in rare instances. Early ligation of the internal iliac (hypogastric) arteries may help avoid hysterectomy or reduce blood loss.

■ FETAL & NEONATAL RESUSCITATION

FETAL RESUSCITATION

Resuscitation of the neonate starts during labor. Any compromise of the uteroplacental circulation readily produces fetal asphyxia. Intrauterine asphyxia during labor is the most common cause of neonatal depression. Fetal monitoring throughout labor is helpful in identifying which babies may be at risk, detecting fetal distress, and evaluating the effect of acute interventions. These include correcting hypotension with fluids or vasopressors, supplemental oxygen, decreasing uterine contraction (stopping oxytocin or administering tocolytics). Some studies suggest that the normal fetus can compensate for up to 45 minutes of fetal hypoxia, a period termed "fetal stress"; the latter is associated with a marked redistribution of blood flow primarily to the heart, brain, and adrenal glands. With time, however, progressive lactic acidosis and asphyxia produce increasing fetal distress that necessitates immediate delivery.

1. Fetal Heart Rate Monitoring

Fetal heart rate monitoring, supplemented by fetal scalp blood sampling, is presently the most useful technique. Correct interpretation of heart rate patterns is crucial.

Three parameters are evaluated: baseline heart rate, baseline variability, and the relationship to uterine contractions (deceleration patterns). Heart rate monitoring is most accurate when fetal scalp electrodes are used, but the latter may require rupture of the membranes and is not without complications (ie, amnionitis or fetal injury).

Baseline Heart Rate

The mature fetus normally has a baseline heart rate of 120–160 beats/min. An increased baseline heart rate may be due to prematurity, mild fetal hypoxia, chorioamnionitis, maternal fever, maternally administered drugs (anticholinergics or β-agonists) or, rarely, hyperthyroidism. A decreased baseline heart rate may be due to a postterm pregnancy, fetal heart block, or fetal asphyxia.

Baseline Variability

The healthy mature fetus normally displays a baseline beat-to-beat (R wave to R wave) variability of 3–6 beats/min. Baseline, **short-term variability**, which is best assessed with scalp electrodes, has become an important sign of fetal well-being and represents a normally functioning autonomic system. Sustained decreased baseline variability is a prominent sign of fetal asphyxia. Central nervous system depressants (opioids, barbiturates, benzodiazepines, or magnesium sulfate) and parasympatholytics (atropine) also decrease baseline variability, as do prematurity, fetal dysrhythmias, and anencephaly. A sinusoidal pattern that resembles a smooth sine wave is associated with fetal depression (hypoxia, drugs, and anemia secondary to Rh isoimmunization).

Long-term variability consists of periodic **accelerations** that are usually related to fetal movements and responses to uterine pressure. Such accelerations are generally considered reassuring. By 32 weeks, fetuses display periodic increases in baseline heart rate that are associated with fetal movements. Normal fetuses have 15–40 accelerations per hour. The mechanism is thought to be increases in catecholamine secretion with decreases in vagal tone. Accelerations diminish with fetal sleep, some drugs (opioids, magnesium, and atropine), as well as fetal hypoxia. Accelerations to fetal scalp or vibroacoustic stimulation are considered a reassuring sign of fetal well-being. The absence of both baseline and long-term variability can be an important sign of fetal distress.

Deceleration Patterns

A. EARLY (TYPE I) DECELERATIONS:

(Figure 43–3A.) This type of deceleration (usually 10–40 beats/min) is thought to be a vagal response to

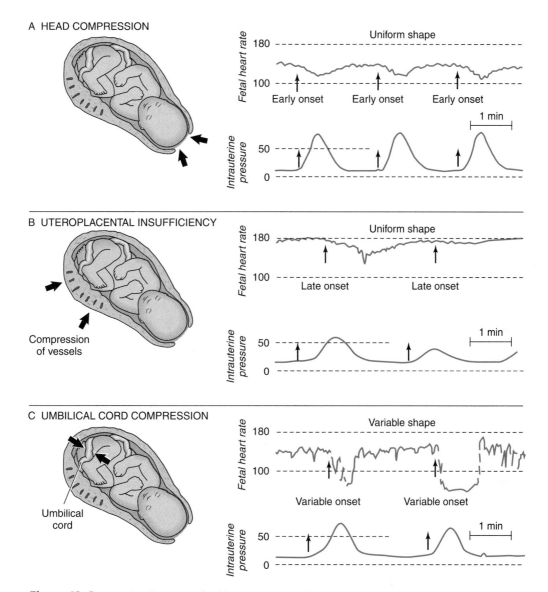

Figure 43–3. Periodic changes in fetal heart rate related to uterine contraction. ***A:*** Early (type I) decelerations. ***B:*** Late (type II) decelerations. ***C:*** Variable (type III) decelerations. (Modified and reproduced, with permission, from Danforth DN, Scott JR: *Obstetrics and Gynecology,* 5th ed. Lippincott, 1986.)

compression of the fetal head or stretching of the neck during uterine contractions. The heart rate forms a smooth mirror image of the contraction. Early decelerations are generally not associated with fetal distress.

B. LATE (TYPE II) DECELERATIONS:

(Figure 43–3B) Late decelerations are associated with fetal compromise and are characterized by a decrease in heart rate at or following the peak of uterine contrac-

tions. Late decelerations may be as few as 5 beats/min and are thought to be due to the effect of a decrease in arterial oxygen tension on chemoreceptors or the sinoatrial node. Late decelerations with normal variability may be observed following acute insults (maternal hypotension or hypoxemia) and are usually reversible with treatment. Late decelerations with decreased variability are associated with prolonged asphyxia and are an indication for fetal scalp sampling (see below section on fetal blood sampling). Complete abolition of variability in this setting is an ominous sign signifying severe decompensation and the need for immediate delivery.

C. VARIABLE (TYPE III) DECELERATIONS:

(Figure 43–3C) These decelerations are variable in onset, duration, and magnitude (often > 30 beats/min). They are typically abrupt in onset and are thought to be related to umbilical cord compression and acute intermittent decreases in umbilical blood flow. Variable decelerations are typically associated with fetal asphyxia when they are greater than 70 beats/min, last more than 60 seconds, or occur in a pattern that persists for more than 30 minutes.

2. Fetal Blood Sampling

Fetal blood can be obtained and analyzed via a small scalp puncture once the membranes are ruptured. A pH higher than 7.20 is usually associated with a vigorous neonate, whereas a pH less than 7.20 is often but not always associated with a depressed neonate. Because of wide overlap, fetal blood sampling can be interpreted correctly only in conjunction with heart rate monitoring. Experience with fetal pulse oximetry is limited but promising.

3. Treatment of the Fetus

Aggressive treatment of intrauterine fetal asphyxia is necessary to prevent fetal demise or permanent neurologic damage. All interventions are directed at restoring an adequate uteroplacental circulation. Aortocaval compression, maternal hypoxemia or hypotension, or excessive uterine activity (during oxytocin infusions) must be corrected. Changes in maternal position, supplemental oxygen, intravenous ephedrine or fluid, or adjustments in an oxytocin infusion often correct the problem. Failure to relieve fetal stress as well as progressive acidosis and asphyxia necessitate immediate delivery.

NEONATAL RESUSCITATION

1. General Care of the Neonate

One person whose sole responsibility is to care for the neonate and is capable of providing resuscitation should attend every delivery. As the head is delivered, the nose, mouth, and pharynx are suctioned with a bulb syringe. After the remainder of the body is delivered, the skin is dried with a sterile towel. Once the umbilical cord stops pulsating or breathing is initiated, the cord is then clamped and the neonate is placed in a radiant warmer with the bed tilted in slight Trendelenburg position. Evaluation and treatment are carried out

simultaneously (Figure 43–4). If the neonate is obviously depressed, the cord is clamped early and resuscitation is initiated immediately. Breathing normally begins within 30 seconds and is sustained within 90 seconds. Respirations should be 30–60 breaths/min and the heart rate 120–160 beats/min. Respirations are assessed by auscultation of the chest, while heart rate is determined by palpation of the pulse at the base of the umbilical cord or auscultation of the precordium. It is critically important to keep the neonate warm.

In addition to respirations and heart rate, color, tone, and reflex irritability should be evaluated. The **Apgar score** (Table 43–7), recorded at 1 minute and again at 5 minutes after delivery, remains the most valuable assessment of the neonate. The 1-minute score correlates with survival, while the 5-minute score is related to neurologic outcome.

Neonates with Apgar scores of 8–10 are vigorous and may only require gentle stimulation (flicking the foot, rubbing the back, and additional drying). A catheter should first be gently passed through each nostril to rule-out choanal atresia, and then through the mouth to suction the stomach and rule out esophageal atresia.

2. Meconium-Stained Neonates

The presence or absence of meconium in the amniotic fluid (about 10–12% of deliveries) dictates the immediate management of the neonate at birth. Fetal distress, especially after 42 weeks of gestation, is often associated with release of thick meconium into the fluid. Fetal gasping during stress results in entry of a large amount of meconium-tainted amniotic fluid into the lungs.

Table 43–7. Apgar Score.

	Points		
Sign	*0*	*1*	*2*
Heart rate (beats/min)	Absent	< 100	> 100
Respiratory effort	Absent	Slow, irregular	Good, crying
Muscle tone	Flaccid	Some flexion	Active motion
Reflex irritability	No response	Grimace	Crying
Color	Blue or pale	Body pink, extremities blue	All pink

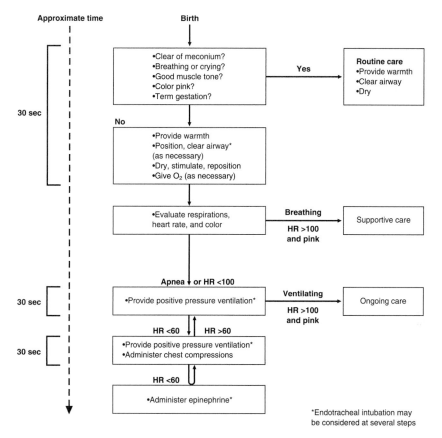

Approximate time

Birth

30 sec

•Clear of meconium?
•Breathing or crying?
•Good muscle tone?
•Color pink?
•Term gestation?

Yes

Routine care
•Provide warmth
•Clear airway
•Dry

No

•Provide warmth
•Position, clear airway*
(as necessary)
•Dry, stimulate, reposition
•Give O₂ (as necessary)

•Evaluate respirations,
heart rate, and color

Breathing

**HR >100
and pink**

Supportive care

Apnea or HR <100

30 sec

•Provide positive pressure ventilation*

Ventilating

**HR >100
and pink**

Ongoing care

HR <60   **HR >60**

30 sec

•Provide positive pressure ventilation*
•Administer chest compressions

HR <60

•Administer epinephrine*

*Endotracheal intubation may
be considered at several steps

Figure 43–4. An algorithm for resuscitation of the newly born infant. (Reproduced, with permission, from the American Heart Association.)

When the neonate initiates respiration at birth, the meconium moves from the trachea and large airways down toward the periphery of the lung. Thick or particulate meconium obstructs small airways and causes severe respiratory distress in 15% of meconium-stained neonates. Moreover, these infants can develop persistent fetal circulation (see Chapter 42). Amnioinfusion prior to delivery can reduce the severity of meconium aspiration syndrome.

Unless the neonate has absent or depressed respirations, thin watery meconium does not require suctioning beyond careful suctioning of the oropharynx when the head emerges from the perineum (or from the uterus at cesarean section). When thick (pea soup) meconium is present in the amniotic fluid, however, some clinicians intubate and suction the trachea immediately after delivery but before the first breath is taken. Tracheal suctioning of the thick meconium is accomplished by a special suctioning device attached to the endotracheal tube as the tube is withdrawn. If meco-

nium is aspirated from the trachea, the procedure should be repeated until no meconium is obtained—but no more than three times, after which it is usually of no further benefit. The infant should then be given supplemental oxygen by face mask and observed closely. The stomach should also be suctioned to prevent passive regurgitation of any meconium. Newborns with meconium aspiration have an increased incidence of pneumothorax (10% compared with 1% for all vaginal deliveries).

3. Care of the Depressed Neonate

Approximately 6% of newborns require some form of advanced life support, most of whom weigh less than 1500 g. Resuscitation of the depressed neonate requires two or more persons—one to manage the airway and ventilation and another to perform chest compressions, if necessary. A third person greatly facilitates the placement of intravascular catheters and the administration of fluids or drugs. The anesthesiologist caring for the mother can only render brief assistance and only when it does not jeopardize the mother; other personnel are, therefore, generally responsible for neonatal resuscitation.

Because the most common cause of neonatal depression is intrauterine asphyxia, the emphasis in resuscitation is on respiration. Hypovolemia is also a contributing factor in a significant number of neonates. Factors associated with hypovolemia include early clamping of the umbilical cord, holding the neonate above the introitus prior to clamping, prematurity, maternal hemorrhage, placental transection during cesarean section, sepsis, and twin-to-twin transfusion.

Failure of the neonate to quickly respond to respiratory resuscitative efforts mandates vascular access and blood gas analysis; pneumothorax (1% incidence) and congenital anomalies of the airway, including tracheoesophageal fistula (1:3000–5000 live births); and congenital diaphragmatic hernia (1:2000–4000) should also be considered.

Grouping by the 1-minute Apgar score greatly facilitates resuscitation: (1) mildly asphyxiated neonates (Apgar score of 5–7) usually need only stimulation while 100% oxygen is blown across the face; (2) moderately asphyxiated neonates (Apgar score of 3–4) require temporary assisted positive pressure ventilation with mask and bag; and (3) severely depressed neonates (Apgar score of 0–2) should be immediately intubated, and chest compressions may be required.

Guidelines for Ventilation

Indications for positive pressure ventilation include (1) apnea, (2) gasping respirations, (3) persistent central cyanosis with 100% oxygen, and (4) heart rate less than 100 beats/min. Excessive flexion or extension of the neck can cause airway obstruction. A 1-inch high towel under the shoulders may be helpful in maintaining proper head position. Assisted ventilation by bag and mask should be at a rate of 40–60 breaths/min with 100% oxygen. Initial breaths may require peak pressures of up to 40 cm H_2O, but pressures should not exceed 30 cm H_2O subsequently. Adequacy of ventilation should be checked by auscultation and chest excursions. Gastric decompression with an 8F tube often facilitates ventilation. If after 30 seconds the heart rate is over 100 beats/min and spontaneous ventilations become adequate, assisted ventilation is no longer necessary. If the heart rate is less than 60 beats/min or is 60–80 beats/min and not rising, the neonate is intubated and chest compressions are started. If the heart rate is 60–80 beats/min and rising, assisted ventilation is continued and the neonate is observed. Failure of the heart rate to rise above 80 beats/min is an indication for chest compressions. Indications for endotracheal in-

tubation include ineffective ventilation, prolonged mask ventilation, and the need to administer medications.

Intubation (Figure 43–5) is performed with a Miller 00, 0, or 1 laryngoscope blade, using a 2.5-, 3-, or 3.5-mm endotracheal tube (for neonates < 1 kg, 1–2 kg, and > 2 kg, respectively). Correct endotracheal tube size is indicated by a small leak with 20 cm H_2O pressure. Right endobronchial intubation should be excluded by chest auscultation. The correct depth of the endotracheal tube ("tip to lip") is usually 6 cm plus the weight in kilograms. Oxygen saturation can usually be measured by a pulse oximeter probe applied to the palm. Capnography is also very useful in confirming endotracheal intubation. Transcutaneous oxygen sensors are useful for measuring tissue oxygenation but unfortunately require time for initial equilibration. Use of a laryngeal mask airway (LMA#1) has been reported in neonates > 2.5 kg and may be useful if endotracheal intubation is difficult (eg, Pierre Robin syndrome).

Guidelines for Chest Compressions

Indications for chest compressions are a heart rate that is less than 60 beats/min or 60–80 beats/min and not rising after 30 seconds of adequate ventilation with 100% oxygen.

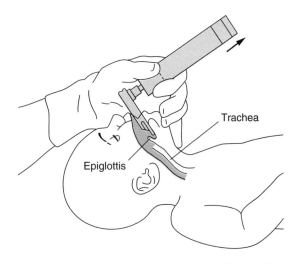

Figure 43–5. Intubation of the neonate. The head is placed in neutral position, and the laryngoscope handle is held with the thumb and index finger as the chin is supported with the remaining fingers. Pressure applied over the hyoid bone with the little finger will bring the larynx into view. A straight blade such as a Miller 0 or 1 usually provides the best view.

Cardiac compressions should be provided at a rate of 120/min. The 2 thumb-encircling hands (Figure 43–6) technique is generally preferred because it appears to generate higher peak systolic and coronary perfusion pressures. Alternatively, the 2-finger technique can be used (Figure 43–7). The depth of compressions should be approximately one-third of the anterior-posterior diameter of the chest and enough to generate a palpable pulse.

Compressions should be interposed with ventilation in a 3:1 ratio, such that 90 compressions and 30 ventilations are given per minute. The heart rate should be checked periodically. Chest compressions should be stopped when the spontaneous heart rate exceeds 80 beats/min.

Vascular Access

Cannulation of the umbilical vein with a 3.5F or 5F umbilical catheter is easiest and the preferred technique. The tip of the catheter should be just below skin level and allow free backflow of blood; further advancement may result in infusion of hypertonic solutions directly into the liver.

Cannulation of one of the two umbilical arteries allows measurement of blood pressure and facilitates blood gas measurements but may be more difficult. Specially designed umbilical artery catheters allow continuous PaO_2 or oxygen saturation monitoring as well as blood pressure. Care must be taken not to introduce any air into either the artery or the vein.

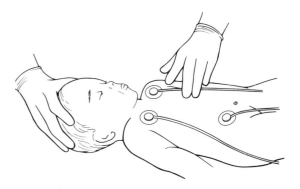

Figure 43–7. The alternative technique for neonatal chest compressions: two fingers are placed on the lower third of the sternum at right angles to the chest. The chest is compressed approximately 1 cm at a rate of 120/min.

Volume Resuscitation

Some neonates at term and nearly two-thirds of premature infants requiring resuscitation are hypovolemic at birth. Diagnosis is based on physical examination (low blood pressure and pallor) and a poor response to resuscitation. Neonatal blood pressure generally correlates with intravascular volume, and should therefore routinely be measured. Normal blood pressure depends on birth weight and varies from 50/25 mm Hg for neonates weighing 1–2 kg to 70/40 mm Hg for those weighing over 3 kg. A low blood pressure suggests hypovolemia. Volume expansion may be accomplished with 10 mL/kg of either lactated Ringer's injection, normal saline, or type O-negative blood crossmatched with maternal blood. Less common causes of hypotension include hypocalcemia, hypermagnesemia, and hypoglycemia.

Drug Therapy

A. EPINEPHRINE:

Epinephrine, 0.01–0.03 mg/kg (0.1–0.3 mL/kg of a 1:10,000 solution), should be given for asystole or a spontaneous heart rate of less than 60 beats/min in spite of adequate ventilation and chest compressions. It may be repeated every 3–5 minutes. Epinephrine may be given in 1 mL of saline down the endotracheal tube if venous access is not available.

B. NALOXONE:

Naloxone, 0.1 mg/kg IV or 0.2 mg/kg IM, is given to reverse the respiratory depressant effect of opioids given to the mother in the last 4 hours of labor. Withdrawal

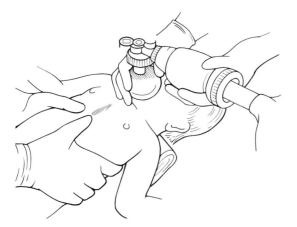

Figure 43–6. Chest compressions in the neonate. The neonate is held with both hands as each thumb is placed just beneath a line connecting nipples and the remaining fingers encircle the chest. The sternum is compressed ½ to ¾ inches (1-cm) at a rate of 120/min. (Reproduced, with permission, from the American Heart Association.)

symptoms may be precipitated in babies of opioid addicts.

C. OTHER DRUGS:

Other drugs may be indicated only in specific settings. Sodium bicarbonate (2 mEq/kg of a 0.5 mEq/mL solution) should generally be given only for a severe metabolic acidosis documented by blood gas measurements and when ventilation is adequate. It may also be administered during prolonged resuscitation (> 5 min)—particularly if blood gas measurements are not readily available. The infusion rate should not exceed 1 mEq/kg/min to avoid hypertonicity and intracranial hemorrhage. Moreover, to prevent hypertonicity-induced hepatic injury, the catheter tip should not be in the liver. Calcium gluconate 100 mg/kg ($CaCl_2$, 30 mg/kg) should only be given to neonates with documented hypocalcemia or those with suspected magnesium intoxication (from maternal magnesium therapy); these neonates are usually hypotensive, hypotonic, and appear vasodilated. Glucose (200 mg/kg of a 10% solution) is given only for documented hypoglycemia because hyperglycemia worsens hypoxic neurologic deficits. Blood glucose should be measured because up to 10% of neonates may have hypoglycemia (glucose < 35 mg/dL), especially those delivered by cesarean section. Dopamine may be started at 5 μg/kg/min to support arterial blood pressure. Lastly, surfactant may be given through the endotracheal tube to premature neonates with respiratory distress syndrome.

CASE DISCUSSION: APPENDICITIS IN A PREGNANT WOMAN

A 31-year-old woman with a 24-week gestation presents for an appendectomy.

How does pregnancy complicate the management of this patient?

Nearly 1–2% of pregnant patients require surgery during their pregnancy. The most common procedure during the first trimester is laparoscopy; appendectomy (1:1500 pregnancies) and cholecystectomy (1:2000–10,000 pregnancies) are the most commonly performed open abdominal procedures. The physiologic effects of pregnancy can alter the manifestations of the disease process and make diagnosis difficult. Patients may therefore present with advanced or complicated disease. The physiologic changes associated with pregnancy (see Chapter 42) further predispose the patient to increased morbidity and mor-

tality. Moreover, both the surgery and the anesthesia can adversely affect the fetus.

What are the potentially detrimental effects of surgery and anesthesia on the fetus?

The procedure can have both immediate and long-term undesirable effects on the fetus. Hypotension, hypovolemia, severe anemia, hypoxemia, and marked increases in sympathetic tone can seriously compromise the transfer of oxygen and other nutrients across the uteroplacental circulation and promote intrauterine fetal asphyxia. The stress of the procedure and underlying process may also precipitate preterm labor. Preterm labor often follows intra-abdominal surgery near the uterus. Laparoscopy may be safely performed but the CO_2 insufflation has the potential to cause fetal respiratory acidosis. Mild to moderate maternal hyperventilation and limiting both insufflation pressure and duration of the procedure limits the degree of acidosis. Long-term detrimental effects relate to possible teratogenic effects on the developing fetus.

When is the fetus most sensitive to teratogenic influences?

Three stages of susceptibility are generally recognized. In the first 2 weeks of intrauterine life, teratogens have either a lethal or no effect on the embryo. The third to eighth weeks are the most critical period, when organogenesis takes place; drug exposure during this period can produce major developmental abnormalities. From the eighth week onward, organogenesis is complete, and organ growth takes place. Teratogen exposure during this last period usually results in only minor morphologic abnormalities but can produce significant physiologic abnormalities and growth retardation. Although the teratogenic influences of anesthetic agents have been extensively studied in animals, retrospective human studies have not been conclusive. A notable exception is the benzodiazepine group, which has been linked to congenital anomalies. Nonetheless, as with all drugs, exposure to anesthetic agents should be kept to a minimum in terms of the number of agents, dosage, and duration of exposure.

What would be the ideal anesthetic technique in this patient?

Towards the end of the second trimester (after 20 weeks' gestation), most of the physiologic changes associated with pregnancy have taken place. Regional anesthesia may therefore be preferable to general anesthesia to decrease the risks of pulmonary aspiration and failed intubation and to minimize drug exposure to the fetus. The patient should be transported and maintained with left lateral uterine displacement when supine. Drug exposure is least (probably negligible) with spinal anesthesia. Moreover, spinal anesthesia may be preferable to epidural anesthesia because it is not associated with unintentional intravascular injections or potentially large intrathecal doses of local anesthetic. On the other hand, general anesthesia guarantees patient comfort and, when a volatile agent is used, may even suppress preterm labor (see Chapter 42). Nitrous oxide without concomitant administration of a halogenated anesthetic is reported to reduce uterine blood flow.

Although regional anesthesia is preferable in most instances, the choice between regional and general anesthesia must be individualized according to the patient, the anesthesiologist, and the type of surgery. Spinal anesthesia is usually satisfactory for appendectomies, while general anesthesia is more satisfactory for cholecystectomies. The same techniques and doses used for the parturient should be followed.

Are any special monitors indicated perioperatively?

In addition to standard monitors, fetal heart rate and uterine activity should be monitored with a Doppler and tocodynamometer during induction of anesthesia, emergence, and recovery and, whenever possible, during surgery in a woman who is 20 weeks pregnant. When regular organized uterine activity is detected, early treatment with a β-adrenergic agonist such as ritodrine usually aborts the preterm labor. Magnesium sulfate and oral or rectal indomethacin may also be used as tocolytics.

When should elective operations be performed during pregnancy?

All elective operations should be postponed until 6 weeks after delivery. Only emergency procedures that pose an immediate threat to the mother or fetus should be routinely performed. The timing of semielective procedures, such as those for cancer, valvular heart disease, or intracranial aneurysms, must be individualized and must balance the threat to maternal health versus fetal well-being. Controlled (deliberate) hypotensive anesthesia may be necessary to reduce blood loss during extensive cancer operations; nitroprusside, nitroglycerin, and hydralazine have been used during pregnancy without apparent fetal

compromise. Nonetheless, large doses and prolonged infusions of nitroprusside should be avoided because the immature liver of the fetus may have a limited ability to metabolize the cyanide breakdown product. Cardiopulmonary bypass has been employed in pregnant patients successfully without adverse fetal outcome, but should probably be carried out only with continuous fetal echocardiography. Circulatory arrest during pregnancy is not recommended.

SUGGESTED READING

American Heart Association: Neonatal Resuscitation. Circulation 2000;102(8)Supplement:I-343-57.

Beilin Y, Leibowitz AB, Bernstein HH, Abramovitz SE: Controversies of labor epidural analgesia. Anesth Analg 1999;89:969-978.

Birnbach DJ, Datta S, Gatt SP: *Textbook of Obstetric Anesthesia.* Churchill Livingstone, 2000.

Bloom RS, Cropley C: *Textbook of Neonatal Resuscitation.* American Heart Association/American Academy of Pediatrics, 1995.

Chestnut DH: *Obstetric Anesthesia,* 2nd ed. Mosby, 1999.

Dahl JB, Jeppesen IS, Jørgensen H, Wetterslev J, Møiniche S: Intraoperative and postoperative analgesic efficacy and adverse effects of intrathecal opioids in patients undergoing cesarean section with spinal anesthesia: A qualitative and quantitative systematic review of randomized controlled trials. Anesthesiology 1999;91:1919-1927.

Datta S: *The Obstetric Anesthesia Handbook,* 3rd ed. Mosby, 2000.

Denny NM, Selander DE: Continuous spinal anaesthesia. Br J Anaesth 1998;81:590-597.

Eisenach JC: Combined spinal-epidural analgesia in obstetrics. Anesthesiology 1999;91:299-302.

Gambling DR, Douglas MJ: *Obstetric Anesthesia and Uncommon Disorders.* WB Saunders and Company, 1998.

Guidelines for Perinatal Care, 4th ed. American Academy of Pediatrics, American College of Obstetricians and Gynecologists, 1997.

Hawkins JL, Koonin LM, Palmer SK, Gibbs CP: Anesthesia-related deaths during obstetric delivery in the United States, 1979-1990. Anesthesiology 1997;86:277-284.

Hawthorne L, Wilson R, Lyons G, Dresser M: Failed intubation revisited: 17 year experience in a teaching maternal unit. Br J Anaesth 1996;76:680-684.

Holdcroft TT: *Principles and Practice of Obstetric Anaesthesia.* Blackwell, 2000.

Koren G, Pastuszak A, Ito S: Drugs in pregnancy. N Engl J Med 1998;338:1128-1137.

Lapinsky SE, Kruczynski K, Seaward GR, Farine D, Grossman RF: Critical care management of the obstetric patient. Can J Anaesth 1997;44:325-329.

Macario A, Scibettaa WC, Navarro J, Riley E: Analgesia for labor pain. A cost model. Anesthesiology 2000;92:841-850.

Morgan P: Spinal anaesthesia in obstetrics. Can J Anaesth 1995;42:1145-1163.

Norris MC: *Handbook of Obstetric Anesthesia.* Lippincott-Williams & Wilkins, 2000.

Norris MC: *Obstetric Anesthesia,* 2nd ed. Lippincott Williams & Wilkins, 1998.

Practice guidelines for obstetric anesthesia. A report by the American Society of Anesthesiologists Task Force on Obstetrical Anesthesia. Anesthesiology 1999;90:600-611.

Rawal N, Van Zundert A, Holmstrom B, Crowhurst JA: Combined spinal-epidural technique. Regional Anesthesia 1997;22:406-423.

Rosen MA: Management of anesthesia for the pregnant surgical patient. Anesthesiology 1999;91:1159-1163.

Zideman DA: Paediatric and neonatal life support. Br J Anaesth 1997;79:178-187.

Pediatric Anesthesia

44

KEY CONCEPTS

 The small and limited number of alveoli in neonates and infants reduces lung compliance; in contrast, their cartilaginous rib cage makes their chest wall very compliant. The combination of these two characteristics promotes chest wall collapse during inspiration and relatively low residual lung volumes at expiration. The resulting decrease in functional residual capacity (FRC) is important because it limits oxygen reserves during periods of apnea (eg, intubation) and readily predisposes them to atelectasis and hypoxemia.

 Neonates and infants have a proportionately larger head and tongue, narrow nasal passages, an anterior and cephalad larynx, a long epiglottis, and a short trachea and neck. These features make them obligate nasal breathers until about 5 months of age. The cricoid cartilage is the narrowest point of the airway in children younger than 5 years of age.

 Stroke volume is relatively fixed by a noncompliant and poorly developed left ventricle in neonates and infants. The cardiac output is therefore very dependent on heart rate.

 Thin skin, low fat content, and a higher surface relative to weight allow greater heat loss in neonates. This problem is compounded by cold operating rooms, wound exposure, intravenous fluid administration, dry anesthetic gases, and the direct effect of anesthetic agents on temperature regulation. Hypothermia has been associated with delayed awakening from anesthesia, cardiac irritability, respiratory depression, increased pulmonary vascular resistance, and altered drug responses.

 Neonates, infants, and young children have relatively higher alveolar ventilation and lower FRC compared with older children and adults. This higher minute ventilation to FRC ratio with relatively higher blood flow to vessel-rich organs contributes to a rapid rise in alveolar anesthetic concentration. These factors result in rapid induction and recovery from general anesthesia.

 Minimum alveolar concentration is higher in infants than in neonates and adults for halogenated agents.

 Children are more susceptible than adults to cardiac arrhythmias, hyperkalemia, rhabdomyolysis, myoglobinemia, masseter spasm, and malignant hyperthermia (MH) after succinylcholine administration. If a child unexpectedly experiences cardiac arrest after succinylcholine administration, immediate treatment for hyperkalemia should be started.

 Unlike in adults, profound bradycardia and sinus node arrest develop in pediatric patients following the first dose of succinylcholine without atropine pretreatment.

 A viral infection within 2–4 weeks before general anesthesia and endotracheal intubation appears to increase the child's risk of perioperative pulmonary complications, such as wheezing, laryngospasm, hypoxemia, and atelectasis.

 Temperature must be closely monitored in pediatric patients because of their higher risk for MH and the potential for both iatrogenic hypothermia and hyperthermia.

(continued)

(continued)

 Meticulous fluid management is required in small pediatric patients because of extremely limited margins of error. A programmable infusion pump or a buret with a microdrip chamber should be used for accurate measurements. Drugs are flushed through low dead-space tubing to minimize unnecessary fluid administration.

 Laryngospasm can usually be avoided by extubating the patient either awake or while deeply anesthetized; both techniques have advocates. Extubation during the interval between these extremes, however, is generally recognized as hazardous.

 Postintubation croup is associated with early childhood (age 1–4 years), repeated intubation attempts, large endotracheal tubes, prolonged surgery, head and neck procedures, and excessive movement of the tube.

 Retinopathy of prematurity, a fibrovascular proliferation overlying the retina, deserves special consideration. Oxygenation should be continuously monitored with pulse oximetry or transcutaneous oxygen analysis, with particular attention given to infants younger than 44 weeks postconception.

 Patients with scoliosis due to muscular dystrophy are predisposed to MH, cardiac dysrhythmias, and untoward effects of succinylcholine (hyperkalemia, myoglobinuria, and sustained muscular contractures).

Neonates (less than 30 days of age), infants (1–12 months of age), and children (1–12 years of age) are not merely small adults. Their successful anesthetic management depends on an appreciation of the physiologic, anatomic, and pharmacologic characteristics of each group (Table 44–1). These characteristics, which differentiate them from each other and adults, necessitate modification of anesthetic equipment and techniques. Indeed infants are at increased risk for anesthetic morbidity and mortality than are older children; risk is generally inversely proportional to age, neonates being at highest risk. In addition, pediatric patients are prone to illnesses that require unique surgical and anesthetic strategies.

ANATOMIC & PHYSIOLOGIC DEVELOPMENT

Respiratory System

The transition from fetal to neonatal physiology is reviewed in Chapter 42. Compared with older children and adults, neonates and infants have less efficient ventilation because of weak intercostal and diaphragmatic musculature, which is due to a paucity of type I fibers, horizontal and more pliable ribs, and a protuberant abdomen. Respiratory rate is elevated in neonates and gradually falls to adult levels by adolescence. Tidal volume and dead space per kilogram remain constant during development. A relative paucity of small airways increases airway resistance. Alveolar maturation is not complete until late childhood (about 8 years of age). The work of breathing is increased and respiratory muscles easily fatigue. The small and limited number of alveoli in neonates and infants reduces lung compliance; in contrast, their cartilaginous rib cage makes their chest wall very compliant. The combination of these two characteristics promotes chest wall collapse during inspiration and relatively low residual lung volumes at expiration. The resulting decrease in functional residual capacity (FRC) is important because it limits oxygen reserves during periods of apnea (eg, intubation) and readily predisposes neonates and infants to atelectasis and hypoxemia. This may be exaggerated by their relatively higher rate of oxygen consumption. Moreover, hypoxic and hypercapnic ventilatory drives are not well developed in neonates and infants. In fact, hypoxia and hypercapnia depress respiration in these patients, unlike in adults.

Neonates and infants have a proportionately larger head and tongue, narrow nasal passages, an anterior and cephalad larynx (at a vertebral level of C4 versus C6 in adults), a long epiglottis, and a short trachea and neck (Figure 44–1). These anatomic features make neonates and most young infants obligate nasal breathers until about 5 months of age. The cricoid cartilage is the narrowest point of the airway in children younger than 5 years of age; in adults, the narrowest point is the glottis. One millimeter of edema will have a proportionately greater effect in children because of their smaller tracheal diameters.

Table 44–1. Characteristics of neonates and infants that differentiate them from adult patients.

Physiologic
  Heart-rate-dependent cardiac output
  Faster heart rate
  Lower blood pressure
  Faster respiratory rate
  Lower lung compliance
  Greater chest wall compliance
  Lower functional residual capacity
  Higher ratio of body surface area to body weight
  Higher total body water content
Anatomic
  Noncompliant left ventricle
  Residual fetal circulation
  Difficult venous and arterial cannulation
  Large head and tongue
  Narrow nasal passages
  Anterior and cephalad larynx
  Long epiglottis
  Short trachea and neck
  Prominent adenoids and tonsils
  Weak intercostal and diaphragmatic muscles
  High resistance to airflow
Pharmacologic
  Immature hepatic biotransformation
  Decreased protein binding
  Rapid rise in F_A/F_I
  Rapid induction and recovery
  Increased minimum alveolar concentration
  Larger volume of distribution for water-soluble drugs
  Immature neuromuscular junction

F_A/F_I = Fractional alveolar concentration/fractional inspired concentration.

Cardiovascular System

 Stroke volume is relatively fixed by a noncompliant and poorly developed left ventricle in neonates and infants. The cardiac output is therefore very dependent on heart rate (see Chapter 19). Although basal heart rate is higher than in adults (Table 44–2), activation of the parasympathetic nervous system, anesthetic overdose, or hypoxia can cause bradycardia and profound reductions in cardiac output. Sick infants undergoing emergency or prolonged surgical procedures appear especially prone to episodes of bradycardia that can lead to hypotension, asystole, and intraoperative death. The sympathetic nervous system and baroreceptor reflexes are not fully mature. The infant cardiovascular system maintains lower catecholamine stores and displays a blunted response to exogenous catecholamines. The vascular tree is less able to respond to hypovolemia with vasoconstriction. The hallmark of intravascular fluid depletion in neonates and infants is therefore hypotension without tachycardia.

Metabolism & Temperature Regulation

Pediatric patients have a larger surface area per kilogram than adults (increased surface area/weight ratio). Metabolism and its associated parameters (oxygen consumption, CO_2 production, cardiac output, and alveolar ventilation) correlate better with surface area than with weight.

 Thin skin, low fat content, and a higher surface relative to weight allow greater heat loss to the environment in neonates. This problem is compounded by cold operating rooms, wound exposure, intravenous fluid administration, dry anesthetic gases, and the direct effect of anesthetic agents on temperature regulation. Hypothermia is a serious problem that has been associated with delayed awakening from anesthesia, cardiac irritability, respiratory depression, increased pulmonary vascular resistance, and altered drug responses. The major mechanism for heat production in neonates is **nonshivering thermogenesis** by metabolism of brown fat. Even this is severely limited in premature infants and in sick neonates who are deficient in fat stores. Furthermore, volatile anesthetics inhibit thermogenesis in brown adipocytes.

Renal & Gastrointestinal Function

Normal kidney function is not present until 6 months of age; function may not achieve levels similar to adults until the child is 2 years old. Premature neonates often possess multiple renal defects, including decreased creatinine clearance; impaired sodium retention, glucose excretion, and bicarbonate reabsorption; and poor di-

Table 44–2. Age-related changes in vital signs.*

| | | | Arterial Blood Pressure | |
Age	Respiratory Rate	Heart Rate	Systolic	Diastolic
Neonate	40	140	65	40
12 months	30	120	95	65
3 years	25	100	100	70
12 years	20	80	110	60

*Values are mean averages derived from numerous sources. Normal ranges vary by as much as 25–50%.

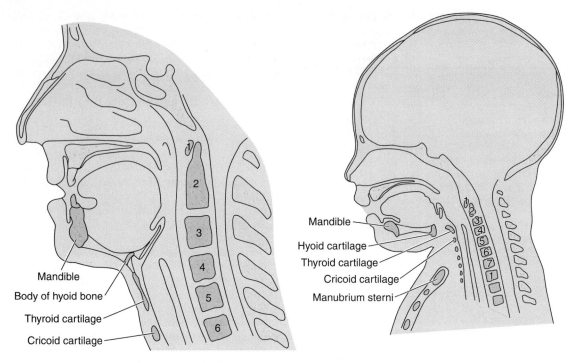

Figure 44–1. Sagittal section of the adult (**A**) and infant (**B**) airway. (Reproduced, with permission, from Snell RS, Katz J: *Clinical Anatomy for Anesthesiologists.* Appleton & Lange, 1988.)

luting and concentrating ability. These abnormalities increase the importance of meticulous attention to fluid administration in the early days of life.

Neonates have also a relatively high incidence of gastroesophageal reflux. A relatively immature liver causes impaired hepatic conjugation early in life.

Glucose Homeostasis

Neonates have low glycogen stores that predispose them to hypoglycemia. Impaired glucose excretion by the kidneys may partially offset this tendency. Neonates at greatest risk for hypoglycemia are those who are premature or small for gestational age, those who have been receiving hyperalimentation, and those born to diabetic mothers.

PHARMACOLOGIC DIFFERENCES

Pediatric drug dosing is typically based on a per-kilogram recommendation (Table 44–3). A child's weight can be roughly estimated based on age:

50th percentile weight (kg) = (Age × 2) + 9

Weight, however, does not take into account the disproportionately larger pediatric intravascular and extracellular fluid compartments, the immaturity of hepatic biotransformation pathways, increased organ blood flow, decreased protein binding, or higher metabolic rate. These variables must be considered on an individual basis. Neonates and infants have a proportionately higher total water content (70–75%) than adults (50–60%).

Inhalational Anesthetics

 Neonates, infants, and young children have relatively higher alveolar ventilation and lower FRC compared with older children and adults. This higher minute ventilation to FRC ratio with relatively higher blood flow to vessel-rich organs contributes to a rapid rise in alveolar anesthetic concentration. Furthermore, the blood/gas coefficients of isoflurane and halothane are lower in neonates than in adults. These factors result in rapid induction and recovery from general anesthesia. The rate of emergence from halothane and isoflurane anesthesia appears to the similar for procedures lasting less than 1 hour. Minimum alveolar concentration (MAC) is higher in infants than in neonates

Table 44–3. Pediatric drug dosages.

Drug	Comment	Dosage*
Acetaminophen	Rectal	40 mg/kg
	PO	15–20 mg/kg
	Maximum (per day)	60 mg/kg
Adenosine	Rapid IV bolus	0.1 mg/kg
	Repeat dose	0.2 mg/kg
	Maximum dose	12 mg
Alfentanil	Anesthetic supplement (IV)	20–25 µg/kg
	Maintenance infusion	1–3 µg/kg/min
Amiodarone	Loading dose (IV)	5 mg/kg
	Repeat dose (slowly)	5 mg/kg
	Maximum dose	15 mg/kg/day
Aminophylline	Loading dose administered over 20 minutes (IV)	5–6 mg/kg
	Maintenance dose (therapeutic level: 10–20 mg/mL)	0.5–0.9 mg/kg/h
Amrinone	Loading (IV)	0.75–1 mg/kg
	Maintenance	5–10 µg/kg/min
Atropine	IV	0.01–0.02 mg/kg
	IM	0.02 mg/kg
	Minimum dose	0.1 mg
	Premedication (PO)	0.03–0.05 mg/kg
Atracurium	Intubation (IV)	0.5 mg/kg
Bretylium	Loading dose (IV)	5 mg/kg
Calcium chloride	IV (slowly)	5–20 mg/kg
Calcium gluconate	IV (slowly)	15–100 mg/kg
Cardioversion	See Table 43–3	0.5–2 J/kg
Chloral hydrate	Oral administration	50–100 mg/kg
Cimetidine	IV or PO	5–10 mg/kg
Cisatracurium	Intubation (IV)	0.15 mg/kg
Dantrolene	Initial dose (10 mg/kg maximum) (IV)	2.5 mg/kg
Defibrillation	First attempt	2 J/kg
	Subsequent attempts	4 J/kg
Dexamethasone	IV	0.1–0.5 mg/kg
Dextrose	$D_{25}W$ or $D_{50}W$ (IV)	0.5–1 g/kg
Diazepam	Sedation	0.1–0.2 mg/kg
Digoxin	Three divided doses over 24 hours (IV)	15–30 µg/kg
Diltiazem	IV over 2 minutes	0.25 mg/kg
Diphenhydramine	IV, IM, or PO	1 mg/kg
Dobutamine	Infusion	2–20 µg/kg/min
Dolasetron	IV	35 µg/kg
Dopamine	Infusion	2–20 µg/kg/min
Droperidol	IV	50–75 µg/kg
Edrophonium	Depends on degree of paralysis (IV)	0.5–1 mg/kg
Ephedrine	IV	0.1–0.3 mg/kg
Epinephrine	IV bolus	0.01 mg/kg
	Endotracheal dose	0.1 mg/kg
	Infusion	0.1–1.0 µg/kg/min
Famotidine	IV	0.15 mg/kg

(*continued*)

Table 44–3. Pediatric drug dosages. (continued)

Drug	Comment	Dosage*
Fentanyl	Pain relief (IV)	1–2 μg/kg
	Pain relief (Intranasal)	2 μg/kg
	Premedication (Oralet)	10–15 μg/kg
	Anesthetic adjunct (IV)	1–5 μg/kg
	Maintenance infusion	2–4 μg/kg/h
	Main anesthetic (IV)	50–100 μg/kg
Flumazinil	IV	0.1 mg/kg
Furosemide	IV	0.2–1 mg/kg
Glucose	IV	0.5–1 g/kg
Glucagon	IV	0.5–1 mg
Glycopyrrolate	IV	0.01 mg/kg
Hydrocortisone	IV	1 mg/kg
Hydromorphone	IV	15–20 μg/kg
Insulin	Infusion	0.02–0.1 U/kg/h
Isoproterenol	Infusion	0.1–1 μg/kg/min
Ketamine	Induction (IV)	1–2 mg/kg
	(IM)	6–10 mg/kg
	(per rectum)	10 mg/kg
	Maintenance infusion	25–75 μg/kg/min
	Premedication (PO)	6–10 mg/kg
Ketorolac	IV	0.5–0.75 mg/kg
Labetalol	IV	0.25 mg/kg
Lidocaine	Loading	1 mg/kg
	Maintenance	20–50 μg/kg/min
Magnesium	IV (slowly)	25–50 mg/kg
	Maximum single dose	2 g
Mannitol	IV	0.25–1 g/kg
Meperidine	Pain relief (IV)	0.2–0.5 mg/kg
	Premedication (IM)	1 mg/kg
Methohexital	Induction (IV)	1–2 mg/kg
	(per rectum)	25–30 mg/kg
	(IM)	10 mg/kg
Methylprednisolone	IV	2–4 mg/kg
Metoclopramide	IV	0.15 mg/kg
Midazolam	Premedication (PO)	0.5 mg/kg
	Maximum dose	20 mg
	Sedation (IM)	0.1–0.15 mg/kg
	Maximum dose	7.5 mg
Milrinone	Loading (IV)	50–70 μg/kg
	Maintenance	0.5–0.75 μg/kg/min
Mivacurium	Intubation (IV)	0.2–0.3 mg/kg
	Infusion	3–24 μg/kg/min
Morphine	Pain relief (IV)	0.02–0.05 mg/kg
	Premedication (IM)	0.1 mg/kg
Naloxone	IV	0.01 mg/kg
Neostigmine	Depends on degree of paralysis (IV)	0.04–0.07 mg/kg
Nitroprusside	Infusion	0.5–8 μg/kg/min
Norepinephrine	Infusion	0.1–2 μg/kg/min
Ondansetron	IV	0.1 mg/kg
Pentobarbital	Premedication (IM)	4–6 mg/kg
Phenobarbital	Sedation (IV or IM)	1–3 mg/kg
	Anticonvulsant dose (IV)	5–20 mg/kg

(continued)

Table 44–3. Pediatric drug dosages. (continued)

Drug	Comment	Dosage*
Phentolamine	IV	30 μg/kg
Phenylephrine	IV	1–2 μg/kg
Phenytoin	Slowly IV	5–20 mg/kg
Physostigmine	IV	0.01–0.3 mg/kg
Procainamide	Loading dose (IV)	15 mg/kg
Propanolol	IV	10–25 μg/kg
Propofol	Induction (IV)	2–3 mg/kg
	Maintenance infusion	60–300 μg/kg/min
Prostaglandin E₁	Infusion	0.05–0.1 μg/kg/min
Ranitidine	IV	0.25–1.0 mg/kg
Rocuronium	Intubation (IV)	0.6–1.2 mg/kg
Sodium bicarbonate	IV	1 mEq/kg
Succinylcholine	Intubation (IV)	2–3 mg/kg
	(IM)	4–6 mg/kg
Sufentanil	Premedication (Intranasal)	2 μg/kg
	Anesthetic adjunct (IV)	1–2 μg/kg
	Maintenance infusion	1–3 μg/kg/h
	Main anesthetic (IV)	10–15 μg/kg
Thipental	Induction (IV)	5–6 mg/kg
	(per rectum)	25–30 mg/kg
Verapamil	IV	0.1–0.3 mg/kg

*Dosages are for intravenous administration if not otherwise specified.

and adults for halogenated agents (Table 44–4); nitrous oxide may not contribute significantly to the MAC of desflurane as it does for other agents. The blood pressure of neonates and infants tends to be more sensitive to volatile anesthetics, probably because of undeveloped compensatory mechanisms (eg, vasoconstriction, tachycardia) and exaggerated myocardial depression. Prepubertal children are at much less risk for halothane-induced hepatic dysfunction than are adults. As with adults, halothane sensitizes the heart to catecholamines; the maximum recommended dose of epinephrine in local anesthetic solutions is 10 μg/kg. Sevoflurane and desflurane may be associated with an increased incidence of agitation or delirium upon emergence, especially in young children.

Nonvolatile Anesthetics

Some barbiturates and opioids appear to be more potent in neonates than in adults. Possible explanations include easier entry across the blood-brain barrier, decreased metabolic capability, or increased sensitivity of the respiratory centers. Morphine sulfate should be used with caution, if at all, in neonates because hepatic conjugation is reduced and renal clearance of morphine metabolites is decreased. In contrast, neonates and infants appear to be more resistant to the effects of ketamine. The cytochrome P-450 pathway is mature at 1 month. Pediatric patients have relatively high rates of biotransformation and elimination as a result of high hepatic blood flow. Sufentanil, alfentanil and, possibly, fentanyl clearances may be higher in children than in adults. Because of higher volume distribution and increased clearances for propofol, children may require significantly higher rates (150–250 μg/kg/min) of infusion during total intravenous anesthesia.

Table 44–4. Approximate MAC values for pediatric patients.*

Agent	Neonates	Infants	Small Children	Adults
Halothane	0.87	1.1–1.2	0.87	0.75
Sevoflurane	3.2	3.2	2.5	2.0
Isoflurane	1.60	1.8–1.9	1.3–1.6	1.2
Desflurane	8–9	9–10	7–8	6.0

MAC = minimum alveolar concentration.
*Values are derived from various sources.

Muscle Relaxants

⑦ Children are more susceptible than adults to cardiac arrhythmias, hyperkalemia, rhabdomyolysis, myoglobinemia, masseter spasm, and malignant hyperthermia after succinylcholine administration. If a child unexpectedly experiences cardiac arrest following succinylcholine administration, immediate treatment for hyperkalemia should be instituted. Prolonged and heroic (eg, cardiopulmonary bypass) resuscitative efforts may be required. For this reason, succinylcholine is best avoided for routine elective surgery in children and adolescents. Generally accepted indications for succinylcholine in children are rapid-sequence induction with a full stomach, laryngospasm, and rapid muscle relaxation prior to intravenous access.

⑧ Unlike in adult patients, profound bradycardia and sinus node arrest develop in pediatric patients following the first dose of succinylcholine without atropine pretreatment. Infants require higher doses of succinylcholine (2 mg/kg) than adults because of a relatively larger volume of distribution (extracellular space). This discrepancy disappears if dosage is based on body surface area.

Rocuronium (0.6 mg/kg) has become the drug of choice for routine intubation in pediatric patients with intravenous access (see Chapter 9). Higher doses of rocuronium (0.9–1.2 mg/kg) may be used for rapid-sequence induction but a prolonged duration (up to 90 minutes) should be expected. Rapacuronium* (1.5–2.0 mg/kg) has also been recommended for rapid-sequence induction because of its shorter latency and duration. Some clinicians feel that the only pediatric indication for succinylcholine is its intramuscular administration (4–6 mg/kg) for immediately securing the airway in a patient without intravenous access. In this situation, atropine (0.02 mg/kg IM) should precede the succinylcholine to prevent bradycardia. Rocuronium can be given intramuscularly (1.0–1.5 mg/kg) but requires 3–4 minutes for onset.

The response of neonates to nondepolarizing muscle relaxants is quite variable. Immaturity of the neuromuscular junction (particularly in premature neonates) tends to increase sensitivity, while a disproportionately large extracellular compartment dilutes drug concentration. Duration of action will be prolonged in neonates if the drug depends on hepatic metabolism (eg, vecuronium). In contrast, atracurium does not depend on hepatic biotransformation and has a shorter duration of effect in infants. Mivacurium, atracurium and cisatracurium may be the preferred agents in neonates. As with adults, the effect of incremental doses of muscle relaxant should be monitored with a peripheral nerve stimulator. Nondepolarizing blockade can be reversed with neostigmine (up to 70 µg/kg) or edrophonium (1 mg/kg) along with an anticholinergic agent.

PEDIATRIC ANESTHETIC TECHNIQUES

Preoperative Considerations

A. Preoperative Interview:

Depending on age, past surgical experiences, and maturity, children suffer from varying degrees of terror when faced with the prospect of surgery. In contrast to adults, who are usually most concerned about the possibility of death, children are principally worried about pain and separation from their parents. Presurgical preparation programs—such as brochures, videos, or tours—can be very helpful in preparing many children and parents. Unfortunately, outpatient and morning-of-admission surgery together with a busy operating room schedule, often make it difficult for an anesthesiologist to have enough time to break through the barriers erected by pediatric patients. For this reason, premedication (below) can be extremely helpful. A key strategy is to demystify the process of anesthesia and surgery by explaining in age-appropriate terms what lies ahead. For example, one might bring an anesthesia mask for the child to play with during the interview and describe it as something the astronauts use. Alternatively, in some centers, someone who the child trusts (eg, a parent, nurse, other physician) may be allowed in attendance during preanesthetic preparations and induction of anesthesia. This can have a particularly calming influence on children undergoing repeated procedures (eg, examination under anesthesia following glaucoma surgery).

B. Recent Upper Respiratory Tract Infection:

Children frequently present for surgery with evidence—a runny nose with fever, cough, or sore throat—of a coincidental viral upper respiratory tract infection (URTI). Attempts should be made to differentiate between an infectious cause of rhinorrhea and an allergic or vasomotor cause. A viral infection within 2–4 weeks before general anesthesia and endotracheal intubation appears to place the child at an increased risk for perioperative pulmonary complications, such as wheezing (10-fold), laryngospasm (5-fold), hypoxemia, and atelectasis. This is especially likely if the child has a severe cough, high fever, or a family history of reactive airway disease. The decision to anesthetize children with URTIs remains controversial and depends on the presence of other coexisting illnesses, the severity of URTI

---

* At the time of publication, rapacuronium had been voluntarily withdrawn by the manufacturer. See Chapter 9 for details.

symptoms, and the urgency of the surgery. If surgery cannot be deferred, consideration should be given to an anticholinergic premedication, mask ventilation, humidification of inspired gases, and a longer-than-usual stay in the recovery room.

C. LABORATORY TESTS:

Few, if any, preoperative laboratory results have been deemed cost-effective. Some pediatric centers require *no* preoperative laboratory tests in *healthy* children undergoing *minor* procedures. Obviously, this places more responsibility on the anesthesiologist, surgeon, and pediatrician to correctly identify those patients who should have preoperative testing for specific surgical procedures.

D. PREOPERATIVE FASTING:

Because pediatric patients are more prone to dehydration, their preoperative fluid restriction has always been more lenient. Several studies, however, have documented low gastric pH (< 2.5) and relatively high residual volumes in pediatric patients scheduled for surgery, suggesting that children may be at a higher risk for aspiration than previously thought. The incidence of aspiration is reported to be approximately 1:1000. Prolonged fasting does not necessarily decrease this risk. In fact, several studies have demonstrated lower residual volumes and higher gastric pH in pediatric patients who received clear fluids a few hours before induction. Depending on age, regular formula feedings or solid foods are continued until 4–8 hours before surgery. More specifically, infants younger than 6 months are fed formula up to 4 hours before induction, while infants 6 to 36 months of age can be given formula or solids up to 6 hours before induction. Clear fluids are offered until 2–3 hours before induction. These recommendations are for healthy neonates, infants, and children without risk factors for decreased gastric emptying or aspiration.

E. PREMEDICATION:

There is great variation in the recommendations for premedication of pediatric patients. Sedative premedication is generally omitted for neonates and sick infants. Children who appear likely to exhibit uncontrollable separation anxiety can be given a sedative, such as midazolam (0.3–0.5 mg/kg). The oral route is generally preferred because it is less traumatic than intramuscular injection but requires 20–45 minutes for effect. Smaller doses of midazolam may be used with the addition of oral ketamine (4–6 mg/kg), but the combination may not be suitable for outpatients. For uncooperative patients, intramuscular midazolam (0.1–0.15 mg/kg) and/or ketamine (2–3 mg/kg) may be helpful. Rectal methohexital (25–30 mg/kg of 10% solution) may also

be administered in such cases while the child is in the parent's arms. The nasal route can be used with some drugs (eg, ketamine 3–6 mg/kg, midazolam 0.2 mg/kg, sufentanil 1–2 µg/kg) but is unpleasant, and some concerns exist over toxicity of midazolam. Fentanyl can also be administered as a lollipop (Oralet 5–15 µg/kg); fentanyl levels continue to rise intraoperatively and can contribute to postoperative analgesia. Older agents such as chloral hydrate and pentobarbital are rarely used. Other premedication considerations are discussed in the case study presented in Chapter 8.

Many anesthesiologists routinely premedicate young children with anticholinergic drugs (eg, atropine 0.02 mg/kg) to lessen the likelihood of bradycardia during induction. Atropine reduces the incidence of hypotension during induction in neonates and infants less than 3 months. Atropine can also prevent accumulation of secretions that can be life threatening in small airways and endotracheal tubes. Secretions can especially be problematic for patients with URTIs or those who have been given ketamine. Atropine is often administered orally (0.05 mg/kg), intramuscularly, or occasionally rectally. Many anesthesiologists prefer to give atropine intravenously at or shortly after induction.

Monitoring

Monitoring requirements for infants and children are generally similar to adults with some minor modifications. Alarm limits should be appropriately adjusted. Smaller electrocardiographic electrode pads may be necessary so that they do not encroach on sterile surgical areas. Blood pressure cuffs must be properly fitted (see Figure 6–10). Noninvasive blood pressure monitors have proved to very reliable. A precordial stethoscope provides an inexpensive means of monitoring heart rate, quality of heart sounds, and airway patency.

Small pediatric patients have a smaller allowable margin of error. Pulse oximetry and capnography assume an even greater monitoring role in pediatric patients because hypoxia from inadequate ventilation is a major cause of perioperative morbidity and mortality in pediatric patients. In neonates, the pulse oximeter probe should preferably be placed on the right hand or ear lobe to measure preductal oxygen saturation. End-tidal CO_2 analysis allows assessment of the adequacy of ventilation, confirmation of endotracheal tube placement, and early warning of malignant hyperthermia. Nonetheless, the small tidal volumes and rapid respiratory rates of small infants can present difficulties with some capnograph models. Flow-through (mainstream) analyzers are usually less accurate in patients weighing less than 10 kg. Even with aspiration (sidestream) capnographs, the inspired (baseline) CO_2 can appear falsely elevated and the expired (peak) CO_2 can be

PROFILES IN ANESTHETIC PRACTICE

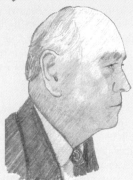

John F. Ryan, MD, MEd

Heart Rate Response to Surgical Incision in Children

In addressing the question of cardiac arrest in children and especially infants, the traditional hallmark of etiology (as repetitious as the realtors' cry: location, location, location) has been airway, airway, airway. However, a recent compilation by the Society of Pediatric Anesthesia[1,2] has identified a different cause—an overdose of anesthetic drugs—as the most frequent one in cardiac arrest. A review of vol-

untarily submitted cases in the past decade shows that an inappropriate level of anesthesia is the prime etiologic factor.

How do we know the status of our patients while they are anesthetized? One way is to monitor inspired and expired concentrations of inhalational gases. However, this information does not tell us anything about a child's or infant's dose–response curve. How do we know whether we are near the level of marked depression of the myocardium? One of the truest of facts regarding children is that variability of response to administered drugs is predominant. For muscle relaxants, for example, the variability of dose response is widest in the youngest patients. For inhalational drugs the mean anesthetic concentrations change with age and variability is still a constant phenomenon. In other words, some children will need one quarter minimum alveolar concentration (MAC), and some will need one MAC to obtain satisfactory but not deep levels of reflex suppression.

One clinically notable event that can help us derive a dose–response curve for general inhalational anesthetics is to assess the response of the infant or

falsely low. The degree of error depends on many factors but can be minimized by placing the sampling site as close as possible to the tip of the endotracheal tube, using a short length of sampling line, and lowering gas-sampling flow rates (100–150 mL/min). Furthermore, the size of some flow-through sensors may lead to kinking of the endotracheal tube or hypercapnia as a result of increased equipment dead space.

Temperature must be closely monitored in pediatric patients because of their higher risk for malignant hyperthermia and the potential for both iatrogenic hypothermia and hyperthermia. There are several ways to prevent hypothermia, including maintaining a warm operating room environment (26 °C or higher), warming and humidifying inspired gases, using a warming blanket and warming lights, and warming all intravenous fluids. The room temperature required for a neutral thermal environment varies with age; it is highest in premature newborns. Note that care must be taken to prevent unintentional skin burns and iatrogenic hyperthermia from overzealous warming efforts.

Invasive monitoring (eg, arterial cannulation, central venous catheterization) requires considerable expertise. Pulmonary artery catheters are usually not used in pediatric patients because of the predictable relationship between right- and left-sided filling pressures in most patients. The right radial artery is often chosen for cannulation in the neonate because its preductal location mirrors the oxygen content of the carotid and retinal arteries. Urinary output is an important measure of volume status.

Neonates who are premature or small for gestational age, have received hyperalimentation, or whose mothers are diabetic may be prone to hypoglycemia. All these infants should have frequent serum glucose determinations. Hypoglycemia is defined as < 30 mg/dL in the neonate and < 40 mg/dL in older children.

Induction

General anesthesia is usually induced by an intravenous or inhalational technique. Induction with intramuscular ketamine (5–10 mg/kg) is reserved for specific situa-

child to the initial surgical incision. Over the years I have noted that if the heart rate of an infant or child does not increase following the first stroke of the knife then for this patient the level of anesthesia is too deep. This does not mean that we should have our patients so lightly anesthetized that they move or that their pulse increases dramatically with a concomitant increase in blood pressure. It does mean that we utilize the reaction of either no change or an increase in heart rate at incision. A modest rise in heart rate that subsides over the next minute or so suggests that the depth of anesthesia is adequate. If the heart rate does not change with incision, it is a good sign that the anesthetic depth is excessive. If this is the case, I recommend a gradual decrease in inspired concentration of volatile anesthetic by 0.1% every 10 minutes until an increase in heart rate is elicited. This strategy makes each anesthetic not just an automatic pilot event but a tailored pharmacologic exercise. This practice is not only safer for infants and children, since we are developing a dose–response curve in real time, but it rewards us with the joy of using our pharmacologic and physiologic expertise.

There is a well-known, direct relationship between heart rate and cardiac output in children.[3,4] This does not mean that every increase in heart rate is effica-cious. For example, as the myocardium is depressed by a relative overdose of anesthetic, the heart of a child will respond by initially attempting to maintain a normal cardiac output by increasing its rate of beating. This is often seen prior to the bradycardia and hypotension that presage a cardiac arrest. However, this special circumstance aside, the reaction of the heart rate to surgical incision has been a valuable guide for me in avoiding levels of anesthesia that would lead to myocardial depression.

1. Morray JP, Geiduschek JM, Caplan RA, et al: A comparison of pediatric and adult anesthesia closed malpractice claims. Anesthesiology 1993;78:461–467.

(http://www/depts.washington.edu/asaccp/POCA/anesth78 461.shtml)

2. Morray JP, Geiduschek JM, Ramamoorthy MB, et al: Anesthesia-related cardiac arrest in children. Anesthesiology 2000;93:6–14.

3. Southhall DP, Richards JM, Johnston PGB, Shinebourne EA: Study of cardiac rhythm in healthy newborn infants. Br Heart J 1979;41:382.

4. DeSwiet M, Fayers P, Swinebourne EA: Systolic blood pressure in a population of infants in the first year of life: The Brompton Study. Pediatrics 1979;65: 1028–1035.

tions, such as those involving combative children. Intravenous induction is preferred if the patient comes to the operating room with an intravenous catheter or is cooperative enough to allow awake venous cannulation. Prior application of EMLA (eutectic [easily melted] mixture of local anesthetic) cream (see Chapter 14) may make intravenous cannulation less stressful for the patient, parent, and anesthesiologist. EMLA cream is not a perfect solution, however. Some children become very anxious at the mere sight of a needle, especially those who have had multiple needle punctures in the past. Furthermore, it can be difficult to anticipate in which extremity intravenous cannulation will prove to be successful. Finally, in order to be effective, EMLA cream must remain in contact with the skin for at least 1 hour.

IV Induction

The same induction sequence can be used as in adults: a rapid-acting barbiturate (eg, thiopental, 3 mg/kg in neonates, 5–6 mg/kg in infants and children) or propofol (2–3 mg/kg) followed by a nondepolarizing muscle relaxant (eg, rapacuronium,* rocuronium, atracurium, mivacurium, or succinylcholine). Atropine should be given intravenously prior to succinylcholine. Propofol may be associated with less hypertension during intubation, faster awakening, and less postoperative nausea and vomiting. The advantages of an intravenous technique include familiarity with the agents, availability of intravenous access if emergency drugs need to be administered, and rapidity of induction in the child at risk for aspiration.

Inhalational Induction

Most children do not arrive in the operating room with an intravenous line in place and dread the prospect of being stuck with a needle. Fortunately, modern potent volatile anesthetics can render small children uncon-

---

* At the time of publication, rapacuronium had been voluntarily withdrawn by the manufacturer. See Chapter 9 for details.

scious within minutes. This is usually easier in children who have been sedated prior to entering the operating room and who are sleepy enough to be anesthetized without ever knowing what has happened (**steal induction**). Alternatives to frightening a child with a black mask include insufflation of the anesthetic gases over the face, substituting a clear face mask, placing a drop of food flavoring on the inside of the mask (eg, oil of orange), and allowing the child to sit during the early stages of induction. Specially contoured masks minimize dead space (see Figure 5–7).

There are many differences between adult and pediatric anatomy that affect mask ventilation and intubation. Equipment appropriate for age and size should be selected (Table 44–5). Neonates and most young infants are obligate nasal breathers and obstruct easily. Oral airways often help displace an oversized tongue, while nasal airways can traumatize small nares or prominent adenoids. Compression of submandibular soft tissues should be avoided during mask ventilation to prevent upper airway obstruction.

Typically, the child is coaxed into breathing an odorless mixture of nitrous oxide (70%) and oxygen (30%). Sevoflurane or halothane is added to the anesthetic gas mixture in 0.5% increments every 3–5 breaths. Desflurane and isoflurane are more pungent and are associated with more coughing, breath-holding, and laryngospasm during an inhalational induction. Some clinicians use a single breath induction technique with sevoflurane (7–8% sevoflurane in 60% nitrous oxide) to speed up induction. After an adequate depth of anesthesia has been achieved, an intravenous line can be started and a muscle relaxant administered. Patients typically pass through an excitement stage during

which any stimulation can induce laryngospasm. Breath holding must be distinguished from laryngospasm. Steady application of 10 cm of positive end-expiratory pressure can help overcome laryngospasm. Alternatively, the anesthesiologist can deepen the level of anesthesia by increasing the concentration of volatile anesthetic, and place a laryngeal mask airway (LMA) or, less commonly, intubating the patient without a muscle relaxant. Because greater anesthetic depth is required for tracheal intubation with the latter technique, the possibility of severe cardiac depression, bradycardia, or laryngospasm occurring without intravenous access detracts from this technique. Intramuscular succinylcholine (4–6 mg/kg, not to exceed 150 mg) and atropine (0.02 mg/kg, not to exceed 0.4 mg) should be available if laryngospasm or bradycardia occurs before an intravenous line is established.

Positive pressure ventilation during mask induction and prior to intubation sometimes causes gastric distention, resulting in impairment of lung expansion. Suctioning with an orogastric or nasogastric tube will decompress the stomach, but it must be done without traumatizing fragile mucous membranes.

IV Access

Cannulation of tiny pediatric veins can be a trying ordeal. This is particularly true for infants who have spent weeks in a neonatal intensive care unit and have few veins left unscarred. Even healthy 1-year-old children can prove a challenge because of extensive subcutaneous fat. The saphenous vein has a consistent location at the ankle and, with experience, the practitioner can usually cannulate it even if it is not visible or palpable. Twenty-

Table 44–5. Airway equipment for pediatric patients.

	Premature	Neonate	Infant	Toddler	Small Child	Large Child
Age	0–1 month	0–1 month	1–12 months	1–3 years	3–8 years	8–12 years
Weight (kg)	0.5–3	3–5	4–10	8–16	14–30	25–50
Tracheal (ET) tube (mm ID)	2.5–3	3–3.5	3.5–4	4–4.5	4.5–5.5	5.5–6 (cuffed)
ET depth (cm at lips)	6–9	9–10	10–12	12–14	14–16	16–18
Suction catheter (F)	6	6	8	8	10	12
Laryngoscope blade	00	0	1	1.5	2	3
Mask size	00	0	0	1	2	3
Oral airway	000–00	00	0 (40 mm)	1 (50 mm)	2 (70 mm)	3 (80 mm)
Laryngeal mask airway (LMA#)	–	1	1	2	2.5	3

ET = endotracheal tube.

four-gauge over-the-needle catheters are adequate in neonates and infants when blood transfusions are not anticipated. All air bubbles should be removed from the intravenous line, since a high incidence of patent foramen ovale increases the risk of **paradoxical air embolism.** In emergency situations where intravenous access is impossible, fluids can be effectively infused through an 18-gauge needle inserted into the medullary sinusoids within the tibial bone. This **intraosseous infusion** can be used for all medications normally given intravenously with virtually as rapid results (see Chapter 48).

Tracheal Intubation

Following inhalational induction, nitrous oxide should be discontinued prior to intubation so that the patient's lungs will contain a high inspired oxygen concentration that allows adequate arterial oxygen saturation during this period of apnea. The choice of muscle relaxant is discussed above.

A prominent occiput tends to place the head in a flexed position prior to intubation. This is easily corrected by slightly elevating the shoulders with towels and placing the head on a doughnut-shaped pillow. In older children, prominent adenoidal and tonsillar tissue can obstruct visualization of the larynx. Straight laryngoscope blades aid intubation of the anterior larynx in infants and young children. Endotracheal tubes that pass through the glottis may still impinge upon the cricoid cartilage; the cricoid cartilage is the narrowest point of the airway in children younger than 5 years of age. Mucosal trauma from trying to force a tube through the cricoid cartilage can cause postoperative edema, stridor, croup, and airway obstruction. Uncuffed endotracheal tubes are usually selected for children between the ages of 8 and 10 years in order to decrease the risk of postintubation croup and to provide a leak to minimize the risk of accidental barotrauma.

The appropriate diameter of inside the endotracheal tube can be estimated by a formula based on age:

$$4 + Age/4 = Tube\ diameter\ (in\ mm)$$

For example, a 4-year-old child would be predicted to require a 5-mm tube. This formula provides only a rough guideline, however. Exceptions include premature neonates (a 2.5–3 mm tube) and full-term neonates (a 3–3.5 mm tube). Endotracheal tubes 0.5 mm larger and smaller than predicted should be readily available. Correct tube size is confirmed by easy passage into the larynx and the development of a gas leak at 15–20 cm H_2O pressure. No leak indicates an oversized tube that should be replaced to prevent postoperative edema, while an excessive leak may preclude adequate

ventilation and contaminate the operating room with anesthetic gases. There is also a formula to estimate endotracheal length:

$$12 + Age/2 = Length\ of\ tube\ (in\ cm)$$

Again, this formula provides only a guideline, and the result must be confirmed by auscultation and clinical judgment. To avoid endobronchial intubation, the tip of the endotracheal tube should pass only 1–2 cm beyond an infant's glottis. An alternative technique is to intentionally place the tip of the endotracheal tube into the right main-stem bronchus and then withdraw it until breath sounds are equal.

Maintenance

Ventilation is usually controlled during anesthesia of neonates and infants. During spontaneous ventilation, even the low resistance of a circle system can become a significant obstacle for a sick neonate to overcome. Unidirectional valves, breathing tubes, and absorbers account for most of this resistance. For patients weighing less than 10 kg, some anesthesiologists prefer the Mapleson D circuit or the Bain system because of their low resistance and light weight (see Chapter 3). Nonetheless, because breathing-circuit resistance is easily overcome by positive pressure ventilation, the circle system can be safely used in patients of all ages if ventilation is controlled.

Airway pressure monitoring may provide early evidence of obstruction caused by a kinked endotracheal tube or advancement of the tube into a main-stem bronchus. Many anesthesia ventilators designed for adult patients, however, cannot reliably provide the low tidal volumes and rapid rates required by neonates and infants. Unintentional delivery of large tidal volumes to a small child can generate enormous peak airway pressures and cause extensive barotrauma.

Small tidal volumes can be manually delivered with greater sensitivity with a 1-L breathing bag than with a 3-L adult bag. For children < 10 kg, adequate tidal volumes are achieved with peak inspiratory pressures of 15–18 cm H_2O. For larger children, tidal volumes may set at 8–10 mL/kg. Most spirometers are less accurate at lower tidal volumes. In addition, the gas lost in long, highly compliant breathing circuits becomes quite significant relative to a child's small tidal volume. For this reason, pediatric tubing is usually shorter and stiffer (less compliant). Equipment dead space, a critical determinant of rebreathing in children, is minimized by a septum that divides the inspiratory and expiratory gas in the Y-piece.

Anesthesia is maintained in pediatric patients with the same agents as in adults. Although the MAC is higher in children than in adults (see Table 44–4), neonates may be particularly susceptible to the cardiodepressant effects of general anesthetics. Nondepolarizing muscle relaxants are often required for optimal surgical conditions; this is especially true in neonates and sick infants who may not tolerate higher doses of volatile agents.

Perioperative Fluid Requirements

 Meticulous fluid management is required in small pediatric patients because of extremely limited margins of error. A programmable infusion pump or a buret with a microdrip chamber should be used for accurate measurements. Drugs are flushed through low dead-space tubing to minimize unnecessary fluid administration. Fluid overload is diagnosed by prominent veins, flushed skin, increased blood pressure, decreased serum sodium, and a loss of the folds in the upper eyelids.

Fluid therapy can be divided into maintenance, deficit, and replacement requirements.

A. MAINTENANCE FLUID REQUIREMENTS:

Maintenance requirements for pediatric patients can be determined by the formula presented in Chapter 29, the 4:2:1 rule: 4 mL/kg/hour for the first 10 kg of weight; 2 mL/kg/hour for the second 10 kg; and 1 mL/kg/hour for each remaining kg. The choice of maintenance fluid remains controversial. A solution such as $D_5\frac{1}{2}NS$ with 20 mEq/L of potassium chloride provides adequate dextrose and electrolytes at these maintenance infusion rates. $D_5\frac{1}{4}NS$ may be a better choice in neonates because of their limited ability to handle sodium loads.

B. DEFICITS:

In addition to a maintenance infusion, any preoperative fluid deficits must be replaced. For example, if a 5-kg infant has not received oral or intravenous fluids for 4 hours prior to surgery, a deficit of 80 mL has accrued (5 kg × 4 mL/kg/hour × 4 hours). In contrast to adults, infants respond to dehydration with decreased blood pressure but without increased heart rate. Preoperative fluid deficits are typically administered with hourly maintenance requirements in aliquots of 50% in the first hour and 25% in the second and third hours. In the example above, a total of 60 mL would be given the first hour (80/2 + 20), and 40 mL in the second and third hours (80/4 + 20). Large quantities of dextrose-containing solutions are avoided to prevent hyperglycemia. Preoperative fluid deficits are usually replaced with a balanced salt solution (eg, lactated Ringer's injection) or ½ normal saline. Compared with lactated Ringer's injection, normal saline has the disadvantage of promoting hyperchloremic acidosis.

C. REPLACEMENT REQUIREMENTS:

Replacement can be subdivided into blood loss and third-space loss.

1. Blood loss—The blood volume of premature neonates (100 mL/kg), full-term neonates (85–90 mL/kg), and infants (80 mL/kg) is proportionately higher than that of adults (65–75 mL/kg). An initial hematocrit of 55% in the healthy full-term neonate gradually falls to as low as 30% in the 3-month-old infant before rising to 35% by 6 months. Hemoglobin (Hb) type is also changing during this period: from a 75% concentration of HbF (high oxygen affinity, low PaO_2, poor tissue unloading) at birth to almost 100% HbA (low oxygen affinity, high PaO_2, good tissue unloading) by 6 months.

Blood loss is typically replaced with nonglucose-containing crystalloid (eg, 3 mL of lactated Ringer's injection for each mL of blood lost) or colloid solutions (eg, 1 mL of 5% albumin per mL of blood lost) until the patient's hematocrit reaches a predetermined lower limit. In premature and sick neonates, this may be as high as 40% or 50%, while in healthy older children a hematocrit of 20–26% is generally well tolerated. Because of their small intravascular volume, neonates and infants are at an increased risk for electrolyte disturbances (eg, hyperglycemia, hyperkalemia, and hypocalcemia) that can accompany rapid blood transfusion. Dosing of packed red blood cell transfusions is discussed in Chapter 29. Platelets and fresh frozen plasma 10–15 mL/kg should be given when blood loss exceeds 1–2 blood volumes. One unit of platelets per 10 kg weight raises the platelet count by about 50,000/μL. The pediatric dose of cryoprecipitate is 1 U/10 kg weight.

2. Third-space loss—such losses are impossible to measure and must be estimated by the extent of the surgical procedure. One popular guideline is 0–2 mL/kg/hour for relatively atraumatic surgery (eg, strabismus correction) and up to 6–10 mL/kg/hour for traumatic procedures (eg, abdominal abscess). Third-space loss is usually replaced with lactated Ringer's injection (see Chapter 29).

Regional Anesthesia

The primary uses of regional techniques in pediatric anesthesia has been to supplement and lower general anesthetic requirements and provide good postoperative pain relief. The complexity of blocks range from the relatively simple peripheral nerve blocks described in Chapter 17 (eg, penile block, ilioinguinal block) to major conduction blocks (eg, spinal anesthesia).

Caudal blocks have proved useful in a variety of surgeries, including circumcision, inguinal herniorrhaphy, hypospadias repair, anal surgery, clubfoot repair, and other subumbilical procedures. Contraindications include infection around the sacral hiatus, coagulopathy, or anatomic abnormalities. The patient is usually lightly anesthetized or sedated and placed in the lateral position.

The technique of caudal anesthesia for adults is described in Chapter 16. For pediatric caudal anesthesia, a short bevel 22-gauge needle can be used. Loss of resistance should be assessed with saline, not air, because of the latter's possible association with hemodynamically significant air embolism. After the characteristic "pop" that signals penetration of the sacrococcygeal membrane, the needle is lowered and advanced only a few more millimeters to avoid entering the dural sac or the anterior body of the sacrum. Aspiration is used to check for blood or cerebrospinal fluid; local anesthetic can then be slowly injected; a 2-mL test dose of local anesthetic with epinephrine (1:200,000) helps exclude intravascular placement.

Many anesthetic agents have been used for caudal anesthesia in pediatric patients, with 1% lidocaine and 0.125–0.25% bupivacaine being most common. Ropivacaine 0.2% can provide analgesia similar to bupivacaine but with less motor blockade. Morphine sulfate (25 μg/kg) or hydromorphone (6 μg/kg) may be added to the local anesthetic solution to prolong postoperative analgesia for inpatients but increases the risk of delayed postoperative respiratory depression. The volume of local anesthetic required depends on the level of blockade desired, ranging from 0.5 mL/kg for a sacral block to 1.25 mL/kg for a midthoracic block. Single shot injections generally last 4–12 hours. Placement of 20-gauge caudal catheters with continuous infusion of local anesthetic (eg, 0.125% bupivacaine at 0.2–0.4 mg/kg/hour) or an opioid (eg, fentanyl 2 μg/mL at 0.6 μg/kg/hour) allows prolonged anesthesia and postoperative analgesia. Complications are rare but include local anesthetic toxicity from prolonged continuous infusions or intravascular injection (eg, seizures, hypotension, dysrhythmias), spinal blockade, and respiratory depression. Postoperative urinary retention does not appear to be a problem following single-dose caudal anesthesia.

Emergence & Recovery

Pediatric patients are particularly vulnerable to two postanesthetic complications: laryngospasm and postintubation croup. As with adult patients, postoperative pain should be aggressively managed.

A. LARYNGOSPASM:

Laryngospasm is a forceful, involuntary spasm of laryngeal musculature caused by stimulation of the superior laryngeal nerve (see Chap-

ter 5). It can usually be avoided by extubating the patient either awake (opening the eyes) or while deeply anesthetized (spontaneously breathing but not coughing); both techniques have advocates. Extubation during the interval between these extremes, however, is generally recognized as hazardous. A recent URTI or exposure to secondhand, tobacco smoke predispose patients to laryngospasm on emergence. Treatment of laryngospasm includes gentle positive pressure ventilation, forward jaw thrust, intravenous lidocaine (1–1.5 mg/kg), or paralysis with intravenous succinylcholine (0.5–1 mg/kg) or rocuronium (0.4 mg/kg) and controlled ventilation. Intramuscular succinylcholine (4–6 mg/kg) remains an acceptable alternative in patients without intravenous access and in whom more conservative measures have failed. Laryngospasm is usually an immediate postoperative event but may occur in the recovery room as the patient wakes up and chokes on pharyngeal secretions. For this reason, recovering pediatric patients should be positioned in the lateral position so that oral secretions pool and drain away from the vocal cords. As the child begins to regain consciousness, it is comforting to have the parents at the bedside.

B. POSTINTUBATION CROUP:

Croup is due to glottic or tracheal edema. Because the narrowest part of the pediatric airway is the cricoid cartilage, this is the most susceptible area. Croup is less common with endotracheal tubes that are uncuffed and small enough to allow a slight gas leak at 10–25 cm H_2O. Postintubation croup is associated with early childhood (age 1–4 years), repeated intubation attempts, large endotracheal tubes, prolonged surgery, head and neck procedures, and excessive movement of the tube (eg, coughing with the tube in place, moving the patient's head). Intravenous dexamethasone (0.25–0.5 mg/kg) may prevent edema formation, while inhalation of nebulized racemic epinephrine (0.25–0.5 mL of a 2.25% solution in 2.5 mL normal saline) is effective treatment. Although postintubation croup is a later complication than laryngospasm, it almost always appears within 3 hours after extubation.

C. POSTOPERATIVE PAIN MANAGEMENT:

Pain in pediatric patients has received considerable attention in recent years, especially the use of regional anesthetic techniques (above). Patient-controlled analgesia (see Chapter 18) can also be successfully used in patients as young as 6 years old, depending on their maturity and preoperative preparation. Commonly used parenteral opioids include fentanyl 1–2 μg/kg and meperidine 0.5 mg/kg. Ketorolac (0.75 mg/kg) lowers opioid requirements. Rectal acetaminophen (40 mg/kg) may also be helpful.

■ PATHOPHYSIOLOGY & ANESTHETIC CONSIDERATIONS IN SPECIFIC PEDIATRIC DISORDERS

PREMATURITY

Pathophysiology

Prematurity is defined as birth before 37 weeks of gestation. This is in contrast to "small for gestational age," which describes an infant (full-term or premature) whose age-adjusted weight is less than the fifth percentile. The multiple medical problems of premature neonates are usually due to immaturity of major organ systems or to intrauterine asphyxia. Pulmonary complications include hyaline membrane disease, apneic spells, and bronchopulmonary dysplasia. Exogenous pulmonary surfactant has proved to be an effective treatment for respiratory distress syndrome in premature infants. A patent ductus arteriosus leads to shunting, pulmonary edema, and congestive heart failure. Persistent hypoxia or shock may result in an ischemic gut and necrotizing enterocolitis. Prematurity increases susceptibility to infection, hypothermia, intracranial hemorrhage, and kernicterus. Premature neonates also have an increased incidence of congenital anomalies.

Anesthetic Considerations

The small size (often less than 1000 g) and fragile medical condition of premature neonates demand meticulous anesthetic technique. Obviously, special attention must be paid to airway control, fluid management, and temperature regulation. The problem of the **retinopathy of prematurity,** a fibrovascular proliferation overlying the retina, deserves special consideration. While hyperoxia is associated with this blinding disease, the presence of fetal hemoglobin and treatment with vitamin E may be protective. Oxygenation should be continuously monitored with pulse oximetry or transcutaneous oxygen analysis, with particular attention given to infants younger than 44 weeks postconception. Normal PaO_2 is 60–80 mm Hg in neonates. Excessive inspired oxygen concentrations are avoided by blending oxygen with air or nitrous oxide. Other risk factors associated with the retinopathy of prematurity include multiple blood transfusions, apnea requiring artificial ventilation, parenteral nutrition, hypoxia, hypercapnia, and hypocapnia.

Anesthetic requirements of premature neonates are reduced. Opioid agonists, such as fentanyl, are often fa-

vored over volatile anesthetics because of the latter's tendency to cause myocardial depression. Even nitrous oxide can cause significant cardiovascular depression. Muscle relaxants provide good surgical conditions, and ventilation is controlled.

Premature infants who are less than 50 (some authorities would say 60) weeks postconceptional age at the time of surgery are prone to postoperative episodes of obstructive and central apnea for up to 24 hours. In fact, even term infants can experience—albeit rarely—apneic spells following general anesthesia. Risk factors for postanesthetic apnea include a low gestational age at birth, anemia (< 30%), hypothermia, sepsis, and neurologic abnormalities. The risk of postanesthetic apnea may be decreased by intravenous administration of caffeine (10 mg/kg) or aminophylline.

Nonetheless, elective or outpatient procedures should be deferred until the preterm infant reaches the age of at least 50 weeks postconception. A 6-month symptom-free interval has been suggested for infants with a history of apneic episodes or bronchopulmonary dysplasia. If surgery must be performed earlier, monitoring with pulse oximetry for 12–24 hours postoperatively is mandatory for infants less than 50 weeks postconception; infants between 50 and 60 weeks postconception should be closely observed in the postanesthesia recovery unit for at least 2 hours.

Sick, premature neonates often receive multiple aliquots of blood during their stay in the pediatric intensive care unit. Their immunocompromised status predisposes them to clinically significant cytomegalovirus infection following transfusion. Signs of infection include generalized lymphadenopathy, fever, pneumonia, hepatitis, hemolytic anemia, and thrombocytopenia. Preventive measures include using cytomegalovirus-seronegative donor blood or frozen blood cells.

CONGENITAL DIAPHRAGMATIC HERNIA

Pathophysiology

During fetal development, the gut can herniate into the thorax through one of three possible diaphragmatic defects: the left or right posterolateral foramen of Bochdalek or the anterior foramen of Morgagni. The reported incidence of diaphragmatic hernia is 1 in 5000 live births. Left-sided herniation is the most common type (90%). Hallmarks of **diaphragmatic herniation** include hypoxia, a scaphoid abdomen, and evidence of bowel in the thorax by auscultation or radiography. Congenital diaphragmatic hernia is often diagnosed antenatally as a result of a routine ultrasound examination. A reduction in alveoli and bronchioli (**pulmonary hypoplasia**) and malrotation of the intestines are almost always present. While the ipsilateral lung is especially impaired, the herniated gut can compress and retard the maturation of both lungs. Diaphragmatic hernia is often accompanied by marked pulmonary hypertension and is associated with 40–50% mortality. Cardiopulmonary compromise is generally thought to be primarily due to the pulmonary hypoplasia and hypertension rather than the mass effect of the herniated viscera.

Treatment is aimed at immediate stabilization with sedation, paralysis, and moderate hyperventilation; some centers also employ permissive hypercapnia. If the pulmonary hypertension stabilizes and there is little right-to-left shunting, early surgical repair may be undertaken. If the patient fails to stabilize extracorporeal membrane oxygenation (ECMO) is undertaken. ECMO usually involves pumping blood from the right atrium through a membrane oxygenator and countercurrent heat exchanger before returning it to the ascending aorta (venoarterial ECMO). Alternatively, blood can be returned to the femoral vein (venoveno ECMO). Timing of the repair following ECMO is controversial. Use of nitric oxide, pulmonary surfactant and high-frequency jet ventilation or high frequency oscillation have had limited success in these patients. Treatment with prenatal intrauterine surgery appears promising.

Anesthetic Considerations

Gastric distention must be minimized by placement of a nasogastric tube and avoidance of high levels of positive pressure ventilation. The neonate is preoxygenated and intubated awake, often without the aid of muscle relaxants. Anesthesia is maintained with low concentrations of volatile agents or opioids, muscle relaxants, and air as tolerated. Hypoxia and expansion of air in the bowel contraindicate the use of nitrous oxide. If possible, peak inspiratory airway pressures should be less than 30 cm H_2O. A sudden fall in lung compliance, blood pressure, or oxygenation may signal a *contralateral* (usually right-sided) pneumothorax and necessitate placement of a chest tube. Arterial blood gases are monitored by sampling a preductal artery. Aggressive attempts at expansion of the ipsilateral lung following surgical decompression are detrimental. Postoperative prognosis parallels the extent of pulmonary hypoplasia and the presence of other congenital defects.

TRACHEOESOPHAGEAL FISTULA

Pathophysiology

There are several types of tracheoesophageal fistula (Figure 44–2). The most common (type III B) is the combination of an upper esophagus that ends in a blind pouch and a lower esophagus that connects to the trachea. Breathing results in gastric distention, while feeding leads to choking and coughing. The diagnosis is suspected by failure to pass a catheter into the stomach and confirmed by visualization of the catheter coiled in a blind, upper esophageal pouch. Aspiration pneumonia and the coexistence of other congenital anomalies (eg, cardiac) are common. These may also include the nonrandom association of *v*ertebral defects, *a*nal atresia, *t*racheoesophageal fistula with *e*sophageal atresia, and *r*adial dysplasia, known as the VATER syndrome.

Anesthetic Considerations

These neonates tend to have copious pharyngeal secretions that require frequent suctioning before and dur-

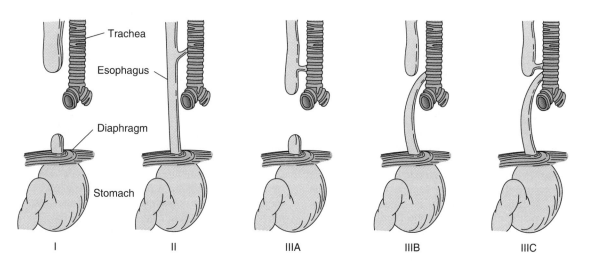

Figure 44–2. Of the five types of tracheoesophageal fistula, type IIIB represents 90% of cases.

ing surgery. Positive pressure ventilation is avoided prior to intubation, since the resulting gastric distention may interfere with lung expansion. Intubation is often performed awake and without muscle relaxants. These neonates are often dehydrated and malnourished due to poor oral intake.

The key to successful management is correct endotracheal tube position. Ideally, the tip of the tube lies between the fistula and the carina, so that anesthetic gases pass into the lungs instead of the stomach. This is impossible if the fistula connects to the carina or a main-stem bronchus. In these situations, intermittent venting of a gastrostomy tube that has been placed preoperatively may permit positive pressure ventilation without excessive gastric distention. Suctioning of the gastrostomy tube and upper esophageal pouch tube helps prevent aspiration pneumonia. Surgical division of the fistula and esophageal anastomosis is performed with the patient in the left lateral position. A precordial stethoscope should be placed in the dependent (left) axilla, since obstruction of the main-stem bronchus during surgical retraction is not uncommon. A drop in oxygen saturation indicates that the retracted lung needs to be reexpanded. Surgical retraction can also compress the great vessels, trachea, heart, and vagus nerve. Blood pressure should be continuously monitored with an arterial line. These infants usually require ventilation with 100% oxygen, despite the risk of the retinopathy of prematurity. Blood should be immediately available for transfusion. Postoperative complications include gastroesophageal reflux, aspiration pneumonia, tracheal compression, and anastomotic leakage. Most patients continue to require intubation and positive pressure ventilation in the immediate postoperative period. Neck extension and instrumentation (eg, suctioning) of the esophagus may disrupt the surgical repair and should be avoided.

GASTROSCHISIS & OMPHALOCELE

Pathophysiology

Gastroschisis and omphalocele are congenital disorders characterized by defects in the abdominal wall that allow external herniation of viscera. Omphaloceles occur at the base of the umbilicus, have a hernia sac and are often associated with other congenital anomalies such as Trisomy 21, diaphragmatic hernia, and cardiac and bladder malformations. In contrast, the gastroschisis defect is usually lateral to the umbilicus, does not have a hernia sac and is often an isolated finding. Antenatal diagnosis by ultrasound can be followed by elective cesarean section at 38 weeks and immediate surgical repair. Perioperative management centers around preventing hypothermia, infection, and dehydration.

These problems are usually more serious in gastroschisis, since the protective hernial sac is absent.

Anesthetic Considerations

The stomach is decompressed with a nasogastric tube before induction. Intubation can be accomplished with the patient awake or asleep and with or without muscle relaxation. Nitrous oxide should be avoided to prevent further bowel distention. Muscle relaxation is required for replacing the bowel into the abdominal cavity. A one-stage closure (primary repair) is not always advisable, since it can decrease pulmonary compliance and reduce blood flow in the lower extremities. Third-space fluid losses are aggressively replaced with a balanced salt solution and 5% albumin. The neonate remains intubated after the procedure and is weaned from the ventilator over the next 1–2 days in the intensive care unit.

PRUNE-BELLY SYNDROME

Pathophysiology

Prune-belly syndrome is caused by agenesis of the abdominal musculature, which results in a thin-walled, protuberant abdomen. Associated anomalies include club feet, cryptorchidism, and other genitourinary tract abnormalities.

Anesthetic Considerations

Patients with prune-belly syndrome have multiple pulmonary complications associated with their inability to cough effectively. They are at risk for aspiration and are often intubated awake. Muscle relaxants are not necessary. If renal anomalies are present, overhydration must be avoided.

HYPERTROPHIC PYLORIC STENOSIS

Pathophysiology

Hypertrophic pyloric stenosis interferes with emptying of gastric contents. Persistent vomiting depletes sodium, potassium, chloride, and hydrogen ions, causing **hypochloremic metabolic alkalosis.** Initially, the kidney tries to compensate for the alkalosis by excreting sodium bicarbonate in the urine. Later, as hyponatremia and dehydration worsen, the kidneys must conserve sodium even at the expense of hydrogen ion excretion (**paradoxic aciduria**). Correction of the volume deficit and metabolic alkalosis requires hydration with a sodium chloride solution supplemented with potassium. Because lactate is metabolized to bicarbonate, lactated Ringer's injection should not be used.

Anesthetic Considerations

Surgery should be postponed until fluid and electrolyte abnormalities have been corrected. The stomach should be emptied with a large nasogastric or orogastric tube. Techniques of intubation and induction may vary, but in all cases one must consider the patient's high risk of aspiration. Pyloromyotomy is a short procedure that requires muscle relaxation. These neonates may be at increased risk for respiratory depression and hypoventilation in the recovery room because of persistent metabolic or cerebrospinal fluid alkalosis.

INFECTIOUS CROUP, FOREIGN BODY ASPIRATION, & ACUTE EPIGLOTTITIS

Pathophysiology

Croup is obstruction of the airway characterized by a barking cough. One type of croup, postintubation croup, has already been discussed. Another type is due to viral infection. **Infectious croup** usually follows a viral, URTI in children aged 3 months to 3 years. The airway *below* the epiglottis is involved (laryngotracheobronchitis). Infectious croup progresses slowly and rarely requires intubation. **Foreign body aspiration** is typically encountered in children aged 6 months to 5 years. Commonly aspirated objects include peanuts, coins, and small pieces of toys. Onset is typically acute and the obstruction may be supraglottic, glottic, or subglottic. Stridor is prominent with the first two, while wheezing is more common with the latter. A clear history of an aspiration may be absent. **Acute epiglottitis** is a bacterial infection (most commonly *Haemophilus influenzae* type B) classically affecting 2- to 6-year-old children. It rapidly progresses from a sore throat to dysphagia and complete airway obstruction. The term supraglottitis has been suggested because the inflammation typically involves all supraglottic structures. Endotracheal intubation and antibiotic therapy can be lifesaving. Epiglottitis has increasing become a disease of adults because of the widespread use of *H influenza* vaccines in children.

Anesthetic Considerations

Patients with croup are managed conservatively with oxygen and mist therapy. Nebulized racemic epinephrine (0.5 mL of a 2.25% solution in 2.5 mL normal saline) and intravenous dexamethasone (0.25–0.5 mg/kg) are used. Indications for intubation include progressive intercostal retractions, obvious respiratory fatigue, and central cyanosis.

Anesthetic management of a foreign body aspiration is challenging, particularly with supraglottic and glottic obstruction. Minor manipulation of the airway can convert partial into complete obstruction. Experts rec-

ommend careful inhalational induction for supraglottic object and gentle upper airway endoscopy to remove the object and/or secure the airway. When the object is subglottic, a rapid-sequence or inhalational induction is followed by prompt endotracheal intubation. Depending on age, flexible or rigid bronchoscopy is then used to remove the object.

Children with impending airway obstruction from epiglottitis present in the operating room for definitive diagnosis by laryngoscopy followed by intubation. A preoperative lateral neck radiograph may show a characteristic thumblike epiglottic shadow, which is very specific but often absent. The radiograph is also helpful in revealing other causes of obstruction, such as foreign bodies. Stridor, drooling, hoarseness, rapid onset and progression, tachypnea, chest retractions, and a preference for the upright position are predictive of airway obstruction. Total obstruction can occur at any moment, and adequate preparations for a possible tracheostomy must be made prior to induction of general anesthesia. Laryngoscopy should not be performed before induction of anesthesia because of the possibility of laryngospasm. In most cases, an inhalational induction is performed with the patient in the sitting position, using a volatile anesthetic and a high concentration of oxygen. Oral intubation with an endotracheal tube one-half to one size smaller than usual is attempted as soon as an adequate depth of anesthesia is established. The oral tube may be replaced with a well-secured nasal endotracheal tube at the end of the procedure, since the latter is better tolerated in the postoperative period. If intubation is impossible, rigid bronchoscopy or emergency tracheostomy must be performed.

TONSILLECTOMY & ADENOIDECTOMY

Pathophysiology

Lymphoid hyperplasia can lead to upper airway obstruction, obligate mouth breathing, and even pulmonary hypertension with cor pulmonale. Although these extremes of pathology are unusual, all children undergoing tonsillectomy or adenoidectomy should be considered to be at increased risk for perioperative airway problems.

Anesthetic Considerations

Surgery should be postponed if there is evidence of acute infection or suspicion of a clotting dysfunction (eg, recent aspirin ingestion). Preoperative administration of an anticholinergic will decrease pharyngeal secretions. A history of airway obstruction or apnea suggests an inhalational induction without paralysis until the ability to ventilate with positive pressure is established. A reinforced or preformed endotracheal tube (eg, RAE tube) lessens the risk of kinking by the surgeon's self-retaining mouth gag. Blood transfusion is usually not necessary, but the anesthesiologist must be wary of occult blood loss. Meticulous but gentle inspection and suctioning of the pharynx precedes extubation. Although deep extubation lessens the chance of laryngospasm and may prevent blood clot dislodgment from coughing, most anesthesiologists prefer an awake extubation because of the risks of aspiration. Postoperative vomiting is common. The anesthesiologist must be alert in the recovery room for postoperative bleeding, which may be evidenced by restlessness, pallor, tachycardia, or hypotension. If reoperation is necessary to control bleeding, intravascular volume must first be restored. Evacuation of stomach contents with a nasogastric tube is followed by a rapid-sequence induction with cricoid pressure. Because of the possibility of bleeding and airway obstruction, children younger than 3 years old are usually hospitalized for the first postoperative night. Sleep apnea and recent infection increase the risk of postoperative complications.

MYRINGOTOMY & INSERTION OF TYMPANOSTOMY TUBES

Pathophysiology

Children presenting for myringotomy and insertion of tympanostomy tubes have a long history of upper respiratory infections that have spread through the eustachian tube, causing episodes of otitis media. Causative organisms are usually bacterial and include *Pneumococcus, H influenza, Streptococcus,* and *Mycoplasma pneumoniae.* Myringotomy, a radial incision in the tympanic membrane, releases any fluid that has accumulated in the middle ear. Tympanostomy tubes provide long-term ventilation and drainage. Because of the chronic and recurring nature of this illness, it is not surprising that these patients often have symptoms of an URTI on the day of scheduled surgery (see Recent Upper Respiratory Tract Infection, above).

Anesthetic Considerations

These are typically very short (10–15 minutes) outpatient procedures. An inhalational induction with nitrous oxide, oxygen, and halothane is a common technique. Unlike tympanoplasty surgery, nitrous oxide diffusion into the middle ear is not a problem during myringotomy because of the brief period of anesthetic exposure before the middle ear is vented. Because most of these patients are otherwise healthy and there is no blood loss, intravenous access is usually not necessary. Ventilation with a face mask or LMA minimizes the

risk of perioperative respiratory complications (eg, laryngospasm) associated with intubation.

TRISOMY 21 SYNDROME (DOWN SYNDROME)

Pathophysiology

An additional chromosome 21—part or whole—results in the most common congenital pattern of human malformation: Down syndrome. Characteristic abnormalities of interest to the anesthesiologist include a short neck, irregular dentition, mental retardation, hypotonia, and a large tongue. Associated abnormalities include congenital heart disease in 40% of patients (especially endocardial cushion defects and ventricular septal defect), subglottic stenosis, tracheoesophageal fistula, chronic pulmonary infections, and seizures. These neonates are often premature and small for their gestational age. Later in life many patients with Down syndrome often require multiple procedures requiring general anesthesia.

Anesthetic Considerations

Because of anatomic differences, these patients often have difficult airways, especially during infancy. The size of endotracheal tube required is typically smaller than that predicted by age. Respiratory complications such as postoperative stridor and apnea are common. Neck flexion during laryngoscopy and intubation may result in atlanto-occipital dislocation because of the congenital laxity of these ligaments. The possibility of associated congenital diseases must always be considered. As in all pediatric patients, care must be taken to avoid air bubbles in the intravenous line because of possible right-to-left shunts (paradoxic air embolus).

CYSTIC FIBROSIS

Pathophysiology

Cystic fibrosis is a hereditary disease of exocrine glands primarily affecting the pulmonary and gastrointestinal systems. Abnormally thick and viscous secretions coupled with decreased ciliary activity lead to pneumonia, wheezing, and bronchiectasis. Pulmonary function studies reveal increased residual volume and airway resistance with decreased vital capacity and expiratory flow rate. Malabsorption syndrome may lead to dehydration and electrolyte abnormalities.

Anesthetic Considerations

Premedication should not include respiratory depressants. Anticholinergic drugs are controversial, but they have been used in large series without ill effects. Induction with inhalational anesthetics may be prolonged in patients with severe pulmonary disease. Intubation should not be performed until the patient is deeply anesthetized in order to avoid coughing and stimulation of mucus secretions. Aggressive suctioning throughout the anesthesia and before extubation minimizes the accumulation of pulmonary secretions. Intraoperative hyperventilation will cause shallow respirations postoperatively and should be avoided. Outcome is favorably influenced by aggressive preoperative and postoperative respiratory therapy that includes bronchodilators, incentive spirometry, postural drainage, and pathogen-specific antibiotic therapy.

SCOLIOSIS

Pathophysiology

Scoliosis is lateral rotation and curvature of the vertebrae and a deformity of the rib cage. It is classified by etiology: idiopathic, congenital, neuromuscular, traumatic, and so on. Scoliosis can affect cardiac and respiratory function. Elevated pulmonary vascular resistance from chronic hypoxia causes pulmonary hypertension and right ventricular hypertrophy. Respiratory abnormalities include reduced lung volumes and chest wall compliance. PaO_2 is reduced as a result of ventilation/perfusion mismatching, while an increased $PaCO_2$ signals severe disease.

Anesthetic Considerations

Preoperative evaluation should include pulmonary function tests, arterial blood gases, and electrocardiography. Corrective surgery is complicated by the prone position, significant blood loss, and the possibility of paraplegia. Spinal cord function can be monitored with somatosensory evoked potentials (see Chapter 6) or by waking the patient intraoperatively to test lower limb muscle strength. Patients with severe respiratory disease are often left intubated postoperatively. Patients with scoliosis due to muscular dystrophy are predisposed to malignant hyperthermia, cardiac dysrhythmias, and untoward effects of succinylcholine (hyperkalemia, myoglobinuria, and sustained muscular contractures).

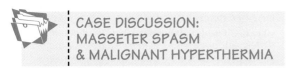

CASE DISCUSSION:
MASSETER SPASM
& MALIGNANT HYPERTHERMIA

A 4-year-old boy is scheduled for strabismus correction. Inhalational induction with nitrous oxide

and halothane is followed by the intravenous administration of atropine and succinylcholine. Rigidity of the masseter muscle prevents mouth opening and intubation.

What is malignant hyperthermia?

Malignant hyperthermia (MH) *is a rare (1:15,000 in pediatric patients and 1:40,000 adult patients) myopathy, characterized by an acute hypermetabolic state within muscle tissue following induction of general anesthesia. It can also present in the postoperative period and even without exposure to known triggering agents, albeit rarely. Although most cases are reported in pediatric patients, all ages can be affected. The earliest signs reported during anesthesia are masseter muscle rigidity (MMR), tachycardia, and hypercarbia due to increased CO_2 production (Table 44–6). Two or more of these signs greatly increase the likelihood of MH. Tachypnea is prominent when muscle relaxants are not used. Sympathetic system overactivity produces tachycardia, arrhythmias, hypertension, and mottled cyanosis. Hyperthermia may be a late sign, but when it occurs, core temperature can rise as much as 1 °C every 5 minutes. Generalized muscle rigidity is not consistently present. Hypertension may be rapidly followed by hypoten-*

Table 44–6. Signs of malignant hyperthermia.

Hypermetabolism
Increased carbon dioxide production
Increased oxygen consumption
Low mixed venous oxygen tension
Metabolic acidosis
Cyanosis
Mottling
Increased sympathetic activity
Tachycardia
Initial hypertension
Arrhythmias
Muscle damage
Masseter spasm
Generalized rigidity
Elevated serum creatine kinase
Hyperkalemia
Hypernatremia
Hyperphosphatemia
Myoglobinemia
Myglobinuria
Hyperthermia
Fever
Sweating

sion as cardiac depression occurs. Dark colored urine reflects myoglobinemia and myoglobinuria.

Laboratory evaluation reveals a mixed metabolic and respiratory acidosis, a marked base deficit, hyperkalemia, hypermagnesemia, and a very low mixed venous oxygen saturation. Serum ionized calcium concentration may initially increase before it falls. Patients also typically have increased serum myoglobin, creatine kinase (CK), lactic dehydrogenase, and aldolase levels. Serum CK levels usually exceed 20,000 IU/L. It should be noted that both serum myoglobin and CK levels can increase markedly in some normal patients after succinylcholine administration without MH.

Part of the problem in diagnosing MH is its variable presentation during or after an anesthetic. For instance, fever is an inconsistent and often late sign. The unanticipated doubling or tripling of end-tidal carbon dioxide is one of the earliest and most sensitive indicators of MH. Ventricular fibrillation can follow the onset of MH within minutes and is the most common cause of death. If the patient survives the first few minutes acute renal failure and DIC can develop rapidly. Other complications of hyperthermia include cerebral edema with seizures and hepatic failure.

What is the pathophysiology of malignant hyperthermia?

Succinylcholine or a halogenated anesthetic agent alone may trigger an MH episode (Table 44–7). In 80% of reported cases, both succinylcholine and a halogenated anesthetic agent were used. Nearly 50% of patients with an episode of MH have had a previous uneventful anesthetic where they were exposed to a triggering agent. Why MH does not occur after every exposure to a triggering agent is poorly understood. Although the precise cellular origin of MH remains poorly understood, investigations reveal an uncontrolled increase in intracellular calcium in skeletal muscle. The sudden release of calcium from sarcoplasmic reticulum removes the inhibition of troponin, resulting in intense muscle contractions. Markedly enhanced and sustained adenosine triphosphatase activity results in an uncontrolled increase in aerobic and anaerobic metabolism. The hypermetabolic state rapidly progresses markedly increasing oxygen consumption and CO_2 production and producing severe lactic acidosis and hyperthermia. As muscle membranes breakdown, an efflux of potassium from muscle cells together with systemic acidosis produces hyperkalemia. Increased sympathetic tone, acidosis, and hyperkalemia all predispose patients to ventricular fibrillation and sudden death, which may occur in as little as 15 minutes.

The initial focus of investigations was on an abnormal ryanodine Ryr_1 receptor in patients with MH. This calcium channel receptor is responsible for calcium release from the sarcoplasmic reticulum and plays a critical role in muscle depolarization. However, further studies have revealed that many MH patients have a normal ryanodine receptor and that abnormalities in secondary messengers and modulators of calcium release, such as fatty acids and phosphatidylinositol, may be present. An abnormal sodium channel in skeletal muscle may also play a role in some patients.

How should an episode of MH be treated?

Treatment is directed at terminating the episode and treating complications such as acidosis and hyperkalemia. The triggering agent must be stopped and dantrolene must be given immediately. The mortality of MH even with prompt treatment may still be as high as 5–30%.

Since succinylcholine and volatile anesthetics are considered to be the principal triggering agents, they should be discontinued immediately. Even trace amounts of anesthetics absorbed by soda lime, breathing tubes, and breathing bags may be detrimental. The patient should be aggressively ventilated with 100% oxygen to minimize the effects of hypercapnia, metabolic acidosis, and increased oxygen consumption. If fever is present, cooling measures should also be instituted immediately. Surface cooling with ice packs over major arteries, cold air convection, and cooling blankets are used. Iced saline lavage of the stomach and body cavities (whenever possible) should also be instituted. Cold dialysis and cardiopulmonary by-

Table 44–7. Drugs known to trigger malignant hyperthermia.

Halogenated general anesthetics
Ether
Cyclopropane
Halothane
Methoxyflurane
Enflurane
Isoflurane
Desflurane
Sevoflurane
Nondepolarizing muscle relaxants
Succinylcholine

pass may also be appropriate if other measures fail.

An arterial line will provide precise blood pressure monitoring and access to serial arterial blood gas measurements. Acidosis should be treated aggressively with intravenous sodium bicarbonate 1–2 mEq/kg. Hyperkalemia should be treated with insulin and glucose, and diuresis. Intravenous calcium should be used cautiously, if at all. Antiarrhythmic agents and catecholamine vasopressors and inotropes are considered safe if used appropriately. Calcium channel blockers should not be used with dantrolene because this combination appears to promote hyperkalemia. Mannitol infusion 0.5 g/kg and/or furosemide should be used to establish a diuresis and prevent acute renal failure from myoglobinuria. Nonetheless, the mainstay of therapy for an MH crisis is immediate administration of intravenous dantrolene.

Describe the mechanism of action of dantrolene, its recommended dosage, and its possible side effects.

Dantrolene, a hydantoin derivative, directly interferes with muscle contraction by binding the Ryr_1 receptor calcium channel and inhibiting calcium ion release from the sarcoplasmic reticulum. This **intracellular** dissociation of excitation-contraction coupling contrasts with the depolarizing and nondepolarizing muscle relaxants that antagonize the **extracellular** neuromuscular junction. The dose is 2.5 mg/kg intravenously every 5 minutes until the episode is terminated. The upper limit of dantrolene therapy is generally 10 mg/kg. Dantrolene is packaged as 20 mg of lyophilized powder to be dissolved in 60 mL of sterile water. Depending on the dose required, reconstitution can be time-consuming. Dantrolene's effective half-life is about 6 hours. After initial control, dantrolene 1 mg/kg intravenously is recommended every 6 hours for 24–48 hours to prevent relapse because MH can recur within 24 hours. It should be noted that dantrolene is not specific for MH; it also decreases temperature in thyroid storm and neuroleptic malignant syndrome. Dantrolene is a relatively safe drug. Although chronic therapy for spastic disorders has been associated with hepatic dysfunction, the most serious complication following acute administration is generalized muscle weakness that may result in respiratory insufficiency or aspiration pneumonia. Dantrolene can cause phlebitis in small peripheral veins and should be given through a central venous line if one is available. The safety and efficacy of dantro-

lene call for its immediate use in this potentially life-threatening disease.

What is the differential diagnosis of masseter spasm during intubation?

Masseter muscle spasm, also known as **MMR, or trismus,** is a forceful contraction of the jaw musculature that prevents full mouth opening. This contrasts with incomplete jaw relaxation, which is a fairly common finding. Both myotonia and MH can cause masseter spasm. The two disorders can be differentiated by the medical history, neurologic examination, and electromyography. The incidence of masseter spasm following succinylcholine administration in pediatric patients at some medical centers may be higher than 1%. Isolated MMR occurs in only 15–30% of true MH episodes. Moreover, less than 50% of patients in whom MMR develops prove to be susceptible to MH by muscle testing. The safest course is to assume that masseter spasm is due to MH and to postpone elective surgery. However, if there are no other signs of MH, and if monitoring and treatment capabilities are readily available, some anesthesiologists will allow surgery to continue and use a safe (nontriggering) anesthetic. Serum CK levels should be followed for 24 hours after an episode of MMR, because an elevation of this enzyme may indicate an underlying myopathy.

Which patients should be considered at increased risk for developing MH?

Several musculoskeletal diseases are associated with a relatively high incidence of MH. These include Duchenne's muscular dystrophy, central-core disease, and osteogenesis imperfecta. King-Denborough syndrome is consistently associated with MH. This syndrome is seen primarily in young boys who exhibit short stature, mental retardation, cryptorchidism, kyphoscoliosis, pectus deformity, slanted eyes, low-set ears, webbed neck, and winged scapulae.

Operations associated with an increased incidence of MH include orthopedic cases (joint-dislocation repair), ophthalmic surgery (ptosis and strabismus correction), and head and neck procedures (cleft palate repair, tonsillectomy and adenoidectomy, dental surgery). Other possible clues to susceptibility include a family history of anesthetic complications, intolerance to caffeine-containing foods, or a history of unexplained fevers or muscular cramps. Prior uneventful anesthesia and absence of a positive family history are notoriously unreliable predictors of susceptibility to MH, however. As previously mentioned, any patient in whom trismus develops during induction of anesthesia should be considered to be susceptible to MH.

What type of hereditary pattern does MH follow?

Although sporadic cases are described, most patients with an episode of MH have a history of relatives with a similar episode or an abnormal halothane-caffeine contracture test. An autosomal pattern of dominance with variable penetrance occurs in about 50% of susceptible families. The complexity of genetic inheritance patterns in families reflects the fact that MH is a heterogenous genetic disorder; it can be caused by mutations of one or more genes on more than one chromosome. Thus, genes on chromosomes 1, 3, 7, 17, and 19 have been linked with MH in different families. The earliest reports linked MH with mutations in the gene for the skeletal muscle, ryanodine (Ryr$_1$) receptor, calcium release channel on chromosome 19 in humans. Subsequent reports on other families linked MH with mutations in the adult muscle, sodium channel, alpha subunit gene on chromosome 17. An autosomal recessive form of MH has been associated with the King-Denborough syndrome. Reports of MH vary greatly from country to country and even in different geographic localities within a country, reflecting varying gene pools. The Midwest appears to have the highest incidence of MH in the United States.

How is susceptibility to MH confirmed?

Patients who have survived an unequivocal episode of MH are considered susceptible. If the diagnosis remains in doubt postoperatively, a biopsy of a fresh section of living skeletal muscle is obtained and exposed to a caffeine, halothane, or combination caffeine-halothane bath. The halothane-caffeine contracture test may have a 10–20% false-positive rate, but the false-negative rate is close to zero. Because of the relative complexity of this test, only a few centers worldwide perform it. Both European and North American MH registries have been established to help physicians identify and treat patients with suspected MH, as well as provide standardization between testing centers. The Malignant Hyperthermia Association of the United States (MHAUS, telephone 1-800-98-MHAUS) operates a 24-hour hotline (1-800-MH-HYPER), an on-demand fax service (1-800-440-9990), and a Web site (www.mhaus. org). If the halothane-caffeine contracture test is positive, genetic counseling and testing of family members is appropriate. Baseline CK may be ele-

vated chronically in 50–70% of people at risk for MH, but the only reliable way to diagnose MH susceptibility is by muscle testing.

How does MH differ from neuroleptic malignant syndrome?

Neuroleptic malignant syndrome (NMS) is characterized by hyperthermia, muscle rigidity with extrapyramidal signs (dyskinesia), altered consciousness and autonomic lability in patients receiving antidopaminergic agents. The syndrome is caused by an imbalance of neurotransmitters in the central nervous system. A functional dopamine deficiency results in hyperactivity of excitatory amino acids in the basal ganglia and hypothalamus. It can occur either during drug therapy with antidopaminergic agents (phenothiazines, butyrophenones, thioxanthines, dibenzoxapines, or metoclopramide) or less commonly following the withdrawal of dopaminergic agonists (levodopa or amantadine) in patients with Parkinson's disease. Thus, it appears to involve abnormal central dopaminergic activity, as opposed to the altered peripheral calcium release seen in MH. These differing mechanisms probably explain why nondepolarizing relaxants reverse the rigidity of NMS, but not the rigidity associated with MH. NMS does not appear to be inherited and typically takes hours to weeks to develop; the majority of episodes develop within 2 weeks of a dose adjustment. Hyperthermia generally tends to be mild, and appears to be proportional to the amount of rigidity. Autonomic dysfunction results in tachycardia, labile blood pressure, diaphoresis, dyspnea, increased secretions and urinary incontinence. Muscle rigidity can produce respiratory distress and together with the increased secretions can promote aspiration pneumonia. CK levels are typically elevated; some patients may develop rhabdomyolysis resulting in myoglobinemia, myoglobinuria, and renal failure.

Mild forms of the NMS promptly resolve after withdrawal of the causative drug (or reinstitution of antiparkinsonian therapy). Initial treatment of more severe forms of NMS should include oxygen therapy and endotracheal intubation for respiratory distress or altered consciousness. Marked muscle rigidity can be controlled with muscle paralysis, dantrolene, or a dopaminergic agonist (amantadine, bromocriptine, or levodopa), depending on the severity and acuity of the syndrome. Resolution of the muscle rigidity usually decreases body temperature.

Although this syndrome is considered a separate entity from MH, many clinicians feel NMS may predispose patients to MH. Patients with NMS should probably not receive succinylcholine or a volatile anesthetic; however, patients susceptible to MH can safely receive phenothiazines.

What other diseases can present like MH?

A number of other disorders may resemble MH (Table 44–8). Surgery and anesthesia can precipitate **thyroid storm** in undiagnosed or poorly controlled hyperthyroid patients. Its signs include tachycardia, tachyarrhythmias (especially atrial fibrillation), hyperthermia (often > 40 °C), hypotension, and in some cases congestive heart failure. In contrast to MH, hypokalemia is very common. Also unlike the typical intraoperative presentation of MH, thyroid storm generally develops postoperatively, (see Chapter 36 and Case Discussion, Chapter 49). **Pheochromocytoma** is associated with dramatic increases in heart rate and blood pressure but not end-tidal CO_2 (see Chapter 36) or temperature. Cardiac manifestations such as arrhythmias, ischemia, or congestive heart failure may also be prominent. Rarely, some patients may present with significant hyperthermia (> 38°C), which is generally thought to be due to increased heat production from catecholamine-mediated increases in metabolic rate together with decreased heat elimination from intense vasoconstriction. **Sepsis** shares several characteristics with MH, including fever, tachypnea, tachycardia, and metabolic acidosis (see Chapter 50). This can be a difficult differential diagnosis if there is no obvious primary site of infection. Less commonly, **drug-induced hyperthermia** may be encountered in the perioperative period with some drug combinations as well as in patients who have been taking certain illicit drugs. These drugs appear to markedly increase serotonin activity in the brain, causing hyperthermia, confusion, shivering, diaphoresis, hyperreflexia, and myoclonus. Combinations associated with this "**serotonin syndrome**" include monoamine oxidase inhibitors (MAOIs) and meperidine, and MAOIs and selective serotonin reuptake inhibitors (SSRIs). Hyperthermia can also be caused by some illicit drugs, including 3,4-methylenedioxymethamphetamine (MDMA or "ecstasy'), "crack" cocaine, amphetamines, phenylcyclidine (PCP), and lysergic acid diethylamine (LSD). **Iatrogenic hyperthermia** is not uncommon especially in pediatric patients. Common sources of excessive heat in the operating room include humidifiers on ventilators, warming blankets, heat lamps, as well as ambient temperature. **Brainstem or hypothalamic injury** near the hypothalamus and brainstem can be associated with marked hyperthermia, but this diagnosis requires exclusion of all other causes.

MH, however, is associated with more dramatic degrees of metabolic acidosis and venous desaturation than are any of these diseases.

What constitutes a *safe* anesthetic in patients who are susceptible to MH?

Thiopental and pancuronium appear to be protective, since they raise the triggering threshold for MH. Other safe drugs include nitrous oxide, propofol, etomidate, benzodiazepines, ketamine, opiates, droperidol, and all local anesthetics. An adequate supply of dantrolene should always be available wherever general anesthesia is provided. Prophylactic use of intravenous dantrolene prior to induction of general anesthesia in susceptible patients is probably not necessary if a safe anesthetic is administered. A minimum recovery room stay of 4 hours has been recommended for patients who are susceptible to MH.

Table 44–8. Differential diagnosis of hyperthermia in the intraoperative and immediate postoperative periods.

Malignant hyperthermia
Neuroleptic malignant syndrome
Thyroid storm
Pheochromocytoma
Drug-induced hyperthermia
Serotonin syndrome
Iatrogenic hyperthermia
Brainstem/hypothalamic injury
Sepsis
Transfusion reaction

SUGGESTED READING

Allen GC, Larach MG, Kunselman AR: The sensitivity and specificity of the caffeine-halothane contracture test: A report from the North American Malignant Hyperthermia Registry. Anesthesiology 1998;88:579.

American Academy of Pediatrics—Section on Anesthesiology: Guidelines for the pediatric anesthesia environment. Pediatrics 1999;103:512.

American Society of Anesthesiologists Task Force on Preoperative Fasting: Practice Guidelines for preoperative fasting and the use of pharmacologic agents to reduce the risk of pulmonary aspiration: Application to healthy patient undergoing elective procedures. Anesthesiology 1999;90:896.

MALIGNANT HYPERTHERMIA PROTOCOL

1. Discontinue volatile anesthetic and succinylcholine. *Call for help!*

2. Hyperventilate with 100% O_2 at high flows.

3. Administer sodium bicarbonate, 1–2 mEq/kg IV.

4. Mix dantrolene sodium with sterile distilled water and administer 2.5 mg/kg IV *as soon as possible.*

5. Institute cooling measures (lavage, cooling blanket, cold intravenous solutions).

6. Administer inotropes and antiarrhythmic agents as necessary.

7. Administer additional doses of dantrolene if needed.

8. Change anesthetic tubing and soda lime.

9. Monitor urinary output, K^+, Ca^{2+}, blood gases, end-tidal carbon dioxide; perform clotting studies.

10. Treat severe hyperkalemia with dextrose, 25–50 g IV, and regular insulin, 10–20 U IV (adult dose).

11. Consider invasive monitoring of arterial blood pressure and central venous pressure.

12. If necessary, consult on-call physicians at the 24-hour MHAUS hotline, **1-800-MH-HYPER.**

Badgwell JM: *Clinical Pediatric Anesthesia.* Lippincott Williams & Wilkins, 1997.

Bell C, Kain ZN: *The Pediatric Anesthesia Handbook,* 2nd ed. Mosby, 1997.

Bissonnette B, Dalens B: *Principles & Practice of Pediatric Anesthesia.* McGraw-Hill, 2001.

Bloch EC, Ginsberg B: *Pediatric Anesthesia. A Quick Pocket Reference,* 2nd ed. Butterworth-Heinemann, 1999.

Brandom BW: Neuromuscular blocking drugs in pediatric patients. Anesth Analg 2000;90:S14.

Butler MG, Hayes BG, Hathaway MM, Begleiter ML: Specific genetic diseases at risk sedation/anesthesia complications. Anesth Analg 2000;91:837.

Cote CJ, Todres ID, Goudsouzian NG, Ryan JF. *A Practice of Anesthesia for Infants and Children,* 3rd ed. WB Saunders and Company, 2001.

Gregory GA (editor): *Pediatric Anesthesia,* 4th ed. Churchill Livingstone, 2001.

Hatch DJ, Hunter JM (editors): The paediatric patient. Br J Anaesth 1999;83:1.

Hopkins PM: Malignant hyperthermia: Advances in clinical management and diagnosis. Br J Anaesth 2000;85:118.

Krauss B, Brustowicz RM: *Pediatric Procedural Sedation and Analgesia.* Lippincott Williams & Wilkins, 1999.

Mazurek AJ, Rae B, Hann S, et al: Rocuroniun versus succinylcholine: Are they equally effective during rapid sequence induction of anesthesia? Anesth Analg 1998;87:1259.

Mellor DJ, Lerman J: Anesthesia for neonatal surgical emergencies. Semin Perinatol 1998;22:363.

Morton NS: *Acute Paediatric Pain Management.* WB Saunders and Company, 1998.

Motoyama EK, Davis PJ (editors): *Smith's Anesthesia for Infants and Children,* 6th ed. Mosby Year Book, 1996.

Peutrell JM: *Regional Anaesthesia for Babies and Children.* Oxford University Press, 1997.

Politis GD, Tobin JR, Morell RC, James RL, Cantwell MF: Tracheal intubation of healthy pediatric patients with muscle relaxant: A survey of technique utilization and perceptions of safety. Anesth Analg 1999;88:737.

Ross AK, Eck JB, Tobias JD: Pediatric regional anesthesia: Beyond the caudal. Anesth Analg 2000;91:16.

Salvo I, Vidyasagar D: *Anaesthesia and Intensive Care in Neonates and Children.* Springer-Verlag, 1999.

Skoulakis CE, Doxas PG, Papadakis CE, et al: Bronchoscopy for foreign body removal in children. A review and analysis of 210 cases. Int J Ped Otorhinolaryngol 2000;53:143.

Splinter WM, Schreiner MS: Preoperative fasting in children. Anesth Analg 1999;89:80.

Steward DJ, Lerman J: *Manual of Pediatric Anesthesia,* 5th ed. Churchill Livingstone, 2001.

Yaster M, Cote CJ, Kaplan RF, Krane EJ, Lappe D: *Pediatric Pain Management and Sedation Handbook.* Mosby, 1998.

Geriatric Anesthesia

KEY CONCEPTS

 In the absence of disease, resting systolic cardiac function appears to be preserved even in octogenarians. Increased vagal tone and decreased sensitivity of adrenergic receptors lead to a decline in heart rate.

 Elderly patients undergoing evaluation for surgery have a high incidence of diastolic dysfunction that can be detected with Doppler echocardiography.

 Diminished cardiac reserve in many elderly patients may be manifested as exaggerated drops in blood pressure during induction of general anesthesia. A prolonged circulation time delays the onset of intravenous drugs but speeds induction with inhalational agents.

 Elasticity is decreased in lung tissue, allowing overdistention of alveoli and collapse of small airways. Airway collapse increases residual volume and closing capacity. Even in normal persons, closing capacity exceeds functional residual capacity at age 45 in the supine position and age 65 in the sitting position. When this happens, some airways close during part of normal tidal breathing, resulting in a mismatch of ventilation and perfusion.

 Aging is associated with a decreasing response to β-adrenergic agents ("endogenous β-blockade").

 Impairment of sodium handling, concentrating ability, and diluting capacity predisposes elderly patients to dehydration or fluid overload. As renal function declines, so does the kidney's ability to excrete drugs.

 Hepatic function (reserves) declines in proportion to the decrease in liver mass.

 Dosage requirements for local (minimum anesthetic concentration) and general (minimum alveolar concentration) anesthetics are reduced in elderly patients. A given volume of epidural anesthetic tends to result in more extensive cephalad spread, but with a shorter duration of analgesia and motor block. A longer duration of action should be expected from a spinal anesthetic.

 Many elderly patients experience varying degrees of an acute confusional state, delirium, or cognitive dysfunction postoperatively.

 Aging produces both pharmacokinetic and pharmacodynamic changes. Disease-related changes and wide inter-individual variations even in similar populations lead to inconsistent generalizations.

 Elderly patients display a lower dose requirement for barbiturates, opioid agonists, and benzodiazepines.

By the year 2040, people aged 65 or older are expected to make up 24% of the population and account for 50% of health care expenditures. Half these individuals will require surgery before they die, despite being at a 3-fold increased risk for perioperative death compared with younger patients. Emergency surgery, surgical site, and physical status defined by the American Society of Anesthesiologists increase anesthetic risk (see Chapter 1). Operations associated with increased risk of perioperative mortality and morbidity for elderly patients include thoracic, intraperitoneal (especially colon surgery), and major vascular procedures.

As with pediatric patients, optimal anesthetic management of geriatric patients depends on an understanding of the normal changes in physiology, anatomy, and response to pharmacologic agents that accompany aging. In fact, there are many similarities between elderly and pediatric patients (Table 45–1). Compared with pediatric patients, however, older people show a wider range of variation in these parameters. The relatively high frequency of serious physiologic abnormalities in elderly patients demands an especially careful preoperative evaluation.

■ AGE-RELATED ANATOMIC & PHYSIOLOGIC CHANGES

CARDIOVASCULAR SYSTEM

It is important to distinguish between changes in physiology that normally accompany aging and the pathophysiology of diseases common in the geriatric population (Table 45–2). For example, atherosclerosis is pathologic—it is not present in healthy elderly patients. On the other hand, a reduction in arterial elasticity caused by fibrosis of the media is part of the normal aging process. Reduced arterial compliance results in increased afterload, elevated systolic blood pressure, and

Table 45–1. Similarities between elderly people and infants, compared with the general population.

Decrease ability to increase heart rate in response to hypovolemia, hypotension, or hypoxia
Decreased lung compliance
Decreased arterial oxygen tension
Impaired ability to cough
Decreased renal tubular function
Increased susceptibility to hypothermia

left ventricular hypertrophy. The left ventricular wall thickens at the expense of the left ventricular cavity. Some myocardial fibrosis and calcification of the valves are common. In the absence of coexisting disease, diastolic blood pressure remains unchanged or decreases. Baroreceptor function is depressed. Similarly, while cardiac output typically declines with age, it appears to be maintained in well-conditioned healthy individuals. In the absence of disease, resting systolic cardiac function appears to be preserved even in octogenarians. Increased vagal tone and decreased sensitivity of adrenergic receptors lead to a decline in heart rate; maximal heart rate declines by approximately one beat per minute per year of age over 50. Fibrosis of the conduction system and loss of sinoatrial node cells increase the incidence of dysrhythmias.

Elderly patients undergoing evaluation for surgery have a high incidence of diastolic dysfunction that can be detected with Doppler echocardiography. Marked diastolic dysfunction may be seen with systemic hypertension, coronary artery disease, cardiomyopathies, and valvular heart disease, especially aortic stenosis. Patients may be asymptomatic or complain of exercise intolerance, dyspnea, cough or fatigue. Diastolic dysfunction results in relatively large increases in ventricular end-diastolic pressure with small changes of left ventricular volume; the atrial contribution to ventricular filling becomes even more important than in younger patients (see Chapter 19). Atrial enlargement predisposes patients to supraventricular tachycardias, especially atrial fibrillation. Patients are at increased risk for developing congestive heart failure.

Diminished cardiac reserve in many elderly patients may be manifested as exaggerated drops in blood pressure during induction of general anesthesia. A prolonged circulation time delays the onset of intravenous drugs but speeds induction with inhalational agents. Like infants, elderly patients have a lesser ability to respond to hypovolemia, hypotension, or hypoxia with an increase in heart rate.

RESPIRATORY SYSTEM

Elasticity is decreased in lung tissue also, allowing overdistention of alveoli and collapse of small airways. The former reduces the alveolar surface area, which decreases the efficiency of gas exchange. Airway collapse increases **residual volume** (the volume of air remaining in the lungs at the end of a forced expiration) and **closing capacity** (the volume of air in the lungs at which small airways begin to close). Even in normal persons, closing capacity exceeds **functional residual capacity** (the volume of air remaining in the lungs at the end of a normal ex-

Table 45–2. Age-related physiologic changes and common diseases of the elderly.

Normal Physiologic Changes	Common Pathophysiology
Cardiovascular	
Decreased arterial elasticity	Atherosclerosis
Elevated afterload	Coronary artery disease
Elevated systolic blood pressure	Essential hypertension
Left ventricular hypertrophy	Congestive heart failure
Decreased adrenergic activity	Cardiac arrhythmias
Decreased resting heart rate	Aortic stenosis
Decreased maximal heart rate	
Decreased baroreceptor reflex	
Respiratory	
Decreased pulmonary elasticity	Emphysema
Decreased alveolar surface area	Chronic bronchitis
Increased residual volume	Pneumonia
Increased closing capacity	Lung cancer
Ventilation/perfusion mismatching	
Decreased arterial oxygen tension	
Increased chest wall rigidity	
Decreased muscle strength	
Decreased cough	
Decreased maximal breathing capacity	
Blunted response to hypercapnia and hypoxia	
Renal	
Decreased renal blood flow	Diabetic nephropathy
Decreased renal plasma flow	Hypertensive nephropathy
Decreased glomerular filtration rate	Prostatic obstruction
Decreased renal mass	Congestive heart failure
Decreased tubular function	
Impaired sodium handling	
Decreased concentrating ability	
Decreased diluting capacity	
Impaired fluid handling	
Decreased drug excretion	
Decreased renin-aldosterone responsiveness	
Impaired potassium excretion	

piration) at age 45 in the supine position and age 65 in the sitting position. When this happens, some airways close during part of normal tidal breathing, resulting in a mismatch of ventilation and perfusion. The additive effect of these emphysema-like changes is said to decrease arterial oxygen tension by an average rate of 0.35 mm Hg per year. There is a wide range of arterial oxygen tensions in elderly preoperative patients, however (Figure 45–1). Both anatomic and physiologic dead space increase. Other pulmonary effects of aging are summarized in Table 45–2.

Mask ventilation may be more difficult in edentulous patients, while arthritis of the temporomandibular joint or cervical spine may make intubation challenging. On the other hand, the absence of upper teeth

often improves visualization of the vocal cords during laryngoscopy.

Prevention of perioperative hypoxia includes higher inspired oxygen concentrations, small increments of positive end-expiratory pressure, and aggressive pulmonary toilet. Aspiration pneumonia is a common and potentially life-threatening complication in elderly patients. One reason for this predisposition is a progressive decrease in protective laryngeal reflexes with age. Ventilatory impairment in the recovery room is more common in elderly patients. Therefore, patients with severe preexisting respiratory disease and those who have just had major abdominal surgery should generally be left intubated postoperatively. In addition, pain control techniques that facilitate postoperative pulmonary

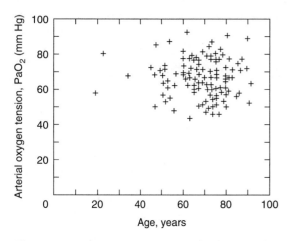

Figure 45–1. There is a wide range of arterial oxygen tensions in elderly preoperative patients. (Redrawn and reproduced, with permission, from Del Guercio LRM, Cohn JD: Monitoring operative risk in elderly. JAMA 1980;243:1350.)

function should be seriously considered (eg, epidural opioids, intercostal nerve blocks).

METABOLIC AND ENDOCRINE FUNCTION

Basal and maximal oxygen consumption declines with age. After reaching peak weight at about age 60, most men and women begin losing weight; the average elderly man and woman weigh less than younger counterparts. Heat production decreases, heat loss increases, and hypothalamic temperature regulating centers may reset at a lower level. Increasing insulin resistance leads to a progressive decrease in the ability to handle glucose loads. The neuroendocrine response to stress appears to be preserved or slightly decreased in most healthy elderly patients. Aging is associated with a decreasing response to β-adrenergic agents ("endogenous β-blockade"). Circulating norepinephrine levels are reported to be elevated in elderly patients.

RENAL FUNCTION

Renal blood flow and kidney mass (eg, glomerular number and tubular length) decrease with age. These changes are particularly prominent in the renal cortex where they are replaced by fat and fibrotic tissue. Renal function as determined by glomerular filtration rate and creatinine clearance is reduced (Table 45–2). Serum creatinine level is unchanged because of a decrease in muscle mass and creatinine production, while

blood urea nitrogen gradually increases (0.2 mg/dL per year). Impairment of sodium handling, concentrating ability, and diluting capacity predisposes elderly patients to dehydration or fluid overload. The response to antidiuretic hormone and aldosterone are reduced. The ability to reabsorb glucose is decreased. The combination of reduced renal blood flow and decreased nephron mass increases the risk of elderly patients for acute renal failure in the postoperative period.

As renal function declines, so does the kidney's ability to excrete drugs. The decreased capacity to handle water and electrolyte loads makes proper fluid management more critical; elderly patients are more predisposed to developing hypokalemia and hyperkalemia. This is further complicated by the common use of diuretics in the elderly population. To this end, serum electrolytes, cardiac filling pressures and urinary output are more frequently monitored.

GASTROINTESTINAL FUNCTION

Liver mass declines as a person ages with a corresponding decrease in hepatic blood flow. Hepatic function (reserves) declines in proportion to the decrease in liver mass. Thus, the rate of biotransformation and albumin production decrease. Plasma cholinesterase levels are reduced in elderly men. Gastric pH tends to rise, while gastric emptying is prolonged, although some studies suggest elderly patients have lower gastric volumes than younger patients.

NERVOUS SYSTEM

Cerebral blood flow and brain mass decrease with age; neuronal loss is prominent in the cerebral cortex, especially the frontal lobes. Neurons decrease in size and lose some complexity of their dendritic tree and number of synapses. The synthesis of some neurotransmitters, such as dopamine, and the number of their receptors are reduced. Astrocytes and microglial cells increase. Cerebral blood flow decreases in proportion to loss of neural tissue. Cerebral autoregulation of blood flow is preserved. In the absence of disease, decreases in cognitive function are normally modest but variable. Physical activity appears to have a positive effect on preservation of cognitive functions. Degeneration of peripheral nerve cells results in prolonged conduction velocity and skeletal muscle atrophy. Aging is associated with an increasing threshold for nearly all sensory modalities, including touch, temperature sensation, proprioception, hearing and vision. Changes in pain perception are complex and poorly understood; central and peripheral processing mechanisms are likely altered.

 Dosage requirements for local (Cm: minimum anesthetic concentration) and general (MAC: minimum alveolar concentration) anesthetics are reduced. Administration of a given volume of epidural anesthetic tends to result in more extensive cephalad spread in elderly patients, but with a shorter duration of analgesia and motor block. In contrast, a longer duration of action should be expected from a spinal anesthetic. Elderly patients often take more time to recover completely from the central nervous system effects of general anesthesia, especially if they were confused or disoriented preoperatively. This is particularly important in geriatric outpatient surgery, where socioeconomic factors such as the lack of a caretaker at home necessitate a higher level of self-care.

Many elderly patients experience varying degrees of an acute confusional state, delirium, or cognitive dysfunction postoperatively. The etiology of the latter is likely multifactorial and includes, drug effects, pain, underlying dementia, hypoxemia, and metabolic disturbances. Low levels of certain neurotransmitters, such as acetylcholine, may be contributory. Elderly patients are especially sensitive to centrally acting anticholinergic agents such as scopolamine and atropine. Interestingly, the incidence of postoperative delirium appears similar with both regional and general anesthesia; it may be less following regional anesthesia without any sedation. Some patients suffer from prolonged or permanent cognitive deficits after surgery and anesthesia. Although the etiology is usually unclear, nonanesthetic factors are likely responsible.

MUSCULOSKELETAL

Muscle mass is reduced. At the microscopic level, neuromuscular junctions thicken. There also appears to be some extrajunctional spread of acetylcholine receptors. Skin atrophies with age and is prone to trauma from adhesive tape, electrocautery pads, and electrocardiographic electrodes. Veins are often frail and easily ruptured by intravenous infusions. Arthritic joints may interfere with positioning (eg, lithotomy) or regional anesthesia (eg, subarachnoid block).

■ AGE-RELATED PHARMACOLOGIC CHANGES

Aging produces both pharmacokinetic (the relationship between drug dose and plasma concentration) and pharmacodynamic (the relationship between plasma concentration and clinical effect) changes. Unfortunately, disease-related changes and wide inter-individual variations even in similar populations lead to inconsistent generalizations.

A progressive decrease in muscle mass and increase in body fat (more pronounced in older women) results in decreased total body water. The reduced volume of distribution for water-soluble drugs can lead to higher plasma concentrations; conversely, an increased volume of distribution for lipid-soluble drugs can lower their plasma concentration. These changes in volume of distribution may affect elimination half-life. If a drug's volume of distribution expands, its elimination half-life will be prolonged unless the rate of clearance is also increased. However, because renal and hepatic functions decline with age, reductions in clearance prolong the duration of action for many drugs. Studies suggest that unlike those who are ill, healthy, active, elderly patients have little or no change in plasma volume.

Distribution and elimination are also affected by altered plasma protein binding (see Chapter 8). Albumin, which tends to bind acidic drugs (eg, barbiturates, benzodiazepines, opioid agonists), typically decreases with age. α_1-Acid glycoprotein, which binds basic drugs (eg, local anesthetics), is increased. Protein-bound drugs cannot interact with end-organ receptors and are unavailable for metabolism or excretion.

The principal pharmacodynamic change associated with aging is a reduced anesthetic requirement, represented by a lower MAC. Careful titration of anesthetic agents to effect helps avoid adverse side effects and prolonged duration; short-acting agents such as propofol, desflurane, remifentanil, and succinylcholine may especially be useful in elderly patients. Drugs that are not significantly dependent on hepatic or renal function or blood flow, such as mivacurium, atracurium, and cisatracurium, may also be useful.

INHALATIONAL ANESTHETICS

The MAC for inhalational agents is reduced by 4% per decade of age over 40 years. For example, the MAC of halothane in an 80-year-old person would be expected to be 0.65 (0.77 − [0.77 × 4% × 4]). Onset of action will be more rapid if cardiac output is depressed, while it will be delayed if there is a significant ventilation/perfusion abnormality (see Chapter 7). The myocardial depressant effects of volatile anesthetics are exaggerated in elderly patients, while the tachycardiac tendencies of isoflurane and desflurane are attenuated. Thus, in contrast to its effects on younger patients, isoflurane reduces cardiac output and heart rate in elderly patients. Recovery from anesthesia with a volatile anesthetic may be prolonged because of an increased volume of distribution (increased body fat), decreased hepatic function (decreased halothane metabolism), and decreased pulmonary gas exchange.

NONVOLATILE ANESTHETIC AGENTS

In general, elderly patients display a lower dose requirement for barbiturates, opioid agonists, and benzodiazepines. For example, the typical octogenarian requires less than half the induction dose of thiopental than that required by a 20-year-old. This probably is the result of peak thiopental levels not decreasing as rapidly in geriatric patients because of a slower distribution from the central compartment to the rapidly equilibrating compartment. In any event, pharmacokinetic and not pharmacodynamic differences are responsible. This is in contrast to opioid agonists, which display pharmacokinetic (smaller initial volume of distribution, prolonged elimination half-life) and pharmacodynamic (increased brain sensitivity) alterations. Because diazepam tends to accumulate in fat stores, its volume of distribution is larger in older patients and its elimination from the body is therefore slowed. A half-life of more than 36 hours can thus cause confusion for days following diazepam administration. Although midazolam is water-soluble at acidic pH, it is lipid-soluble at physiologic pH and undergoes similar pharmacokinetic changes. Furthermore, aging increases the pharmacodynamic sensitivity to midazolam, independent of any pharmacokinetic enhancement. Lorazepam is less lipid-soluble than diazepam, and its elimination half-life remains relatively unchanged.

MUSCLE RELAXANTS

The response to succinylcholine and nondepolarizing agents is unaltered with aging. Decreased cardiac output and slow muscle blood flow, however, may cause up to a 2-fold prolongation in onset of neuromuscular blockade in elderly patients. Recovery from nondepolarizing muscle relaxants that depend on renal excretion (eg, metocurine, pancuronium, doxacurium, tubocurarine) may be delayed owing to decreased drug clearance. Likewise, decreased hepatic excretion from a loss of liver mass prolongs the elimination half-life and duration of action of rocuronium and vecuronium. The pharmacologic profiles of atracurium and pipecuronium are not significantly affected by age. Elderly men—but not elderly women—may display a slightly prolonged effect from succinylcholine owing to their lower plasma cholinesterase levels.

CASE DISCUSSION: THE ELDERLY PATIENT WITH A FRACTURED HIP

An 86-year-old nursing home patient is scheduled for open reduction and internal fixation of a subtrochanteric fracture of the femur.

How should this patient be evaluated for the risk of perioperative morbidity?

Anesthetic risk correlates much better with the presence of coexisting disease than chronologic age. Therefore, preanesthetic evaluation should concentrate on the identification of age-related diseases (Table 45–2) and an estimation of physiologic reserve. There is a tremendous physiologic difference between a patient who walks three blocks to a grocery store on a regular basis and one who is bedridden, even though both may be the same age. Obviously, any condition that may be amenable to preoperative therapy (eg, bronchodilator administration) must be identified and addressed. At the same time, lengthy delays may compromise surgical repair and increase overall morbidity.

What are some of the considerations in selection of premedication for this patient?

In general, elderly patients require lower doses of premedication. Nonetheless, hip fractures are painful, particularly during movement to the operating room. Unless contraindicated by severe concomitant disease, an opioid premedication may be valuable. Anticholinergic medication is rarely needed, since aging is accompanied by atrophy of the salivary glands. These patients may be at risk for aspiration, since opioid premedication and pain from the injury will decrease gastric emptying. Therefore, pretreatment with an H_2 antagonist or an oral nonparticulate antacid should be considered (see Chapter 15). Metoclopramide can also be used to promote gastric emptying but elderly patients may be at increased risk for extrapyramidal side effects, such as rigidity.

What factors might influence the choice between regional and general anesthesia?

Advancing age is not a contraindication for either regional or general anesthesia. Each technique, however, has its advantages and disadvantages in the elderly population. For hip surgery, regional anesthesia can be achieved with a subarachnoid or epidural block extending to the T8 sensory level. Both these blocks require patient cooperation and the ability to lie still for the duration of the surgery. A paramedian approach is helpful when optimal positioning is not possible (see Chapter 16). Unless regional anesthesia is accompanied by heavy sedation, postoperative confusion and disorientation are less troublesome than after general anesthesia. Cardiovascular changes are usually limited to a fall in arterial blood pressure as sympathetic block is established. While this fall can be minimized by prophylactic fluid loading, a patient with borderline heart function may develop congestive heart failure when the block dissipates and sympathetic tone returns. Reduced afterload can result in profound hypotension in patients with aortic stenosis, a common valvular lesion in the elderly population. Patients with coronary artery disease may experience an increase in myocardial oxygen demand as a result of reflex tachycardia or a decrease in supply caused by lower coronary artery perfusion.

Are there any specific advantages or disadvantages to a regional technique in elderly patients having hip surgery?

A major advantage in regional anesthesia—particularly for hip surgery—is a lower incidence of postoperative thromboembolism (see Chapter 40). This is presumably due to peripheral vasodilation and maintenance of venous blood flow in the lower extremities. In addition, local anesthetics inhibit platelet aggregation and stabilize endothelial cells. Regional anesthesia is considered by many anesthesiologists to maintain respiratory function better than general anesthesia does. Unless the anesthetic level involves the intercostal musculature, ventilation and the cough reflex are well maintained.

Technical problems associated with regional anesthesia in the elderly include altered landmarks as a result of degeneration of the vertebral column and the difficulty of obtaining adequate patient positioning. To avoid having the patient lie on the fracture, a hypobaric solution can be injected intrathecally. Postpuncture headache is less of a problem in the elderly population.

If the patient refuses regional anesthesia, is general anesthesia acceptable?

General anesthesia is an acceptable alternative to regional block. One advantage is that the patient can be induced in bed and moved to the operating room table after intubation, avoiding the pain of positioning. A disadvantage is that the patient is unable to provide feedback regarding pressure points on the unpadded orthopedic table.

What specific factors should be considered during induction and maintenance of general anesthesia with this patient?

Intravenous induction agents should be administered slowly, since slow blood circulation will delay the onset of action. It is important to remember that because a subtrochanteric fracture can be associated with more than 1 L of occult blood loss, induction with sodium thiopental or propofol may lead to an exaggerated drop in arterial blood pressure. Thus, although the patient may be at risk for aspiration, the usual rapid-sequence induction should be modified to minimize cardiovascular changes. An acceptable compromise allows slower drug administration and gentle mask ventilation while maintaining firm cricoid pressure until satisfactory endotracheal tube position is confirmed. Initial hypotension may be replaced by hypertension and tachycardia during laryngoscopy and intubation. This roller-coaster volatility in blood pressure increases the risk of myocardial ischemia and can be avoided by preceding airway instrumentation with lidocaine (1.5 mg/kg), esmolol (0.3 mg/kg), or alfentanil (5–15 µg/kg).

Intraoperative paralysis with a nondepolarizing muscle relaxant improves surgical conditions and allows maintenance of a lighter plane of anesthesia. Deliberate hypotension may lessen intraoperative blood loss and is not contraindicated solely on the basis of age (see Case Discussion, Chapter 13).

SUGGESTED READING

Dodds C, Allison J: Postoperative cognitive deficit in the elderly surgical patient. Br J Anaesth 1998;81:449.

Ferrell BR, Ferrell BA (editors): *Pain in the Elderly.* IASP Press, 1996.

McLeskey CH (editor): *Geriatric Anesthesiology.* Williams & Wilkins, 1997.

Muravchick S: *Geroanesthesia. Principles for Management of the Elderly Patient.* Mosby-Year Book, Inc., 1997.

O'Keeffe ST, Chonchubhair AN: Postoperative delirium in the elderly. Br J Anaesth 1994;73:673.

Parikh SS, Chung F: Postoperative delirium in the elderly. Anesth Analg 1995;80:1223.

Priebe H-J. The aged cardiovascular risk patient. Br J Anaesth 2000;85:763.

Smith RB, Gurkowski MA, Bracken CA (editors): *Anesthesia and Pain Control in the Geriatric Patient.* McGraw-Hill, 1995.

Wright PMC: Population based pharmacokinetic analysis: Why do we need it; What is it; and what has it told us about anaesthetics? Br J Anaesth 1998;80:488.

Outpatient Anesthesia

Stuart Ackerman, MD*

KEY CONCEPTS

 The appropriateness of performing a particular surgical procedure on an outpatient basis depends on the resources of the facility, the estimated duration of the procedure, and the level of postoperative care the patient will probably require.

 The same level of perioperative care, including laboratory testing, is required for outpatients and inpatients.

 Intraoperative monitoring standards for outpatient and inpatient anesthesia are identical.

 Problems associated with spinal or epidural anesthesia that can delay discharge include orthostatic hypotension, prolonged motor or sensory blockade, and urinary retention.

 One method to reduce the incidence of postoperative nausea and vomiting is to order no oral intake, including fluids, until the patient feels hungry.

 All outpatients must be discharged home in the company of a responsible adult who will stay with them overnight.

One of the most dramatic transformations in health care delivery during the past two decades has been a shift from inpatient to outpatient surgery (also called *ambulatory surgery*). It is estimated that 60–70% of all surgical procedures in the United States are done on an outpatient basis. The primary impetus for this change was the economic savings afforded by not admitting patients the night before surgery or keeping them in hospital the night after surgery. Other advantages of outpatient surgery include earlier ambulation, patient convenience, and a lessened risk of nosocomial infection. As would be expected, the trend toward outpatient surgery has affected the practice of anesthesia.

The tremendous success of outpatient surgery has also led to advances in surgical and anesthetic techniques. A whole new spectrum of minimally invasive and endoscopic approaches to surgery has made outpatient surgery or early hospital discharge practical for an increasing number of operations. Outpatient surgery has also led to an increasing interest in the development of short- and ultra-short-acting anesthetic agents and regional anesthetic techniques. The speed of these de-

velopments and their application have led to controversies over which surgical procedures can be done safely on an outpatient basis and where they should be done—in a hospital's outpatient area, free-standing surgery center, or a physician's office.

In this chapter, the special constraints and considerations involved in the safe and efficient administration of anesthesia for outpatient surgery will be explored. Preoperative, intraoperative, and postoperative considerations are presented.

▓ PREOPERATIVE CONSIDERATIONS

SITE CONSIDERATIONS

Surgery performed on an outpatient basis usually takes place in one of three settings: typical hospital setting, free-standing surgery center, and doctor's office. Each of these settings gives rise to specific considerations. First, the typical hospital setting offers both inpatient and outpatient accommodations and equipment. Second, a free-standing surgery center is designed for short daytime

* Attending Anesthesiologist, San Fernando Valley Heart Institute, Encino-Tarzana Regional Medical Center, Los Angeles, California.

882

stays; some centers may offer overnight facilities. Third, one estimate is that 15–20% of all outpatient procedures are performed in an office-based setting.

Regardless of location, it is incumbent upon the anesthesiologist to ascertain that all drugs and equipment are immediately available and in good working order to provide a safe environment for patients.

SURGICAL CASE SELECTION

 The appropriateness of performing a particular surgical procedure on an outpatient, or ambulatory, basis depends on the resources of the facility, the estimated duration of the procedure, and the level of postoperative care the patient will probably require. For example, a free-standing surgical facility may not allow a potentially complex operation because the facility may not be able to accommodate a patient who needs postoperative admission, whereas an outpatient department in a hospital is obviously equipped to handle such a case. Furthermore, inpatient facilities typically provide both more comprehensive laboratory resources and greater access to specialized consultants. Since recovery room time is relatively independent of the duration of surgery and anesthesia, most centers now feel comfortable in accepting patients for outpatient surgery that extends beyond the traditional recommendation of a 2-hour maximum. Clearly, outpatient surgery is inappropriate if a patient will require extensive postoperative care because of the nature of the surgery or because of a preexisting medical condition. Some outpatient surgical centers do not accept cases complicated by infection because of the lack of isolation facilities. Finally, economics often necessitate that surgery be performed in an outpatient setting. Many third-party payers will not pay for cosmetic surgical procedures or may mandate outpatient surgery to avoid the expense of "unnecessary" inpatient care. A "compromise" situation has resulted in many hospitals offering a 23-hour overnight unit. In this setting, the patients are observed overnight and discharged the next morning—providing extended care and observation while delivering the service on the "outpatient" basis that is mandated by many insurance plans.

The controversy surrounding outpatient case selection is typified by tonsillectomies and adenoidectomies. Approximately 3% of patients requiring these procedures experience postoperative bleeding; many patients will need transfusion and reoperation. It should be noted that post-tonsillectomy hemorrhage often does not occur until more than 12 hours after surgery. For these reasons, many centers schedule these operations in the morning to allow maximal in-facility observation, while some may not allow tonsillectomies to be performed in the outpatient setting.

PATIENT SELECTION

As with surgical procedures, the guidelines for patient selection have progressively become much more liberal. While only American Society of Anesthesiologists (ASA) class 1 or class 2 patients were formerly considered candidates for outpatient surgery, many centers currently allow medically stable ASA class 3 patients. Some centers allow ASA class 4 patients to have procedures that are limited in nature or when hospital admission would place the patient at increased risk. An example of this situation would be an immunosuppressed cancer patient requiring insertion of a Hickman catheter for chemotherapy. Patients with serious systemic diseases (eg, morbid obesity, poorly controlled type I diabetes mellitus, steroid-dependent asthma, myasthenia gravis) need to be evaluated on a case-by-case basis, with consideration of both the extent of the disease and the nature of the surgical procedure.

The ability of a patient to cooperate with written preoperative and postoperative instructions and the availability of a responsible adult to accompany the patient home are often as important as the patient's medical condition in determining the suitability of outpatient surgery. The possibility of overnight hospital admission must be understood and accepted by the patient.

Age is not a contraindication to outpatient surgery with the following exceptions:

- Premature infants younger than 50 weeks postconception (some centers use 60 weeks as the cutoff time).
- Infants with a history of bronchopulmonary dysplasia or apneic episodes who have been symptomatic within the last 6 months.
- Siblings of infants who have died of sudden infant death syndrome.

These groups of patients are at increased risk for postoperative apnea and should be monitored for at least 24 hours after surgery. Elderly patients may require more time than do young adults to recover psychomotor skills fully. Nonetheless, they—and children—benefit most from outpatient surgery because they are most susceptible to the adverse psychological effects associated with hospital admission.

LABORATORY TESTING & PREOPERATIVE EVALUATION

The need for laboratory testing does not depend on whether surgery is performed on an outpatient or inpatient basis. The same level of perioperative care, including laboratory testing, is required 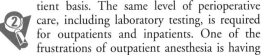 for outpatients and inpatients. One of the frustrations of outpatient anesthesia is having to cancel a scheduled procedure because of an inadequate preoperative workup, unexpected laboratory abnormalities, or the patient's failure to follow preoperative instructions (eg, nothing by mouth orders). Because of the logistical problems often encountered in evaluating an outpatient prior to the day of surgery, physicians often order excessive laboratory testing. Much of this confusion and expense can be eliminated by having the anesthesiologist evaluate patients before the day of surgery. This might take the form of the usual preoperative history and physical examination, a telephone interview, or a screening questionnaire. Multiple studies have demonstrated that a history and a physical examination are more effective screening procedures for disease than are a battery of routine laboratory tests.

PREMEDICATION

The considerations for outpatient premedication are similar to those for inpatients except for the added goal of rapid emergence (see Case Discussion, Chapter 8). Intramuscular injection of long-acting agents such as morphine sulfate or lorazepam can easily be switched to intravenous administration of shorter-acting drugs such as fentanyl or midazolam. In general, judicious use of short-acting agents does not significantly prolong recovery time. Of course, withholding all sedative premedication is an alternative for many patients. As is true with inpatients, the most effective premedication is an informative preoperative interview.

In some studies, outpatients have been shown to be at increased risk for aspiration pneumonia because of increased acidity and volume of gastric secretions. However, the routine administration of H_2 histamine antagonists or other protective drugs is not recommended by most authorities.

■ INTRAOPERATIVE CONSIDERATIONS

ANESTHETIC TECHNIQUES & PHARMACOLOGIC CONSIDERATIONS

1. General Anesthesia

Most common induction techniques do not interfere with wake-up times except following the shortest of cases. Specifically, propofol, thiopental, etomidate, methohexital, and inhalational inductions are acceptable. Ketamine has been associated with prolonged emergence in some patients. Propofol may be the best choice of induction agent in most outpatients because of its tendency to provide a rapid, clear-headed wake-up with a low incidence of nausea or vomiting. Outpatient surgery is not itself a contraindication to intubation, but many cases are brief enough to allow the use of a face mask or laryngeal mask airway (LMA).

Anesthesia can be maintained with volatile agents, small boluses of short-acting opioids, or continuous infusions of intravenous anesthetics. Enflurane appears to be an exception to the lack of correlation between anesthesia time and recovery time and should probably be avoided during cases exceeding 2 hours. Desflurane and sevoflurane provide the fastest wake-up time of the currently available volatile anesthetics because of their low blood/gas partition coefficients (see Chapter 7). Numerous intravenous anesthetics and combinations of anesthetics have been used in total intravenous anesthetic techniques during outpatient anesthesia. Propofol, remifentanil, alfentanil, and sufentanil have short durations of action and are popular outpatient anesthetics. Because shorter-acting drugs tend to be costly to administer during a case of moderate duration, an alternative would be to switch techniques during the procedure. For example, the anesthetic could begin with a propofol induction, followed by maintenance with isoflurane or sevoflurane and changed to a propofol infusion or desflurane at the end for a rapid emergence. Anesthesia may be supplemented with nitrous oxide.

The choice of muscle relaxant depends on many variables, including the anticipated duration of anesthesia, coexisting medical problems, and the cost of the drug (see Chapter 9). Mivacurium provides a moderate onset of action, but it has the shortest duration of action of any nondepolarizing muscle relaxant. Atracurium, vecuronium, and rocuronium are intermediate-acting muscle relaxants. Routine use of a nerve stimulator helps avoid overdosage and problems with residual muscle paralysis. A continuous infusion of succinylcholine may be a reasonable choice for cases requiring an ultra-short period of profound muscle relaxation (eg, esophagoscopy). Outpatients appear to be at increased risk for postoperative myalgias following succinylcholine. Whether or not this complication can be prevented by pretreatment with a nondepolarizing muscle relaxant is controversial.

Intraoperative monitoring standards for outpatient and inpatient anesthesia are identical; the *minimum* standards for intraoperative monitoring adopted by the ASA can be found in Chapter 6.

2. Regional Anesthesia

The advantages of regional anesthesia in outpatient surgery include less alteration in central nervous system function and a degree of postoperative pain relief. Depending on the type of regional block, some postoperative complications (eg, emesis, drowsiness) appear to be reduced, compared with general anesthesia. A potential disadvantage of regional anesthesia in a busy outpatient setting is the amount of time required to perform some blocks. Possible techniques range from spinal or epidural anesthesia to peripheral nerve blocks (retrobulbar block) or local infiltration. Problems associated with spinal or epidural anesthesia that can delay discharge include orthostatic hypotension, prolonged motor or sensory blockade, and urinary retention. Post-dural puncture headache appears to be more common in outpatients than in inpatients. Techniques that may be associated with occult complications should be avoided; for example, supraclavicular block may result in a pneumothorax. Local anesthetic agents should be chosen carefully to prevent prolonged muscle relaxation in the postoperative period. Even with regional anesthesia, psychomotor function may be impaired for several hours after surgery if sedative drugs are also administered.

3. Monitored Anesthesia Care

Many relatively minor procedures can be safely performed using local anesthesia (eg, a field block given by the surgeon) in combination with intravenous sedation. Surgical procedures such as minor plastic surgical procedures, ophthalmic procedures, and breast biopsies can all be smoothly accomplished using this technique. Monitoring is the same as for any general anesthetic. Oxygen can be administered by nasal cannula or clear plastic mask—sometimes cut to allow greater surgical assess for eye or facial surgery. A common technique is initial sedation and anxiolysis with a benzodiazepine (midazolam 1–3 mg) followed by propofol. A small propofol bolus can be given just before the surgeon injects local anesthetic so that the patient is briefly unconscious and does not recall the initial burning associated with local anesthetic injection. Monitored anesthesia care is discussed further in the Case Discussion at the end of this chapter.

■ POSTOPERATIVE CONSIDERATIONS

COMPLICATIONS

Postoperative complications that are relatively insignificant for an inpatient can prevent an outpatient from becoming "home ready" and jeopardize discharge from an ambulatory surgical unit. Factors that have been associated with postoperative complications include female gender, no previous exposure to general anesthesia, endotracheal intubation, abdominal surgery, and surgical time in excess of 20 minutes.

Emesis is a common problem that, if protracted, can require hospital admission. Its incidence is increased with anesthetic techniques that require high doses of opioids, certain types of surgery, postoperative pain, and a predisposition to motion sickness (Table 46–1). Patients at increased risk benefit from routine prophylaxis with an antiemetic agent. Serotonin 5-HT$_3$ receptor blocking drugs such as ondansetron (4 mg IV) or dolasetron (12.5 mg IV) are widely used and extremely well tolerated. Droperidol (0.01–0.05 mg/kg IV) is also an effective agent, but its adult dose should be limited to less than 1.25 mg to prevent postoperative drowsiness. Even this small dose has been implicated in postoperative anxiety and dysphoria. Metoclopramide (10 mg IV) has the advantage of not prolonging the recovery from general anesthesia and may decrease residual gastric volume. In patients at high risk for emesis two agents can be given in combination. Clinical studies suggest that ondansetron is equallly effective as the combination of droperidol and metoclopramide. Dexamethasone (10–12 mg IV) has been shown to be useful in patients with refractory nausea and vomiting. Application of a transdermal scopolamine patch 2 hours before surgery may reduce the incidence of postoperative nausea and vomiting, but

Table 46–1. Risk factors for postoperative nausea and vomiting.

Patient factors
Young age
Female gender, particularly if menstruating on day of surgery or in first trimester of pregnancy
History of prior postoperative emesis
History of motion sickness
Delayed gastric emptying (eg, obesity)
Anesthetic techniques
Opioid administration
General anesthesia
Anesthetic drugs (? neostigmine, ketamine, volatile agents)
Postoperative pain
Hypotension
Surgical procedures
Strabismus surgery
Ear surgery
Laparoscopy
Orchiopexy
Ovum retrieval
Tonsillectomy

anticholinergic side effects (eg, dry mouth, loss of near vision, urinary retention, disorientation, somnolence) limit its usefulness. One method to reduce the incidence of postoperative nausea and vomiting is to order *no* oral intake, including fluids, until the patient feels *hungry.* Complaints of thirst in the absence of hunger can be relieved by gargling water, but swallowing should be avoided. Forcing oral fluids onto a nauseated patient has predictably disappointing results.

Postoperative pain can be controlled with intravenous analgesics or local nerve block. Although intraoperative administration of short-acting opioid agonists may increase the incidence of postoperative nausea and vomiting, recovery from anesthesia is not prolonged by low doses (eg, 2 μg/kg of fentanyl). Even lower doses are often effective at controlling pain in the recovery room (fentanyl, 0.5 μg/kg). Intramuscular or intravenous ketorolac (30–60 mg) given prior to the end of surgery usually provides some degree of analgesia without predisposing the patient to respiratory depression or emesis. A less expensive alternative is preoperative administration of a generic oral nonsteroidal antiinflammatory agent. Infiltration with local anesthetic during surgery may effectively decrease postoperative discomfort following inguinal hernia repair, circumcision, and tubal ligation. After discharge from the recovery room, most patients can be given oral pain medications (eg, acetaminophen) if they have regained their appetites.

Prolonged somnolence is unusual unless long-acting anesthetic agents have been administered (see Case Discussion, Chapter 9). **Headache** is a common postoperative problem and appears to be increased following administration of volatile anesthetic agents. **Urinary retention** can follow general anesthesia as well as spinal or epidural blockade. This is especially a problem in elderly men with prostatic hypertrophy. Simple bladder catheterization may prove to be traumatic and require consultation with a urologist. **Sore throat** and **hoarseness** are common complaints following endotracheal intubation, but they can also occur after mask ventilation, LMA, or regional anesthesia with sedation. **Postintubation croup** is usually limited to pediatric patients and is discussed in Chapter 44.

DISCHARGE CRITERIA

Recovery from anesthesia can be divided into at least three stages: emergence and awakening, home readiness, and complete psychomotor recovery.

Discharge from an outpatient surgical center is conditioned upon achieving a minimum level of home readiness (Table 46–2). Current cognitive and psychomotor tests (Trieger test, digit symbol substitution

Table 46–2. Criteria defining home readiness.*

Orientation to person, place, and time
Stable vital signs for 30–60 minutes
Ability to ambulate unassisted
Ability to tolerate oral fluids[†]
Ability to void[†]
Absence of significant pain or bleeding

*These criteria assume normal preoperative function.
[†]These may not be mandatory in all patients.

test) are not routinely recommended for this purpose. Recovery of proprioception, sympathetic tone, bladder function, and motor strength are additional criteria following regional anesthesia. For example, intact proprioception of the big toe, minimal orthostatic changes, and normal plantar flexion of the foot are important signals of recovery following spinal anesthesia.

All outpatients must be discharged home in the company of a responsible adult who will stay with them overnight. Patients must be provided with written postoperative instructions on how to obtain emergency help and to perform routine follow-up care. The assessment of home readiness is the responsibility of the physician, preferably an anesthesiologist, who is familiar with the patient. The authority to discharge a patient home can be delegated to a nurse if preapproved discharge criteria are rigorously applied.

Home readiness does not imply that the patient has the ability to make important decisions, to drive, or to return to work. These activities require complete psychomotor recovery, which is often not achieved until 24–72 hours postoperatively. In some free-standing centers, or office-based surgery centers, arrangements can be made with nearby care facilities to provide 1- or 2-day post-recovery management. This should be considered when additional pain control, wound care, or skilled nursing assistance is indicated.

All outpatient centers must use some system of postoperative follow-up involving the use of patient questionnaires or phone contacts the day after discharge.

CASE DISCUSSION:
MONITORED ANESTHESIA
CARE FOR EYE SURGERY

A healthy 70-year-old retired physician presents to an outpatient surgery center for a cataract extraction and insertion of an intraocular lens. Surgery is scheduled as "monitored anesthesia care."

What considerations help determine the choice of sedative agents and technique for administration?

Although almost any form of sedation may be satisfactory, a few factors should receive special attention. Because this is an outpatient procedure, short-acting agents are preferable to long-acting ones. Furthermore, a continuous infusion, as opposed to intermittent boluses, can often provide an equivalent level of sedation with a smaller total drug dose. Surgical manipulation of the eyes may lead to nausea, so a drug with antiemetic properties would be desirable. An analgesic agent might also be valuable during anticipated periods of painful stimulation (eg, during injection of the retrobulbar or peribulbar block). Supplemental oxygen is always administered by nasal cannula or a face mask in which the nose piece has been removed to avoid the surgical field.

One possible technique is the administration of propofol using an infusion pump: a bolus of 20–40 mg followed by an infusion of 25–100 µg/kg/min. The dose of propofol can be easily titrated to the desired depth of sedation. Moreover, its short duration of action makes propofol desirable for short procedures, particularly in an outpatient setting. Alternate hypnotic-sedative agents include midazolam 1–3 mg, thiopental 25–50 mg, or methohexital 10–30 mg. Just prior to the injection of local anesthetic, a small bolus of alfentanil (5–10 µg/kg) or remifentanil (0.5–2 µg/kg) produces a brief period of intense analgesia. Premedication with a 5-HT$_3$ antagonist (ondansetron 4 mg or dolasetron 12.5 mg) helps avoid opioid-induced nausea.

What level of sedation is appropriate following the retrobulbar block for this patient and procedure?

Surgical site is an important consideration when using intravenous sedation to supplement regional or local anesthesia. (See chapter 8, Profiles in Anesthetic Practice: Rational Administration of Intravenous Anesthesia.) A still patient is an absolute necessity in ocular surgery where a microscope is used and sharp instruments are placed within the eye; even small sudden movement at a critical moment can injure the eye and have potentially disastrous consequences. The patient should therefore generally be awake and oriented, or completely anesthetized. Moreover, it is important to be able to communicate with the awake patient. In the case of a confused patient or one who cannot communicate with the surgical team,

a general anesthetic with endotracheal intubation may be preferable. It is important to discuss the plan for monitored anesthesia care preoperatively with the patient and make sure that his or her expectations are realistic. Patients may be misinformed and not understand just how monitored anesthesia with sedation "works." They may have concerns about either being completely awake, or may complain later about some periods of awareness—believing they were supposed to be unconscious.

Ten minutes following incision, the patient becomes increasingly agitated and restless. How would you proceed?

Agitation and restlessness in the sedated patient should immediately alert the anesthesiologist to the possibility of hypoxia. Adequacy of oxygenation can be quickly assessed by pulse oximetry. Ventilation can be grossly monitored in the nonintubated patient by connecting the aspiration tubing of a sidestream capnograph to the patient's face mask. After ensuring adequate oxygenation and ventilation, disorientation or inadequate analgesia from the retrobulbar block are likely explanations. The latter may be treated with topical local anesthetic on the eye.

It often is difficult to predict which patients will remain cooperative and oriented during the procedure and who will become confused or restless following some sedation. Many elderly patients and some younger patients may initially be cooperative but later become increasingly disoriented, restless, and uncooperative once the procedure is well underway. In such cases, one of two approaches may be helpful depending on the adequacy of the airway, ventilation, and oxygen saturation. The first approach is to stop all sedation and allow the patient to become reoriented. If airway patency, ventilation, and oxygen saturation are adequate, the second approach is to increase the level of sedation; insertion of a nasal airway (well lubricated with lidocaine jelly) may be helpful.

What are potential pitfalls associated with the use of an infusion pump for sedation or total intravenous anesthesia (TIVA)?

The safe and continuous administration of intravenous anesthetics or vasoactive agents critically depends on a reliable delivery system. Although a simple gravity intravenous infusion can be "piggy-backed" to a carrier line, a pump offers the advantages of more precise dose selection, a lower risk of unintentional drug bolusing, and minimal flow variation from changes in venous pressure or bag height. Pumps can be categorized into two types: syringe and volumetric.

Syringe pumps *use a driver that pushes fluid out of a syringe by advancing its plunger while the barrel is kept stationary. These units tend to be small, lightweight, cordless, and accurate at very low flow rates. Some models recognize and automatically compensate for the type and size of syringe being used. Other possible features include a program memory (library) of frequently used drugs and their usual concentration, initial infusion rate, and bolus size. Small dead-space tubing minimizes the amount of wasted drug, but can increase resistance to flow and the frequency of occlusion false alarms. Because the small capacity of a syringe pump requires high drug concentrations to minimize the frequency of syringe replacement, an infusion rate error can be quite serious. Syringe pumps can also be prone to gravitational infusion of fluid if exposed to large changes in height relative to the patient. The pump line must be properly primed with the purge button before connecting to the patient to avoid delays caused by system compliance (eg, the rubber tip of the plunger), mechanical slack (eg, engagement of the driver), or air in the tubing. Similarly, the source of any occlusion should be gradually released to avoid an unintentional drug bolus from pressure buildup within the line.*

Volumetric pumps *require a disposable cassette within an intravenous set that controls flow rate by a variety of methods. In contrast to syringe pumps, the higher capacity of volumetric pumps allows them to deliver a lower concentration of drug, and their cassette design does not allow any significant degree of gravitational infusion. Disadvantages include the added cost of the disposable cassettes, a susceptibility to air bubbles, and the inconvenience associated with their larger size and power requirements. Newer volumetric pumps also incorporate dose-rate calculators so that drips may be controlled either by flow rate or the desired dose rate.*

Regardless of pump design, some general recommendations for continuous infusion of intravenous anesthetics can be made. Continuous monitoring of the pump and the intravenous line is critical because the entire anesthetic management may depend on their proper functioning. For example, disconnection of the pump line, occlusion and retrograde flow up the carrier line, or misassembly of the pump system can result in unwanted patient awakening and awareness. Digital keypads present the possibility for easily entering the wrong number (eg, 550 mL/min instead of 50 mL/min). To minimize the effects of changes in the carrier-fluid flow rate on anesthetic delivery, an infusion of anesthetic agents should receive generally a dedicated intravenous line or should be placed as close to the patient as possible (eg, at the intravenous catheter hub).

SUGGESTED READING

Aldrete JA: The post-anesthesia recovery score revisited. J Clin Anesth 1995;7:89.

Chung F, Mezei G: Adverse outcomes in ambulatory anesthesia. Can J Anaesth 1999;46:R18.

Chung F: Recovery pattern and home readiness after ambulatory surgery. Anesth Analg 1996:896.

Kovac AL: Prevention and treatment of postoperative nausea and vomiting. Drugs 2000;59:213.

Marshall SI, Chung F: Discharge criteria and complications after ambulatory surgery. Anaesth Analg 1999;88:508.

Padfield NL: *Total Intravenous Anaesthesia*. Butterworth-Heinemann, 2000.

Pavlin DJ, Rapp SE, Polissar NL, et al: Factors affecting discharge times in adult outpatients. Anesth Analg 1998;87:816.

Peacock JE, Philip BK: Ambulatory anesthesia experience with remifentanil. Anesth Analg 1999;89:S22.

White P: *Ambulatory Anesthesia & Surgery*. Lippincott Williams & Wilkins, 1997.

White P: *Textbook of Intravenous Anesthesia*. Lippincott Williams & Wilkins, 1997.

SECTION V
Special Problems

Anesthetic Complications

47

Joseph T. Nitti, MD, and Gary J. Nitti, MD*

KEY CONCEPTS

1 Complications related to the delivery of anesthesia care are inevitable. Even the most experienced, diligent, and careful practitioners will have to manage complications despite acting well within the standard of care.

2 Anesthetic mishaps can be categorized as preventable or unpreventable. Of the preventable incidents, most involve human error, as opposed to equipment malfunctions.

3 Most serious anesthetic complications are associated with adverse respiratory events.

4 Many anesthetic fatalities occur only after a series of coincidental circumstances, misjudgments, and technical errors (mishap chain).

5 Although the mechanisms differ, anaphylactic and anaphylactoid reactions can be clinically indistinguishable and equally life-threatening.

6 Patients with spina bifida, spinal cord injury, and congenital abnormalities of the genitourinary tract have a very high incidence of latex allergy.

7 Although there is no clear evidence that exposure to trace amounts of anesthetic agents present a health hazard to operating room personnel, the US Occupational Health and Safety Administration continues to set maximum acceptable trace concentrations of less than 25 ppm for nitrous oxide and 0.5 for ppm halogenated anesthetics (2 ppm if the halogenated agent is used alone).

8 The risk of transmission of a blood-borne infectious disease can be estimated if three factors are known: the prevalence of the infection within the patient population, the incidence of exposure (eg, frequency of needlestick), and the rate of seroconversion after a single exposure.

9 Anesthesiology is a high-risk medical specialty for drug addiction.

10 The two most important methods of minimizing radiation exposure are using proper barriers and maximizing one's distance from the source of radiation.

---

* Both coauthors are affiliated with San Fernando Valley Heart Institute, Encino-Tarzana Regional Medical Center, Los Angeles, California. Dr. Joseph T. Nitti is attending anesthesiologist, and Dr. Gary J. Nitti is chief of anesthesiology.

INTRODUCTION

 Complications related to the delivery of anesthesia care are inevitable. Even the most experienced, diligent, and careful practitioners will have to manage complications despite acting well within the standard of care. These complications will range from minor (such an infiltrated intravenous line) to catastrophic (such hypoxic brain injury or even death).

When complications do occur, appropriate evaluation, management, and documentation are critical in minimizing or eliminating negative outcomes. A good example of such a complication is the unanticipated difficult airway. While a comprehensive preanesthetic airway evaluation will help the clinician anticipate and prepare for most difficult intubations, it will still fail to predict problems in a few patients who cannot be intubated except by specialized techniques (see Chapter 6). In these cases of an unrecognized difficult airway, despite preoxygenation and cricoid pressure (if appropriate), the risk of aspiration, airway obstruction, and hypoxia are high and extraordinary measures to secure the airway (cricothyrotomy, or surgical tracheostomy) may become necessary. Although establishing a surgical airway is a lifesaving procedure and if done properly will avoid aspiration, pulmonary edema, or hypoxic brain injury, it will inevitably be considered a "complication." Also, the patient will likely spend additional time on a mechanical ventilator and in the hospital, may require a second surgical procedure, and might be left with a small but unsightly scar. These "complications" will trigger institutional review, peer review, and potential legal action.

Litigation may occur in the example cited above despite the best efforts to communicate with the patient and family about the intraoperative events, management decisions, and the catastrophic complications that were avoided. It is essential to document the preoperative airway examination, to record maneuvers to preoxygenate and provide cricoid pressure, and to write a complete postanesthesia note so that the appropriate, standard-of-care of the patient can be defended should litigation occur.

Earlier chapters have discussed the risks and alternative anesthetic techniques associated with specific procedures. *Complications caused by errors in anesthetic management can still occur despite an adequate knowledge of didactic material.* This chapter reviews the incidences, causes, and prevention of both common and catastrophic anesthetic complications. The discussion includes important aspects of documentation that may make perioperative management and decision-making processes clearer to consultants when they review the medical record following complications. Documentation is also discussed in Chapter 1. Because of the rela-

tively low rate of anesthetic complications, we relied on large-scale studies, particularly the American Society of Anesthesiologists (ASA) Closed Claims Project. The Project is a collection of 4459 completed malpractice claims that span over two decades (1970–1994); it therefore provides a "snapshot" of anesthesia liability rather than a study of the incidence of anesthetic complications. These claims are grouped by subject area (eg, awareness and eye injury) and were independently reviewed to determine patterns of causation and liability. After a discussion of hypersensitivity reactions, anaphylaxis, and latex allergy, the chapter concludes with an examination of occupational hazards in anesthesiology, including trace exposure to anesthetic agents, infections, substance abuse, and radiation exposure.

ANESTHETIC ACCIDENTS

Incidence

There are several reasons why it is difficult to measure the incidence of anesthetic accidents accurately. First, it is often impossible to assign the responsibility for a poor outcome to the patient's inherent disease, the surgical procedure, or the anesthetic management. In fact, all three can contribute to a poor outcome. It is also difficult to define a measurable event. Death is a clear end point, but perioperative death is so rare that a very large series of patients must be studied in order to assemble conclusions that have statistical significance. Finally, medicolegal fears hinder accurate reporting.

Nonetheless, many studies have attempted to determine the incidence of deaths attributable to anesthesia complications. It is clear that most perioperative fatalities are due to the patient's preoperative disease or the surgical procedure. The mortality rate attributable primarily to anesthesia *appears* to have dropped during the last 30 years from one or two deaths per 3000 anesthetic experiences to a current rate of one or two deaths per 20,000 experiences. However, these statistics should be viewed with considerable skepticism, since they are derived from different countries using different methodologies. Recent studies indicate that the anesthetic mortality rate in some institutions may be even less than 1:20,000. This decline may be due to the availability and utilization of new monitoring equipment, greater knowledge of anesthetic physiology and pharmacology, or improved surgical and medical care. Indeed, in one large study, the mortality that was attributed solely due to anesthesia was 1 in 185,000.

Causes

Anesthetic mishaps can be categorized as preventable or unpreventable. Examples of the latter include sudden death syndrome, fatal

Table 47–1. Common human errors leading to preventable anesthetic accidents.

Unrecognized breathing circuit disconnection
Mistaken drug administration
Airway mismanagement
Anesthesia machine misuse
Fluid mismanagement
Intravenous line disconnection

Table 47–2. Common equipment malfunctions leading to preventable anesthetic accidents.

Breathing circuit
Monitoring device
Ventilator
Anesthesia machine
Laryngoscope

idiosyncratic drug reactions, or any poor outcome that occurs despite proper management. However, studies of anesthetic-related deaths or near misses demonstrate that most accidents are preventable. Of these preventable incidents, most involve human error (Table 47–1), as opposed to equipment malfunctions (Table 47–2). Unfortunately, some rate of human error is inevitable, and a preventable accident is not synonymous with incompetence. For the most recent period (1990–1994), the top three causes for claims in the ASA Closed Claims Project are death (22%), nerve injury (18%), and brain damage (9%).

Most serious anesthetic complications are associated with adverse respiratory events. Even in the most recent reporting period, respiratory events still accounted for the largest number of malpractice claims (38%) involving death or brain damage in ASA Closed Claims Project; cardiac events and equipment problems accounted for 25% and 8%, respectively.

Problems of airway management include inadequate ventilation, premature extubation, and unrecognized esophageal intubation. Breathing-circuit disconnection is a problem, especially with mechanical ventilation, and usually occurs at the endotracheal tube connector. Anesthesia machines with built-in low-circuit-pressure alarms and end-tidal CO_2 analysis should reduce the likelihood of this problem. Hypoxia from failing to ventilate a paralyzed patient has probably been the most common cause of intraoperative cardiac arrest. Aspiration pneumonia is discussed in the Case Discussion in Chapter 15.

Most accidents related to the anesthesia machine also involve an element of human error: gas flow control changes, vaporizer errors, gas supply problems, and unnoticed fail-safe activation. Unintentional administration of the wrong drug (**syringe swap**) often involves muscle relaxants or their reversal agents; look-alike prefilled syringes containing resuscitation drugs are also easily confused. The administration of an inappropriate dose of the correct drug is also hazardous. Drug syringes and ampules in the work area should be restricted to only those needed for the current, specific

case. They should be consistently diluted to the same concentration for each use and clearly labeled. Another type of human error occurs when the most critical problem is ignored because attention is inappropriately focused on a less important problem or an incorrect solution (**fixation error**).

Another generalization about serious anesthetic accidents is that there are usually other factors associated with their occurrence (Table 47–3). For instance, the impact of most equipment failures is lessened or totally avoided by routine preoperative checkouts and personnel training. Many anesthetic fatalities occur only after a series of coincidental circumstances, misjudgments, and technical errors (**mishap chain**).

Prevention

Strategies to reduce the incidence of serious anesthetic complications include better monitoring and anesthetic technique, improved education, more comprehensive protocols and standards of practice, and active risk management programs. Better monitoring and anes-

Table 47–3. Factors associated with human errors and equipment misuse.

Factor	Example
Inadequate preparation	No machine checkout or preoperative evaluation; haste and carelessness
Inadequate experience and training	Unfamiliarity with anesthetic technique or equipment
Environmental limitations	Inability to visualize surgical field: poor communication with surgeons
Physical and emotional factors	Fatigue; personal problems

thetic techniques imply closer patient contact, more comprehensive monitoring equipment, and better designed anesthesia machines and workspaces. The fact that most accidents occur during the maintenance phase of anesthesia—rather than during induction or emergence—implies a failure of vigilance. Inspection, auscultation, and palpation of the patient are a constant responsibility. Instruments should supplement but never replace the anesthesiologist's own senses.

A major goal of the Society for Education in Anesthesia is to improve resident training. Of course, education must continue beyond residency as new drugs, techniques, and equipment are developed. Part of this continuing education requirement includes awareness of recommended monitoring standards, equipment checkouts, preoperative evaluation, postoperative follow-up, and relief exchanges. The medicolegal obligations that accompany the establishment of specific standards are part of the cost of patient safety.

Risk management and continuous quality improvement programs at the departmental level may possibly reduce anesthetic morbidity and mortality rates by addressing equipment, continuing education, and staffing issues. Specific responsibilities of peer-review committees include identifying and preventing potential problems, formulating departmental policies, ensuring the availability of properly functioning anesthetic equipment, enforcing standards required for clinical privileges, and evaluating the appropriateness of patient care. A quality improvement system impartially reviews complications, ensures physician compliance, and continuously monitors quality indicators.

AIRWAY INJURY

Injury to airway structures is a constant concern to practicing anesthesiologists. The daily insertion of endotracheal tubes, laryngeal mask airways, oral/nasal airways, gastric tubes, transesophageal echocardiogram (TEE) probes, esophageal (boogie) dilators, and emergency airways all pose the risk of airway structure damage. Common morbidities such as sore throat and dysphagia are usually self-limiting but may also be nonspecific symptoms of more ominous complications.

The most common permanent airway injury is dental trauma. In a retrospective study of 600,000 surgical cases, the incidence of injury requiring dental intervention and repair was approximately 1 in 4500. In most cases, laryngoscopy and endotracheal intubation were involved, and the upper incisors were the most frequently injured. Dental trauma may occur less commonly from oral airways. Major risk factors for dental trauma included tracheal intubation, preexisting

poor dentition, and patient characteristics associated with difficult airway management (including limited neck motion, previous head and neck surgery, craniofacial abnormalities, and a history of difficult intubation).

Other types of airway trauma are rare. Although there are scattered case reports in the literature, the most comprehensive analysis is the ASA Closed Claims project. This report describes 266 claims, which were grouped by the site of injury. In general, the least serious were temporomandibular joint (TMJ) injuries, which were all associated with otherwise uncomplicated intubations and occurred mostly in females younger than 60 years. Approximately one-fourth of these patients had previous TMJ disease. Laryngeal injuries primarily included vocal cord paralysis, granuloma, and arytenoid dislocation. These were also generally associated with routine intubations and possibly related to tube movement or pressure necrosis. Most tracheal injuries were associated with emergency surgical tracheotomy, but a few were related to endotracheal intubation. These latter perforations contributed to death in 5 of 13 patients, who most often presented with delayed-onset subcutaneous emphysema or pneumothorax. Finally, pharyngoesophageal perforation was clearly associated with difficult intubation, age over 60 years, and female gender. As in tracheal perforation, obvious signs were often delayed in onset. Instead, initial sore throat, cervical pain, and cough often progress to fever, dysphagia, and dyspnea as mediastinitis, abscess, or pneumonia develop. Mortality rates of 25–50% after esophageal perforation have been reported, with the lower percentage being due to rapid detection and treatment.

Minimizing the risk of airway injury begins with the preoperative assessment. A thorough airway examination will help determine the risk for difficulty (see Chapter 5). Documentation of current dentition (including all dental work) should be included. Many practitioners believe preoperative consent should include a discussion of the risk of dental, oral, vocal cord, and esophageal trauma in every patient that could potentially need any airway manipulation. If a difficult airway is suspected, a more detailed discussion of risks (eg, emergency tracheostomy), is appropriate. In such cases, emergency airway supplies and experienced help should be immediately available, and the ASA algorithm for difficult airway management should be utilized (see Figure 5–21). Follow-up should occur to assess for latent signs of perforation when there is evidence of airway trauma. If intubation cannot be accomplished by conventional means, the patient or guardian should be informed in case of the future need for airway intervention.

PERIPHERAL NERVE INJURY

Perioperative nerve injury is a known complication of both regional and general anesthesia. Neuraxial (spinal cord or spinal root) injury is discussed in Chapter 16. Peripheral nerve injury, however, is a more frequent and oftentimes debilitating problem. In most cases, these injuries resolve within 6 to 12 weeks, but some persist for months or even years. Because peripheral neuropathies are commonly associated (sometimes incorrectly!) with patient positioning, a review of mechanisms and prevention is necessary.

The most common peripheral nerve injury is ulnar neuropathy. In a retrospective study of over 1 million patients, persistent ulnar neuropathy (greater than 3 months' duration) occurred in approximately 1 in 2700 patients. Interestingly, initial symptoms were most frequently noted more than 24 hours after a surgical procedure and may have occurred while the patient was on the hospital ward sleeping. Risk factors included male gender, hospital stay greater than 14 days, and very thin or obese body habitus. More than half of these patients regained full sensory and motor function within 1 year. Anesthetic technique was not implicated as a risk factor; one-fourth of patients with ulnar neuropathy underwent monitored care or lower extremity regional technique. This casts doubt that a stretch or compression mechanism caused the injury, because awake patients would likely respond to discomfort. The ASA Closed Claims Project findings support most of these findings, particularly the delayed onset of symptoms and the lack of relationship between anesthesia technique and injury. This study also noted that many neuropathies occurred despite notation of extra padding over the elbow area, further negating compression as a possible mechanism of injury.

The Role of Positioning

Other peripheral nerve injuries appear to be more closely related to positioning or surgical procedure. They may involve the peroneal nerve, the brachial plexus, or the femoral and sciatic nerves. External pressure on a nerve could compromise its perfusion, disrupt its cellular integrity, and eventually result in edema, ischemia, and necrosis. Pressure injuries are particularly likely when nerves pass through closed compartments formed by dense osseofascial membranes or take a superficial course (eg, the perineal nerve around the fibula). Lower extremity neuropathies, especially involving the peroneal nerve, have been associated with improper lithotomy positioning, extreme (high) lithotomy position, and especially prolonged duration (greater than 2 hours). Patient risk factors for this complication include hypotension; thin body habitus; old age; and history of vascular disease, diabetes, or smoking. Ulnar nerve injuries are associated with cardiac surgery because rib retraction may promote stretch on the brachial plexus. Similarly, the long thoracic nerve may be severed during pneumonectomy or axillary lymph node dissection, resulting in paralysis of the serratus anterior muscle and winging of the scapula. Some brachial plexus injuries following lateral decubitus positioning may be related to improper positioning of the axillary roll. This roll should be caudad to the axilla to prevent direct pressure on the brachial plexus, and large enough to relieve any pressure from the mattress on the lower shoulder.

The data suggest that some peripheral nerve injury is not preventable. Patient, procedure, and position factors contribute a significant amount of risk. While the risk of peripheral neuropathy should be discussed during informed consent, especially in patients to be placed in a nonsupine position, other practices may be helpful. Whenever possible, patients can be positioned before induction of anesthesia to check for discomfort. Final positioning should be evaluated carefully prior to draping. The upper extremities should not be extended greater than 90 degrees at any joint and should be supinated to protect the ulnar tunnel. Prolonged pronation of the forearm can compress the ulnar nerve in the cubital tunnel (Figure 47–1). Lower extremities should not have any obvious pressure points. Although injuries can occur despite the presence of padding, additional padding may be helpful in vulnerable areas. Documentation should include positioning information, including the presence of padding. Finally, if a patient complains of sensory or motor dysfunction in the postoperative period, he or she should be reassured that this is frequently a temporary condition. Motor and sensory function should be documented and the patient should be referred for neurologic evaluation and physiologic testing, such as nerve conduction and electromyographic studies.

OTHER COMPLICATIONS RELATED TO POSITIONING

Changes of body position have physiologic consequences that can be exaggerated in disease states. General and regional anesthesia may limit the cardiovascular response to such a change. Even positions that are safe for short periods may eventually lead to complications in persons who are not able to move in response to pain. For example, the alcoholic patient who passes out on a hard floor may waken with a brachial plexus injury. Similarly, regional and general anesthesia abolish protective reflexes and predispose patients to injury.

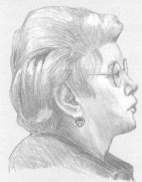

M. Jane Matjasko, MD

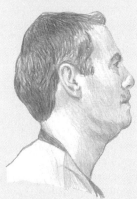

Douglas G. Martz, MD

THE SEATED POSITION—GONE FOREVER?

For patients who are undergoing posterior midline cranial and cervical procedures, the seated position appears to be ideal because surgical venous bleeding is decreased, surgical visibility is improved, and the surgeon sees structures in anatomically normal relationships. However, morbidity and mortality from complications associated with this position, such as venous air embolism (VAE), quadriplegia, peripheral nerve injury, arterial air embolism, and airway and tongue edema, are of great concern.

Beginning in the 1970s early detection of air embolism became possible because of the realization that precordial Doppler monitoring detected air volumes as low as 0.125 ml.[1] The possibility of aspiration of air via a central venous pressure catheter placed at the superior vena cava–right atrial junction was a promising method for treating venous air embolism and decreasing morbidity and mortality.

However, arterial air embolism became known to occur both in the presence of a patent or probe-patent foramen ovale (23% of the general population) and in its absence.[2] It was also postulated that under some circumstances air might traverse the pulmonary vessels and be dispersed to all major organs, most importantly the cerebral and coronary arteries. Because of concern about VAE and quadriplegia from excessive neck flexion or inadequate spinal cord perfusion, as well as the argument that access to a hyperbaric chamber was necessary to treat arterial air embolism should it occur, most surgeons and anesthesiologists abandoned the seated position. Teaching centers also stopped using the seated position. As a result, surgery and anesthesia residents did not encounter a single case during their training, nor did their bedside and classroom teaching include much regarding the seated position.

In the 1980s, several large retrospective and prospective series that evaluated the complications of the seated position were published.[3] The inci-

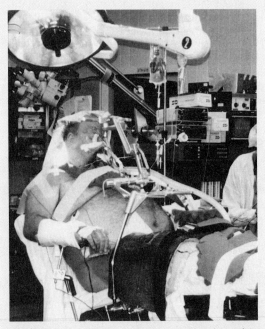

Figure 1. Patient in seated position. Note that the neck is not excessively flexed, The abdomen is free, and the arms supported.

dence of VAE was about 25% in most studies (about 10% in cervical procedures); use of nitrous oxide was not associated with more severe cardiovascular instability if it was discontinued at the first Doppler sign of air entry;[4] and there was no difference in morbidity or mortality in matched patients with surgery performed in the seated (n=100) versus the supine (n=100) position. However, there was greater blood loss and less satisfactory surgical exposure in the horizontal group.[5] In both retrospective and prospective studies after the mid-1970s, morbidity and mortality approached zero. Clinically available and reliable mass spectrometers, capable of end-tidal nitrogen monitoring, were more sensitive to early detection of air embolism than to either a decrease in end-tidal carbon dioxide or an increase in pulmonary artery pressure. Attention to the details of positioning and to maintaining adequate blood pressure and presumably blood flow to the spinal cord significantly decreased the risk of quadriplegia. Surgical hemostasis became more vigorous and complete.

In the meantime, authors published case reports of other rare sources of VAE, such as bladder irrigation after transurethral resection of the prostate, hysteroscopy, arthroscopy, Cesarean section, pulmonary barotrauma, prone position, caudal catheter placement in infants, and liver tumor resection, to name a few. The very low incidence of serious complications from VAE, and a particular patient encounter led us to realize that those training in anesthesiology should know how to position and monitor patients in the seated position, recognize when a VAE is occurring, know the treatment, and be able to provide appropriate operating conditions for unusual patients such as the one presented here.

The patient referred to above is a 47-year-old, 212-kg man who had progressive cervical stenosis related to osteoarthritis as evidenced by myelopathy and a narrow cervical canal on magnetic resonance imaging. Progressive inactivity due to myelopathy would not permit exercise and weight reduction. As the myelopathy worsened (3/5 in both arms and legs); the patient became more sedentary. Surgery was necessary to stabilize at least, if not improve, his neurologic status. Pertinent medical history included hypertension, type II diabetes mellitus, and obstructive sleep apnea. Electrocardiographic findings and laboratory values were normal.

The prone position was not possible due to excessive abdominal girth causing probable respiratory compromise. The airway anatomy was Mallampati III, the neck was short, and good mask fit was tenuous. The opinion of the anesthesiologist was that awake fiberoptic intubation was required and the only acceptable position for surgery, in consultation with the surgeon, was the seated one. Only three individuals in the department were familiar with use of the seated position for patients during surgery, and no current resident had seen one. After detailed informed consent, the patient was brought to the operating room and placed on the operating table in the seated position. Sequential pressure stockings were placed on the legs. After administration of midazolam, 1 mg, intravenously, routine monitoring, left subclavian access, and a left radial arterial catheter were inserted after local infiltration. A mul-

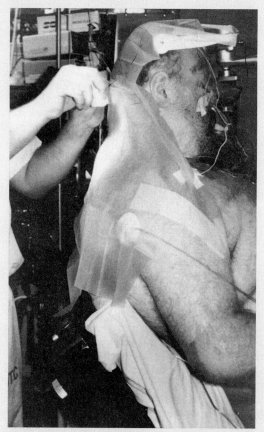

Figure 2. Lateral view. Surgical access optimal.

(continued on next page)

(continued from previous page)

tiorificed central venous catheter was inserted through the introducer and the tip positioned at the superior vena cava–right atrial junction with electrocardiographic confirmation.

With the patient in the seated position, the airway was anesthetized with nebulized lidocaine, 4%, via mask. Glycopyrrolate, 0.4 mg, and midazolam, 2 mg, were given. After nasal administration of neosynephrine, 0.25%, the left nares was serially dilated, with 6.5–8.0 mm naso-pharyngeal airways. An 8.0 endotracheal tube was inserted through the left nares and positioned 3 cm above the carina under fiberoptic guidance. General anesthesia was then induced with etomidate, 20 mg, and fentanyl, 250 mg, and maintained with isoflurane-air-oxygen. Muscle relaxation was maintained with rocuronium. After induction, upper and lower extremity somatosensory evoked potential (SSEP) monitoring was established, a precordial Doppler ultrasonographic monitor was placed at the right fourth intercostal space, and the legs and arms were positioned without pressure points. The patient's head was stabilized in a three-point Mayfield clamp after local infiltration of the pin sites (Figure 1). The neck was mildly flexed (Figure 2), and SSEPs remained at baseline after final positioning.

A C3–7 laminectomy proceeded uneventfully. During the surgery no Doppler changes were noted, and the SSEPs remained unchanged. Blood loss was estimated at 300 mL; 2500 mL of crystalloid was administered. The patient met extubation criteria at the end of the procedure.

In the postanesthesia care unit, his blood pressure was 140/85 mm Hg, pulse, 80 beats/min, and SpO_2, 97% with supplemental nasal oxygen. The patient was discharged to a rehabilitation facility after an uneventful 4-day postoperative course.

Familiarity with the indications for the seated position, understanding of and proper application of positioning techniques, careful attention to hemostasis, and communication between the anesthesiologist and surgeon decrease the rate and severity of complications. This case demonstrates that a cervical laminectomy can be performed safely in a high-risk patient in the seated position with no morbidity or mortality, while providing optimal surgical exposure. Because of cases such as this one, we believe that it is important to teach and provide practical experience (even simulated experience) with use of the seated position.

1. Edmonds-Seal J, Maroon JC: Air embolism diagnosed with ultrasound. Anaesthesia 1969;24:438.
2. Marquez J, Sladen A, Gendell H, et al: Paradoxical cerebral air embolism without an intracardiac defect. J Neurosurg 1986; 55:97.
3. Matjasko J, Petrozza P, Cohen M, et al: Anesthesia and surgery in the seated position: Analysis of 554 cases. Neurosurgery 1985;17:695.
4. Losasso TJ, Black S, Muzzi DA, et al: Detection and hemodynamic consequences of venous air embolism: Does nitrous oxide make a difference? Anesthesiology 1992;77:148.
5. Black S, Ockert DP, Oliver WC, et al: Outcome following posterior fossa craniotomy in patients in the sitting or horizontal positions. Anesthesiology 1988;69:49.

Postural hypotension, the most common physiologic consequence of positioning, can be minimized by avoiding abrupt or extreme position changes (eg, sitting up quickly), reversing the position if vital signs deteriorate, keeping the patient as well hydrated as possible, and having drugs available to counter any anticipated reaction. While maintaining a minimal level of anesthesia will lessen the likelihood of hypotension, coincidental movement of the endotracheal tube during positioning may cause the patient to cough and become hypertensive. Table 47–4 summarizes the major physiologic effects of common patient positions. Note that these effects are generalizations that can vary with the patient's volume status and cardiac reserve.

Many complications, including air embolism caused by the physiologic changes described above, nerve damage as a result of ischemic injury, and the need for finger amputation following a crush injury, have been associated with improper patient positioning (Table 47–5). These complications are best prevented by evaluating the patient's postural limitations during the preanesthetic visit; padding pressure points, susceptible nerves, and any area of the body that will *possibly* be in contact with the operating table or its attachments; avoiding flexion or extension of a joint to its limit; having an awake patient assume the position to ensure comfort; and understanding the potential complications of each position. Periods of patient transport pose

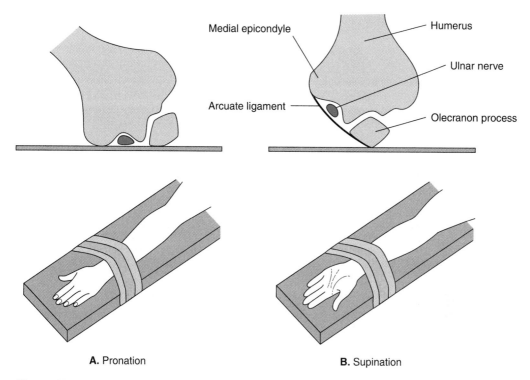

Figure 47–1. Pronation of the forearm can cause external compression of the ulnar nerve in the cubital tunnel (**A**). Forearm supination avoids this problem (**B**). (Modified and reproduced, with permission, from Wadsworth TG: The cubital tunnel and the external compression syndrome. Anesth Analg 1974;53:303.)

a particular threat if monitoring is interrupted for any reason. Similarly, monitors often must be disconnected during patient repositioning.

Compartment syndromes can result from hemorrhage into a closed space following a vascular puncture or prolonged venous outflow obstruction, especially when associated with hypotension. In severe cases, this may lead to muscle necrosis, myoglobinuria, and renal damage unless the pressure within the compartment is relieved by surgical decompression (fasciotomy).

AWARENESS

A series of media reports have imprinted the fear of awareness under anesthesia into the psyche of the general population. Accounts of recall and helplessness while paralyzed have made unconsciousness a primary concern to patients undergoing general anesthesia. Some reports may appear overdramatized; however, when awareness does occur, patients may exhibit symptoms ranging from mild anxiety to post-traumatic stress disorder (eg, sleep disturbances, nightmares, and social difficulties).

Although the incidence is difficult to document, certain patterns are clear. Evidence of awareness under general anesthesia was found in 0.2–0.4% to be the most quoted studies. Certain types of surgical settings are most frequently associated with awareness, including major trauma, obstetrics, and cardiac surgery. In many instances, awareness may be related to the depth of anesthesia that can be tolerated. In early studies, recall rates for intraoperative events during major trauma surgery have been reported as high as 43%; the incidence of awareness during cardiac surgery and cesarean sections is 1.5% and 0.4%, respectively. As of 1999, the ASA Closed Claims Project reported 79 awareness claims; approximately 20% for awake paralysis and the remainder for recall under general anesthesia. Most claims for awake paralysis were thought to be due to errors in drug labeling and administration. Recall under general anesthesia was found to be more likely in women and when anesthesia relying on opioids and

Table 47–4. Physiologic effects of common patient positions.

Position	Organ System	Effects
Supine		
Horizontal[1]	Cardiac	Equalization of pressures throughout the arterial system; increased right-sided filling and cardiac output; decreased heart rate and peripheral vascular resistance.
	Respiratory	Gravity increases perfusion of dependent (posterior) lung segments; abdominal viscera displace diaphragm cephalad. Spontaneous ventilation favors dependent lung segments, while controlled ventilation favors independent (anterior) segments. Functional residual capacity decreases and may fall below closing volume in older patients.
Trendelenburg	Cardiac	Activation of baroreceptors, generally causing decreased cardiac output, peripheral vascular resistance, heart rate, and blood pressure.
	Respiratory	Marked decreases in lung capacities from shift of abdominal viscera; increased ventilation/perfusion mismatching and atelectasis; increased likelihood of regurgitation.
	Other	Increase in intracranial pressure and decrease in cerebral blood flow because of cerebral venous congestion; increased intraocular pressure in patients with glaucoma.
Reverse Trendelenburg	Cardiac	Preload, cardiac output, and arterial pressure decrease. Baroreflexes increase sympathetic tone, heart rate, and peripheral vascular resistance.
	Respiratory	Spontaneous respiration requires less work; functional residual capacity increases.
	Other	Cerebral perfusion pressure and blood flow may decrease.
Lithotomy	Cardiac	Autotransfusion from leg vessels increases circulating blood volume and preload; lowering legs has opposite effect. Effect on blood pressure and cardiac output depends on volume status.
	Respiratory	Decreases vital capacity; increases likelihood of aspiration.
Prone	Cardiac	Pooling of blood in extremities and compression of abdominal muscles may decrease preload, cardiac output, and blood pressure.[2]
	Respiratory	Compression of abdomen and thorax decreases total lung compliance and increases work of breathing.
	Other	Extreme head rotation may decrease cerebral venous drainage and cerebral blood flow.
Lateral decubitus	Cardiac	Cardiac output unchanged unless venous return obstructed (eg, kidney rest). Arterial blood pressure may fall as a result of decreased vascular resistance (right side > left side).
	Respiratory	Decreased volume of dependent lung; increased perfusion of dependent lung. Increased ventilation of dependent lung in awake patients (no $\dot{V}/\dot{Q}$ mismatch); decreased ventilation of dependent lung in anesthetized patients $\dot{V}/\dot{Q}$ mismatch). Further decreases in dependent lung ventilation with paralysis and an open chest (see Chapter 24).
Sitting	Cardiac	Pooling blood in lower body decreases central blood volume. Cardiac output and arterial blood pressure fall despite rise in heart rate and systemic vascular resistance.
	Respiratory	Lung volumes and functional residual capacity increase; work of breathing increases.
	Other	Cerebral blood flow decreases.

[1]The effects described for the horizontal position are in comparison with a patient standing erect. All other positions are compared with the horizontal position.
[2]Changes associated with the prone position are exaggerated by the convex saddle frame used in posterior spinal surgery and minimized by the prone jackknife position.

Table 47–5. Complications associated with patient positioning.

Complication	Position	Prevention
Air embolism	Sitting, prone, reverse Trendelenburg	Maintain venous pressure above 0 at the wound (see Chapter 26).
Alopecia	Supine, lithotomy, Trendelenburg	Normotension, padding, and occasional head turning.
Backache	Any	Lumbar support, padding, and slight hip flexion.
Compartment syndrome	Especially lithotomy	Maintain perfusion pressure and avoid external compression.
Corneal abrasion	Especially prone	Taping and lubricating eye.
Digit amputation	Any	Check for protruding digits before changing table configuration.
Nerve palsies		
Brachial plexus	Any	Avoid stretching or direct compression at neck or axilla.
Common peroneal	Lithotomy, lateral decubitus	Pad lateral aspect of upper fibula.
Radial	Any	Avoid compression of lateral humerus.
Ulnar	Any	Padding at elbow, forearm supination.
Retinal ischemia	Prone, sitting	Avoid pressure on globe.
Skin necrosis	Any	Padding over bony prominences.

muscle relaxants without volatile anesthetic was used. Besides poor tolerance of anesthesia and medication errors, certain patients have been shown to have an increased anesthetic requirement; younger age, smoking, and long-term use of certain drugs (alcohol, opiates, or amphetamines) may increase the anesthetic requirements for unconsciousness.

The studies referenced above provide clues on how to minimize the chance of awareness and how to deal with it should it occur. Some clinicians routinely discuss recall as part of informed consent for general anesthesia and discuss the steps that will be taken to minimize that possibility. It is advisable to also remind patients who are undergoing monitored anesthesia care with sedation that awareness is a strong possibility, since these patients oftentimes think that they will be "out" for the procedure. Volatile anesthetics should be used at a level consistent with amnesia (at least 0.6 minimum alveolar concentration [MAC] when combined with opiates and nitrous oxide or 0.8–1.0 MAC when used alone). If this is not possible, consider the use of benzodiazepines (and/or scopolamine) to ensure amnesia. Movement of an unparalyzed patient may be indicative of inadequate anesthetic depth. Documentation should include end-tidal concentrations of anesthetic gases (when available) and accurate dosages of amnesic drugs. Use of a bispectral analysis (BIS) monitor may be helpful (see Chapter 6). Finally, if there is evidence of intraoperative awareness during follow-up, the practitioner should obtain a detailed account of the experience, be very sympathetic, answer patient questions, and refer the patient for psychological counseling if appropriate.

EYE INJURY

A wide range of conditions from simple corneal abrasion to blindness has been reported. Corneal abrasion is by far the most common and transient eye injury. The ASA Closed Claims Project identified a small number of claims for abrasion; even in this subset that prompted litigation, the cause was rarely identified (20%) and the incidence of permanent injury was low (16%). The project also identified a subset of claims concerning blindness that resulted from patient movement during ophthalmologic surgery. Both general anesthesia and monitored anesthesia care were used in those instances.

The causation and implications of each subset is quite different. Even though the cause of corneal abrasion may not be obvious, properly securing the eyes with tape after loss of consciousness but prior to intubation during general anesthesia and avoiding any direct contact with oxygen masks, drapes, lines, and pillows (especially during monitored anesthesia care, in transport, and nonsupine positions) can help minimize the possibility of injury. Paralysis and/or adequate anesthetic depth should be maintained to prevent movement during ophthalmologic surgery under general anesthesia. A clear understanding should be reached with the patient that movement under monitored care is hazardous, and minimal sedation to facilitate patient motor control should be considered.

Recently, a devastating eye injury called ischemic optic neuropathy (ION) has been described. ION is now the most common cause of postoperative vision loss. This syndrome results from optic nerve infarction due to decreased oxygen delivery via one or more small arterioles supplying the nerve head. It is most commonly reported after cardiopulmonary bypass, radical neck dissection, abdominal and hip procedures, and spinal surgeries in the prone position. Both preoperative and intraoperative factors may be contributory. Many of the case reports implicate preexisting hypertension, diabetes, coronary artery disease, and smoking, suggesting that preoperative vascular abnormalities may play a role. Intraoperative deliberate hypotension and anemia have also been implicated, perhaps because of their potential to reduce oxygen delivery. Finally, prolonged surgical time in positions that compromise venous outflow (prone, head down, compressed abdomen) have also been found to be factors. Symptoms are usually immediate but have been reported within the first 12 days postoperatively and range from decreased visual acuity to complete blindness. Recommendations to prevent this complication are difficult because risk factors for ION are often unavoidable due to the nature of the surgery. Steps that might be taken include (1) enhancing venous outflow by positioning the patient head up and minimizing abdominal constriction, (2) monitoring blood pressure carefully with an arterial line, (3) limiting the degree and duration of hypotension during controlled (deliberate) hypotension, (4) administering a transfusion to anemic patients who appear at risk for ION early enough to avoid severe anemia, and (5) discussing with the surgeon the possibility of staged operations in high-risk patients to limit prolonged procedures.

CARDIOPULMONARY ARREST DURING SPINAL ANESTHESIA

Sudden cardiac arrest during an otherwise routine administration of spinal anesthetic is an uncommon but catastrophic complication. The initial published report was a closed claims analysis of 14 patients who experienced cardiac arrest during spinal anesthesia. The cases involved primarily young (average age 36 years), relatively healthy (ASA physical status I–II) patients who were given appropriate doses of local anesthetic with the high level of block prior to arrest (T4 level). Subclinical respiratory insufficiency with hypercarbia due to sedatives was thought to be a potential contributing factor. The average time from spinal administration to arrest was 36 ± 18 minutes, and in all cases, arrest was preceded by a gradual decline in heart rate and blood pressure to 20% below baseline values. Just prior to arrest the most common signs were bradycardia, hypotension, and cyanosis. Treatment consisted of ventilatory support, ephedrine, atropine, cardiopulmonary resuscitation (average duration 10.9 minutes) and finally epinephrine (on average given 5 minutes into arrest period). Despite these interventions, 10 patients remained comatose and 4 regained consciousness with significant neurologic deficits. A subsequent study concluded that such arrests had little relationship to sedation but were more related to high sympathetic blockade, leading to high vagal tone and profound bradycardia. Most authorities have concluded that rapid, aggressive treatment of bradycardia and hypotension is essential in minimizing the risk of arrest. Early, rapid reversal of volume deficits and prophylactic treatment of bradycardia with atropine may prevent a downward spiral. Stepwise doses of ephedrine should be given to treat hypotension. Moreover, practitioners should not hesitate to use epinephrine for bradycardia or hypotension that is unresponsive to atropine and ephedrine. If cardiopulmonary arrest occurs, ventilatory support, cardiopulmonary resuscitation, and full resuscitation doses of atropine and epinephrine should be administered without any delay.

α-AGONIST/β-BLOCKER INTERACTION LEADING TO CARDIAC ARREST

The anesthesia literature from the 1980s describes several instances of severe hypertension leading to congestive heart failure and cardiac arrest in adult patients receiving long-term β-blocker therapy and undergoing ear, nose, and throat procedures. Patients were generally middle aged and all received 8–40 mL of local anesthetic containing 1:100,000 to 1:200,000 epinephrine. A hypertensive/bradycardic response ensued almost immediately and up to 15 minutes postinjection. The initial recommendation was for treatment with an α-blocker or hydralazine during the acute crisis phase. Subsequently, an editorial in Archives of Otolaryngology postulated that in patients being treated with nonselective β-blockers, the primary effect of epinephrine would be α-receptor activation. This would result in profound hypertension and bradycardia due to activation of the carotid baroreceptors and secondary increase in parasympathetic tone. Since β_1-cardiac-receptors are blocked, the tachycardia normally induced by epinephrine is not seen, and β_2-receptor blockade of peripheral vasodilation results in an unopposed α-constrictor response.

Since that time, physicians have substituted other topical vasoconstrictors to improve the conditions of the surgical field in various procedures. In March 2000, the Phenylephrine Advisory Committee of New York State reported on the mirror image of this problem—patients receiving vasoconstrictors who were treated for secondary hypertension with β-blockers. A review of 22 cases indicated a recurring pattern: topical vasoconstrictor caused profound hypertension, which was treated with a β-blocker that resulted in pulmonary edema and cardiac arrest. The report strongly implied that the use of β-blockers was responsible for poor patient outcome.

Treatment of hypertension secondary to α-agonists depends on the severity of the patient response. Mild to moderate hypertension may be left untreated, because it is well understood that the hypertension is transient. Severe hypertension, however, can lead to rapid end-organ damage, especially myocardial ischemia, and as such should be treated immediately with α-blocking agents, such as phentolamine, or a direct vasodilator, such as nitroprusside. The immediate use of β-blockers in this setting is not indicated and may be potentially catastrophic.

DOCUMENTATION ISSUES

All anesthesia documentation regarding preoperative evaluation, intraoperative management, invasive procedures, and postoperative care is "patient driven." It will differ with each patient and may change significantly for the same patient within a short period of time due to different surgical procedures and changes in patient status. For example, a 55-year-old patient (status, ASA I) who comes in for an elective laparoscopic cholecystectomy will require an entirely different evaluation and anesthetic plan than when he returns 15 hours later with an acute abdomen, suspected hepatic bleeding, severe anemia, and new onset of unstable angina with electrocardiographic changes. It is important to customize the evaluation to each patient's particular medical problems and anesthetic needs. However, some general aspects of documentation are important to review. It is critical for clinicians to clearly and legibly document their actions in these areas so that other specialists can clearly understand the rationale for anesthetic management and how it was carried out.

The preoperative anesthesia evaluation should indicate that an airway examination was performed and document its results, such as the Mallampati score, thyro-mental distance, neck extension, and dentition examination findings. Other evaluation systems are acceptable, but writing or checking "normal" may leave doubt to subsequent reviewers that a rigorous evaluation was performed. The airway management process should also be outlined; "intubation × 2" does not provide the same level of detail as:

"PreO$_2$, smooth IV induction, eyes taped, easy mask, laryngoscopy w/MAC 3, grade III view, change head position, Miller 2, grade II view, 7.0 oral endotracheal tube first pass, no blood or trauma noted, cuff up, +ETCO$_2$, cuff position checked."

Similarly, at extubation, instead of "ETT out" more informative documentation is provided by:

"Patient suctioned, cuff down, patient extubated, no evidence trauma, good airway."

If a patient subsequently developed such problems as dental trauma, altered voice, vocal cord trauma, granuloma, or pharyngoesophageal laceration, the more detailed documentation would better support that the standard-of-care for anesthetic management was met (see Chapter 1).

Eye trauma during surgery may be caused by a variety of factors. Since it is assumed that the unsedated/unanesthetized patient retains protective reflexes, eye trauma is frequently, but by no means appropriately, attributed to defects in anesthesia management. Although awakening patients in the recovery room are far more likely to suffer a corneal abrasion while scratching their noses and pushing the oxygen mask into their eye than to have the same trauma occur when their eyes are taped shut, the anesthesiologist will be called to assess purported "intraoperative eye trauma." It is important to document when the eyes were taped during anesthesia (as noted above, eyes were taped before intubation attempts to rule out corneal abrasion during laryngoscopy), and how the eyes were protected from pressure when the patient is positioned prone or lateral:

"patient's head in Richard's headrest, eyes/nose/ETT checked, no pressure points."

Neuraxial and peripheral nerve blocks, even with atraumatic placement, have the potential for catastrophic complications including high spinal, subdural injection, epidural hematoma, cauda equina syndrome, radiculopathies, neuropathies, and arachnoiditis. Without adequate documentation, a retrospective review of the chart may attribute these complications to a substandard technique. The written record should include notation of sterile technique, needle type, interspace or approach, number of passes, the presence or absence of blood/paresthesia/cerebrospinal fluid (CSF), and the type and effect of any test dose given. For example,

"Spinal in lateral position, back prepped/draped, L3–L4 interspace approximated, 1% lido local/25 g Whitacre, 1st pass +CSF, no heme/paresthesia, tetracaine 1% 10 mg plus 1 mL D$_{10}$, clear CSF aspirated before and after administration, block to T6 at 15 minutes."

and

"Lumbar epidural in lateral position, back prepped/draped, L3–L4 interspace approximated, 1% lido

local/17 g Tuohy, 1st pass LOR w/NS, no heme/CSF/ paresthesia, cath threaded 4 cm space/7 cm skin, no paresthesia, test dose lido 2% w/epi 3 mL, no evidence subarachnoid placement." (LOR = loss of resistance)

The eventual highest level of the block and length of time it took to achieve it should be recorded.

Placement of central venous lines, arterial lines, nasogastric or orogastric tubes, and TEE probes should also be well documented. With pulmonary artery catheters and central venous lines, sterile technique, number of passes, and lack of pulsatile flow through the needle and respiratory variation of a column of blood in IV tubing open to air before the wire is passed all serve to reaffirm proper positioning. The arterial line should be documented with the number of sticks and quality of waveform after the catheter is placed. When placing gastric tubes and TEE probes, use of lubricant, ease of placement, and presence of gastric aspirate (for gastric tubes) or adequate image (TEE) should be noted. If studies such as chest films are ordered, device location and lack of possible complications should be documented. It is very important that a legible, detailed, and accurate record be completed for every case. Sudden hemodynamic changes in catastrophes, such as pulmonary embolism (thrombus, air, or amniotic fluid) and cardiac arrhythmias, are often not preceded by warning signs. A well-documented record of stable hemodynamics with normal physiologic variations may be the only indication of adequate anesthesia care prior to these events and substantiate the contention that these type of events were not anesthetic mishaps.

Table 47–6 lists eight of the most common errors of documentation in anesthetic practice. It is important to remember that the anesthesia record and any subsequent notes are the only information that will be available should litigation occur. In some instances, the clinician may not be aware of an adverse outcome (or perceived adverse outcome) until weeks or months later. Although it can save time, writing an early entry in the anesthesia record before the event (eg, "patient extubated to recovery, vitals stable") *severely* undercuts the practitioner's credibility if the patient subsequently suffers an adverse event. Events and procedures should be recorded only after they occur. Moreover, notations should be sufficiently descriptive to make it clear that anesthetic management was within standard of care. *Patient care always supersedes record keeping,* but it is important to note times for critical events. Even in the middle of a crisis, one should attempt to periodically record hemodynamic variables and time of event so that treatment modalities can be accurately reconstructed later. In the event of cardiac arrest, one person (the anesthesiologist) should decide which clock or watch is to be used for all records. *Records, such cardiopulmonary resuscitation ("code") sheets, should not be signed before they are read and verified for accuracy.* Whenever feasible, save and retrieve important information, such as vital signs, before monitors are turned off. If possible, review the sequence of care with present personnel immediately after the event to ensure accurate documentation in all records. Following an adverse event, it is important to take the time to write a well thought-out note that describes relevant issues and conveys the thought processes and actions involved in the patient's management. In the emotional atmosphere that occurs after a critical adverse event, a well-intentioned visit to explain events and to comfort a patient's family may be misunderstood and mistakenly recollected 2 years later as an admission of liability or substandard care. It is always important to discuss events openly and answer questions but prudent to have a witness present. Moreover, such meetings should be documented in the medical record and the witness should cosign the note.

Table 47–6. Common documentation pitfalls to avoid.

---

1. Completing entries for events prior to when they occur.
2. Incomplete descriptions of procedures or management.
3. Inaccurate or conflicting times between different records.
4. Lost critical patient data.
5. Incomplete or poorly thought-out notes following an adverse event.
6. Signing inaccurate documents or documents without reading them.
7. Failure to document meetings with the patient/family, leaving open the possibility of conflicting recollections.
8. Failure to obtain supporting documentation from others.

ALLERGIC REACTIONS

Hypersensitivity (or allergic) reactions are exaggerated immunologic responses to antigenic stimulation in previously sensitized persons. The antigen, or allergen, may be a protein, polypeptide, or smaller molecule that is covalently bound to a carrier protein. Moreover, the allergen may be the substance itself, a metabolite, or breakdown product. Patients may be exposed to antigens through the nose, lungs, eyes, skin, gastrointestinal tract, as well as parenterally (intravenously or intramuscularly) and transperitoneally. Specialized classes of monocytes/macrophages process antigens and present them on their cell membrane surface protein to CD4+ helper T lymphocytes. The latter can induce a TH1 delayed hypersensitivity, TH2 immediate hypersensitivity, or TH0 anergic (no) response.

Depending on the antigen and the immune system components involved, hypersensitivity reactions are

Table 47–7. Hypersensitivity reactions.

Type I (immediate)
    Atopy
    Urticaria—angioedema
    Anaphylaxis
Type II (cytotoxic)
    Hemolytic transfusion reactions
    Autoimmune hemolytic anemia
    Heparin-induced thrombocytopenia
Type III (immune complex)
    Arthus reaction
    Serum sickness
    Acute hypersensitivity pneumonitis
Type IV (delayed, cell-mediated)
    Contact dermatitis
    Tuberculin-type hypersensitivity
    Chronic hypersensitivity pneumonitis

---

classically divided into four types (Table 47–7). In many cases an allergen, eg, latex, may cause more than one type of hypersensitivity reaction. Type I reactions involve antigens that cross-link immunoglobulin (Ig) E antibodies triggering the release inflammatory mediators from mast cells. In type II reactions, complement-fixing (C1-binding) IgG antibodies bind to antigens on cell surfaces, activating the classic complement pathway and lysing the cells. Examples of type II reactions include hemolytic transfusion reactions (see Chapter 29) and heparin-induced thrombocytopenia (see Chapter 21). Type III reactions occur when antigen-antibody (IgG or IgM) immune complexes are deposited in tissues, activating complement and generating chemotactic factors which attract neutrophils to the area. The activated neutrophils cause tissue injury by releasing lysosomal enzymes and toxic products. Type III reactions include serum sickness reactions and acute hypersensitivity pneumonitis. Type IV reactions, often referred to as delayed hypersensitivity, are mediated by CD4+ T lymphocytes that have been sensitized to a specific antigen by prior exposure. Prior TH1 response causes expression of a T cell receptor protein that is specific for the antigen. Reexposure to the antigen causes these lymphocytes to produce lymphokines—interleukins (IL), interferon (IFN), and tumor necrosis factor-γ (TNFγ)—that attract and activate inflammatory mononuclear cells over 48–72 hours. Production of IL-1 and IL-6 by antigen processing cells amplifies clonal expression of the specific sensitized T cells and attracts other types of T cells. IL-2 secretion transforms CD8+ cytotoxic T cells into killer cells; IL-4 and IFNγ cause macrophages to undergo epithelioid transformation, often producing granuloma. Examples of type IV reactions are those associated with tuberculosis, histo-plasmosis, schistosomiasis, and hypersensitivity pneumonitis as well as some autoimmune disorders such as rheumatoid arthritis and Wegener's granulomatosis.

1. Immediate Hypersensitivity Reactions

Initial exposure of a susceptible person to an antigen induces CD4+ T cells to produce IL-4, IL-5, IL-6, IL-10, and granulocyte-macrophage colony-stimulating factor (GM-CSF). These lymphokines activate and transform specific B lymphocytes into plasma cells, which produce allergen-specific IgE antibodies (Figure 47–2). The Fc portion of these antibodies then associates with high affinity receptors on the cell surface of tissue mast cells and circulating basophils. During subsequent reexposure to the antigen, it binds Fab portion of adjacent IgE antibodies on the mast cell surface, inducing degranulation and release of inflammatory lipid mediators and additional cytokines from the mast cell. The end result is an increase in intracellular calcium that causes degranulation of the mast cells, releasing histamine, tryptase, proteoglycans (heparin and chondroitin sulfate), and carboxypeptidases. The increase in intracellular calcium also activates prostaglandin (mainly prostaglandin D_2) and leukotriene (B_4, C_4, D_4, E_4, and platelet activating factor) synthesis. Leukotrienes were previously referred to as slow reacting substance of anaphylaxis. Additional mediators include neutrophil chemotactic factors (NCF), eosinophil chemotactic factor of anaphylaxis (ECF-A), and basophil kallikrein of anaphylaxis (BK-A). Mast cells may also release IL-3, IL-4, IL-5, IL-6, IFNγ, TNFα, and GM-CSF. The combined effects of these mediators can produce arteriolar vasodilatation, increased vascular permeability, increased mucus secretion, smooth muscle contraction, and other clinical manifestations of type I reactions.

Type I hypersensitivity reactions are classified as atopic or nonatopic. Atopic disorders typically affect the skin or respiratory tract and include allergic rhinitis, atopic dermatitis, and allergic asthma. Nonatopic hypersensitivity disorders include urticaria, angioedema, and anaphylaxis; when these reactions are mild they are confined to the skin (urticaria) or subcutaneous tissue (angioedema), but when they are severe, they become generalized and a life-threatening medical emergency (anaphylaxis). Urticarial lesions are characteristically well-circumscribed, skin wheals with raised erythematous borders and blanched centers; they are intensely pruritic and may be localized or generalized. Angioedema presents as deep nonpitting cutaneous edema resulting from marked vasodilation and increased permeability of subcutaneous blood vessels. When angioedema is extensive, it can be associated with large fluid shifts; when it is localized to the pharyngeal or laryngeal mucosa, it can rapidly compromise the airway.

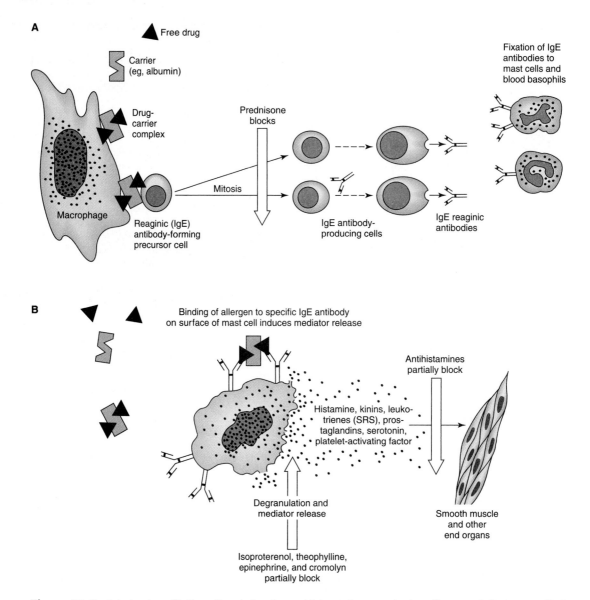

Figure 47–2. ***A:*** Induction of IgE-mediated allergic sensitivity to drugs and other allergens. ***B:*** Response of IgE sensitized cells to subsequent exposure to allergens. (Ig = immunoglobulin.) (Reproduced, with permission, from Katzung BG (editor): *Basic & Clinical Pharmacology,* 8th ed. McGraw-Hill, 2001.)

2. Anaphylactic Reactions

Anaphylaxis is an exaggerated response to an allergen (eg, antibiotic) that is mediated by a type I hypersensitivity reaction. The syndrome appears within minutes following exposure to a specific antigen in a sensitized person and characteristically presents as acute respiratory distress, circulatory shock, or both. Death usually occurs from asphyxiation or irreversible circulatory shock. The incidence of anaphylactic reactions during anesthesia has been estimated at a rate of 1:5000 to 1:25,000 anesthetics. Antibiotics are the most common cause of anaphylactic reactions, but latex has also become an increasingly important cause.

The most important mediators of anaphylaxis are histamine, leukotrienes, BK-A, and platelet activating factor. They increase vascular permeability and contract smooth muscle. H_1-receptor activation contracts bronchial smooth muscle, while H_2-receptor activation causes vasodilation, enhanced mucus secretion, tachycardia, and increased myocardial contractility. BK-A cleaves bradykinin from kininogen; bradykinin increases vascular permeability and vasodilation, and contracts smooth muscle. Activation of Hageman factor can initiate intravascular coagulation in some patients. ECF-A, NCF, and leukotriene B_4 attract inflammatory cells that mediate additional tissue injury. Angioedema of the pharynx, larynx, and trachea produce upper airway obstruction, while bronchospasm and mucosal edema result in lower airway obstruction. Histamine may preferentially constrict large airways, while leukotrienes primarily affect smaller peripheral airways. Transudation of fluid into the skin (angioedema) and viscera produces hypovolemia and shock, while arteriolar vasodilation decreases systemic vascular resistance. Coronary hypoperfusion and hypoxemia promote arrhythmias and myocardial ischemia. Leukotriene and prostaglandin mediators may also cause coronary vasospasm. Prolonged circulatory shock results in progressive lactic acidosis and ischemic damage to other vital organs. Table 47–8 summarizes important manifestations of anaphylactic reactions.

Anaphylactoid reactions resemble anaphylaxis but do not depend on IgE antibody interaction with antigen. A drug can directly release histamine from mast cells (eg, urticaria following high-dose morphine sulfate) or activate complement. Although the mechanisms differ, anaphylactic and anaphylactoid reactions can be clinically indistinguishable and equally life-threatening. Table 47–9 lists common causes of anaphylactic and anaphylactoid reactions.

Factors that may predispose patients to these reactions include youth, pregnancy, known atopy, and previous drug exposure. Laboratory identification of patients who have experienced an adverse allergic reaction or who may be particularly susceptible is often aided by intradermal skin testing, leukocyte or basophil degranu-

Table 47–9. Causes of anaphylactic and anaphylactoid reactions.

Anaphylactic reactions against polypeptides	Venoms (Hymenoptera, fire ant, snake, jellyfish)
	Airborne allergens (pollen, molds, danders)
	Foods (peanuts, milk, egg, seafood, grain)
	Enzymes (trypsin, streptokinase, chymopapain, asparaginase)
	Heterologous serum (tetanus antitoxin, antilymphocyte globulin, antivenin)
	Human proteins (insulin, corticotropin, vasopressin, serum and seminal proteins)
	Latex
Anaphylactic reactions against hapten-carrier	Antibiotics (penicillin, cephalosporins, sulfonamides)
	Disinfectants (ethylene oxide, chlorhexidine)
	Local anesthetics (procaine)
Anaphylactoid reactions	Polyionic solutions (radiocontrast medium, polymyxin B)
	Opioids (morphine, meperidine)
	Hypnotics (thiopental, propofol)
	Muscle relaxants (curare, succinylcholine, atracurium)
	Synthetic membranes (dialysis)
	Nonsteroidal anti-inflammatory drugs
	Preservatives (sulfites, benzoates)
	Protamine
	Dextran
	Steroids
	Exercise
	Idiopathic

Adapted, with permission, from Bochner BS, Lichtenstein LM: N Engl J Med 1991;324:1786.

lation testing (histamine release test), or radioallergosorbent testing (RAST). The latter is capable of measuring the level of drug-specific IgE antibody in the serum. Prophylactic pretreatment with histamine-receptor antagonists and corticosteroids decreases the severity of the reaction. Treatment must be immediate and tailored to the severity of the reaction (Table 47–10).

3. Latex Allergy

The severity of allergic reactions to latex-containing products ranges from mild contact dermatitis to life-

Table 47–8. Clinical manifestations of anaphylaxis.

Organ System	Signs and Symptoms
Cardiovascular	Hypotension,* tachycardia, arrhythmias
Pulmonary	Bronchospasm,* cough, dyspnea, pulmonary edema, laryngeal edema, hypoxia
Dermatologic	Urticaria,* facial edema, pruritus

*Key signs during general anesthesia.

Table 47–10. Treatment of anaphylactic and anaphylactoid reactions.

Discontinue drug administration
Administer 100% oxygen
Epinephrine (0.01–0.5 mg IV or IM)*
Consider intubation or tracheostomy
Intravenous fluids (1–2 L lactated Ringer's injection)
Diphenhydramine (50–75 mg IV)
Hydrocortisone (up to 200 mg IV) or methylprednisolone
(1–2 mg/kg)

---

*The dose and route of epinephrine depend on the severity of the reaction.

threatening anaphylaxis. Most serious reactions appear to involve a direct IgE-mediated immune response to polypeptides in natural latex, although some cases of contact dermatitis may be due to a type IV sensitivity reaction to chemicals introduced in the manufacturing process. Nonetheless, a relationship between the occurrence of contact dermatitis and the probability of future anaphylaxis has been suggested. Chronic exposure to latex and a history of atopy increases the risk of sensitization. Health care workers and patients undergoing frequent procedures with latex items (eg, repeated urinary bladder catheterization, barium enema examinations) should therefore be considered at increased risk. Between 5% and 17% of health care workers are estimated to be allergic to latex. Patients with spina bifida, spinal cord injury, and congenital abnormalities of the genitourinary tract have a very high incidence of latex allergy. The incidence of latex anaphylaxis in children is estimated to be 1 in 10,000. A history of allergic symptoms to latex should probably be sought in all patients during the preanesthetic interview.

Anaphylactic reactions to latex may be confused with reactions to other substances (eg, drugs, blood products) because the onset of symptoms can be delayed for more than an hour after initial exposure. Treatment is the same as for other forms of anaphylactic reactions. Skin-prick tests, intradermal tests, basophil histamine-release tests, and RAST have been used to evaluate high-risk patients. Preventing a reaction in sensitized patients includes pharmacologic prophylaxis and absolute avoidance of latex. Preoperative administration of H_1 and H_2 histamine antagonists (see Chapter 15) and steroids may provide some protection, although their use is controversial. Many pieces of anesthetic equipment contain latex: gloves, tourniquets, some endotracheal tubes, ventilator bellows, intravenous injection ports, blood pressure cuffs, and some

face masks. An allergic reaction has even been documented from inhalation of latex antigen contained within aerosolized glove powder. Manufacturers of latex-containing medical products must label their products accordingly. Only devices specifically known not to contain latex (eg, polyvinyl or neoprene gloves, silicone endotracheal tubes or laryngeal masks, plastic face masks) can be used in these patients. Rubber stoppers should be removed from drug vials prior to use and injections should be made through plastic stopcocks.

4. Allergic Reactions to Anesthetic Agents

True anaphylaxis due to anesthetic agents is rare; anaphylactoid reactions are much more common (see Table 47–9). Risk factors associated with hypersensitivity to anesthetics include female gender, atopic history, preexisting allergies, and previous anesthetic exposures. Hypnotic agents (thiopental and propofol) and muscle relaxants (succinylcholine, curare, and atracurium) are most often responsible. Anti-thiopental IgE antibodies have been demonstrated in some patients, and IgE-mediated reactions following exposure to succinylcholine, atracurium, vecuronium, and pancuronium have also been described. The IgE antibodies in these latter instances are directed against tertiary or quaternary ion epitopes. True anaphylactic reactions due to opiates are very rare. Anaphylactic reactions to local anesthetics are also rare. Vasovagal reactions, toxic reactions, and side effects from epinephrine are much more common. IgE-mediated reactions to ester-type local anesthetics, however, are well described. Because they all share common antigenicity with *p*-aminobenzoic acid, cross-reactivity should be expected between ester-type local anesthetics. In contrast, anaphylaxis due to amide-type local anesthetics is very rare; in most instances, the preservative (paraben or methylparaben) was believed to be responsible; moreover, the cross-reactivity between amide-type local anesthetics appears to be low.

5. Allergies to Antibiotics

Nearly one-half of true drug allergies in surgical patients are due to antibiotics, mainly β-lactam antibiotics, such as penicillins and cephalosporins. Although 1–4% of β-lactams administrations result in allergic reactions, only 0.004–0.015% of these reactions produce anaphylaxis. To put things in perspective, up to 2% of the general population is allergic to penicillin, but only 0.01% of penicillin administrations result in anaphylaxis. Cephalosporin cross-sensitivity in patients with penicillin allergy is estimated to be 2–7%, but a history of an anaphylactic reaction to penicillin increases the cross-reactivity rate up to 50%. Patients with a prior history of an anaphylactic reaction to penicillin should therefore not receive a cephalosporin. While imipenem exhibits similar cross-sensitivity, aztreonam appears to be antigenically distinct and reportedly does not cross-react with other β-lactams. Sulfonamide allergy is also relatively common in surgical patients. Sulfa drugs include sulfonamide antibiotics, furosemide, hydrochlorothiazide, and captopril. Fortunately, the frequency of cross-reactivity between these agents is low.

Like cephalosporins, vancomycin is commonly used for antibiotic prophylaxis in surgical patients. Unfortunately, it is commonly associated with adverse reactions. An anaphylactoid-type reaction, "red man's syndrome," consists of intense pruritus, flushing, and erythema of the head and upper torso, often with arterial hypotension; this syndrome may be more related to a rapid rate of administration rather than dose or a true allergy. Isolated systemic hypotension is a much more frequent side effect and appears to be primarily mediated by histamine release because pretreatment with H_1 and H_2 antihistamines can prevent hypotension even with rapid rates of administration.

OCCUPATIONAL HAZARDS IN ANESTHESIOLOGY

1. Chronic Exposure to Anesthetic Gases

Chapter 2 began with the statement that anesthesiologists spend more time in operating rooms than do any other group of physicians. This results in greater exposure to the risks of the operating room environment, such as the potential long-term effects of trace anesthetic gases. Fortunately, there is no clear evidence that exposure to trace amounts of anesthetic agents present a health hazard to operating room personnel. However, because previous studies examining this issue have been flawed or have produced conflicting results, the US Occupational Health and Safety Administration continues to set maximum acceptable trace concentrations of less than 25 ppm for nitrous oxide and 0.5 for ppm halogenated anesthetics (2 ppm if the halogenated agent is used alone). Achieving these low levels depends on efficient scavenging equipment, adequate operating room ventilation, and conscientious anesthetic technique. Most people cannot detect the odor of volatile agents at a concentration of less than 30 ppm (nitrous oxide is essentially odorless). Without a properly functioning scavenging system, anesthetic gases concentrations are about 3000 ppm for nitrous oxide and 50 ppm for volatile agents.

2. Infectious Diseases

Hospital workers are exposed to many infectious diseases prevalent in the community (eg, respiratory viral infections, rubella, and tuberculosis).

Herpetic whitlow is infection of the finger with herpes simplex virus type 1 or 2 and usually involves direct contact of previously traumatized skin with contaminated oral secretions. Painful vesicles appear at the site of infection. The diagnosis is confirmed by the appearance of giant epithelial cells or nuclear inclusion bodies in a smear taken from the base of a vesicle, the presence of a rise in herpes simplex virus titer, or identification of the virus with antiserum. Treatment is conservative and includes topical application of 5% acyclovir ointment. Prevention rests upon wearing gloves when contacting oral secretions. Patients at risk for harboring the virus include those suffering from other infections, immunosuppression, cancer, and malnutrition.

Viral DNA has been identified in the smoke plume generated during laser treatment of condyloma. The theoretical possibility of viral transmission from this source can be minimized by using smoke evacuators, gloves, and high-efficiency masks.

More disturbing is the potential of acquiring serious blood-borne infections such as **hepatitis B**; **hepatitis C**; or **human immunodeficiency virus (HIV)**. Although parenteral transmission of these diseases can occur following mucous membrane, cutaneous, or percutaneous exposure to infected body fluids, accidental injury with a needle contaminated with infected blood represents the most common occupational mechanism.

The risk of transmission can be estimated if three factors are known: the prevalence of the infection within the patient population, the incidence of exposure (eg, frequency of needlestick), and the rate of seroconversion after a single exposure. The seroconversion rate after a specific exposure depends on several factors, including the infectivity of the organism, the stage of the patient's disease (extent of viremia), the size of the inoculum, and the immune status of the health care provider. Rates of seroconversion following a single needlestick are estimated to range between 0.3% and 30%. It should be noted that hollow (hypodermic) needles pose a greater risk than solid (surgical) needles because of the potentially larger inoculum. The use of gloves, needleless systems, or protected needle devices may decrease the incidence of some (but not all) types of injury.

Initial management of needlesticks involves cleaning the wound and notifying the appropriate authority within the health care facility. The serologic status of the health care worker and, if possible, the source patient should be established. Ig may be partially effective in preventing hepatitis B. Prophylactic IFN (with or without ribovirin) following a high-risk inoculation from a hepatitis C patient is highly controversial because of considerable drug side effects. Although prophylactic administration of zidovudine alone reduces the risk HIV infection following a contaminated needlestick, concerns over rising drug-resistance have caused many experts to recommend multidrug prophylaxis regimens.

The prevalence of hepatitis B serologic markers is several times higher in anesthesia personnel (15–50%) than in the general population (3–5%). The risk of infection is proportional to the number of years in practice. Fulminant hepatitis (1% of acute infections) carries a 60% mortality rate. Chronic active hepatitis (< 5% of all cases) is associated with an increased incidence of cirrhosis of the liver and hepatocellular carcinoma. Transmission of the virus is chiefly through contact with blood products or body fluids. The diagnosis is confirmed by detection of hepatitis B surface antigen (HBsAg). Uncomplicated recovery is signaled by the disappearance of HBsAg and the appearance of antibody to the surface antigen (anti-HBs). A hepatitis vaccine is available and is strongly recommended prophylactically for anesthesia personnel. The appearance of anti-HBs after a three-dose regimen indicates successful immunization.

Hepatitis C is another important occupational hazard in anesthesiology; 4–8% of hepatitis C infections occur in health care workers. Most (50–90%) of these infections lead to chronic hepatitis which, although often asymptomatic, can progress to liver failure and death. In fact, hepatitis C is the most common cause of nonalcoholic cirrhosis in the United States. There is currently no vaccine to protect against hepatitis C infection. Screening donor blood for antibodies to hepatitis C has decreased but not eliminated the incidence of hepatitis C infections following blood transfusion.

Anesthesia personnel appear to be at a low but real risk of the occupational contraction of AIDS. The risk of acquiring HIV infection following a single needlestick contaminated with blood from an HIV-infected patient has been estimated at 0.4–0.5%. Because there are documented reports of transmission of HIV from infected patients to health care workers (including anesthesiologists), the Centers for Disease Control and Prevention has proposed guidelines that apply to all categories of patient contact. These **universal precautions,** which are equally valid for protection against hepatitis B or C infection, are as follows:

- Needle precautions, including no recapping and immediate disposal of contaminated needles.
- Use of gloves and other barriers during contact with open wounds and body fluids.

- Frequent hand-washing.
- Proper techniques for disinfection or disposal of contaminated materials.
- Particular caution by pregnant health care workers, and no contact with patients by workers who have exudative or weeping dermatitis.

3. Substance Abuse

 Anesthesiology is a high-risk medical specialty for drug addiction. Reasons for this include the stress of anesthetic practice, the easy availability of drugs with addiction potential, and curiosity aroused by a patient's euphoria after receiving opioids and sedatives. The likelihood of developing a substance abuse problem is increased by coexisting personal problems (eg, marital, financial difficulties) and a family history of alcoholism or drug addiction.

The voluntary use of mood-altering drugs is a disease. If left untreated, substance abuse often leads to death from drug overdose—intentional or unintentional. One of the greatest challenges in treating this illness is identifying the afflicted individual, since denial is a consistent feature. Unfortunately, changes evident to an outside observer are often both vague and late: reduced involvement in social activities, subtle changes in appearance, extreme mood swings, and altered work habits. Treatment begins with an intervention plan of enrolling the individual in a formal rehabilitation program. The possibility of retaining one's medical license and reentering the mainstream of practice provides powerful motivation. Some diversion programs report a success rate of approximately 70%. Long-term compliance often involves continued participation in support groups (eg, Narcotics Anonymous), random urine testing, and oral naltrexone therapy (a long-acting opioid antagonist). Effective prevention strategies are difficult to formulate but may include better control of drug availability and education about the severe consequences of substance abuse.

4. Radiation Exposure

The intraoperative use of imaging equipment (eg, fluoroscopy) and attendance during radiologic procedures (eg, interventional radiology) expose the anesthesiologist to the potential risks of ionizing radiation. The two most important methods of minimizing exposure are using proper barriers and maximizing one's distance from the source of radiation. Lead glass partitions or lead aprons with thyroid shields are mandatory protection for all personnel working in an imaging environment. The inverse square law states that the amount of radiation changes inversely with the square of the distance. Thus, the exposure at 4 meters will be one-sixteenth that at 1 meter. The maximum recommended occupational whole-body exposure to radiation is 5 rem/year. This can be monitored by wearing an exposure badge.

CASE DISCUSSION: UNEXPLAINED INTRAOPERATIVE TACHYCARDIA & HYPERTENSION

A 73-year-old man is scheduled for emergency relief of an intestinal obstruction with strangulation from a volvulus at midnight. The patient had a myocardial infarction 1 month ago that was complicated by intermittent congestive heart failure. His blood pressure is 160/90 mm Hg; pulse, 110 beats/min; respiratory rate, 22/min; temperature, 38.8 °C.

Why is this case an emergency?

Strangulation of the bowel begins with venous obstruction but can quickly progress to arterial occlusion, ischemia, infarction, and perforation. Acute peritonitis could lead to severe dehydration, sepsis, shock, and multiorgan failure—obviously a poor prognosis in this elderly patient. Nonetheless, a few hours could be well spent optimizing the patient's fluid status and cardiovascular parameters before rushing to the operating room. Furthermore, a complex and high-risk case such as this requires extra operating room setup time in preparing medications, monitors, and other anesthetic equipment.

The patient is immediately rushed to an available operating room that has been set up for possible open-heart surgery.

What special monitoring is appropriate for this patient?

Because of the history of recent myocardial infarction and congestive heart failure, an arterial line and a pulmonary artery catheter would be useful. Large fluid shifts should be anticipated, and a beat-to-beat monitor of blood pressure is needed. Furthermore, information regarding myocardial supply (diastolic blood pressure) and demand (systolic blood pressure, left ventricular wall stress, and heart rate) should be continuously available. A central venous pressure may give misleading information because of the potential discrepancy between right- and left-sided pressures in a patient with significant left ventricular dysfunction. Further monitoring might include transesophageal echocardiography for early detection

of myocardial ischemia and assessment of ventricular wall motion.

An arterial line is easily placed, but the pulmonary artery catheter gives only an intermittent pulmonary artery tracing.

What cardiovascular medications might be useful during induction and maintenance of general anesthesia?

A continuous intravenous infusion of nitroglycerin could beneficially alter the myocardial supply/demand balance. Esmolol might be useful in decreasing the heart rate, but caution is suggested by the history of congestive heart failure. Drugs causing tachycardia or extremes in arterial blood pressure should obviously be avoided.

A nitroglycerin drip is begun, and the patient's vital signs remain stable throughout a standard thiopental induction. During the laparotomy, gradual increases in heart rate and blood pressure are noted. The rate of administration of nitroglycerin is increased, and ST-segment elevations appear on the electrocardiogram (ECG). The heart rate is now 130/min and the blood pressure 220/140 mm Hg. The pulmonary artery catheter tracing is consistent with a right ventricular location. The concentration of volatile anesthetic is increased, and propranolol is administered intravenously in 1-mg increments. This results in a decline in heart rate to 115 beats/min but a rise in blood pressure to 250/160 mm Hg. Suddenly, the rhythm converts to ventricular tachycardia, with a profound drop in blood pressure. As lidocaine is being administered and the defibrillation unit prepared, the rhythm degenerates into ventricular fibrillation.

What can explain this series of events?

A differential diagnosis of pronounced tachycardia and hypertension might include pheochromocytoma, malignant hyperthermia, or thyroid storm. In this case, further inspection of the nitroglycerin infusion reveals that the intravenous tubing had been mislabeled. In fact, while the tubing was labeled nitroglycerin, *the infusion bag was labeled* epinephrine.

How does this explain the paradoxic response to propranolol?

Propranolol is a nonselective β-adrenergic antagonist. It blocks the tachycardia because of epinephrine's β$_1$-stimulation and the dilatation of blood vessels as a result of β$_2$-stimulation, but it does not affect α-induced vasoconstriction. The *net result is a decrease in heart rate but an increase in blood pressure.*

Why wasn't the patient hypotensive during induction?

It was surprising that a standard thiopental induction would not result in profound hypotension in this dehydrated elderly patient with a history of heart disease. The epinephrine infusion may have masked the hypotensive effects of induction, resulting in relatively stable vital signs.

What is the cause of the ventricular tachycardia?

An overdose of epinephrine can cause life-threatening ventricular dysrhythmias. A high concentration of volatile anesthetic could have further sensitized the myocardium to the dysrhythmogenic effects of epinephrine. In addition, the malpositioned tip of the pulmonary artery catheter could have irritated the endothelium and conduction pathways in the right ventricle.

What other factors may have contributed to this anesthetic mishap?

Many factors may have indirectly contributed to this end result, including the midnight timing of the case (eg, physician fatigue), the lack of preparation (eg, patient fine-tuning), the use of drugs prepared by another anesthesiologist, and the decision to proceed with induction and surgery despite unsatisfactory positioning of the pulmonary artery catheter. The end result of this chain of coincidence, misjudgment, and an unhealthy patient was a poor outcome.

SUGGESTED READING

Atlee AL: *Complications in Anesthesia.* WB Saunders and Company, 1999.

Benumof JL, Saidman LJ: *Anesthesia & Perioperative Complications,* 2nd ed. Mosby, 1999.

Bogner MS: *Human Error in Medicine.* Lawrence Erlbaum, 1994.

Brown RH et al: Anemia and hypotension as contributors to perioperative loss of vision. Anesthesiology 1994;80:222.

Brummet R: Warning to otolaryngologists using local anesthetics containing epinephrine. Arch of Otolaryngology 1984;110:72.

Caplan RA, Posner KL, Ward RJ, Cheney FW: Adverse respiratory events in anesthesia: A closed claims analysis. Anesthesiology 1990;72:828.

Caplan RA, Vistica MF, Posner KL, Cheney FW: Adverse anesthetic outcomes arising from gas delivery equipment: A closed claims analysis. Anesthesiology 1997;87:741.

Caplan RA, Ward RJ, Posner K, Cheney FW: Unexpected cardiac arrest during spinal anesthesia: A closed claims analysis of predisposing factors. Anesthesiology 1988;68:5.

Chadwick HS, Posner K, Caplan RA, et al: A comparison of obstetric and nonobstetric anesthesia malpractice claims. Anesthesiology 1991;74:242.

Chadwick HS: An analysis of obstetric anesthesia cases from the American Society of Anesthesiologists closed claims project database. Int J Obstet Anesth 1996;5:258.

Cheney FW: The American Society of Anesthesiologists closed claims project: What have we learned, how has it affected practice, and how will it affect practice in the future? Anesthesiology 1999;91:552.

Cheney FW et al: Nerve injury associated with anesthesia: A closed claims analysis. Anesthesiology 1999;90:1062.

Cheney FW et al: Standard of care and anesthesia liability. JAMA 1989;261:1599. Review of more than 1000 malpractice actions for anesthesia-related injuries.

Cheney FW, Posner KL, Caplan RA: Adverse respiratory events infrequently leading to malpractice suits. Anesthesiology 1991;75:932.

Cheney FW, Posner KL, Caplan RA, Gild WM: Burns from warming devices in anesthesia. Anesthesiology 1994;80:806.

Domino KB et al: Awareness during anesthesia: A closed claims analysis. Anesthesiology 1999;90:1053.

Domino KB, Posner KL, Caplan RA, Cheney FW: Airway injury during anesthesia: A closed claims analysis. Anesthesiology 1999;91:1703.

Edbril SD, Lagasse RS: Relationship between malpractice litigation and human errors. Anesthesiology 1999;91:848.

Finucane BT: Complications of Regional Anesthesia. Churchill Livingstone, 1999.

Fisher DM: New York State guidelines on the topical use of phenylephrine in operating rooms. Anesthesiology 2000;92:858.

Foster CA et al: Propranolol-epinephrine interaction: A potential disaster. Plast Reconstr Surg 1983;72:72.

Ghoneim MM: Awareness during anesthesia. Anesthesiology 2000;92:597.

Gild WM et al: Eye injuries associated with anesthesia. Anesthesiology 1992;76:204.

Holzman RS: Latex allergy: An emerging operating room problem. Anesth Analg 1993;76:635.

Kroll DA, Caplan RA, Posner K, et al: Nerve injury associated with anesthesia. Anesthesiology 1990;73:202.

Lee LA: Postoperative visual loss data gathered and analyzed. ASA Newsletter 2000;64(9):25.

Levy JH: *Anaphylactic Reactions in Anesthesia and Intensive Care,* 2nd ed. Butterworth-Heinemann, 1992.

Liu WHD et al: Incidence of awareness with recall during general anesthesia. Anaesthesia 1991;46:435.

Lyons G, Macdonald R: Awareness during caesarean section. Anaesthesia 1991;46:62.

Martin JT: *Positioning in Anesthesia & Surgery,* 3rd ed. WB Saunders and Company, 1997.

Martin JT: Compartment syndromes: Concept and perspectives for the anesthesiologist. Anesth Analg 1992;75:275.

McLeskey CH: Awareness during anesthesia. Can J Anaesth 1999;46:R80.

Morray JP, Geiduschek JM, Caplan RA et al: A comparison of pediatric and adult anesthesia closed malpractice claims. Anesthesiology 1993;78:461.

Phillips AA et al: Recall of intraoperative events after general anaesthesia and cardiopulmonary bypass. Can J Anaesth 1993;40:922.

Pollard JB: Cardiac arrest during spinal anesthesia: common mechanisms and strategies for prevention. Anesth Analg 2001;92:252.

Practice advisory for the prevention of perioperative peripheral neuropathies: A report by the American Society of Anesthesiologists Task Force on prevention of peripheral neuropathies. Anesthesiology 2000;92:1168.

Ranta SOV et al: Awareness with recall during general anesthesia: Incidence and risk factors. Anesth Analg 1998;86:1084.

Sharma AD, Parmley CL, Sreeram G, Grocott HP: Peripheral nerve injuries during cardiac surgery: Risk factors, diagnosis, prognosis, and prevention. Anesth Analg 2000;91:1358.

Silverstein JH, Silva DA, Iberti TJ: Opioid addiction in anesthesiology. Anesthesiology 1993;79:354.

Tait AR: Occupational transmission of tuberculosis: Implications for anesthesiologists. Anesth Analg 1997;85:444.

Warner MA et al: Lower extremity neuropathies associated with lithotomy positions. Anesthesiology 2000;93:938.

Warner MA et al: Ulnar neuropathy. Incidence, outcome, and risk factors in sedated or anesthetized patients. Anesthesiology 1994;81:1332.

Warner ME et al: Perianesthetic dental injuries. Anesthesiology 1999;90:1302.

Weinger MB, Englund CE: Ergonomic and human factors affecting anesthetic vigilance and monitoring performance in the operating room environment. Anesthesiology 1990;73:995.

Williams EL et al: Postoperative ischemic optic neuropathy. Anesth Analg 1995;80:1018.

Withington DE: Allergy, anaphylaxis and anaesthesia. Can J Anaesth 1994;41:1133.

Cardiopulmonary Resuscitation

KEY CONCEPTS

① Cardiopulmonary resuscitation and emergency cardiac care should be considered any time an individual cannot adequately oxygenate or perfuse vital organs—not only following cardiac or respiratory arrest.

② Regardless of which transtracheal jet ventilation system is chosen, it must be readily available, use low-compliance tubing, and have secure connections.

③ Ventilation should not be delayed for intubation if a patent airway is established by a jaw-thrust maneuver.

④ Attempts at intubation should not interrupt ventilation for more than 30 seconds.

⑤ Chest compressions should be immediately initiated in the pulseless patient.

⑥ Lidocaine, epinephrine, atropine, and vasopressin should be delivered down a catheter

whose tip extends past the endotracheal tube bevel. Dosages 2–2½ times higher than recommended for intravenous use, diluted in 10 mL of normal saline or distilled water, are recommended for adult patients.

⑦ If intravenous cannulation is difficult, an intraosseous infusion can provide emergency vascular access in children.

⑧ Because carbon dioxide, but not bicarbonate, readily crosses cell membranes and the blood-brain barrier, the resulting arterial hypercapnia will cause intracellular tissue acidosis.

⑨ A wide QRS complex following a pacing spike signals electrical *capture*, but mechanical (ventricular) capture must be confirmed by an improving pulse or blood pressure.

One goal of anesthesiology is to maintain the function of vital organ systems during surgery. It is not surprising, therefore, that anesthesiologists have played a major role in the development of cardiopulmonary resuscitation techniques outside the operating room. Cardiopulmonary resuscitation and emergency cardiac care (CPR-ECC) should be considered any time an individual cannot adequately oxygenate or perfuse vital organs—not only following cardiac or respiratory arrest.

This chapter presents an overview of the American Heart Association and the International Liaison Committee on Resuscitation (ILCOR) Year 2000 recommendations for establishing and maintaining the **ABCD**s of cardiopulmonary resuscitation: **A**irway,

Breathing, **C**irculation, and **D**efibrillation. The best outcomes, however, come from instituting ECC (Table 48–1, Figures 48–1 and 48–2). The guidelines have been updated for 2000 and are now more than ever evidence-based and international. Major changes for the layperson are that the pulse should not be checked, and chest compression without ventilation may be as effective as compression with ventilation for the first several minutes. If a lay-bystander is unwilling to perform mouth-to-mouth ventilation, chest compressions alone are preferred to doing nothing. For the health care provider, defibrillation using biphasic electrical current works best, endotracheal tube (ETT) placement should be confirmed with a qualitative end-tidal CO_2 device, bretylium is no longer recommended but vasopressin

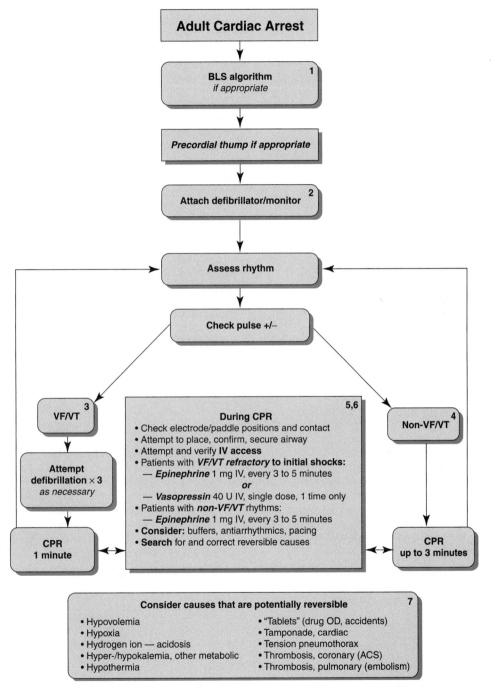

Figure 48–1. Universal algorithm for adult emergency cardiac care. BLS = basic life support, VF/VT = ventricular fibrillation and pulseless ventricular tachycardia, CPR = cardiopulmonary resuscitation. [Reproduced, with permission, from The American Heart Association in Collaboration with the International Liaison Committee on Resuscitation (ILCOR): Guidelines 2000 for cardiopulmonary resuscitation and emergency cardiovascular care. Circulation 2000;102:1.]

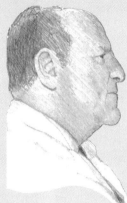

David J. Cullen, MD, MS

MANAGEMENT OF THE DIFFICULT AIRWAY BY ANESTHESIOLOGISTS

When called to the emergency department, intensive care unit, or other patient care unit for emergency management of a patient's airway, and a difficult intubation is encountered, what are the options for immediately securing the airway? The term "difficult airway" is used to identify a situation in which three or more unsuccessful attempts at direct laryngoscopy have been made by an individual skilled in airway management. Assuming that mask ventilation is unsuccessful or inadequate, placement of a laryngeal mask airway should be attempted immediately. Combitubes, airway exchange catheters, tongue sutures, and various other devices may also be tried. However, a so-called surgical airway should be considered and requested as soon as it is apparent that airway difficulties are mounting.

By definition, a surgical airway procedure involves a cricothyrotomy or emergency tracheotomy, which should only be performed by a surgeon specifically skilled to do so. The vast majority of anesthesiologists are not trained to perform a surgical airway procedure under actual conditions or conditions simulating an emergency airway problem in patients in whom emergency intubation by highly skilled operators has already failed.

Needle cricothyrotomy by anesthesiologists has been advocated as an alternative approach to provide at least a temporary source of oxygen while additional help or equipment is being sought. However, because of the high complication rate and the likelihood it will interfere with the option of a surgical airway procedure when a qualified surgeon arrives to do so, needle cricothyrotomies should not be placed. Common sense indicates that only those patients with very abnormal anatomy or pathology, whether internal or external to the airway, are likely to need an emergency surgical airway. Were their anatomy more normal, the airway would likely have been secured by other means in almost all cases. Therefore, the rare situations requiring a surgical airway procedure are usually those in which the basic internal or external anatomy is distorted or abnormal. This makes the performance of a surgical airway procedure by one who has never done it almost impossible to accomplish successfully.

The use of a needle cricothyrotomy connected to jet ventilation, an Ambu bag, or other oxygen delivery system was carefully considered and determined to be contraindicated by the Emergency Airway Committee of the Harvard Anaesthesia Depart-

---

Table 48–1. Emergency cardiac care (ECC).

1. Recognition of impending event
2. Activation of emergency response system
3. Basic life support
4. Defibrillation
5. Ventilation
6. Pharmacotherapy

has been added to the algorithms, and amiodarone has gained new emphasis in these newest guidelines. This chapter is not, however, intended as a substitute for a formal course in either life support without the use of special equipment (Basic Life Support [BLS]) or with the use of special equipment and drugs (Advanced Cardiac Life Support [ACLS]).

Resuscitation of neonates is discussed in Chapter 43.

ments.[1] Its use was mentioned as being appropriate only as the final attempt to save a life when all else fails, including the failure to obtain the services of a surgeon to perform a surgical airway procedure.

Complications from needle cricothyrotomy with jet ventilation include subcutaneous emphysema, pneumothorax, and bleeding. More important, these complications will interfere with the ability of the surgeon to obtain a surgical airway. Certainly, there have been successful case reports of needle cricothyrotomy, but there are also many unsuccessful reports and intolerable complications resulting from needle cricothyrotomy.

Reported difficulties with transtracheal jet ventilation include the following six problems. First, catheter dislodgment occurs frequently and easily, producing massive subcutaneous emphysema and thereby preventing surgical access to the airway. Second, catheters kink easily, particularly in patients with abnormal neck anatomy in whom access to the neck is already abnormal, a condition usually encountered when dealing with a difficult airway. Third, exhalation from the airway is difficult to control and overinflation with jet ventilation may easily occur, producing a pneumothorax. The same condition that renders intubation impossible may make exhalation of jet-ventilated oxygen inadequate or impossible. When using airway exchange catheters, barotrauma can result from air entry exceeding air exit. If the air exit space surrounding the airway exchange catheter is less than a 4-mm internal diameter, ventilation will not be possible because exhalation time will be too prolonged.[2] Certainly in cases of upper airway obstruction that result in a "can't intubate, can't ventilate" situation, it is likely that one of the major causes is limited airway size. Otherwise, ventilation by bag and mask would likely have been satisfactory. In addition, Candido et al. suggest there is a blast effect of air impacting on intact human tissue, another cause of barotrauma to the tracheobronchial tree.[3] A blast effect may also occur with needle cricothyrotomy, in which the air entry lumen is even smaller than an airway exchange catheter. It is suggested that jet ventilation be performed with no more than 25 psi and no more than half-a-second inspiratory time, which requires adjustment of most jet ventilation systems.[2] In the middle of an airway catastrophe, such adjustments may not occur.

Fourth, a substantial amount of time is required to activate a jet ventilation system, for one is rarely instantly available. Fifth, significant tracheal damage may occur to both the anterior and posterior tracheal walls, especially in pediatric patients or patients with small or narrowed airways, during insertion of a cricothyrotomy needle. Abnormal airways may very well be present when severe airway obstruction cannot be relieved by those skilled in airway management who are using familiar techniques. Sixth, it is impossible to gain appreciable hands-on experience for a procedure that is rarely performed, cannot be simulated with animal models or mannequins, and is not allowed to be practiced on cadavers.

Surgical cricothyrotomy should be reserved for someone skilled in the procedure, usually a surgeon. A needle cricothyrotomy should be delayed until no other option exists.

1. Report of the Airway Management Committee, Harvard Departments of Anaesthesia, Boston, 1996.
2. Benumof JL: Airway exchange catheters: Simple concept, potentially great danger. Anesthesiology 1999;91:342.
3. Candido KD, Saatee S, Appavu SK, Khorasani A: Revisiting the ASA guidelines for management of a difficult airway. Anesthesiology 2000;93:295.

AIRWAY

Although the *A* of the mnemonic *ABC* stands for *airway*, it should also stand for the initial *a*ssessment of the patient. Before CPR is initiated, unresponsiveness is established and the emergency response system activated.

The airway is then evaluated. The patient is positioned supine on a firm surface. The airway is most commonly obstructed by posterior displacement of the tongue or epiglottis. If there is no evidence of cervical spine instability, a **head-tilt chin-lift** should be tried first (Figure 48–3). One hand (palm) is placed on the patient's forehead applying pressure to tilt the head back while lifting the chin with the fore and index finger of the opposite hand. The **jaw-thrust** may be more effective in opening the airway and is executed by placing both hands on either side of the patient's head, grasping the angles of the jaw, and lifting.

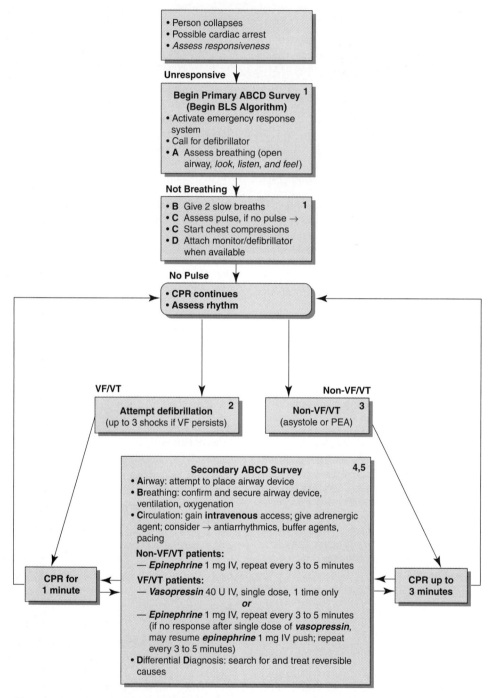

Figure 48–2. Comprehensive emergency cardiac care algorithm. BLS = basic life support, VF/VT = ventricular fibrillation and pulseless ventricular tachycardia, PEA = pulseless electrical activity, CPR = cardiopulmonary resuscitation. [Reproduced, with permission, from The American Heart Association in Collaboration with the International Liaison Committee on Resuscitation (ILCOR): Guidelines 2000 for cardiopulmonary resuscitation and emergency cardiovascular care. Circulation 2000;102:1.]

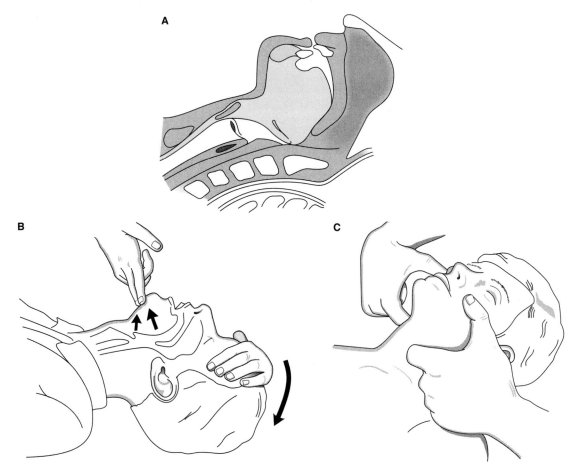

A

B

C

Figure 48–3. Loss of consciousness is often accompanied by loss of submandibular muscle tone (**A**). Occlusion of the airway by the tongue can be relieved by a head-tilt chin-lift (**B**) or a jaw thrust (**C**). In patients with possible cervical spine injury, the angles of the jaw should be lifted anteriorly without hyperextending the neck. (Courtesy American Heart Association.)

Basic airway management is discussed in detail in Chapter 5, and the trauma patient is considered in Chapter 41.

If vomitus or a foreign body is visible in the mouth of an unconscious patient, it should be swept out with a hooked index finger. If the patient is conscious or if the foreign body cannot be removed by a finger sweep, the **Heimlich maneuver** is recommended. This subdiaphragmatic abdominal thrust elevates the diaphragm, expelling a blast of air from the lungs that displaces the foreign body (Figure 48–4). Complications of the Heimlich maneuver include rib fracture, trauma to the internal viscera, and regurgitation. A combination of back blows and chest thrusts are recommended to clear foreign body obstruction in infants (Table 48–2).

If after opening the airway there is no evidence of adequate breathing, the rescuer should initiate assisted ventilation; inflating the victim's lungs with each breath by mouth-to-mouth, mouth-to-nose, mouth-to-stoma, mouth-to-barrier device, mouth-to-face shield, or mouth-to-mask rescue breathing or by using a bag-mask device (see Chapter 5). Breaths are delivered slowly (inspiratory time of ½–1 second) with a smaller tidal volume [V_T] (approximately 700–1000 mL, smaller [400–600 mL] if supplemental O_2 is used) than was recommended in the past.

With positive pressure ventilation, even with a small V_T, gastric inflation with subsequent regurgitation and aspiration are possible. Therefore, as soon as it is feasible, the airway should be secured with an ETT or, if

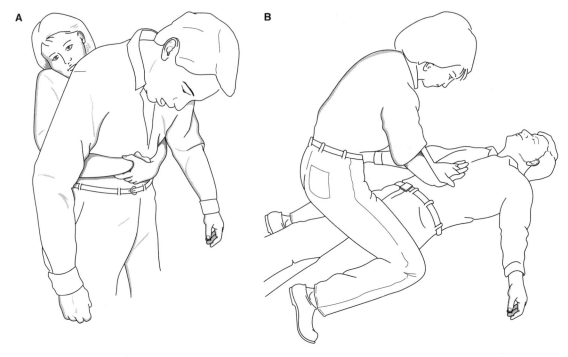

A **B**

Figure 48–4. The Heimlich maneuver can be performed with the victim standing (**A**) or lying down (**B**). The hands are positioned slightly above the navel and well below the xiphoid process and then pressed into the abdomen with a quick upward thrust. The maneuver may need to be repeated. (Courtesy American Heart Association.)

not possible, an alternative airway should be inserted. Alternative airways include the esophageal-tracheal Combitube (ETC), the laryngeal mask airway (LMA), the pharyngotracheal lumen airway, and the cuffed oropharyngeal airway. The ETC and LMA along with the oral and nasopharyngeal airways, face masks, laryngoscopes, and ETTs are discussed in Chapter 5. The new 2000 CPR-ECC guidelines recommend an ETT as the airway adjunct of choice.

Independent of which airway adjunct is used, the new guidelines state that rescuers must confirm ETT placement with an end-tidal CO_2 detector—an indicator, a capnograph, or a capnometric device. Once an artificial airway is successfully placed, *it must be* carefully secured with a tie or tape.

Some causes of airway obstruction, however, may not be relieved by conventional methods. Furthermore, endotracheal intubation may be technically impossible

Table 48–2. Summary of recommended basic life support techniques.

	Infant (1–12 mo)	Child (> 12 mo)	Adult
Breathing rate	20 breaths/min	20 breaths/min	10–12 breaths/min
Pulse check	Brachial	Carotid	Carotid
Compression rate	> 100/min	100/min	100/min
Compression method	Two or three fingers	Heel of one hand	Hands interlaced
Compression/ventilation ratio	5:1	5:1	15:2*
Foreign body obstruction	Back blows and chest thrusts	Heimlich maneuver	Heimlich maneuver

*Decrease to 5:1 if airway secured with endotracheal tube.

to perform (eg, severe facial trauma), or repeated attempts may be unwise (cervical spine trauma). In these circumstances, cricothyrotomy or tracheotomy may be necessary. **Cricothyrotomy** involves placing a large intravenous catheter or a commercially available cannula into the trachea through the midline of the cricothyroid membrane (Figure 48–5). Proper location is confirmed

by aspiration of air. A 12- or 14-gauge catheter requires a driving pressure of 50 psi to generate sufficient gas flow (**transtracheal jet ventilation**).

Various systems are available that connect a high-pressure source of oxygen (eg, central wall oxygen, tank oxygen, or the anesthesia machine fresh gas outlet) to the catheter (Figure 48–6). A hand-operated jet injector

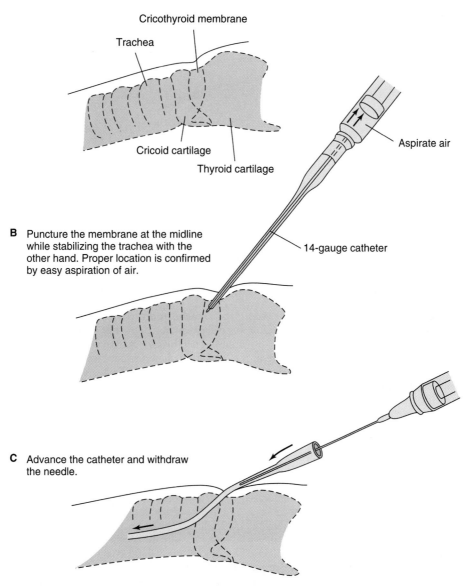

A Locate the cricothyroid membrane.

Cricothyroid membrane

Trachea

Cricoid cartilage

Thyroid cartilage

Aspirate air

14-gauge catheter

B Puncture the membrane at the midline while stabilizing the trachea with the other hand. Proper location is confirmed by easy aspiration of air.

C Advance the catheter and withdraw the needle.

Figure 48–5. Percutaneous cricothyrotomy with a 14-gauge over-the-needle intravenous catheter.

A

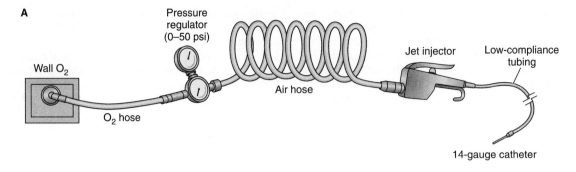

Wall O₂

O₂ hose

Pressure regulator (0–50 psi)

Air hose

Jet injector

Low-compliance tubing

14-gauge catheter

B

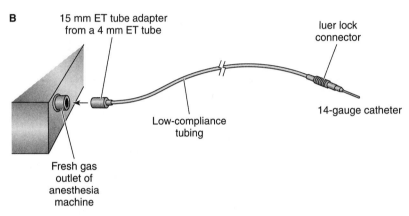

15 mm ET tube adapter from a 4 mm ET tube

luer lock connector

Low-compliance tubing

14-gauge catheter

Fresh gas outlet of anesthesia machine

Figure 48–6. Two systems for transtracheal jet ventilation after cricothyrotomy (see Figure 48–5). A jet ventilator and pressure regulator (as shown in *A*) provide better control of the inspiratory cycle. Both systems use low-compliance tubing and a high-pressure source of oxygen.

or the oxygen flush valve of an anesthesia machine controls ventilation. The addition of a pressure regulator minimizes the risk of barotrauma.

Regardless of which transtracheal jet ventilation system is chosen, it must be readily available, use low-compliance tubing, and have secure connections. Direct connection of a 12- or 14-gauge intravenous catheter to the anesthesia circle system does not allow adequate ventilation, owing to the high compliance of the corrugated breathing tubing and breathing bag. It is also impossible to reliably deliver acceptable ventilation through a 12- or 14-gauge catheter with a self-inflating resuscitation bag.

Adequacy of ventilation—particularly expiration—is judged by observation of chest wall movement and auscultation of breath sounds. Acute complications include pneumothorax, subcutaneous emphysema, mediastinal emphysema, bleeding, esophageal puncture, aspiration, and respiratory acidosis. Long-term complications include tracheomalacia, subglottic stenosis, and vocal cord changes. Cricothyrotomy is not generally recommended in children under 10 years of age.

Tracheotomy can be performed in a more controlled environment after oxygenation has been secured by cricothyrotomy. A detailed description of tracheotomy, however, is beyond the scope of this text.

BREATHING

Assessment of spontaneous breathing should immediately follow the opening or the establishment of the airway. Ventilation should not be delayed for intubation if a patent airway is established by a jaw-thrust maneuver. Apnea is confirmed by observing no chest movement, absence of breath sounds, and lack of airflow. Regardless of the airway and breathing methods employed, a specific regimen of ventilation has been proposed for the apneic patient. Initially, two breaths are slowly administered (2 seconds per breath in adults, 1–1½ seconds in infants and children). If these breaths cannot be delivered, the airway is still obstructed and the head and neck need repositioning, or a foreign body is present that must be removed.

Mouth-to-mouth or **mouth-to-mask (mouth-to-barrier-device)** rescue breathing must be immediately instituted in the breathless patient, even in the hospital setting when the crash cart is on its way. Pinching the nose allows formation of an airtight seal between the rescuer's lips and the outside of the victim's mouth. Successful rescue breathing (700–1000 mL V_T, 10–12 times per minute in an adult) is confirmed by observing the chest rising and falling with each breath and hearing and feeling the escape of air during expiration. The most common cause of inadequate mouth-to-mouth ventilation is insufficient airway control. **Mouth-to-mouth-and-nose** breathing is more effective in infants and small children than in adults.

A rescuer's exhaled air has an oxygen concentration of only 16–17%, but even that is far better than no oxygen at all. This low inspired oxygen concentration, combined with low cardiac output and intrapulmonary shunting during resuscitation, invariably results in hypoxia. **Supplemental oxygen,** preferably 100%, should always be used if available. If supplemental oxygen is used, a smaller V_T of 400–700 mL is recommended.

Mouth-to-mask or barrier device breathing has a hygienic advantage over mouth-to-mouth breathing since the rescuer's lips form a seal with an intervening device. Devices that avoid mouth-to-mouth contact should be immediately available everywhere in the hospital. Ventilation with a mask may be performed more easily in some patients because the rescuer may be able to adjust the airway or make an airtight seal more effectively. Furthermore, some mouth-to-mask devices allow the delivery of supplemental oxygen.

A self-inflating **bag-valve-mask** device is described in Chapter 3 (see Resuscitation Breathing Systems). These devices can be less effective than mouth-to-mask or **bag-valve-endotracheal tube** ventilation because of the difficulty inexperienced personnel may have in maintaining an airway and seal with one hand while simultaneously delivering an adequate V_T with the other. If additional personnel are available, cricoid pressure should be considered to prevent regurgitation.

Endotracheal intubation should be attempted as soon as practical. Attempts at intubation should not interrupt ventilation for more than 30 seconds. Cricoid pressure lessens the possibility of regurgitation and aspiration during intubation. After intubation, the patient can be ventilated with a self-inflating bag capable of delivering high oxygen concentrations. Since two hands are now available to squeeze the bag, ventilation should be satisfactory.

Automatic transport ventilators, used in Europe since the 1980s, are now recommended in the United States for prehospital care and transport of intubated patients. When choosing a ventilator for a hospitalized patient undergoing CPR-ECC, avoid pressure-cycled ventilator modes in favor of volume- or time-cycled ventilators.

The ratio of physiologic dead space to tidal volume (V_D/V_T) reflects the efficiency of CO_2 elimination. V_D/V_T increases during CPR as a result of low pulmonary blood flow and high alveolar pressures. Thus, minute ventilation may need to be increased by 50–100% once circulation is restored as CO_2 from the periphery is brought back to the lungs.

CIRCULATION

After successful delivery of two initial breaths (each 2 seconds in duration), the circulation must be rapidly assessed—health care providers are advised in the 2000 guidelines to continue to check for a pulse (the lay rescuer should not). If the patient has an adequate pulse (carotid artery in an adult or child, brachial or femoral artery in an infant) or blood pressure, breathing is continued at 10–12 breaths/min for an adult or a child older than 8 years, and 20 breaths/min for an infant or a child up to 8 years of age (Table 48–2). If the patient is pulseless or severely hypotensive, the circulatory system must be supported by a combination of external chest compressions, intravenous drug administration, and defibrillation when appropriate. Initiation of chest compressions is mandated by the inadequacy of peripheral perfusion, while drug choices and defibrillation energy levels often depend on electrocardiographic diagnosis of dysrhythmias.

External Chest Compression

Chest compressions should be *immediately* initiated in the pulseless patient. The xiphoid process is located and the heel of the rescuer's hand is placed over the lower half of the sternum. The other hand is placed over the hand on the sternum with the fingers either interlaced or extended, but off the chest. The rescuer's shoulders should be positioned directly over the hands with the elbows locked into position and arms extended, so that the weight of the upper body is used for compressions. With a straight downward thrust, the sternum is depressed 1½–2 inches (4–5 cm) in adults, 1–1½ inches (2–4 cm) in children, and then allowed to return to its normal position. For an infant, compressions ½–1 inch (1½–2½ cm) in depth are made with the middle and ring fingers on the sternum one finger-breadth below the nipple line. Compression and release times should be equal.

Whether or not adult resuscitation is performed by a single rescuer or two rescuers, 2 breaths are administered every 15 compressions (15:2), allowing 2 seconds for each breath. The cardiac compression rate should be

100/min regardless of the number of rescuers. A slightly higher compression rate of > 100/min is suggested for infants, with 1 breath delivered every 5 compressions. Note that the compression rate refers to the speed of compression (slightly less than 2/sec) and not the number of compressions delivered in 1 minute. The number of compressions per minute may be less if there is a single rescuer who pauses to ventilate the patient during BLS maneuvers. The adequacy of cardiac output can be estimated by monitoring end-tidal CO_2 or arterial pulsations.

Chest compressions force blood to flow either by increasing intrathoracic pressure (**thoracic pump**) or by directly compressing the heart (**cardiac pump**). During CPR of short duration, blood flow is created more by the cardiac pump mechanism; as CPR continues, the heart becomes less compliant and the thoracic pump mechanism becomes more important. As important as the rate and force of compression is for maintaining blood flow, effective perfusion of the heart and brain are best achieved when chest compression consumes 50% of the duty cycle, with the remaining 50% devoted to the relaxation phase (allowing blood to flow into the chest and heart).

DEFIBRILLATION

Ventricular fibrillation is found most commonly in adults who experience nontraumatic cardiac arrest. The time from collapse to defibrillation is the single most important determinant of survival. The chances for survival decline 7–10% for every minute without defibrillation. Therefore, patients who have cardiac arrest should be defibrillated at the earliest possible moment. Health care personnel working in hospitals and ambulatory care facilities must be able to provide early defibrillation to collapsed patients with ventricular fibrillation as soon as possible. Shock should be delivered within 3 minutes (± 1 minute) of arrest.

There is no definite relationship between the energy requirement for successful defibrillation and body size; a shock with too low an energy level will not successfully cardiovert; conversely, too high an energy level will result in functional and morphologic injury.

Defibrillators deliver energy in either monophasic or biphasic waveforms. Increasingly, biphasic waveforms are recommended for successful cardioversion.

In many institutions, automated external defibrillators (AEDs) are available. Such devices are increasingly being used in the community by police, firefighters, security personnel, sports marshalls, ski patrol members, airline flight attendants, etc. AEDs are technologically advanced, microprocessor-based devices that are capable of electrocardiographic analysis, with excellent recognition of cardiac rhythm and ventricular fibrillation. The device will rarely (< 0.1%) deliver an inap-

propriate electric counter shock. The majority of AEDs built since 1996 will deliver a biphasic shock. Biphasic shocks deliver energy in two directions with equivalent efficacy at lower energy levels compared with monophasic shocks, perhaps with less myocardial injury. These devices deliver an impedance-compensating, biphasic, truncated exponential (BTE) shocks. Such 150 joule BTE shocks have been found to be as effective as 200 joule or greater monophasic damped sine (MDS) waveform shocks that have been the norm in the past. When using the AED, one electropad is placed on the upper right sternal border, just below the clavicle and the other pad is placed just lateral to the left nipple, with the top of the pad a few inches below the axilla.

Current recommendations for cardioversion for atrial fibrillation (Table 48–3) are initially for 100–200 joules-MDS. For atrial flutter or paroxysmal supraventricular tachycardia (PSVT), an initial energy level of 50–100 J-MDS is often adequate. Energy level is increased if initial shocks are unsuccessful.

Ventricular tachycardia, especially monomorphic ventricular tachycardia, responds well to shocks at initial energy levels of 100 J-MDS. For polymorphic ventricular tachycardia or for ventricular fibrillation, initial energy should be 200 joules-MDS. Step-wise increases in energy levels should be used if the first shock fails (Table 48–3).

Cardioversion should be synchronized with the QRS complex and is recommended for hemodynamically stable, wide complex tachycardia requiring cardioversion, PSVT, atrial fibrillation, and atrial flutter. Ventricular fibrillation requires unsynchronized defibrillation.

Invasive Cardiopulmonary Resuscitation

Thoracotomy and open-chest cardiac massage are not part of routine CPR because of the high incidence of severe complications. Nonetheless, these invasive techniques can be helpful in specific life-threatening circumstances that preclude effective closed-chest massage. Possible indications include cardiac arrest associated with penetrating or blunt chest trauma, penetrating abdominal trauma, severe chest deformity, pericardial tamponade, or pulmonary embolism.

Intravenous Access

Some resuscitation drugs are fairly well absorbed following administration through an endotracheal tube (eg, lidocaine, epinephrine, atropine, vasopressin, but *not* sodium bicarbonate). These drugs should be delivered down a catheter whose tip extends past the endotracheal tube bevel. Furthermore, dosages 2–2½ times higher than rec-

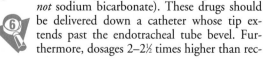

Table 48–3. Energy requirements for cardioversion and defibrillation using monophasic damped sinusoidal waveform shocks.*

Indications	Shocks (joules)			
	First	Second	Third	Subsequent
Unstable atrial fibrillation (adult)†	100–200	100–200	100–300	360
Unstable paroxysmal atrial tachycardia/atrial flutter				
Adult	50	100	200	360
Child	0.5–1/kg	2/kg	4/kg	4/kg
Monomorphic ventricular tachycardia	100	200	200–300	360
Ventricular fibrillation‡				
Adult	200	200–300	200–360	360
Child	2/kg	4/kg	4/kg	4/kg

*If biphasic truncated exponential (BTE) waveform shocks are used, energy level is usually < 200 joules.
†BTE waveform shocks ≥ 120 joules.
‡BTE waveform shocks ≥ 150 joules.

ommended for intravenous use, diluted in 10 mL of normal saline or distilled water, are recommended for adult patients. Even though establishing reliable intravenous access is a high priority, it *should not take precedence* over initial airway management, chest compressions, or defibrillation. A preexisting internal jugular or subclavian line is ideal for venous access during resuscitation. If there is no central line access, then one should attempt to establish peripheral intravenous access, either in the antecubital or external jugular vein. Peripheral intravenous sites are associated with a significant delay of between 1 and 2 minutes between drug administration and delivery to the heart, since peripheral blood flow is drastically reduced during resuscitation. Administration of drugs given through a peripheral intravenous line should be followed by an intravenous flush (eg, a 20-mL fluid bolus in adults) and elevation of the extremity for 10–20 seconds. Cardiac chest compressions may have to be briefly interrupted to establish an internal jugular line if the response to peripherally administered drugs is inadequate.

If intravenous cannulation is difficult, an intraosseous infusion can provide emergency vascular access in children. The success rate is lower in older children, but intraosseous cannulas have been successfully placed even in adults in the tibia and in the distal radius and ulna. A rigid 18-gauge spinal needle with a stylet or a small bone marrow trephine needle can be inserted into the distal femur or proximal tibia. If the tibia is chosen, a needle is inserted 2–3 cm below the tibial tuberosity at a 45-degree angle away from the epiphyseal plate (Figure 48–7). Once the

needle is advanced through the cortex, it should stand upright without support. Proper placement is confirmed by the ability to aspirate marrow through the needle and a smooth infusion of fluid. A network of venous sinusoids within the medullary cavity of long bones drains into the systemic circulation by way of nu-

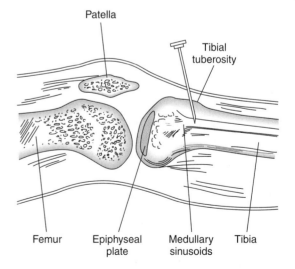

Figure 48–7. Intraosseous infusions provide emergency access to the venous circulation in pediatric patients by way of the large medullary venous channels. The needle is directed away from the epiphyseal plate to minimize the risk of injury.

trient or emissary veins. This route is very effective for administration of drugs, crystalloids, colloids, and blood and can achieve flow rates exceeding 100 mL/hour under gravity. Much higher flow rates are possible if the fluid is placed under pressure (eg, 300 mm Hg) with an infusion bag. The onset of drug action will be slightly delayed compared with intravenous or endotracheal administration. The interosseous route may require a higher dose of some drugs (eg, epinephrine) than recommended for intravenous administration. The use of intraosseous infusion for induction and maintenance of general anesthesia, antibiotic therapy, seizure control, and inotropic support has been described. Because of the risks of osteomyelitis and compartment syndrome, however, intraosseous infusions should be replaced by a conventional intravenous route as soon as possible. In addition, because of the theoretical risk of bone marrow or fat emboli, intraosseous infusions should be avoided in patients with right-to-left shunts, pulmonary hypertension, or severe pulmonary insufficiency.

Dysrhythmia Recognition

Successful pharmacologic and electrical treatment of cardiac arrest (Figure 48–8) depends on definitive identification of the underlying dysrhythmia. Interpreting rhythm strips in the midst of a resuscitation situation is complicated by artifacts and variations in monitoring techniques (eg, lead systems, equipment).

Drug Administration

Many of the drugs administered during CPR have been described elsewhere in this text. Table 48–4 summarizes the cardiovascular actions, indications, and dosages of drugs commonly used during resuscitation.

Calcium chloride, sodium bicarbonate, and bretylium are conspicuously absent from this table. Calcium (2–4 mg/kg of the chloride salt) is helpful in the treatment of documented hypocalcemia, hyperkalemia, hypermagnesemia, or a calcium channel blocker overdose. When used, 10% calcium chloride can be given at 2–4 mg/kg every 10 minutes. Sodium bicarbonate (0.5–1 mEq/kg) is not recommended in the ACLS guidelines and should be considered only in specific situations such as preexisting metabolic acidosis, hyperkalemia, or in the treatment of tricyclic antidepressant or barbiturate overdose. Sodium bicarbonate elevates plasma pH by combining with hydrogen ions to form carbonic acid, which readily dissociates into carbon dioxide and water. Because carbon dioxide, but not bicarbonate, readily crosses cell membranes and the blood-brain barrier, the resulting arterial hypercapnia will cause intracellular

tissue acidosis. Although successful defibrillation is not related to *arterial* pH, increased *intramyocardial* carbon dioxide may reduce the possibility of cardiac resuscitation. Furthermore, bicarbonate administration can lead to detrimental alterations in osmolality and the oxygen-hemoglobin dissociation curve. Therefore, effective alveolar ventilation and adequate tissue perfusion are the treatments of choice for the respiratory and metabolic acidosis that accompany resuscitation.

Bretylium tosylate is a quaternary compound used to treat ventricular tachycardia and fibrillation. A national shortage stimulated an assessment of its role in managing these rhythms. Based on this review, bretylium was removed from the ACLS guidelines because of a high incidence of serious adverse events associated with its use, the availability of equally effective drugs, and its national shortage.

Intravenous fluid therapy with either colloid or balanced salt solutions (eg, normal saline) is indicated in patients with intravascular volume depletion (eg, acute blood loss, diabetic ketoacidosis, thermal burns). Dextrose-containing solutions may lead to a hyperosmotic diuresis and may worsen neurologic outcome. They should be avoided unless hypoglycemia is suspected. Likewise, free water administration (eg, D_5W) may lead to cerebral edema.

Emergency Pacemaker Therapy

Transcutaneous cardiac pacing (TCP) is a noninvasive method of rapidly treating dysrhythmias caused by conduction disorders or abnormal impulse. These may include asystole, bradycardia caused by heart block, or tachycardia from a reentrant mechanism. If there is worry about the use of atropine in high-grade block, TCP is always appropriate. If the patient is unstable with marked bradycardia, TCP should be implemented immediately. The pacer unit has become a built-in feature of some defibrillator models. Disposable pacing electrodes are usually positioned on the patient in an anterior-posterior manner. The placement of the negative electrode corresponds to a V_2 electrocardiograph position, while the positive electrode is placed on the left posterior chest beneath the scapula and lateral to the spine. Note that this positioning does not interfere with paddle placement during defibrillation. Failure to capture may be due to electrode misplacement, poor electrode-to-skin contact, or increased transthoracic impedance (eg, barrel-shaped chest, pericardial effusion). Current output is slowly increased until the pacing stimuli obtain electrical and mechanical capture. A wide QRS complex following a pacing spike signals *electrical* capture, but *mechanical* (ventricular) capture must be confirmed by an

Table 48–5. Steps for synchronized cardioversion.

---

1. Consider sedation.
2. Turn on defibrillator (monophasic or biphasic).
3. Attach monitor leads to the patient ("white to right, red to ribs, what's left over to the left shoulder") and ensure proper display of the patient's rhythm.
4. Engage the synchronization mode by pressing the "sync" control button.
5. Look for markers on R waves indicating sync mode.
6. If necessary, adjust monitor gain until sync markers occur with each R wave.
7. Select appropriate energy level.
8. Position conductor pads on patient (or apply gel to paddles).
9. Position paddle on patient (sternum-apex).
10. Announce to team members: *"Charging defibrillator—stand clear!"*
11. Press "charge" button on apex paddle (right hand).
12. When the defibrillator is charged, begin the final clearing chant. State firmly in a forceful voice the following chant before each shock:
    - *"I am going to shock on three. One, I'm clear."* (Check to make sure you are clear of contact with the patient, the stretcher, and the equipment.
    - *"Two, you are clear."* (Make a visual check to ensure that no one continues to touch the patient or stretcher. In particular, do not forget about the person providing ventilation. That person's hands should not be touching the ventilatory adjuncts, including the tracheal tube!).
    - *"Three, everybody's clear."* (Check yourself one more time before pressing the "shock" buttons.)
13. Apply 25 lb pressure on both paddles.
14. Press the "discharge" buttons simultaneously.
15. Check the monitor. If tachycardia persists, increase the joules according to the electrical cardioversion algorithm.
16. **Reset the sync mode after each synchronized cardioversion because most defibrillators default back to unsynchronized mode.** This default allows an immediate defibrillation if the cardioversion produces ventricular fibrillation.

Reproduced with permission from: The American Heart Association in Collaboration with the International Liaison Committee on Resuscitation (ILCOR): Guidelines 2000 for cardiopulmonary resuscitation and emergency cardiovascular care. *Circulation* 2000;102:1.

improving pulse or blood pressure. Conscious patients may require sedation to tolerate the discomfort of skeletal muscle contractions. Transcutaneous pacing can provide effective temporizing therapy until transvenous pacing or other definitive treatment can be initiated. TCP has many advantages over transvenous pacing be-

cause it can be used by almost all ECC providers and can be started quickly and conveniently at the bedside.

RECOMMENDED RESUSCITATION PROTOCOLS

A resuscitation team leader integrates the assessment of the patient, including electrocardiographic diagnosis, with the electrical and pharmacologic therapy (Table 48–5). This person must have a firm grasp of the guidelines for cardiac arrest presented in the ACLS algorithms (Figures 48–8 to 48–12).

CASE DISCUSSION: INTRAOPERATIVE HYPOTENSION & CARDIAC ARREST

A 16-year-old boy is rushed to the operating room for emergency laparotomy and thoracotomy after suffering multiple abdominal and thoracic stab wounds. In the field, paramedics intubated the patient, started two large-bore intravenous lines, began fluid resuscitation, and inflated a pneumatic antishock garment. Upon arrival in the operating room, the patient's blood pressure is unobtainable, heart rate is 128 beats per minute (sinus tachycardia), and respirations are being controlled by a bag-valve device.

What should be done immediately?

Cardiopulmonary resuscitation must be initiated immediately: external chest compressions should be started as soon as the arterial blood pressure is found to be inadequate for vital organ perfusion. Because the patient is already intubated, the location of the endotracheal tube should be confirmed with chest auscultation, and 100% oxygen should be delivered.

Which cardiopulmonary resuscitation sequence best fits this situation?

Pulselessness in the presence of sinus rhythm suggests severe hypovolemia, cardiac tamponade, ventricular rupture, dissecting aortic aneurysm, tension pneumothorax, profound hypoxemia and acidosis, or pulmonary embolism. Epinephrine, 1 mg, should be administered intravenously.

What is the most likely cause of this patient's profound hypotension?

The presence of multiple stab wounds strongly suggests hypovolemia. Fluids, preferably warmed, should be rapidly administered. Additional venous

Table 48–4. Cardiovascular effects, indications, and dosages of resuscitation drugs.

Drug	Cardiovascular Effects	Indications	Initial Dose — Adult	Initial Dose — Pediatric	Comments
Adenosine	Slows AV nodal conduction	Narrow complex tachycardias, stable supraventricular tachycardia and wide complex tachycardias if supraventricular in origin	6 mg over 1–3 sec; 12 mg repeat dose	Initial dose 0.1–0.2 mg/kg; subsequent doses doubled to maximum single dose of 12 mg	Recommended as diagnostic or therapeutic maneuver for supraventricular tachycardias; give as rapid IV bolus. Vasodilates, BP may decrease. Theoretical risk of angina, bronchospasm, proarrhythmic action. Drug-drug interaction with theophylline, dipyridamole
Atropine	Anticholinergic (parasympatholytic). Increases sinoatrial node rate and automaticity; increases AV node conduction	Symptomatic brachycardia, AV block	0.5–1.0 mg repeated every 3–5 min	0.02 mg/kg	Repeat atropine doses every 5 min to a total dose of 3 mg in adults or 0.5 mg in children, 1.0 mg in adolescents. The minimum pediatric dose is 0.1 mg. Do not use for infranodal (Mobitz II) block.
		Ventricular asystole	1 mg	0.02 mg/kg	
Epinephrine	α-Adrenergic effects increase myocardial and cerebral blood flow. β-Adrenergic effects may increase myocardial work and decrease subendocardial perfusion and cerebral blood flow.	VF/VT, electromechanical dissociation, ventricular asystole, severe bradycardia unresponsive to atropine or pacing	1 mg IV	Initial dose 0.01 mg/kg IV; repeat same for subsequent doses or up to 0.1–0.2 mg/kg IV	Repeat doses every 3–5 min as necessary. An infusion of epinephrine (eg., 1 mg in 250 mL D₅W or NS, 4 µg/mL) can be titrated to effect in adults (1–4 µg/min) or children (0.1–1 µg/kg/min). Administration down an endotracheal tube requires higher doses (2–2.5 mg in adults, 0.1 mg/kg in children). High-dose epinephrine (0.1 mg/kg) in adults is recommended only after standard therapy has failed.
		Severe hypotension	1 µg/min in an infusion increased to effect	1 µg/kg	
Lidocaine	Decreases rate of phase 4 depolarization (decreases automaticity); depresses conduction in reentry pathways. Elevates VF threshold. Reduces disparity in action potential dura-	VT that has not responded to defibrillation; premature ventricular contractions.	1–1.5 mg/kg	1 mg/kg	Doses of 0.5 to 1.5 mg/kg can be repeated every 5–10 minutes to a total dose of 3 mg/kg. After infarction or successful resuscitation, a continuous infusion (eg, 1 g in 500 mL D₅, 2 mg/mL) should be run at a rate of 20–50 µg/kg/min (2–4 mg/min in most adults). Therapeutic blood levels are usually 1.5–6 µg/mL.

Lidocaine (continued)

	tion between normal and ischemic tissue. Reduces action potential and effective refractory period duration.	Postinfarction dysrhythmia prophylaxis	1.5 mg/kg	Not applicable	Newly recommended as alternative to epinephrine; used only one time; has a 10- to 20-min half-life.
Vasopressin	Nonadrenergic peripheral vasoconstrictor; direct stimulation of V₁ receptors	Bleeding esophageal varices; adult shock-refractory VF; hemodynamic support in vasodilatory (septic) shock	40 U IV, single dose, 1 time only	Not recommended	
Procainamide	Suppresses both atrial and ventricular dysrhythmias	AF/flutter; preexcited atrial arrhythmias with rapid ventricular response; wide complex tachycardia that cannot be distinguished as SVT or VT.	20 mg/min until arrhythmia suppressed, hypotension develops, QRS complex increases by > 50%, or total dose of 17 mg/kg has infused.In urgent situation, 50 mg/min may beused to maximum of 17 mg/kg. Maintenance infusion, 1–4 mg/min	Loading dose: 15 mg/kg; infusion over 30–60 minutes; routine use in combination with drugs that prolong QTs is not recommended	Contraindicated in overdose of tricyclic antidepressants or other antiarrhythmic drugs. Bolus doses can result in toxicity. Should not be used in preexisting QT prolongation or torsades de pointes. Blood levels should be monitored in patients with impaired renal function and when constant infusion > 3 mg/min for >24 h
Amiodarone	Complex drug with effects on sodium, potassium, and calcium channels as well as α- and β-adrenergic blocking properties	SVT with accessory pathway conduction; unstable VT and VF; stable VT, polymorphic VT, wide-complex tachycardia of uncertain origin; AF/flutter with CHF; preexcited AF/flutter; adjunct to electrical cardioversion in refractory PSVTs, atrial tachycardia, and AF	150 mg over 10 min, followed by 1 mg/min for 6 hrs, then 0.5 mg/min, with supplementary infusion of 150 mg as necessary up to 2 g. For pulseless VT or VF, initial administration is 300 mg rapid infusion diluted in 20–30 mL of saline or dextrose in water.	5 mg/kg for pulseless VT/VF; For perfusing tachycardia loading dose, 5 mg/kg IV/IO; maximum dose, 15 mg/kg/d	Antiarrhythmic of choice if cardiac function is impaired, EF < 40%, or CHF. Routine use in combination with drugs prolonging QT interval is not recommended. Most frequent side effects are hypotension and bradycardia.

(continued)

Table 48–4. Cardiovascular effects, indications, and dosages of resuscitation drugs. (continued)

Drug	Cardiovascular Effects	Indications	Initial Dose		Comments
			Adult	Pediatric	
Verapamil	Calcium channel blocking agent used to slow conduction and increase refractoriness in AV node, terminating reentrant arrhythmias that require AV nodal conduction for continuation.	Controls ventricular response rate in AF/flutter and MAT; rate control in AF; terminating narrow-complex PSVT	2.5–5 mg IV over 2 min; without response, repeat dose with 5–10 mg q 15–30 min to a max of 20 mg		Use only in patients with narrow-complex PSVT or supraventricular arrhythmia. Do not use in presence of impaired ventricular function or CHF
Diltiazem	Calcium channel blocking agent used to slow conduction and increase refractoriness in AV node, terminating reentrant arrhythmias that require AV nodal conduction for continuation.	Slows conduction and increases refractoriness in AV node. May terminate reentrant arrhythmias. Controls ventricular response rate in AF/flutter and MAT.	0.25 mg/kg, followed by second dose of 35 mg/kg if necessary; maintenance infusion of 5–15 mg/h in AF/flutter		May exacerbate CHF in severe LV dysfunction; may decrease myocardial contractility, but less so than verapamil.
Dobutamine	Synthetic catecholamine and potent inotropic agent with predominant β-adrenergic receptor-stimulating effects that increase cardiac contractility in a dose-dependent manner, accompanied by a decrease in LV filling pressures.	Severe systolic heart failure	5–20 µg/kg/min		Hemodynamic end points rather than specific dose is goal. Elderly have significantly reduced response. May induce or exacerbate myocardial ischemia with doses > 20 µg/kg per min with increases in heart rate > 10%
Flecainide	Potent sodium channel blocker with significant conduction-slowing effects	AF/flutter, ventricular arrhythmias and supraventricular arrhythmias with structural heart disease, ectopic atrial heart disease, AV nodal reentrant tachycardia, SVTs associated with an accessory pathway, including preexcited AF	2 mg/kg at 10 mg/min (IV use not approved in the United States)		Should not be used in patients with impaired LV function, or when coronary artery disease is suspected

Drug	Properties	Indication	Dose		Comments
Ibutilide	Short-acting antiarrhythmic, prolongs the action potential duration and increases refractory period	Acute conversion or adjunct to electrical cardioversion of AF/flutter of short duration	In patients > 60 kg, 1 mg (10 mL) over 10 min; a second similar dose may be repeated in 10 min. In patients < 60 kg, initial dose is 0.01 mg/kg		Patients should be monitored for arrhythmias for 4–6 h, and longer in those with hepatic dysfunction
Magnesium	Hypomagnesemia associated with arrhythmias, cardiac insufficiency, and sudden death; can precipitate refractory VF; can hinder K^+ replacement	Torsades de pointes even with normal serum levels of magnesium	1–2 g in 50–100 mL D_5W over 5–60 min, follow with infusion of 0.5–1 g/h	500 mg/mL–IV/IO: 25–50 mg/kg; maximum dose: 2 g per dose	Rapid IV infusion for torsades de pointes or suspected hypomagnesemia not recommended in cardiac arrest except when arrhythmia suspected. 10- to 20-min infusion for asthma poorly responsive to β-adrenergic blockers
Propafenone	Significant conduction-slowing and negative inotropic effects. Nonselective β-adrenergic blocking properties	AF/flutter, ventricular arrhythmias and supraventricular arrhythmias with structural heart disease, ectopic atrial tachycardia, AV nodal reentrant tachycardia, SVTs associated with an accessory pathway	2.0 mg/kg at 10 mg/min (IV use not approved in the United States)		Should be avoided with impaired LV function or when CAD suspected
Sotalol	Prolongs action potential duration and increases cardiac tissue refractoriness. Nonselective β-adrenergic blocking properties	Preexcited AF/flutter, ventricular and supraventricular arrhythmias	1.0–1.5 mg/kg at a rate of 10 mg/min (IV use not approved in the United States)		Limited by need to be infused slowly

AV = atrioventricular, BP = blood pressure, VF = ventricular fibrillation, VT = ventricular tachycardia, AF = atrial fibrillation, SVT = supraventricular tachycardia, CHF = congestive heart failure, PSVT = paroxysmal supraventricular tachycardia, IV/IO = intravenous/intraosseous, EF = ejection fraction, MAT = multifocal atrial tachycardia, LV = left ventricular, CAD = coronary artery disease.

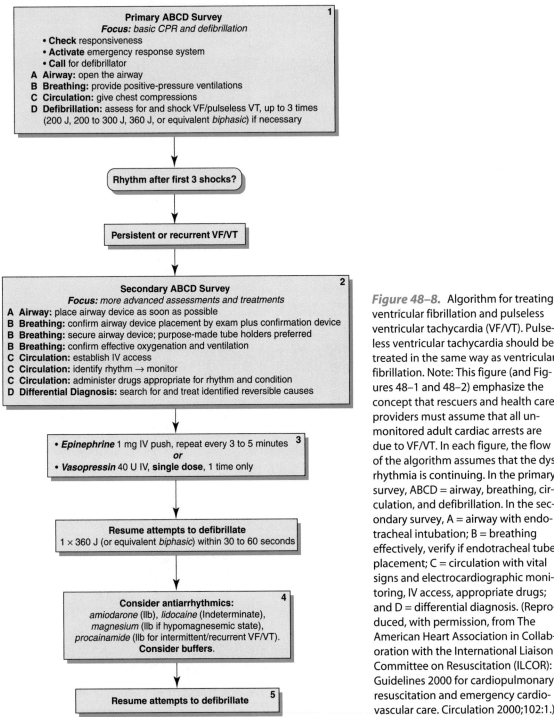

Figure 48–8. Algorithm for treating ventricular fibrillation and pulseless ventricular tachycardia (VF/VT). Pulseless ventricular tachycardia should be treated in the same way as ventricular fibrillation. Note: This figure (and Figures 48–1 and 48–2) emphasize the concept that rescuers and health care providers must assume that all unmonitored adult cardiac arrests are due to VF/VT. In each figure, the flow of the algorithm assumes that the dysrhythmia is continuing. In the primary survey, ABCD = airway, breathing, circulation, and defibrillation. In the secondary survey, A = airway with endotracheal intubation; B = breathing effectively, verify if endotracheal tube placement; C = circulation with vital signs and electrocardiographic monitoring, IV access, appropriate drugs; and D = differential diagnosis. (Reproduced, with permission, from The American Heart Association in Collaboration with the International Liaison Committee on Resuscitation (ILCOR): Guidelines 2000 for cardiopulmonary resuscitation and emergency cardiovascular care. Circulation 2000;102:1.)

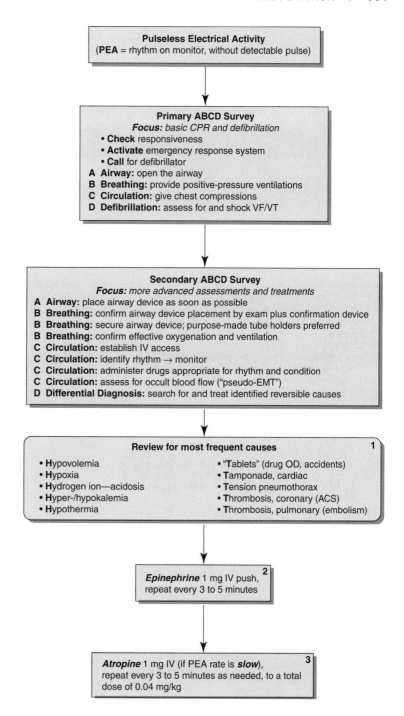

Figure 48–9. Pulseless electrical activity algorithm. VF/VT = ventricular fibrillation and pulseless ventricular tachycardia. (Reproduced, with permission, from The American Heart Association in Collaboration with the International Liaison Committee on Resuscitation (ILCOR): Guidelines 2000 for cardiopulmonary resuscitation and emergency cardiovascular care. Circulation 2000;102:1.)

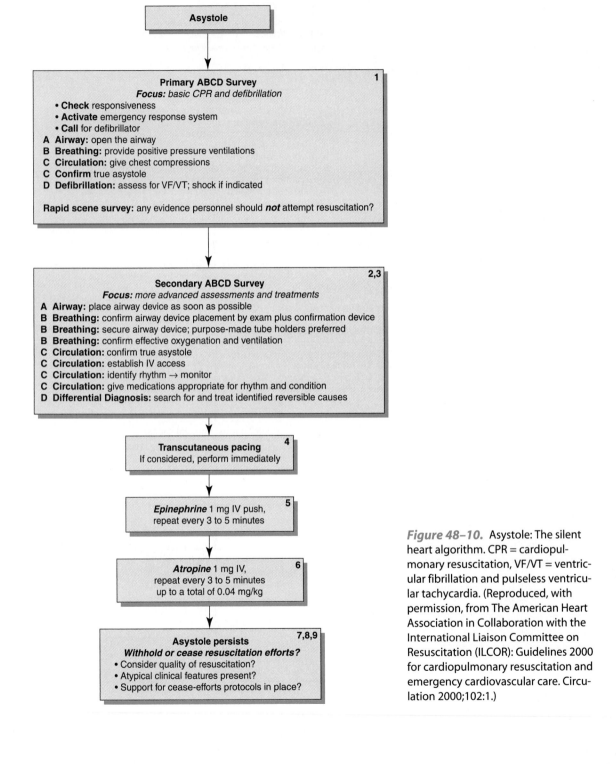

Figure 48–10. Asystole: The silent heart algorithm. CPR = cardiopulmonary resuscitation, VF/VT = ventricular fibrillation and pulseless ventricular tachycardia. (Reproduced, with permission, from The American Heart Association in Collaboration with the International Liaison Committee on Resuscitation (ILCOR): Guidelines 2000 for cardiopulmonary resuscitation and emergency cardiovascular care. Circulation 2000;102:1.)

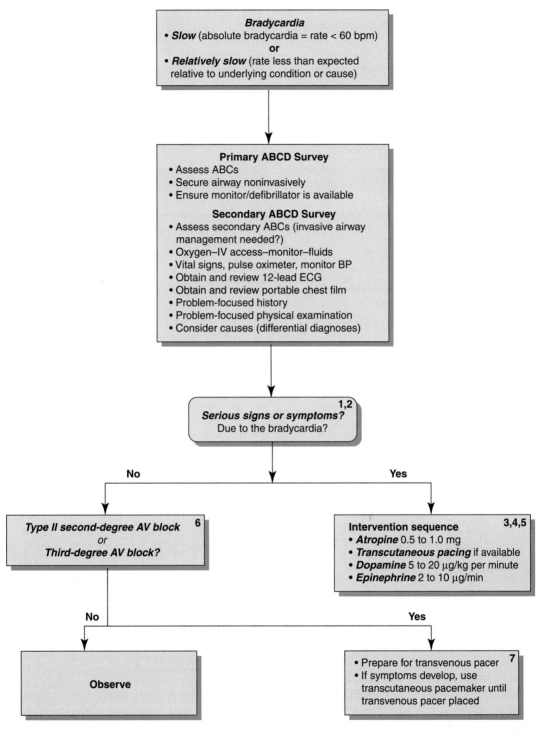

Figure 48–11. Bradycardia algorithm. AV = atrioventricular. (Reproduced, with permission, from The American Heart Association in Collaboration with the International Liaison Committee on Resuscitation (ILCOR): Guidelines 2000 for cardiopulmonary resuscitation and emergency cardiovascular care. Circulation 2000;102:1.)

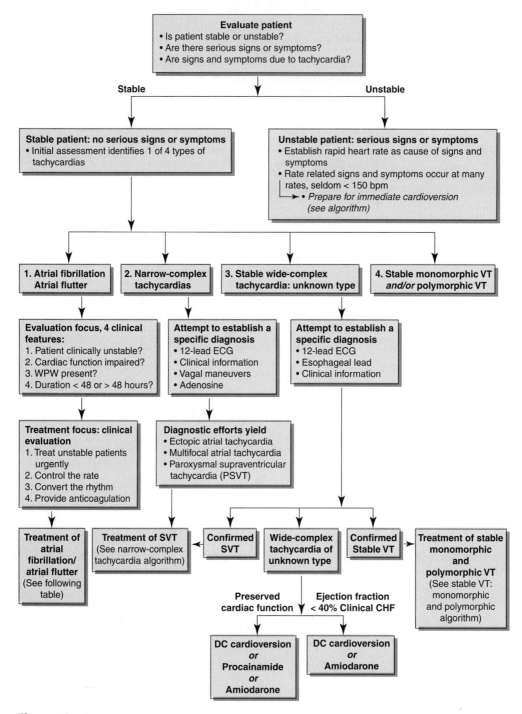

Figure 48–12. Tachycardia overview algorithm. VT = ventricular tachycardia, CHF = congestive heart failure. (Reproduced, with permission, from: The American Heart Association in Collaboration with the International Liaison Committee on Resuscitation (ILCOR): Guidelines 2000 for cardiopulmonary resuscitation and emergency cardiovascular care. Circulation 2000;102:1.)

access can be sought as other members of the operating room team administer fluid through blood pumps or other rapid infusion devices. Five percent albumin or lactated Ringer's solution is acceptable until blood products are available.

What are the signs of tension pneumothorax and pericardial tamponade?

The signs of **tension pneumothorax**—the presence of air under pressure in the pleural space—include increasing peak inspiratory pressures, tachycardia and hypotension (decreased venous return), hypoxia (atelectasis), distended neck veins, unequal breath sounds, tracheal deviation, and mediastinal shift away from the pneumothorax.

Pericardial tamponade (cardiac compression from pericardial contents) should be suspected in any patient with narrow pulse pressure; pulsus paradoxus (a > 10 mm Hg drop in systolic blood pressure with inspiration); elevated central venous pressure with neck vein distention; equalization of central venous pressure, atrial pressures, and ventricular end-diastolic pressures; distant heart sounds; tachycardia; and hypotension. Many of these signs may be masked by concurrent hypovolemic shock.

Aggressive fluid administration and properly performed external cardiac compressions do not result in satisfactory carotid or femoral pulsations. What else should be done?

Because external chest compressions are often ineffective in trauma patients, an emergency thoracotomy should be performed as soon as possible in order to clamp the thoracic aorta, relieve a tension pneumothorax or pericardial tamponade, identify possible intrathoracic hemorrhage, and perform open-chest cardiac compressions. Cross-clamping of the thoracic aorta increases brain and heart perfusion while decreasing subdiaphragmatic hemorrhage. Lack of response to cross-clamping is a good predictor of demise. Direct cardiac massage is more effective than external chest compressions, particularly in the presence of pericardial tamponade.

What is the function of the pneumatic antishock garment, and how should it be removed?

Inflation of the bladders within a pneumatic antishock garment increases arterial blood pressure by elevating peripheral vascular resistance. Functionally, the suit has the same effect as thoracic aorta cross-clamping by decreasing blood flow and hemorrhage in the lower half of the body. Complications of inflating the abdominal section of the pneumatic antishock garment include renal dysfunction, altered lung volumes, and visceral injury during external chest compressions. The suit should be deflated only after restoration of hemodynamic parameters. Even then, deflation should be gradual, since it may be accompanied by marked hypotension and metabolic acidosis caused by reperfusion of ischemic tissues.

SUGGESTED READING

The American Heart Association in Collaboration with the International Liaison Committee on Resuscitation (ILCOR): Guidelines 2000 for cardiopulmonary resuscitation and emergency cardiovascular care. Circulation 2000;102:1.

Kern KB, Halperin RH, Field J: New guidelines for cardiopulmonary resuscitation and emergency cardiac care. Changes in the management of cardiac arrest. JAMA 2001;285:1267.

Otto CW: Current concepts in cardiopulmonary resuscitation. In: Murray MJ, Coursin DB, Pearl RG, Prough DS (editors). *Critical Care Medicine: Perioperative Management,* 2nd ed. Lippincott Williams & Wilkins, 2002.

White RD: Acute therapy in patients with cardiac arrhythmias. In: Murray MJ, Coursin DB, Pearl RG, Prough DS (editors). *Critical Care Medicine: Perioperative Management,* 2nd ed. Lippincott Williams & Wilkins, 2002.

Postanesthesia Care

49

KEY CONCEPTS

 1 Patients should not leave the operating room unless they have a stable and patent airway, have adequate ventilation and oxygenation, and are hemodynamically stable.

2 Before the patient is fully responsive, pain is often manifested as postoperative restlessness. Serious systemic disturbances (such as hypoxemia, acidosis, or hypotension), bladder distention or a surgical complication (such as occult intra-abdominal hemorrhage) should always be considered as well.

 3 Intense shivering causes precipitous rises in oxygen consumption, CO_2 production, and cardiac output. These physiologic effects are often poorly tolerated by patients with preexisting cardiac or pulmonary impairment.

4 Hypoventilation in the postanesthesia care unit (PACU) is most commonly due to the residual depressant effects of anesthetic agents on respiratory drive.

 5 Obtundation, circulatory depression, or severe acidosis (arterial blood pH < 7.15) are indications for immediate endotracheal intubation in patients suffering from hypoventilation.

 6 Following naloxone administration to increase respiration, patients should be watched carefully for recurrence of the opioid-induced respiratory depression (renarcotization), since naloxone has a shorter duration than most opioids.

 7 Increased intrapulmonary shunting from a decreased functional residual capacity relative to closing capacity is the most common cause of hypoxemia following general anesthesia.

 8 The possibility of a postoperative pneumothorax should always be considered following central line placement, intercostal blocks, rib fractures, neck dissections, tracheostomy, nephrectomies, or other retroperitoneal or intra-abdominal procedures (including laparoscopy), especially when the diaphragm might be penetrated.

 9 Hypovolemia is by far the most common cause of hypotension in the PACU.

 10 Noxious stimulation from incisional pain, endotracheal intubation, or bladder distention is usually responsible for cases of postoperative hypertension.

Recovery rooms have been in existence for less than 40 years in most medical centers. Prior to that time, many early postoperative deaths occurred immediately after anesthesia and surgery. The realization that many of these deaths were preventable emphasized the need for specialized nursing care immediately following surgery. A nursing shortage in the United States following World War II may have also contributed to centralization of this care in the form of recovery rooms where one or more nurses could pay close attention to several patients at one time. As surgical procedures became increasingly complex and were performed on sicker patients, recovery room care was often extended beyond the first few hours after surgery, and some critically ill patients were kept in the recovery room overnight. The success of these early recovery rooms was a major factor in the evolution of modern surgical intensive care units (see Chapter 50). Ironically, the recovery rooms only recently received intensive care status in most hospitals, where they are now referred to as postanesthesia care units (PACUs).

At the conclusion of most operations, anesthetic agents are discontinued, monitors are disconnected, and the patient (often still anesthetized) is taken to the PACU. Following general anesthesia, if the patient was intubated and if ventilation was judged adequate, the endotracheal tube is also usually removed prior to transport. Patients are also routinely observed in the PACU following regional anesthesia, and in most instances following monitored anesthesia care (local anesthesia with sedation). Most guidelines require that a patient be admitted to the PACU following any type of anesthesia, except by specific order of the attending anesthesiologist. After a brief verbal report to the PACU nurse, the patient is left in the PACU until the major effects of anesthesia are judged to have worn off. This period is characterized by a relatively high incidence of potentially life-threatening respiratory and circulatory complications. This chapter discusses the essential components of a modern PACU, the general care of patients recovering from anesthesia, and the most commonly encountered respiratory and circulatory complications.

In some centers, outpatients are discharged home directly from the PACU, while others have a separate PACU and outpatient area. The latter functions as preoperative holding area and a second level postanesthesia recovery (predischarge) area. Thus, two phases of recovery are generally recognized for outpatient surgery. **Phase 1** is the immediate intensive care level recovery that continues until standard PACU criteria are met (see Discharge Criteria below), while **Phase 2** is a lower level care that ensures the patient is ready to go home. **"Fasting-tracking"** of selected outpatients, may allow them to safely bypass phase 1 recovery and go directly to the phase 2 area. Discharge criteria for outpatients are discussed in Chapter 46.

THE POSTANESTHESIA CARE UNIT

Design

The PACU should be located near the operating rooms. A central location in the operating room area itself is desirable, since it ensures that the patient can be rushed back to surgery if needed or that members of the operating room staff can quickly attend to patients. Proximity to radiographic, laboratory, and other intensive care facilities on the same floor is also highly desirable. The transfer of critically ill patients in elevators or through long corridors can jeopardize their care, because emergencies may arise along the way.

An open ward design facilitates observation of all patients simultaneously. At least one enclosed patient space is desirable for patients needing isolation for infection control. A ratio of 1.5 PACU beds per operating room is customary. Each patient space should be well lighted and large enough to allow easy access to patients in spite of poles for intravenous infusion pumps, a ventilator, or radiographic equipment; construction guidelines dictate a minimum of 7 ft between beds and 120 sq ft/patient. Multiple electrical outlets and at least one outlet for oxygen, air, and suction should be present at each space.

Equipment

Pulse oximetry (SpO_2) as well as electrocardiographic and automated blood pressure monitors for each space are desirable but not mandatory. However, all three monitors should be used for every patient in the initial phase of recovery from anesthesia (phase 1 care). Lesser monitoring may be appropriate subsequently. Guidelines requiring a minimum of one set of monitors for every two beds are probably no longer acceptable, particularly since most PACU incidents leading to serious morbidity are related to inadequate monitoring. Mercury or aneroid sphygmomanometers should also be readily available as back-ups for noninvasive blood pressure monitors. Monitors with the capability for transducing at least two pressures simultaneously should be available for direct arterial, central venous, pulmonary artery, or intracranial pressure monitoring. Capnography may be useful for intubated patients. Temperature-sensitive strips may be used to measure temperature in the PACU but are generally not sufficiently accurate to follow hypothermia or hyperthermia; mercury or electronic thermometers should be used if an abnormality in temperature is suspected. A forced-air warming device, heating lamps, and warming/cooling blanket should be available.

The PACU should have its own supplies of basic and emergency equipment, separate from that of the operating room. This includes oxygen cannulae, a selection of masks, oral and nasal airways, laryngoscopes, endotracheal tubes, laryngeal mask airways, and self-inflating bags for ventilation. An ample supply of catheters for vascular cannulation (venous, arterial, central venous, or pulmonary artery) is mandatory. Transvenous pacing catheters and a generator should also be available. A transthoracic pacing capability is also desirable. A defibrillation device with transcutaneous pacing capabilities and an emergency cart with drugs and supplies for advanced life support (see Chapter 48) and infusion pumps should be present and periodically inspected. Tracheostomy, chest tube, and vascular cutdown trays are also mandatory.

Respiratory therapy equipment for aerosol bronchodilator treatments, continuous positive airway pressure (CPAP), and ventilators should be in close proximity to the recovery room. A bronchoscope for the PACU is desirable but not mandatory.

Staffing

The PACU should be staffed only by nurses specifically trained in the care of patients emerging from anesthesia. They should have expertise in airway management and advanced cardiac life support as well as problems commonly encountered in surgical patients relating to wound care, drainage catheters, and postoperative bleeding.

The PACU should be under the medical direction of an anesthesiologist. A physician assigned full-time to the PACU is desirable in busy centers but is not mandatory in smaller facilities. The management of the patient in the PACU should not differ from that in the operating room and should reflect a coordinated effort between the anesthesiologist, surgeon, and any consultants. The anesthesiologist still manages the analgesia as well as airway, cardiac, pulmonary, and metabolic problems, whereas the surgeon manages any problems directly related to the surgical procedure itself. Based on the assumptions that the average PACU stay is 1 hour and the average procedure lasts 2 hours, a ratio of one recovery nurse for two patients is generally satisfactory. Staffing for nursing care should be tailored for each facility's unique requirements. A minimum of two nurses generally ensures that if one patient requires continuous 1:1 nursing care, other patients will still be cared for adequately. The latter is also important medicolegally, because inadequate staffing is often cited as a major contributing factor to mishaps in the PACU. When the operating room schedule regularly includes pediatric patients or frequent short procedures, a ratio of one nurse to one patient is often needed. A charge nurse should be assigned to ensure optimal staffing at all times.

■ CARE OF THE PATIENT

EMERGENCE FROM GENERAL ANESTHESIA

Recovery from general or regional anesthesia is a time of great physiologic stress for many patients. Emergence from general anesthesia should ideally be a smooth and gradual awakening in a controlled environment. Unfortunately, it often begins in the operating room or during transport to the recovery room and is frequently characterized by airway obstruction, shivering, agita-

tion, delirium, pain, nausea and vomiting, hypothermia, and autonomic lability. Even patients receiving spinal or epidural anesthesia can experience marked decreases in blood pressure during transport or recovery; the sympatholytic effects of regional blocks prevent compensatory reflex vasoconstriction when patients are moved or when they sit up.

Following an inhalational-based anesthetic, the speed of emergence is directly proportional to alveolar ventilation but inversely proportionate to the agent's blood solubility (see Chapter 7). As the duration of anesthesia increases, emergence also becomes increasingly dependent on total tissue uptake, which is a function of agent solubility, the average concentration used, and the duration of exposure to the anesthetic. Recovery is therefore fastest with desflurane and nitrous oxide and slowest from prolonged deep anesthesia with halothane and enflurane. Hypoventilation delays emergence from inhalational anesthesia.

Emergence from an intravenous anesthetic is a function of its pharmacokinetics. Recovery from most intravenous anesthetic agents is dependent chiefly on redistribution rather than on elimination half-life. As the total administered dose increases, however, cumulative effects become apparent in the form of prolonged emergence; the termination of action becomes increasingly dependent on the elimination or metabolic half-life. Under these conditions, advanced age or renal or hepatic disease can prolong emergence (see Chapter 8). Patients receiving propofol for induction and maintenance notably recover faster than those receiving other agents.

The speed of emergence can also be influenced by preoperative medications. Premedication with agents that outlast the procedure may be expected to prolong emergence. The short duration of action of midazolam makes it a suitable premedication agent for short procedures. The effects of preoperative sleep deprivation or drug ingestion (alcohol, sedatives) can also be additive to those of anesthetic agents and can prolong emergence.

Delayed Emergence

The most frequent cause of delayed emergence (when the patient fails to regain consciousness 30–60 minutes after general anesthesia) is residual anesthetic, sedative, and analgesic drug effect. Delayed emergence might occur as a result of absolute or relative drug overdose, or potentiation of anesthetic agents by prior drug ingestion (alcohol). Administration of naloxone (0.04 mg increments) and flumazenil (0.2 mg increments) readily reverses and can exclude the effects of an opioid and benzodiazepine, respectively. Physostigmine 1–2 mg may partially reverse the effect of other agents. A nerve stimulator can be used to exclude significant neuromuscular blockade in patients on a mechanical ventilator who have inadequate spontaneous tidal volumes.

Less common causes of delayed emergence include hypothermia, marked metabolic disturbances, and perioperative stroke. Core temperatures less than 33 °C have an anesthetic effect, and greatly potentiate the effects of central nervous system depressants. Forced-air warming devices are most effective in raising body temperature. Hypoxemia and hypercarbia are readily excluded by blood gas analysis. Hypercalcemia, hypermagnesemia, hyponatremia, and hypoglycemia and hyperglycemia are rare causes that require laboratory measurements for diagnosis. Perioperative stroke is rare except following neurologic, cardiac, and cerebrovascular surgery (see Chapter 27); diagnosis requires neurologic consultation and radiologic imaging.

TRANSPORT FROM THE OPERATING ROOM

This period is usually complicated by the lack of adequate monitors, access to drugs, or resuscitative equipment. Patients should not leave the operating room unless they have a stable and patent airway, have adequate ventilation and oxygenation, and are hemodynamically stable. Most if not all patients should be transported with oxygen supplementation because transient hypoxemia ($SpO_2 <$ 90%) may develop in as many as 30–50% of otherwise "normal" patients during transport while breathing room air. Unstable patients should be left intubated and transported with a portable monitor (electrocardiograph [ECG], SpO_2, and blood pressure) and a supply of emergency drugs.

All patients should be taken to the PACU on a bed or gurney that can be placed in either the head-down (Trendelenburg) or head-up position. The head-down position is useful for hypovolemic patients, while the head-up position is useful for patients with underlying pulmonary dysfunction (see Chapter 22). Those at high risk for vomiting or upper airway bleeding, such as following tonsillectomy, should be transported in the lateral position. This position also helps prevent airway obstruction and facilitates drainage of secretions.

ROUTINE RECOVERY

General Anesthesia

Vital signs and oxygenation should be checked immediately on arrival. Subsequent blood pressure, pulse rate, and respiratory rate measurements are routinely made at least every 5 minutes for 15 minutes or until stable, and every 15 minutes thereafter. Although the occurrence of hypoxemia does not necessarily correlate with the level of consciousness, pulse oximetry should be monitored continuously in all patients recovering from general anesthesia, at least until they regain consciousness. At least one temperature measurement should also be obtained. After initial vital signs have been recorded, the anesthesiologist should give a brief report to the PACU nurse that includes the preoperative history (including mental status and any communication problems such as language barriers, deafness, blindness, or mental retardation), pertinent intraoperative events (type of anesthesia, the surgical procedure, blood loss, fluid replacement, and any complications), expected postoperative problems, and postanesthesia orders (epidural catheter care, transfusion, postoperative ventilation, etc).

All patients recovering from general anesthesia should receive 30–40% oxygen during emergence because transient hypoxemia can develop in healthy patients. Patients at increased risk for hypoxemia, such as those with underlying pulmonary dysfunction or those undergoing upper abdominal or thoracic procedures, should continue to be monitored with a pulse oximeter even after emergence and may need oxygen supplementation for longer periods. A rational decision regarding continuing supplemental oxygen therapy at the time of discharge from the PACU can be made based on SpO_2 readings on room air. Arterial blood gas measurements can be obtained to confirm abnormal oximetry readings. Oxygen therapy should be carefully controlled in patients with chronic obstructive pulmonary disease and a history of CO_2 retention. Patients should generally be nursed in the head-up position whenever possible to optimize oxygenation. Elevating the head of the bed, however, before the patient is responsive, can lead to airway obstruction. In such cases, the oral or nasal airway should be left in place until the patient is awake. Deep breathing and coughing should be encouraged periodically.

Regional Anesthesia

Patients who are heavily sedated or hemodynamically unstable following regional anesthesia should also receive supplemental oxygen in the PACU. Sensory and motor levels should be periodically recorded following regional anesthesia to document dissipation of the block. Precautions in the form of padding or repeated warning may be necessary to prevent self-injury from uncoordinated arm movements following brachial plexus blocks. Blood pressure should be closely monitored following spinal and epidural anesthesia. Bladder catheterization may be necessary in patients who have had spinal or epidural anesthesia for longer than 4 hours.

Pain Control

Moderate to severe postoperative pain in the PACU can be managed with parenteral or intraspinal opioids, regional anesthesia, or specific nerve blocks (see Chapter 18). When opioids are used, titration of small intravenous doses is generally safest. Although considerable variability may be encountered, most patients are quite sensitive to opioids within the first hour after general anesthesia. Adequate analgesia must be balanced against excessive sedation. Opioids of intermediate to long duration, such as meperidine, 10–20 mg (0.25–0.5 mg/kg in children), hydromorphone 0.25–0.5 mg (0.015–0.02 mg/kg in children), or morphine, 2–4 mg (0.025–0.05 mg/kg in children), are most commonly used. Analgesic effects usually peak within 4–5 minutes. Maximal respiratory depression, especially with morphine, may not be seen until 20–30 minutes later. When the patient is fully awake, patient-controlled analgesia (PCA) can be instituted (see Chapter 18). Intramuscular administration of opioids has the disadvantage of delayed and variable onset (10–20 minutes) and delayed respiratory depression (up to 1 hour).

When an epidural catheter has been placed, epidural administration of fentanyl, 50–100 μg, sufentanil, 20–30 μg, or morphine, 3–5 mg, can provide excellent pain relief in adults; however, the risk of delayed respiratory depression with morphine mandates special monitoring precautions for 12–24 hours afterward (see Chapter 18). Wound infiltration with local anesthetic or intercostal, interscalene, epidural, or caudal anesthesia is often helpful when opioid analgesia alone is unsatisfactory (see Chapter 18).

Mild to moderate pain can be treated intravenously with an opioid agonist-antagonist (butorphanol, 1–2 mg, or nalbuphine, 5–10 mg) or ketorolac tromethamine, 30 mg (a parenteral nonsteroidal anti-inflammatory agent). The latter is especially useful following orthopedic and gynecologic procedures.

Agitation

Before the patient is fully responsive, pain is often manifested as postoperative restlessness. Serious systemic disturbances (such as hypoxemia, acidosis, or hypotension), bladder distention or a surgical complication (such as occult intra-abdominal hemorrhage) should always be considered as well. Marked agitation may necessitate arm and leg restraints to avoid self-injury, particularly in children. When serious physiologic disturbances have been excluded in children, cuddling and kind words from a sympathetic attendant or the parents (if they are allowed in the PACU) often calm the pediatric patient. Other contributory factors include marked preoperative anxiety and fear, and adverse drug effects (large doses of central anticholinergic agents, phenothiazines, or ketamine). Physostigmine, 1–2 mg intravenously (0.05 mg/kg in children), is most effective in treating delirium due to atropine and scopolamine but may also be useful in other cases. If serious systemic disturbances and pain can be excluded, persistent agitation may require sedation with intermittent intravenous doses of midazolam, 0.5–1 mg (0.05 mg/kg in children).

Nausea & Vomiting

Postoperative nausea and vomiting are the common problem following general anesthesia. Nausea may also be seen with hypotension from spinal or epidural anesthesia. An increased incidence of nausea is reported following opioid and possibly nitrous oxide anesthesia, intraperitoneal surgery (especially laparoscopy), and strabismus surgery. The highest incidence appears to be in young women; studies suggest nausea is more common during menstruation. Increased vagal tone manifested as sudden bradycardia commonly precedes or coincides with emesis. Propofol anesthesia decreases the incidence of postoperative nausea and vomiting. Intravenous droperidol 0.625–1.25 mg (0.05–0.075 mg/kg in children), when given intraoperatively, significantly decreases the likelihood of postoperative nausea without significantly prolonging emergence; a second dose may be necessary if nausea occurs in the PACU. Metoclopramide, 0.15 mg/kg intravenously, may be as effective as droperidol and causes less drowsiness. Some studies suggest that when propofol is not used during anesthesia, droperidol may be more effective than metoclopramide. Selective 5-hydroxytryptamine (serotonin) receptor 3 (5-HT$_3$) antagonists such as ondansetron 4 mg (0.1 mg/kg in children), granisetron 0.01–0.04 mg/kg, and dolasetron 12.5 mg (0.035 mg/kg in children) are also extremely effective. 5-HT$_3$ antagonists are not associated with the sedation, acute extrapyramidal (dystonic) manifestations, and dysphoric reactions that may be encountered with other agents. Ondansetron may be more effective than other agents in children. Dexamethasone, 8–10 mg (0.10 mg/kg in children), when combined with another antiemetic is especially effective for refractory nausea and vomiting. Low-dose propofol (20-mg bolus, or a 10-mg bolus followed by 10 μg/kg/min) has also been reported to be effective for postoperative nausea and vomiting.

Shivering & Hypothermia

Shivering can occur in the PACU as a result of intraoperative hypothermia or the effects of anesthetic agents. It is also common in the immediate postpartum period.

The most important cause of hypothermia is a redistribution of heat from the body core to the peripheral compartments (see Chapter 6). A cold ambient temperature in the operating room, prolonged exposure of a large wound, and the use of large amounts of unwarmed intravenous fluids or high flows of unhumidified gases can also be contributory. Nearly all anesthetics, especially volatile agents, decrease the normal vasoconstrictive response to hypothermia. Although anesthetic agents also decrease the shivering threshold, shivering is commonly observed during or after emergence from general anesthesia. Shivering in such instances represents the body's effort to increase heat production and raise body temperature and may be associated with intense vasoconstriction. Emergence from even brief general anesthesia is sometimes also associated with shivering. Although the shivering can be part of nonspecific neurologic signs (posturing, clonus, or Babinski's sign) that are sometimes observed during emergence, it is most often due to hypothermia and most commonly associated with volatile anesthetics. Regardless of the mechanism, its incidence appears related to duration of surgery and the use of high concentrations of a volatile agent. The shivering occasionally can be intense enough to cause hyperthermia (38–39°C) and a significant metabolic acidosis, both of which promptly resolve when the shivering stops. Both spinal and epidural anesthesia also lower the shivering threshold and vasoconstrictive response to hypothermia; shivering may also be encountered in the recovery room following regional anesthesia. Other causes of shivering should be excluded, such as sepsis, drug allergy, or a transfusion reaction.

Hypothermia should be treated with a forced-air warming device, or (less satisfactorily) with warming lights or heating blankets, to raise body temperature to normal. Intense shivering causes precipitous rises in oxygen consumption, CO_2 production, and cardiac output. These physiologic effects are often poorly tolerated by patients with preexisting cardiac or pulmonary impairment. Hypothermia has been associated with an increased incidence of myocardial ischemia, arrhythmias, increased transfusion requirements, and increased duration of muscle relaxant effects. Small intravenous doses of meperidine, 10–50 mg, can dramatically reduce or even stop shivering. Intubated and mechanically ventilated patients can also be sedated and given a muscle relaxant until normothermia is reestablished and the effects of anesthesia have dissipated.

Discharge Criteria

All patients must be evaluated by an anesthesiologist prior to discharge from the PACU unless strict discharge criteria are adopted. Criteria for discharging patients from the PACU are established by the department of anesthesiology and the hospital's medical staff. They may allow PACU nurses to determine when patients may be transferred without the presence of a physician provided all criteria have been met. Criteria can vary according to whether the patient is going to be discharged to an intensive care unit, a regular ward, the outpatient department (phase 2 recovery), or directly home (see Chapter 46).

Before discharge, patients should have been observed for respiratory depression for at least 30 minutes after the last dose of parenteral narcotic. Other minimum discharge criteria for patients recovering from general anesthesia usually include the following:

(1) Easy arousability
(2) Full orientation
(3) The ability to maintain and protect the airway
(4) Stable vital signs for at least 30–60 minutes
(5) The ability to call for help if necessary
(6) No obvious surgical complications (such as active bleeding).

Controlling postoperative pain and reestablishing normothermia prior to discharge are also highly desirable. Scoring systems are widely used. Most assess SpO_2 (or color), consciousness, circulation, respiration, and motor activity (Table 49–1). The majority of patients can meet discharge criteria within 60 minutes in the PACU. Patients to be transferred to other intensive care facilities need not meet all requirements.

In addition to the above criteria, patients receiving regional anesthesia should also show signs of resolution of both sensory and motor blockade. Complete resolution of the block is generally desirable to avoid inadvertent injuries due to motor weakness or sensory deficits; some medical centers have nursing protocols that allow earlier discharge to appropriately staffed areas. Documenting resolution of the block is also critically important. Failure of a spinal or epidural block to resolve after 6 hours raises the possibility of spinal cord or epidural hematoma, which should be excluded by radiologic imaging.

In some centers, outpatients who meet the above discharge criteria when they come out of the operating room may be "fast-tracked" and taken directly to the phase 2 recovery area. Similarly, inpatients who meet the same criteria may be transferred directly from the operating room to their ward. Criteria for discharging ambulatory surgery patients to home care are discussed in Chapter 46.

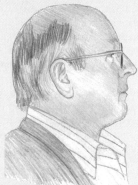

Frederic A. Berry, MD

ROUTINE POSTOPERATIVE SUCTIONING: A BAD IDEA

One of the major challenges for the anesthesiologist occurs at the end of the surgical procedure when it is time for the patient to recover their protective airway reflexes such as coughing and swallowing that were obliterated by general anesthesia. The question is, "How should these reflexes be activated without the patient developing laryngospasm?" Postoperative laryngospasm continues to be a major problem for the anesthesiologist. One report suggested that

1 in 1,000 patients develops negative-pressure pulmonary edema from laryngospasm at the end of surgery. One technique for assisting a patient in recovering protective reflexes is to allow him to spontaneously awaken fully from anesthesia before removing the endotracheal tube. However, this approach is in direct conflict with the practice of many anesthesiologists who routinely perform deep hypopharyngeal suctioning just before removing an endotracheal tube.

If deep hypopharyngeal suctioning is done while a patient is still anesthetized and paralyzed, it has no effect on airway reflexes. However, if it is done at the end of the anesthetized period as the patient is regaining protective airway reflexes, it may stimulate the patient and result in coughing, breathholding, or efforts at self-removal of the tube. While these events may suggest that the patient is sufficiently recovered from anesthesia to permit endotracheal extubation, there are case reports of severe laryngospasm with negative-pressure pulmonary edema following this scenario. Every year at the University of Virginia Health System there are 4 or 5 cases of negative-pressure pulmonary edema subsequent to laryngospasm. Most cases occur in young, healthy pa-

■ MANAGEMENT OF COMPLICATIONS

RESPIRATORY COMPLICATIONS

Respiratory problems are the most frequently encountered serious complications in the PACU. The overwhelming majority are related to airway obstruction, hypoventilation, or hypoxemia. Because hypoxemia is the final common pathway to serious morbidity and mortality, routine monitoring of pulse oximetry in the PACU leads to earlier recognition of these complications and fewer adverse outcomes.

Airway Obstruction

Airway obstruction in unconscious patients is most commonly due to the tongue falling back against the posterior pharynx (see Chapter 5). Other causes include

laryngospasm; glottic edema; secretions, vomitus, or blood in the airway; or external pressure on the trachea (most commonly from a neck hematoma). Partial airway obstruction usually presents as sonorous respiration. Total obstruction causes cessation of airflow, an absence of breath sounds, and marked paradoxic (rocking) movement of the chest. The abdomen and chest should normally rise together during inspiration; however, with airway obstruction, the chest descends as the abdomen rises during each inspiration (paradoxic chest movement). Patients with airway obstruction should receive supplemental oxygen while corrective measures are undertaken. A combined jaw-thrust and head-tilt maneuver pulls the tongue forward and opens the airway. Insertion of an oral or nasal airway also often alleviates the problem. Nasal airways may be better tolerated than oral airways by patients during emergence and lessen the likelihood of trauma to the teeth when the patient bites down.

If the above maneuvers fail, laryngospasm should be considered. Laryngospasm is usually characterized by tients in their second or third decade of life. Larson has described a very effective technique for treating the laryngospasm that occurs at the time of extubation.[1] However, it is still better to avoid laryngospasm, rather than having to treat it.

THE SPONTANEOUS AWAKENING FROM ANESTHESIA

What are the options during emergence from anesthesia if the patient has bloody secretions or saliva in the hypopharynx? There are two ways to manage this. One is to perform suctioning while the patient is still anesthetized and not reactive. The second is to ignore the secretions or blood and place the patient in the lateral position at the end of surgery, allowing gravity to remove the secretions. The secret to peaceful awakening is to avoid stimulating the patient. I administer lidocaine, 1.5 mg/kg, intravenously just before the patient is moved from the operating table to the stretcher to go to the postanesthesia care unit (PACU). If necessary, this dose can be repeated one time in a 5-minute period. Sometimes the patient stirs, coughs, moves, and reaches toward the endotracheal tube. This creates a difficult quandary for the anesthesiologist. It is accepted practice to infer that when a patient has purposeful movements he is sufficiently recovered from anesthesia to maintain his airway. At times it is very difficult to tell exactly when that point has arrived. If a patient opens her eyes, follows command, and reaches for the endotracheal tube, these are thought to be sound indicators of appropriateness for extubation. However, if the PACU nurse suctions the hypopharynx while the patient is spontaneously recovering from anesthesia, the patient may give the appearance of arousal, suggesting that extubation is needed. However, doing so may be inappropriate. In this setting, laryngospasm followed by pulmonary edema and hemorrhage has been reported.[2]

Because much of the recovery process takes place in the PACU, it is important that the PACU nurses be aware of the technique of spontaneous awakening from anesthesia. Without undergoing oropharyngeal suctioning, the patient is kept on her side until awake enough to pull out her own tube. Using this technique, I have never seen a patient develop postoperative laryngospasm that was not easily managed with mild airway maneuvers.

1. Dolinski SY, MacGregor DA, Scuderi PE:Pulmonary hemorrhage associated with negative-pressure pulmonary edema. Anesthesiology 2000;93:888.
2. Larson CP Jr.:Laryngospasm—the best treatment. Anesthesiology 1998;89:1293.

high-pitched crowing noises but may be silent, with complete glottic closure. Spasm of the vocal cords is more apt to occur following airway trauma, or repeated instrumentation, or stimulation from secretions or blood in the airway. The jaw-thrust maneuver, especially when combined with gentle positive airway pressure via a tight-fitting face mask, usually breaks laryngospasm. Insertion of an oral or nasal airway is also helpful in ensuring a patent airway down to the level of the vocal cords. Any secretions or blood in the hypopharynx should be suctioned to prevent recurrence. Refractory laryngospasm should be treated aggressively with a small dose of succinylcholine (10–20 mg) and temporary positive pressure ventilation with 100% oxygen to prevent severe hypoxemia or negative pressure pulmonary edema. Endotracheal intubation may occasionally be necessary to reestablish ventilation; cricothyrotomy or transtracheal jet ventilation is indicated if intubation is unsuccessful in such instances.

Glottic edema following airway instrumentation is an important cause of airway obstruction in infants and young children. Intravenous corticosteroids (dexamethasone, 0.5 mg/kg) or aerosolized racemic epinephrine (0.5 mL of a 2.25% solution with 3 mL of normal saline) may be useful in such cases. Postoperative wound hematomas following head and neck, thyroid, and carotid procedures can quickly compromise the airway; opening the wound immediately relieves tracheal compression. Rarely, gauze packing may be unintentionally left in the hypopharynx following oral surgery and can cause immediate or delayed complete airway obstruction.

Hypoventilation

Hypoventilation, which is generally defined as a $PaCO_2$ greater than 45 mm Hg, is a common occurrence following general anesthesia. In most instances, the hypoventilation is mild, and many cases are overlooked. Significant hypoventilation is usually only clinically apparent when the $PaCO_2$ is greater than 60 mm Hg or arterial blood pH is less than 7.25. Signs are varied and

Table 49–1. Postanesthetic Aldrete recovery score.[1] (Ideally, the patient should be discharged when the total score is 10 but a minimum of 9 is required)

Original Criteria	Modified Criteria	Point Value
Color	**Oxygenation**	
Pink	$SpO_2 > 92\%$ on room air	2
Pale or dusky	$SpO_2 > 90\%$ on oxygen	1
Cyanotic	$SpO_2 < 90\%$ on oxygen	0
Respiration		
Can breathe deeply and cough	Breathes deeply and coughs freely	2
Shallow but adequate exchange	Dyspneic, shallow or limited breathing	1
Apnea or obstruction	Apnea	0
Circulation		
Blood pressure within 20% of normal	Blood pressure $\pm$ 20 mm Hg of normal	2
Blood pressure within 20–50% of normal	Blood pressure $\pm$ 20–50 mm Hg of normal	1
Blood pressure deviating > 50% from normal	Blood pressure more than $\pm$ 50 mm Hg of normal	0
Consciousness		
Awake, alert, and oriented	Fully awake	2
Arousable but readily drifts back to sleep	Arousable on calling	1
No response	Not responsive	0
Activity		
Moves all extremities	Same	2
Moves two extremities	Same	1
No movement	Same	0

[1]Based on Aldrete JA, Kronlik D: A postanesthetic recovery score. Anesth Analg 1970;49:924 and Aldrete JA: The post-anesthesia recovery score revisited. J Clin Anesth 1995;7:89.

include excessive or prolonged somnolence, airway obstruction, slow respiratory rate, tachypnea with shallow breathing, or labored breathing. Mild to moderate respiratory acidosis causes tachycardia and hypertension or cardiac irritability (via sympathetic stimulation), but a more severe acidosis produces circulatory depression (see Chapter 30). If significant hypoventilation is suspected, arterial blood gas measurements should be obtained to assess its severity and guide further management.

Hypoventilation in the PACU is most commonly due to the residual depressant effects of anesthetic agents on respiratory drive. Opioid-induced respiratory depression characteristically produces a slow respiratory rate, often with large tidal volumes. Excessive sedation is also often present, but the patient may be responsive and able to increase breathing on command. Biphasic or recurring patterns of respiratory depression have been reported with all opioids. Proposed mechanisms include variations in the intensity of stimulation during recovery and delayed release of the opioid from peripheral compartments such as skeletal muscle (or possibly the lungs with fentanyl) as the patient rewarms or begins to move. Secretion of intravenously administered opioids into gastric fluid followed by reabsorption has also been described but appears to be an unlikely explanation because of high hepatic extraction for most opioids.

Inadequate reversal, overdose, hypothermia, pharmacologic interactions (such as with "mycin" antibiotics or magnesium therapy), altered pharmacokinetics (due to hypothermia, altered volumes of distribution, renal or hepatic dysfunction), or metabolic factors (such as hypokalemia or respiratory acidosis) can be responsible for residual muscle paralysis in the PACU. Regardless of the cause, discoordinated breathing movements with shallow tidal volumes and tachypnea are usually apparent. The diagnosis can be made with a nerve stimulator in unconscious patients; awake patients can be asked to lift their head. The ability to sustain a head-lift for 5 seconds may be the most sensitive test for assessing the adequacy of reversal.

Splinting due to incisional pain and diaphragmatic dysfunction following upper abdominal or thoracic surgery, abdominal distention, or tight abdominal dressings are other factors that can contribute to hypoventilation. Increased CO_2 production from shivering, hyperthermia, or sepsis can also increase $PaCO_2$

even in normal patients recovering from general anesthesia. Marked hypoventilation and respiratory acidosis can result when these factors are superimposed on an impaired ventilatory reserve due to underlying pulmonary, neuromuscular, or neurologic disease.

TREATMENT:

Treatment should generally be directed at the underlying cause, but marked hypoventilation always requires controlled ventilation until contributory factors are identified and corrected. Obtundation, circulatory depression, or severe acidosis (arterial blood pH < 7.15) are indications for immediate endotracheal intubation. Antagonism of opioid-induced depression with naloxone is a two-edged sword; the abrupt increase in alveolar ventilation is usually also associated with sudden pain and sympathetic discharge. The latter can precipitate a hypertensive crisis, pulmonary edema, and myocardial ischemia or infarction. If naloxone is used to increase respiration, titration with small increments (0.04 mg in adults) may avoid complications by allowing partial reversal of the respiratory depression without significant reversal of the analgesia. Following naloxone, patients should be watched carefully for recurrence of the opioid-induced respiratory depression (renarcotization), since naloxone has a shorter duration than most opioids. Alternatively, doxapram, 60–100 mg, followed by 1–2 mg/min intravenously, may be used; doxapram does not reverse the analgesia, but can cause hypertension and tachycardia. If residual muscle paralysis is present, additional cholinesterase inhibitor may be given. Residual paralysis in spite of a full dose of a cholinesterase inhibitor necessitates controlled ventilation until spontaneous recovery occurs. Judicious opioid analgesia (intravenous or intraspinal), epidural anesthesia, or intercostal nerve blocks are often beneficial in alleviating splinting following upper abdominal or thoracic procedures.

Hypoxemia

Mild hypoxemia is common in patients recovering from anesthesia unless supplemental oxygen is given during emergence. Mild to moderate hypoxemia (PaO_2 50–60 mm Hg) in young healthy patients may be well tolerated initially, but with increasing duration or severity the initial sympathetic stimulation often seen is replaced with progressive acidosis and circulatory depression. Obvious cyanosis may be absent if the hemoglobin concentration is reduced. Clinically, hypoxemia may also be suspected from restlessness, tachycardia, or cardiac irritability (ventricular or atrial). Obtundation, bradycardia, hypotension, and cardiac arrest are late signs. The routine use of a pulse oximeter in the PACU

facilitates early detection. Arterial blood gas measurements should be performed to confirm the diagnosis and guide therapy.

Hypoxemia in the PACU is usually caused by hypoventilation, increased right-to-left intrapulmonary shunting, or both. A decrease in cardiac output or an increase in oxygen consumption (as with shivering) will accentuate the hypoxemia. Diffusion hypoxia (see Chapter 7) is an uncommon cause of hypoxemia when recovering patients are given supplemental oxygen. Hypoxemia due to pure hypoventilation is also unusual in patients receiving supplemental oxygen unless marked hypercapnia or a concomitant increase in intrapulmonary shunting is present. Increased intrapulmonary shunting from a decreased functional residual capacity (FRC) relative to closing capacity is the most common cause of hypoxemia following general anesthesia. The greatest reductions in FRC occur following upper abdominal and thoracic surgery. The loss of lung volume is often attributed to microatelectasis, since visible atelectasis is often not evident on a chest film. A semi-upright position helps maintain FRC.

Marked right-to-left intrapulmonary shunting ($\dot{Q}_s/\dot{Q}_t > 15\%$) is usually associated with radiographically discernible findings such as pulmonary atelectasis, parenchymal infiltrates, or a large pneumothorax. Causes include prolonged intraoperative hypoventilation with low tidal volumes, unintentional endobronchial intubation, lobar collapse from bronchial obstruction by secretions or blood, pulmonary aspiration, or pulmonary edema. Postoperative pulmonary edema most often presents as wheezing within the first 60 minutes after surgery; it may be due to left ventricular failure (cardiogenic), the acute respiratory distress syndrome (ARDS), or the sudden relief of prolonged airway obstruction. In contrast to that associated with pulmonary edema, wheezing due to primary obstructive lung disease, which also often results in large increases in intrapulmonary shunting, is not associated with auscultatory crackles, edema fluid in the airway, or infiltrates on the chest film. The possibility of a postoperative pneumothorax should always be considered following central line placement, intercostal blocks, rib fractures, neck dissections, tracheostomy, nephrectomies, or other retroperitoneal or intra-abdominal procedures (including laparoscopy) especially when the diaphragm might be penetrated. Patients with subpleural blebs or large bullae can also develop pneumothorax during positive pressure ventilation.

TREATMENT:

Oxygen therapy with or without positive airway pressure is the cornerstone of treatment. Routine administration of 30–60% oxygen is usually enough to prevent hypoxemia with even moderate hypoventilation and hypercapnia. Patients with underlying pulmonary or cardiac disease may require higher concentrations of oxygen; oxygen therapy should be guided by SpO_2 or arterial blood gas measurements. Oxygen concentration must be closely controlled in patients with chronic CO_2 retention to avoid precipitating acute respiratory failure. Patients with severe or persistent hypoxemia should be given 100% oxygen via a nonrebreathing mask or an endotracheal tube until the cause is established and other therapies are instituted; controlled or assisted mechanical ventilation may also be necessary. The chest film (preferably an upright film) is invaluable in assessing lung volume and heart size and demonstrating a pneumothorax or pulmonary infiltrates. Infiltrates may initially be absent immediately following aspiration.

Additional treatment should be directed at the underlying cause. A chest tube should be inserted for any symptomatic pneumothorax or one that is greater than 15–20%. Bronchospasm should be treated with aerosolized bronchodilators and perhaps intravenous aminophylline. Diuretics should be given for circulatory fluid overload. Cardiac function should be optimized. Persistent hypoxemia in spite of 50% oxygen generally is an indication for positive end-expiratory pressure (PEEP) or CPAP. Bronchoscopy is often useful in reexpanding lobar atelectasis caused by bronchial plugs or particulate aspiration.

CIRCULATORY COMPLICATIONS

The most common circulatory disturbances in the PACU are hypotension, hypertension, and arrhythmias. The possibility that the circulatory abnormality is secondary to an underlying respiratory disturbance should always be considered before any other intervention.

Hypotension

Hypotension is usually due to decreased venous return to the heart, left ventricular dysfunction, or less commonly excessive arterial vasodilation. Hypovolemia is by far the most common cause of hypotension in the PACU. Absolute hypovolemia can result from inadequate intraoperative fluid replacement, continuing fluid sequestration by tissues ("third-spacing") or wound drainage, or postoperative bleeding. Venoconstriction during hypothermia may mask the hypovolemia until the patient's temperature begins to rise again; subsequent venodilatation results in delayed hypotension. Relative hypovolemia is responsible for the hypotension associated with spinal

or epidural anesthesia, venodilators, and α-adrenergic blockade; the increase in venous capacitance reduces venous return in spite of a previously normal intravascular volume in such instances. Hypotension associated with sepsis and allergic reactions is usually the result of both hypovolemia and vasodilatation. Hypotension following a tension pneumothorax or cardiac tamponade is the result of impaired cardiac filling.

Left ventricular dysfunction in previously healthy persons is unusual unless it is associated with severe metabolic disturbances (hypoxemia, acidosis, or sepsis). Hypotension due to ventricular dysfunction is primarily encountered in patients with underlying coronary artery or valvular heart disease, and is usually precipitated by fluid overload, myocardial ischemia, acute increases in afterload, or dysrhythmias.

TREATMENT:

Mild hypotension during recovery from anesthesia is common and usually reflects the decrease in sympathetic tone normally associated with sleep or residual effects of anesthetic agents; it typically does not require treatment. Significant hypotension is usually defined as a 20–30% reduction of blood pressure below the patient's baseline level and indicates a serious derangement requiring treatment. Treatment depends on the ability to assess intravascular volume. An increase in blood pressure following a fluid bolus (250–500 mL crystalloid or 100–250 mL colloid) generally confirms hypovolemia. With severe hypotension, a vasopressor or inotrope (dopamine or epinephrine) may be necessary to increase arterial blood pressure until the intravascular volume deficit is at least partially corrected. Signs of cardiac dysfunction should be sought in elderly patients and patients with known heart disease. Failure of a patient to promptly respond to treatment mandates invasive hemodynamic monitoring; manipulations of cardiac preload, contractility, and afterload are often necessary. The presence of a tension pneumothorax, as suggested by hypotension with unilaterally decreased breath sounds, hyperresonance, and tracheal deviation, is an indication for immediate pleural aspiration even before radiographic confirmation. Similarly, hypotension due to cardiac tamponade, usually following chest trauma or thoracic surgery, often necessitates immediate pericardiocentesis or thoracotomy.

Hypertension

Postoperative hypertension is common in the PACU and typically occurs within the first 30 minutes after admission. Noxious stimulation from incisional pain, endotracheal intubation, or bladder distention is usually responsible. Postoperative hypertension may also reflect sympathetic activation, which may be part of the neuroendocrine response to surgery or secondary to hypoxemia, hypercapnia, or metabolic acidosis. Patients with a history of systemic hypertension are likely to develop hypertension in the PACU even in the absence of an identifiable cause. The degree of preoperative control over blood pressure bears an inverse relationship to the incidence of postoperative hypertension in such patients. Fluid overload or intracranial hypertension can also occasionally present as postoperative hypertension.

TREATMENT:

Mild hypertension generally does not require treatment, but a reversible cause should be sought. Marked hypertension can precipitate postoperative bleeding, myocardial ischemia, heart failure, or intracranial hemorrhage. The decision about what degree of hypertension should be treated must be individualized. In general, blood pressure elevations greater than 20–30% of the patient's normal baseline or those associated with adverse effects (such as myocardial ischemia, heart failure, or bleeding) should be treated. Mild to moderate elevations can be treated with an intravenous β-adrenergic blocker such as labetalol, esmolol, or propranolol; calcium channel blocker nicardipine; or nitroglycerin paste. Sublingual nifedipine and hydralazine are also effective but frequently causes reflex tachycardia and have been associated with myocardial ischemia and infarction. Marked hypertension in patients with limited cardiac reserve requires direct intra-arterial pressure monitoring and should be treated with an intravenous infusion of nitroprusside, nitroglycerin, nicardipine, or fenoldopam. The end point for treatment should be consistent with the patient's own normal blood pressure.

Arrhythmias

The role of respiratory disturbances, especially hypoxemia, hypercarbia, and acidosis, in promoting cardiac arrhythmias cannot be overemphasized. Residual effects from anesthetic agents, increased sympathetic nervous system activity, other metabolic abnormalities, and preexisting cardiac or pulmonary disease also predispose patients to arrhythmias in the PACU.

Bradycardia often represents the residual effects of a cholinesterase inhibitor (neostigmine), a potent synthetic opioid (sufentanil), or β-adrenergic blockers (propranolol). Tachycardia may represent the effect of an anticholinergic agent (atropine), a vagolytic drug (pancuronium or meperidine), a β-agonist (albuterol), reflex tachycardia (hydralazine), in addition to more common causes such as pain, fever, hypovolemia, and anemia. Moreover, anesthetic-induced depression of

baroreceptor function makes heart rate an unreliable monitor of intravascular volume in the PACU.

Premature atrial and ventricular beats usually represent hypokalemia, hypomagnesemia, increased sympathetic tone, or less commonly, myocardial ischemia. The latter can be diagnosed with a 12-lead ECG. Supraventricular tachyarrhythmias including paroxysmal supraventricular tachycardia, atrial flutter, and atrial fibrillation are typically encountered in patients with a history of these arrhythmias, and are more commonly encountered following thoracic surgery. The management of arrhythmias is discussed in Chapters 19 and 48.

CASE DISCUSSION: FEVER & TACHYCARDIA IN A YOUNG ADULT MALE

A 19-year-old man sustains a closed fracture of the femur in a motor vehicle accident. He is placed in traction for 3 days prior to surgery. During that time, a persistent low-grade fever (37.5–38.7 °C orally), mild hypertension (150–170/70–90 mm Hg), and tachycardia (100–126 beats/min) are noted. His hematocrit remains between 30% and 32.5%. Broad-spectrum antibiotic coverage is initiated. He is scheduled for open reduction and internal fixation of the fracture. When the patient is brought into the operating room, vital signs are as follows: blood pressure 162/95 mm Hg, pulse 150 beats/min, respirations 20 breaths/min, and oral temperature 38.1 °C. He is sweating and appears anxious in spite of intramuscular premedication with meperidine, 75 mg, and promethazine, 25 mg. On close examination, he is noted to have a slightly enlarged thyroid gland.

Should the surgical team proceed with the operation?

The proposed operation is elective; therefore, significant abnormalities should be diagnosed and properly treated preoperatively, if possible, to make the patient optimally ready for surgery. If the patient had an open fracture, the risk of infection would clearly mandate immediate operation. Even with a closed femoral fracture, needless cancellations or delays should be avoided because nonoperative treatment entails the risks of prolonged bed rest (with traction), including atelectasis, pneumonia, deep venous thrombosis, and potentially lethal pulmonary thromboembolism. In deciding whether to proceed with the surgery, the anesthesiologist must ask the following questions:

(1) *What are the most likely causes of the abnormalities based on the clinical presentation?*

(2) *What, if any, additional investigations or consultations might be helpful?*

(3) *How would these or other commonly associated abnormalities affect anesthetic management?*

(4) *Are the potential anesthetic interactions serious enough to delay surgery until a suspected cause is conclusively excluded? The tachycardia of 150 beats/min and the low-grade fever therefore require further evaluation prior to surgery.*

What are the likely causes of the tachycardia and fever in this patient?

These two abnormalities may reflect one process or separate entities (Tables 49–2 and 49–3). Moreover, although multiple factors can often be simultaneously identified, their relative contribution is usually not readily apparent. Fever commonly follows major trauma; contributory factors can include the inflammatory reaction to the tissue trauma, superimposed infection (most

Table 49–2. Perioperative causes of tachycardia.

Anxiety
Pain
Fever (see Table 49–3)
Respiratory
  Hypoxemia
  Hypercapnia
Circulatory
  Hypotension
  Anemia
  Hypovolemia
  Congestive heart failure
  Cardiac tamponade
  Tension pneumothorax
  Thromboembolism
Drug-induced
  Antimuscarinic agents
  β-Adrenergic agonists
  Vasodilators
  Allergy
  Drug withdrawal
Metabolic disorders
  Hypoglycemia
  Thyrotoxicosis
  Pheochromocytoma
  Adrenal (addisonian) crisis
  Carcinoid syndrome
  Acute porphyria

Table 49–3. Perioperative causes of fever.

Infections
Immunologically mediated processes
  Drug reactions
  Blood reactions
  Tissue destruction (rejection)
  Connective tissue disorders
  Granulomatous disorders
Tissue damage
  Trauma
  Infarction
  Thrombosis
Neoplastic disorders
Metabolic disorders
  Thyroid storm (thyroid crisis)
  Adrenal (addisonian) crisis
  Pheochromocytoma
  Malignant hyperthermia
  Neuroleptic malignant syndrome
  Acute gout
  Acute porphyria

commonly wound, pulmonary, or urinary), antibiotic therapy (drug reaction), or thrombophlebitis. Infection must be seriously considered in this patient because of the risk of bacteria seeding and infecting the metal fixation device placed during surgery. Although tachycardia is commonly associated with a low-grade fever, it is usually not of this magnitude in a 19-year-old patient. Moderate to severe pain, anxiety, hypovolemia, or anemia may be other contributory factors. Pulmonary fat embolism should also be considered in any patient with long bone fracture, especially when hypoxemia, tachypnea, or mental status changes are present. Lastly, the possibly enlarged thyroid gland, sweating, and anxious appearance together with both fever and tachycardia suggest thyrotoxicosis.

What (if any) additional measures may be helpful in evaluating the fever and tachycardia?

Arterial blood gas measurements and a chest film would be helpful in excluding fat embolism. A repeat hematocrit or hemoglobin concentration measurement would exclude worsening anemia; significant tachycardia may be expected when the hematocrit is below 25–27% (hemoglobin < 8 g/dL) in most patients. The response to an intravenous fluid challenge with 250–500 mL of a colloid solution may be helpful; a decrease in heart rate after the fluid bolus is strongly suggestive of hypovolemia. Similarly, response of the heart rate to sedation and additional opioid analgesia can be helpful in excluding anxiety and pain, respectively, as causes. Although a tentative diagnosis of hyperthyroidism can be made based on clinical grounds, confirmation requires measurement of serum thyroid hormones; the latter usually requires 24–48 hours in most hospitals. Signs of infection—such as increased inflammation or purulence in a wound, purulent sputum, an infiltrate on the chest film, pyuria, or leukocytosis with premature white cells on a blood smear (shift to the left)—should prompt cultures and a delay of surgery until the results are obtained and correct antibiotic coverage is confirmed.

The patient is transferred to the PACU for further evaluation. A 12-lead ECG confirms sinus tachycardia of 150 beats/min. A chest film is normal. Arterial blood gas measurements on room air are normal (pH 7.44, $PaCO_2$ 41 mm Hg, PaO_2 87 mm Hg, HCO_3^- 27 mEq/L). The hemoglobin concentration is found to be 11 g/dL. Blood for thyroid function tests is sent to the laboratory. The patient is sedated intravenously with midazolam, 2 mg, and fentanyl, 50 mg, and is given 500 mL of 5% albumin. He appears relaxed and pain-free, but the heart rate decreases only to 144 beats/min. The decision is made to proceed with surgery using continuous lumbar epidural anesthesia with 2% lidocaine. Esmolol, 100 mg, is administered slowly until his pulse decreases to 120 beats/min, and a continuous esmolol infusion is administered at a rate of 300 µg/kg/hour.

The procedure is completed in 3½ hours. Although the patient did not complain of any pain during the procedure and was given only minimal additional sedation (midazolam, 2 mg), he is delirious upon admission to the PACU. The esmolol infusion is proceeding at a rate of 500 µg/kg/min. He has also received propranolol, 24 mg intravenously. Estimated blood loss was 500 mL, and fluid replacement consisted of 2 units of packed red blood cells, 1000 mL of hetastarch, and 9000 mL of lactated Ringer's injection. Vital signs are as follows: blood pressure 105/40 mm Hg, pulse 124 beats/min, respirations 30 breaths/min, and rectal temperature 38.8 °C. Arterial blood gas measurements are reported as follows: pH 7.37, $PaCO_2$ 37 mm Hg, PaO_2 91 mm Hg, HCO_3^- 22 mEq/L.

What is the most likely diagnosis?

The patient is now obviously in a hypermetabolic state manifested by excessive adrenergic activity, fever, markedly increased fluid requirements, and a worsening mental status. The

absence of major metabolic acidosis and lack of exposure to a known triggering agent exclude malignant hyperthermia (see Chapter 44). Other possibilities include a transfusion reaction, sepsis, or an undiagnosed pheochromocytoma. The sequence of events makes the first two unlikely, while the decreasing prominence of hypertension (now replaced with relative hypotension) and increasing fever make the latter unlikely as well. The clinical presentation now strongly suggests thyroid storm.

Emergency consultation is obtained with an endocrinologist, who concurs with the diagnosis of thyroid storm. How is thyroid storm managed?

Thyroid storm (crisis) is a medical emergency that carries a 10–50% mortality rate. It is usually encountered in patients with poorly controlled or undiagnosed Graves disease. Precipitating factors include (1) the stress of surgery and anesthesia, (2) labor and delivery, (3) severe infection, and, rarely, (4) thyroiditis 1–2 weeks following radioactive iodine administration. Manifestations usually include mental status changes (irritability, delirium, or coma), fever, tachycardia, and hypotension. Both atrial and ventricular arrhythmias are common, especially atrial fibrillation. Congestive heart failure develops in 25% of patients. Hypertension that often precedes hypotension, heat intolerance with profuse sweating, nausea and vomiting, and diarrhea may be prominent initially. Hypokalemia is present in up to 50% of patients. Levels of thyroid hormones are high in plasma but correlate poorly with the severity of the crisis. The sudden exacerbation of thyrotoxicosis may represent a rapid shift of the hormone from the protein-bound to the free state or increased responsiveness to thyroid hormones at the cellular level.

Treatment is directed toward reversing the crisis as well as its complications. Large doses of corticosteroids (dexamethasone intravenously, 10 mg followed by 2 mg every 6 hours), inhibit the synthesis, release, and peripheral conversion of thyroxine (T_4) to triiodothyronine (T_3). Corticosteroids also prevent relative adrenal insufficiency secondary to the hypermetabolic state. Propylthiouracil, 200–400 mg, followed by 100 mg every 2 hours, is used to inhibit thyroid hormone synthesis. Although methimazole inhibits thyroid hormone production and has a longer half-life, propylthiouracil is preferred because it also inhibits peripheral conversion of T_4. Intravenous preparations are not available for either agent, so they must be administered orally or via nasogastric tube. Iodide is given to inhibit release of thyroid *hormones from the gland. The iodide may be given intravenously as sodium iodide, 1 g over 24 hours, or enterally as potassium iodide, 100–200 mg every 8 hours; the x-ray contrast agent sodium ipodate 1 g/d can alternatively be used. Propranolol not only antagonizes the peripheral effects of the thyrotoxicosis but may also inhibit peripheral conversion of T_4. Combined β_1- and β_2-blockade is preferable to selective β_1-antagonism (esmolol or metoprolol) because excessive β_2-receptor activity is responsible for the metabolic effects. β_2-Receptor blockade also reduces muscle blood flow and may decrease heat production. Supportive measures include surface cooling (cooling blanket), acetaminophen (aspirin is not recommended because it may displace thyroid hormone from plasma carrier proteins), and generous intravenous fluid replacement. Vasopressors are often necessary to support arterial blood pressure. Digoxin is indicated in patients with atrial fibrillation to control the ventricular rate (see Chapter 19) and those with congestive heart failure. A pulmonary artery catheter greatly facilitates management in patients with signs of congestive heart failure or persistent hypotension by allowing measurements of cardiac output and indices of ventricular filling pressures. β-Adrenergic blockade is contraindicated in patients with low cardiac output.*

Propranolol, dexamethasone, propylthiouracil, and sodium iodide are given; the patient is admitted to the ICU, where treatment is continued. Over the next 3 days, his mental status markedly improves. The T_3 and total thyroxine levels on the day of surgery were both elevated to 250 ng/dL and 18.5 mg/dL, respectively. He was discharged home 6 days later on a regimen of propranolol and propylthiouracil with a blood pressure of 124/80 mm Hg, a pulse of 92 beats/min, and an oral temperature of 37.3 °C.

SUGGESTED READING

Aldrete JA: The post-anesthesia recovery score revisited. J Clin Anesth 1995;7:89.

Cohen MM, O'Brian-Pallas LL, Copplestone C, et al: Nursing work load associated with adverse events in the postanesthesia care unit. Anesthesiology 1999;91:1882.

Chung F: Recovery pattern and home readiness after ambulatory surgery. Anesth Analg 1996:896.

Dexter F, Tinker JH: Analysis of strategies to decrease postanesthesia care costs. Anesthesiology 1995;82:941.

Hines R, Barash PG, Watrous G, O'Connor T: Complications occurring in the postanesthesia care unit: A survey. Anesth Analg 1992;74:503.

Kovac AL: Prevention and treatment of postoperative nausea and vomiting. Drugs 2000;59:213.

Marshall SI, Chung F: Discharge criteria and complications after ambulatory surgery. Anesth Analg 1999;88:508.

Pavlin DJ, Rapp SE, Polissar NL, et al: Factors affecting discharge times in adult outpatients. Anesth Analg 1998;87:816.

Rose DK, Cohen MM, DeBoer DP: Cardiovascular events in the postanesthesia care unit: Contribution of risk factors. Anesthesiology 1996;84:772.

Critical Care

KEY CONCEPTS

Brain death criteria can only be applied in the absence of hypothermia, hypotension, metabolic or endocrine abnormalities, neuromuscular blockade, or drugs known to depress brain function.

In contrast to pulmonary toxicity, retrolental fibroplasia correlates better with arterial than with alveolar O_2 tension.

The principal advantages of pressure support ventilation are its ability to augment spontaneous tidal volume (VT), decrease the work of breathing, and increase patient comfort.

The disadvantage of pressure control ventilation is that VT is not guaranteed.

Compared with oral intubation, nasal intubation may be more comfortable for the patient, more secure (fewer instances of accidental extubation), and less likely to cause laryngeal damage. Nasal intubation, however, can result in significant nasal bleeding, transient bacteremia, submucosal dissection of the nasopharynx or oropharynx, and sinusitis or otitis media (from obstruction of the auditory tubes).

When left in place for more than 2 to 3 weeks, both oral and nasal translaryngeal endotracheal tubes predispose patients to subglottic stenosis.

A higher incidence of pulmonary barotrauma is observed when excessive positive end-expiratory or continuous positive airway pressure is added, especially at levels greater than 20 cm H_2O.

Maneuvers that produce sustained maximum lung inflation such as the use of an incentive spirometer can be helpful in inducing cough as well as preventing atelectasis and preserving normal lung volume.

Early elective endotracheal intubation is advisable when there are obvious signs of heat injury to the airway.

Continuous renal replacement therapy—continuous venovenous hemofiltration and continuous venovenous hemodialysis—is increasingly used in critically ill patients with acute renal failure.

Advanced age (> 70 years), corticosteroid therapy, chemotherapy, prolonged use of invasive devices, respiratory failure, renal failure, head trauma, and burns are established risk factors for nosocomial infections.

Systemic venodilation and transudation of fluid into tissues results in a relative hypovolemia in patients with sepsis.

In contrast to nonstressed patients, who require about 0.5 g/kg/d of protein, critically ill patients generally require 1.0–1.5 g/kg/d.

The gastrointestinal tract is the route of choice for nutritional support when its functional integrity is intact.

Abrupt withdrawal of total parenteral nutrition can precipitate hypoglycemia due to high circulating insulin levels, but this is not a common problem if the patient is not overfed; in these instances, 10% glucose can be temporarily used and gradually decreased.

Critical care medicine—also referred to as intensive care medicine—deals with potentially life-threatening illnesses. Anesthesiologists have played a major role in the development of this multidisciplinary subspecialty. Expertise in airway management, mechanical ventilation, administering potent fast-acting drugs, fluid resuscitation, and monitoring techniques gives the anesthesiologist the technical skills required. Moreover, the emphasis in anesthesia on physiology, pathophysiology, and pharmacology as well as the ability to make a rapid diagnosis and treat abrupt physiologic derangements provides an excellent foundation for dealing with critically ill patients. The critical care practitioner (intensivist) also requires a broad base of knowledge that crosses subspecialties in internal medicine, surgery, pediatrics, neurology, and emergency medicine. Unlike traditional training in these subspecialties, which tends to emphasize single organ systems, intensive care training also provides experience in treating patients with multiple organ dysfunction syndrome (MODS). The American Boards of Anesthesiology, Internal Medicine, Pediatrics, and Surgery recognize these requirements and now require specialized training for certification in critical care medicine. Clinicians who have such certification are increasingly recognized by multinational corporations and organizations as making important contributions to the outcomes of hospitalized patients.

The purpose of this chapter is only to provide a survey of critical care medicine. Many items have already been covered in other chapters. Only important topics not previously discussed will be presented.

■ ECONOMIC, ETHICAL, & LEGAL ISSUES IN CRITICAL CARE

COST

Critical care is very expensive. Intensive care unit (ICU) beds constitute only 8–10% of all beds in most hospitals yet account for over 20% of hospital expenditures. One percent of the U.S. gross national product is used to provide care in ICUs. To justify this cost, clear benefits in terms of reductions in morbidity or mortality should be readily demonstrable. Unfortunately, supporting studies are few and often flawed by the use of historical controls. Disease severity, reversibility, previous health status, and age are major determinants of outcome. A method of reliably predicting which patients benefit most from intensive care is needed. Several scoring systems based on the severity of physiologic derangements and preexisting health have been pro-

posed, such as the Acute Physiology and Chronic Health Evaluation (APACHE) and Therapeutic Intervention Scoring System (TISS), but none is entirely satisfactory. Survival is generally inversely related to the severity of illness and number of organ systems affected. The Society of Critical Care Medicine has recently established Project Impact, a system that allows ICUs to compare their outcomes and the care they provide against a national and international network of ICUs.

ETHICAL & LEGAL ISSUES

The high cost and economic constraints increasingly applied by governments and third-party payers, together with an increased awareness of ethical issues and legal precedents, have changed the practice of critical care medicine. Until recently, nearly all patients in the United States—even those who were clearly terminal—received maximal treatment (often contrary to the patient's or family's wishes) for fear of the possible legal repercussions of withholding treatment. "Heroic" measures such as cardiopulmonary resuscitation, mechanical ventilation, and vasoactive infusions were continued until the patient died.

Decisions about when to initiate or terminate treatment can be difficult. Generally, any treatment that can reasonably be expected to reverse illness or restore health is justified, while withholding that treatment requires specific ethical justification. Conversely, if treatment will definitely not reverse a disease process or restore health, then the decision to initiate such treatment may not be justified and may be unethical. These complex decisions must involve the patient (or guardian) and the family and must be consistent with hospital policies and state and federal law.

Fortunately, the legal guidelines that can be used by the practitioner in arriving at these decisions are available in nearly all states; although laws vary from state to state, they tend to be similar. The greatest problems are related to withholding treatment and discontinuing artificial life-support systems. Competent patients have the right to refuse treatment, and the right to have life-support machines or devices turned off when they so request. Most states allow competent individuals to prepare an advanced directive, usually either a "living will" or a "durable power of attorney for health care" to prevent needless prolongation of life if they become incompetent (eg, irreversible coma). Withholding treatment or discontinuing life support from **incompetent** minors and adults requires permission of the spouse, guardian, or next of kin; in some cases, clarification from the courts may be necessary. "Do not resuscitate" (DNR) or Allow Natural Death (AND) orders have been upheld by the courts in cases where resuscitation clearly offers no hope of curing or reversing the disease process responsible for imminent death.

Artificial support of respiration and the circulation complicates legal definitions of death. Until recently, most states required only a determination by a physician that irreversible cessation of respiratory and circulatory function had occurred. Nearly all states have added the concept of brain death to that definition.

Brain Death

Brain death is defined as irreversible cessation of all brain function. Spinal cord function below C1 may still be present. Establishing brain death gives relief from unjustifiable hope, prolonged anxiety, and financial burdens on families and society. It also allows more efficient utilization of medical resources and potentially allows the harvesting of organs for transplantation.

Brain death criteria can only be applied in the absence of hypothermia, hypotension, metabolic or endocrine abnormalities, neuromuscular blockade, or drugs known to depress brain function. A toxicology screen is necessary if sufficient time since admission (at least 3 days) has not elapsed to exclude a drug effect. Moreover, the patient should be observed long enough to establish with reasonable certainty the irreversible nature of the injury. Generally accepted clinical criteria for brain death include the following:

(1) Coma

(2) Absent motor activity, including decerebrate and decorticate posturing (spinal cord reflexes may be preserved in some patients)

(3) Absent brainstem reflexes, including the pupillary, corneal, vestibulo-ocular (caloric), and gag (and/or cough) reflexes

(4) Absence of respiratory effort with the arterial CO_2 tension 60 mm Hg or 20 mm Hg above the pretest level.

Repeating the examination (not less than 2 hours apart) is optional. The number of physician observers varies by state (Florida requires two), as does the level of expertise (Virginia requires a neurologist or neurosurgeon). The apnea test should be reserved for last because of its detrimental effects on intracranial pressure (ICP). Confirmatory tests that may be helpful but are not required include an isoelectric electroencephalogram, absent brainstem auditory evoked potentials, and absence of cerebral perfusion as documented by angiographic, transcranial Doppler, or radioisotopic studies.

■ RESPIRATORY CARE

Respiratory care (also called respiratory therapy) refers both to the delivery of pulmonary therapy and diagnostic tests and to the allied health profession that has evolved since the 1950s to become an integral part of cardiopulmonary diagnostics and critical care. Respiratory therapists' scope of practice encompasses medical gas therapy, airway management, mechanical ventilation, positive airway pressure therapy, and the application of various techniques collectively termed chest physical therapy. The latter includes administering aerosolized bronchodilators, clearing pulmonary secretions, reexpansion of atelectatic lung, and preserving normal lung function postoperatively or during illness. Diagnostic services may include pulmonary function testing, arterial blood gas analysis, electrocardiography testing, and evaluation of sleep disordered breathing.

MEDICAL GAS THERAPY

The therapeutic medical gases include supplemental ambient or hyperbaric oxygen, helium-oxygen mixtures, and nitric oxide. Oxygen is medically indicated for both pulmonary and nonpulmonary disorders. Oxygen is made available in high-pressure cylinders, via pipeline systems, from oxygen concentrators, as well as in liquid form. Heliox is occasionally used to treat the increased work of breathing (WOB) due to upper airway obstructing lesions. Nitric oxide is administered for its dilating effect on the pulmonary vasculature.

The primary goal of oxygen therapy is to prevent or correct hypoxemia and/or tissue hypoxia. Table 50–1 identifies classic categories of hypoxia. Oxygen therapy alone may not correct hypoxemia, hypoxia, or both. Continuous positive airway pressure (CPAP) or positive end-expiratory pressure (PEEP) may be required to recruit collapsed alveoli. Patients with profound hypercapnia may require ventilatory assistance. High concentrations of oxygen may be indicated for conditions requiring removal of entrapped gas (eg, nitrogen) from body cavities or vessels. The short-term application of high concentrations of oxygen is relatively free of complications.

Supplemental oxygen is indicated for adults, children, and infants (older than 1 month) when PaO_2 is less than 60 mm Hg (7.98 kPa) or SaO_2 or SpO_2 is less than 90% while at rest breathing room air. In neonates, therapy is recommended if PaO_2 is less than 50 mm Hg (6.7 kPa) or SaO_2 less than 88% (or capillary PCO_2 of less than 40 mm Hg [5.33 kPa]). Therapy may be re-

Table 50–1. Classification of hypoxias.

Hypoxia	Pathophysiologic Category	Clinical Example
Hypoxic hypoxia	$\downarrow P_{Barom}$ or $\downarrow FiO_2$ (< 0.21) Alveolar hypoventilation Pulmonary diffusion defect Pulmonary $\dot{V}/\dot{Q}$ mismatch $R \rightarrow L$ shunt	Altitude, O_2 equipment error Drug overdose, COPD exacerbation Emphysema, pulmonary fibrosis Asthma, pulmonary emboli Atelectasis, cyanotic congenital heart disease
Circulatory hypoxia	Reduced cardiac output	Congestive heart failure, myocardial infarction, dehydration
Hemic hypoxia	Reduced hemoglobin content Reduced hemoglobin function	Anemias Carboxyhemoglobinemia, methemoglobinemia
Demand hypoxia	$\uparrow$ Oxygen consumption	Fever, seizures
Histotoxic hypoxia	Inability of cells to utilize oxygen	Cyanide toxicity

P_{Barom} = barometric pressure, COPD = chronic obstructive pulmonary disease, $\dot{V}/\dot{Q}$ = ventilation/perfusion, $R \rightarrow L$ = right to left.

quired for patients when clinicians suspect hypoxia based on a review of cardiopulmonary problems or on physical examination. Patients with myocardial infarction, cardiogenic pulmonary edema, acute respiratory distress syndrome (ARDS), pulmonary fibrosis, cyanide poisoning, or carbon monoxide inhalation all require supplemental oxygen. Supplemental oxygen is given during the perioperative period because general anesthesia commonly causes a decrease in PaO_2 secondary to increased pulmonary ventilation/perfusion mismatching and decreased functional residual capacity (FRC). Supplemental oxygen should be provided before such procedures as tracheal suctioning or bronchoscopy, which commonly cause arterial desaturation. Lower than "normal" tensions may be acceptable for patients with chronic hypoxemia and CO_2 retention that may occur with exacerbations of chronic obstructive pulmonary disease (COPD).

AMBIENT OXYGEN THERAPY EQUIPMENT

Classifying Oxygen Therapy Equipment

Oxygen given alone or in a gas (mixed with air, helium or nitric oxide) can be administered as a partial supplement to patients' tidal or minute volume or as the entire source of the inspired volume. This approach provides the basis for classifying devices or systems according to their ability to provide adequate flow levels and a range of fraction of inspired oxygen (FiO_2). Other considerations in selecting therapy include patient compliance, the presence and type of artificial airway, and the need for humidification or an aerosol delivery system.

LOW-FLOW OR VARIABLE-PERFORMANCE EQUIPMENT:

Oxygen (usually 100%) is supplied at a fixed flow that is only a portion of inspired gas. Such devices are usually intended for patients with stable breathing patterns. As ventilatory demands change, variable amounts of room air will dilute the oxygen flow. Low-flow systems are adequate for patients with:

- Minute ventilation less than ~ 8 to 10 L/min
- Breathing frequencies less than ~ 20 breaths/mm
- Tidal volumes (V_T) less than ~ 0.8 L
- Normal inspiratory flow (10 to 30 L/min).

HIGH-FLOW OR FIXED-PERFORMANCE EQUIPMENT:

Inspired gas at a preset FiO_2 is supplied continuously at high flow or by providing a sufficiently large reservoir of premixed gas. Ideally, the delivered FiO_2 is not affected by variations in ventilatory level or breathing pattern. Profoundly dyspneic and hypoxemic patients may need flows of 100% oxygen in excess of 100 L/min. High-flow systems are indicated for patients who require:

- Consistent FiO_2 and/or
- Large inspiratory flows of gas (> 40 L/min).

1. Variable Performance Equipment (Table 50–2)

Nasal Cannulas

The nasal cannula is available as either a blind-ended soft plastic tube with an over-the-ear head-elastic or dual-flow with under-the-chin lariat adjustment. Sizing is available for adults, children, and infants. Cannulas

Table 50–2. Oxygen delivery devices and systems.

Device/System	Oxygen Flow Rate (L/min)	FiO₂ Range
Nasal cannula	1	0.21–0.24
	2	0.23–0.28
	3	0.27–0.34
	4	0.31–0.38
	5–6	0.32–0.44
Simple masks	5–6	0.30–0.45
	7–8	0.40–0.60
Masks with reservoirs	5	0.35–0.50
Partial rebreathing mask-bag	7	0.35–0.75
	15	0.65–1.00
Nonrebreathing mask-bag	7–15	0.40–1.00
Venturi masks and jet nebulizers	4–6 (total flow = 15)	0.24
	4–6 (total flow = 45)	0.28
	8–10 (total flow = 45)	0.35
	8–10 (total flow = 33)	0.40
	8–12 (total flow = 33)	0.50

are connected to flowmeters with small-bore tubing and may be used with a bubble humidifier. The nasal cannula can be rapidly and comfortably placed on most patients. The tension of attachment should be firm yet comfortable enough to avoid pressure sores on the ears, cheeks, and nose. Patients on long-term oxygen therapy most commonly use a nasal cannula. The appliance is usually well tolerated and allows speech and eating/drinking, and is non-claustrophobic. Cannulas can be combined with spectacle frames for convenience or to improve acceptance by improving cosmesis. Oxygen-conserving cannulas equipped with inlet reservoirs are available for patients receiving long-term oxygen. Since oxygen flows continuously, approximately 80% of the gas is wasted during expiration. This concept has resulted in the use of valved reservoir devices to allow storage of incoming oxygen until inspiration occurs.

The actual FiO₂ delivered to adults with nasal cannulas is determined by oxygen flow, nasopharyngeal volume, and the patient's inspiratory flow (which depends both on VT and inspiratory time). Oxygen from the cannula can fill the nasopharynx during exhalation, yet with inspiration, oxygen and entrained air is drawn into the trachea. The inspired percent oxygen increases by approximately 1–2% (above 21%) per liter of oxygen flow with quiet breathing in adults. Cannulas can be expected to provide inspired oxygen concentrations up to 30–35% with normal breathing and oxygen flows of 3–4 L/min. However, levels of 40–50% can be attained with oxygen flows of greater than 10 L/min for short periods. Usually flows greater than 5 L/min are poorly tolerated because of the discomfort of gas jetting into the nasal cavity and because of drying and crusting of the nasal mucosa.

Data from "normal breathing subjects" may not be accurate for acutely ill tachypneic patients. Increasing VT and short inspiratory time will dilute the small flow of oxygen. Different levels of mouth-only versus nasal-only breathing patterns and varied inspiratory flow can vary FiO₂ by up to 40%. In clinical practice, flow should be titrated according to vital signs and pulse oximetric and arterial blood gas measurements. Some patients with COPD tend to hypoventilate with even modest oxygen flows, yet are hypoxemic on room air. They may do well with the cannula at flows of less than 1 to 2 L/min.

Pediatric-sized nasal cannulas are available and their clinical use has become increasingly common. Some special cannulas allow babies to nurse and subject them to less trauma of the face and nose than do oxygen masks. Because of the inherently reduced minute ventilation of infants, flow requirements to the cannula must be proportionately reduced. This generally requires a pressure-compensated flowmeter accurate to deliver oxygen flows in the less than 1 to 3 L/min range. Hypopharyngeal oxygen sampling from infants breathing with cannulas has demonstrated mean FiO₂s of 0.35, 0.45, 0.6, and 0.68 with flows of 0.25, 0.5, 0.75, and 1.0 L/min, respectively.

Nasal Mask

The nasal mask is a hybrid of the nasal cannula and a face mask. It can be applied to the face either by over-the-ear lariat or headband strap. The lower edge of the mask's flanges rest on the upper lip, surrounding the external nose. Nasal masks have been shown to provide supplemental oxygen equivalent to the nasal cannula under low-flow conditions for adult patients. The primary advantage of the nasal mask appears to be patient comfort. Sores can develop around the external nares of long-term nasal cannula wearers. Oxygen is not "jetted" into the nasal cavity as with the cannula. The nasal mask should be considered if it improves patient comfort and compliance.

Nonreservoir Oxygen Mask

The "simple" or nonreservoir oxygen-free mask is a disposable lightweight plastic device that covers both nose and mouth. Masks are fastened to the patient's face by adjustment of an elastic headband; some manufacturers provide a malleable metal nose-bridge adjustment device. The face seal is rarely free of "inboard" leaking; therefore, patients receive a mixture of pure oxygen and secondarily entrained room air. This varies depending on size of leak, oxygen flow, and breathing pattern. Some brands of the simple mask connect tubing to a standard tapered fitting; others have a small room air-entrainment hole at the connection.

The body of the mask functions as a reservoir for both oxygen and expired carbon dioxide. A minimum oxygen flow of approximately 5 L/min is applied to the mask in order to avoid rebreathing and excessive respiratory work. Wearing any mask appliance for long periods of time is uncomfortable. Speech is muffled and drinking and eating are difficult.

The amount of oxygen enrichment of the inspired air depends on mask volume, pattern of ventilation, and the oxygen flow to the mask. It is difficult to predict delivered FIO_2 at specific flows. During normal breathing, it is reasonable to expect an FIO_2 of 0.3 to 0.6 with flows of 5 to 10 L/min, respectively. Oxygen levels can be higher with small V_T or slow breathing rates. With higher flows and ideal conditions, FIO_2 may approach 0.7 or 0.8.

The nonreservoir mask may be best suited for patients who require higher levels of oxygen than cannulas provide, yet need oxygen therapy for fairly short periods of time. Examples would include medical transport or interim therapy in the postanesthesia recovery or emergency room. It is not the device of choice for patients with severe respiratory disease who are profoundly hypoxemic, tachypneic, or are unable to protect their airway from aspiration.

Reservoir Masks

Incorporating some type of gas reservoir is a logical adaptation to the simple mask. Two types of reservoir mask are commonly used: the partial rebreathing mask and the nonrebreathing mask. Both are disposable, lightweight, transparent plastic under-the-chin reservoirs. The difference between the two relates to use of valves on the mask and between the mask and the bag reservoir. Mask reservoirs commonly hold approximately 600 mL or less. The term "partial rebreather" refers to "part" of the patient's expired V_T refilling the bag. Usually that gas is largely dead space that should not result in significant rebreathing of carbon dioxide.

The nonrebreather uses the same basic system as the partial rebreather but incorporates flap-type valves between the bag and mask and on at least one of the mask's exhalation ports. Inboard leaking is common, and room air will enter during brisk inspiratory flows,

even when the bag contains gas. The lack of a good facial seal system and a relatively small reservoir, can affect delivered oxygen concentration. The key factor to successful application of the masks is to use sufficient flow of oxygen, so the reservoir bag is at least partially full during inspiration. Typical minimum flows of oxygen are 10 to 15 L/min. Well-fitting partial rebreathing masks provide a range of FIO_2 from 0.35 to 0.60 with oxygen flows up to 10 L/min. With inlet flows of 15 or more and ideal breathing conditions, FIO_2 may approach 1.0. Either style of mask is indicated for patients suspected of significant hypoxemia, with relatively normal spontaneous minute ventilation. Such patients may include victims of trauma, myocardial infarction, or carbon monoxide exposure. Profoundly dyspneic patients with gasping respiration may be better suited with a fixed-performance, high-flow, oxygen system.

2. Fixed Performance (High-Flow) Equipment

Anesthesia Bag or Bag-Mask-Valve Systems

The basic design follows that of the nonrebreathing reservoir mask but with more "capable" components. Self-inflating bags consist of a football-sized bladder, usually with oxygen inlet reservoir. Anesthesia bags are 1-, 2-, or 3-L nonself-inflating reservoirs with a tail-piece gas inlet. Masks (see Figure 5–6) are designed to provide a comfortable leak-free seal for manual ventilation. The inspiratory/expiratory valve systems may vary. The flow to the reservoir should be kept high so that the bags do not deflate substantially. When using an anesthesia bag, operators may have to frequently adjust the oxygen flow and exhaust valve spring tension to respond to changing breathing patterns or demands.

The most common system for disposable and permanent self-inflating resuscitation bags uses a unidirectional gas flow. Although these devices offer the potential for a constant FIO_2, it may not occur in all clinical situations. If these situations are not recognized, clinicians might be misled into thinking the patient is receiving a specific concentration of oxygen when the contrary is true. There are limits to the ability of each system to maintain its fixed-performance characteristics. Delivered FIO_2 can equal or approach 1.0 with either anesthesia or self-inflating bag. Spontaneously breathing patients are allowed to breathe only the contents of the system if the mask seal is tight and reservoir adequately maintained. Operators must adjust gas flow to the bag to accommodate for any changes in ventilation demand; observation of patient and reservoir provides that information.

A primary concern for clinicians using mask-bag systems is aspiration. Failure to maintain an adequate oxygen supply in the reservoir and inlet flow is another concern. Adjustment of the spring-loaded valve of anesthesia bags must be done properly to prevent overdistention of the bag. Self-inflating bags do not look different when oxygen flow to the unit is inadequate and they will entrain room air into the bag, thus lowering the delivered FIO_2.

Air-Entrainment Venturi Masks

The gas delivery approach with air-entrainment masks is somewhat different than with an oxygen reservoir. The goal is to create an open-system with high flow about the nose and mouth, with a fixed FIO_2. Masks are known as "Venturi" or "Venti-" masks, or high airflow with oxygen-entrainment (HAFOE) systems. Oxygen is directed by small-bore tubing to a mixing-jet; the final oxygen concentration depends on the ratio of air drawn-in through entrainment ports. Manufacturers have developed both fixed and adjustable entrainment selections over an FIO_2 range. Most provide instructions for the operator to set a minimum flow of oxygen. Table 50–3 identifies total flow at various inlet flows and FIO_2.

Despite the high-flow concept, FIO_2 can vary up to 6% per setting. The air-entrainment masks are a logical choice for patients whose hypoxemia cannot be controlled on lower FIO_2 devices such as the cannula. Patients with COPD who tend to hypoventilate with a moderate FIO_2 are candidates for the Venturi mask. Clinicians providing oxygen therapy by HAFOE therapy should be aware of the previously mentioned problems involving the mask itself. FIO_2 can increase if the entrainment ports are obstructed by the patient's hands, bed sheets, or water condensate. Clinicians

should encourage the patient and caregivers to keep the mask on the face continuously. Interruption of oxygen is a serious problem in unstable patients with hypoxemia and or hypercarbia.

Direct analysis of the FIO_2 during air-entrainment mask breathing is possible but difficult to perform accurately. Correlating blood gases with some index of inspiratory flow demand, such as breathing rate, should allow clinicians to know when to suspect that the patient's demands may not be met by the mask's flow. If that occurs, then inlet oxygen flows may need to be increased or an alternate device selected.

Air-Entrainment Nebulizers

Large-volume, high-output or "all-purpose" nebulizers have been used in respiratory care for many years to provide bland mist therapy with some control of the FIO_2. These units are commonly placed on patients following extubation for their aerosol-producing properties. Like the entrainment masks, nebulizers use a jet and an adjustable orifice to vary entrained air for various FIO_2 levels at fixed setting points or are continuously adjustable from 0.24 to 1.0. Most commercial devices have an inlet orifice diameter that maximally allows only 15 L/min when the source pressure is 50 psi. This means that on the 100% setting (no air entrainment) output flow is only 15 L/min. Only patients breathing at slow rates and small VT will receive 100% oxygen. For the typical device, more room air is entrained as the FIO_2 is reduced, increasing the total flow output.

Knowledge of the air/oxygen ratio and the input flow rate of oxygen allow the total outflow to be calculated. Nebulizer systems can be applied to the patient with many different devices including aerosol, tracheostomy dome/collar, face tent, and T-piece adapter. These appliances can all be attached via large-bore tubing to the nebulizer. This open system freely vents inspiratory and expiratory gases around the patient's face or out a distal port of a Briggs adapter. Unfortunately, the lack of any valves allows patients to secondarily entrain room air. It is common practice to use either a reservoir bag before the "T" or a reservoir tube on the distal side of the "T" in order to provide a larger volume of gas than that coming from the nebulizer. The major concern of those applying air-entrainment aerosol therapy with controlled oxygen concentration is that the system provide adequate flow. Clinicians should observe the mist like a tracer to determine adequacy of flow. If a T-piece is used and if the visible mist (exiting the distal port) disappears during inspiration, the flow is inadequate.

Another concern in clinical practice is that excess water in the tubing collects and can obstruct gas flow completely or offer increased resistance to flow. The

Table 50–3. Air-entrainment mask input flow versus total flow at varying FIO_2.

FIO_2	Inlet Oxygen Flow (minimum)	Total Flow (L/min)
0.24	4	97
0.28	6	68
0.3	6	54
0.35	8	45
0.40	12	50
0.50	12	33
0.70	12	19
0.80	12	16
1.0	12	12

FIO_2 = fraction of inspired oxygen.

latter may increase the FIO_2 above the desired setting. Another complication is bronchospasm in some patients as the sterile water aerosol can be irritating. In such circumstances, a nonaerosol humidification system should be substituted.

High-Flow Air/Oxygen Systems

Dual air-oxygen flowmeters, air-oxygen blenders, or the Down's flow generator are commonly used for oxygen administration as are free-standing CPAP and "add-on" ventilator systems. These systems contrast to the air-entrainment nebulizer, which can be flow-limiting at high FIO_2 settings. With high-flow systems, the total flow to the patient can be independently set (versus FIO_2) to meet or exceed patient needs. This can be done using a large reservoir bag or constant flows in the 50 to more than 100 L/min range. Clinicians can use a variety of appliances with any of these systems, including aerosol masks, face tents, or well-fitted nonrebreathing system masks with blenders. Face-sealing mask systems can also be constructed but require a reservoir bag with a safety valve to allow breathing if the blender fails. The high flows of gas require use of heated humidifiers of the type commonly used on mechanical ventilators. Humidification offers an advantage for patients with hyperreactive airways. Because of the high flows, such systems are used to apply CPAP for spontaneously breathing patients.

Oxygen Hoods

Although many of the devices previously described have pediatric-sized options, such as cannulas and masks, many young infants and neonates will not tolerate facial appliances. Oxygen hoods cover only the head, allowing access to the infant's lower body while still permitting use of a standard incubator or radiant warmer. The hood is ideal for relatively short-term oxygen therapy for newborns and inactive infants. However, for mobile infants requiring longer term therapy, for example, the nasal cannula, facemask, or full-bed enclosure affords greater mobility.

Normally, oxygen and air are premixed by an air/oxygen blending device and passed through a heated humidifier. Nebulizers should be avoided as the gas source. Most pneumatic jet-type nebulizers create noise levels (> 65 dB) that may cause newborn hearing loss, and cold gas can induce an increase in oxygen consumption. Hoods come in different sizes to accommodate a variety of infants. Some are simple Plexiglas boxes; others have elaborate systems for sealing the neck opening. There is no attempt to completely seal the system, since a constant flow of gas is needed to remove

carbon dioxide (minimum flow > 7 L/min). Hood inlet flows of 10 to 15 L/min are adequate for a majority of patients.

Helium-Oxygen Therapy

Helium-oxygen (heliox) mixtures have a notable, yet limited clinical role. Other than its uses in industry and deep sea diving, there are a number of medical applications for heliox. Helium is premixed with oxygen in several standard blends. The most popular mixtures are the 80%/20% and 70%/30% helium-oxygen, which have densities that are 1.805 and 1.586 times less dense respectively, compared with pure oxygen. They are available in large-sized compressed gas cylinders.

In anesthetic practice, pressures needed to ventilate patients with small diameter endotracheal tubes (ETTs) can be substantially reduced (halved) when 80%/20% mixture is used. Patients with acute distress from upper airway obstructing lesions such as subglottic edema, foreign bodies, and tracheal tumors, may obtain relief until more definitive care can be delivered. Clinicians have reported variable benefits in treating lower airway obstruction in COPD and acute asthma. Helium mixtures may also be used as supplemental gas for bronchodilator nebulization in asthma therapy. Inspiratory driving pressures can be reduced when heliox is delivered via the mechanical ventilator. Nonintubated patients commonly receive heliox therapy via mask with reservoir bag. Accurate flows are not required in administering helium/oxygen mixtures.

Hyperbaric Oxygen

Hyperbaric oxygen therapy uses a pressurized chamber to expose the patient to oxygen tensions exceeding ambient barometric pressure (usually > 760 mm Hg). With a one-person (monoplace) hyperbaric chamber, 100% oxygen is usually used to pressurize the chamber. Larger multi-place chambers allow for the treatment of multiple patients at one time and for medical personnel to be in the chamber with patients. Multiple chambers use air to pressurize the chamber while patients receive 100% oxygen by mask, hood, or ETT. Commonly established indications for hyperbaric oxygen include decompression sickness, gas embolism, gas gangrene, carbon monoxide poisoning, and to treat certain complicated wounds.

3. Hazards of Oxygen Therapy

Oxygen therapy can result in both respiratory and nonrespiratory toxicity. Important factors include patient susceptibility, the FIO_2, and duration of therapy.

Hypoventilation

This complication is primarily seen in patients with COPD who have chronic CO_2 retention. These patients may have an altered respiratory drive that becomes at least partly dependent on the maintenance of relative hypoxemia. Alternatively, oxygen-mediated release of hypoxic vasoconstriction can result in greater blood flow to areas of high ventilation/perfusion ($\dot{V}/\dot{Q}$) (see Chapter 23). Elevation of arterial oxygen tension to "normal" can therefore cause severe hypoventilation in these patients.

Absorption Atelectasis

High concentrations of oxygen can cause pulmonary atelectasis in areas of low $\dot{V}/\dot{Q}$ ratios. When the more insoluble nitrogen is replaced by oxygen in these areas, alveolar volume decreases because of greater uptake of oxygen, causing alveolar collapse (absorption atelectasis). If the area remains perfused but nonventilated, the resultant intrapulmonary shunt can lead to progressive widening of the alveolar-to-arterial (A-a) gradient.

Pulmonary Toxicity

Prolonged high concentrations of oxygen are known to damage the lungs. Toxicity is dependent both on the partial pressure of oxygen in the inspired gas and the duration of exposure. Alveolar rather than arterial oxygen tension is most important in the development of oxygen toxicity. Although 100% oxygen for up to 10–20 hours is generally considered safe (at sea level), concentrations greater than 50–60% for longer periods may lead to toxicity and are undesirable.

Molecular oxygen (O_2) is unusual in that each atom has unpaired electrons in its outer (2P) shell. This gives the molecule the paramagnetic property that allows precise measurements of oxygen concentration (see Chapter 4). Notably, internal rearrangement of these electrons or their interaction with other atoms (iron) or molecules (xanthine) can produce potentially toxic chemical species. Oxygen toxicity is thought to be due to intracellular generation of highly reactive O_2 metabolites (free radicals) such as superoxide and activated hydroxyl ions, singlet O_2, and hydrogen peroxide. A high concentration of O_2 increases the likelihood of generating toxic species. These metabolites are cytotoxic because they readily react with cellular DNA, sulfhydryl proteins, and lipids. Two cellular enzymes, superoxide dismutase and catalase, provide some protection by sequentially converting superoxide first to hydrogen peroxide and then to water. Additional protection may be provided by antioxidants and free radi-

cal scavengers such as glutathione peroxidase, ascorbic acid (vitamin C), α-tocopherol (vitamin E), acetylcysteine, and possibly mannitol; however, clinical evidence supporting the use of these agents in preventing pulmonary toxicity is lacking.

Oxygen-mediated injury of the alveolar-capillary membrane produces a syndrome that is pathologically and clinically indistinguishable from ARDS. Pulmonary capillary permeability increases and the membrane thickens as type I alveolar cells decrease and type II cells proliferate. Tracheobronchitis may also be present initially in some patients. Pulmonary O_2 toxicity in newborn infants is manifested as bronchopulmonary dysplasia.

Retrolental Fibroplasia

Oxygen therapy in neonates with immature retinas can lead to disorganized vascular proliferation and fibrosis, retinal detachment, and eventual blindness. Neonates of less than 36 weeks gestational age are at greatest risk, but even those up to 44 weeks gestational age may be at risk (see Chapter 44). In contrast to pulmonary toxicity, retrolental fibroplasia correlates better with arterial than with alveolar O_2 tension. Arterial O_2 tensions below 140 mm Hg are generally considered safe.

Hyperbaric Oxygen Toxicity

The high inspired O_2 tensions associated with hyperbaric O_2 therapy greatly accelerate O_2 toxicity. The risk and expected degree of toxicity is directly related to the pressures employed as well as the duration of exposure. Prolonged exposure to O_2 partial pressures in excess of 0.5 atmospheres absolute (ATA) can cause pulmonary O_2 toxicity. This may present initially with retrosternal burning, cough, and chest tightness, and will result in progressive impairment of pulmonary function with continued exposure. Patients exposed to O_2 at 2 ATA or greater are also at risk for central nervous system toxicity. Behavior changes, nausea, vertigo, and/or muscular twitching may or may not precede frank convulsions.

Fire Hazard

Oxygen vigorously supports combustion. Its potential for causing fires and explosions is discussed in Chapter 2.

MECHANICAL VENTILATION

Despite early intervention and aggressive respiratory care, patients in an ICU will often require mechanical ventilation. Mechanical ventilation replaces or supplements normal ventilation by the pulmonary system. In most instances, the problem is primarily that of impaired CO_2 elimination (ventilatory failure). In other instances, mechanical ventilation may be used as an adjunct (usually to positive pressure therapy; see below) in the treatment of hypoxemia (hypoxemic respiratory failure). The decision to initiate mechanical ventilation is a clinical one, but certain parameters have been suggested as guidelines (Table 50–4).

Of the two available techniques, positive pressure ventilation and negative pressure ventilation, the former has much wider applications and is almost universally used. Although negative pressure ventilation does not require endotracheal intubation, it cannot overcome substantial increases in airway resistance or decreases in pulmonary compliance, and it also limits access to the patient.

During positive pressure ventilation, lung inflation is achieved by periodically applying positive pressure to the upper airway through a tight-fitting mask (**noninvasive mechanical ventilation**) or through an endotracheal or tracheostomy tube. Increased airway resistance and decreased lung compliance can be overcome by manipulating inspiratory gas flow and pressure. The major disadvantages of positive pressure ventilation are altered ventilation-to-perfusion relationships, potentially adverse circulatory effects, and the risk of pulmonary **barotrauma** and **volutrauma.** Positive pressure ventilation increases physiologic dead space because gas flow is preferentially directed to the more compliant, nondependent areas of the lungs while blood flow (which is affected by gravity) favors dependent areas. Reductions in cardiac output are primarily

due to decreased venous return to the heart because of the elevated intrathoracic pressure. Barotrauma is closely related to repetitive high peak inflation pressures and underlying lung disease, while volutrauma is related to the repetitive collapse and reexpansion of normal or diseased lung.

1. Positive Pressure Ventilators

Positive pressure ventilators periodically create a pressure gradient between the machine circuit and alveoli that results in inspiratory gas flow. Exhalation occurs passively. Ventilators and their control mechanisms can be powered pneumatically (by a pressurized gas source), electrically, or by both mechanisms. Gas flow is either derived directly from the pressurized gas source or produced by the action of a rotary or linear piston. This gas flow then either goes directly to the patient (single-circuit system) or, as commonly occurs on operating room ventilators, compresses a reservoir bag or bellows that is part of the patient circuit (double-circuit system).

All ventilators have four phases: inspiration, the changeover from inspiration to expiration, expiration, and the changeover from expiration to inspiration (see Chapter 4). Manipulation of these phases determines VT, ventilatory rate, inspiratory time, inspiratory gas flow, and expiratory time.

Classification of Ventilators

The complexity of modern ventilators defies simple classification. Incorporation of microprocessor technology into the newest generation of ventilators has further complicated this task. Nonetheless, ventilators are most commonly classified according to their inspiratory phase characteristics and their method of cycling from inspiration to expiration.

A. INSPIRATORY CHARACTERISTICS:

Most modern ventilators behave like flow generators. **Constant flow generators** deliver a constant inspiratory gas flow regardless of airway circuit pressure. Constant flow is produced by the use of either a solenoid (on-off) valve with a high-pressure gas source (5–50 psi) or via a gas injector (Venturi) with a lower-pressure source. Machines with high-pressure gas sources allow inspiratory gas flow to remain constant in spite of large changes in airway resistance or pulmonary compliance. The performance of ventilators with gas injectors varies more with airway pressure. **Nonconstant flow generators** consistently vary inspiratory flow with each inspiratory cycle (such as by a rotary piston); a sine wave pattern is most common.

Constant-pressure generators maintain airway pressure constant throughout inspiration and irrespec-

Table 50–4. Guidelines suggesting the need for mechanical ventilation.

Respiratory gas tensions	Direct indices Arterial oxygen tension < 50 mm Hg on room air, or arterial CO_2 tension > 50 mm Hg in the absence of metabolic alkalosis Derived indices PaO_2/FiO_2 ratio < 300 mm Hg $PA\text{-}aO_2$ gradient > 350 mm Hg VD/VT > 0.6
Clinical indices	Respiratory rate > 35 breaths/min
Mechanical indices	Tidal volume < 5 mL/kg Vital capacity < 15 mL/kg Maximum inspiratory force < –25 cm H_2O, ie, –15 cm H_2O

tive of inspiratory gas flow. Gas flow ceases when airway pressure equals the set inspiratory pressure. Pressure generators typically operate at low gas pressures (just above peak inspiratory pressure).

B. CYCLING (CHANGEOVER FROM INSPIRATION TO EXPIRATION):

Time-cycled ventilators cycle to the expiratory phase once a predetermined interval elapses from the start of inspiration. VT is the product of the set inspiratory time and inspiratory flow rate. Time-cycled ventilators are commonly used for neonates and in the operating room.

Volume-cycled ventilators terminate inspiration when a preselected volume is delivered. Many adult ventilators are volume-cycled but also have secondary limits on inspiratory pressure to guard against pulmonary barotrauma. If inspiratory pressure exceeds the pressure limit, the machine cycles into expiration even if the selected volume has not been delivered. In reality, properly functioning volume-cycled ventilators still do not deliver the set volume to the patient. A percentage of the set VT is always lost owing to expansion of the breathing circuit during inspiration. Circuit compliance is usually about 3–5 mL/cm H_2O; thus, if a pressure of 30 cm H_2O is generated during inspiration, 90–150 mL of the set VT is lost to the circuit. Loss of VT to the breathing circuit is therefore inversely related to lung compliance. For accurate measurement of the exhaled VT, the spirometer must be placed at the ETT rather than the exhalation valve of the ventilator.

Pressure-cycled ventilators cycle into the expiratory phase when airway pressure reaches a predetermined level. VT and inspiratory time vary, being related to airway resistance and pulmonary and circuit compliance. A significant leak in the patient circuit can prevent the necessary rise in circuit pressure and machine cycling. Conversely, an acute increase in airway resistance, or decrease in pulmonary compliance, or circuit compliance (kink) causes premature cycling and decreases the delivered VT. Pressure-cycled ventilators are generally most useful for short-term use only (transport).

Flow-cycled ventilators have pressure and flow sensors that allow the ventilator to monitor inspiratory flow at a preselected fixed inspiratory pressure; when this flow reaches a predetermined level (usually 25% of the initial peak mechanical inspiratory flow rate), the ventilator cycles from inspiration into expiration (see Pressure Support/Pressure Control Ventilation).

C. MICROPROCESSOR-CONTROLLED VENTILATORS:

These versatile machines can be set to function in any one of a variety of inspiratory flow and cycling patterns. The microprocessor allows closed-loop control over the ventilator's performance characteristics. Microproces-

sor-controlled ventilators include the Puritan-Bennett 7200 and 840, Seimens Servo 300, Respironics Espirit and Hamilton Veolar ventilators, and the ventilators on the Ohmeda 7600 and the Drager 6000 anesthesia machines.

Ventilatory Modes

Ventilatory mode is defined by the method by which the ventilator cycles from expiration to inspiration as well as whether the patient is able to breathe spontaneously (see Table 50–5 and Figure 50–1). Most modern ventilators are capable of more than one ventilatory mode, and some (microprocessor-controlled ventilators) can combine modes simultaneously.

A. CONTROLLED MECHANICAL VENTILATION (CMV):

In this mode, the ventilator cycles from expiration to inspiration after a fixed time interval. The interval determines the ventilatory rate. Settings on this mode provide a fixed VT and fixed rate (and, therefore, minute ventilation) regardless of patient effort, because the patient cannot breathe spontaneously. Settings to limit inspiratory pressure guard against pulmonary barotrauma. Controlled ventilation is best reserved for patients capable of little or no ventilatory effort. Awake patients with active respiratory effort require sedation or muscle paralysis.

B. ASSIST-CONTROL VENTILATION (AC):

By incorporating a pressure sensor in the breathing circuit, the patient's inspiratory effort can be used to trigger inspiration. A sensitivity control allows selection of the inspiratory effort required. The ventilator can be set for a fixed ventilatory rate, but each patient effort of sufficient magnitude will trigger the set VT. If spontaneous inspiratory efforts are not detected, the machine functions as if in the control mode.

C. INTERMITTENT MANDATORY VENTILATION (IMV):

IMV allows spontaneous respirations while the patient is on the ventilator. A selected number of mechanical breaths (with fixed VT) is given to supplement spontaneous breathing. At high mandatory rates (10–12 breaths/min), IMV essentially provides all of the patient's ventilation; while at low rates (1–2 breaths/min), it provides minimal mechanical ventilation and allows patients to breathe relatively independently. The VT and frequency of spontaneous breaths are determined by the patient's respiratory drive and muscle strength. The IMV rate can be adjusted to maintain a desired minute ventilation. IMV has found greatest use as a weaning technique.

Synchronized intermittent mandatory ventilation (SIMV) times the mechanical breath, whenever possi-

Table 50–5. Ventilatory modes.

| Mode | I to E Cycling | | | | E to I Cycling | | Allows Spontaneous Ventilation | Weaning Mode |
	Volume	Time	Pressure	Flow	Time	Pressure		
CMV	+				+			
AC	+				+	+		
IMV	+				+		+	+
SIMV	+				+	+	+	+
PSV				+		+	+	+
PCV			+		+			
MMV							+	
PC-IRV			+		+			
APRV		+			+		+	
HFJV		+			+		+	

CMV = controlled mechanical ventilation, AC = assist-control ventilation, IMV = intermittent mandatory ventilation, SIMV = synchronized intermittent mandatory ventilation, PSV = pressure support ventilation, PCV = pressure control ventilation, MMV = mandatory minute ventilation, IRV = inverse I:E ratio ventilation, APRV = airway pressure release ventilation, HFJV = high-frequency jet ventilation.

ble, to coincide with the beginning of a spontaneous effort. Proper synchronization prevents superimposing (stacking) a mechanical breath in the middle of a spontaneous breath, resulting in a very large V_T. As with CMV and AC, settings to limit inspiratory pressure guard against pulmonary barotrauma. The advantages of SIMV include patient comfort, and if used for weaning, the machine breaths provide a backup if the patient becomes fatigued. However, if the rate is too low (4 breaths/min) the backup may be too low, especially for weak patients who may not be able to overcome the added WOB superimposed by the ventilator during spontaneous breaths.

IMV circuits provide a continuous supply of gas flow for spontaneous ventilation between mechanical breaths. Modern ventilators incorporate SIMV into their design, but older models must be modified by a parallel circuit, a continuous flow system, or a demand flow valve. Regardless of the system, proper functioning of one-way valves and sufficient gas flow are necessary to prevent an increase in the patient's WOB, especially when PEEP is also used.

D. MANDATORY MINUTE VENTILATION (MMV):

The patient is able to breathe spontaneously and receives mechanical breaths also, while the machine monitors the exhaled minute ventilation. In this mode, the machine then continuously adjusts the number of mechanical breaths so that the sum of spontaneous plus mechanical breaths equals the desired set minute ventilation. The role of this mode in weaning remains to be defined.

E. PRESSURE SUPPORT VENTILATION (PSV):

Pressure support ventilation was designed to augment the V_T of spontaneously breathing patients and overcome any increased inspiratory resistance from the ETT, breathing circuit (tubing, connectors, and humidifier), and ventilator (pneumatic circuitry and valves). Microprocessor-controlled machines have this mode, which delivers sufficient gas flow with every inspiratory effort to maintain a predetermined positive pressure throughout inspiration. When inspiratory flow decreases to a predetermined level, the ventilator's feedback (servo) loop cycles the machine into the expiratory phase, and airway pressure returns to baseline (Figure 50–2). The only setting in this mode is inspiratory pressure. The patient determines the respiratory rate and V_T varies according to inspiratory gas flow, lung mechanics, and the patient's own inspiratory effort. Low levels of PSV (5–10 cm H_2O) are usually sufficient to overcome any added resistance imposed by the breathing apparatus. Higher levels (10–40 cm H_2O) can function as a stand-alone ventilatory mode if the patient has sufficient spontaneous ventilatory drive and stable lung mechanics. The principal advantages of PSV are its ability to augment spontaneous V_T, decrease the WOB, and increase patient comfort. However, if the patient fa-

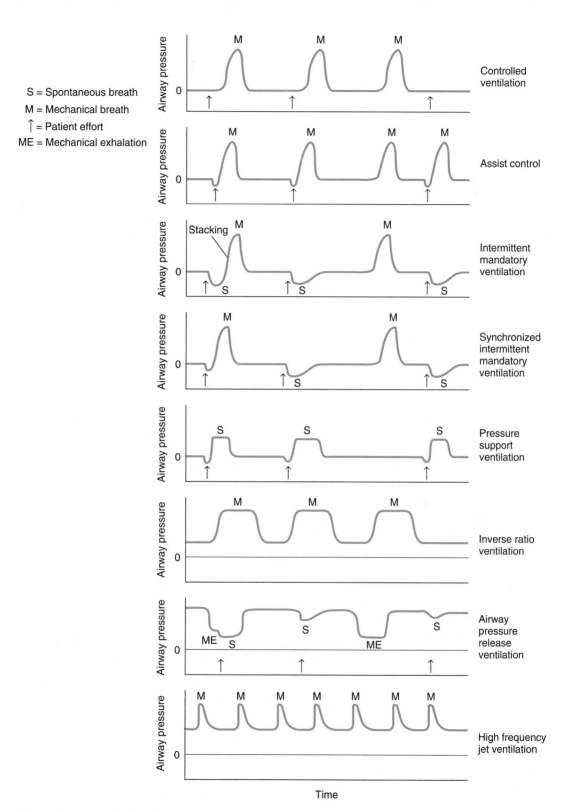

Figure 50–1. Airway pressure waveforms of ventilatory modes.

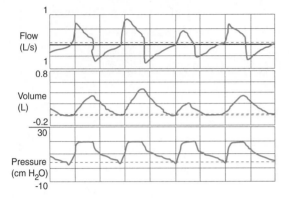

Figure 50–2. Pressure support ventilation. Patient initiates breath; machine set to deliver 15 cm H_2O pressure (above 5 cm H_2O of continuous positive airway pressure [CPAP]). When flow ceases, the machine cycles into the expiratory mode.

tigues or lung mechanics change, V_T may be inadequate and there is no backup rate if the patients' intrinsic respiratory rate decreases or the patient becomes apneic. Pressure support is often used in conjunction with IMV (Figure 50–3). The IMV machine breaths provide backup and a low level of pressure support is used to offset the WOB superimposed by the breathing circuit and machine.

F. PRESSURE CONTROL VENTILATION (PCV):

This is similar to pressure support ventilation in that peak airway pressure is set, but different in that a mandatory rate is set. As with pressure support, gas ceases when flow ceases, cycling the ventilator into the expiratory phase. PCV may be used in both the AC and in the IMV modes. In AC, all breaths (either machine initiated or patient initiated) are time cycled. The inspiratory time is set and the breaths are pressure limited. In IMV mode, machine-initiated breaths are time cycled and pressure limited. The advantage of PCV is that the rate is set and by pressure limiting breaths, the risks of barotrauma and volutrauma are decreased compared with breaths that are volume set. Combining PCV with an adequate level of PEEP may recruit collapsed and flooded alveoli. The disadvantage of PCV is that V_T is not guaranteed. This is a major issue in patients with acute lung injury (ALI) because if the compliance changes without augmenting the pressure, the V_T will decrease. PCV is increasingly being used for patients with ALI and in patients with ARDS. Often times it is combined with inverse I:E ratio ventilation (IRV) (see below) which helps recruit collapsed and flooded alveoli. The disadvantage of using IRV with PCV is that the patient

needs to be heavily sedated or paralyzed to tolerate this particular ventilatory mode.

With PCV, pressure and inspiratory time are preset, airflow and volume are variable and dependent on the patient's resistance and compliance. With volume ventilation, on the other hand, inspiratory time is also preset but flow and V_T are also preset, and in this circumstance the pressure can be very high.

G. INVERSE I:E RATIO VENTILATION:

This mode reverses the normal inspiratory to expiratory time ratio of 1:3 or greater, to a ratio of 1:1 to 1.5:1. This may be achieved by an end-inspiratory pause or by decreasing peak inspiratory flow during volume-cycled ventilation (CMV), or by prolonging inspiratory time such that inspiration is longer than expiration during PCV (PC-IRV). **Intrinsic PEEP** may be produced because when this technique is initiated, each new breath may begin prior to the complete exhalation of the last; air trapping increases FRC until a new equilibrium is reached. This mode does not allow spontaneous breathing and requires heavy sedation or muscle paralysis. IRV with PEEP is effective for improving oxygenation in patients with decreased FRC. Oxygenation is generally directly proportional to mean airway pressure.

H. AIRWAY PRESSURE RELEASE VENTILATION (APRV):

APRV is a ventilatory mode in which a high CPAP level is used, and the patient is allowed to breath spontaneously. Intermittently, the CPAP level decreases to help eliminate CO_2 (Figure 50–4). Periodic release of CPAP to a lower level allows exhalation that augments

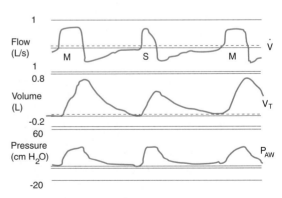

Figure 50–3. Intermittent mechanical ventilation with pressure support. M = machine breath → set tidal volume (V_T) delivered. S = spontaneous breath, 15 cm of pressure support over 5 of PEEP. V_T depends on patient effort and lung mechanics. V̇ = flow, Paw = partial airway pressure, PEEP = positive end-expiratory pressure.

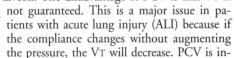

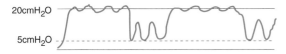

Figure 50–4. Airway pressure release ventilation.

spontaneous ventilation. The inspiratory and expiratory times, duration of CPAP release, and spontaneous respiratory activity determine minute ventilation. Initial settings include a minimum CPAP of 10–12 cm H_2O and a release level of 5–10 cm H_2O. An advantage of APRV appears to be less circulatory depression and pulmonary barotrauma. This technique appears to be an attractive alternative to PC-IRV for overcoming problems with high peak inspiratory pressures in patients with reduced lung compliance.

I. High-Frequency Ventilation (HFV):

Three forms of HFV are available. High-frequency positive pressure ventilation (HFPPV) involves delivering a small "conventional" V_T at a rate of 60–120 breaths/min. High-frequency jet ventilation (HFJV) utilizes a small cannula at or in the airway through which a pulsed jet of high pressure gas is delivered at a set frequency of 120–600 times/min (2–10 Hz). The jet of gas may entrain air (Bernoulli effect) which may augment V_T. High-frequency oscillation (HFO) employs a driver (usually a piston) that creates to-and-fro gas movement in the airway at rates of 600–3000 times/min (10–50 Hz).

The mechanism of gas exchange with these techniques, which employ V_T below anatomic dead space, is not clear, but it is often described as augmented diffusion. HFJV has found widest use in the operating room. It may be used for laryngeal, tracheal, and bronchial procedures, and can be extremely useful in emergency management of the airway when endotracheal intubation and conventional positive pressure ventilation are unsuccessful (see Chapter 5). In the ICU, HFJV may be useful in managing some patients with bronchopleural and tracheoesophageal fistulas when conventional ventilation has failed. Occasionally, it or HFO are used in patients with ARDS to try to improve oxygenation. Inadequate heating and humidification of inspired gases during prolonged HFV, however, can be a problem. Initial settings for HFJV in the operating room are typically a rate of 120–240 breaths/min, an inspiratory time of 33%, and a drive pressure of 15–30 psi. Mean airway pressure should be measured in the trachea at least 5 cm below the injector to avoid an artifactual error from gas entrainment. Carbon dioxide elimination is generally directly proportional to drive pressure, while oxygenation is directly propor-

tional to mean airway pressure. An intrinsic PEEP-effect is seen during HFJV at high drive pressures and inspiratory times greater than 40%.

J. Differential Lung Ventilation (DLV):

This technique, also referred to as independent lung ventilation (ILV) may be used in patients with severe unilateral lung disease or in patients with bronchopleural fistula. Use of conventional positive pressure ventilation and PEEP in such instances can aggravate ventilation/perfusion mismatching, or in patients with fistula, result in inadequate ventilation of the unaffected lung. In patients with restrictive disease of one lung, overdistention of the normal lung can lead to worsening hypoxemia or barotrauma. After separation of the lungs with a double lumen endobronchial tube, differential positive pressure ventilation with two ventilators is applied to each lung independently. When two ventilators are used, the timing of mechanical breaths is usually synchronized with one ventilator, the "master," setting the rate for the "slave" ventilator.

2. Care of Patients Requiring Mechanical Ventilation

Endotracheal Intubation

Endotracheal intubation for mechanical ventilation is most commonly undertaken in ICU patients to manage respiratory failure. Both nasal and oral (translaryngeal) endotracheal intubation appear to be relatively safe for at least 2–3 weeks. When compared with oral intubation, nasal intubation may be more comfortable for the patient, more secure (fewer instances of accidental extubation), and less likely to cause laryngeal damage. Nasal intubation, however, can result in significant nasal bleeding, transient bacteremia, submucosal dissection of the nasopharynx or oropharynx, and sinusitis or otitis media (from obstruction of the auditory tubes).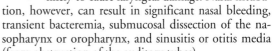

Intubation can often be carried out without the use of sedation or muscle paralysis in agonal and unconscious patients. Topical anesthesia of the airway or sedation, however, are helpful in patients who still have active airway reflexes. Airway management for patients with head trauma is discussed in Chapter 26. More vigorous and uncooperative patients require varying degrees of sedation; administration of a neuromuscular blocking agent (also called a muscle relaxant) also greatly facilitates orotracheal intubation. Small doses of relatively short-acting agents are generally used; popular agents include midazolam, etomidate, propofol, and methohexital. Succinylcholine or a nondepolarizing relaxant (mivacuronium or rocuronium) can be used for paralysis after a hypnotic is given.

The time of endotracheal intubation and initiation of mechanical ventilation is often a period of great hemodynamic instability. Hypertension or hypotension and bradycardia or tachycardia may be encountered. Responsible factors include activation of autonomic reflexes from stimulation of the airway, myocardial depression and vasodilation from sedative-hypnotic agents, straining by the patient, withdrawal of intense sympathetic activity, and reduced venous return due to positive pressure in the airways. Careful monitoring is therefore required during and immediately following intubation.

 When left in place for more than 2 to 3 weeks, both oral and nasal translaryngeal ETTs predispose patients to subglottic stenosis. If longer periods of mechanical ventilation are necessary, the ETT should generally be replaced by a cuffed tracheostomy tube. If it is anticipated that an ETT will be required for more than 2 to 3 weeks, a tracheostomy should be performed sooner rather than later.

Initial Ventilator Settings

Depending on the type of respiratory failure, mechanical ventilation is used to provide either partial or full ventilatory support. For full ventilatory support, CMV, AC, or PCV is generally employed with a respiratory rate of 10–12 breaths/min and a V_T of 8–10 mL/kg; lower V_T (6–8 mL/kg) may be necessary to avoid high peak inflation pressures (> 35–40 cm H_2O), and pulmonary barotrauma and volutrauma. High airway pressures that overdistend alveoli (transalveolar pressure > 35 cm H_2O) have been shown experimentally to promote lung injury. Likewise, V_T greater than 10 mL have been associated with increased mortality in patients with ARDS. Partial ventilatory support is usually provided by low SIMV settings (< 8 breaths/min), either with or without pressure support. Lower mean airway pressures (< 20–30 cm H_2O) can help preserve cardiac output and may be less likely to alter normal ventilation/perfusion relationships.

Patients breathing spontaneously on SIMV must overcome the additional resistances of the ETT, demand valves, and breathing circuit of the ventilator. These imposed resistances increase the WOB. Small ETTs (< 7.0–7.5 mm ID) should therefore be avoided whenever possible. The simultaneous use of pressure support 5–15 cm H_2O during SIMV can compensate for ETT and circuit resistance.

The addition of 5–8 cm H_2O of PEEP during positive pressure ventilation preserves FRC and gas exchange. This "physiologic" PEEP is purported to compensate for the loss a similar amount of intrinsic PEEP (and decrease in FRC) in patients following endotra-

cheal intubation. Periodic large V_T (sigh breaths) are not necessary when physiologic PEEP (approximately 5 cm H_2O) and a V_T of 6–10 mL/kg are used.

Sedation & Paralysis

Heavy sedation or paralysis may be necessary in patients who become agitated and "fight" the ventilator. Repetitive coughing ("bucking") and straining can have adverse hemodynamic effects, can interfere with gas exchange, and may predispose to pulmonary barotrauma and to self-inflicted injury. Sedation with or without paralysis may also be desirable when patients continue to be tachypneic in spite of high mechanical respiratory rates (> 16–18 breaths/min).

Commonly used sedatives include opioids (morphine or fentanyl), benzodiazepines (diazepam, midazolam, or lorazepam), propofol, and dexmedetomidine. These agents may be used alone or in combination, and are most effectively administered by continuous infusion. Nondepolarizing muscle relaxants are used for paralysis when all other means to ventilate the patient have failed.

Monitoring

Patients on mechanical ventilation require continuous monitoring for adverse hemodynamic and pulmonary effects resulting from positive pressure in the airways. Continuous electrocardiographic, pulse oximetry, and direct intra-arterial pressure monitoring are extremely useful. The latter also allows frequent sampling of arterial blood for respiratory gas analysis. Careful recording of fluid intake and output are necessary to accurately assess fluid balance. An indwelling urinary catheter is very helpful. Central venous and/or pulmonary artery pressure monitoring are indicated in hemodynamically unstable patients and those with a low urinary output. Daily chest radiographs are commonly obtained to assess ETT and central line positions, look for evidence of pulmonary barotrauma, help evaluate fluid balance, and follow the progression of pulmonary disease.

Airway pressures (baseline, peak, and mean), inhaled and exhaled V_T (mechanical and spontaneous), and fractional concentration of oxygen should be closely followed. Monitoring these parameters not only allows optimal adjustment of ventilator settings but helps detect problems with the ETT, breathing circuit, and ventilator. Inadequate periodic suctioning of airway secretions and the presence of large mucus plugs are often manifested as increasing peak inflation pressures and decreasing exhaled V_T. Moreover, an abrupt increase in peak inflation pressure together with sudden hypotension strongly suggests a pneumothorax.

3. Discontinuing Mechanical Ventilation

The ease of weaning a patient from a ventilator is generally inversely related to the duration of the mechanical ventilation. The process that necessitated mechanical ventilation must be reversed or under control before weaning is attempted. Complicating factors should also be adequately treated, including bronchospasm, heart failure, infection, malnutrition, metabolic acidosis or alkalosis, anemia, increased CO_2 production due to high carbohydrate loads, altered mental status, and sleep deprivation. Underlying lung disease and respiratory muscle wasting from prolonged disuse are often major factors that complicate weaning.

Weaning from mechanical ventilation may be considered when patients no longer meet general criteria for mechanical ventilation (see Table 50–4). Additional mechanical indices have also been suggested (Table 50–6). Clinical signs of improvement should be supported by laboratory and radiographic findings. The most useful weaning parameters are arterial blood gas tensions, the respiratory rate, and the **rapid shallow breathing index (RSBI)**. Intact airway reflexes and a cooperative patient are also mandatory prior to completion of the weaning process unless the patient has a cuffed tracheostomy tube. Similarly, adequate oxygenation (arterial hemoglobin saturation > 90%) on 40–50% oxygen with less than 5 cm H_2O of PEEP is imperative prior to extubation. When the patient is weaned from the ventilator and extubation is planned, the RSBI is frequently used to help predict who can be successfully weaned from mechanical ventilation and extubated. With the patient breathing spontaneously on a T-piece, the VT and respiratory rate (f) are measured:

$$RSBI = \frac{f(breaths/min)}{V_t(L)}$$

Patients with an RSBI less than 100 can be successfully extubated. Patients with an RSBI greater than 120

Table 50–6. Mechanical criteria for weaning/extubation.

Criterion	Measurement
Inspiratory pressure	<–25 cm H_2O
Tidal volume	> 5 mL/kg
Vital capacity	> 10 mL/kg
Minute ventilation	< 10 mL
Rapid shallow breathing index	< 100

should remain on some degree of mechanical ventilation.

The most common techniques to wean a patient from the ventilator include IMV, pressure support, or periods of spontaneous breathing alone on a T-piece or on low levels of CPAP. Mandatory minute ventilation has also been suggested as an ideal weaning technique but experience with it is more limited.

Weaning With IMV

With IMV the number of mechanical breaths is progressively decreased (by 1–2 breaths/min) as long as the arterial CO_2 tension and respiratory rate remain acceptable (generally < 45–50 mm Hg and < 30 breaths/min, respectively). If pressure support is concomitantly used, it should generally be reduced to 5–8 cm H_2O. In patients with acid-base disturbances or chronic CO_2 retention, arterial blood pH (> 7.35) is more useful than CO_2 tension. Blood gas measurements can be checked after a minimum of 15–30 minutes at each setting. When an IMV of 2–4 breaths is reached, mechanical ventilation is discontinued if arterial oxygenation remains acceptable.

Weaning With PSV

Weaning with PSV alone is accomplished by gradually decreasing the pressure support level by 2–3 cm H_2O while VT, arterial blood gas tensions, and respiratory rate are monitored (using the same criteria as for IMV). The goal is to assure a VT of 4–6 mL/kg and a f of less than 30 with acceptable PaO_2 and $PaCO_2$. When a pressure support level of 5–8 cm H_2O is reached, the patient is considered weaned.

Weaning With a T-Piece or CPAP

T-piece trials allow observation while the patient breathes spontaneously without any mechanical breaths. The T-piece attaches directly to the ETT or tracheostomy tube and has corrugated tubing on the other two limbs. A humidified oxygen-air mixture flows into the proximal limb and exits from the distal limb. Sufficient gas flow must be given in the proximal limb to prevent the mist from being completely drawn back at the distal limb during inspiration; this ensures that the patient is receiving the desired oxygen concentration. The patient is observed closely during this period; obvious signs of fatigue, chest retractions, tachypnea, marked tachycardia, dysrhythmias, or hypertension or hypotension should terminate the trial. If the patient appears to tolerate the trial period and the RSBI is less than 100, mechanical ventilation can be discontinued permanently. If the patient can also protect and clear his or her airway, the ETT can be removed.

If the patient has been intubated for a prolonged period or has severe underlying lung disease, sequential T-piece trials may be necessary: periodic trials of 10–30 minutes are initiated and progressively increased by 5–10 minutes per trial until the patient appears comfortable and maintains acceptable arterial blood gases.

Many patients develop progressive atelectasis during prolonged T-piece trials. The latter may reflect the absence of a normal "physiologic" PEEP when the larynx is bypassed by an ETT. If this is a concern, the patient can be tried on spontaneous breathing trials on low levels (5 cm H_2O) of CPAP. The CPAP helps prevent atelectasis and maintain FRC.

POSITIVE AIRWAY PRESSURE THERAPY

Positive airway pressure therapy can be used in patients breathing spontaneously as well as those receiving mechanical ventilation. The principal indication for positive airway pressure therapy is a symptomatic decrease in FRC, resulting in absolute or relative hypoxemia. By increasing transpulmonary distending pressure, positive airway pressure therapy can increase lung volume, improve (increase) lung compliance, and reverse ventilation/perfusion mismatching. The latter is reflected in a decrease in venous admixture and an improvement in arterial O_2 tension.

Positive End-Expiratory Pressure

When the positive pressure is applied during expiration as an adjunct to a mechanically delivered breath, this form of therapy is referred to as **PEEP.** The ventilator's PEEP valve provides a pressure threshold that allows expiratory flow to occur only when airway pressure equals or exceeds the selected PEEP level. This threshold usually is provided by a pressurized expiratory valve or diaphragm.

Continuous Positive Airway Pressure

When a positive pressure threshold is applied during both inspiration and expiration during spontaneous breathing, this form of therapy is referred to as CPAP. Constant levels of pressure can only be attained if a high flow (inspiratory) gas source is provided. When the patient does not have an artificial airway, tightly fitting full-face masks, nasal masks, nasal "pillows" (ADAM circuit), or nasal prongs (neonatal) can be used. Because of the risks of gastric distention and regurgitation, CPAP masks should be used only on alert patients with intact airway reflexes and with CPAP levels less than 15 cm H_2O (less than lower esophageal

sphincter pressure in normal persons). Expiratory pressures above 15 cm H_2O require an artificial airway.

CPAP Versus PEEP

The distinction between PEEP and CPAP is often blurred in the clinical setting since patients may breathe with a combination of mechanical and spontaneous breaths. Therefore, the two terms are often used interchangeably. In the strictest sense, "pure" PEEP is provided as a ventilator-cycled breath. In contrast, a "pure" CPAP system only provides sufficient continuous or "on-demand" gas flows (60–90 L/min) to prevent inspiratory airway pressure from falling perceptibly below the expiratory level during spontaneous breaths (Figure 50–5). Thus, when compared with PEEP, CPAP breathing provides less support but with reduced mean airway pressure. Some ventilators with demand valve-based CPAP systems may not be adequately responsive and result in increased inspiratory WOB. This situation can be corrected by adding low levels of (inspiratory) PSV, if in a volume-targeted mode or changing to a pressure-targeted mode. In clinical practice, the application of controlled ventilation, PSV and CPAP/PEEP support can be delivered by most modern ICU ventilators. Manufacturers have also developed specific devices to deliver bilevel inspiratory positive airway pressure [IPAP] with expiratory positive airway pressure [EPAP] in either a spontaneous or time-cycled fashion. The term "bilevel positive airway pressure (BiPAP)" has become a commonly used phrase, adding to the confusion of airway pressure terminology.

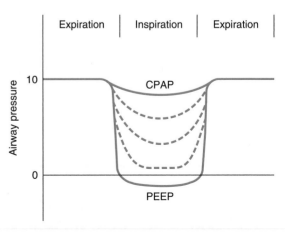

Figure 50–5. Airway pressure during positive end-expiratory pressure (PEEP) and continuous positive airway pressure (CPAP). Note that by increasing inspiratory gas flows, PEEP progressively becomes CPAP.

Pulmonary Effects of PEEP & CPAP

The major effect of positive expiratory pressure on the lungs is to increase FRC. In patients with decreased lung volume, both PEEP and CPAP increase FRC and tidal ventilation above closing capacity, improve lung compliance, and correct ventilation/perfusion abnormalities. The resulting decrease in intrapulmonary shunting improves arterial oxygenation. Their principal mechanism of action appears to be stabilization and expansion of partially collapsed alveoli. Recruitment (reexpansion) of collapsed alveoli occurs at PEEP or CPAP levels above the inflection point, defined as the pressure level on a pressure-volume curve at which collapsed alveoli are recruited (open); with small changes in pressure there are large changes in volume (Figure 50–6). Although neither PEEP nor CPAP decreases total extravascular lung water, studies suggest that they do redistribute extravascular lung water from the interstitial space between alveoli and endothelial cells toward peribronchial and perihilar areas. Both effects can potentially improve arterial oxygenation.

Excessive PEEP or CPAP, however, can overdistend alveoli (and bronchi), increasing dead space ventilation and reducing lung compliance; both effects can significantly increase the WOB. By compressing alveolar capillaries, overdistention of normal alveoli can also increase pulmonary vascular resistance and right ventricular afterload.

A higher incidence of pulmonary barotrauma is observed when excessive PEEP or CPAP is added, especially at levels greater than 20 cm H_2O. Disruption of alveoli allows air to track interstitially along bronchi into the mediastinum (pneumomediastinum). From the mediastinum, air can then rupture into the pleural space (pneumothorax) or the pericardium (pneumopericardium), or dissect along tissue planes subcutaneously (subcutaneous emphysema) or into the abdomen (pneumoperitoneum or pneumoretroperitoneum). Failure of an air leak to seal results in a bronchopleural fistula. Barotrauma may be more closely associated with the higher peak inspiratory pressures that result as the level of PEEP or CPAP increases. Other factors that may increase the risk of barotrauma include underlying lung disease, a high rate of mechanical breaths such that there is stacking of breaths so that intrinsic PEEP develops, large VT (> 10–15 mL/kg), and young age.

Adverse Nonpulmonary Effects of PEEP & CPAP

These adverse effects are primarily circulatory and are related to transmission of the elevated airway pressure to the contents of the chest. Fortunately, transmission is directly related to lung compliance; thus, patients with decreased lung compliance (most patients requiring PEEP) are least affected.

Progressive reductions in cardiac output are often seen as mean airway pressure and, secondarily, mean intrathoracic pressure rise. The principal mechanism appears to be a progressive decrease in venous return to the heart. Other mechanisms may include leftward displacement of the interventricular septum (interfering with left ventricular filling) because of the increase in pulmonary vascular resistance (increased right ventricular afterload) from overdistention of alveoli, leading to an increase in right ventricular volume. Left ventricular compliance may therefore be reduced; when this occurs, the same preload requires a higher filling pressure. Intravenous fluid administration usually at least partially offsets the effects of CPAP and PEEP on cardiac output. Circulatory depression is most often associated with end-expiratory pressures greater than 15 cm H_2O.

PEEP-induced elevations in central venous pressure and reductions in cardiac output decrease both renal and hepatic blood flow (see Chapters 31 and 34). Circulating levels of antidiuretic hormone and angiotensin are usually elevated. Urinary output, glomerular filtration, and free water clearance decrease.

The increases in central venous pressure also aggravate intracranial hypertension (see Chapter 25). Increased end-expiratory pressures, because they decrease venous return, may also manifest as an increase in ICP in patients whose ventricular compliance is decreased. Therefore, in patients on mechanical ventilation for ALI and with evidence of raised ICP, the level of PEEP

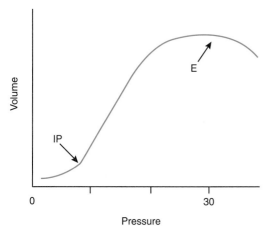

Figure 50–6. Pressure-volume curve for pulmonary system (lung, thoracic, etc). Inflection point (IP) above which majority of alveoli are recruited. E = result of excessive pressure when alveoli are over-distended and pulmonary compliance decreases.

must be carefully chosen to balance oxygenation requirements against effects on the ICP.

Optimum Use of PEEP & CPAP

The goal of positive pressure therapy is ultimately to increase oxygen delivery to tissues, while avoiding the adverse sequelae of high (> 0.5) FIO₂. The latter is optimally accomplished only if adequate cardiac output and a hemoglobin concentration greater than 8–10 g/dL are maintained as well. Ideally, mixed venous oxygen tensions or the arteriovenous oxygen content difference should be followed (see Chapter 22). The salutary effect of PEEP (or CPAP) on arterial oxygen tension must be balanced against any detrimental effect on cardiac output. PEEP or CPAP levels exceeding 15 cm H₂O usually require pulmonary artery pressure monitoring to properly assess circulatory function and allow measurement of mixed venous oxygen tension and calculation of the venous admixture. Volume infusion or inotropic support may be necessary and should be guided by hemodynamic measurements.

Optimal PEEP is that amount at which the maximum beneficial effects of PEEP overshadow any detrimental effect. Practically, PEEP is usually added in increments of 3–5 cm H₂O until the desired therapeutic end point is reached. The most commonly suggested end point is an arterial oxygen saturation of hemoglobin of greater than 88–90% on a nontoxic inspired oxygen concentration (< 50%). Many clinicians favor reducing the inspired oxygen concentration to 50% or less because of the potentially adverse effect of higher oxygen concentrations on the lung. Alternatively, PEEP may be titrated to the mixed venous artery oxygen saturation ($S\bar{v}O_2 > 50$–60%). Monitoring lung compliance and dead space has also been suggested.

OTHER TECHNIQUES

These techniques preserve or improve pulmonary function. They include administering aerosolized water or bronchodilators and clearing pulmonary secretions.

An aerosol mist is a gas or gas mixture containing a suspension of liquid particles. Aerosolized water may be administered to loosen inspissated secretions and facilitate their removal from the tracheobronchial tree. Aerosol mists are also used to administer bronchodilators, mucolytic agents, or vasoconstrictors, although metered-dose inhalers are preferred for administration of bronchodilators. A normal cough requires an adequate inspiratory capacity, an intact glottis, and adequate muscle strength (abdominal muscles and diaphragm). Aerosol mist therapy with or without bronchodilators may induce cough as well as loosen secretions. Additional effective measures include chest percussion or vibration therapy, and postural drainage of the various lung lobes.

 Maneuvers that produce sustained maximum lung inflation such as the use of an incentive spirometer can be helpful in inducing cough as well as preventing atelectasis and preserving normal lung volume. Patients should be instructed to inhale approximately 15–20 mL/kg and to hold it for 2 to 3 seconds before exhalation.

When thick and copious secretions are associated with obvious atelectasis and hypoxemia, more aggressive measures may be indicated. These include suctioning via a nasopharyngeal catheter, flexible bronchoscope, or through an ETT. When atelectasis is not associated with retention of secretions, a brief period of CPAP by mask or positive pressure ventilation through an ETT is often very effective.

■ RESPIRATORY FAILURE

Respiratory failure may be defined as impairment of normal gas exchange severe enough to require acute therapeutic intervention. Definitions based on arterial blood gases (see Table 50–1) may not apply to patients with chronic pulmonary diseases; dyspnea and progressive respiratory acidosis must also be present in patients with chronic CO₂ retention. Arterial blood gases typically follow one of several patterns in patients with respiratory failure (Figure 50–7). At one extreme, the derangement primarily affects oxygen transfer from the alveoli into blood, giving rise to hypoxemia (hypoxic respiratory failure); unless severe ventilation/perfusion mismatching is present, CO₂ elimination in these instances is typically normal or even enhanced. At the other extreme, the disorder primarily affects carbon dioxide elimination (pure ventilatory failure), resulting in hypercapnia; mismatching of ventilation to perfusion is typically absent or minimal. Hypoxemia, however, can occur with pure ventilatory failure when arterial CO₂ tension reaches 75–80 mm Hg in patients breathing room air (see the alveolar gas equation in Chapter 22). Most patients with respiratory failure display a pattern between these extremes.

Treatment

Regardless of the disorder, the treatment of respiratory failure is primarily supportive while the reversible components of underlying disease are being treated. Hypoxemia is treated with oxygen therapy and positive airway pressure (if FRC is decreased), while hypercarbia (ventilatory failure) is treated with mechanical ventilation. Other general measures may include aerosolized bron-

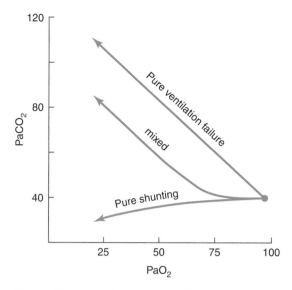

Figure 50–7. Arterial gas tension (room air) patterns during acute respiratory failure.

chodilators, intravenous antibiotics, diuretics for fluid overload, optimizing cardiac function, and adequate nutritional support. Some patients may benefit from aminophylline infusions, which can improve diaphragmatic function.

PULMONARY EDEMA

Pathophysiology

Pulmonary edema results from transudation of fluid, first from pulmonary capillaries into interstitial spaces and then from the interstitial spaces into alveoli. Fluid within the interstitial space and alveoli is collectively referred to as extravascular lung water. The movement of water across the pulmonary capillaries is similar to what occurs in other capillary beds (see Chapter 28) and can be expressed by the Starling equation:

$$Q = K \times [(P\acute{c} - Pi) - \sigma(\Pi\acute{c} - \Pi i)]$$

where Q is net flow across the capillary; P$\acute{c}$ and Pi are capillary and interstitial hydrostatic pressures, respectively; and $\pi\acute{c}$ and πi are capillary and interstitial oncotic pressures, respectively; K is a filtration coefficient related to effective capillary surface area per mass of tissue; and σ is a reflection coefficient that expresses the permeability of the capillary endothelium to albumin. A σ with a value of 1 implies that the endothelium is completely impermeable to albumin, while a value of 0 indicates free passage. The pulmonary en-

dothelium normally is partially permeable to albumin, such that interstitial albumin concentration is approximately one-half that of plasma; therefore, πi must be about 14 mm Hg (one-half that of plasma). Pulmonary capillary hydrostatic pressure is dependent on vertical height in the lung (gravity) and normally varies from 0 to 15 mm Hg (average: 7 mm Hg). Since Pi is thought to be normally about −4 to −8 mm Hg, the forces favoring transudation of fluid (P$\acute{c}$, Pi, and πi) are normally almost balanced by the forces favoring reabsorption ($\pi\acute{c}$). The net amount of fluid that normally moves out of pulmonary capillaries is small (about 10–20 mL/hour in adults) and is rapidly removed by pulmonary lymphatics, which return it into the central venous system.

The alveolar epithelial membrane is normally permeable to water and gases but is impermeable to albumin (and other proteins). A net movement of water from the interstitium into alveoli occurs only when the normally negative Pi becomes positive (relative to atmospheric pressure). Fortunately, because of the lung's unique ultrastructure and its capacity to increase lymph flow, the pulmonary interstitium normally accommodates large increases in capillary transudation before Pi becomes positive. When this reserve capacity is exceeded, pulmonary edema develops.

Pulmonary edema is often divided into four stages:

Stage I: Only interstitial pulmonary edema is present. Patients often become tachypneic as pulmonary compliance begins to decrease. The chest radiograph reveals increased interstitial markings and peribronchial cuffing.

Stage II: Fluid fills the interstitium and begins to fill the alveoli, being initially confined to the angles between adjacent septa (crescentic filling). Gas exchange may remain relatively preserved.

Stage III: Alveolar flooding occurs such that many alveoli are completely flooded and no longer contain air. Flooding is most prominent in dependent areas of the lungs. Blood flow through the capillaries of flooded alveoli results in a large increase in intrapulmonary shunting. Hypoxemia and hypocapnia (due to dyspnea and hyperventilation) are characteristic.

Stage IV: Marked alveolar flooding spills over into the airways as froth. Gas exchange is severely compromised owing to both shunting and airway obstruction. Progressive hypercapnia and severe hypoxemia follow.

Causes of Pulmonary Edema

Pulmonary edema usually results from either an increase in the net hydrostatic pressure across the capillaries (hemodynamic edema) or an increase in the permeability of the alveolar-capillary membrane (permeability edema). The distinction can often be based on the pulmonary artery occlusion pressure (PAOP), which if greater than 18 mm Hg, indicates that hydrostatic pressure is involved in forcing fluid across the capillaries into the interstitium and alveoli. The protein content of the edema fluid can also help differentiate the two. Edema fluid from the hemodynamic causes has a low protein content, while fluid due to permeability edema has a high protein content.

Less common causes of edema include prolonged severe airway obstruction, sudden reexpansion of a collapsed lung, high altitude, pulmonary lymphatic obstruction, or severe head injury, although the same mechanisms, ie, changes in hemodynamic parameters or capillary permeability, also account for these diagnoses. Pulmonary edema associated with airway obstruction may result from an increase in the transmural pressure across pulmonary capillaries associated with a markedly negative interstitial hydrostatic pressure. Neurogenic pulmonary edema appears to be related to a marked increase in sympathetic tone, which causes severe pulmonary hypertension. The latter can disrupt the alveolar-capillary membrane.

1. Hemodynamic Pulmonary Edema

Significant elevations in $P\acute{c}$ can increase extravascular lung water and result in pulmonary edema. As can be seen from the Starling equation, a decrease in $\pi\acute{c}$ may accentuate the effects of any increase in $P\acute{c}$. Two major mechanisms increase $P\acute{c}$, namely, pulmonary venous hypertension or a markedly increased pulmonary blood flow. Any elevation of pulmonary venous pressure is transmitted passively backward to the pulmonary capillaries and secondarily increases $P\acute{c}$. Pulmonary venous hypertension usually results from left ventricular failure, mitral stenosis, or left atrial obstruction. Increases in pulmonary blood flow that exceed the capacity of the pulmonary vasculature will also raise $P\acute{c}$. Marked increases in pulmonary blood flow can be the result of large left-to-right cardiac or peripheral shunts, hypervolemia (fluid overload), severe anemia, or exercise.

Treatment

Management of hemodynamic pulmonary edema is aimed at decreasing the pressure in the pulmonary capillaries. Generally, this includes measures to improve left ventricular function, correcting fluid overload with diuretics, or reducing pulmonary blood flow. Pharmacologic treatments include morphine, diuretics, vasodilators, and inotropes. Vasodilators, particularly ni-

trates, have proved extremely useful. By reducing preload, pulmonary congestion is relieved; and by reducing afterload, cardiac output may be improved. Positive airway pressure therapy is also a useful adjunct for improving oxygenation.

2. Permeability Pulmonary Edema: ALI & ARDS

Extravascular lung water increases in permeability pulmonary edema owing to enhanced permeability or disruption of the capillary-alveolar membrane. The protective effect of plasma oncotic pressure is lost as increased amounts of albumin "leak" into the pulmonary interstitium; normal—or even low—capillary hydrostatic pressures are unopposed and result in transudation of fluid into the lungs. Permeability edema is seen with ALI (P:F ratio $\leq$ 300 [P = PaO_2 and F = FIO_2]) and is often associated with sepsis, trauma, and pulmonary aspiration; when severe (P:F ratio < 200), it is referred to as ARDS.

Pathophysiology

This syndrome represents the pulmonary manifestation of the systemic inflammatory response syndrome (SIRS). Central to the pathophysiology of ARDS is severe injury of the capillary-alveolar membrane. Regardless of the type of injury, the lung responds to the ensuing inflammatory response in a similar fashion. The inflammatory response includes the release of large amounts of cytokines and other secondary mediators, and activation of the complement, coagulation, fibrinolytic, and kinin cascades. Initial mediators include tumor necrosis factor (TNF), interleukins 1 and 6 (IL-1 and IL-6), platelet activating factor, as well as various prostaglandins and leukotrienes. Activation of neutrophils and macrophages in the lung exposes the pulmonary parenchyma to oxygen-derived free radicals and proteases. The released mediators increase pulmonary capillary permeability, induce pulmonary vasoconstriction, and alter vascular reactivity such that hypoxic pulmonary vasoconstriction is abolished. Destruction of alveolar epithelial cell (types I and II) is prominent. Alveolar flooding, together with decrease in surfactant production (due to loss of type II pneumocytes), results in collapse. The exudative phase of ARDS may rapidly resolve or persist for a varying period; it is often followed by a fibrotic phase (fibrosing alveolitis), which in some cases leads to permanent scarring.

Clinical Manifestations

The diagnosis of ARDS requires the exclusion of significant underlying left ventricular dysfunction (PAOP

< 18 mm Hg) combined with a **P:F ratio of < 200** and the presence of **diffuse infiltrates** on a chest radiograph. The lung is often affected in a nonhomogenous pattern, although dependent areas tend to be most affected.

ARDS is most commonly seen in the setting of sepsis and trauma. Patients present with severe dyspnea and labored respirations. Hypoxemia due to intrapulmonary shunting is a universal finding. Although dead space ventilation is increased, arterial CO_2 tension is typically decreased because of a marked increase in minute ventilation. Ventilatory failure may be seen initially in severe cases or may eventually develop owing to respiratory muscle fatigue or marked destruction of the capillary-alveolar membrane. Pulmonary hypertension and low or normal left ventricular filling pressures are characteristic hemodynamic findings.

Treatment

In addition to intensive respiratory care, treatment should also be directed at reversible processes such as sepsis or hypotension. Hypoxemia is treated with oxygen therapy. Milder cases may be treated with a CPAP mask, but most patients require intubation and at least some degree of mechanical ventilatory support. High peak inflation pressures (> 35 cm H_2O) and high V_T (> 8–10 mL/kg), however, should also be avoided, because overdistention of alveoli (high Paw or high V_T) can induce iatrogenic lung injury, as can high FIO_2 (> 0.5). The latter has not been conclusively demonstrated in humans, but V_T of > 10 mL/kg is associated with increased mortality.

If possible, the FIO_2 should be maintained at ≤ 0.5, primarily by increasing PEEP above the inflection point (Figure 50–7). Other maneuvers to improve oxygenation include the use of inhaled nitric oxide, inhaled prostacyclin or PGE_1, or ventilation in the prone position. These three techniques improve oxygenation in a majority of patients with ALI but are not risk free and have not been associated with an improvement in survival. Steroids early in ARDS are associated with an increased mortality but are often used (day 4–10) during the fibroproliferative phase of ARDS.

Morbidity and mortality from ARDS are usually due to the precipitating cause or complications rather than the respiratory failure itself. The most common serious complications are sepsis, renal failure, gastrointestinal (GI) hemorrhage, etc. [multiple-organ dysfunction syndrome (MODS)]. Nosocomial pneumonia is especially common in patients with a protracted course. Nosocomial pneumonia is often difficult to diagnose; antibiotics are generally indicated when there is a high index of suspicion (fever, purulent secretions, leukocytosis, and change in chest radiograph). Protected speci-

men brushings and bronchoalveolar lavage sampling via a flexible bronchoscope may be useful in selected patients. Colonization by gram-negative organisms, breach of mucocutaneous barriers by various catheters, malnutrition, and altered host immunity contribute to a high incidence of infection. Renal failure is usually due to volume depletion, sepsis, or nephrotoxins and substantially increases the mortality rate (to > 60%). Prophylaxis for GI hemorrhage with sucralfate, antacids, H_2 blockers, or proton pump inhibitors is recommended.

DROWNING & NEAR-DROWNING

Drowning, with or without aspiration of water, is death while submerged in water. Near-drowning, with or without aspiration, is to suffocate while submerged and to survive at least temporarily. Both drowning and near-drowning can occur whether or not inhalation (aspiration) of water occurs. If water does not enter the airways, the patient primarily suffers from asphyxia, but if the patient inhales water, marked intrapulmonary shunting also takes place. Survival depends on the intensity and duration of the hypoxia as well as the temperature of the water.

Pathophysiology

Ninety percent of drowning patients aspirate fresh water, seawater, brackish water, or other fluids. Although the amount of liquid aspirated is generally small, marked ventilation/perfusion mismatching can result from fluids in the airways and alveoli, reflex bronchospasm, and loss of pulmonary surfactant. Aspiration of gastric contents can also complicate drowning before or after loss of consciousness, or during resuscitation.

The hypotonic water aspirated following fresh water drowning is rapidly absorbed by the pulmonary circulation; water cannot usually be recovered from the airways. If a significant amount is absorbed (> 800 mL in a 70-kg adult) transient hemodilution, hyponatremia, and even hemolysis may occur. In contrast, aspiration of salt water, which is hypertonic, draws out water from the pulmonary circulation into the alveoli, flooding them. Hemoconcentration and hypernatremia can occur following saltwater drowning but are uncommon. Hypermagnesemia and hypercalcemia have also been reported following near-drowning in salt water.

Patients who suffer from cold water drowning lose consciousness when body temperature decreases below 32 °C. Ventricular fibrillation occurs at about 28–30 °C, but the hypothermia has a protective effect on the brain (see Chapter 25) and may improve outcome providing resuscitation measures are successful.

Clinical Manifestations

Nearly all patients with a significant near-drowning episode have hypoxemia, hypercarbia, and metabolic acidosis. Patients may also suffer from other injuries, such as spine fractures, following diving accidents. Neurologic impairment is generally related to the duration of the submersion and the severity of the asphyxia. Cerebral edema complicates prolonged asphyxia (see Chapter 25). ARDS develops in a significant number of patients following resuscitation.

Treatment

Initial treatment of near-drowning is directed at restoring ventilation, perfusion, oxygenation, an acid-base balance as quickly as possible. Immediate measures include clearing and establishing an airway, administering oxygen, and initiating cardiopulmonary resuscitation. In-line stabilization of the cervical spine is necessary while intubating patients who suffer from near-drowning following a dive. Although salt water can often be drained out of the lungs by gravity, this practice should not delay institution of cardiopulmonary resuscitation; abdominal thrusts may promote aspiration of gastric contents. Resuscitation efforts are always continued until the patient is fully assessed and under treatment in a hospital, especially following cold water drowning. Complete recovery is possible in such instances even after prolonged periods of asphyxia. Management includes endotracheal intubation, positive pressure ventilation, and PEEP. Bronchospasm should be treated with bronchodilators, electrolyte abnormalities corrected, and ALI treated as discussed above. If the patient is hypothermic, rewarming should be undertaken over a few hours.

SMOKE INHALATION

Smoke inhalation is the leading cause of death from fires. Affected persons may or may not have sustained a burn. Burn victims who suffer from smoke inhalation have a mortality rate significantly higher than other burn patients. Any exposure to smoke in a fire requires a presumptive diagnosis of smoke inhalation until proved otherwise. A history of loss of consciousness or disorientation, or a burn acquired in a closed space is suggestive.

Pathophysiology

The consequences of smoke inhalation are complex because they can involve three types of injuries: heat injury to the airways, exposure to toxic gases, and a chemical burn with deposition of carbonaceous particulates into the lower airways. The pulmonary response to smoke inhalation is equally complex and depends on the duration of the exposure, the composition of the material that burned, and the presence of any underlying lung disease. Combustion of many synthetic materials produces highly toxic gases such as carbon monoxide, hydrogen cyanide, hydrogen sulfide, hydrogen chloride, ammonia, chlorine, benzene, and aldehydes. When these gases react with water in the airways, they can produce hydrochloric, acetic, formic, and sulfuric acids. Carbon monoxide and cyanide poisoning are common.

Pathologic correlates of smoke inhalation include direct mucosal injury resulting in edema, inflammation, and sloughing. Loss of ciliary activity impairs the clearance of mucus and bacteria. Manifestations of ARDS typically occur 2–3 days after the injury and appear to be more related to the delayed development of SIRS rather than the acute smoke inhalation itself.

Clinical Manifestations

Patients may initially have few if any symptoms of smoke inhalation. Suggestive physical findings include facial or intraoral burns, singed nasal hairs, cough, carbonaceous sputum, and wheezing. The diagnosis can usually be made with flexible bronchoscopy of the upper airway and the tracheobronchial tree. Bronchoscopy reveals erythema, edema, mucosal ulcerations, and carbonaceous deposits. Arterial blood gases may initially be normal or reveal only mild hypoxemia and metabolic acidosis due to carbon monoxide. The chest radiograph is often also initially normal.

Heat injury to the airways is usually confined to supraglottic structures, unless there was prolonged exposure to steam. Progressive hoarseness and stridor are ominous signs of impending airway obstruction, which may develop over 12–18 hours. Fluid resuscitation of the patient frequently aggravates the edema.

Carbon monoxide poisoning is usually defined as greater than 15% carboxyhemoglobin in the blood. The diagnosis is made by cooximetric measurements of blood. Carbon monoxide has 200–300 times the affinity of oxygen for hemoglobin. When a carbon monoxide molecule combines with hemoglobin to form carboxyhemoglobin, it decreases the affinity of the other binding sites for oxygen, shifting the hemoglobin dissociation curve to the right. The net result is a marked reduction in the oxygen-carrying capacity of blood. Moreover, the rate of dissociation for carbon monoxide from hemoglobin is slow with a half-life of approximately 2–4 hours. Clinical manifestations are due to tissue hypoxia from impaired oxygen delivery. Levels greater than 20–40% carboxyhemoglobin are associated with neurologic impairment, nausea, fatigue, disorientation, and shock. Lower levels may also produce significant symptoms because carbon monoxide also binds cytochrome c and myoglobin. Compensatory mechanisms include increased cardiac output and peripheral vasodilation.

Cyanide toxicity may occur in patients exposed to fumes from fires that contain synthetic materials, especially those containing polyurethane. The cyanide, which may be inhaled or absorbed through mucosal surfaces and skin, binds the cytochrome system of enzymes and inhibits cellular production of adenosine triphosphate (ATP). Patients present with neurologic impairment and lactic acidosis; they typically have arrhythmias, a high cardiac output, and marked vasodilation.

A **chemical burn** of the respiratory mucosa follows inhalation of large amounts of carbonaceous material, especially when combined with toxic fumes. Inflammation of the airways results in bronchorrhea and wheezing. Bronchial edema and sloughing of the mucosa leads to obstruction of the lower airways and atelectasis. Progressive ventilation/perfusion mismatching can lead to marked hypoxemia over the course of 24–48 hours. Development of SIRS can lead to ARDS.

Treatment

Fiberoptic bronchoscopy usually establishes the diagnosis of an inhalation injury. Bronchoscopy is usually carried out with an ETT over the bronchoscope so that in-

tubation can readily be accomplished if edema threatens the patency of the airway. Early elective endotracheal intubation is advisable when there are obvious signs of heat injury. Patients with hoarseness and stridor require immediate intubation; emergency cricothyrotomy or tracheostomy is necessary if oral or nasal intubation is unsuccessful.

The presence of clinically significant carbon monoxide or cyanide poisoning, as evidenced by obtundation or coma, also requires prompt endotracheal intubation and a high inspired oxygen concentration. The diagnosis of carbon monoxide poisoning requires cooximetry measurements because pulse oximeters cannot reliably differentiate between carboxyhemoglobin and oxyhemoglobin (see Chapter 6). The half-life of carboxyhemoglobin is reduced to 1 hour with 100% oxygen; some clinicians advocate hyperbaric oxygen therapy if the patient does not respond to 100% oxygen. The diagnosis of cyanide poisoning is more difficult to make because reliable measurements of cyanide levels are not readily available (normally < 0.1 mg/L). The enzyme rhodanase normally converts cyanide to thiocyanate, which is subsequently eliminated by the kidneys. Treatment for severe cyanide toxicity consists of administering sodium nitrite 300 mg IV as a 3% solution over 3–5 minutes, followed by sodium thiosulfate 12.5 g IV

in the form of a 25% solution over 1–2 minutes. Sodium nitrite converts hemoglobin to methemoglobin, which has a higher affinity for cyanide than cytochrome oxidase; the cyanide which is slowly released from cyanomethemoglobin is converted by thiosulfate to the less toxic thiocyanate.

Marked hypoxemia due to intrapulmonary shunting should be managed with endotracheal intubation, oxygen therapy, bronchodilators, positive pressure ventilation, and PEEP. Corticosteroids are ineffective and increase the rate of infections. As with other forms of ARDS, nosocomial infectious pneumonias are common.

■ ACUTE MYOCARDIAL INFARCTION

Acute myocardial infarction (AMI) is a serious complication of ischemic heart disease (see Chapter 20), with an overall mortality rate of 25%. Over one-half of deaths are estimated to occur within the first hour and are usually due to arrhythmias (ventricular fibrillation). With recent advances in interventional cardiology, the hospital mortality rate has been reduced to less than 10–15%. Pump (ventricular) failure is now the leading cause of death in hospitalized patients.

Most myocardial infarctions occur in patients with more than one severely narrowed (> 75%) coronary artery. A transmural infarction occurs in an area distal to a complete occlusion. The occlusion is nearly always due to thrombosis at a stenotic atheromatous plaque. Coronary emboli or severe spasm is less commonly the cause. The size and location of the infarct depend on the distribution of the obstructed vessel and whether collateral vessels have formed. Anterior, apical, and septal infarcts of the left ventricle are usually due to thrombosis in the left anterior descending circulation; lateral and posterior left ventricular infarcts result from occlusions in the left circumflex system, while right ventricular and posterior-inferior left ventricular infarcts are from thrombosis in the right coronary artery. In contrast, subendocardial (nontransmural, or "non–Q wave") infarctions usually occur in the setting of a sustained and severe increased myocardial demand in patients with severe stenosis, but can also be due to coronary thrombosis.

Following even brief episodes of severe ischemia, prolonged myocardial dysfunction with only slow and gradual return of contractile function can be observed. This phenomenon of "stunning" is often thought to occur in areas adjacent to infarcted myocardium and can contribute to ventricular dysfunction following AMI. Relief of the ischemia in these areas can restore contractile function. When this phenomenon is observed in the setting of severe chronic ischemia, the myocardium in these noninfarcted but poorly contractile areas is often said to have been "hibernating." Stunning and hibernation are commonly observed in the settings of ischemic cardiac arrest during cardiopulmonary bypass and following myocardial revascularization, respectively.

The immediate treatment of AMI is the administration of oxygen (4–6 L/min), aspirin (160–325 mg), nitroglycerin (sublingual or spray), and morphine (2–4 mg IV every 5 min) until the pain is relieved. Remember the acronym: MONA (morphine, oxygen, nitroglycerin, and aspirin) greets all patients. Because the prognosis following AMI is generally inversely proportionate to the extent of necrosis, the current emphasis in management of an evolving myocardial infarction is reperfusion. Based on local resources and timing, angiography with angioplasty and/or a stent with coronary artery bypass surgery backup may be preferred. Alternately, front-loaded alteplase or streptokinase, anisoylated plasminogen streptokinase activator complex (APSAC), or reteplase or tenecteplase will improve survival. The greatest benefit is if treatment is given within the first hour, but benefit can be seen if treatment is given within 12 hours of the AMI.

Patients with ST-segment depression or dynamic T-wave changes (non–Q wave infarction; unstable angina) benefit from antithrombin (heparin) and antiplatelet (aspirin) therapy. All patients without contraindications should receive β-blockers. Patients who have recurrent angina should be given nitrates. If angina persists or if there is a contraindication to β-blockers, calcium channel blockers should be administered.

Intra-aortic balloon counterpulsation is usually reserved for hemodynamically compromised patients with refractory ischemia. Temporary pacing following AMI is indicated for Mobitz type II and complete heart block, a new bifascicular block, and bradycardia with hypotension. Stable monomorphic ventricular tachycardia, if treated medically and the patient's ejection fraction is normal, is best managed with procainamide or sotalol. If the ejection fraction is poor, amiodarone at 150 mg IV bolus over 10 minutes is administered. If ventricular tachycardia is polymorphic and the QT interval is normal, correct abnormal electrolytes, treat ischemia, and administer β-blockers (amiodarone, procainamide, or sotalol can also be given). If the QT interval is prolonged, then in addition to correcting electrolytes, magnesium, overdrive pacing, isoproterenol, phenytoin, or lidocaine is recommended. Lidocaine is the second tier choice for all four of these indications. Patients with a stable narrow complex supraventricular tachycardia should be treated with amiodarone. Patients with paroxysmal supraventricular tachycardia, whose ejection fraction is preserved, should be treated with a calcium channel blocker, a β-blocker, digoxin, or DC cardioversion. If the ejection fraction is less than 40%, DC cardioversion should be avoided in deference to digoxin, amiodarone, or diltiazem.

Patients with ectopic or multifocal atrial tachycardia should not receive DC cardioversion, but instead should be treated with calcium channel blockers, a β-blocker, or amiodarone. If the ejection fraction is less than 40%, diltiazem could also be considered in addition to amiodarone.

RENAL FAILURE

Acute renal failure (ARF) is a rapid deterioration in renal function that is not immediately reversible by altering extrarenal factors, such as blood pressure, intravascular volume, cardiac output, or urinary flow. The hallmark of renal failure is azotemia and often times oliguria (see Chapter 32). However, not all patients with acute azotemia have acute renal failure. Likewise, greater than 500 mL of urine per day does not imply that renal function is normal. Basing the diagnosis of ARF on creatinine levels or an increase in blood urea nitrogen (BUN) is also problematic because creatinine clearance is not always a good measure of glomerular filtration rate.

Typically then, ARF is diagnosed by documenting an increase in BUN and plasma creatinine over several days. In 50% of patients, ARF is secondary to ischemia; in 35% of patients, ARF is due to nephrotoxic causes; and in the remaining 15%, patients have acute tubular interstitial nephritis or acute glomerular nephritis.

Azotemia may be classified as prerenal, renal, and postrenal. Moreover, the diagnosis of ARF (renal azotemia) is one of exclusion; thus, prerenal and postrenal causes must always be excluded.

PRERENAL AZOTEMIA

Prerenal azotemia occurs as a result of hypoperfusion of the kidneys; if untreated, it progresses to ARF. Renal hypoperfusion is most commonly the result of a decrease in arterial perfusion pressure, a marked increase in venous pressure, or renal vasoconstriction (Table 50–7). Decreased perfusion pressure is usually associated with the release of norepinephrine, angiotensin II, arginine vasopressin (AVP, also called antidiuretic hormone), and endothelin. These hormones constrict cutaneous muscle and splanchnic vasculature and promote salt and water retention. The synthesis of vasodilating prostaglandins (prostacyclin and PGE_2) and nitric

Table 50–7. Reversible causes of azotemia.

> Prerenal
> > Decreased renal perfusion pressure
> > > Hypovolemia
> > > Decreased cardiac output
> > > Hypotension
> > Increased renal vascular resistance
> > > Neural
> > > Humoral
> > > Pharmacologic
> > > Thromboembolic
> Postrenal
> > Urethral obstruction
> > Bladder outlet obstruction
> > > Prostatic
> > > Bladder tumor
> > > Cystitis
> > > Neurogenic bladder
> > Bilateral ureteral obstruction
> > > Intrinsic
> > > > Calculi
> > > > Tumor
> > > > Blood clots
> > > > Papillary necrosis
> > > Extrinsic
> > > > Abdominal or pelvic tumor
> > > > Retroperitoneal fibrosis
> > > > Inadvertent ureteral ligations

---

oxide in the kidneys, and the intrarenal action of angiotensin II help maintain glomerular filtration. Use of cyclooxygenase inhibitors or angiotensin-converting enzyme inhibitors in the setting of marked prerenal azotemia can precipitate ARF. The diagnosis of prerenal azotemia is usually suspected from the clinical setting and confirmed by urinary laboratory indices (Table 50–8). Treatment of prerenal azotemia is directed at correcting intravascular volume deficits, improving cardiac function, restoring a normal blood pressure, and reversing increases in renal vascular resistance. The hepatorenal syndrome is discussed in Chapter 35.

POSTRENAL AZOTEMIA

Azotemia due to urinary tract obstruction is referred to as postrenal azotemia. Obstruction of urinary flow from both kidneys is usually necessary for azotemia and oliguria/anuria in these conditions. Complete obstruction eventually develops into ARF, while prolonged partial obstruction leads to chronic renal impairment. Rapid diagnosis and relief of acute obstruction usually restores normal renal function. Obstruction may be suggested by a physical examination (distended bladder) or a plain radiograph of the abdomen (revealing bilateral renal calculi) but is confirmed by demonstrating dilation of the urinary tract proximal to the site of obstruction. Renal ultrasonography, computerized tomography, or cystoscopy with retrograde urograms are most commonly used. Treatment depends on the site of obstruction. Obstruction at the bladder outlet can be relieved with a catheterization of the bladder or suprapubic cystostomy, while ureteral obstruction requires nephrostomy or ureteral stents.

REVERSIBLE AZOTEMIA VERSUS ACUTE RENAL FAILURE

The ability to differentiate prerenal and postrenal azotemia from ARF (renal azotemia) is critical. Exclusion of postrenal azotemia requires visualization of the urinary tract, while exclusion of prerenal azotemia depends on the response to treatments aimed at improving renal perfusion. The latter may be facilitated by analysis of urinary composition (Table 50–8); urinary

Table 50–8. Urinary indices in azotemia.

Index	Prerenal	Renal	Postrenal
Specific gravity	> 1.018	< 0.012	Variable
Osmolality (mmol/kg)	> 500	< 350	Variable
Urine/plasma urea nitrogen ratio	> 8	< 3	Variable
Urine/plasma creatinine ratio	> 40	< 20	Variable
Urine/sodium (mEq/L)	< 10	> 40	Variable
Fractional excretion of sodium (%)	< 1	> 3	Variable
Renal failure index	< 1	> 1	Variable

composition in postrenal azotemia is variable and depends on the duration and severity of obstruction. In prerenal azotemia, tubular concentrating ability is preserved and reflected by a low urinary sodium concentration and high urine/serum creatinine ratio. Calculation of the fractional excretion of filtered sodium (FE_{Na^+}) may also be extremely useful in the setting of oliguria:

$$FE_{Na^+} = \frac{\text{Urine sodium}/\text{serum sodium}}{\text{Urine creatinine}/\text{serum creatinine}} \times 100\%$$

FE_{Na^+} is less than 1% in oliguric patients with prerenal azotemia but typically exceeds 3% in patients with oliguric ARF. Values of 1–3% may be present in patients with nonoliguric ARF. The renal failure index, which is the urinary sodium concentration divided by the urine/plasma creatinine ratio, is the most sensitive index for diagnosing renal failure. The use of diuretics increases urinary sodium excretion and invalidates indices that rely on urinary sodium concentration as a measure of tubular function. Moreover, intrinsic renal diseases that primarily affect renal vasculature or glomeruli may not affect tubular function and therefore are associated with indices that are similar to prerenal azotemia. Measurement of a 3-hour creatinine clearance test (see Chapter 32) can be used to estimate the residual glomerular filtration rate, but there are several factors that must be taken into account. For there to be a good correlation, the increasing serum creatinine must have plateaued.

Etiology of ARF

Causes of ARF are listed in Table 50–9. Up to 50% of cases follow major trauma or surgery; in the majority of instances, ischemia and nephrotoxins are responsible. ARF associated with ischemia and nephrotoxins is generally referred to as acute tubular necrosis. The latter term, however, is inaccurate because intrinsic renal diseases, such as glomerulonephritis and interstitial nephritis, can cause renal failure without tubular necrosis. Moreover, many patients who develop ischemic or nephrotoxic renal failure do not have tubular necrosis on pathologic examination. Aminoglycosides, amphotericin B, radiographic contrast dyes, cyclosporine, and cisplatin are the most commonly implicated exogenous nephrotoxins. Amphotericin B, contrast dyes, and cyclosporine also appear to produce direct intrarenal vasoconstriction. Hemoglobin and myoglobin are potent nephrotoxins when they are released during intravascular hemolysis and rhabdomyolysis, respectively. Cyclooxygenase inhibitors, especially nonsteroidal anti-inflammatory drugs (NSAIDs), may play an important

Table 50–9. Causes of acute renal failure.

Renal ischemia (50%)
  Hypotension
  Hypovolemia
  Impaired cardiac output
Nephrotoxins (35%)
  Endogenous pigments
    Hemoglobulin (hemolysis)
    Myoglobin (rhabdomyolysis from crush injury and burns)
  Radiographic contrast agents
  Drugs
    Antibiotics (aminoglycosides, amphotericin)
    Nonsteroidal anti-inflammatory drugs
    Chemotherapeutic agents (cisplatin, methotrexate)
  Tubular crystals
    Uric acid
    Oxalate
    Sulfonamides
  Heavy metal poisoning
  Organic solvents
  Myeloma protein
Intrinsic renal disease (15%)
  Glomerular disease
  Interstitial nephritis

role at least in some patients. Inhibition of prostaglandin synthesis by the latter group of agents decreases prostaglandin-mediated renal vasodilation, allowing unopposed renal vasoconstriction. Other factors predisposing to ARF include preexisting renal impairment, advanced age, atherosclerotic vascular disease, diabetes, and dehydration.

Pathogenesis of ARF

The sensitivity of the kidneys to injury may be explained by their very high metabolic rate and ability to concentrate potentially toxic substances. The pathogenesis of ARF is complex and probably has both a vascular and a tubular basis. Afferent arteriolar constriction, decreased glomerular permeability, direct epithelial cell injury and tubular obstruction from intraluminal debris or edema can all decrease glomerular filtration (see Chapter 31). A backleak of filtered solutes through damaged portions of renal tubules may allow reabsorption of creatinine, urea, and other nitrogenous wastes.

Renal ischemia or hypoxia is the likely triggering event in many instances. An imbalance between ATP production and demand in epithelial cells leads to altered ion transport, cellular swelling, altered metabolism of phospholipids and an accumulation of intracellular calcium. Free radical-mediated cell injury can also occur during reperfusion and reoxygenation.

Oliguric Versus Nonoliguric ARF

ARF is often classified as oliguric (urinary volume < 400 mL/d), anuric (< 100 mL/d), or nonoliguric (urinary volume > 400 mL/d). Nonoliguric ARF accounts for up to 50% of all cases. Patients with nonoliguric ARF typically have lower urinary sodium concentrations than oliguric patients. Moreover, they also appear to have a lower complication rate and to require shorter hospitalizations. Nonoliguric ARF may therefore represent less severe renal injury. In some instances, it may be possible to convert oliguric ARF into nonoliguric ARF by administering mannitol, furosemide, or "renal" doses of dopamine (1–2 μg/kg/min). The resulting increase in urinary output may be therapeutic by preventing tubular obstruction. Mannitol may also decrease cellular swelling and has a free radical scavenging action. Alternatively, the response to diuretic therapy may help identify patients with lesser degrees of renal impairment.

Treatment of ARF

The course of ARF is described in Chapter 32. Management is primarily supportive. Diuretics and mannitol may be used to maintain urinary output in nonoliguric patients. Dopamine has not been shown to be effective in ARF. ARF due to glomerulonephritis or vasculitis may respond to glucocorticoids. Standard treatment for oliguric and anuric patients, who do not increase their urinary output following diuretics, includes restriction of fluid, sodium, potassium, and phosphorus. Daily weight measurements help guide fluid therapy. Fluid intake should generally equal 500 mL plus urinary output. Sodium and potassium intake is limited to 1 mEq/kg/d, while protein intake is less than 0.7 g/kg/d and consists mainly of high biologic value protein. Hyponatremia can be treated with water restriction. Hyperkalemia may require use of an ion-exchange resin (sodium polystyrene), glucose and insulin, calcium gluconate, or sodium bicarbonate administration. Sodium bicarbonate therapy may also be necessary for metabolic acidosis when the serum bicarbonate falls below 15 mEq/L. Hyperphosphatemia requires dietary phosphate restriction and phosphate-binding antacid (aluminum hydroxide). The dosages of renally excreted drugs should be adjusted to the estimated glomerular filtration rate or measured creatinine clearance to prevent accumulation.

Dialysis may be employed to treat or prevent uremic complications (see Table 32–4). A double-lumen catheter placed in the internal jugular, subclavian, or femoral vein is usually used. The high morbidity and mortality rates associated with ARF favor early dialysis, but supporting studies are controversial. Dialysis does not appear to hasten recovery but may in fact aggravate renal injury if hypotension occurs or too much fluid is removed.

Because of concern that intermittent dialysis associated with hypotension may perpetuate the renal injury, continuous renal replacement therapy (CRRT), continuous venovenous hemofiltration (CVVHF) and continuous venovenous hemodialysis (CVVHD), which removes fluid and solutes at a slow controlled rate, is increasingly used in critically ill patients with ARF who do not tolerate the hemodynamic effects of intermittent hemodialysis. The main problem associated with CRRT is the expense, since the membrane is prone to clot formation and, therefore, must be periodically replaced. Despite this limitation, many experts believe CRRT is the best way to manage ICU patients with ARF.

Another change in the management of ARF is that whereas protein was withheld or limited to less than 0.4–0.6 g/kg/d, most nephrologists now believe that nutrition supplementation should not be withheld, and 1.0–1.5 g/kg/d of protein can be given, especially for patients on CRRT.

■ SEPSIS & SEPTIC SHOCK

The systemic inflammatory response to infection is commonly termed sepsis. This response is not unique to severe infections because similar manifestations may be encountered with noninfectious illnesses (Figure 50–8). Moreover, it does not necessarily indicate the presence of bacteremia. The term systemic inflammatory response syndrome (SIRS) has been suggested by an American College of Chest Physicians/Society of Critical Care Medicine Consensus Conference (Table 50–10). Severe sepsis exists when the response is associated with organ dysfunction or generalized hypoperfusion. The term MODS has been suggested to describe progressive dysfunction of two or more organs that is associated with sepsis.

PATHOPHYSIOLOGY OF SIRS

A mild systemic inflammatory response to any bodily insult may normally have some salutatory effects. However, a marked or prolonged response, such as that associated with severe infections, is often deleterious and can result in widespread organ dysfunction. Although gram-negative organisms account for a majority of infection-related SIRS, many other infectious agents are capable of inducing the same syndrome. These organisms either elaborate toxins or stimulate release of substances that trigger this response. The most commonly

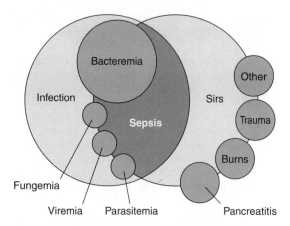

Figure 50–8. The relationship between infection, sepsis, and the systemic inflammatory response system (SIRS). (Modified from the American College of Chest Physicians/Society of Critical Care Medicine Consensus Conference: Definitions for sepsis and organ failure and guidelines for the use of innovative therapies in sepsis. Crit Care Med 1992;20:864.)

recognized initiators are the lipopolysaccharides (LPSs), which are released by gram-negative bacteria. LPS is composed of an O polysaccharide, a core, and lipid A. The O polysaccharide distinguishes between different types of gram-negative bacteria, while lipid A, an endotoxin, is responsible for the compound's toxicity. The resulting response to endotoxin involves a complex interaction between macrophages/monocytes, neutrophils, lymphocytes, platelets, and endothelial cells that can affect nearly every organ.

The central mechanism in initiating SIRS appears to be the abnormal secretion of cytokines. These low molecular weight peptides and glycoproteins function as intercellular mediators and normally regulate many biologic processes including local and systemic immune responses, inflammation, wound healing, and hematopoiesis. The most important cytokines released during SIRS are TNF and IL-1, IL-6, and IL-8. Macrophages synthesize and release TNF following exposure to triggering substances. Both TNF and IL-1 enhance their own secretion and induce the formation of other cytokines (such as IL-6, IL-8 and γ-interferon). The resulting inflammatory response involves release of potentially harmful phospholipids, attraction of neutrophils, and activation of the complement, kinin and coagulation cascades.

Increased phospholipase A_2 levels release arachidonic acid from cell membrane phospholipids. Cyclooxygenase converts arachidonic acid to thromboxane and prostaglandins, while lipoxygenase converts arachidonic acid into leukotrienes (slow reacting substances of anaphylaxis). Increased phospholipase A_2 and acetyltransferase activities result in the formation of another potent proinflammatory compound, platelet-activating factor (PAF). Attraction and activation of neutrophils release a variety of proteases and free radical compounds that damage vascular endothelium. TNF and IL-1 additionally induce endothelial cells to form abnormally large amounts of nitric oxide. Activation of monocytes causes them to express increased amounts of tissue factor, which in turn can activate both the intrinsic and extrinsic coagulation cascades.

INFECTIONS IN THE ICU

Infections are a leading cause of death in ICUs. Serious infections may be acquired outside the hospital (community-acquired) or subsequent to admission for an unrelated illness (nosocomial). The term "nosocomial infection" describes hospital-acquired infections that develop at least 48 hours following admission. The reported incidence of nosocomial infections in ICU patients ranges between 10 and 50%. Strains of bacteria resistant to commonly used antibiotics are often responsible. Host immunity plays an important role not only in determining the course of an infection but also the types of organisms that can cause infection. Thus, organisms that normally do not cause serious infections in immunocompetent patients can produce life-threatening infections in those who are immunocompromised (Table 50–11).

Critically ill patients frequently have demonstrable abnormal host defenses, including defective chemotaxis and phagocytosis, altered helper:suppressor T lymphocyte ratios, and impaired humoral immunity. Other host factors include age, drug therapy, integrity of mucosal and skin barriers, and underlying disease. Thus, advanced age (> 70 years), corticosteroid therapy, chemotherapy, prolonged use of invasive devices, respiratory failure, renal

Table 50–10. Definition of the systemic inflammatory response syndrome.

Criterion	Measurement
Altered body temperature	> 38° or 36° C
Tachycardia	> 100 beats/min
Tachypnea or hypocapnia	> 20 breaths/min < 32 mm Hg
Leukocytosis	> 12,000/μL
Leukopenia or immature leukocyte (band) forms	< 4000/μL

Table 50–11. Conditions associated with immunocompromise.

Hereditary disorders
   Defects in phagocytosis
   Defects in antibody-mediated (B cell) immunity
   Defects in cell-mediated (T cell) immunity
   Defects in complement
   Combined defects
Acquired disorders
   Neutropenia
   Splenectomy
   Acquired immunodeficiency syndrome (AIDS)
   Bone marrow transplantation
   Immunosuppressive therapy
      Organ transplantation
      Autoimmune disorders
   Cytotoxic chemotherapy
   Glucocorticoid therapy
   Radiation therapy
   Malignancies
      Multiple myeloma
      Leukemias
      Lymphomas
   Multiple transfusions

---

failure, head trauma, and burns are established risk factors for nosocomial infections. Patients with burns involving greater than 40% of body surface area have significantly increased mortality from infections. Use of topical antibiotics such as sodium mafenide, silver sulfadiazine and nystatin delays but does not prevent wound infections. Early removal of the necrotic eschar followed by skin grafting and wound closure appears to reverse immunologic defects and reduce infections.

Most nosocomial infections arise from the endogenous bacterial flora. Furthermore, many critically ill patients eventually become colonized with resistant bacterial strains. The urinary tract accounts for up to 35–40% of nosocomial infections. Urinary infections are usually due to gram-negative organisms and are associated with the use of indwelling catheters or urinary obstruction. Wound infections are the second most common cause, accounting for up to 25–30%, while pneumonia accounts for another 20–25%. Intravascular catheter-related infections are responsible for 5–10% of ICU infections.

Nosocomial pneumonias are usually caused by gram-negative organisms and are the leading cause of death in many ICUs. GI bacterial overgrowth with translocation into the portal circulation versus retrograde colonization of the upper airway from the GI tract followed by aspiration are possible mechanisms for entry for these bacteria. Preservation of gastric acidity may inhibit overgrowth of gram-negative organisms in the stomach and their migration up into the oropharynx. Endotracheal intubation does not appear to provide effective protection because patients commonly aspirate gastric fluid containing bacteria in spite of a properly functioning ETT cuff; nebulizers and humidifiers can also be sources of infection. Selective decontamination of the gut with nonabsorbable antibiotics may reduce the incidence of infection, but does not change outcome.

Wounds are common sources of sepsis in postoperative and trauma patients; limited antibiotic prophylaxis appears to decrease the incidence of postoperative infections in some groups of patients. Although more commonly seen in postoperative patients, intra-abdominal infections due to perforated ulcer, diverticulitis, appendicitis, and acalculous cholecystitis, can also develop in critically ill nonsurgical patients. Intravascular catheter-related infections are most commonly due to *Staphylococcus epidermidis, Staphylococcus aureus,* streptococci, *Candida* species and gram-negative rods. Bacterial sinusitis may be an unrecognized source of sepsis in nasally intubated patients. The diagnosis is suspected from purulent drainage and confirmed by radiographs and cultures.

SEPTIC SHOCK

An American College of Chest Physicians/Society of Critical Care Medicine Consensus Conference defined **septic shock** as sepsis associated with hypotension (systolic blood pressure < 90 mm Hg) and signs of hypoperfusion despite adequate fluid resuscitation. Septic shock is usually characterized by inadequate tissue perfusion and widespread cellular dysfunction. In contrast to other forms of shock (hypovolemic, cardiogenic, neurogenic, or anaphylactic), cellular dysfunction in septic shock is not necessarily related to the hypoperfusion. Instead, there may be a metabolic block at the cellular level that contributes to impaired cellular oxidation.

Pathophysiology

A severe or protracted SIRS can result in septic shock. Septic shock is most commonly due to gram-negative infections arising from the genitourinary tract or from the lungs in hospitalized patients, but identical presentations are also seen with other pathogens. Bacteremia is usually present, but may be absent. Increased levels of TNF and IL-1 cause generalized vasodilation and increased capillary permeability. Increased nitric oxide levels may be responsible for the vasodilation. The hypotension is also due to a decreased circulating intravascular volume resulting from a diffuse capillary leak.

Many patients also manifest evidence of myocardial depression. Activation of platelets and the coagulation cascade can lead to the formation of fibrin-platelet aggregates, which further compromise tissue blood flow. Hypoxemia resulting from ARDS accentuates tissue hypoxia. The release of vasoactive substances, formation of microthrombi in the pulmonary circulation, or both together, increase pulmonary vascular resistance.

Hemodynamic Subsets:

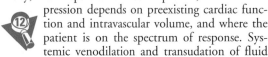

The circulation in patients with septic shock is often described as either hyperdynamic or hypodynamic. In reality, both represent the same process, but their expression depends on preexisting cardiac function and intravascular volume, and where the patient is on the spectrum of response. Systemic venodilation and transudation of fluid into tissues results in a relative hypovolemia in all patients.

Hyperdynamic septic shock is characterized by normal or elevated cardiac output and profound vasodilation (low systemic vascular resistance). Decreased myocardial contractility is often demonstrable even in hyperdynamic patients. Mixed venous oxygen saturation is characteristically high in the absence of hypoxemia and likely reflects the high cardiac output and the cellular metabolic defect in oxygen utilization.

Hypodynamic septic shock, usually seen later in the course of shock, is characterized by decreased cardiac output with low or normal systemic vascular resistance. It is more likely to be seen in severely hypovolemic patients and those with underlying cardiac disease. Myocardial depression is a prominent feature. Mixed venous oxygen saturation may be low in these patients. Pulmonary hypertension is also often prominent in septic shock. Elevation of pulmonary vascular resistance widens the normal pulmonary artery diastolic to wedge pressure gradient; large gradients have been associated with a higher mortality rate. The increase in pulmonary vascular resistance may contribute to right ventricular dysfunction.

Clinical Manifestations

Manifestations of septic shock appear to be primarily related to host response rather than the infective agent. Septic shock classically presents with an abrupt onset of chills, fever, nausea (and often vomiting), decreased mental status, tachypnea, hypotension, and tachycardia. The patient may appear flushed and feel warm (hyperdynamic) or pale with cool and often cyanotic extremities (hypodynamic); in the latter case, a high index of suspicion is required. In old, debilitated patients and in infants, the diagnosis often is less obvious and hypothermia may be seen.

Leukocytosis with a leftward shift to premature cell forms is typical, but leukopenia can be seen with overwhelming sepsis and is an ominous sign. Progressive metabolic acidosis (usually lactic acidosis) is typically partially compensated by a concomitant respiratory alkalosis. Elevated lactate levels reflect both increased production resulting from poor tissue perfusion and decreased uptake by the liver and kidneys. Hypoxemia may herald the onset of ARDS. Oliguria is most commonly due to the combination of hypovolemia, hypotension, and a systemic inflammatory insult and often progresses to ARF. Elevations in serum aminotransferases and bilirubin are due to hepatic dysfunction. Insulin resistance is uniformly present and produces hyperglycemia. Thrombocytopenia is common and often an early sign of sepsis. Laboratory evidence of disseminated intravascular coagulation (DIC) is often present but is rarely associated with a bleeding diathesis. The latter only responds to control of the sepsis. Gastric mucosal stress ulceration is common. Respiratory and renal failure are the leading causes of death.

Neutropenic patients (absolute neutrophil count 500/μL) may develop macular or papular lesions that can ulcerate and become gangrenous (ecthyma gangrenosum). These lesions are commonly associated with *Pseudomonas* septicemia but can be caused by other organisms. Perirectal abscesses can develop very quickly in neutropenic patients with few external signs; patients may only complain of perirectal pain.

Treatment

Septic shock is a medical emergency that requires immediate and aggressive intervention. Treatment is threefold: (1) control and eradication of the infection by appropriate and timely intravenous antibiotics, drainage of abscesses, debridement of necrotic tissues, and removal of infected foreign bodies; (2) maintenance of adequate perfusion with intravenous fluids and inotropic agents; and (3) supportive treatment of complications such as ARDS, ARF, GI bleeding, and DIC.

Antibiotic treatment must be initiated before pathogens are identified but after adequate cultures are obtained (usually of blood, urine, wounds, and sputum). Combination therapy with two or more antibiotics is generally indicated until pathogens are known. In most instances, the combination of a penicillin/β-lactamase inhibitor or third-generation cephalosporin with an aminoglycoside is adequate (Table 50–12). Additional diagnostic studies may be indicated, eg, thoracentesis, paracentesis, lumbar puncture, or computed tomographic scans. Debridement and drainage of infections and abscesses should be undertaken expeditiously.

Empiric antibiotic therapy in immunocompromised patients should be based on pathogens that are gener-

Table 50–12. Initial Antibiotic Therapy for Life-threatening Infectious Disease Syndromes.

Syndrome	Pathogens	Initial Empiric Regimens
Cryptogenic sepsis *without* identifiable local infection Community-acquired		
Immunocompetent	*Staphylococcus aureus* *Neisseria meningitidis* Group A streptococci	Ceftriaxone or cefotaxime (levofloxicin or gatifloxi-cin[1]) *plus* vancomycin (*if* MRSA in community-acquired infections or has long-term CVC)
A child or elderly adult, or immunocompromised	Same as above *plus* *Streptococcus pneumoniae* (including PRP) *Salmonella* *Listeria*	Ceftriaxone or cefotaxime *plus* ampicillin (vancomycin[1])
Nosocomial	*S. aureus* (including MRSA) Enterococcus (possible VRE) *Pseudomonas aeruginosa* and other resistant gram-negative bacilli	Cefepime, carbapenem or anti-pseudomonal penicillin (aztreonam[1]) *plus* ciprofloxacin or tobramycin plus vancomycin (*if* risk MRSA/MRCNS) plus drug for VRE *only* if known culture-positive
Granulocytopenic fever	Same as above	Cefepime or carbapenem *Add* vancomycin (*if* cellulitis, CVC spesis, septic shock or known MRSA-positive) Ciprofloxacin *plus* vancomycin[1]
Acute bacterial endocarditis		
Native valve	*S. aureus* Group A streptococci Gram-negative bacilli *Enterococcus*	Penicillin *plus* nafcillin (vancomycin[1]) plus gentamicin
Prosthetic Valve	Same as above *plus* coagulase-negative Staphylococcus MRSA Nosocmial gram-negative bacilli *Candida*	Vancomycin *plus* gentamicin
Susptected IV line spesis	Same as above	Vancomycin *plus* ciprofloxacin or gentamicin
Presumed bacterial pneumonia, Community-acquired	*S. pneumoniae* *S. aureus* Oral anaerobes Enteric gram-negative bacilli *Legionella* *Chlamydia pneumoniae*	Ceftriaxone or cefotaxime plus azithromycin Levofloxicin or gatifloxicin[1]
Nosocomial or severe community-acquired requiring ICU care	Same as above *plus* *P. aeruginosa* MRSA	Cefepime or piperacillin-tazobactam or carbapenem (aztreonam[1]) *plus* ciprofloxacin, *plus* vancomycin (*if* risk MRSA)
Sinusitis		
Community-acquired	*S. pneumoniae* *Haemophilus influenzae* *S. aureus*	Cefotaxime or ceftriaxone Levofloxicin or gatifloxicin[1] *Add* vancomyucin (if risk MRSA)
Nosocomial	*S. aureus* (including MRSA) Gram-negative bacilli Fungi	Same as nosocomial pneumonia

(continued)

Table 50–12. Initial Antibiotic Therapy for Life-threatening Infectious Disease Syndromes. (continued)

Syndrome	Pathogens	Initial Empiric Regimens
Nosocomial	S. aureus (including MRSA) Gram-negative bacilli Fungi	Same as nosocomial pneumonia

Presumed bacterial meningitis
Community-acquired
	S. pneumoniae
	Haemophilus influenzae
	  Type B
	Neisseria meningitidis
	Listeria monocytogenes
		Ceftriaxone, cefotaxime or cefepime *and*
		  vancomycin,
		    add rifampin (if also giving corticosteroids)

Nosocomial	Enteric gram-negative bacilli
	P. aeruginosa
	S. aureus (including MRSA)
	  coagulase-negative
	  Staphylococcus
		Cefepime or piperacillin-tazobactam *plus*
		  ciprofloxacin *plus* vancomycin

Intra-abdominal infections
Cholangitis
	Enteric gram-negative
	  bacilli
	Enterococci
	Clostridium
		Ciprofloxacin or gentamicin plus ampicillin
		  (vancomycin[1])
		Third-generation cephalosporin *plus* ampillicin
		  (vancomycin)
		Carbapenem
		Aztreonam *plus* vancomycin[1]

Secondary peritonitis or intra- abdominal abscess, granulo- cytopenic typhlitis	Same as above *plus Bacteroides fragilis* Other anaerobes	Metronidazole or clindamycin, *plus* gentamicin or ciprofloxacin *plus* ampicillin (vancomycin[1]) Ampicillin-sulbactam *and* gentamicin Piperacillin-tazobactam *and* gentamicin Carbapenem
Spontaneous bacterial peritonitis	Gram-negative bacilli S. pneumoniae	Ceftriaxone or cefotaxime Ciprofloxacin *and* vancomycin[1] Levofloxicin or gatifloxicin[1]
Urosepsis[2] Community-acquired	Enteric gram-negative bacilli Enterococcus	Ciprofloxacin *and* ampicillin (vancomycin[1]) Gentamicin (tobramycin) *and* ampicillin (vancomycin[1])
Nosocomial	Same as above *plus* P. aeruginosa VRE	Same Carbapenem Give quinupristin or linezolid *only* for documented VRE
Skin and soft tissue Uncomplicated, without granulocytopenia	S. aureus Beta-hemolytic streptococci	Nafcillin *with* or *without* penicillin (vancomycin[1]) Vancomycin[1] Ceftriaxone or cefotaxime (children)

Granulocytopenia	S. aureus
	Gram-negative bacilli,
	  including P. aeruginosa
		Cefepime or ticarcillin-claviculate or piperacillin-
		  tazobactam *and* ciprofloxacin or tobramycin *plus*
		  vancomycin

Necrotizing fasciitis	Gram-negative bacilli Clostridia and B. fragilis S. aureus Group A streptococci Vibrio vulnificans	Same as secondary peritonitis Doxycycline Ceftriaxone or cefotaxime

(continued)

Table 50–12. Initial Antibiotic Therapy for Life-threatening Infectious Disease Syndromes. (continued)

Syndrome	Pathogens	Initial Empiric Regimens
Streptococcal toxic shock syndrome with necrotizing cellulitis	Toxigenic Group A streptococci	Penicillin (vancomycin) *plus* clindamycin
Enteric infection		
Bacterial pathogens	*Salmonella* *Shigella* *Campylobacter* Enteropathogenic *Escherichia coli* *Vibrio*	Ciprofloxacin *orally* Ceftriaxone or cefotaxime IV
Antibiotic-associated colitis	*C. difficile*	Metronidazole (mild or moderately severe) Vancomycin (severe), *also* give IV metronidazole (if ileus)
Toxic shock syndrome	*S. aureus* Group A streptococci	Nafcillin *and* clindamycin Penicillin G *and* clindamycin
Malaria		
Non-falciparum species	*Plasmodium vivax* *Plasmodium malariae* *Plasmodium ovale*	Chloroquine, followed by primaquine[3]
Falciparum	*Plasmodium falciparum*[4]	Quinine orally (Quinine IV) *plus* doxycycline or clindamycin Atrovaquone-proguanil Mefloquine[5] Artesunate *plus* mefloquine
Rickettsial infections	*Ricketssia rickettsii* *Ricketssia typi* *Ricketssia prowazeki* *Ricketssia akari* *Coxiella burnetii* *Ehrlichia chaffeensis* and *Ehrlichia phagocytophilia*	Doxycycline Chloramphenicol

[1]For serious penicillin hypersensitivity.
[2]Gram stain of the urine will show organisms and allow determination, with >98% reliability, whether a drug regimen is needed for gram-negative bacilli alone, for gram-positive cocci alone, or both.
[3]Check for G-6 PD deficiency before giving primaquine.
[4]Assume all falciparum infections are caused by chloroquine-resistant strain.
[5]Mefloquine resistance is growing.
MRSA, methicillin-resistant staphylococcus aureus; CVC, central venous catheter; PRP, penicillin-resistant pneumococcus; VRE, vancomycin-resistant enterococci; MRCNS, methicillin-resistant coagulase-negative staphylococcus.

Reproduced with permission from Maki D. 2002. Management of life threatening infections in the ICU. In Murray MJ, Coursin DB, Pearl R, Pough D (eds). *Critical Care Medicine: Perioperative Management.* Philadelphia: Lippincott Williams & Wilkins.

ally associated with the immune defect (Table 50–13). Vancomycin is added if intravascular catheter-related infection is suspected. Clindamycin or metronidazole should be given to neutropenic patients if a rectal abscess is suspected. Many clinicians initiate amphotericin B or fluconazole therapy for a presumed fungal infection, or when an immunocompromised patient continues to experience fever after 96 hours of antibiotic therapy. Granulocyte colony stimulating factor or granulocyte macrophage colony stimulating factor may be used to shorten the period of neutropenia; granulocyte transfusion may occasionally be used in refractory gram-negative bacteremia. Diffuse interstitial infiltrates on a chest radiograph may suggest unusual bacterial, parasitic, or viral pathogens; many clinicians initiate empiric therapy with trimethoprim-sulfamethoxazole and erythromycin in such instances. Nodular infiltrates on a radiograph suggest a fungal pneumonia and may warrant amphotericin B therapy. Antiviral therapy should be considered in septic patients who are more

Table 50–13. Infections Associated with Altered Host Immunity

| Host Defect | Pathogens Encountered at the Site of Infection | | | |
	Bloodstream or Disseminated	Pulmonary	Central Nervous System	Gastrointestinal
Hypogammaglobulinemia	Streptococcus pneumoniae Haemophilus influenzae Neisseria meningitidis	S. pneumoniae H. influenzae Branhamella catarrhalis	S. pneumoniae H. influenzae	Giardia lamblia
Splenectomy	Same as above, plus Bartonella, Plasmodium, Babesia,	as above	as above	
Cell-mediated immunity	Listeria monocytogenes Salmonella Mycobacterium tuberculosis Coccidioides immitis Histoplasma capsulatum Cryptococcus neoformans Cytomegalovirus Varicella-zoster virus Herpes simplex virus	Legionella Nocardia Mycobacteria C. immitis H. capsulatum Pneumocystis carinii Cytomegalovirus	Listeria M. tuberculosis C. neoformans Toxoplasma gondii Herpes simplex virus Cytomegalo- virus	Salmonella Campylobacter Candida Cryptosporidium Entamoeba histolytica Strongyloides stercoralis Cytomegalovirus Herpes simplex virus

Tumorous obstruction	Cholangitis:
	  Gram-negative bacilli
	  Enterococcus
	  Clostridium
	Urosepsis:
	  Gram-negative bacilli
	  Enterococcus
	  Candida
	Pneumonia:
	  Staphylococcus
	  S. aureus
	  Oral anaerobes
		S. pneumoniae
		S. aureus
		Oral anaerobes
				Gram-negative bacilli
				Enterococci
				Clostridium
				Bacteroides fragilis

Granulocytopenia	Gram-negative bacilli, especially Pseudomonas aeruginosa Staphylococci Fusarium spp. Candida spp.	Gram-negative Staphylococci Aspergillus	Aspergillus Candida	Candida Clostridium difficile Other clostridia Herpes simplex virus
Reactivation of latent infections	H. capsultaum C. immitis Plasmodium	M. tuberculosis	M. tuberculosis H. capsulatum C. immitis Toxoplasma gondii	S. stercoralis
Central venous catheter	Staphylococcus epidermidis S. aureus Corynebacterium JK Mycobacterium Bacillus Candida Fusarium Trichosporan			

than 1 month status-post bone marrow or solid organ transplantation.

Tissue oxygenation and perfusion are maintained with oxygen therapy, intravenous fluids, inotropes, and packed red blood cell transfusions to keep hemoglobin levels > 8–10 g/dL. Marked "third spacing" is characteristic of septic shock. An inotrope should be used if intravenous fluids fail to quickly restore adequate perfusion. Colloid solutions more rapidly restore intravascular volume compared with crystalloid solutions. Inotropic therapy is generally initiated if 1–3 L of intravenous fluids does not correct the hypotension. Hematocrit should probably be maintained at or above 24–30% to enhance oxygen delivery. Pulmonary artery catheterization greatly facilitates management in such instances because it allows measurement of PAOP, and cardiac output. Most clinicians generally select dopamine as the initial inotrope, while others use dobutamine because the latter more effectively increases cardiac output and oxygen delivery (Table 50–14). Some studies suggest that patient mortality may be lower if oxygen delivery can be increased. When either dopamine or dobutamine is ineffective in increasing blood pressure and cardiac output, epinephrine (2–18 μg/min) is the agent of choice. In patients with refractory hypotension, vasopressin is increasingly administered with a good improvement in blood pressure but without evidence that it affects outcome. Severe acidosis may decrease the efficacy of inotropes and should therefore generally be corrected (pH > 7.20) with bicarbonate therapy in patients with refractory hypotension. Even in the absence of arterial hypotension, "renal" doses of dopamine may be helpful in maintaining urinary output and preventing renal failure in oliguric patients. The use of corticosteroids, naloxone, opsonins (fibronectin) and monoclonal antibodies directed against lipopolysaccharide in septic shock has been disappointing, but inhibitors of the coagulation cascade show promise. One such agent (Protein C) has been approved by the U.S. Food and Drug Administration for use during sepsis.

■ GASTROINTESTINAL HEMORRHAGE

Acute GI hemorrhage is a common reason for admission to the ICU. Advanced age (> 60 years), comorbid conditions, hypotension, marked blood loss (> 5 units), and recurrent hemorrhage (rebleeding) after 72 hours increase mortality. Management consists of simultaneous and rapid evaluation and identification of the site of bleeding and stabilization. Although volume resuscitation is similar, the clinician must attempt to differentiate between upper GI and lower GI bleeding. A history of hematemesis indicates bleeding proximal to the ligament of Treitz. Melena often indicates bleeding proximal to the cecum. Hematochezia (bright red blood from the rectum) indicates either very brisk upper GI bleeding or more commonly lower GI bleeding. The former is likely to be associated with hypotension. Maroon stools usually localizes the bleeding to the area between the distal small bowel and the right colon.

At least two large-bore (14–16 gauge) intravenous cannulas should be placed and blood should be sent for laboratory analysis (including hematocrit, hemoglobin, platelet count, prothrombin time, and activated partial thromboplastin time). The patient should also be typed and crossed for at least 4–6 units. Fluid resuscitation guidelines are discussed in Chapter 29. Serial hematocrits are useful but may not accurately reflect true blood loss. Intra-arterial blood pressure monitoring is very helpful. Central venous cannulation is useful for both venous access and pressure measurements. Placement of a nasogastric tube may help identify an upper GI source if bright red blood or "coffee grounds" material can be aspirated; inability to aspirate blood, however, does not rule out an upper GI source.

Upper GI Bleeding

Lavage through a nasogastric tube can help assess the rate of bleeding and facilitate esophagoduodenoscopy (EGD). EGD should be performed whenever possible to diagnose the cause of bleeding. Failure to visualize the source by endoscopy because of brisk bleeding requires arteriography. Both EGD and arteriography can also be used therapeutically to stop the bleeding. The most common causes of upper GI bleeding, in decreasing frequency, are duodenal ulcer, gastric ulcer, erosive gastritis, and esophageal varices. Erosive gastritis may

Table 50–14. Effects of inotropes in septic patients.

Agent	Blood Pressure	Cardiac Output	Oxygen Delivery
Dopamine	↑↑	↑	↑
Dobutamine	0 or ↑	↑↑	↑↑
Norepinephrine	↑↑	0	0
Epinephrine	↑↑↑	↑↑↑	↑↑↑
Vasopressin	↑↑	0	0

be due to stress, alcohol, aspirin, NSAIDs, and possibly corticosteroids. Less common causes include angiodysplasia, erosive esophagitis, Mallory-Weiss tear, gastric tumor, and aortoenteric fistula.

Bleeding from peptic ulcers (gastric or duodenal) can be coagulated via EGD. Surgery is generally indicated for severe hemorrhage (> 5 units) and recurrent bleeding. H_2 receptor blockers are ineffective in stopping the bleeding but may reduce the likelihood of rebleeding. Selective arteriography of the bleeding vessel allows localized infusion of vasopressin (0.15–0.20 units/min) or arterial embolization.

The most effective treatment for erosive gastritis is prevention. Proton pump inhibitors, H_2 receptor blockers, antacids, and sucralfate are all effective for prevention. Many gastroenterologists advocate the routine administration of a proton pump inhibitor. Currently, they are only available by mouth in the United States, but intravenous pantoprazole should be available soon. Once bleeding has occurred, there is generally no specific therapy.

Endoscopic therapy, either with bipolar electrocoagulation or heater probes, is the most effective nonsurgical treatment that reduces blood transfusions, rebleeding, hospital stay, and the need for urgent surgery. Intravenous vasopressin infusions (0.3–0.8 units/min) are generally not as effective; concomitant infusion of nitroglycerin can help reduce portal pressure and may reduce the incidence of cardiac complications. Intravenous propranolol can also lower portal venous pressure and may reduce variceal bleeding. Balloon tamponade (Sengstaken-Blakemore, Minnesota, or Linton tubes) may be used as adjunctive therapy, but usually require elective endotracheal intubation to protect the airway against aspiration.

Lower GI Bleeding

Common causes of lower GI bleeding include diverticulosis, angiodysplasia, neoplasms, inflammatory bowel disease, ischemic colitis, infectious colitis, and anorectal disease (hemorrhoids, fissure, or fistula). Rectal examination, anoscopy, and sigmoidoscopy can usually diagnose very distal lesions. As with EGD, colonoscopy usually allows definitive diagnosis and is often useful therapeutically. A technetium-99 labeled red blood scan can be used to identify the source of bleeding when colonoscopy cannot be carried out because of inadequate preparation.

Cauterization of the site of bleeding is often possible via colonoscopy. When colonoscopy is unavailable or not possible because of brisk bleeding, selective arteriography can be used to identify the source which is either embolized or infused with vasopressin. Surgical

treatment is reserved for severe or recurrent hemorrhage.

■ NUTRITIONAL SUPPORT

The importance of maintaining adequate nutrition in critically ill patients cannot be overemphasized. Severe malnutrition causes widespread organ dysfunction and increases perioperative morbidity and mortality rates. Nutritional repletion may improve wound healing, restore immune competence, and reduce morbidity and mortality rates in critically ill patients.

OVERVIEW OF NUTRITION

Maintenance of normal body mass, composition, structure, and function requires the periodic intake of water, energy substrates, and specific nutrients. Nutrients that cannot be synthesized from other nutrients are characterized as "essential." Remarkably, relatively few essential nutrients are required to form the thousands of compounds that make up the body. Known essential nutrients include 8–10 amino acids, two fatty acids, 13 vitamins, and approximately 16 minerals.

Energy is normally derived from dietary or endogenous carbohydrates, fats, and protein. Metabolic breakdown of these substrates yields the ATP required for normal cellular function. Dietary fats and carbohydrates normally supply most of the body's energy requirements. Dietary proteins provide amino acids for protein synthesis; however, when their supply exceeds both essential and nonessential amino acid requirements, they also function as energy substrates. The metabolic pathways of carbohydrate, fat, and amino acid substrates overlap such that some interconversions can occur through metabolic intermediates (see Figure 34–3). Excess amino acids can therefore be converted to carbohydrate or fatty acid precursors. Excess carbohydrates are stored as glycogen in the liver and skeletal muscle. When glycogen stores are saturated (200–400 g in adults), excess carbohydrate is converted to fatty acids stored as triglycerides primarily in fat cells.

Normal Energy Requirements

Total energy requirements vary widely and depend on the basal metabolic rate (BMR), specific dynamic action (energy required for digestion of meals), and a person's activity level. BMR is energy expenditure measured in the morning immediately after awakening, 12 hours after the last meal, and in a state of thermal neutrality. Clinically, basal energy expenditure (BEE) in kilocalories can be estimated by the Harris-Benedict equation, using weight in kilograms, height in centimeters, and age in years:

Males: BEE = 66 + (13.7 × weight [kg]) + (5 × height [cm])
    − (6.8 × age)
Females: BEE = 655 + (9.6 × weight [kg]) + (1.8 × height
    [cm]) − (4.7 × age)

BEE is increased by temperature (13% per °C), and degree of stress (see below).

Organ-Specific Substrate Utilization

Variations in the ability to store glycogen and triglycerides, enzyme pathways, and membrane transport mechanisms result in differing substrate utilizations between organs. Neurons, red cells, and cells of the renal medulla normally utilize only glucose. The liver, heart, skeletal muscle, and renal cortex preferentially rely on fatty acid metabolism for energy.

Starvation

The physiology of starvation is such that the protein content of essential tissues is spared. As blood glucose concentration begins to fall during fasting, insulin secretion decreases while glucagon increases. Hepatic and, to a lesser extent, renal glycogenolysis and gluconeogenesis are enhanced (see Chapter 34). Because glycogen supplies are depleted within 24 hours, gluconeogenesis becomes increasingly important. The liver uses chiefly deaminated amino acids (alanine and glutamine) as precursors for glucose synthesis. Only neural tissue, renal medullary cells, and erythrocytes continue to utilize glucose, in effect sparing tissue proteins. Lipolysis in adipose tissue is enhanced, so that fats become the principal energy source. Glycerol from the triglycerides enters the glycolytic pathway, while fatty acids are broken down to acetyl-CoA. Excess acetyl-CoA results in the formation of ketone bodies (ketosis). Some fatty acids can contribute to gluconeogenesis. If starvation is prolonged, the brain, kidneys, and muscle also begin to utilize ketone bodies efficiently.

NUTRITION IN CRITICAL ILLNESS

Perioperative critical illnesses are usually characterized by tissue injury, a neuroendocrine stress response, and starvation. The response to injury involves increases in the secretion of catecholamines, cortisol, glucagon, thyroxine, angiotensin, aldosterone, growth hormone, ACTH, ADH, and TSH. Insulin secretion is at least initially decreased but may subsequently rise due to increasing levels of growth hormone.

Catecholamines, glucagon, and perhaps growth hormone promote glycogenolysis, while glucagon and possibly cortisol induce gluconeogenesis. Hyperglycemia is characteristic and reflects increased hepatic production as well as decreased utilization by peripheral tissues. Moreover, decreased tolerance to glucose loads occurs, apparently as a result of both decreased insulin secretion and peripheral resistance to its actions. Both effects are probably due to increased catecholamine secretion, which also enhances lipolysis. Both protein synthesis and breakdown are increased, but the latter exceeds the former, so that there is a net loss of tissue protein. During sepsis, muscle utilization of fat and carbohydrate is impaired resulting in increased protein breakdown. Moreover, cells appear to rely more on branched-chain amino acids. Circulating levels of glutamine are decreased. Glutamine is the most prevalent free amino acid in the body. It is an important intermediate in a large number of metabolic pathways. Moreover, rapidly proliferating cells, such as those of the immune system and the GI tract, utilize this amino acid as an energy source.

Glucose administration during acute illnesses fails to suppress protein breakdown. An adequate intake of calories and proteins can decrease but not prevent protein catabolism in a stressed patient.

Nutritional Assessment of Patients

Evaluation of nutritional status is central to nutritional support of critically ill patients. With the subjective global assessment, a clinician takes a history to detect weight loss, dietary habits, and symptoms of hypoproteinemia (edema) and examines the patient for evidence of loss of skeletal mass or fat stores, edema, or jaundice. He or she would then classify the patient as being normally nourished or mildly or severely malnourished. Alternately, one can use anthropometric measurements, cutaneous hypersensitivity tests, and laboratory determinations to classify a patient's degree of malnutrition. Patients requiring close assessment include those with less than 80% acceptable body weight or weight loss exceeding 10% in the preceding 6 months; those with serum albumin < 3 g/dL or serum transferrin < 150 mg/dL; those with skin anergy; and those with low total lymphocyte counts (< 1200 cells/μL).

Comparison of body weight to acceptable body weight criteria and measurement of skinfolds are generally indicative of body fat stores. Midarm muscle circumference measurements and the urinary creatinine excretion to height index reflect skeletal protein muscle mass. Serum albumin and transferrin measurements generally indicate protein synthetic ability, although the serum albumin is a better marker of severity of illness. Prealbumin, because of its shorter half-life, is occasionally followed to try to help assess adequacy of anabolism.

Calculating Energy Requirements

Caloric requirements are usually derived by means of the Harris-Benedict equation (see above). Some clinicians multiply the BMR by a stress factor according to the degree of tissue injury and severity of illness:

Stress factor = 1–1.25 for mild starvation
= 1.25–1.5 for moderate to severe illness
= 1.5–1.75 for severe illness

Most nutritionists, however, give critically ill patients only 20–30 kcal/kg/d as such patients have impaired cellular metabolism—glucose and fatty acids are not completely oxidized. Instead, metabolic intermediates are transported from the cells back to the liver where they are recycled (substrate cycling), increasing metabolic rate even further.

Calculating Energy Expenditure

The resting energy expenditure (REE [not truly basal as the patient is stressed]) can be calculated using indirect calorimetry. This technique relies on measuring oxygen consumption and carbon dioxide production, according to the formula:

$$REE = (3.94 \times \dot{V}O_2) + (1.11 \times \dot{V}CO_2)$$

This calculation is not accurate during gluconeogenesis and lipogenesis.

The respiratory quotient, $\dot{V}O_2/\dot{V}CO_2$, may indicate the primary fuel utilized: an RQ of 1 reflects glucose utilization; a quotient of 0.7 reflects lipid oxidation. Values above 1 reflect lipogenesis.

Calculating Protein Requirements

In contrast to nonstressed patients, who require about 0.5 g/kg/d of protein, critically ill patients generally require 1.0–1.5 g/kg/d. Increasing protein intake to > 1.5 g/kg/d increases anabolism and catabolism such that there is not an increase in net protein balance.

ENTERAL NUTRITION

The GI tract is the route of choice for nutritional support when its functional integrity is intact. Enteral feedings can be used to provide complete or supplemental nutrition. Enteral nutrition is simpler, cheaper, less complicated, and associated with fewer complications than parenteral nutrition. Moreover, enteral nutrition appears to better preserve GI structure and function than the parenteral route, especially when glutamine-rich preparations are used; studies also suggest that early (1–3 days) enteral nutrition may blunt the hypermetabolic response to improve the host response to infection.

Enteral feedings are most often given as a continuous infusion through a small-bore nasogastric or nasoduodenal tube, gastrostomy, or feeding jejunostomy tube. Therapy is usually initiated at a rate of 25 mL/hour and is increased slowly over the course of a few days until the desired caloric and protein goals are reached. Most enteral formulas contain polymeric mixtures of proteins, fats, and carbohydrates. Numerous preparations are available. Selection is based on osmolality, and fat content. Some formulas are composed of elemental low-residue formulas. Elemental formulas are indicated in patients with short bowel syndrome, GI fistula, inflammatory bowel disease, and those who have been NPO (nothing by mouth) for weeks; they are readily absorbed and have low residues. Medium-chain triglycerides (MCT) are composed of 8 to 10 carbon-chain fatty acids that do not require bile salts or pancreatic enzymes for absorption; MCT oils are indicated for patients with pancreatic insufficiency and cholestasis.

Diarrhea is one of the most common problems with enteral feedings and is usually related either to hyperosmolarity of the solution or lactose intolerance. Gastric distention is another complication that increases the risk of regurgitation and pulmonary aspiration; duodenal or jejunostomy tubes should decrease its incidence. Progressive abdominal distention or large gastric residual volumes are indicative of ileus and should prompt discontinuation of enteral feedings.

PARENTERAL NUTRITION

Total parenteral nutrition (TPN) is indicated if the GI tract cannot be used or if absorption is inadequate. TPN formulas utilize hyperosmolar solutions of amino acids and glucose mixed together. The hypertonic nature of these solutions requires central venous access. Electrolytes, trace elements, and a multivitamin preparation are added. Parenteral glucose solutions provide only 3.4 kcal/g (compared with 4 kcal/g for dry carbohydrate) because their glucose concentration is expressed as the monohydrate. Fats are given in the form of a fat emulsion that can be infused separately or mixed with the glucose-amino acid solution. Fat emulsions are available as either 10% (1.1 kcal/mL) or 20% (2 kcal/mL). Failure to give fat at least once a week may result in essential fatty acid deficiency, which is manifested as dermatitis, alopecia, hepatomegaly (fatty liver), and defective immunity. In order to infuse an adequate amount of calories in the least volume, fat is often given on a daily basis.

The amount of amino acids given is determined by estimated protein requirements (see above), while glucose and fat are given to the desired caloric requirements (see above). Fat calories generally should account for 30–40% of desired caloric requirements. Excessive reliance on glucose exacerbates problems with hyperglycemia and increases CO_2 production. The latter may be a problem in weaning patients with a compromised pulmonary reserve from mechanical ventilation.

Complications of TPN are either metabolic or related to central venous access (Table 50–15). Overfeeding with excess amounts of glucose can increase energy requirements and carbon dioxide production; the respiratory quotient can exceed 1 because of lipogenesis (RQ 2.75). Overfeeding can lead to reversible cholestatic jaundice. Mild elevations of serum transaminases and alkaline phosphatase may reflect fatty infiltration of the liver resulting from overfeeding.

TPN can be modified for patients with significant hepatic or renal impairment. Altering the amino acid load may be beneficial in patients with hepatic encephalopathy (see Chapter 34). Plasma amino acid concentrations tend to be altered in these patients: phenylalanine and methionine are usually elevated, while branched-chain amino acids (leucine, isoleucine, and valine) are reduced. Amino acid formulations for patients with liver disease (Hepatamine) are therefore rich in branched-chain amino acids but low in aromatic amino acids. Patients with hepatic encephalopathy can be tried on Hepatamine, which is continued if there is evidence of improvement in the mental status.

Protein content is no longer reduced in patients with ARF. With the availability of CRRT, it is better to feed these patients adequate amounts of protein (1.0–1.5 g of protein/kg/d). Total TPN volume, acid-base balance, and potassium content must be altered based on patient assessment.

Monitoring Patients on TPN

Initiation of TPN requires close metabolic monitoring. The most common problem is hyperglycemia. A gradual increase in the infusion rate lessens the severity of hyperglycemia and allows sufficient time for enhanced endogenous insulin secretion. Stressed patients often require the addition of insulin to the TPN solution. Abrupt withdrawal of TPN can precipitate hypoglycemia due to high circulating insulin levels, but this is not a common problem if the

Table 50–15. Complications of total parenteral nutrition.

Catheter-related
  Pneumothorax
  Hemothorax
  Chylothorax
  Hydothorax
  Air embolism
  Cardiac tamponade
  Thrombosis
    Subclavian vein
    Vena cava
    Pulmonary thromboembolism
  Catheter sepsis
Metabolic
  Azotemia
  Hepatic dysfunction
  Cholestasis
  Hyperglycemia
    Hyperosmolar coma
    Diabetic ketoacidosis
  Excessive CO_2 production
  Hypoglycemia (due to interruption of infusion)
  Metabolic acidosis or alkalosis
  Hypernatremia
  Hyperkalemia
  Hypokalemia
  Hypocalcemia
  Hypophosphatemia
  Hyperlipidemia
  Pancreatitis
  Fat embolism syndrome
  Anemia
    Iron
    Folate
    B_{12}
    ? Copper
  Vitamin D deficiency
  Vitamin K deficiency
  Essential fatty acid deficiency
  Hypervitaminosis A
  Hypervitaminosis D

patient is not overfed; in these instances, 10% glucose can be temporarily used and gradually decreased. Serum glucose measurements should generally be measured every 4 hours until they stabilize. Other measurements (serum electrolytes, BUN, creatinine) are obtained daily. Calcium, phosphate, and magnesium concentrations and liver tests (including prealbumin) can be checked weekly. The complete blood cell count (including a differential count) should also be followed. Lipid clearance can be checked by measuring a serum triglyceride level if there is any evidence of lipemia or concern about pancreatitis, or in patients with a history of abnormal lipoprotein concentrations. Twenty-four-hour nitrogen balance studies are sometimes used in checking the efficacy of nutritional support:

$$\text{Nitrogen balance} = \text{input} - \text{output},$$
$$\text{Nitrogen output} = (\text{UUN} \times 1.2 \times \text{urinary volume}) + 2\,g$$

where UUN = urinary urea nitrogen concentration (g/L). The 2 g in the above equation represents fecal and integumentary nitrogen losses. UUN is multiplied by 1.2, since urea nitrogen represents only 80% of urinary nitrogen losses. Ideally, TPN should result in a positive nitrogen balance but is rarely, if ever, achieved in critically ill patients.

Anesthetic Management of Patients Receiving TPN

Patients who are receiving TPN often require surgical procedures. They require careful preoperative evaluation because of the large number of potentially serious complications that can be associated with TPN (Table 50–15). Metabolic abnormalities are relatively common and should generally be corrected preoperatively. Hypophosphatemia is a serious and often unrecognized complication that can contribute to postoperative muscle weakness and respiratory failure (see Chapter 28).

When TPN infusions are suddenly stopped or decreased perioperatively, hypoglycemia may develop. Frequent measurements of blood glucose concentration are therefore required in such instances during general anesthesia. On the other hand, if the TPN solution is continued unchanged, excessive hyperglycemia resulting in hyperosmolar nonketotic coma or ketoacidosis (in diabetics) is also possible. The neuroendocrine stress response to surgery frequently aggravates glucose intolerance. Some clinicians routinely reduce the rate of the TPN infusion, while others substitute a 10% dextrose solution, although with the current practice of not overfeeding patients, it is safe to discontinue TPN completely. Regardless of whether the TPN infusion is continued, reduced, replaced with 10% dextrose, or stopped, subsequent therapy should be based on blood glucose measurements. Blood glucose concentration should generally be maintained between 100–180 mg/dL. Lastly, to decrease the likelihood of catheter sepsis, the integrity of the TPN infusion-catheter system generally should not be violated with drug injections. Separate infusions should be used for injection of

anesthetic agents and administration of other perioperative fluids and blood.

PERIPHERAL PARENTERAL NUTRITION

When a 3–4% amino acid solution is added to a 5–10% dextrose solution, the resulting solution is still hypertonic but can generally be infused through a peripheral vein without irritation. Simultaneous infusion of a 1% fat emulsion through the same intravenous catheter further reduces the concentration and provides additional calories. Volume constraints limit caloric intake with peripheral parenteral nutrition to a maximum of 800–1200 kcal/d, which is satisfactory in a majority of patients.

 CASE DISCUSSION:
AN OBTUNDED YOUNG WOMAN

A 23-year-old woman is admitted to the hospital obtunded with slow respirations (7 breaths/min). Blood pressure is 90/60 mm Hg and the pulse is 90 beats/min. She was found at home in bed with empty bottles of diazepam, acetaminophen with codeine, and fluoxetine lying next to her.

How is the diagnosis of a drug overdose made?

The presumptive diagnosis of a drug overdose usually must be made from the history, circumstantial evidence, and any witnesses. Signs and symptoms may not be helpful. Confirmation of a suspected drug overdose or poison ingestion usually requires delayed laboratory testing for the suspected agent in body fluids. Intentional overdoses (self-poisoning) are the most common mechanism and typically occur in young adults who are depressed. Ingestion of multiple drugs is common. Benzodiazepines, antidepressants, aspirin, acetaminophen, and alcohol are the most commonly ingested agents.

Accidental overdoses frequently occur in intravenous drug abusers. Commonly abused substances include opioids, stimulants (cocaine and amphetamine), and hallucinogens (phencyclidine, PCP). Younger children occasionally accidentally ingest caustic household alkali (such as drain cleaner), acids, and hydrocarbons (such as petroleum products). Organophosphate poisoning (parathion and malathion) usually occur in adults following agricultural exposure. Overdoses and poisoning less commonly occur as an attempted homicide.

What are appropriate steps in managing this patient?

Regardless of the type of drug or poison ingested, the principles of initial supportive care are the same. Airway patency and adequate ventilation and oxygenation must be established. Unless otherwise indicated, oxygen therapy (100%) should probably be administered. Hypoventilation and obtunded airway reflexes require endotracheal intubation and mechanical ventilation. Many clinicians routinely administer naloxone (up to 2 mg), dextrose 50% (50 mL), and thiamine 100 mg intravenously to all obtunded or comatose patients until a diagnosis is established; this may help exclude or treat opioid overdose, hypoglycemia, and Wernicke-Korsakoff syndrome, respectively. The dextrose can be omitted if a glucose determination can be obtained by a fingerstick. In this case, intubation should be performed prior to naloxone because the respiratory depression is likely due to both the codeine and the diazepam.

Blood, urine, and gastric fluid should be obtained and sent for drug screening. Blood is also sent for routine hematologic and chemistry studies (including liver function). Urine is usually obtained, by bladder catheterization, while gastric fluid can be aspirated from a nasogastric tube; the latter should be placed after intubation to avoid pulmonary aspiration. Alternatively, emesis material may be tested for drugs in conscious persons.

Hypotension should generally be treated with intravenous fluids unless the patient is obviously in pulmonary edema; an inotrope may be necessary in some instances. Seizure activity may be the result of hypoxia or a pharmacologic action of a drug (tricyclic antidepressants) or poison. Seizure activity is unlikely in this patient because she ingested diazepam, a commonly used anticonvulsant.

Should flumazenil be administered?

Flumazenil should generally not be administered to patients who overdose on both a benzodiazepine and an antidepressant, or those who have a history of seizures. Reversal of the benzodiazepine's anticonvulsant action can precipitate seizure activity in such instances. Moreover, as is the case with naloxone and opioids, the half-life of flumazenil is shorter than benzodiazepines. Thus it is often preferable to ventilate the patient until the benzodiazepine effect dissipates, the patient regains consciousness, and the respiratory depression resolves.

Should any other antidotes be given?

Since the patient also ingested an unknown quantity of acetaminophen (paracetamol) administration of acetylcysteine (Mucomyst) should be considered. Acetaminophen toxicity is due to depletion of hepatic glutathione, resulting in the accumulation of toxic metabolic intermediates. Hepatic toxicity is usually associated with ingestion of more than 140 mg/kg of acetaminophen. Acetylcysteine prevents hepatic damage by acting as a sulfhydryl donor and restoring hepatic glutathione levels. If the patient is suspected of having ingested a toxic dose of acetaminophen, an initial dosage of acetylcysteine (140 mg/kg orally or by nasogastric tube) should be administered even before plasma acetaminophen levels are obtained; additional doses are given according to the measured plasma level.

What measures might limit drug toxicity?

Toxicity may be reduced by decreasing drug absorption or enhancing elimination. GI absorption of an ingested substance can be reduced by emptying stomach contents and administering activated charcoal. Both methods can be effective up to 12 hours following an ingestion. If the patient is intubated, the stomach is lavaged carefully to avoid pulmonary aspiration. Emesis may be induced in conscious patients with syrup of ipecac 30 mL (15 mL in a child). Gastric lavage and induced emesis are generally contraindicated for patients who ingest caustic substances or hydrocarbons because of a high risk of aspiration and worsening mucosal injury.

Activated charcoal 1–2 g/kg is administered orally or by nasogastric tube with a diluent. The charcoal irreversibly binds most drugs and poisons in the gut, allowing them to be eliminated in stools. In fact, charcoal can create a negative diffusion gradient between the gut and the circulation allowing the drug or poison to be effectively removed from the body.

Alkalinization of the serum with sodium bicarbonate for tricyclic antidepressant overdose is beneficial because by increasing pH, protein binding is enhanced; the sodium decreases sodium channel inhibition, and if seizures occur, the alkalinization prevents acidosis-induced cardiotoxicity.

What other methods can enhance drug elimination?

The easiest method of increasing drug elimination is forced diuresis. Unfortunately, this method is of limited use for drugs that are highly protein-bound or have large volumes of distribution. Mannitol or furosemide with saline may be used. Concomitant administration of alkali (sodium bicarbonate) enhances the elimination of weakly acidic drugs such as salicylates and barbiturates; alkalization of the urine traps the ionized form of these drugs in the renal tubules and enhances urinary elimination. Hemodialysis generally has a limited role in this type of setting; it is usually reserved for patients with severe toxicity who continue to deteriorate despite aggressive supportive therapy.

SUGGESTED READING

American Heart Association: Guidelines 2000 for Cardiopulmonary Resuscitation and Emergency Cardiovascular Care. *Circulation* (Suppl) 102:I-1-I-384, 2000.

Murray MJ, Coursin DB, Pearl RG, Prough DS: *Critical Care Medicine. Perioperative Medicine.* Lippincott Williams & Wilkins, New York, 2002.

Parillo JE, Dellinger RP (editors): *Critical Care Medicine. Principles of Diagnosis and Management.* WB Saunders and Company, New York, 2001.

Star RA: Treatment of acute renal failure. *Kidney Int* 1998;54: 1817.

Ward JJ: Medical gas therapy. In: Burton GG, Hodgkin JE, Ward JJ (editors). *Respiratory Care: A Guide to Clinical Practice,* 4th ed. Lippincott-Raven, Philadelphia, 1997:335-404.

Index

NOTE: Page numbers in **boldface** type indicate a major discussion. A *t* following a page number indicates tabular material and *f* following a page number indicates a figure. Drugs are listed under their generic names. When a drug trade name is listed, the reader is referred to the generic name.

A-a gradient. *See* **Alveolar-arterial gradient**
Aα fibers, 260*t*
Aβ fibers, 260*t*
Aδ fibers, 260*t*
  in pain sensation, 310, 313, 313*f*, 315
    cornea/tooth pulp innervation and, 316
Aγ fibers, 260*t*
A₁ receptors, segmental pain inhibition and, 319
A₂ receptors, segmental pain inhibition and, 319
a wave, 102, 102*f*, 366, 367*f*
AAG. *See* α₁-Acid glycoprotein
ABCD's of cardiopulmonary resuscitation, 912. *See also* Cardiopulmonary resuscitation
Abdominal aorta, surgery on, 469
Abdominal compartment syndrome, 800
Abdominal muscles, neuraxial anesthesia affecting, 261
Abdominal trauma, **799–800**
ABO incompatibility, 633–634
  acute hemolytic reactions caused by, 626, 636
ABO system, for blood typing, 633, 633*t*
  testing before blood transfusion and, 633–634
Abruptio placentae, 835
Absence (petit mal) seizures, 585, 585*t*. *See also* Seizures
Absolute humidity, 54
Absolute intrapulmonary shunt, 494
Absorbent granules, carbon dioxide, in circle system, 33–34, 33*t*, 34*t*
Absorbers, carbon dioxide, for circle system, 27, 34–35, 34*f*
Absorption, drug, 152–153. *See also specific agent*
  of inhalation anesthetics, alveolar gas concentration (FA) and, 129–131, 130*t*, 131*f*, 132*f*
  of nonvolatile anesthetics, 152–153
Absorption atelectasis, 496, 959
AC. *See* Assist-control ventilation
Acadesine, for cerebral protection, 562
Accelerations, in fetal heart rate monitoring, 842
Accessory muscles of respiration, neuraxial anesthesia affecting, 261
ACE inhibitors. *See* Angiotensin-converting enzyme (ACE) inhibitors
Acebutolol, 399*t*
Acetaminophen
  hepatic disease caused by, 724
  overdose/toxicity of, 991
  pediatric dosing and, 853*t*
  for postoperative pain management, 341, 341*t*
    with opioid analgesics, 342*t*
Acetate, in crystalloid solutions, 629*t*
Acetazolamide, 676
  carbon dioxide transport affected by, 505
  ophthalmic, systemic effects of, 764*t*
Acetylcholine, 199, **199–200**
  anticholinergic drugs affecting, 207
  cholinesterase inhibitors affecting, 200–202
  in neuromuscular transmission, 179–181, 180*f*, 199, 200
    hypermagnesemia and, 623
  ophthalmic, systemic effects of, 764*t*
  pain mediation/modulation and, 316*t*
  pharmacology of, **199–200**, 200*f*, 200*t*, 201*f*, 203*f*
  receptors for, 179, 180*f*, 200, 201*t*. *See also* Cholinergic receptors
    cardiac, 366
    mechanism of action of neuromuscular blocking agents and, 181
    in myasthenia gravis, 752, 753
    succinylcholine affecting, 186
  structure of, 184*f*
  synthesis/hydrolysis of, 199–200, 200*f*
Acetylcholinesterase (specific cholinesterase/true cholinesterase), 180–181, 200, 200*f*
  cholinesterase inhibitors affecting, 200
Acetylcholinesterase inhibitors. *See* Cholinesterase inhibitors
Acetylcysteine
  for acetaminophen overdose/poisoning, 991

  in radiocontrast dye-induced renal failure prophylaxis, 673
Acetylsalicylic acid (ASA), for postoperative pain management, 341–342, 341*t*
Achalasia, surgical management of, 548
Acid-base balance, **644–661**
  acids and, 645
  bases and, 645
  bicarbonate in maintenance of, 646–648, 647*t*
  buffers and, 645–646, **646–648**
  chemistry of, **644–646**
  compensatory mechanisms and, **646–650**
  conjugate pairs and, 645–646
  definition of terms related to, **644–646**
  disorders of, 646, 646*t*. *See also* Acidosis; Alkalosis
    diagnosis of, **658–660**, 658*f*, 659*t*
    mixed, 660–661
    definition of, 646
  hemoglobin in maintenance of, 648
  hydrogen ion concentration/pH relationship and, 644–645, 645*f*, 647*t*
  massive transfusion affecting, 639
  neuromuscular blocking agents affected by, 189
  pulmonary compensation in maintenance of, **648**
  renal compensation in maintenance of, 648–650, 649*f*, 650*f*, 651*f*
α₁-Acid glycoprotein (AAG), drugs bound by, 153
Acidemia. *See also* Acidosis
  definition of, 646
  physiologic effects of, **650**
Acidosis, 646, 646*t*, **650–656**. *See also* Metabolic acidosis; Respiratory acidosis
  anesthesia in patients with, **656**
  atracurium duration of action and, 192
  burn injuries and, 802
  definition of, 646, 646*t*
  in diabetes (diabetic ketoacidosis), 737–738
  diagnosis of, **658–660**, 658*f*, 659*t*
  massive transfusion causing, 639
  in mixed acid-base disorder, 660–661
  neuromuscular blocking agents affected by, 189
  physiologic effects of, **650**
  potassium concentration affected by, 612
  pulmonary compensation during, 648
  renal compensation during, 648–649, 649*f*, 650*f*
  in septic shock, 982
  after thoracotomy, 539
  urinary diversion and, 624–625
Acids. *See also* Acid-base balance
  definition of, 645
  titratable, excretion of in renal compensation, 649, 649*f*
Aciduria, paradoxic, in hypertrophic pyloric stenosis, 866
Acinus, hepatic, 709
Acquired immune deficiency syndrome (HIV infection/AIDS)
  transfusion-related, 626, 638
  transmission of to health care worker, 907–908
ACT. *See* Activated clotting time
ACTH. *See* Adrenocorticotropic hormone
Actif. *See* Fentanyl lozenges
Actin, in myocardial contraction, 364, 365*f*
Action potential
  cardiac, 359, **360–361**, 361*t*, 362*f*, 363*t*
  local anesthetic action and, 234
  in neuromuscular transmission, 179
    muscle relaxation and, 181
Activated charcoal, for drug overdose/poisoning, 991–992
Activated clotting time
  anticoagulation for cardiopulmonary bypass and, 449
  monitoring in cardiac surgery, 441, 449, 452, 452*f*
Activated partial thromboplastin time, 720
Active phase, of labor, 812, 812*f*
Active transport, placental exchange by, 808
Acupuncture, for pain management, **339–340**
Acute angle-closure glaucoma, anticholinergic drugs and, 209

Acute intermittent porphyria, barbiturate enzyme induction causing, 159
Acute lung injury (ALI), **972–973**
  pressure control ventilation in, 964
Acute myocardial infarction (AMI), **975–976**. *See also* Myocardial infarction
Acute pain, 311–312. *See also* Pain
  systemic responses to, 320–321
Acute renal failure (ARF), 683, 951, **976–979**. *See also* Renal failure
Acute respiratory distress syndrome (ARDS), 518–519, **972–973**
  infection/sepsis and, 972, 973
  in trauma patient, 799
    head trauma and, 577
ADAM circuit, for CPAP, 968
Adamkiewicz, artery of (arteria radicularis magna), 258, 259*f*
Adapin. *See* Doxepin
Addisonian crisis, 746
Addison's disease, 746
Adenoidectomy, **867–868**
  as outpatient procedure, 883
Adenopathy, mediastinal, 550–551
Adenosine, 224, 225*f*, 226*t*, **230**
  in cardiopulmonary resuscitation, 926*t*
  pain mediation/modulation and, 316*t*
    segmental inhibition and, 319
  for paroxysmal supraventricular tachycardia (PSVT), 230, 385
  pediatric dosing and, 853*t*
  for Wolff-Parkinson-White (WPW) syndrome, 230, 385
Adenosine triphosphate (ATP), pain mediation/modulation and, 316*t*
Adenylate cyclase
  α₂ adrenoceptor activation and, 215
  β₁ adrenoceptor activation and, 215
  β₂ adrenoceptor activation and, 215
ADH. *See* Antidiuretic hormone
Adrenal cortex, 745
Adrenal gland, **745–748**
  physiology of, 745
Adrenal insufficiency, 746–747
  etomidate causing, 152, 173, 746
Adrenal medulla, 745
Adrenergic, definition of, 199, 212
Adrenergic drugs, **212–223**. *See also specific agent*
  adrenoceptor physiology and, **212–215**, 213*f*, 214*f*, 215*f*
  aging affecting response to (endogenous β-blockade), 875, 878
  agonists, **215–220**, 215*t*, 216*f*, 217*t*
    α₂, 216*t*, **217**
      adverse effects of, 391*t*
      for hypertension, 390*t*
      preoperative, 393
    β, for asthma, 513, 514*t*
    direct, 207, 216
    indirect, 207, 216
    receptor selectivity of, 215–216, 216*t*
  antagonists, **220–222**, 220*t*, 221*t*
    for hypertension, 389, 390, 390*t*
    receptor selectivity of, 220, 220*t*
  myocardial contraction affected by, 364
  supraspinal pain inhibition and, 319
Adrenoceptors, 212
  adrenergic agonist selectivity and, 215–216, 216*t*
  adrenergic antagonist selectivity and, 220, 220*t*
  α₁, 214, 216*t*, 220*t*
  α₂, 215, 216*t*, 220*t*
  β₁, 215, 216*t*, 220*t*
  β₂, 215, 216*t*, 220*t*
  cardiac, 366
  in heart failure, 380
  in hepatic blood flow regulation, 710
  physiology of, **212–215**, 213*f*, 214*f*, 215*f*
  in renal blood flow regulation, 671

Adrenocortical suppression, etomidate causing, 152, 173, 746
Adrenocorticotropic hormone (ACTH), 581, 745
Adsol. *See* AS-1 preservative
Advanced directive, 952
AEDs. *See* Automated external defibrillators
Aerobic metabolism, 476–477
Aerosol mist/gas therapy, 970
Afferent arteriole, glomerulus supplied by, 663, 664*f*, 669
Afterload, 369–370, 371*f*
  adenosine affecting, 226*t*, 230
  antianginal agents affecting, 397*t*
  calcium channel blockers affecting, 397, 397*t*
  cardiac output and, 360, 370, 371*f*
  hydralazine affecting, 226*t*, 228
  hypotensive agents affecting, 226*t*
  nitroglycerine affecting, 226*t*, 228
  nitroprusside affecting, 226*t*, 227
  stroke volume affected by, 369–370, 371*f*
Age. *See also* Geriatric anesthesia; Pediatric anesthesia
  level of block after epidural anesthesia affected by, 271
  minimum alveolar concentration affected by, 136*t*, 137
  neuromuscular blocking agent sensitivity affected by, 189
  patient selection for outpatient procedures and, 883
Agent-specific theory, of anesthetic action, 133
Agent-specific vaporizers, for anesthesia machine, 49, 49*f*
Agitation, in postanesthesia care unit, 936, 940
Agonists (drug), 155
AICD. *See* Automatic internal cardiac defibrillator
AIDS. *See* Acquired immune deficiency syndrome
Air
  intravitreal injection of, intraocular gas expansion and, 761, 763–764
  residual, transesophageal echocardiography for intraoperative assessment of, 446
  storage of for anesthesiology, 18*t*, 19
Air embolism, 521
  arterial, sitting position and, 894–895
  paradoxical, 574
    liver transplant and, 734
    in pediatric patient, 861
  patient positioning and, 894–895, 899*t*
  venous, 567, 574–575
    liver transplant and, 734
    sitting position and, 894–895
Air-entrainment nebulizers, for oxygen therapy, 957–958
Air-entrainment Venturi masks, for oxygen therapy, 955*t*, 957, 957*t*
Air leaks, 541–542
  after lung resection, 525, 540–542
Air-oxygen blenders, 958
Air/oxygen systems, high-flow, 958
Airflow resistance. *See also* Airway resistance
  in obstructive pulmonary disease, 512
Airway. *See also* Airway management
  anatomy of, 59–61, 60*f*, 61*f*
    in pediatric patient, 849, 850, 852*f*
  assessment of, preoperative, 7
  injury to
    as anesthetic complication, 891, **892**
    heat causing, 801, 951, 974
  laser surgery and, 773–774, 774*t*
  sensory nerve supply of, 60, 62*f*
  trauma to during intubation, 78–79
Airway collapse
  flow-related, 487, 488*f*
  volume-related, 487, 487*f*
Airway fire, during laser surgery, 771, 773–774, 774*t*
Airway management, **59–85.** *See also* Difficult airway; Intubation
  anatomic considerations and, **59–61,** 60*f*, 61*f*
  anesthetic accidents and, 891
  in asthma, 515
  in cardiopulmonary resuscitation, 915–920, 917*f*, 918*t*, 918*t*, 919*f*, 920*f*
  complications related to, 891, **892**
  for craniofacial reconstruction, 777, 777*f*, 778*f*
  for difficult airway, 73, 75*f*, 80–84, 81*t*, 82*f*, 83*f*, 84*f*, 84*t*
  documenting, 901
  for endoscopy, 772–773
  equipment used in, **61–70.** *See also specific type*
  extubation techniques and, 77
  for head and neck cancer surgery, 776
  intubation complications and, **77–84,** 77*t*
  intubation techniques and, **70–76**
  laryngoscopy techniques and, **70–72**

mediastinal adenopathy and, 550–551
  in obese patient, 736, 749
  for tracheal resection, 543, 544*f*
  for trauma patient, 794
Airway obstruction
  in burn injury/smoke inhalation, 801, 974, 975
  in mediastinal adenopathy, 550, 551
  in postanesthesia care unit, 942–943
Airway pressure release ventilation (APRV), 962*t*, 963*f*, 964–965, 965*f*
Airway pressures
  graphic display of on anesthesia machine, 46*f*, 47
  monitoring in pediatric patient, 861
Airway resistance, 485–488, 486*t*, 487*f*, 488*f*, 489*f*
  anesthesia affecting, 490
  in asthma, 513
  flow-related collapse and, 487, 488*f*
  forced vital capacity and, 487–488, 489*f*
  in pediatric patient, 850
  volume-related collapse and, 487, 487*f*
Akinesis, 371, 433, 444, 444*f*
  transesophageal echocardiography for intraoperative assessment of, 444, 444*f*
Aladin Cassette, for electronically controlled vaporizer, 50, 51*f*
Alanine aminotransferase (ALT/SGPT), 714*t*, 715
Albumin
  drugs bound by, 153
    geriatric anesthesia and, 879
  in fluid management, 630
  hepatic production of, 712
  plasma concentration of, calcium concentration affected by, 618
  serum levels of, 708, 714*t*, 715
Albuterol, for asthma, 514*t*
Alcohol blocks, in pain management, **336**
Alcohol use/abuse
  anesthetic requirements affected by, 594*t*
  hepatitis and, 724
    surgery in patient with, 725–726
  liver disease/cirrhosis caused by, 726
    coagulopathy and, 717–722, 718*t*, 719*f*, 721*t*
  minimum alveolar concentration affected by, 136*t*
Alcuronium, altered renal function and, 683
Aldactone. *See* Spironolactone
Aldosterone, 745
  in blood pressure control, 375–376
  cortical collecting tubule affected by, 668, 745
  hyperkalemia and, 616, 745
  in volume regulation, 610, 745
Aldosterone antagonists, **676,** 745
Aldosteronism, 745–746
  in renovascular hypertension, 690
  spironolactone for, 676, 746
Aldosteronoma, 745
Alfentanil, 166*f*. *See also* Opioids
  altered renal function and, 682
  biotransformation of, 165, 167*f*
  cardiovascular effects of, 167, 171*t*
  context-sensitive half time of, 167*f*
  distribution of, 165, 167*f*
  drug interactions and, 169
  for electroconvulsive therapy, 595
  history of use of, 4
  for infusion anesthesia, 162
  intraspinal, 346
  organ system effects of, 171*t*
  for outpatient procedures, 884
  in pediatric anesthesia, 855
  pediatric dosing and, 853*t*
  placental transfer of, 811
  stress response affected by, 169
  uses and doses of, 168*t*
ALI. *See* Acute lung injury
Alkalemia. *See also* Alkalosis
  anesthesia in patients with, **658**
  definition of, 646
Alkaline phosphatase, serum levels of, 714*t*, 715
  in pregnancy, 807
Alkalosis, 646, 646*t*, **656–658.** *See also* Metabolic alkalosis; Respiratory alkalosis
  anesthesia in patients with, **658**
  definition of, 646, 646*t*
  diagnosis of, 658–660, 658*f*, 659*t*
  hypokalemia and, 614–615, 614*t*
  massive transfusion causing, 626, 639
  in mixed acid-base disorder, 660–661
  physiologic effects of, 656

potassium concentration affected by, 612
  pulmonary compensation during, 648
  renal compensation during, 649–650
  in septic shock, 982
Allen's test, 92
Allergic (extrinsic) asthma, 513. *See also* Asthma
Allergic reactions, **902–907,** 903*t*
  anaphylactic, **904–905,** 905*t*, 906*t*
  to anesthetic agents, **906**
  as anesthetic complication, **902–907,** 903*t*, 904*f*, 905*t*, 906*t*
  to antibiotics, **906–907**
  anticholinergic drugs and, 209
  antihistamines in management of, 243, 244
  barbiturates and, 159
  histamine causing, 243
  immediate hypersensitivity reactions, 902–903, **903,** 903*t*, 904*f*
  to latex, 889, **905–906**
  local anesthetics and, 240
  opioids causing, 345
  pancuronium and, 195
  to penicillin, **906–907**
  preoperative identification of, 6
Allodynia
  definition of, 311*t*
  glycine and GABA inhibition producing, 318–319
Allow Natural Death (AND) orders, 952–953
Alopecia, patient positioning and, 899*t*
Alpha₁-acid glycoprotein (AAG), drugs bound by, 153
Alpha (α)-agonists, interaction of with β-blockers, cardiac arrest caused by, **900–901**
Alpha₂ (α₂)-agonists, 216*t*, **217.** *See also specific agent*
  adverse effects of, 392*t*
  for hypertension, 390*t*
  preoperative, 393
Alpha₁ (α₁)-antitrypsin
  in emphysema, 516–517
  hepatic formation of, 712
Alpha (α) blockers, **220**
  adverse effects of, 391*t*
  for hypertension, 390*t*
  before pheochromocytoma surgery, 747
Alpha (α/distribution) phase, of two-compartment model, 154–155, 154*f*
Alpha₁ (α₁)-receptors, 214
  adrenergic agonist selectivity and, 215–216, 216*t*
  adrenergic antagonist selectivity and, 220, 220*t*
  in hepatic blood flow regulation, 710
  in renal blood flow regulation, 671
Alpha₂ (α₂)-receptors, 215
  adrenergic agonist selectivity and, 215–216, 216*t*
  adrenergic antagonist selectivity and, 220, 220*t*
  supraspinal pain inhibition and, 319
Alpha residues, 453
Alpha (α≥-stat management, during cardiopulmonary bypass, 453
Alpha (α≥-thalassemia, 642
Alprenolol, 399*t*
ALS. *See* Amyotrophic lateral sclerosis
Alteplase, for acute myocardial infarction, 976
Alupent. *See* Metaproterenol
Alveolar-arterial gradient, 498, 499, 499*f*
Alveolar blood flow, uptake affected by, 130
Alveolar carbon dioxide tension (PACO₂), 500, 500*f*
Alveolar collapse
  in ARDS, 972
  surface tension and, 482
Alveolar concentration (FA), of inhalational anesthetic, **129–132,** 130*t*, 131*f*, 132*f*
  inspired concentration and, 131–132
  minimum (MAC), 127, **135–137,** 135*f*, 136*t*
    in geriatric patient, 875, 879
    local anesthetics affecting, 239
    in pediatric patient, 849, 852–855, 855*t*
    during pregnancy, 804, 805, 805*t*
  in pediatric patient, 849, 852
  uptake affecting, 127, 129–131, 130*t*, 131*f*, 132*f*
  ventilation affecting, 131
Alveolar dead space, 490, 493. *See also* Dead space
  end-tidal carbon dioxide analysis in monitoring, 112
Alveolar gas tensions, **496–501**
Alveolar nerve, inferior, blocking, 325–326, 325*f*
Alveolar oxygen tension, 496–498
Alveolar pressure, during normal breathing, 480, 481*f*
Alveolar ventilation, distribution of, 491, 493*f*

Alveoli, respiratory, 478, 479f
  in ARDS, 972
  in pediatric patient, 849, 850
  PEEP/CPAP affecting, 969
Alveolitis, fibrosing, in ARDS, 972
Alzheimer's disease, **587**
Amantadine, for Parkinson's disease, 587
Amaurosis fugax, in stroke, 470
Ambient light, pulse oximetry artifacts caused by, 110
Ambu bags, for resuscitation, 37
Ambulatory surgery, **882–888**. *See also* Outpatient
    anesthesia
American Society of Anesthesiologists (ASA), physical
    status classification of, 7–8, 8t
AMI. *See* Acute myocardial infarction
Amide local anesthetics, 234, 236–237t
  metabolism and excretion of, 233, 238
Amiloride, 676
Amino acids. *See also specific type*
  accumulation of, in high anion gap metabolic acidosis,
    654
  hepatic deamination of, 712
  pain mediation/modulation and, central sensitization
    and, 318
p-Aminobenzoic acid, allergic reaction to, 238, 240
γ-Aminobutyric acid (GABA)
  anesthetic mechanism of action and, 134
  benzodiazepines affecting binding of, 160
  etomidate affecting binding of, 172
  pain mediation/modulation and, 316t
    central inhibition and, 318–319
  receptors for. *See* GABA receptors
ε-Aminocaproic acid
  for bleeding prophylaxis in cardiopulmonary bypass, 450
  for persistent bleeding after cardiopulmonary bypass, 458
p-Aminohippurate clearance, in renal plasma flow
    measurement, 669
Aminophylline, pediatric dosing and, 853t
Aminotransferases, serum levels of, 714t, 715
Amiodarone
  for acute myocardial infarction, 976
  in cardiopulmonary resuscitation, 914, 927t
  pediatric dosing and, 853t
Amitriptyline
  for depression, 591, 592t
  for pain management, 337t
Amlodipine, 397, 398t
Ammonia
  blood, 715
  formation of in renal compensation, 649, 650f
Amnesia, antegrade, benzodiazepines producing, 164
Amniotic fluid, meconium-staining of, **843–844**
Amniotic fluid embolism, **839**
Amniotomy, for primary dysfunctional labor, 834
Amoxapine, for depression, 591
Amphetamines
  abuse of, anesthetic requirements affected by, 594t
  minimum alveolar concentration affected by, 136t
Amrinone, 456t
  after cardiopulmonary bypass, 456t, 457
  pediatric dosing and, 853t
Amsorb. *See* Calcium hydroxide and calcium chloride
Amyotrophic lateral sclerosis (ALS), **588**
  neuromuscular blocking agent response affected in, 190t
Anaerobic metabolism, 477
Anafranil. *See* Clomipramine
Analgesia. *See also* Pain management
  definition of, 311t
  preemptive, **319**
Anaphylactic/anaphylactoid reactions, **904–905**, 905t, 906t
  to barbiturates, 159
  blood transfusion causing, 637
  epinephrine for management of, 218
  to latex, 906
"Anaphylactoid syndrome of pregnancy" (amniotic fluid
    embolism), **839**
Anaprox. *See* Naproxen sodium
Anatomic dead space, 490. *See also* Dead space
AND (Allow Natural Death) orders, 952–953
Anemia
  in cirrhosis, 727–728
  minimum alveolar concentration affected by, 136t
  nitrous oxide causing, 127, 139
  physiologic effects of, 790–791
  in pregnancy, 806, 807
  in renal failure, 685
Anesthesia/anesthetics. *See also* Inhalational (volatile)
    anesthesia/anesthetics; Local (regional)

anesthesia/anesthetics; Nonvolatile
    (intravenous) anesthesia/anesthetics
adjuncts to, **242–252**
  cerebral effects of, 560
  placental transfer of, 811
allergic reactions to, **906**
antacids used with, **245**
aspiration pneumonia risk/prevention and, 242, 244t,
    245, 250–252
balanced, 4
in cerebral protection, 562
complications associated with, **889–911**. *See also*
    Anesthetic complications
definition of, 1, 311t
dissociative, 169
doxapram used with, **248–249**
emergence from, **938–939**, 943. *See also* Emergence
    from anesthesia
flumazenil used with, **249–250**
histamine-receptor antagonists used with, **242–245**,
    243t, 244t
history of, **2–5**
5-HT₃ receptor antagonists used with, **247–248**, 247f
inadequate level of, 37–39, 39f
ketorolac used with, **248**
for magnetic resonance imaging studies, 123–124
metoclopramide used with, **245–246**
monitored care, 8, 124, 886–888. *See also* Monitored
    anesthesia care
naloxone used with, **249**
occupational hazards and, 889, **907–909**
open drop, **28–29**, 33t
outpatient, **882–888**
  pediatric drug dosing and, 852, 853–855t
  placental transfer and, 804, 810–811
preoperative patient evaluation and, **5–8**, 6t, 7t, 8t
proton pump inhibitors used with, **246**
scope of, 2t, **5**
slow recovery from, 197–198
spontaneous awakening from, **943**
Anesthesia bag, for oxygen therapy, 956–957
Anesthesia dolorosa, definition of, 311t
Anesthesia machine, **40–58**, 41f, 43f
  breathing-circuit pressure gauges for, 41, **44–47**, 46f,
    47t
  breathing system/patient relationship and, 28f
  checkout list for, **55–56**, 56–57t
  components of, 41–42, 41–42f, 43f
  flow-control valves/flowmeters/electronic flow control
    and, 41, **43–44**, 44f, 45f
  fresh gas outlet for, 41
  gas inlets for, 41, **42**
  humidifiers/nebulizers for, 41, **54–55**, 55f
  malfunction of, 40, 56–58, 891, 891t
    cardiovascular changes during surgery and, 38, 39f
    inspection routine for prevention of, **55–56**, 56–57t
  oxygen analyzers for, 41, **55**, 55t
  oxygen-pressure-failure devices/oxygen flush valves for,
    41, **42–43**, 44f
  pressure regulators for, 41, **42**, 43f
  spirometers for, 41, 44–47, 45f, 46f, 47t
  vaporizers for, 41, **47–50**, 48f, 49f, 51f
  ventilators/ventilatory cycle of, 41, **50–54**, 52f, 53f
    disconnect alarms for, 41, 53, 57
    malfunction/leak in, 56–58, 891, 891t
      inspection routine for prevention of, **55–56**,
      56–57t
  waste-gas scavengers for, 41, **54**, 54f
Anesthesia ventilators, 41, **50–54**, 52f, 53f. *See also*
    Mechanical ventilation
  disconnect alarms for, 41, 53, 57
  malfunction/leak in, 56–58, 891, 891t
    inspection routine for prevention of, **55–56**, 56–57t
Anesthesiology
  documentation and, **8–13**, 9f, 11f, 12f, **901–902**, 902t
  evolution of as specialty, **4–5**
  official recognition of as specialty, 5
  practice of, **1–14**
    definition of, 1, 2t
    scope of, 2t, **5**
Anesthetic accidents/mishaps, 889, **890–892**, 891t. *See also*
    Anesthetic complications
  medication errors and, 909–910
Anesthetic complications, **889–911**
  accidents, 889, **890–892**, 891t
  airway injury/mismanagement, 891, **892**
  allergic reactions, **902–907**, 903t, 904f, 905t, 906t

awareness, **897–899**
  bispectral index (BIS) monitoring in prevention of,
    118
cardiac arrest
  α-agonist/β-blocker interactions causing, **900–901**
  during spinal anesthesia, 277, **900**
documentation issues and, **901–902**, 902t
equipment misuse/failure and, 40, 56–58, 891, 891t
  cardiovascular changes during surgery and, 38, 39f
  inspection routine for prevention of, **55–56**, 56–57t
eye injury, **899–900**
intraoperative hypertension and tachycardia, 909–910
medication errors causing, 909–910
patient positioning and, 893–897, 897f, 898t, 899t
  seated position and, 894–896, 894f, 895f, 898t, 899t
peripheral nerve injury, **893–897**, 897f, 899t
prevention of, 891–892
Anesthetic gas analysis, intraoperative, **113–114**, 113f
Anesthetic-gas scavenging, 20
  active, 54
  by anesthesia machine, 41, **54**, 54f
  breathing circuits and, 33t
  passive, 54
Anesthetic plan, 1, **5–8**, 6t, 7t, 8t
  for cardiac surgery, 440
Aneurysms
  aortic, 467
  cerebral, 567, **578–579**
Angina, 396. *See also* Ischemic heart disease
  treatment of, 396–399, 397t, 398t, 399t
  unstable, 396, 976
Anginal equivalent, 396
Angioedema, 903
Angiography, coronary
  for acute myocardial infarction, 976
  preoperative, in ischemic heart disease, 401–402
Angioplasty, for acute myocardial infarction, 976
Angiotensin
  in blood pressure control, 375–376
  pain mediation/modulation and, central sensitization
    and, 318
  in renal blood flow regulation, 671
Angiotensin-converting enzyme (ACE) inhibitors
  adverse effects of, 392t
  for hypertension, 389, 390, 391t
    preoperative discontinuation of, 391, 393
  renal effects of, 673
Angiotensin-receptor antagonists
  adverse effects of, 392t
  for hypertension, 391t
Angle-closure glaucoma, anticholinergic drugs and, 209
Anhepatic phase of liver transplant, 733
  physiologic derangements associated with, 734
Anion gap, 653–654
  metabolic acidosis and
    in diabetes (diabetic ketoacidosis), 737–738
    high anion gap, 654
    normal anion gap, 654–655
Anisoylated plasminogen streptokinase activator complex
    (APSAC), for acute myocardial infarction, 976
Ankle block, 283, 303, 304f, 305f
Ankylosing spondylitis, back pain caused by, 355
Annulus fibrosus, disk herniation and, 353
ANP. *See* Atrial natriuretic peptide
Antacids, **245**
  for aspiration pneumonia prophylaxis, 244t,
    245
  cesarean section and, 830
  labor and delivery and, 820
  open eye surgery in full stomach patient and, 769
Antagonists (drug), 155–156
Antecubital space
  median nerve block in, 295, 296f
  radial nerve block in, 294, 295f
Antegrade amnesia, benzodiazepines producing, 164
Antepartum hemorrhage, **835–836**
Anterior chamber surgery, regional anesthesia for, 767
Anterior ethmoidal nerve, 60, 62f
Anterior (motor) horn, 314, 315t
Anterior spinal artery, 257, 259f
Anterior spinal artery syndrome, 258
Antianalgesic effect, of barbiturates, 159
Antianginal agents, 396–399, 397t, 398t, 399t
Antiarrhythmic agents, 384t, 385
  neuromuscular blocking agent interactions and, 185t
  in Wolff-Parkinson-White (WPW) syndrome, 385
Antibiotic prophylaxis, in valvular heart disease, 407,
    408–409t

Antibiotics
allergic reactions to, **906–907**
anaphylaxis, 904
neuromuscular blocking agent interactions and, 185t
Antibody-mediated immunity, impaired. *See also*
Immunocompromised host
septic shock and, 985t
Antibody screen, for blood transfusion, 634
Anticholinergic drugs, **207–210**, 208t
altered renal function and, 682
for asthma, 514
cholinesterase inhibitor administration and, 202, 204t
in geriatric patient, 879
intraocular pressure affected by, 762
mechanisms of action of, **207**, 208t
in oculocardiac reflex prevention, 763
overdose/toxicity of, 210–211
for Parkinson's disease, 587
pharmacology of, **208–209**, 208t
Anticholinergic syndrome, 210–211
Anticholinesterase drugs. *See also* Cholinesterase inhibitors
for myasthenia gravis, 753
Anticoagulant therapy. *See also* Anticoagulation
neuraxial anesthesia in setting of, 279–280
for pulmonary embolism, 521
in valvular heart disease, 407–408
Anticoagulation. *See also* Anticoagulant therapy
for cardiopulmonary bypass, 433, 434, 449–450
reversal of, 434, 457–458
Anticonvulsants, 586, 586t
neuromuscular blocking agent interactions and, 185t
for pain management, 309, 337–338, 338t
Antidepressants, 583, 591–593, 592t
atypical, 593, 593t
for pain management, 309, 337, 337t
Antidiuretic hormone (ADH/arginine vasopressin), 456t,
581
in blood pressure control, 375–376
after cardiopulmonary bypass, 456t, 457
in cardiopulmonary resuscitation, 912, 912–914, 913f,
916f, 927t, 930f
in heart failure, 380
medullary collecting tubule affected by, 668
nonosmotic release of, 604
in plasma osmolality control, 604
for septic shock, 986t
in urine concentration, 668
in volume control, 611
Antidysrhythmics. *See* Antiarrhythmic agents
Antiemetics
droperidol as, 152, 175
5HT₃-receptor antagonists as, 247–248, 885, 940
for outpatients, 885
Antifibrinolytic agents, for bleeding prophylaxis for
cardiopulmonary bypass, 450
Antiglobulin (Coombs) test, for blood transfusion, 634
delayed hemolytic transfusion reaction and, 637
Antihemophilic factor, 718t
deficiency of (hemophilia A), 722
Antihistamines, **242–245**, 243t, 244t. *See also specific agent*
Antihypertensive therapy, 389–390, 390–391t. *See also*
Hypotensive agents
adverse effects of, 392, 392t
neuromuscular blocking agent interactions and, 185t
in pregnancy-induced hypertension, 838
preoperative continuation of, 391, 393
for renovascular hypertension, 690–691
Antimuscarinic drugs, **207–211**. *See also* Anticholinergic
drugs
Antiplatelet therapy
for acute myocardial infarction, 976
neuraxial anesthesia in setting of, 279–280
Antipsychotic agents (neuroleptics), 593
neuroleptic malignant syndrome and, **593–594**,
872–873
in pain management, 338
Antireflux surgery, 548
Anti-shock garment, pneumatic, 935
Antisialagogue effects, of anticholinergic drugs, 208t, 209
Antithrombin III, 720
Antithrombin III deficiency, heparin resistance and, 450
Antithrombin therapy, for acute myocardial infarction,
976
Antithyroid medications, 741
preoperative, 742
α₁-Antitrypsin
in emphysema, 516–517
hepatic formation of, 712

Anxiety
pain causing, 321
premedication for minimizing, 175–176
Aorta. *See also under* Aortic
abdominal, clamping, for hemorrhage control, 799–800
coarctation of, 467
cross-clamping, 466
for abdominal aorta surgery, 469
for descending aorta surgery, 468
paraplegia and, 468–469
occlusive disease of, 467
surgery on, **466–470**
abdominal aorta and, 469
aortic arch and, 468
thoracic aorta and
ascending, 467–468
descending, 468–469
Aortic aneurysms, 467
Aortic arch, surgery involving, 468
Aortic baroreceptors, 375
Aortic bodies, in breathing regulation, 507
Aortic cannulation, for cardiopulmonary bypass, 450
Aortic dissection, 467
Aortic regurgitation, 387, **419–420**
choice of anesthetic agent in patient with, 420
heart murmur in, preoperative evaluation of, 407t
Aortic stenosis, 387, **416–418**
choice of anesthetic agent in patient with, 387, 417–418
heart murmur in, preoperative evaluation of, 407t
Aortic transection, 799
Aortic trauma, 467
Aortic valve area, calculation of, 416–417
Aortic valve flow, calculation of, 416–417
Aortocaval compression, during pregnancy, 806–807
Apgar score, 842, 842t
Aplastic crises, in sickle cell anemia, 641
Apnea. *See also* Ventilation/ventilatory drive
after retrobulbar block, 761, 766
sleep, obesity and, 748
Apnea test, of brain death, 953
Apneic oxygenation
for endoscopy, 773
as one-lung ventilation alternative, 539
for rigid bronchoscopy, 544
Apneic threshold, 507
halothane affecting, 140
opioids affecting, 167
Apneustic center, 506
Apparatus dead space. *See also* Dead space
in circle system, 27, 35–36
closed-circuit anesthesia and, 148
condenser humidifiers and, 54
open drop anesthesia and, 29
pediatric masks minimizing, 62, 860
pediatric patient and, 861
Apparent volume of distribution. *See* Volume of
distribution
Appendicitis/appendectomy, during pregnancy, 846–847
Aprotinin
cardiopulmonary bypass and, 434, 449, 450
descending aorta surgery and, 468
APRV. *See* Airway pressure release ventilation
APSAC. *See* Anisoylated plasminogen streptokinase
activator complex
aPTT. *See* Activated partial thromboplastin time
Arachnoid, spinal cord, 255, 258f
Arachnoiditis, neuraxial anesthesia and, 278
Arcuate arteries, 669, 670f
ARDS. *See* Acute respiratory distress syndrome
ARF. *See* Acute renal failure
Arginine vasopressin (AVP/antidiuretic hormone), 456t,
581
in blood pressure control, 375–376
after cardiopulmonary bypass, 456t, 457
in cardiopulmonary resuscitation, 912–914, 913f, 916f,
927t, 930f
in heart failure, 380
medullary collecting tubule affected by, 668
nonosmotic release of, 604
in plasma osmolality control, 604
for septic shock, 986t
in urine concentration, 668
in volume control, 611
Aristocort. *See* Triamcinolone
Arnold-Chiari malformation, 589
Arrhythmias. *See* Dysrhythmias
Arteria radicularis magna (artery of Adamkiewicz), 258,
259f

Arterial air embolism, sitting position and, 894–895
Arterial blood gases
in acid-base disorders, 658–659, 658f, **659**, 659t
monitoring
intraoperative
in COPD patients, 518
for craniotomy, 569
management during cardiopulmonary bypass and,
453
via intra-arterial catheter, 95–97
in postanesthesia care, 945
pneumonectomy criteria and, 535–536, 535t
preoperative, in valvular heart disease patient, 406
in respiratory failure, 970, 971f
Arterial blood pressure, **375–376**
adenosine affecting, 230
adrenergic agonists affecting, 217t, 389–390, 390t
barbiturates affecting, 158, 171t
benzodiazepines affecting, 161, 171t
cardiopulmonary bypass and, 451
cocaine affecting, 239
control of, 375–376
desflurane affecting, 128, 138t, 144
dobutamine affecting, 217t, 219
droperidol affecting, 175
enflurane affecting, 138t, 142
ephedrine affecting, 217t, 218
epinephrine affecting, 217t, 218
esmolol affecting, 221
etomidate affecting, 171t, 172
fenoldopam affecting, 217t, 220, 231
halothane affecting, 138t, 139
histamine affecting, 243
hydralazine affecting, 228–229
hypotensive agents for intraoperative control of, **224–232**
in hypovolemia evaluation, 627t
inhalational anesthetics affecting, 138t
intraocular pressure and, 762, 762t
isoflurane affecting, 138t, 143
labetalol affecting, 220
local anesthetics affecting, 238–239
methoxyflurane affecting, 138t, 141
minimum alveolar concentration affected by, 136t
mivacurium affecting, 194
monitoring
intraoperative, **87–97**, 87f, 88f, 92f
in aortic stenosis, 417
auscultation for, 89, 90f
axillary artery catheterization for, 87f, 93
brachial artery catheterization for, 87f, 93
for cardiac surgery, 441
for carotid endarterectomy, 470–471
controlled hypotension and, 232
for craniotomy, 569
descending aorta surgery and, 468
Doppler probe for, 89, 89f
dorsalis pedis artery catheterization for, 87f, 93
femoral artery catheterization for, 87f, 93
for head and neck cancer surgery, 776
invasive, **91–97**
for lung resection, 537
noninvasive, **88–91**
oscillometry for, 89–90, 90f
palpation techniques for, 88–89, 89f
in pediatric patient, 857
plethysmography for, 90
posterior tibial artery catheterization for, 93
radial artery catheterization for, 87f, 92, 93, 96f
sample site and, 87, 87f, 88f
tonometry for, 91, 91f
ulnar artery catheterization for, 93
in postanesthesia care, 937
in neonate, volume resuscitation and, 845
neuraxial anesthesia affecting, 260
nitroglycerine affecting, 228
nitroprusside affecting, 227
nonvolatile anesthetics affecting, 171t
norepinephrine affecting, 217t, 219
opioids affecting, 167, 171t
in pediatric patient, 851t
phentolamine affecting, 220
phenylephrine affecting, 207, 216, 217t
propofol affecting, 171t, 174, 175
propranolol affecting, 222
rapacuronium affecting, 197
in renal failure, 685
succinylcholine affecting, 186
trimethaphan affecting, 229

Arterial carbon dioxide tension (PaCO₂), 500
  bicarbonate buffering and, 647–648
  central chemoreceptors in regulation of, 476, 507
  cerebral blood flow affected by, 554, 554f
  desflurane affecting, 144
  enflurane affecting, 138t, 142
  halothane affecting, 138t, 140
  inhalational anesthetics affecting, 138t
  intracranial compliance affected by, 556
  intraocular pressure and, 762, 762t
  labor and delivery affecting, 812
  in metabolic acidosis, 646t, 648, 658–659, 658f, 659t
  in metabolic alkalosis, 646t, 648
  methoxyflurane affecting, 138t, 141
  minimum alveolar concentration affected by, 136t
  nitrous oxide affecting, 137, 138t
  opioids affecting, 167, 168f, 344
  pneumonectomy criteria and, 535t
  pregnancy affecting, 805, 805t
  P$_{tc}$CO₂ (P$_{a}$CO₂) as measure of, 113
  pulmonary compensation and, 648
  in respiratory acidosis, 646t, 650–653
  in respiratory alkalosis, 646t, 656, 658–659, 658f, 659t
Arterial concentration (FA), of inhalational anesthetic, **132**
Arterial filter, for cardiopulmonary bypass machine, 435f, 436–437
Arterial gas tensions, **496–501**. *See also specific type*
Arterial lines. *See* Intra-arterial monitoring
Arterial oxygen tension (PaO₂), 475, 498–499, 498t, 499f
  cerebral blood flow affected by, 554, 554f
  endobronchial intubation affecting, 510
  of fetal blood, 809
  in geriatric patient, 877, 878f
  intraocular pressure and, 762, 762t
  minimum alveolar concentration affected by, 136t
  peripheral chemoreceptors in regulation of, 507, 508f
  pneumonectomy criteria and, 535t
  pregnancy affecting, 805, 805t
  P$_{tc}$O₂ (P$_{a}$O₂) as measure of, 113
  shunting affecting, 499, 499f
Arterial pulsations, oxygen saturation of (SpO₂), pulse
      oximetry for monitoring, 108–109
Arterial switch procedure, for transposition of great arteries, 426
Arterial tonometry, for arterial blood pressure monitoring, 91, 91f
Arteriolar gas tensions. *See also specific type*
Arteriovenous malformation (AVM), **579–580**
Artery of Adamkiewicz (arteria radicularis magna), 258, 259f
Arthritis
  back pain caused by, 355
  cricoarytenoid, 785
  degenerative (osteoarthritis), 784
  rheumatoid, 784–785, 784t, 785f
Arthroplasty, total
  hip, **784–787**, 784t, 785f
  knee, **788**
Arthroscopy, knee, **787–788**
Articular processes, vertebral, 255, 256f, 352
Articulating arms, for medical gas delivery, 18f
Artificial airways, oral and nasal, 62, 63f
Arytenoid cartilage, 60, 61f
AS-1 preservative, for blood storage, 634
AS-3 preservative, for blood storage, 634
ASA. *See* Acetylsalicylic acid
ASA physical status classification, 7–8, 8t
Ascendin. *See* Amoxapine
Ascending aorta, surgery on, 367–368
Ascending (standing) bellows, for anesthesia ventilators, 52, 53f
Ascites, in cirrhosis, 728
  respiratory effects of, 728
ASDs. *See* Atrial septal defect
Aspartate, pain mediation/modulation and, 316t
  central sensitization and, 318
Aspartate aminotransferase (AST/SGOT), 714t, 715
Asphyxia, fetal, treatment of, **842**
Aspiration
  foreign body
    Heimlich maneuver for, 917, 918f, 918t
    in pediatric patient, **867**, 917, 918t
  pulmonary/aspiration pneumonia, 518–519
    esophageal surgery and, 525, 548
    management of, 252
    open eye surgery and, 768, 769t
    pathophysiology/clinical findings in, 252
    risk/prevention of, 242, 244t, 250–252, 769t

antacids and, 245
cardiac transplantation and, 463
cesarean section and, 830
H₂-receptor antagonists and, 242, 244
metoclopramide and, 225–226, 242
obesity and, 748
pregnancy/labor and delivery and, 804, 807, 819, 820
  postpartum tubal ligation and, 816–817
proton pump inhibitors and, 246
of water, in drowning/near drowning, 973
Aspiration (sidestream) capnographs, 111
  in pediatric patient, 857–858
Aspirin
  for acute myocardial infarction, 976
  platelet function affected by, 721
  for postoperative pain management, 341–342, 341t
    with opioid analgesics, 342t
Assist-control ventilation, 961, 962t, 963f
Asthma, 511, **513–516**
  acute, 513
  anesthesia in patient with, 514–516, 515f
  chronic, 513
  extrinsic (allergic), 513
  intrinsic (idiosyncratic), 513
  pathophysiology of, 513
  treatment of, 513–514, 514t
Asthmatic bronchitis, chronic, 516
Asymmetric septal hypertrophy. *See* Hypertrophic cardiomyopathy
Asystole, algorithm for management of, 932f
Atarax. *See* Hydroxyzine
Atelectasis
  absorption, 496, 959
  burn injuries and, 801
  postoperative
    risk factors for, 512
    after thoracotomy, 540
Atenolol, 221t, 399t
Atheroma, transesophageal echocardiography for assessment of, 446
Atherosclerosis, coronary, ischemic heart disease caused by, 395–396
Atkinson facial nerve block, 766, 768f
Atlantoaxial subluxation, in rheumatoid arthritis, 782, 784–785, 785f
Atlas, 255
Atopic hypersensitivity reactions, 903
ATP, pain mediation/modulation and, 316t
Atracurium, 179, 184f, 188t, **191–192**
  altered renal function and, 683
  histamine release caused by, 187, 188t, 191
  in ischemic heart disease patients, 405
  for outpatient procedures, 884
  in pediatric anesthesia, 856
  pediatric dosing and, 853t
  seizure activity and, 586
Atrial compliance, mitral regurgitation and, 412
Atrial contraction, abnormal, preload affected by, 368
Atrial fibrillation
  cardioversion for, 472–473, 922, 923t
  in Wolff-Parkinson-White (WPW) syndrome, 383
Atrial natriuretic peptide
  in heart failure, 380
  in renal blood flow regulation, 671
  in volume control, 610
Atrial pressure, 366, 367f
Atrial septal defect, 424
Atrial stretch receptors, antidiuretic hormone secretion and, 604
Atrial switch (Senning) procedure, for transposition of great arteries, 426
Atrioventricular (AV) conduction abnormalities. *See also* Heart block
  appearance of on electrocardiogram, 428
  significance of, 429
Atrioventricular (AV) dissociation, 429
Atrioventricular (AV) nodal reentrant tachycardia,
      paroxysmal supraventricular tachycardia
      (PSVT) caused by, 383
Atrioventricular (AV) node, 362f, 363
  antianginal agents affecting, 397t
  blood supply to, 363
Atrioventricular (AV) reentrant tachycardia, paroxysmal
      supraventricular tachycardia (PSVT) caused
      by, 383
Atrioventricular (AV) septal defects, 425
Atrioventricular (AV) sequential pacing, 431

Atropine, 207, 208f, 208t, **209–210**
  in cardiopulmonary resuscitation, 912, 926t, 931f, 932f, 933f
  cholinesterase inhibitor administration and, 202, 204t, 209
    edrophonium, 204t, 205
  intraocular pressure affected by, 762
  in oculocardiac reflex prevention, 763
  ophthalmic, systemic effects of, 210, 764t
  overdose/toxicity of, 210–211
    physostigmine for, 205, 211
  pediatric dosing and, 853t
  preoperative, in pediatric patient, 857
    for cardiac surgery, 460
Atropine fever, 209
Atropine flush, 209
Auditory evoked potentials, for intraoperative monitoring, 115–116, 116t
  anesthetic agents affecting, 563t, 564
Augmented inflow effect, 132
Auscultation
  for arterial blood pressure monitoring, 89, 90f
  after intubation, 72–73, 74f
Auscultatory gap, 89
Autoimmune disease
  hypothyroidism caused by, 742
  neuromuscular blocking agent response affected in, 190t
Autologous muscle grafts (free flaps), 789–790
Autologous transfusions, **639**
Automated external defibrillators (AEDs), 922
Automatic internal cardiac defibrillator (AICD),
      extracorporeal shock wave lithotripsy in
      patients with, 692, 697–698
Automatic transport ventilators, 921
Autonomic dysfunction (dysautonomia), 583, **589**
Autonomic effects, of nondepolarizing neuromuscular
      blocking agents, 187
Autonomic hyperreflexia, 583, 590, 798
  trimethaphan in management of, 229
Autonomic nervous system
  in arterial blood pressure control, 375
  blockade of, neuraxial anesthesia producing, **260–262**
  cardiac innervation and, 366
  in cerebral blood flow control, 555
  liver supplied by, 709
  systemic vasculature controlled by, **374–375**
Autonomic neuropathy, diabetic, 736, 738–739, 739t
Autoregulation, **372–373**
  cerebral blood flow, 552, **553–554**, 554f
    halothane affecting, 140
    hydralazine affecting, 229
    nitroprusside affecting, 227
    sevoflurane affecting, 145
  renal blood flow, 662, 670–671
    volatile agents affecting, 672
Autosomal recessive muscular dystrophy, 756
AV node. *See* Atrioventricular (AV) node
AVM. *See* Arteriovenous malformation
AVP. *See* Arginine vasopressin
Awake paralysis, 897–899
Awareness under anesthesia, **897–899**
  bispectral index (BIS) monitoring in prevention of, 118
Axid. *See* Nizatidine
Axillary artery
  catheterization of for arterial blood pressure monitoring, 87f, 93
  fixed anatomic relationships and, 285
  transarterial axillary brachial plexus block and, 291
Axillary brachial plexus block, 283, 291–292, 292f
Axillary temperature, intraoperative monitoring of, 119
Axis, 255
Ayre's T-piece, in Mapleson circuits, 30t
Azotemia, 681, 683, 976–978, 977t. *See also* Renal failure
  acute renal failure differentiated from, 977–978, 977t
  postrenal, 683, **977**, 977t
  prerenal, 683, **976–977**, 977t
  renal, 683, 977, 977t
  reversible causes of, 977t

B fibers, 260t
Back, applied anatomy of, **352**
Back blows, for foreign body removal in pediatric patient, 917, 918t
Back pain, **352–355**
  neuraxial anesthesia and, 275, 277
    epidural abscess causing, 279
  patient positioning and, 899t

Bacteremia, pulmonary artery catheterization and, 105
Bacteria
blood transfusion in transmission of infections caused by, 638
circle system contamination by, 36
BAER. *See* Brainstem evoked potentials
Bag-mask-valve system, for oxygen therapy, 955*t*, 956–957
Bag-mask ventilation, for resuscitation, 37, 918, 921
Bag-valve-endotracheal tube ventilation, in cardiopulmonary resuscitation, 921
Bag-valve ventilation
in cardiopulmonary resuscitation, 921
for trauma patient, 795
Bain system, for pediatric patient, 861
Balanced anesthesia, 4
Balloon tamponade, for upper gastrointestinal bleeding, 986
Band leukocytes, in systemic inflammatory response syndrome, 980*t*
Barbiturates, 151, **156–159**, 157*f. See also specific agent*
abuse of, anesthetic requirements affected by, 594*t*
cerebral effects of, 151, 158–159, 171*t*, 558*t*, 559
for cerebral protection, 552, 562
electroencephalogram affected by, 563*t*, 564
evoked potentials affected by, 563*t*, 564
in geriatric anesthesia, 875, 880
for induction, history of use of, 3
intraocular pressure affected by, 763*t*
mechanisms of action of, 156
minimum alveolar concentration affected by, 136*t*
organ system effects of, 158–159, 159*t*, 171*t*
in pediatric anesthesia, 855
pharmacokinetics of, 156–158, 158*f*
renal effects of, 673
altered renal function and, 681
structure-activity relationships of, 156, 157*f*
uses and doses of, 159*t*
uteroplacental blood flow affected by, 811
Barbituric acid, 156, 157*f*
Baricity, neural blockade after spinal anesthesia affected by, 267, 267*t*
Barium hydroxide lime, as carbon dioxide absorbent, 33–34, 33*t*
Baroreceptor reflex, 375
Baroreceptors
in blood pressure control, 375
in volume regulation, 610
Barotrauma
mechanical ventilation and, 960
PEEP/CPAP and, 951, 969
Basal energy expenditure (BEE), energy requirements and, 987
Basal metabolic rate (BMR), energy requirements and, 987
Base excess, 650, 651*f*
Baseline heart rate, in fetal heart rate monitoring, 840
Baseline variability, in fetal heart rate monitoring, 840
Bases. *See also* Acid-base balance
definition of, 645
Basic life support, 913*f*, 916*f*, 918*t. See also* Cardiopulmonary resuscitation
Basilar skull fracture, 576
Basilic vein cannulation, for central venous pressure monitoring, 100*t*
Basophil kallikrein of anaphylaxis, 903–905
Beat-to-beat variability, in fetal heart rate monitoring, 840
Beck Depression Inventory, in pain evaluation, 322
Becker's muscular dystrophy, 755
anesthetic considerations in patients with, 756
Becker's myotonia congenita, 757
BEE. *See* Basal energy expenditure
Behavior therapy, for pain management, 339
Bellows assembly
for anesthesia ventilators, 52, 53*f*
ventilator failure and, 52, 57
Benadryl. *See* Diphenhydramine
Benign prostatic hypertrophy, transurethral resection of prostate for, 694–697
Bentall procedure, 468
Benzodiazepines, **160–164**, 160*f. See also specific agent*
abuse of, anesthetic requirements affected by, 594*t*
altered renal function and, 682
antagonist of. *See* Flumazenil
for cardiac surgery
postbypass, 458
for premedication, 440
cerebral effects of, 164, 171*t*, 558*t*, 560
congenital anomalies caused by, 847
drug interactions and, 164
electroencephalogram affected by, 563*t*, 564

evoked potentials affected by, 563*t*
in geriatric anesthesia, 875, 880
for induction, history of use of, 3
intraocular pressure affected by, 763*t*
mechanisms of action of, 160
minimum alveolar concentration affected by, 136*t*
organ system effects of, 161–164, 171*t*
pharmacokinetics of, 161, 161*t*
placental transfer of, 811, 821
receptors for, 160
structure-activity relationships of, 160, 160*f*
uses and doses of, 161*t*
Benzothiazapine, for hypertension, 391*t*
Bepridil, 398*t*
Bernoulli effect, in high-frequency jet ventilation, 965
Bernoulli equation, in pressure gradient determination, in mitral stenosis, 411
Beta (β)-agonists
for asthma, 513, 514*t*
for hyperkalemia, 617
uterine activity during labor affected by, 813
Beta (β) blockers, 207, **221**, 221*t*, 397*t*, 398, 399*t*
for acute myocardial infarction, 976
adverse effects of, 391*t*
for hypertension, 389, 390, 390*t*
intraoperative, 395
in postanesthesia care unit, 947
interaction of with α-agonists, cardiac arrest caused by, **900–901**
for ischemic heart disease, 397*t*, 398, 399*t*
for thyroid storm, 950
Beta (β) cells, pancreatic, insulin produced by, 737, 737*t*
Beta (β) endorphins. *See also* Endorphins
pain mediation/modulation and, 316*t*
central inhibition, 319
Beta (β/elimination) phase, of two-compartment model, 154*f*, 155
Beta₁ (β₁)-receptors, 215
adrenergic agonist selectivity and, 215–216, 216*t*
adrenergic antagonist selectivity and, 220, 220*t*
cardiac, 366
Beta₂ (β₂)-receptors, 215
adrenergic agonist selectivity and, 215–216, 216*t*
adrenergic antagonist selectivity and, 220, 220*t*
cardiac, 366
in hepatic blood flow regulation, 710
Beta (β)-thalassemia, 642
Betamethasone, for pain management, 338*t*
Betaxolol, 399*t*
Bicarbonate
in body fluid/fluid compartments, 599*t*, 631
buffering action of, 644, 646–648, 647*t*
in carbon dioxide transport, 476, 504–505, 504*t*, 505*t*
in cardioplegia solutions, 438–439, 438*t*
in cardiopulmonary resuscitation, 912, 924
in crystalloid solutions, 629*t*
for drug overdose/poisoning, 992
gastrointestinal loss of, in hyperchloremic acidosis, 655
for hypercalcemia, 617
in metabolic acidosis, 646*t*, 653–656
in metabolic alkalosis, 646*t*, 656–658
for neonatal resuscitation, 846
pediatric dosing and, 855*t*
pregnancy affecting, 805, 805*t*
in renal compensation, 648–650, 649*f*, 650*f*
reabsorption and, 648–649
renal loss of, in hyperchloremic acidosis, 655
in respiratory acidosis, 646*t*, 652, 658–659, 659*t*
in respiratory alkalosis, 646*t*, 656, 658–659, 659*t*
Bicarbonate space, 656
Bicitra. *See* Sodium citrate
Bidirectional Glenn shunt, for tricuspid atresia, 426
Bier block (intravenous regional anesthesia), 283, 284
of arm, **297–298**, 298*f*
for pain management, 335
Bifascicular block, presentation of, 429
Bile, formation/excretion of, **713–714**, 713*f*
anesthesia affecting, 708, 716
Bile acids, formation of, 714
Bile canaliculi, 709, 709*f*
Bile ducts, 709, 709*f*, 713, 713*f*
Bilevel positive airway pressure (BiPAP), 968
Biliary cirrhosis, 726
Biliary colic, opioids causing, 169
Biliary reconstruction, after liver transplant, 733
Biliary secretions, electrolyte content of, 631*t*
Biliary spasm, opioids causing, 169
Biliary system, 713*f*

Bilirubin
excretion of, 714
serum levels of, 714–715, 714*t*
Bioavailability, 152
Biofeedback, for pain management, 339
Bioimpedance
drug interactions and, 159
thoracic, in intraoperative monitoring, 107
Biotransformation, drug, 713. *See also specific agent* and Metabolism
in geriatric patient, 878
of inhalational agents, 132–133
BiPAP. *See* Bilevel positive airway pressure
Bipolar disorder, 593
Bipolar electrodes, for surgical diathermy unit, 23–24
BIS. *See* Bispectral Index
Bisoprolol, 399*t*
Bispectral index (BIS), for intraoperative monitoring, 115, 115*f*, 116*f*
prevention of awareness and, 118
Bisphosphonates, for hypercalcemia, 619–620
Bitolterol, for asthma, 514*t*
Biventricular heart failure, in children, 460
BK-A. *See* Basophil kallikrein of anaphylaxis
Bladder cancer, **701–702**
Bladder catheterization
for neuraxial blocks, 276
for urinary output monitoring, 120, 677
during craniotomy, 569
during head and neck cancer surgery, 776
during renal transplant, 705
Bladder function, neuraxial anesthesia affecting, 261
Bladder perforation, during transurethral resection of prostate, 696
Blalock-Taussig shunt
for tetralogy of Fallot, 425
for tricuspid atresia, 426
Bleeding. *See also* Blood loss; Postoperative bleeding/hemorrhage
antepartum, **835–836**
after cardiopulmonary bypass, persistent, 434, 458
gastroesophageal variceal, in cirrhosis, 723, 727
gastrointestinal, **984–986**
from hip fracture, 783, 783*f*, 881
intra-arterial monitoring and, 93
liver disease and, 717–722, 718*t*, 719*f*, 721*t*
management of, in Jehovah's Witnesses, 790–791
after massive transfusion, dilutional thrombocytopenia causing, 626, 638
after nasal or sinus surgery, 779–780
postpartum, **839–840**
during surgery
estimating loss and, 631
fluid replacement for, 632–633, 632*t*
hip replacement surgery and, 786–787
liver disease and, 717–722, 718*t*, 719*f*, 721*t*
in trauma patient, 795–796, 795*t*, 796*t*
fluid resuscitation and, 795–797
Bleeding prophylaxis, cardiopulmonary bypass and, 450
Bleeding time, 721
Bleomycin, oxygen-induced toxicity and, 520, 692, 703
Blood bank practices, **634–635**
Blood-brain barrier, 153, 552, **555**
cerebral effects of vasopressors and, 560
disruption of, cerebral edema and, 568
Blood clotting. *See* Coagulation
Blood flow. *See specific organ or system*
pulsatile, for cardiopulmonary bypass, 436
Blood/gas partition coefficients. *See* Partition coefficients
Blood gases, arterial. *See* Arterial blood gases
Blood groups, **633**, 633*t*
Blood loss. *See also* Bleeding
during delivery, 806
from hip fracture, 783, 783*f*, 881
management of, in Jehovah's Witnesses, 790–791
during surgery
estimating, 631
fluid replacement for, 632–633, 632*t*
Blood pressure. *See* Arterial blood pressure; Central venous pressure
Blood salvage and reinfusion, **639**
for Jehovah's witnesses, 790
Blood transfusion. *See* Transfusion
Blood urea nitrogen, **680**
in azotemia/renal failure, 976, 977*t*
in geriatric patient, 878
in pregnancy, 807
Blood urea nitrogen:creatinine ratio, **680–681**

Blood viscosity
    cerebral blood flow affected by, 554–555
    in congenital heart disease, 422
Blood volume
    distribution of, 372, 374*t*
    normal values for, 632*t*
    pregnancy affecting, 805*t*, 806
Bloody show, 811
Blue bloater syndrome, 516
BMI. *See* Body mass index
BMR. *See* Basal metabolic rate
Body fluid compartments, **598–601**, 598*t*, 599*t*, 600*f*,
        601*f*
    exchanges between, **600**, 601*f*
Body fluids, electrolyte content of, 631*t*
Body mass index (BMI), 748
Body temperature. *See also* Hyperthermia; Hypothermia
    acid-base disorder diagnosis and, 644, 659
    anticholinergic drugs affecting, 209
    atracurium duration of action and, 192
    cerebral blood flow affected by, 554
    intraoperative monitoring of, **117**, 117*f*, 125
        for cardiac surgery, 441
        in pediatric patient, 849, 851
    minimum alveolar concentration affected by, 136*t*
    neuromuscular blocking agents affected by, 189
    in pediatric patient, 849, 851
    in systemic inflammatory response syndrome, 980*t*
Body weight, in nutritional assessment, 988
Bohr effect, 502
Bohr equation, 490–491
Bone cement implantation syndrome
    hip replacement and, 786
    knee replacement and, 788
Bone marrow depression, nitrous oxide causing, 139
Botulism, neuromuscular blocking agent response affected
        in, 190*t*
Bourdon pressure gauge, on anesthesia machine, 42, 43*f*
Bowel edema, in abdominal trauma, 800
Bowman's capsule, 663, 664*f*
Brachial artery catheterization, for arterial blood pressure
        monitoring, 87*f*, 93
Brachial plexus
    anatomy of, 283, **286–287**, 287*f*, 288*f*
        fixed relationships and, 285–286
    entrapment of, 351*t*
    injury of during surgery, 893, 899*t*
        lithotomy and, 693
Brachial plexus block, 283, 286, 287*f*, **288–292**, 288*f*
    axillary, 283, 291–292, 292*f*
    infraclavicular, 290, 291*f*
    interscalene, 283, 288–289, 289*f*
        dyspnea after, 308
    midhumeral, 292
    in pain evaluation/management, **335–336**
    supraclavicular (subclavian), 289–290, 290*f*
    techniques for, **288–292**
Bradyarrhythmias, sources of, 428
Bradycardia. *See also* Heart rate
    algorithm for management of, 933*f*
    during carotid endarterectomy, 471
    cholinesterase inhibitors causing, 202
    in postanesthesia care unit, 947
    succinylcholine causing, 186
Bradycardia-tachycardia syndrome, 428
Bradykinin, in primary hyperalgesia, 317
Brain. *See also under Cerebral*
    blood supply of, **553**, 564–566, 565*f*. *See also* Cerebral
        circulation/blood flow
    herniation of, elevated intracranial pressure and,
        556–557, 557*f*
    oxygen saturation in, 552–553, 553*f*
        regional (rSO₂), intraoperative oximetry in
            monitoring of, 110
Brain circuit, 30*t*, 32, 33*f*
Brain concussion, 576
Brain contusion, 576
Brain death, 951, 953
Brain injury, 793, 797–798. *See also* Head trauma
Brain mass, in geriatric patient, 878
Brain oximetry, noninvasive, for intraoperative monitoring,
        110
Brain protection. *See* Cerebral protection
Brain stimulation, for pain management, 340
Brainstem evoked potentials (BAER), for intraoperative
        monitoring, anesthetic agents affecting, 563*t*,
        564
Brainstem injury

malignant hyperthermia differentiated from, 873
    posterior fossa craniotomy and, 573
Braxton Hicks contractions, 811, 812
Breath holding, during induction in pediatric patient, 860
Breath sounds, unilaterally diminished, during anesthesia,
        509–510
Breathing. *See also* Respiration; Respiratory physiology;
        Ventilation
    at birth, 816
    in cardiopulmonary resuscitation, 918*t*, **920–921**
    control of, **505–508**
        anesthesia affecting, 508, 509*f*
        central respiratory centers in, **506–507**
        central sensors in, 476, 507, 507*f*
        peripheral receptors in, **507–508**, 508*f*
    mechanical ventilation and, 480
    mechanism of, **480–482**
    pregnancy affecting, 805–806, 805*t*
    rescue, 918*t*, **920–921**
    spontaneous ventilation, 480, 481*f*
    work of, **488–489**, 490*f*, 491*f*
        anesthesia affecting, 490
        in pediatric patient, 850
Breathing bag
    in circle system, 35, 36*f*
    in Mapleson circuits, 30*t*, 31*f*, 32, 32*f*, 33*f*
Breathing-circuit disconnection/leak, 56–58, 891, 891*t*
    alarms signaling, 41, 53, 57
    inspection routine for prevention of, **55–56**, 56–57*t*
Breathing-circuit pressure gauges, for anesthesia machine,
        41, **44–47**, 46*f*, 47*t*
Breathing systems, **27–39**, 28*f*
    characteristics of, 33*t*
    checkout list for, **55–56**, 56–57*t*
    circle system, **32–36**, 33*t*, 34*f*, 34*t*, 35*f*, 36*f*
    insufflation, 15, **28**, 28*f*, 29*f*, 33*t*
    leaks in, 56–58, 891, 891*t*
        alarms signaling, 41, 53, 57
        inspection routine for prevention of, **55–56**, 56–57*t*
    Mapleson circuits/systems, **29–32**, 30*t*, 31*f*, 32*f*, 33*f*, 33*t*
    open drop anesthesia, **28–29**, 33*t*
    for pediatric patient, 861
    resuscitation, **37**, 37*f*
    unexplained light anesthesia and, 37–39, 39*f*
    ventilator use and, 53–54
Breathing tubes, in Mapleson circuits, 15, 30*t*, 31, 31*f*, 33*f*
Breech presentation, 834
Brethaire. *See* Terbutaline
Bretylium
    in cardiopulmonary resuscitation, 924
    for intravenous regional sympathetic blockade, 335
    pediatric dosing and, 853*t*
Brofaromine, for depression, 592*t*
Bronchial adenomas, 534
Bronchial blocker, with single-lumen endotracheal tube
    for one-lung ventilation, **533–534**
    for pulmonary hemorrhage, 541
Bronchial circulation, 478
Bronchiectasis, lung resection for, **536**
Bronchitis, chronic, 516. *See also* Chronic obstructive
        pulmonary disease
Bronchoalveolar lavage, 546
Bronchoconstriction, H₁-receptor stimulation causing, 243
Bronchodilation
    adrenergic agonists causing, 217*t*
    anticholinergic drugs causing, 207, 208*t*, 209
    asthma medications producing, 513–514
    ephedrine causing, 217*t*, 218
    epinephrine causing, 217*t*, 218
    H₂-receptor stimulation causing, 243
    halothane causing, 140
    isoflurane causing, 143
    local anesthetics causing, 239
    methoxyflurane causing, 141
    nitroglycerine causing, 228
    nonvolatile anesthetics causing, 171*t*
Bronchodilators
    for asthma, 513–514, 514*t*
        preoperative use of, 515
    for COPD, 517
Bronchopleural fistula, 541–542
    after lung resection, 525, 540–542
    PEEP/CPAP and, 969
Bronchoscopes/bronchoscopy, 772–773
    flexible fiberoptic, 69–70, 71*f*
        for double-lumen endobronchial tube placement
            confirmation/repositioning, 531–533
        in inhalation injury, 975

for nasal intubation, 74–77, 77*f*
    rigid, 544–545
Bronchospasm
    airway instrumentation causing, 80
        asthma and, 515
        barbiturate induction and, 158
    in asthma, 511, 513–516
    atracurium causing, 191
    cholinesterase inhibitors causing, 202
    intraoperative, in asthma patient, 511, 515–516
    rapacuronium causing, 197
    tubocurarine causing, 191
Bronkosol. *See* Isoetharine
Brönsted-Lowry definitions, 645
Brow presentation, 834
Brown fat, thermoregulation in pediatric patient and, 851
Bruits, cervical, in cerebrovascular disease, 583, 584
Bubble-through humidifier, in breathing circuit, 54–55
Buccal drug administration/absorption, 152
Buffers, in acid-base balance, 644, 645–646, **646–648**
    carbon dioxide transport and, 505
Bullae, pulmonary, lung resection and, 525, 541
Bumetanide, 674–675. *See also* Loop diuretics
Bumex. *See* Bumetanide
BUN. *See* Blood urea nitrogen
Bundle branch block, significance of, 429
Bundle of His, 362*f*, 363
Bundle of Kent, in preexcitation, 381
Bupivacaine, 236*t*
    cardiotoxicity of, 239, 241, 363
    for caudal anesthesia, 273
        in pediatric patient, 863
    for epidural anesthesia, 271, 272, 272*t*
        for labor and delivery, 824, 827, 827*t*
    infiltration of, for postoperative pain management, 342
    intravascular administration of, unintentional, 233, 241
    placental transfer of, 811
    specific gravity of, 267*t*
    for spinal anesthesia, 268, 268*t*
        for labor and delivery, 825, 827, 827*t*
        with opioids, 347, 827, 827*t*
        after thoracotomy, 540
Buprion, for depression, 592*t*, 593
Burns, 800*f*, 801–803, 801*f*
    classification of, 801, 801*f*
    diathermy, 15, **23–24**, 25*f*
    infection and, 981
    neuromuscular blocking agent response affected in, 190*t*
    smoke inhalation injury and, 801, 974–975
Butorphanol, 348
    epidural, 348
    neonate affected by, 811, 821
    in postanesthesia care unit, 940
    for postoperative shivering, 706

C fibers, 260*t*
    in pain sensation, 310, 312–313, 313*f*, 315
        cornea/tooth pulp innervation and, 316
        visceral, 316
c wave, 102, 102*f*, 366, 367*f*
Ca⁺ channels. *See* Calcium channels
CACI. *See* "Computer-assisted continuous infusion"
Calcitonin, 743, 744*t*
    calcium concentration affected by, 619, 743, 744*t*
    for hypercalcemia, 619
    in medullary thyroid carcinoma, 750
Calcitonin gene-related peptide, pain
        mediation/modulation and, 316, 316*t*
    central sensitization and, 318
Calcium
    balance of
        disorders of, **618–621**. *See also* Hypercalcemia;
            Hypocalcemia
        minimum alveolar concentration affected by, 136*t*
        normal, **618**
    parathyroid hormone in maintenance of, 743, 744*t*
    in cardioplegia solutions, 438, 438*t*
    in cerebral ischemia, 561
    as coagulation factor, 718*t*
    in crystalloid solutions, 629*t*
    extracellular ionized, regulation of, 618–619
    in fluid compartments, 599*t*
    for hyperkalemia, 617
    for hypermagnesemia, 623
    for hypocalcemia, 621
    plasma concentration of, 618
    supplemental/replacement, in hypocalcemia, 621

Calcium channel blockers, 364, 397–398, 397t, 398t
  for acute myocardial infarction, 976
  adverse effects of, 392t
  for cerebral protection, 562
  for hypertension, 389, 391t, 398t
  for ischemic heart disease, 397–398, 397t, 398t
Calcium channels
  abnormalities of, periodic paralysis and (voltage-gated
      calcium channelopathy/hypokalemic periodic
      paralysis), 758, 759
  myocardial, 361, 363t
Calcium chloride
  in cardiopulmonary resuscitation, 924
  for hypocalcemia, 621
  pediatric dosing and, 853t
Calcium-dependent calcium release, in excitation-
    contraction coupling, 364
Calcium gluconate
  for hypermagnesemia, 623
  for neonatal resuscitation, 846
  pediatric dosing and, 853t
Calcium hydroxide and calcium chloride, as carbon dioxide
    absorbent, 34
Caldwell-Luc procedure, 774–776, 775f
Canaliculi, bile, 709, 709f
Cancer pain, 348–350
  facial, trigeminal nerve block in management of,
      323–326, 324–325f
  intraspinal, 349
  management of, 348–350
  neurolytic blocks in management of, 336, 349–350
  opioids for
    oral, 348–349
    parenteral, 349
    transdermal, 349
Cannulation, for cardiopulmonary bypass, 450–451
Capillary fluid exchange, 600, 601f
Capillary gas tensions, in acid-base disorder diagnosis, 659
Capillary hydrostatic pressure (Pc), in pulmonary edema,
    971, 972
Capnography
  for detection of tracheal tube placement, 59, 86, 111
  for end-tidal carbon dioxide analysis, 110–112, 111f,
      112f
  in neonate/pediatric patient, 845, 857–858
Caput medusae, 727
Carbamazepine
  for pain management, 337, 338, 338t
  for seizures, 586, 586t
Carbamino compounds, in carbon dioxide transport, 504t,
    505, 505f
Carbicarb, for respiratory acidosis, 652
Carbidopa, with levodopa, for Parkinson's disease, 587
Carbocaine. See Mepivacaine
Carbohydrate metabolism
  in diabetes, 737
  in liver, 710–712, 711f
  pregnancy affecting, 807
Carbon dioxide, 504–505
  absorption spectrum for, capnography and, 110, 111f
  intraoperative monitoring of
    end-tidal analysis of, 110–112, 111f, 112f. See also
        End-tidal carbon dioxide
    transcutaneous, 112–113
  oxygen consumption relationship and, 147
  partial pressures of, 499–501. See also specific type
    in acid-base disorder diagnosis, 660
  production of
    anesthesia affecting, 475, 477
    ratio of to oxygen consumption (respiratory quotient),
        476–477
  rebreathing, 33t. See also Rebreathing
    circle system and, 33–35, 33t, 34f, 34t, 35f
    Mapleson circuits and, 32, 33t
  stores of, 505
  transport of, 504–505, 504t
    across placenta, 810
    bicarbonate and, 476, 504–505, 504t, 505t
    carbamino compounds and, 504t, 505, 505t
    dissolved in blood, 504, 504t, 505t
    hemoglobin buffering and, 505
Carbon dioxide absorbents, in circle system, 33–34, 33t, 34t
Carbon dioxide absorbers, for circle system, 27, 34–35, 34f
Carbon dioxide dissociation curve, 505, 506f
Carbon dioxide laser, 773
Carbon dioxide narcosis, 650
Carbon dioxide tension
  alveolar (PACO$_2$), 500, 500f

  arterial (PaCO$_2$), 500
    bicarbonate buffering and, 647–648
    central chemoreceptors in regulation of, 476, 507
    cerebral blood flow affected by, 554, 554f
    desflurane affecting, 138t, 144
    enflurane affecting, 138t, 142
    halothane affecting, 138t, 140
    inhalational anesthetics affecting, 138t
    intracranial compliance affected by, 556
    intraocular pressure and, 762, 762t
    labor and delivery affecting, 812
    in metabolic acidosis, 646t, 648, 658–659, 658f, 659t
    in metabolic alkalosis, 646t, 648
    methoxyflurane affecting, 138t, 141
    minimum alveolar concentration affected by, 136t
    nitrous oxide affecting, 137, 138t
    opioids affecting, 167, 168f, 344
    pneumonectomy criteria and, 535t
    pregnancy affecting, 805, 805t
    P$_{tc}$CO$_2$ (P$_s$CO$_2$) as measure of, 113
    pulmonary compensation and, 648
    in respiratory acidosis, 646t, 650–653
    in respiratory alkalosis, 646t, 656, 658–659, 658f,
        659t
  end-tidal (PETCO$_2$), 501
    monitoring, during laparoscopy, 523
  hemoglobin dissociation curve affected by, 502
  management of during cardiopulmonary bypass, 453
    during carotid endarterectomy, 471
  mixed venous (Pv̄CO$_2$), 500
Carbon monoxide. See also Carbon monoxide poisoning
  desflurane degradation to, absorbent granule exposure
      causing, 27, 34, 144–145
  oxygen carrying capacity of hemoglobin affected by, 503,
      974
Carbon monoxide diffusion capacity (DLCO), 498
Carbon monoxide poisoning, 801–802, 974–975
  oximetry in, 109, 801, 974, 975
  smoke inhalation/burn injuries and, 801–802, 974–975
Carbonic anhydrase, in carbon dioxide transport, 504–505
Carbonic anhydrase inhibitors, 676–677
Carboxyhemoglobin (COHb)
  in carbon monoxide poisoning, 801–802, 974–975
  light absorption by, oximetry and, 109
Carcinoid syndrome, 736, 749–750, 750t
Carcinoid tumors, 749
  pulmonary, 534
Cardiac action potential, 359, 360–361, 361t, 362f, 363t
Cardiac arrest
  algorithms for management of, 913f, 916f
  α-agonist/β-blocker interactions causing, 900–901
  intraoperative, cardiopulmonary resuscitation for,
      925–935
  neuraxial anesthesia and, 261, 277
  in pediatric patient, 858–859
  during spinal anesthesia, 277, 900
Cardiac catheterization
  in left-to-right shunts, 423
  preoperative, in valvular heart disease, 407
Cardiac cirrhosis, 726
Cardiac compressions
  in cardiopulmonary resuscitation, 918t, 921–922
  for neonatal resuscitation, 845, 845f, 918t
Cardiac conduction, 361–364
  abnormal, preexcitation and, 381
  adenosine affecting, 230
  anticholinergic drugs affecting, 208
  β$_1$ adrenoceptor activation affecting, 215
  inhalational anesthetics affecting, 359, 363
  local anesthetics affecting, 238–239, 363
Cardiac contractility. See Myocardial
    contraction/contractility
Cardiac cycle, 366, 367f
  coronary blood flow during, 376, 378f
Cardiac enzymes, preoperative evaluation of, 400
Cardiac failure. See Heart failure
Cardiac impulse, initiation/conduction of, 361–364. See
    also Cardiac conduction
Cardiac index, 359, 366
  adenosine affecting, 230
  pulmonary artery catheterization monitoring of, 106t
Cardiac induction
  in adults, 447–448
  in children, 460–462
Cardiac massage, open-chest, 922
Cardiac monitoring, intraoperative, 87–108, 125
  arterial blood pressure, 87–97
  cardiac output, 106–108

  central venous catheterization for, 100–102
  electrocardiography, 97–100
  pulmonary artery catheterization for, 102–106
  venous pressure, 100–102
Cardiac output, 359–360, 366. See also Ventricular
    function
  A-a gradient affected by, 499, 499f
  adrenergic agonists affecting, 217t
  afterload and, 360, 370, 371f
  in aortic stenosis, 416
  barbiturates affecting, 158
  benzodiazepines affecting, 161
  in cirrhosis, 728
  desflurane affecting, 138t, 144
  dobutamine affecting, 217t, 219
  dopamine affecting, 217t, 219
  enflurane affecting, 138t, 142
  ephedrine affecting, 217t, 218
  epinephrine affecting, 217t, 218
  in geriatric patient, 876
  halothane affecting, 138t, 140
  in heart failure, 380
  heart rate and, 367, 368f
  hydralazine affecting, 229
  inhalational anesthetics affecting, 138t
  intraoperative monitoring of, 86, 106–108
  isoflurane affecting, 143
  labetalol affecting, 220
  labor and delivery affecting, 804, 813
  measurement of, 359, 366
  methoxyflurane affecting, 138t, 141
  nitroprusside affecting, 227
  obesity affecting, 748
  pain affecting, 320
  PEEP/CPAP affecting, 969
  phenylephrine affecting, 216, 217t
  pregnancy affecting, 805t, 806
  propofol affecting, 174
  propranolol affecting, 222
  in renal failure, 685
  sevoflurane affecting, 138t, 145
  trimethaphan affecting, 229
  venous admixture and, 494–495, 497f
Cardiac pacing. See also Pacemakers
  transcutaneous, in cardiopulmonary resuscitation, 912,
      924–925, 932f, 933f
Cardiac physiology. See Cardiovascular physiology
Cardiac reserve, in geriatric patient, 875, 876
Cardiac surgery, 440–459. See also Cardiopulmonary
    bypass
  for acute myocardial infarction, 976
  anesthesia for
    during bypass, 453–454
    during postbypass period, 458
  anticoagulation for, 433, 434, 449–450
    reversal of, 434, 457–458
  bleeding after bypass and, 458
  bleeding prophylaxis for, 450
  bypass period and, 451–454
  cannulation for cardiopulmonary bypass and, 450–451
  cardioplegia for, 452–453
  cerebral protection during, 454
  choice of anesthetic agent for, 448–449
  hypothermia for, 434, 452–453
  induction of anesthesia for
    in adults, 447–448
    in children, 460–462
  inhalational anesthesia for, 448
    in children, 461, 462
  intravenous anesthesia for
    in adults, 448–449
    in children, 461, 462
  management of respiratory gases during, 453
  monitoring during
    in adults, 441–448
    bypass and, 451–452, 452f
    in children, 461
  muscle relaxants for, 449
  off-pump, 459–460, 459f
  in pediatric patients, 460–463
  postbypass period and
    in adults, 457–458
    in children, 462–463
  postoperative period and, 458–459
  prebypass period and, 449–451
  preinduction period of
    in adults, 440–449
    in children, 460

premedication for, 440
preparation for, 440
stroke after, 454, 584
termination of bypass and, **454–457**, 455*t*, 456*t*, 457*t*
transportation to ICU after, **458**
venous access for, 440–441
ventilation during, 453
Cardiac tamponade, 434, **464–465**, 935
central venous catheterization and, 102, 464
traumatic, 799
Cardiac transplant, **463–464**
for hypoplastic left heart syndrome, 427
surgery in patient with, 387, **427**
Cardiac valves. *See also* Valve replacement; Valvular heart disease
transesophageal echocardiography for intraoperative assessment of, 444–446, 445*f*, 446*f*
Cardiogenic shock, 795*t*
Cardiomyopathy
hypertrophic, **418–419**
heart murmur in, preoperative evaluation of, 407*t*
transesophageal echocardiography for assessment of, 446
ischemic, 396
Cardioplegia, 438–439, 438*t*, 452–453
Cardioplegia pump, for cardiopulmonary bypass machine, 437
Cardiopulmonary arrest. *See* Cardiac arrest
Cardiopulmonary bypass, 433, **435–440**, **451–454**
accessory pump/devices for, 435*f*, 437
in adults, **451–454**
anesthesia for
during bypass, 453–454
after bypass, 458
anticoagulation for, 433, 434, 449–450
reversal of, 434, 457–458
for aortic arch surgery, 468
arterial filter for, 435*f*, 436–437
for ascending aorta surgery, 467–468
basic circuit for, **435–437**, 435*f*
bleeding prophylaxis for, 450
cannulation for, 450–451
for cardiac surgery, **451–454**, 462
for cardiac transplantation, 463–464
cardioplegia for, 438–439, 438*t*, 452–453
cerebral protection and, 454
in children, 462
flow and pressure considerations in, 451
heat exchanger for, 435*f*, 436
hormonal responses to, 439
humoral responses to, 439
hypothermia used for, 434, **437**, 452–453
initiation of, 433, 451
for lung transplant, 547
main pump for, 435*f*, 436
monitoring during, 451–452, 452*f*
myocardial preservation and, **437–439**
oxygenator for, 435*f*, 436
persistent bleeding after, 434, 458
pharmacokinetics affected by, 439–440
physiologic effects of, **439–440**
potassium cardioplegia and, 438–439, 438*t*
in pregnant patient, 847
reservoir for, 435*f*, 436
respiratory gases management during, 453
termination of, **454–457**, 455*t*, 456*t*, 457*t*
transportation to intensive care unit after, 458
ventilation during, 453
weaning from
adults, 455–457, 455*t*, 456*t*, 457*f*
children, 462
Cardiopulmonary resuscitation (CPR), **912–935**, 914*t*. *See also* Neonatal resuscitation
airway management in, 915–920, 917*f*, 918*f*, 918*t*, 919*f*, 920*f*
algorithms/protocols for, 913*f*, 916*f*, **925**, 930–934*f*
breathing in, 918*t*, **920–921**
chest compressions in, 912, 921–922
circulation in, **921–922**
defibrillation in, **922**, 923*t*, 925*t*
drugs used in, 924, 926–929*t*
dysrhythmia recognition and, 924, 930*f*
emergency pacemaker therapy in, 924–925
for intraoperative hypotension and cardiac arrest, 925–935
intravenous access for, 922–924
invasive, 922

Cardiopulmonary resuscitation and emergency care (CPR-ECC), 912, 913*f*, 914*t*, 916*f*
Cardiotomy suction pump, for cardiopulmonary bypass machine, 437
Cardiovascular disease, **386–432**. *See also specific disorder and* Cardiovascular physiology; Cardiovascular surgery
risk factors and, **387–388**, 388*t*
Cardiovascular physiology, **359–385**. *See also specific aspect and under* Cardiac; Circulation; Heart; Myocardial
age-related changes in, 875, **876**, 877*t*
anticholinergic drugs affecting, 208–209
atracurium affecting, 191
atropine affecting, 207, 208*t*, 209
barbiturates affecting, 158, 171*t*
benzodiazepines affecting, 161, 171*t*
burn injuries affecting, 802
in children, 460
cholinesterase inhibitors affecting, 202, 202*t*
desflurane affecting, 138*t*, 144
dobutamine affecting, 217*t*, 219
dopamine affecting, 217*t*, 219
droperidol affecting, 171*t*, 175
endoscopy affecting, 773
enflurane affecting, 138*t*, 142, 363
ephedrine affecting, 217*t*, 218
epinephrine affecting, 217*t*, 218
esmolol affecting, 221
etomidate affecting, 171*t*, 172
fenoldopam affecting, 231
in geriatric patient, 875, **876**, 877*t*
halothane affecting, 138*t*, 139, 363
histamine affecting, 243
hydralazine affecting, 228–229
hyperkalemia affecting, 617
hyperparathyroidism affecting, 744*t*
hyperthyroidism affecting, 741
hypocalcemia affecting, 620–621
hypokalemia affecting, 614, 614*t*
hypoparathyroidism affecting, 745*t*
hypotensive agents affecting, 226*t*
inhalational anesthetics affecting, 138*t*, 363, 364
indirect renal effects and, 672
intraocular pressure and, 762, 762*t*
isoflurane affecting, 138*t*, 143, 363
ketamine affecting, 151, 171–172, 171*t*
labetalol affecting, 220
labor affecting, 804, 812–813
laparoscopy affecting, 522–523
local anesthetics affecting, 233, 238–239, 363, 366
indirect renal effects and, 672
methoxyflurane affecting, 138*t*, 141
neuraxial anesthesia affecting, 253, 260–261
nitroglycerine affecting, 228
nitroprusside affecting, 227
nitrous oxide affecting, 137, 138*t*
nonvolatile anesthetics affecting, 171*t*
indirect renal effects and, 672
obesity affecting, 748
opioids affecting, 167, 171*t*
pain affecting, 320
patient positioning affecting, 898*t*
in pediatric patient, 851, 851*t*
phentolamine affecting, 220
pregnancy affecting, 805*t*, 806–807
propofol affecting, 171*t*, 174
radical neck dissection affecting, 777
renal failure affecting, 685
rheumatoid arthritis affecting, 784*t*
sevoflurane affecting, 138*t*, 145
succinylcholine affecting, 186
trimethaphan affecting, 229
tubocurarine affecting, 190
vecuronium affecting, 195
Cardiovascular surgery, **433–474**. *See also specific procedure and* Vascular surgery
in adults, **440–459**
cardiopulmonary bypass and, **435–440**, **451–454**. *See also* Cardiopulmonary bypass
in adults, **451–454**
anticoagulation for, 433, 434, 449–450
reversal of, 434, 457–458
bleeding prophylaxis for, 450
cannulation for, 450–451
in children, 462
initiation of, 433, 451
termination of, **454–457**, 455*t*, 456*t*, 457*t*

choice of anesthetic agent for, 448–449
heart transplant, **463–464**
inhalational anesthesia for
in adults, 448
in children, 461, 462
intravenous anesthesia for
in adults, 448–449
in children, 461, 462
monitoring during
in adults, 441–448
bypass and, 451–452, 452*f*
in children, 461
muscle relaxants for, 449
off-pump, **459–460**, 459*f*
opioids for
in adults, 448–449
in children, 461, 462
in pediatric patients, **460–463**
for pericardial disease, **464–466**
postbypass period and
in adults, **457–458**
in children, 462–463
postoperative period and, **458–459**
prebypass period and, **449–451**
preinduction period and
in adults, **440–449**
in children, 460
premedication for, 440
preparation for, 440
venous access for, 440–441
Cardioversion, 472–473, 922, 923*t*, 925*t*
for atrial fibrillation, 922, 923*t*
for atrial tachycardia in acute myocardial infarction, 976
in pediatric patient, 853*t*
for ventricular fibrillation, 922, 923*t*
in Wolff-Parkinson-White (WPW) syndrome, 385
Carlens double-lumen endobronchial tube, 529*t*, 530
Carotid arteries
brain supplied by, 564, 565*f*
larynx supplied by branches of, 60–61
obstruction of, in cerebrovascular disease, 584
surgery on, **470–472**
hemiplegia and, 564–566
Carotid baroreceptors, 375
antidiuretic hormone secretion and, 604
Carotid bodies, in breathing regulation, 507
Carotid cross-clamping, cerebral protection during, 471
Carotid endarterectomy, 470–472
Carpal tunnel syndrome, 351*t*
Carpopedal spasm (Trousseau's sign), in hypocalcemia, 620, 745
Carrier state, for hepatitis, 724
Carteolol, 399*t*
Cartilages, of larynx, 60, 61*f*
Carvedilol, 399*t*
Cataract surgery, regional blocks for, 767
Catecholamines, 216, 216*f*, 745
excess of, 736, **747–748**
in heart failure, 360, 380
nitroprusside affecting release of, 227
in renal blood flow regulation, 671
structure of, 216, 216*f*
Catheter-tubing-transducer system
for intra-arterial monitoring, 93–97, 97*f*, 98*f*, 99*f*
damping and, 93–94, 98*f*
Catheters. *See specific type*
Cauda equina, 255
Cauda equina (conus medullaris) syndrome, 239–240, 278, 590
Caudal anesthesia, 253–255, **273–274**, 274*f*, 275*f*. *See also* Neuraxial anesthesia
for labor and delivery, with local anesthetics, 826
in pediatric patient, 862–863
systemic toxicity and, 278
technique for, 273, 275*f*
Caudal steroids, 354
Caudate lobe of liver, 708
Causalgia (CRPS type II), 350
Cautery tip, for surgical diathermy unit, 23
Caval cannulas, for cardiopulmonary bypass, 450–451
Cavitary lesions, pulmonary, lung resection for, 536
CBF (cerebral blood flow). *See* Cerebral circulation/blood flow
CCK. *See* Cholecystokinin
Ceiling hose drops, for medical gas delivery, 18*f*
Celecoxib
for arthritis, 786
for postoperative pain management, 341, 341*t*

Celestone. *See* Betamethasone
Celexa. *See* Citalopram
Celiac plexus block, for pain management, 333–334, 333*f*
Cell-mediated/delayed (type IV) hypersensitivity reactions, 903, 903*t*
Cell-mediated immunity, impaired. *See also* Immunocompromised host
  septic shock and, 984–985*t*
Cell membrane, diffusion through, 600
Cellular respiration, **476–477**
  anesthesia affecting, **477**
Central anticholinergic syndrome, 210–211
Central chemoreceptors, in breathing control, 476, 507, 507*f*
Central compartment, in pharmacokinetic model, 154
Central-core disease, malignant hyperthermia and, 871
Central nervous system. *See* Neurologic system
Central pain modulation, 318–319
  facilitation, 318
  inhibition, 318–319
Central sensors, in breathing control, **507**, 507*f*
Central venous catheterization, **100–102**, 100*t*, 101*f*, 102*f*
  for cardiac surgery
    in adults, 441
    in children, 461
  for craniotomy, 569
  documentation of, 902
  for head and neck cancer surgery, 776
  for lung resection, 537
  for total parenteral nutrition, 989
  venous air embolism and, 102, 574–575
Central venous pressure
  intraocular pressure and, 762, 762*t*
  monitoring
    in hypovolemia evaluation, 627–628
    intraoperative, 100–102, 100*t*, 101*f*, 102*f*
      for cardiac surgery
        in adults, 441
        in children, 461
      controlled hypotension and, 232
      for craniotomy, 569
      for lung resection, 537
      in mitral stenosis, 411
      for renal transplant, 705
      in tricuspid regurgitation, 421
    PEEP/CPAP affecting, 969
Centrifugal pumps, for cardiopulmonary bypass machine, 436
Centrilobular necrosis, halothane causing, 140
Centrilobular vein, 709, 709*f*
Cephalosporins, penicillin allergy and, 906–907
Cerebral aneurysms, 567, **578–579**
Cerebral autoregulation curve, 552, 554, 554*f*. *See also* Autoregulation, cerebral blood flow
Cerebral blood volume, inhalational anesthetics affecting, 557–558, 558*t*
Cerebral circulation/blood flow, **553**, 564–566, 565*f*
  barbiturates affecting, 151, 158–159, 171*t*, 558*t*, 559
  benzodiazepines affecting, 164, 171*t*, 558*t*, 560
  during carotid endarterectomy, maintenance of, 471
  cerebral metabolic rate coupling and, 558
  desflurane affecting, 138*t*, 144, 557, 558*t*
  droperidol affecting, 171*t*, 175, 560
  enflurane affecting, 138*t*, 142, 557, 558*t*
  etomidate affecting, 171*t*, 173, 558*t*, 560
  in geriatric patient, 878
  halothane affecting, 138*t*, 140, 557, 558*t*
  hydralazine affecting, 229
  hypotensive agents affecting, 226*t*
  inhalational anesthetics affecting, 138*t*, 557–558, 558*f*, 558*t*
  isoflurane affecting, 138*t*, 143, 557, 558*t*
  ketamine affecting, 171*t*, 172, 558*t*, 560
  lidocaine affecting, 239, 558*t*, 560
  methoxyflurane affecting, 138*t*, 141
  nitroglycerine affecting, 226*t*, 228
  nitroprusside affecting, 226*t*, 227
  nitrous oxide affecting, 137, 138*t*, 558*t*, 559
  nonvolatile anesthetics affecting, 171*t*
  opioids affecting, 167–168, 171*t*, 558*t*, 559
  propofol affecting, 171*t*, 174
  regulation of, **553–555**
  sevoflurane affecting, 138*t*, 145, 557, 558*t*
Cerebral edema, **568**. *See also* Intracranial pressure
Cerebral function, monitoring, during carotid endarterectomy, 471
Cerebral infarct, hemispheric, carotid cross-clamping and, 566

Cerebral ischemia
  pathophysiology of, **561**
  prevention of, **561–563**. *See also* Cerebral protection
Cerebral metabolic rate. *See* Cerebral oxygen consumption/metabolic rate
Cerebral oxygen consumption/metabolic rate, **552–553**, 552*f*
  barbiturates affecting, 159, 171*t*, 558*t*, 559
  benzodiazepines affecting, 164, 171*t*, 558*t*, 560
  cerebral blood flow coupling and, 558
  desflurane affecting, 138*t*, 144, 557, 558*t*
  etomidate affecting, 171*t*, 173, 558*t*, 560
  halothane affecting, 138*t*, 140, 557, 558*t*
  inhalational anesthetics affecting, 138*t*, 557, 558, 558*t*
  ketamine affecting, 171*t*, 172, 558*t*, 560
  methoxyflurane affecting, 138*t*, 141
  nitrous oxide affecting, 137, 138*t*, 558*t*
  nonvolatile anesthetics affecting, 171*t*
  opioids affecting, 167–168, 171*t*, 558*t*, 559
Cerebral palsy, neuromuscular blocking agent response affected in, 190*t*
Cerebral perfusion pressure (CPP), 552, **553**
  barbiturates affecting, 158–159
  cerebral protection and, 52
  epinephrine affecting, 218
  etomidate affecting, 173
  monitoring, during craniotomy, 569
  opioids affecting, 168, 559
  propofol affecting, 174
  in ruptured aneurysm, 578
Cerebral physiology, **552–557**. *See also specific aspect*
  adjunctive agents affecting, **550**
  anesthetics affecting, **557–561**. *See also specific agent*
  anticholinergic drugs affecting, 209
  barbiturates affecting, 151, 158–159, 171*t*, 558*t*, 559
  benzodiazepines affecting, 164, 171*t*, 558*t*, 560
  blood-brain barrier and, **555**
  cerebral blood flow and, **553**, **553–555**
  cerebral metabolism and, **552–553**, 553*f*
  cerebrospinal fluid and, **555**, 556*f*
  cholinesterase inhibitors affecting, 202, 202*t*
  desflurane affecting, 138*t*, 144
  droperidol affecting, 171*t*, 175
  enflurane affecting, 138*t*, 142
  etomidate affecting, 171*t*, 173, 558*t*, 560
  halothane affecting, 138*t*, 140, 557, 558, 558*t*
  hydralazine affecting, 229
  inhalational anesthetics affecting, 138*t*, **557–559**, 558*f*, 558*t*
  intracranial pressure and, **556–557**, 556*f*, 557*f*
  isoflurane affecting, 138*t*, 143
  ketamine affecting, 171*t*, 172, 558*t*, 560
  methoxyflurane affecting, 138*t*, 141
  neuromuscular blocking agents affecting, **561**
  nitroglycerine affecting, 228
  nitroprusside affecting, 227
  nitrous oxide affecting, 137, 138*t*, 558*t*, **559**
  nonvolatile (intravenous) anesthetics affecting, 171*t*, 552, 558*t*, **559–560**
  opioids affecting, 167–168, 168*t*, 171*t*, 558*t*, 559
  propofol affecting, 171*t*, 174, 558*t*, 560
  sevoflurane affecting, 138*t*, 145
  trimethaphan affecting, 229
  vasodilators affecting, **560**
  vasopressors affecting, 552, **560**
Cerebral protection, 552, **561–562**, 566
  during cardiopulmonary bypass, 454
Cerebral vasospasm
  calcium channel blockers for, 398*t*
  ruptured aneurysm and, 567, **578–579**
Cerebrospinal fluid (CSF), **555**, 556*f*
  absorption of, 555
  barbiturates affecting, 558*t*, 559
  enflurane affecting, 142, 558
  etomidate affecting, 560
  inhalational anesthetics affecting dynamics of, 558–559, 558*t*
  leakage of after dural puncture, headache and, 276
  secretion of, 555
  volume of, level of blockade after spinal anesthesia and, 268
Cerebrovascular disease, **584–585**, 585*f*
  carotid artery surgery for, 470–472
Cervical blocks, 269. *See also* Epidural anesthesia
  paravertebral, for pain management, 328, 329*f*
Cervical bruits, in cerebrovascular disease, 583, 584
Cervical plexus blocks

for carotid surgery, 471–472
  superficial, of, 288*f*, 304–305
Cervical spine fracture, assumption of in trauma patient, 793, 794
Cervical spine mobility, limited, in diabetes, 736, 739
Cervicothoracic (stellate) block, for pain management, 332–333, 332*f*
CES. *See* Cauda equina (conus medullaris) syndrome
Cesarean section, 819, **828–833**, 829*t*
  for abnormal vertex presentations, 834
  for breech presentation, 834
  combined spinal epidural (CSE) anesthesia for, **830**
  emergency, **833**, 833*t*
  epidural anesthesia for, 819, 828–829, **830**
  general anesthesia for, 819, 829, **830–832**, 831*f*, 832*f*
  indications for, 829*t*
  regional anesthesia for, 828–829, **829–830**
  spinal anesthesia for, 819, 828–829, **829–830**
  technique for, 831–832
CGRP. *See* Calcitonin gene-related peptide
Channelopathies
  anesthetic considerations in patients with, 759
  sodium (hyperkalemic periodic paralysis), **758–759**
  voltage-gated calcium (hypokalemic period paralysis), **758**
Charcoal, activated, for drug overdose/poisoning, 991–992
Chassaignac's tubercle, 332
Chemical burn, respiratory, 975
Chemoreceptor trigger zone, opioids affecting, 168
Chemoreceptors, in breathing control
  central, 507
  peripheral, 507, 508*f*
Chest compressions
  in cardiopulmonary resuscitation, 912, 918*t*, 921–922
    without ventilation, 912
  for neonatal resuscitation, 845, 845*f*, 918*t*
Chest film, preoperative, in valvular heart disease, 407, 408*f*
Chest pain, in angina, 396. *See also* Angina; Ischemic heart disease
Chest thrusts, for foreign body removal in pediatric patient, 917, 918*t*
Chest trauma, **798–799**
Chest wall compliance, 483, 483*f*. *See also* Compliance
  anesthesia affecting, 489–490, 492*f*
Chest wall rigidity, opioids causing, 151, 167
Children. *See* Pediatric anesthesia
Child's classification, 727, 728*t*
Chloral hydrate, pediatric dosing and, 853*t*
Chloride
  in body fluid/fluid compartments, 599*t*, 631
  in cardioplegia solutions, 438*t*
  in crystalloid solutions, 629*t*
  reabsorption of
    in loop of Henle, 666–667, 666*f*, 667*f*
    tubular, 665, 666*f*
Chloride channels, abnormalities of, in myotonia congenita, 757
Chloride-resistant metabolic alkalosis, 656, 657–658, 657*t*
Chloride-sensitive metabolic alkalosis, 656, 657, 657*t*
Chloride (Hamburger) shift, 505
Chloroform, 2, 3
Chloroprocaine
  for epidural anesthesia, 271, 272*t*
    for labor and delivery, 824
  neurologic effects of, 239
  systemic administration of, for pain management, 339
Chlorpheniramine, 243*t*
Chlorprocaine, 237*t*
  epidural anesthesia affected by, 271–272
  placental transfer of, 811
Chlorpromazine, 593
  for postoperative shivering, 706
Chlorthalidone, 675. *See also* Thiazide diuretics
Chlor-Trimeton. *See* Chlorpheniramine
Cholangitis, 731
Cholecystectomy, 731
  laparoscopic, 522–524, 731
    during pregnancy, 846
Cholecystitis, 731
Cholecystokinin, 714
  pain mediation/modulation and, central sensitization and, 318
Cholelithiasis, 730–731
Cholestasis, in hepatobiliary disease, 730
Choline acetyltransferase, 200, 200*f*
Choline magnesium trisalicylate, for postoperative pain management, 341*t*

Cholinergic, definition of, 199
Cholinergic crisis, in myasthenia gravis, 753
Cholinergic receptors, 200, 200*t*
  mechanism of action of cholinesterase inhibitors and,
    200–202
  mechanism of action of neuromuscular blocking agents
    and, 181
  muscarinic, 200, 200*t*
    nondepolarizing neuromuscular blocking agents
      affecting, 187
    succinylcholine affecting, 186
  nicotinic, 200, 200*t*
    in neuromuscular transmission, 179, 180*f*
    nondepolarizing neuromuscular blocking agents
      affecting, 187
    succinylcholine affecting, 186
  succinylcholine affecting, 186
Cholinesterase. *See also* Pseudocholinesterase
  atypical, 183
  hepatic production of, 712
  specific/true. *See* Acetylcholinesterase
Cholinesterase inhibitors, **199–206**. *See also specific agent*
  anticholinergic drugs administered with, 202, 204*t*
  cholinergic pharmacology and, **199–200**, 200*f*, 200*t*,
    201*f*, 203*f*
  local anesthetic interactions and, 240
  mechanism of action of, **200–202**
  muscarinic effects of, 202, 202*t*
  for myasthenia gravis, 753
  neuromuscular blocking agent interactions and, 185*t*
  neuromuscular blocking agent reversal and, 182–183,
    199–206
  pharmacology of, **202–203**, 202*t*
  succinylcholine interaction and, 183, 201
Chorioamnionitis, **836**
Christmas factor, 718*t*
  deficiency of (Christmas disease), 722
Chronic asthmatic bronchitis, 516
Chronic bronchitis, 516. *See also* Chronic obstructive
    pulmonary disease
Chronic lobular hepatitis, 726
Chronic obstructive pulmonary disease, 511, **516–518**,
  516*t*
Chronic pain, 309, 312. *See also* Pain
  pathophysiology of, **319–320**, 319*t*, 320*t*
  psychological/environmental factors in, 320, 320*t*, 322
  interventions and, **339**
Chronic persistent hepatitis, 726
Chronotropic effects, of β$_1$ adrenoceptor activation, 215
Chvostek's sign (masseter spasm), in hypocalcemia, 620,
  745
Cigarette smoking
  discontinuing, before surgery in COPD patient, 517
  emphysema and, 516
Cimetidine, 244, 244*t*, 245
  for aspiration pneumonia prophylaxis, 244*t*
  open eye surgery in full stomach patient and, 769
  pediatric dosing and, 853*t*
Circle system, **32–36**, 33*t*, 34*f*, 34*t*, 35*f*, 36*f*
  components of, 33–35
  disadvantages of, 36
  optimization of design of, 35, 36*f*
  for pediatric patient, 861
  performance characteristics of, 35–36
Circuit breaker, ground-leakage (ground-fault circuit
    interrupter), in electrical shock prevention, 22
Circulation, **372–379**. *See also specific organ or system and*
    Arterial blood pressure; Cardiovascular
    physiology; Perfusion
  autonomic control of, **374–375**
  autoregulation and, **372–373**
  blood volume distribution and, 372, 374*t*
  in cardiopulmonary resuscitation, 918*t*, **921–922**
  cirrhosis affecting, 727*t*, 728
  coronary, **376–379**. *See also* Coronary circulation/blood
    flow
  endothelium-derived factors affecting, **373–374**
  intraoperative monitoring of, 87–108, 125. *See also*
    Cardiac monitoring
  postanesthesia care unit complications related to, **946–947**
  pulmonary, **478–480**
  in septic shock, 982
  trauma and, 795–797
  venous clamping for liver transplant and, 733–734
Circulatory arrest, hypothermic, 462
  for aortic arch surgery, 468
Circulatory assist devices, for pump failure after
    cardiopulmonary bypass, 456

Circulatory hypoxia, 954*t*
Circulatory steal phenomenon, 558
Circumflex artery, 376, 377*f*
Circus movement, 383
Cirrhosis, 723, **726–730**, 726*t*. *See also* Hepatic failure
  anesthetic technique in patients with, 729–730
  Child's classification in, 727, 728*t*
  drug response affected in, 729
  nondepolarizing neuromuscular blocking agent
    metabolism affected by, 178, 187–188, 189
  vecuronium metabolism affected by, 195–196
Cisatracurium, 179, 188*t*, **192–193**
  altered renal function and, 683
  in pediatric anesthesia, 856
  pediatric dosing and, 853*t*
  seizure activity and, 586
Citalopram
  for depression, 592*t*
  for pain management, 337*t*
Citanest. *See* Prilocaine
Citrates, for blood preservation, toxicity of in mass
    transfusions, 638–639
Citric acid cycle, 476
CK. *See* Creatine kinase
Clark electrode (polarographic cell), for oxygen
    concentration monitoring, 55, 55*t*, 113
Clayton yellow, as carbon dioxide absorbent indicator dye,
  34*t*
Clearance. *See* Hepatic clearance; Renal clearance
Clomipramine, 591, 592*t*
Clonazepam, for pain management, 337, 338*t*
Clonidine, 207, 217, 218
  epidural, 348
  minimum alveolar concentration affected by, 136*t*
  preoperative, in hypertensive patients, 393
  receptor selectivity of, 216*t*, 217
Closed-circuit anesthesia, 146–150
Closed-loop intravenous and inhalation anesthesia system,
  163, 163*f*
Closed reduction, for hip dislocation, **787**
Closing capacity, 475, 484–485, 485*f*, 486*f*
  anesthesia affecting, 490
  in geriatric patient, 875, 876
Clotting. *See* Coagulation
Clotting time. *See also* Coagulation studies
  anticoagulation for cardiopulmonary bypass and, 449
  monitoring, during cardiac surgery, 441, 449, 452,
    452*f*
Clozapine, 593
Clozaril. *See* Clozapine
Clubbing of fingers, in heart disease in children, 460
Cm (minimum concentration), of local anesthetic, 233,
  234
  in geriatric patient, 875, 879
CMR (cerebral metabolic rate). *See* Cerebral oxygen
    consumption/metabolic rate
CMRO$_2$. *See* Cerebral oxygen consumption
CMV. *See* Controlled mechanical ventilation
CO$_2$. *See* Carbon dioxide
CO$_2$ laser. *See* Carbon dioxide laser
Coagulation
  abnormalities of, 717–722, 718*t*, 719*f*, 721*t*. *See also*
    Coagulopathy
  in cyanotic heart disease, 422
  cardiopulmonary bypass affecting, 439
  disseminated intravascular. *See* Disseminated
    intravascular coagulation
  inhibitors of, 718–720
    for septic shock, 984
  lidocaine affecting, 240
  mechanisms in, 718–720, 719*f*
  pathways of, 718, 719*f*
  pregnancy affecting, 805*t*, 807
Coagulation factors, 708, 718, 718*t*
  depletion of, bleeding after cardiopulmonary bypass and,
    458
  hepatic production of, 708, 712
  in liver disease, 720
  pregnancy affecting, 805*t*, 807
Coagulation pathways, 718, 719*f*
Coagulation studies, 720–721, 721*t*
  intraoperative, during cardiac surgery, 441, 449
  preoperative, in valvular heart disease, 406
Coagulopathy
  in cyanotic heart disease, 422
  in liver disease, 717–722, 718*t*, 719*f*, 721*t*
  posttransfusion, 626, 638
  transurethral resection of prostate and, 696

Coarctation of aorta, 467
Cocaine, 233, 237*t*
  abuse of, anesthetic requirements affected by, 594*t*
  cardiovascular effects of, 239
  history of use of, 284
  intranasal, for nasal and sinus surgery, 775
  minimum alveolar concentration affected by, 136*t*
  neurologic effects of, 239
Codeine, for postoperative pain management, 342, 342*t*
Cognitive dysfunction, postoperative, in geriatric patient,
  875, 879
Cognitive therapy, for pain management, 339
Cold therapy, in pain management, 339
Collecting tubules, 663*t*, 664*f*, 668, 668*f*
Colloid solutions, for fluid management, 626, 628, **630**
  in cardiopulmonary resuscitation, 924
  during craniotomy, 572–573
  in hemorrhagic shock/trauma patient, 796
  intraoperative therapy with, 632
Colonoscopy, in lower gastrointestinal tract bleeding, 986
Color-flow mapping, transesophageal Doppler, for
    intraoperative monitoring, 107
  in mitral regurgitation, 414, 415*t*
Coma, 990–992
  Glasgow Coma Scale (GCS) in evaluation of, 576, 576*t*
  hyperosmolar nonketotic, 738
  myxedema, 743
  overdose/poisoning causing, 990–992
Combined spinal and epidural (CSE) analgesia/anesthesia
  for cesarean section, **830**
  for labor and delivery, 827
Combitube (esophageal-tracheal), 59, 65–67, 68*f*
  for cardiopulmonary resuscitation, 918
Common bile duct, 713, 713*f*
Common bundle of His, 362*f*, 363
Common peroneal nerve, entrapment of, 351*t*
Compartment models, in pharmacokinetics, 154–155, 154*f*
Compartment syndrome
  abdominal, 800
  postoperative, patient positioning and, 893, 897, 899*t*
Compatibility testing, for blood transfusion, **633–634**
Competence, legal issues in critical care and, 952
Competitive antagonists (drug), 155
Complement
  activation of by cardiopulmonary bypass, 439
  defects in. *See also* Immunocompromised host
    septic shock and, 985*t*
Complex regional pain syndrome (CRPS), 350–351
Compliance, 482–483, 483*f*
  anesthesia affecting, 489–490, 492*f*
  chest wall, 483, 483*f*
  dynamic, 482
    peak inspiratory pressure and, 47
  intracranial, 556–557, 556*f*, 557*f*
  lateral decubitus position affecting, 526, 526*f*, 527, 527*f*
  lung, 482–483, 483*f*
  reduced, in restrictive lung disease, 518–519
  static, plateau pressure and, 47
  ventricular, 368–369, 370*f*
Complications of anesthesia, **889–911**. *See also* Anesthetic
    complications
Compound A, sevoflurane metabolism producing, 146,
  662, 672
Compound presentation, 834
Computer-assisted continuous infusion (CACI),
  162–163
Concentrating effect, 131–132
Concentration effect, 131
Concussion, brain, 576
Condensation humidifier, in breathing circuit, 54, 55*f*
Conduction, cardiac. *See* Cardiac conduction
Conduction abnormalities
  appearance of on electrocardiogram, 428
  significance of, 429
Conduction velocity, local anesthetics affecting, 238
Confusion, postoperative, in geriatric patient, 875, 879
Congenital diaphragmatic hernia, **864–865**
Congenital heart disease, 387, **421–427**. *See also specific*
    lesion
  anesthetic management in patient with, 422–423, 423*t*
  classification of, 422, 422*t*
  left-to-right (simple) shunts, 422, 422*t*, **423–425**
  obstructive lesions and, **423**
  pregnancy and, 839
  preoperative considerations in, 421–422, 422*t*
  right-to-left (complex) shunts, 422, 422*t*, **425–427**
  surgical repair of, perioperative problems and, 423, 423*t*
  transesophageal echocardiography for assessment of, 446

Congestive heart failure. *See* Heart failure
Conjugate pairs, in acid base balance, 645–646
Connecting segment, 664*f*, 667–668
Conn's syndrome, 745–746
Consent, informed, 1, 8
Constant-flow generators, for mechanical ventilation, 50, 52*f*, 960
Constant-pressure generators, for mechanical ventilation, 50, 52*f*, 960–961
Constant-pressure variable-orifice flowmeters, 43–44, 44*f*
Constipation, opioids causing, 169
Constrictive pericarditis, **465–466**
Contact thermography, in pain evaluation, 322
Context-sensitive half-time, 165, 167*f*
Continuous ambulatory electrocardiographic (Holter) monitoring, preoperative, in ischemic heart disease, 401
Continuous positive airway pressure (CPAP), 968
  adverse nonpulmonary effects of, 969–970
  for ARDS, 973
  high-flow air/oxygen systems for, 958
  optimum use of, 970
  PEEP compared with, 968, 968*t*
  pulmonary effects of, 969, 969*f*
  weaning from ventilator with, 967–968
Continuous renal replacement therapy (CRRT), 951, 979
Continuous venovenous hemodialysis (CVVHD), 951, 979
Continuous venovenous hemofiltration (CVVHF), 951, 979
Continuous-wave suprasternal Doppler, for intraoperative monitoring, 107
Contractility, myocardial. *See* Myocardial contraction/contractility
Contrast media, renal failure caused by, acetylcysteine in prevention of, 673
Contrecoup lesions, 576
Controlled hypotension
  for cerebral aneurysm surgery, 579
  for hip replacement surgery, 786
  in pregnant patient, 847
Controlled mechanical ventilation (CMV), 961, 962*t*, 963*f*. *See also* Mechanical ventilation
Contusion
  brain, 576
  myocardial, 799
  pulmonary, 798–799
Conus medullaris (cauda equina) syndrome, 239–240, 278, 590
Coombs test, for blood transfusion, 634
  delayed hemolytic transfusion reaction and, 637
Cooximetry, in carbon monoxide poisoning, 801, 974, 975
COPD. *See* Chronic obstructive pulmonary disease
Copper kettle vaporizers, for anesthesia machine, 47–49, 48*f*
Core temperature. *See also* Hyperthermia; Hypothermia
  changes in during anesthesia, 117–118, 117*f*
Corneal abrasion
  as anesthetic complication, 899
    patient positioning and, 899*t*
  face mask positioning and, 64
  prevention of during nasal and sinus surgery, 775
Corniculate cartilage, 60, 61*f*
Coronary angiography
  for acute myocardial infarction, 976
  preoperative, in ischemic heart disease, 401–402
Coronary arteries, 376, 377*f*
  antianginal agents affecting, 397*t*
  atherosclerosis of, 395–396. *See also* Ischemic heart disease
  calcium channel blockers affecting, 397, 397*t*, 398
  in myocardial infarction patients, 975
  nitrates affecting, 397, 397*t*
  transesophageal echocardiography for intraoperative assessment of, 444, 445*f*
Coronary artery bypass surgery. *See also* Cardiac surgery
  off-pump, **459–460**, 459*f*
Coronary artery disease. *See* Ischemic heart disease
Coronary circulation/blood flow, **376–379**
  adenosine affecting, 230
  anatomy of, 376, 377*f*
  during cardiac cycle, 376, 378*f*
  control of, 376–378, 378*f*
  desflurane affecting, 379
  determinants of, 376–378, 378*f*
  dobutamine affecting, 219
  epinephrine affecting, 218
  halothane affecting, 139, 378
  inhalational anesthetics affecting, 378–379
  isoflurane affecting, 128, 143, 378

  myocardial oxygen demand affecting, 376–378, **378–379**, 379*t*
  nitroglycerine affecting, 228
  phenylephrine affecting, 216
Coronary embolism, 975
Coronary perfusion pressure, 376
Coronary sinus oxygen saturation, 378
Coronary steal syndrome
  adenosine causing, 230
  isoflurane causing, 128, 143
Coronary vasospasm, 396, 975
Cortical collecting tubule, 664*f*, 668, 668*f*
Corticosteroids. *See also* Glucocorticoids
  for asthma, 513, 514
  for glucocorticoid deficiency, 736, 747
  for intracranial hypertension, 568
  for pain management, 338–339, 338*t*
  for surgery in patient with heart transplant, 427
  for thyroid storm, 949
Cough reflex, opioids affecting, 345
Counter-regulatory failure, in diabetic patient, 738
Countercurrent multiplier, 667, 667*f*
Coup lesions, 576
Couvelaire uterus, 835
COX (cyclooxygenase)
  inhibition of, by nonsteroidal anti-inflammatory drugs, 318, 341, 785–786
  in primary hyperalgesia, 317–318
COX (cyclooxygenase) inhibitors
  for arthritis, 785–786
  for postoperative pain management, 341–342, 341*t*
    with opioids, 342, 342*t*
  COX-2 inhibitors, 341, 341*t*, 782, 785–786
    for arthritis, 785–786
    for postoperative pain management, 341, 341*t*
CPAP. *See* Continuous positive airway pressure
CPB. *See* Cardiopulmonary bypass
CPDA-1 preservative, for blood storage, 634
  toxicity of in mass transfusions, 638–639
CPP. *See* Cerebral perfusion pressure
Cranial nerves
  airway supplied by, 60, 62*f*
  entrapment of, 351*t*
Craniofacial reconstruction, 771, **777–779**, 777*f*, 778*f*
Craniosacral blockade, neuraxial anesthesia producing, 260–262
Craniotomy
  anesthesia maintenance for, 572–573
  brainstem injury and, 573
  central venous catheterization for, 574–575
  emergence from anesthesia after, 573
  induction for, 571–572
  for mass lesions, 569–573
    in posterior fossa, **573–575**
  neuronavigation and, 570–571, 570*f*, 571*f*
  obstructive hydrocephalus and, 573
  patient monitoring for, 569–571
    venous air embolism and, 575
  patient positioning for, 572–574, 574*f*
  pneumocephalus and, 574
  preoperative management for, **569**
  sitting position for, 573–574, 574*f*
  venous air embolism and, 567, 574–575
Crawford needle, 269, 270*f*
Creatine kinase (CK), plasma levels of, in Duchenne's muscular dystrophy, 755
Creatinine, serum levels of, **680**, 680*f*
  in azotemia/renal failure, 977*t*, 978
  in geriatric patient, 878
  in pregnancy, 807
Creatinine:blood urea nitrogen ratio, **680–681**
Creatinine clearance
  in glomerular filtration rate/renal function evaluation, 670, 679, 680, **681**
  patient classification and, 680*t*
Crescendo angina, 396. *See also* Angina
Cretinism, 742
Cricoarytenoid arthritis, 785
Cricoid cartilage, 60, 61*f*
  in pediatric patient, 849, 850, 852*f*
Cricothyroid artery, larynx supplied by, 60–61
Cricothyrotomy, 914–915, 919–920, 919*f*, 920*f*
Critical care, **951–992**
  brain death and, 953
  cost of, **952**
  for drowning/near-drowning, **973–974**
  for drug overdose, 990–992
  economic issues in, **952**

  ethical issues and, **952–953**
  for gastrointestinal hemorrhage, **984–986**
  infections in intensive care unit and, **980–981**, 981*t*
  legal issues and, **952–953**
  mechanical ventilation and, **959–968**
  medical gas therapy and, **953–959**, 954*t*
  for myocardial infarction (acute), **975–976**
  nutritional support and, **986–990**
  oxygen therapy and, 953–954, **954–959**, 954*t*
  positive airway pressure therapy and, **968–970**
  for pulmonary edema, **971–973**
  for renal failure, **976–979**
  respiratory care and, **953–970**. *See also* Mechanical ventilation; Oxygen therapy
  for respiratory failure, **970–975**, 971*f*
  for sepsis/septic shock, **979–984**, 984–985*t*
  for smoke inhalation, **974–975**
Critical temperature, liquid oxygen storage and, 15, 17
Critical volume hypothesis, of anesthetic action, 133
  local anesthetics and, 234
Cross-tolerance, 713
Crossmatching, for blood transfusion, 634
  with blood typing versus antibody screen, 634
  regulations regarding frequency of, 634
Croup
  infectious, **867**
  postintubation, 78, 850, 863, 886
CRPS. *See* "Complex regional pain syndrome"
CRRT. *See* Continuous renal replacement therapy
Cryoanalgesia/cryoneurolysis, in pain management, **336**
  after thoracotomy, 540
Cryoprecipitate
  for hemophilia, 722
  preparation of, 635
  for von Willebrand's disease, 721
Crystalloid solutions, for fluid management, 626, **628–630**, 629*t*, 630
  during craniotomy, 572–573
  in hemorrhagic shock/trauma patient, 796
  intraoperative therapy with, 632
  for Jehovah's witnesses, 790
CSE. *See* Combined spinal and epidural (CSE) analgesia/anesthesia
CSF. *See* Cerebrospinal fluid
Cubital tunnel syndrome, 351*t*
  postoperative, patient positioning and, 893, 897*f*
Cuffs
  blood pressure, for arterial blood pressure monitoring, 91, 92*f*
    by auscultation method, 89, 90*f*
    by Doppler probe, 89, 89*f*
    by oscillometry, 89–90
    by palpation, 88, 89*f*
  endotracheal tube, 59, 67–69
    inflation system for, 67, 69*f*
Cuneiform cartilage, 60, 61*f*
Curare
  altered renal function and, 683
  history of use of, 3–4
Current flow, leakage, electrocution risk in operating room and, 15, 21
Cushing response, in intracranial hypertension, 568, 577
Cushing triad, 797
Cushing's disease, 746
Cushing's syndrome, 736, 746
Cutaneous nociceptors, 315–316
Cutaneous partial pressures, transcutaneous sensors measuring, 113
cv wave, 366
CVVHD. *See* Continuous venovenous hemodialysis
CVVHF. *See* Continuous venovenous hemofiltration
CX. *See* Circumflex artery
Cyanide toxicity
  nitroprusside causing, 224, 226–227, 226*f*
  in smoke inhalation, 975
Cyanosis, congenital heart disease causing, 422, 460
Cyclooxygenase (COX)
  inhibition of, by nonsteroidal anti-inflammatory drugs, 318, 341, 785–786
  in primary hyperalgesia, 317–318
Cyclooxygenase (COX) inhibitors
  for arthritis, 785–786
  for postoperative pain management, 341–342, 341*t*
    with opioids, 342, 342*t*
Cyclooxygenase-2 (COX-2) inhibitors, 341, 341*t*, 782, 785–786
  for arthritis, 785–786
  for postoperative pain management, 341, 341*t*

Cyclopentolate, ophthalmic, systemic effects of, 764*t*
Cyclophosphamide, pseudocholinesterase affected by, 185
Cycloplegia, anticholinergic drugs causing, 209
Cyclopropane, 3
Cylinders, gas, 18*t*
  for nitrous oxide, 17–19, 18*t*
  for oxygen, 16, 16*f*, 17, 18*t*
  pin index safety system for, 19, 19*f*
  testing/certification of, 25–26
Cystectomy, radical, for bladder cancer, 701–702
Cystic fibrosis, **868–869**
Cystoscopy, 692, **693–694**, 694*f*
Cytochrome P-450, 713
  in barbiturate biotransformation, 159
  in inhalational anesthetic metabolism, 133
    halothane, 140
    methoxyflurane, 128, 141
    sevoflurane, 145–146
    in pediatric patient, 855
Cytokines, in systemic inflammatory response syndrome, 980
Cytomegalovirus (CMV) infection, transfusion-related, 626, 638
Cytotoxic cerebral edema, 568
Cytotoxic (type II) hypersensitivity reactions, 903, 903*t*

D antigen, in Rh system for blood typing, 633
D-lite sensors, for anesthesia machine, 45
D₅W. *See* Dextrose in water
DA. *See* Dopamine
DA₁ receptors, 219
  adrenergic agonist selectivity and, 216*t*
  fenoldopam affecting, 220
DA₂ receptors, adrenergic agonist selectivity and, 216*t*
Damping coefficient, in hyperresonance prevention, 93–94, 98*f*
Dantrolene
  for malignant hyperthermia, 871
  neuromuscular blocking agent interactions and, 185*t*
  pediatric dosing and, 853*t*
Darvocet. *See* Propoxyphene
Darvon. *See* Propoxyphene
DBP. *See* Diastolic arterial blood pressure
DBS. *See* Double-burst stimulation
DC cardioversion. *See* Cardioversion
DDAVP. *See* Desmopressin
Dead space, 490–491
  alveolar, 490, 493
    end-tidal carbon dioxide analysis in monitoring, 112
  anatomic, 490
  in circle system, 27, 35–36
  closed-circuit anesthesia and, 147–148
  condenser humidifiers and, 54
  end-tidal carbon dioxide analysis in monitoring, 112
  factors affecting, 492*t*
  open drop anesthesia and, 29
  pediatric masks minimizing, 62, 860
  in pediatric patient, 850
  PEEP/CPAP therapy and, 969
  physiologic, 490
  tidal volume and, 490–491
Deamination, in protein metabolism, 712
Death, legal definition of, 953
Decadron. *See* Dexamethasone
Decamethonium, altered renal function and, 683
Deceleration patterns, in fetal heart rate monitoring, 840–842, 841*f*
Deep nociceptors, 316
Deep peroneal nerve
  blockade of (ankle block), 303, 304*f*
  entrapment of, 351*t*
Deep venous thrombosis, pulmonary embolism and, **520–522**, 520*t*
Defibrillation, 912, **922**, 923*t*, 925*t*
  in pediatric patient, 853*t*
Deflation reflex, 508
Degenerative neurologic disorders, **586–589**. *See also specific disorder*
Dehydration. *See also* Fluid replacement/management
  in diabetic ketoacidosis, 738
  in hyperosmolar nonketotic coma, 738
Delayed/cell-mediated (type IV) hypersensitivity reactions, 903, 903*t*
Delta (δ) receptors, 164, 164*t*
  supraspinal pain inhibition and, 319
Delta virus (hepatitis D virus), 724
Demadex. *See* Torsemide

Demand hypoxia, 954*t*
Dementia, Alzheimer's, **587**
Demerol. *See* Meperidine
Demyelinating diseases, **586–589**. *See also specific disorder*
Dental malocclusion, orthognathic procedures for, 777–779, 777*f*
Dental trauma, anesthesia-related, 892
Deoxyhemoglobin, light absorption by, oximetry and, 108, 110*f*
Depakene. *See* Valproate/valproic acid
Dependence, opioid, 310
  in cancer pain management, 348
Depo-Medrol. *See* Methylprednisolone
Depolarizing neuromuscular blocking agents, 178, 181*t*, **183–187**, 184*f*, 185*t*. *See also* Succinylcholine
  concurrent disease and, 190*t*
  intraocular pressure affected by, 763*t*
  in Lambert-Eaton myasthenic syndrome, 190*t*, 754
  mechanism of action of, 181
  in muscular dystrophies, 190*t*, 756–757
  in myasthenia gravis, 190*t*, 754
  in myotonias, 190*t*, 757
  in paramyotonia congenita, 190*t*, 757
  in periodic paralysis, 190*t*, 759
  response of to peripheral nerve stimulation, 181–182, 182*f*
  reversal of block caused by, 182–183
  structure of, 184*f*
  versus nondepolarizing agents, **181–183**, 181*t*
Depressed neonate, **844–846**, 844*f*, 845*f*
Depressed skull fracture, 576
Depression, **590–593**
  drugs for management of, 591–593, 592*t*
  electroconvulsive therapy (ECT) for management of, 591, 594–596
  pain and
    acute pain, 321
    antidepressant therapy and, 309, 337, 337*t*
    chronic pain, 321, 322
    evaluation of, 322
Depression (nervous system), anticholinergic drugs causing, 209
Dermal effects
  of histamine, 243
  of rheumatoid arthritis, 784*t*
Dermatomyositis, neuromuscular blocking agent response affected in, 190*t*
Descending (hanging) bellows, for anesthesia ventilators, 52, 53*f*
Desflurane, 3, 128, 135*t*, **144–145**
  absorbent granules causing degradation of, 27, 34, 144–145
  alveolar concentration of, 131*f*, 144
  cardiovascular effects of, 138*t*, 144, 364
  cerebral effects of, 138*t*, 144, 557, 558*t*, 559
  electroencephalogram affected by, 564
  metabolism of, 138*t*
  minimum alveolar concentration of, 135*t*
  organ system effects of, 138*t*
  partition coefficient of, 130*t*
  for pediatric anesthesia, 860
    MAC value for, 855*t*
  uterine activity during labor affected by, 813
  vapor pressure/vaporization of, 50, 144
Desipramine
  for depression, 591, 592*t*
  for pain management, 337*t*
Desmopressin
  for diabetes insipidus, 605
  for persistent bleeding after cardiopulmonary bypass, 458
  for von Willebrand's disease, 721
Desyrel. *See* Trazodone
Dexamethasone
  for outpatients, 885
  for pain management, 338*t*
  pediatric dosing and, 853*t*
  in postanesthesia care unit, 940
  for thyroid storm, 949
Dexmedetomidine, **217–218**
  minimum alveolar concentration affected by, 136*t*
Dextran, in fluid management, 630
  for Jehovah's witnesses, 790
Dextrose, for obtunded/comatose patient, 991
Dextrose in water, for fluid management, 629*t*, 630
  pediatric dosing and, 853*t*
Diabetes insipidus, 605
  central, 605
  in head trauma, 577, 605

hypernatremia and, 605
  nephrogenic, 605
    thiazide diuretics in management of, 675
Diabetes mellitus, 736, **737–740**, 741*t*
  anesthesia recovery time and, 197
  classification of types of, 737, 738*t*
  intraoperative insulin management and, 739–740, 739*t*
  postoperative insulin management and, 739*t*, 740, 741*t*
  preoperative insulin management and, 739*t*
  silent ischemia in, 396, 738
Diabetic autonomic neuropathy, 736, 738–739, 739*t*
Diabetic ketoacidosis, 737–738
Diagnostic tests. *See* Laboratory tests/evaluation
Dialysis
  complications of, 684–685, 684*t*
  determining need for, 686, 686*t*
  for drug overdose/poisoning, 992
  hypokalemia and, 613
  for renal failure, 684–685, 979
Diameter index safety system, in medical gas delivery systems, 18*f*, 19, 42
Diamox. *See* Acetazolamide
Diaphragm, 477
  elevation of during pregnancy
    cardiovascular effects of, 807
    respiratory effects of, 805–806
  innervation of, 480
Diaphragmatic hernia, congenital, **864–865**
Diarrhea
  enteral nutritional support and, 988–989
  hyperchloremic metabolic acidosis caused by, 644, 655
Diarrheal stool, electrolyte content of, 631*t*
Diastole, 366
Diastolic arterial blood pressure, 87, 376. *See also* Arterial blood pressure
Diastolic function, 368–369
  assessment of, 360, **372**, 374*f*
  disorders of
    in aortic stenosis, 416
    in geriatric patient, 875, 876
    in heart failure, 379, 379*f*
    in hypertrophic cardiomyopathy, 418
Diasyst, for arterial blood pressure monitoring, 89, 90*f*
Diathermy, surgical
  electrical burns and, 15, **23–24**, 25*f*
  fires/explosions in operating room and, 25
Diazepam, 160*f*. *See also* Benzodiazepines
  for cardiac surgery premedication, 440
  cardiovascular effects of, 161, 171*t*
  drug interactions and, 164
  in geriatric anesthesia, 880
  for induction, history of use of, 3
  organ system effects of, 171*t*
  pediatric dosing and, 853*t*
  pharmacokinetics of, 161, 161*t*
  structure-activity relationships of, 160, 160*f*
  uses and doses of, 161*t*
Diazoxide, for intraoperative hypertension, 394*t*
Dibucaine, 236*t*
  drug interactions and, 240
  pseudocholinesterase activity affected by, 183
Dibucaine number, 183
DIC. *See* Disseminated intravascular coagulation
Differential blockade, 253, 260, **335–336**
  in pain evaluation/management, 309, 323, **335–336**, 335*t*
  solutions for, 335, 335*t*
Differential lung ventilation (DLV), 965. *See also* One-lung ventilation
Difficult airway
  cesarean section and, 819, 830–831, 831*f*, 832*f*
  complications associated with, 892
  management of, 73, 75*f*, 80–84, 81*t*, 82*f*, 83*f*, 84*t*, 914–915
    face mask technique for, 63–64, 64*f*
    laryngeal mask for, 64–65, 65*f*, 66*f*, 67*t*
    surgical airway for, 914–915
  mediastinal adenopathy and, 550, 551
  obesity and, 736, 749
Diffusion, 600, 601*f*
  placental exchange by, 808
Diffusion hypoxia, nitrous oxide elimination and, 133
Diflunisal, for postoperative pain management, 341*t*
Digit amputation, patient positioning and, 899*t*
Digital nerve block, 297, 298*f*
Digitalis, myocardial contraction affected by, 364

Digoxin
for atrial tachycardia in acute myocardial infarction, 976
pediatric dosing and, 853*t*
for thyroid storm, 950
Dihydropyridines, for hypertension, 391*t*
Dilantin. *See* Phenytoin
Dilaudid. *See* Hydromorphone
Diltiazem, 364, 397–398, 397*t*, 398*t*
for acute myocardial infarction, 976
in cardiopulmonary resuscitation, 928*t*
for ischemic heart disease, 397–398, 397*t*, 398*t*
pediatric dosing and, 853*t*
Dilutional thrombocytopenia
bleeding after transfusion and, 626, 638
transurethral resection of prostate and, 696
Dimenhydrinate, 243*t*
Diphenhydramine, 243–244, 243*t*
pediatric dosing and, 853*t*
2,3-Diphosphoglycerate (2,3-DPG), hemoglobin
dissociation curve affected by, 502–503, 502*f*
Dipyridamole-thallium study, preoperative, in ischemic
heart disease, 401
Direct Coombs test, in delayed hemolytic transfusion
reaction, 637
Direct current cardioversion. *See* Cardioversion
Discharge criteria
after outpatient surgery, 882, 886, 886*t*
for postanesthesia care unit, 941, 944*t*
Disconnect alarms, for anesthesia ventilators, 40, 41, 53, 57
Disequilibrium syndrome, 685
Disse, space of, 709, 709*f*
Disseminated intravascular coagulation (DIC), 720
in head trauma, 577
in septic shock, 982
transurethral resection of prostate and, 696
Dissociation constant, for water, hydrogen ion/pH
relationship and, 645
Dissociative anesthesia, ketamine causing, 169
Distal forearm, radial nerve block at, 294–295, 295*f*
Distal renal tubule, 663*t*, 664*f*, 667–668
Distribution, drug, 153–154, 153*t*. *See also* Volume of
distribution
in geriatric patient, 879
of nonvolatile anesthetics, 153–154, 153*t*
Distribution (alpha/α) phase, of two-compartment model,
154–155, 154*f*
Distributive shock, 795*t*
Diuresis, forced, for drug overdose/poisoning, 992
Diuretics, 673–677, 979. *See also specific type*
adverse effects of, 392*t*
carbonic anhydrase inhibitors as, 676–677
chloride-sensitive metabolic alkalosis caused by, 657
with hydration, for hypercalcemia, 597, 619
for hypermagnesemia, 623
for hypertension, 389–390, 390*t*
hypokalemia caused by, 613, 614
for intracranial hypertension, 568
loop, 674–675
for oliguria/renal failure, 875, 979
osmotic, 673–674. *See also* Mannitol
potassium-sparing, 675–676
thiazide-type, 675
DKA. *See* Diabetic ketoacidosis
D$_L$CO. *See* Carbon monoxide diffusion capacity
DLV. *See* Differential lung ventilation
"Do not resuscitate" (DNR) orders, 952–953
Dobutamine, 207, 217*t*, **219**, 456*t*
after cardiopulmonary bypass, 456–457, 457
in cardiopulmonary resuscitation, 928*t*
organ system effects of, 217*t*
pediatric dosing and, 853*t*
receptor selectivity of, 216*t*, 219
in septic shock, 986*t*
Documentation of anesthesia care, **8–13**, 9*f*, 11*f*, 12*f*,
901–902, 902*t*
Dolasetron, 247
altered renal function and, 682
for outpatients, 885
pediatric dosing and, 853*t*
in postanesthesia care unit, 940
Dolobid. *See* Diflunisal
Dolophine. *See* Methadone
Donor-directed transfusions, **639–640**
Dopamine, 207, 217*t*, **219**, 456*t*
after cardiopulmonary bypass, 456–457, 456*t*
in cardiopulmonary resuscitation, 933*f*
for hypotension in postanesthesia care unit, 946
in neonatal resuscitation, 846

for oliguria/renal failure, 979
organ system effects of, 217*t*
pediatric dosing and, 853*t*
receptor selectivity of, 216*t*, 219
in renal blood flow regulation, 662, 671
renal dose, 689
in septic shock, 983, 984, 986*t*
Dopamine receptors, 219
adrenergic agonist selectivity and, 215–216, 216*t*
droperidol affecting, 174
fenoldopam affecting, 220
in hepatic blood flow regulation, 710
in renal blood flow regulation, 671
Dopamine reuptake inhibitors, for depression, 592*t*
Dopexamine, 217*t*, **219**
organ system effects of, 217*t*
receptor selectivity of, 216*t*
Doppler effect, 89
Doppler imaging
continuous-wave suprasternal, for intraoperative
monitoring, 107
echocardiography
in diastolic function assessment, 360, 372, 374*f*
for intraoperative monitoring, 107
in pressure gradient determination
in aortic stenosis, 417
in mitral stenosis, 411
in regurgitant fraction calculation
in aortic regurgitation, 419
in mitral regurgitation, 412
venous air embolism monitoring and, 575
pulsed, for intraoperative monitoring, 107
transcranial, during cardiac surgery, 447
transesophageal color-flow mapping, for intraoperative
monitoring, 107
in mitral regurgitation, 414, 415*t*
transtracheal, for intraoperative monitoring, 107
Doppler probe, for arterial blood pressure monitoring, 89,
89*f*
Dorsal column, pain fibers in, 314
Dorsal column (spinal cord) stimulation, for pain
management, 309, 340
Dorsal horn, 313
in central pain modulation
facilitation, 318
inhibition, 319
Dorsalis pedis artery catheterization, for arterial blood
pressure monitoring, 87*f*, 93
Dose-response curves, 155, 156*f*
for nonvolatile anesthetics, 155, 156*f*
Double-burst stimulation (DBS), in neuromuscular
monitoring, 121, 122*t*, 181, 182*t*
respiratory failure evaluation and, 206
Double-lumen endobronchial tubes
for bronchopleural fistula, 543
for one-lung ventilation, **529–533**, 529*t*, 531*f*, 532*f*,
533*f*, 533*t*, 965
anatomic considerations and, 530, 530*f*, 531*f*
complications of, 533
malpositioning of, 525, 531–533
placement of, 531–533, 532*f*, 533*f*, 533*t*
for pulmonary hemorrhage, 541
Double lung transplant, 547
Down-regulation, receptor
in heart failure, 380
response to neuromuscular blocking agents and, 181
Down syndrome (trisomy 21), **868**
Down's flow generator, 958
Doxacurium, 188*t*, **194**
in ischemic heart disease patients, 405
renal excretion of, 188, 188*t*
altered renal function and, 683
Doxapram, 242, **248–249**
for hypoventilation in postanesthesia care unit, 945
Doxepin
for depression, 591, 592*t*
for pain management, 337*t*
Doxorubicin, preoperative, anesthetic implications of, 791
dP/dt. *See* Ventricular pressure, change in during systole
2,3-DPG. *See* 2,3-Diphosphoglycerate
Dramamine. *See* Dimenhydrinate
Draw-over vaporizers, for anesthesia administration, 29
Dromotropic effects, of β$_1$ adrenoceptor activation, 215
Droperidol, 152, 170*f*, **174–175**, 593
cerebral effects of, 171*t*, 175, 560
with fentanyl, 175
organ system effects of, 171*t*, 175
for outpatients, 885

pediatric dosing and, 853*t*
pheochromocytoma as contraindication to use of, 175, 223
postoperative nausea and vomiting prevention and, 940
renal effects of, 673
altered renal function and, 682
uses and doses of, 169*t*
Drowning, **973–974**
Drug abuse. *See* Substance abuse
Drug allergies. *See* Allergic reactions
Drug-induced hyperthermia, malignant hyperthermia
differentiated from, 873
Drug intolerance, preoperative identification of, 6
Drug metabolism. *See also specific agent*
in burn patient, 803
hepatic, 713. *See also* Biotransformation; Hepatic
metabolism
in cirrhosis, 729
in obese patient, 749
Drug overdose, 990–992
Drug receptors, 155–156. *See also specific type and under
Receptor*
Drug tolerance
opioid, in cancer pain management, 348
intraspinal administration and, 349
substance abuse and, 594
Dual air-oxygen flowmeters, 958
Duchenne's muscular dystrophy, 754–755
anesthetic considerations in patient with, 756
malignant hyperthermia and, 871
neuromuscular blocking agent response affected in, 190*t*,
756
Ductus arteriosus, 814, 814*f*
Duodenal ulcers, bleeding from, 986
Dura mater, spinal, 255, 258*f*
"Durable power of attorney for health care," 952
Duranest. *See* Etidocaine
D$_5$W. *See* Dextrose in water
Dye dilution technique, for cardiac output determination,
107
Dye indicator curve, 107
Dynamic compliance, 482
peak inspiratory pressure and, 47
Dynorphins, 164
Dyrenium. *See* Triamterene
Dysautonomia (autonomic dysfunction), 583, **589**
Dysesthesia, definition of, 311*t*
Dysfunctional labor, primary, 833–834
Dyskinesia, 371, 433, 444, 444*f*
transesophageal echocardiography for intraoperative
assessment of, 444, 444*f*
Dyspnea
in chronic intrinsic pulmonary disease, 519
after interscalene block, 308
Dysrhythmias. *See also specific type*
anesthesia for patient with, 381–385
anticholinergic drugs affecting, 208
drugs for management of, 384*t*, 385
neuromuscular blocking agent interactions and, 185*t*
epinephrine causing, inhalational anesthetics and, 139,
142, 218
extracorporeal shock wave lithotripsy and, 698
intraoperative, monitoring for, 97–100, 99*f*
lidocaine in management of, 238
local anesthetics causing, 233, 238–239
pancuronium causing, 195
in postanesthesia care unit, 947
pulmonary artery catheterization and, 105
recognition of, cardiopulmonary resuscitation and, 924,
930*f*
in renal failure, 685
Dystocia, **833–834**
shoulder, 834
Dystrophin, abnormal
in Becker's muscular dystrophy, 755
in Duchenne muscular dystrophy, 755

E-cylinders, 18*t*
for nitrous oxide, 17–19, 18*t*
for oxygen, 17, 18*t*
pin index safety system for, 19, 19*f*
EA. *See* Epidural abscess
Eagle's syndrome, 351*t*
Ear surgery, **779**
Early decelerations, in fetal heart rate monitoring,
840–841, 841*f*
ECF. *See* Extracellular fluid
ECF-A. *See* Eosinophil chemotactic factors of anaphylaxis

Echinacea, 7t
Echocardiography
  Doppler
    in diastolic function assessment, 360, 372, 374f
    in pressure gradient determination
      in aortic stenosis, 417
      in mitral stenosis, 411
    in regurgitant fraction calculation
      in aortic regurgitation, 419
      in mitral regurgitation, 412
  intraoperative, in mitral regurgitation, 414, 415f
  in mitral regurgitation, 412
  preoperative
    in hypertension, 392–393
    in hypertrophic cardiomyopathy, 418
    in ischemic heart disease, 401
    in mitral valve prolapse, 414, 415
    in valvular heart disease, 407
  transesophageal (TEE)
    documentation of probe placement and, 902
    intraoperative, 107
      during cardiac surgery, 433, 442–443f, 443–446,
        444f, 445f, 446f
      in children, 461
      in ischemic heart disease patient, 404
      venous air embolism monitoring and, 575
    in mitral regurgitation, 412
Echothiophate
  mechanism of action of, 201
  ophthalmic, systemic effects of, 761, 764, 764t
  pseudocholinesterase affected by, 185
Eclampsia, 837
  magnesium for seizures in, 813
ECMO. See Extracorporeal membrane oxygenation
ECT. See Electroconvulsive therapy
Ecthyma gangrenosum, in septic shock, 982
ED₅₀. See Median effective dose
Edecrin. See Ethacrynic acid
Edema
  carbonic anhydrase inhibitors in management of, 676
  hyponatremia and, 607
  in hypovolemia evaluation, 627t
  loop diuretics in management of, 674
  pulmonary. See Pulmonary edema
  thiazide diuretics in management of, 675
EDP. See End-diastolic point
Edrophonium, 203f, 204–205, 204t
  altered renal function and, 683
  mechanism of action of, 200–202
  pediatric dosing and, 853t
  in pediatric patient, 856
Edrophonium test, in myasthenia gravis, 753
EEG. See Electroencephalography
EF. See Ejection fraction
Efferent arteriole, glomerulus drained by, 663, 664f, 669
Effexor. See Venlafaxine
Efficacy, drug, dose-response curve demonstrating, 155, 156f
EGD. See Esophagoduodenoscopy
Eisenmenger syndrome, 424
Ejection fraction, 372
  in mitral regurgitation, 412
Elastic recoil, 482
Elastic resistance, 482–483, 483f
  in geriatric patient, 875, 876
Elavil. See Amitriptyline
Elbow
  median nerve block at, 295, 296f
  radial nerve block at, 294, 295f
  ulnar nerve block at, 297, 297f
Elderly patients. See Geriatric anesthesia
Electrical burns, 802
Electrical circuit, electrocution risk in operating room and,
    20–22, 21f
  isolation transformer in prevention of, 22, 22f, 23f, 24f
Electrical safety in operating room, 20–24, 21f, 22f, 23f,
    24f, 25f
Electrical shock, in operating room, 15, 20–22, 21f
  electrocution risk and, 20–22, 21f
  protection from, 22–23, 22f, 23f, 24f
Electrical stimulation, for pain management, 340
Electrocardiography (ECG)
  in burn patient, 802
  continuous ambulatory (Holter monitoring), in ischemic
    heart disease, 401
  exercise, in ischemic heart disease, 401, 401t
  in hyperkalemia, 617, 617f
  in hypokalemia, 614–615, 614f, 614t
  intraoperative, 97–100, 99f

in aortic stenosis, 417
  during cardiac surgery, 441
  during carotid endarterectomy, 470–471
  controlled hypotension and, 232
  during extracorporeal shock wave lithotripsy, 698–699
  in hypertensive patient, 393
  in ischemic heart disease patient, 386, 402–403, 403f
  in postanesthesia care, 937
  preoperative
    in hypertension, 392
    in hypertrophic cardiomyopathy, 418
    in ischemic heart disease, 400, 401
    in valvular heart disease, 406–407
Electroconvulsive therapy (ECT), 591, 594–596
Electrocution, in operating room, risk of, 20–22, 21f
Electrodes
  for intraoperative electroencephalography, 114, 114f
  silver chloride, for intraoperative electrocardiographic
    monitoring, 99, 99f
  for surgical diathermy unit, 23–24
Electroencephalography (EEG), intraoperative monitoring
    of, 86, 114–115, 114f, 115f, 116f
  anesthetic agents affecting, 562–564, 563t
  during cardiac surgery, 446–447
Electrolyte balance/imbalance, 597–625. See also
    Fluid/electrolyte disturbances
  burn injury and, 802
  minimum alveolar concentration affected by, 136t
  neuromuscular blocking agents affected by, 189
  preoperative evaluation of, in hypertension, 393
  urinary diversion and, 624–625
Electromyography, in pain evaluation, 322
Electronic flow control, for anesthesia machine, 44
  vaporizers and, 50, 51f
Electrophysiologic studies. See also specific study
  cardiac, preoperative pacing and, 430
  neurologic, anesthesia affecting, 562–564, 563t
Electrosurgical units (surgical diathermy)
  electrical burns and, 15, 23–24, 25f
  fires/explosions in operating room and, 25
Elimination, of inhalational anesthetic, 132–133
Elimination (beta/β) phase, of two-compartment model,
    154t, 155
Embolectomy, pulmonary, 521
Embolic stroke, 584. See also Stroke
Embolism. See also specific type
  air, 521
    arterial, sitting position and, 894–895
    paradoxical, 574
      liver transplant and, 734
      in pediatric patient, 861
    patient positioning and, 894–895, 899t
    venous, 567, 574–575
      liver transplant and, 734
      sitting position and, 894–895
  amniotic fluid, 839
  central venous catheterization and, 102, 574–575
  coronary, 975
  pulmonary, 511, 520–522, 520t
    anesthesia for patient with, 521–522
    intraoperative, 521–522
Emergence from anesthesia, 938–939, 943
  after craniotomy, 573
  delayed, 938–939
    neuromuscular blocking agents and, 197–198
Emergency cardiac care (ECC), 912, 913f, 914t, 916f. See
    also Cardiopulmonary resuscitation
Emergency transfusions, 634
Emesis. See Vomiting
EMLA cream, 235, 461, 859
Emphysema, 516–517. See also Chronic obstructive
    pulmonary disease
  subcutaneous, PEEP/CPAP and, 969
Enalaprilat, 394t
Encephalopathy
  hepatic, 723, 729
    nutritional support in, 989
  uremic, 686
End-capillary oxygen tension, 498
End-diastolic point (EDP), 371, 373f
End-diastolic pressure, left ventricular (LVEDP), 369
  in aortic stenosis, 416
  coronary perfusion pressure affected by, 376
End-diastolic volume, 368, 369f
  measurement of, 368–369
  in mitral regurgitation, 412
End-plate potential, in neuromuscular transmission, 179
  muscle relaxation and, 181

End-systolic point (ESP), 371, 373f
End-systolic volume, in mitral regurgitation, 412
End-tidal carbon dioxide (ETCO₂)
  for endotracheal tube placement confirmation, 73, 918
  intraoperative monitoring of, 110–112, 111f, 112f
    for craniofacial reconstruction and orthognathic
      surgery, 779
    for craniotomy, 569
    in pediatric patient, 857
  venous air embolism affecting, 574
End-tidal carbon dioxide tension (PETCO₂), 501
  monitoring, during laparoscopy, 523
Endarterectomy, carotid, 470–472
Endep. See Amitriptyline
Endobronchial intubation. See also Endobronchial tubes
  unintentional, 59, 73, 80
    capnographs and, 59, 86, 111
    diminished breath sounds and, 509–510
Endobronchial tubes, double-lumen, 543
  for bronchopleural fistula, 543
  for one-lung ventilation, 529–533, 529t, 531f, 532f,
    533f, 533t, 965
    anatomic considerations and, 530, 530f, 531f
    complications of, 533
    malpositioning of, 525, 531–533
    placement of, 531–533, 532f, 533f, 533t
  for pulmonary hemorrhage, 541
Endocardial cushion (AV canal) defects, 425
Endocarditis prophylaxis, in valvular heart disease, 407,
    408–409t
Endocrine system. See also specific gland and Stress response
  age-related changes in, 878
  disorders of, 736–751
    intraoperative cardiovascular changes caused by, 38
  etomidate affecting, 173
  in geriatric patient, 878
  neuraxial anesthesia affecting, 262
  opioids affecting, 151, 169
  pain affecting, 320–321
  in renal failure, 684t, 685–686
  rheumatoid arthritis affecting, 784t
  trimethaphan affecting, 229
Endogenous β-blockade, 875, 878
Endorphins, 164
  pain mediation/modulation and, 316t
    central inhibition, 319
Endoscopy, 771, 772–774. See also Flexible fiberoptic
    bronchoscopes
  for nasal intubation, 74–77, 77f
  for otorhinolaryngologic surgery, 772–774
  for upper gastrointestinal bleeding, 986
Endothelial cells, hepatic, 709
Endothelins, 374
  in pregnancy-induced hypertension, 837
Endothelium-derived factors, circulation affected by,
    373–374
Endotracheal tube fire, during laser surgery, 771, 773–774,
    774f
Endotracheal tubes/endotracheal intubation, 67–69, 69f,
    69t, 965–966. See also Intubation
  for airway obstruction in postanesthesia care unit, 943
  with bronchial blocker
    for one-lung ventilation, 533–534
    for pulmonary hemorrhage, 541
  in cardiopulmonary resuscitation, 917–918, 921
  for cesarean section, 819, 830–831, 831f
  checking/preparation for intubation and, 71–72, 71f
  for craniotomy, 571–572
  for endoscopy, 772–773
  in hypertensive patient, 393–394
  in ischemic heart disease patient, 404
  for laparoscopy, 523
  laryngeal mask airway compared with, 67t
  for laser surgery, 774–775, 774t
  for lung resection, 537
  for mechanical ventilation in critical care unit, 965–966
  nasal intubation and, 73–74, 76f
  "blind," 82–83, 83f
  for neonate, 844–845, 844f
  for one-lung ventilation, with bronchial blocker,
    533–534
  oral intubation and, 72–73, 73f, 74f
  in pediatric patient, 860, 860t, 861
  position of
    errors of, 79–80
    verification of, 59, 72–73, 74f, 118–119
      in cardiopulmonary resuscitation, 918
      in neonate, 844–845

Endotracheal tubes/endotracheal intubation (*cont.*)
removal of (extubation), 77. *See also* Extubation
right-angle
for craniofacial reconstruction and orthognathic surgery, 777, 777*f*
for nasal and sinus surgery, 775, 775*f*
securing tube and, 73, 74*f*
for smoke inhalation, 975
in trauma patient, 794
tube malfunction and, 80
Energy expenditure
basal (BEE), energy requirements and, 987
in critical illness, calculating, 988
Energy requirements
in critical illness, calculating, 988
normal, 987
Enflurane, 135*t*, **142–143**
alveolar concentration curve for, 131*f*
cardiovascular effects of, 138*t*, 142, 359, 363, 364
cerebral effects of, 138*t*, 142, 557, 558, 558*t*, 559
electroencephalogram affected by, 564
evoked potentials affected by, 563*t*, 564
metabolism of, 138*t*
minimum alveolar concentration of, 135*t*
organ system effects of, 138*t*
partition coefficient of, 130*t*
renal effects of, 138*t*, 142, 672, 682
seizure activity and, 138*t*, 142, 559, 586
uterine activity during labor affected by, 813
vapor pressure/vaporization of, 48–49
Enkephalins, 164
pain mediation/modulation and, 316*t*
central inhibition, 319
Enteral nutrition, 951, **988–989**
Enterohepatic recirculation, 154
Entrapment syndromes, **351**, 351*t*
electromyography and nerve conduction studies in evaluation of, 322
Enzyme induction, 713
by barbiturates, 159
Eosinophil chemotactic factors of anaphylaxis, in immediate hypersensitivity reactions, 903
EPAP. *See* Expiratory positive airway pressure
Ephedra, 7*t*
Ephedrine, 207, 217*t*, **218**, 456*t*
after cardiopulmonary bypass, 456*t*
minimum alveolar concentration affected by, 136*t*, 218
organ system effects of, 217*t*
pediatric dosing and, 853*t*
during pregnancy, 804, 813
receptor selectivity of, 216*t*
uterine activity during labor affected by, 804, 813
Epicritic sensation, 310
Epidural abscess, neuraxial anesthesia and, 279
Epidural anesthesia/analgesia, 253–255, **269–273**. *See also* Neuraxial anesthesia
activating, 270–271
agents used for, 271–272, 272*t*
for obstetric anesthesia, 824
pH adjustment and, 272
catheters for, 269–270
for obstetric anesthesia, 824
cervical, 269
for cesarean section, 819, 828–829, **830**
clinical considerations and, **262–266**
complications of, **274–280**, 276*t*
pregnancy/labor and delivery and, 805, 825–826
for cystoscopy, 692, 693–694
differential blockade in pain evaluation and, 335–336, 335*t*
for extracorporeal shock wave lithotripsy, 698
factors affecting level of block and, 271
failed, 272–273
in geriatric patient, 875, 879
for hip fracture repair, 784
incremental dosing and, 271
for labor and delivery
anesthetic sensitivity/dose requirements and, 805
choice of anesthetic for, 824
choice of catheter for, 824
complications and, 805, 813, 825–826
during first stage of labor, 819, 824–825
with local anesthetic, 823–826
with local anesthetic and opioid mixtures, 819, 826–827, 827*t*
with opioids, 823
during second stage of labor, 819, 825
with spinal anesthesia (CSE), 827
technique for, 824

uterine activity affected by, 813
lumbar, 269
for labor and delivery, 823–826
after thoracotomy, 640
misplaced injections and, 270–271, 273, 819, 825, 826
needles for, 269, 270*f*
with opioids, 168
for cancer pain, 349
for outpatient procedures, 882, 885
pheochromocytoma and, 223
in postanesthesia care unit, 940
for postpartum tubal ligation, 817–818
with spinal anesthesia/analgesia (CSE)
for cesarean section, **830**
for labor and delivery, 827
with steroids, for radiculopathy, 354
systemic toxicity and, 278
technique for, 270
for obstetric anesthesia, 824
test dose and, 270–271, 825
in parturients, 825
thoracic, 269
after thoracotomy, 540
for transurethral resection of prostate (TURP), 696–697
uteroplacental blood flow affected by, 811
Epidural blood patch, for post-dural puncture headache, 276
Epidural blood volume, during pregnancy, 805
Epidural hematoma, 576
neuraxial anesthesia and, 279
Epidural space, spinal, 255, 258*f*
Epiglottic cartilage, 60, 61*f*
Epiglottis, 60, 60*f*, 61*f*
Epiglottitis, acute, **867**
Epinephrine, 217*t*, **218**, 456*t*
for asthma, 514*t*
after cardiopulmonary bypass, 456*t*, 457
in cardiopulmonary resuscitation, 912, 913*f*, 916*f*, 926*t*, 930*f*, 932*f*, 933*f*
dysrhythmic effects of, inhalational anesthetics and, 139, 142, 218
for hypotension in postanesthesia care unit, 946
intranasal, for nasal and sinus surgery, 775
with local anesthetic, 235–238, 284
for epidural anesthesia, 271
test dose and, 270
for spinal anesthesia, 268
uterine activity during labor affected by, 813, 824
uteroplacental blood flow affected by, 811
for neonatal resuscitation, 846
ophthalmic, systemic effects of, 764, 764*t*
organ system effects of, 217*t*
pediatric dosing and, 853*t*
pheochromocytoma secreting, 222
receptor selectivity of, 216, 216*t*, 218, 514*t*
in renal blood flow regulation, 671
for septic shock, 983, 986*t*
Epistaxis, after nasal or sinus surgery, 779–780
Epstein-Barr virus, blood transfusion in transmission of, 638
Equal pressure point, 487
Equipment misuse/failures, anesthetic complications caused by, 40, 56–58, 891, 891*t*
cardiovascular changes during surgery and, 38, 39*f*
inspection routine for prevention of, **55–56**, 56–57*t*
Equivalency, 598
Erb's (scapulo-humeral) muscular dystrophy, 756
Ergot alkaloids, uterine activity during labor affected by, 813
ERV. *See* Expiratory reserve volume
Erythrocytosis
compensated, 422
in congenital heart disease, 422
Esmarch bandage
for intravenous regional anesthesia of arm, 297
for knee arthroscopy, 787
Esmolol, 207, **221**, 221*t*, 394*t*, 399*t*
receptor selectivity of, 220*t*, 221, 221*t*, 399*t*
Esophageal intubation, unintentional, 59, 79
capnographs in detection of, 86, 111
Esophageal stethoscope, for intraoperative monitoring, **108**, 109*f*
Esophageal surgery, 525, **548–549**
Esophageal temperature, intraoperative monitoring of, 119–120
Esophageal-tracheal combitube, 59, 65–67, 68*f*
for cardiopulmonary resuscitation, 918
Esophagectomy, 548–549

Esophagitis, in pregnancy, 807
Esophagoduodenoscopy (EGD), in upper gastrointestinal bleeding, 986
Esophagoscopy, 772–773
ESP. *See* End-systolic point
Ester hydrolysis
of atracurium, 191
of local anesthetics, 238
Ester local anesthetics, 234, 237*t*
metabolism and excretion of, 233, 238
ESWL. *See* Extracorporeal shock wave lithotripsy
ETCO₂. *See* End-tidal carbon dioxide
Ethacrynic acid, 674–675. *See also* Loop diuretics
Ether
history of use of, 2, 3
open drop administration of, 28–29
Ethical issues, in critical care, **952–953**
Ethmoid artery, anterior, ligation of in epistaxis control, 780
Ethmoidal nerve, anterior, 60, 62*f*
Ethosuximide, for seizures, 586
Ethrane. *See* Enflurane
Ethyl orange, as carbon dioxide absorbent indicator dye, 34*t*
Ethyl violet, as carbon dioxide absorbent indicator dye, 34*t*
Etidocaine, 236*t*
cardiovascular effects of, 363
for epidural anesthesia, 271
Etomidate, 151, 170*f*, **172–173**
adrenocortical suppression caused by, 152, 173, 746
altered renal function and, 682
cerebral effects of, 171*t*, 173, 558*t*, 560
for cerebral protection, 562
electroencephalogram affected by, 563*t*, 564
evoked potentials affected by, 563*t*, 564
history of use of, 3
organ system effects of, 171*t*, 172–173
for outpatient procedures, 884
uses and doses of, 169*t*
ETT. *See* Endotracheal tubes
Evaporation, intraoperative fluid loss by, 631–632
fluid replacement for, 633, 633*t*
testicular cancer surgery and, 703
Evoked potentials, for intraoperative monitoring, **115–116**, 116*t*
anesthetic agents affecting, 563*t*, **564**
during spinal surgery, 782, 789
Excitation-contraction coupling, in myocardial contraction, 364–366, 365*f*
Excitatory neurotransmitters. *See also* Neurotransmitters
barbiturates affecting, 156
ketamine affecting, 169
opioids affecting, 164
Excretion, drug, 154
of nonvolatile anesthetics, 154
Exercise, rehabilitation in chronic pain and, 339
Exercise electrocardiography, preoperative, in ischemic heart disease, 401, 401*t*
Exophthalmos, in hyperthyroidism, 741
Expiration, pulmonary pressure during, 480, 481*f*
Expiratory positive airway pressure (EPAP), 968
Expiratory reserve volume (ERV), 484*f*, 484*t*
Expiratory valve function, checking, 38, 39*f*
Explosion, in operating room, **24–25**
External jugular vein, cannulation of, for central venous pressure monitoring, 100*t*
External (motor) laryngeal nerve, 60
Extracellular fluid (ECF), 598, 598*t*, **599–600**, 599*t*, 600*f*
osmolality of, plasma sodium concentration and, 503*t*, **602–604**
volume of. *See also* Hypervolemia; Hypovolemia
regulation of, **610–612**, 611*t*
Extracorporeal membrane oxygenation (ECMO), for congenital diaphragmatic hernia, 865
Extracorporeal shock wave lithotripsy, **697–699**, 697*f*
choice of anesthetic agent for, 698
neuraxial anesthesia for, 280–281
Extrapyramidal effects, of droperidol, 152, 175
Extravascular hemolysis, blood transfusion causing, 636–637
Extremity trauma, **800–801**
Extrinsic (allergic) asthma, 513. *See also* Asthma
Extrinsic pathway, of coagulation cascade, 718, 719*f*
Extrinsic restrictive pulmonary disorders, **520**
Extubation, 77
airway obstruction and, 551
after cardiac surgery, 459
after cerebral aneurysm surgery, 579

after craniotomy, 573
  documenting, 901
after nasal or sinus surgery, 779–780
after open eye surgery in full stomach patient, 769
after ophthalmic surgery, **765–766**
superior vena cava syndrome and, 551
before transport to PACU, 937
weaning from mechanical ventilation and, 967–968, 967*t*
Eye. *See also under* Ophthalmic
  anticholinergic drugs affecting, 209
  cholinesterase inhibitors affecting, 202*t*
  fenoldopam affecting, 231
  injury of. as anesthetic complication, **899–900**
    documentation and, 901
Eye surgery. *See* Ophthalmic surgery

FA. *See* Alveolar concentration
FA. *See* Arterial concentration
FABERE sign, 352
Face mask, 59, 61–64, 64*f. See also* Mask ventilation
  for cardiopulmonary resuscitation, 918
  laryngeal mask compared with, 67*t*
  pediatric, 62, 64*f,* 860, 860*t*
Face presentation, 834
Facet joints, spinal, 255, 256*f,* 352
Facet syndrome, **355**
Facial nerve, 60
  blockade of, 326, **766,** 768*f*
  identification of in ear surgery, 779
  mask ventilation causing pressure injury of, 64
  stimulation of, in neuromuscular monitoring, 120, 121*f*
Facial nerve block
  for ophthalmic surgery, **766,** 768*f*
  in pain management, 326
Facial pain, in cancer, trigeminal nerve block in management of, 323–326, 324–325*f*
Facioscapulohumeral dystrophy, 756
  anesthetic considerations in patients with, 757
Factor I (fibrinogen), 718*t*
  serum levels of, testing for, 720, 721*t*
Factor II (prothrombin), 718*t*
Factor III (tissue thromboplastin), 718*t*
Factor IV (calcium), 718*t*
Factor V (proaccelerin), 718*t*
Factor VII (proconvertin), 718*t*
Factor VIII (antihemophilic factor), 718*t*
  deficiency of (hemophilia A), 722
Factor VIII concentrates
  for hemophilia, 722
  for von Willebrand's disease, 721
Factor IX (Christmas factor), 718*t*
  deficiency of (Christmas disease), 722
Factor X (Stuart factor), 718*t*
Factor XI (plasma thromboplastin antecedents), 718*t*
Factor XII (Hageman factor), 718*t,* 720
Factor XIII (fibrin-stabilizing factor), 718*t*
  deficiency of, 722
Fade, in neuromuscular monitoring, 181–182, 182*t*
Fail-safe valve, oxygen, on anesthesia machine, 41, **42–43,** 44*f*
Falciform ligament, 708, 709
Fallot, tetralogy of, 425–426
Familial dysautonomia (Riley-Day syndrome), 589
Familial periodic paralysis, neuromuscular blocking agent response affected in, 190*t*
Famotidine, 244, 244*t,* 245
  for aspiration pneumonia prophylaxis, 244*t*
    open eye surgery in full stomach patient and, 769
  pediatric dosing and, 853*t*
Fasciculations, succinylcholine causing, 186
  nondepolarizing neuromuscular blocking agents for prevention of, 189
    rocuronium, 189, 196
  pheochromocytoma and, 223
Fasting, preoperative, in pediatric patient, 857
  for cardiac surgery, 460
Fat
  absorption of, bile acids and, 714
  brown, thermoregulation in pediatric patient and, 851
  drug distribution and, 153, 153*t*
    absorption of nonvolatile anesthetics and, 153
    uptake of inhalational anesthetics and, 130*t,* 131, 132*f*
  metabolism of
    in liver, 711*f,* 712
    pregnancy affecting, 807

Fat embolism, 782, 783–784, 800
  extremity trauma and, 800
  hip fracture and, 783–784
  intraoperative, 521
Fat embolism syndrome, 782, 783–784
Febrile transfusion reaction, 637
Feeding jejunostomy tube, 988
Feet. *See* Foot
FEF$_{25-75\%}$. *See* Forced midexpiratory flow
Felbamate, for seizures, 586, 586*t*
Felodipine, 398*t*
Felsinoxan, for depression, 592*t*
Femoral artery, catheterization of, for arterial blood pressure monitoring, 87*f,* 93
Femoral nerve
  fixed anatomic relationships and, 285–286
  lateral cutaneous
    blockade of, 300, 301*f*
    entrapment of, 351*t*
Femoral nerve block, 283, 298–299, 299*f*
  lateral cutaneous, 300, 301*f*
Femoral vein, cannulation of, for central venous pressure monitoring, 100*t*
FE$_{Na+}$. *See* Fractional excretion of sodium
Fengamine, for depression, 592*t*
Fenoldopam, 217*t,* **220,** 224, 225*f,* 226*t,* **230–231,** 394*t*
  as hypotensive, 225*f,* 226*t,* 394*t,* 395
  organ system effects of, 217*t,* 226*t*
  for post-cardiopulmonary bypass anesthesia, 458
  receptor selectivity of, 216*t,* 220
Fentanyl, 166*f. See also* Opioids
  absorption of, 165
  altered renal function and, 682
  biotransformation of, 165, 167*f*
  for cancer pain, 348, 349
  for cardiac surgery
    in adults, 448–449
    in children, 461, 462
  cardiovascular effects of, 167, 171*t*
  with caudal anesthesia, 274
  cerebral effects of, 168, 171*t*
  context-sensitive half time of, 167*f*
  distribution of, 165, 167*f*
  with droperidol, 175
  as epidural anesthesia test dose, 270
  excretion of, 165–167
  history of use of, 4
  intraspinal, 346, 347, 347*t*
  for labor and delivery, 821
    epidural, 823, 827, 827*t*
    intrathecal, 823, 827*t*
    neonate affected by, 821
  organ system effects of, 171*t*
  for patient-controlled analgesia, 343*t*
  in pediatric anesthesia, 855
  pediatric dosing and, 854*t*
  placental transfer of, 811, 821
  in postanesthesia care unit, 940
  stress response affected by, 169
  transdermal, 165
    for cancer pain, 349
  uses and doses of, 168*t*
Fentanyl/droperidol, 175
Fentanyl lollipop, 165, 857
Fentanyl lozenges, for cancer pain, 348
Fentanyl patch, 165
  for cancer pain, 349
Ferguson reflex, regional analgesia/anesthesia affecting, 813
Fetal asphyxia, treatment of, **842**
Fetal blood sampling, **842**
Fetal circulation, 814–815, 814*f,* 815*f*
  maternal anesthetics detected in, 810–811
  persistent, 816, 817*f*
  meconium aspiration and, 843
Fetal distress
  baseline heart rate variability and, 840
  emergency cesarean section and, 833, 833*t*
  meconium staining and, 843
Fetal heart rate
  maternal opioids affecting, 821
  monitoring, **840–842,** 841*f*
    for surgery during pregnancy, 847
Fetal hemoglobin, in sickle cell anemia, 640
Fetal lungs
  changes at birth and, 816
  maturation of, 804, 816
Fetal physiology, **814–816,** 814*f,* 815*f*
  transitions at birth and, **816,** 817*f*

Fetal presentation/position, abnormal, **833–834**
Fetal resuscitation, **840–842,** 841*f*
Fetal umbilical artery/umbilical vein concentration (UA/UV), placental transfer of anesthetic agents affected by, 804, 810
Fetal umbilical vein/maternal venous concentration (UV/MV), placental transfer of anesthetic agents affected by, 804, 810
Fetus. *See also under* Fetal
  maternal anesthetics affecting, 810–811, 846–847
  maternal surgery affecting, 846
FEV$_1$. *See* Forced expiratory volume in 1 second
Fever. *See also* Pyrexia
  atropine, 209
  blood transfusion causing, 637
  maternal, epidural analgesia and, 277
  perioperative causes of, 947–950, 948*t*
FF. *See* Filtration fraction
FFP. *See* Fresh frozen plasma
Fi. *See* Inspiratory concentration
Fiberoptic bronchoscopes, flexible, 69–70, 71*f*
Fibrillation
  atrial
    cardioversion for, 472–473
    in Wolff-Parkinson-White (WPW) syndrome, 383
  microshock (microelectrocution), 23
  ventricular, emergency management of, 912, 913*f,* 916*f,* **922,** 923*t,* 925*t,* 930*f*
Fibrin-stabilizing factor (factor XIII), 718*t*
  deficiency of, 722
Fibrinogen, 718*t*
  serum levels of, testing for, 720, 721*t*
Fibrinolytic system/fibrinolysis, 720
  activation of, by cardiopulmonary bypass, 439, 458
  pregnancy affecting, 807
  transurethral resection of prostate and, 696
Fibrinolytic therapy, neuraxial anesthesia in setting of, 280
Fibrosing alveolitis, in ARDS, 972
Fick equation, 503
Fick principle, in cardiac output determination, 107
Field block, 285
  brachial plexus supplemented by, 286, 288*f*
Filgrastim (granulocyte colony-stimulating factor/G-CSF), 636
Filtration fraction, 670
Filum terminale, 257
Finapres plethysmograph, 90
Fingers, digital nerve block for surgery on, 297, 298*f*
FiO$_2$ (inspired oxygen)
  with air-entrainment nebulizer, 957–958
  with air-entrainment Venturi mask, 957
  with bag-mask-valve system, 956–957
  with nasal cannula, 955
  with nonreservoir mask, 956
  with reservoir mask, 956
Fire. *See also* Burns
  in operating room, **24–25**
  oxygen and, 959
  smoke inhalation and, 974–975
First-degree burns, 801
First-order kinetics, 155
First-order neurons, in pain pathway, 312–313
First-pass hepatic metabolism, 152
Fixation error, 891
Fixed-orifice flowmeters, 44
Fixed-performance (high-flow) equipment, for oxygen therapy, 954, **956–958**
Fixed-threshold angina, 396. *See also* Angina
Flail chest, 798
Flecainide, in cardiopulmonary resuscitation, 928*t*
Flexible fiberoptic bronchoscopes, 69–70, 71*f*
  for double-lumen endobronchial tube placement confirmation/repositioning, 531, 532–533
  in inhalation injury, 975
  for nasal intubation, 74–77, 77*f*
Flexion reflexes, hyperexcitability of, in central pain modulation, 318
Flow-control valves, on anesthesia machine, 41, **43–44,** 45*f*
Flow-cycled ventilators, 961
Flow sensors, for anesthesia machine, 45
Flow-through (mainstream) capnographs, 110, 111*f*
  in pediatric patient, 857–858
Flow-volume loops, in tracheal obstruction evaluation, 542*f,* 543
Flowmeters, on anesthesia machine, 40, 41, **43–44,** 44*f*
Fluid administration. *See* Fluid replacement/management
Fluid compartments, **598–601,** 598*t,* 599*t,* 600*f,* 601*f*
  exchanges between, **600,** 601*f*

Fluid/electrolyte disturbances, **597–625**. *See also specific disorder*
  burn injuries and, 802
  calcium balance/imbalance and, **618–621**
  in cirrhosis, 728–729
  fluid compartments and, **598–601**, 598*t*, 599*t*, 600*f*, 601*f*
  magnesium balance/imbalance and, **622–624**
  management of. *See* Fluid replacement/management
  molarity/molality/equivalency and, **598**
  nomenclature of solutions and, **598**
  osmolarity/osmolality/tonicity and, **598**
  phosphorus balance/imbalance and, **621–622**
  potassium balance/imbalance and, **612–618**
  sodium balance/imbalance and, **609–612**, 611*t*
  urinary diversion and, 624–625
  water balance/imbalance and, **602–609**, 603*t*
Fluid loads, water balance affected by, 602, 603*t*
Fluid loss. *See also* Hypovolemia
  blood loss and, 631, 632–633, 632*t*
  chloride-sensitive metabolic alkalosis and, 657, 657*t*
  hypernatremia and, 604–605
  hyponatremia and, 607
  management of. *See* Fluid replacement/management
  redistributive and evaporative, 631–632, 633, 633*t*
    testicular cancer surgery and, 703
  signs of, 627, 627*t*
  surgical, **631–632**
    intraoperative fluid replacement for, **632–633**, 632*t*, 633*t*
    in pediatric patient, 862
Fluid replacement/management, **626–643**
  for abdominal trauma, 799
  for blood loss, 631, 632–633, 632*t*
  in cardiopulmonary resuscitation, 924
  in cirrhosis, 723, 730
  colloid solutions for, 628, **630**
  for craniotomy, 572–573
  crystalloid solutions for, **628–630**, 629*t*
  in diabetic ketoacidosis, 738
  for extracorporeal shock wave lithotripsy, 699
  for hemorrhagic shock, 793, 795, 796–797
  in hyperosmolar nonketotic coma, 738
  for hypotension in postanesthesia care unit, 946
  intraoperative, **632–633**, 632*t*, 633*t*
    blood loss and, 632–633, 632*t*
    in pediatric patient, 850, 862
    redistributive and evaporative losses and, 633, 633*t*
  intravascular volume evaluation and, 527*t*, **626–628**
  intravenous fluid for, **628–633**. *See also* Intravenous fluid therapy
  in Jehovah's Witnesses, 790–791
  during labor and delivery, 820
  in neonatal resuscitation, 845
  normal maintenance requirements and, 630–631, 631*t*
  in pediatric patient, 850, 862
  preexisting deficits and, **631**, 631*t*
  for redistributive and evaporative losses, 631–633, 633*t*
  in renal failure patients, 688
  in renal insufficiency patients (mild to moderate renal impairment), 689
  in septic shock, 983
  surgical fluid loss and, **631–632**
  in testicular cancer surgery, 703
  transfusion for, **633–639**. *See also* Transfusion
    alternatives to, **639–640**
  for trauma patient, 795, 796–797
Fluid requirements, normal, **630**, 631*t*
Fluidization theory of anesthesia, 133–134
Flumazenil, 160, 160*f*, 242, **249–250**
  for delayed emergence, 938
  in drug overdose/poisoning, 991
  pediatric dosing and, 854*t*
Fluoride, plasma levels of
  desflurane anesthesia and, 144
  isoflurane anesthesia and, 143, 145
  methoxyflurane anesthesia and, 662, 672
Fluothane. *See* Halothane
Fluoxetine
  for depression, 592*t*, 593
  for pain management, 337*t*
Fluphenazine, 593
Fluvoxamine, for depression, 592*t*, 593
Focal cerebral ischemia, 561
Focal (partial) seizures, 585, 585*t*. *See also* Seizures
Foley catheter. *See also* Bladder catheterization
  for urinary output monitoring, 120
Follicle-stimulating hormone (FSH), 581

Fontan procedure, for tricuspid atresia, 426
Foot. *See also* Lower extremity
  somatic blockade of, **298–303**, 304*f*, 305*f*
Foramen ovale, 814, 814*f*
Forane. *See* Isoflurane
Forced duction test, 763
Forced expiratory volume in 1 second (FEV₁), 475, 487–488
  pneumonectomy criteria and, 535*t*, 536
Forced midexpiratory flow (FEF₂₅–₇₅%), 475, 488
Forced vital capacity (FVC), 475, 487–488, 489*f*
  pneumonectomy criteria and, 535*t*
Forearm, distal, radial nerve block at, 294–295, 295*f*
Foreign body aspiration
  Heimlich maneuver for, 917, 918, 918*t*
  in pediatric patient, 867, 917, 918*t*
Four-chamber view, for transesophageal echocardiography during cardiac surgery, 442*f*, 443, 444*f*
Fourier analysis, 93
Fractional excretion of sodium, in azotemia/renal failure, 977*t*, 978
FRC. *See* Functional residual capacity
Free flaps (autologous muscle grafts), 789–790
Fresh frozen plasma, transfusion of, 635
Fresh gas inlet
  in circle system, 35, 36*f*
  in Mapleson circuits, 30*t*, 31, 31*f*, 33*f*
Fresh gas outlet, on anesthesia machine, 41
Fresh gas requirements
  in circle system, 35
  in Mapleson circuits, 32
  in resuscitation breathing system, 37
FSH. *See* Follicle-stimulating hormone
Full stomach patient. *See also* Aspiration
  cardiac transplantation and, 463
  intubation of head trauma patient and, 576–577
  local/regional anesthesia for, 251
  obstetric patient as, 819, 820
  open eye surgery and, 761, 768–770, 768*t*, 769*t*
Functional residual capacity (FRC), 475, 483–484, 483*f*, 484*f*, 484*t*
  anesthesia affecting, 475, 489–490
  closing capacity and, 485, 485*f*, 486*f*
  in geriatric patient, 875–877
  in pediatric patient, 849, 850
  PEEP/CPAP affecting, 969
  pregnancy affecting, 805*t*, 806
Furosemide, 674–675. *See also* Loop diuretics
  for drug overdose/poisoning, 992
  for hyperkalemia, 617–618
  for intracranial hypertension, 569
  neuromuscular blocking agent interactions and, 185*t*
  for oliguria/renal failure, 674–675, 979
  pediatric dosing and, 854*t*
FVC. *See* Forced vital capacity

G-CSF. *See* Granulocyte colony-stimulating factor
GABA. *See* γ-Aminobutyric acid
GABA receptors, segmental pain inhibition and, 318–319
GABAmimetics, for depression, 592*t*
Gabapentin
  for pain management, 337, 338*t*
  for seizures, 586*t*
Galanin, pain mediation/modulation and, central sensitization and, 318
Gallamine, 184*f*
  autonomic effects of, 187
  renal excretion of, 188
    altered renal function and, 683
Gallbladder, 713*f*, 714
Gallstones, 730–731
Galvanic cell, for oxygen concentration monitoring, 55, 55*t*
Gamma-aminobutyric acid (GABA)
  anesthetic mechanism of action and, 134
  benzodiazepines affecting binding of, 160
  etomidate affecting binding of, 172
  pain mediation/modulation and, 316*t*
    central inhibition and, 318–319
  receptors for. *See* GABA receptors
Gamma-glutamyl transpeptidase, in liver disease, 714*t*
Ganglion blockers
  adverse effects of, 392*t*
  for hypertension, 391*t*
Ganglion impar (ganglion of Walther) block, for pain management, 335
Garlic, 7*t*
Gas bubbles, intraocular expansion of, 761, **763–764**

Gas columns, for medical gas delivery, 18*f*
Gas cylinders, 18*t*
  for nitrous oxide, 17–19, 18*t*
  for oxygen, 16, 16*f*, 17, 18*t*
  pin index safety system for, 19, 19*f*
  testing/certification of, 25–26
Gas exchange
  across placenta, 809–810
  across respiratory epithelium, 477
  anesthesia affecting, **495–496**
  cirrhosis affecting, 728
  in respiratory failure, 970, 971*f*
Gas inlets, on anesthesia machine, 41, **42**
Gas scavenging, 20
  active, 54
  by anesthesia machine, 41, **54**, 54*f*
  breathing circuits and, 33*t*
  passive, 54
Gas tensions, respiratory, **496–501**
  in acid-base disorder diagnosis, 658–659, 658*f*, **659**, 659*t*
  cerebral blood flow affected by, 554, 554*f*
Gas transport, **501–505**
  oxygen, **501–504**
Gases (medical), **16–19**, 16*f*, 17*f*, 18*f*, 18*t*, 19*f*, 20*f*, 25–26. *See also specific gas*
  characteristics of cylinders for, 17, 18*t*
  delivery systems for, 18*f*, **19**, 19*f*, 20*f*
  sources of, **16–19**
  testing/certification of, 25–26
Gasserian ganglion, 313, 323, 324*f*
Gasserian ganglion block, 323, 324*f*
  complications of, 326
Gastric acid, electrolyte content of, 631*t*
Gastric acid secretion
  aspiration pneumonia risk/prophylaxis and, 242, 244*t*, 250–252
    antacids and, 245, 251
    H₂-receptor antagonists and, 242, 244, 251
    hiatal hernia and, 250
    proton pump inhibitors and, 246
  histamine affecting, 243
  pain affecting, 320
  during pregnancy, 807
  in renal failure, 686
Gastric contents, perioperative aspiration of (Mendelson's syndrome), 250. *See also* Aspiration
  risk/prevention of, 242, 244*t*, 250–252
Gastric emptying time
  anticholinergic drugs affecting, 209
  metoclopramide affecting, 242, 245, 251
  opioids affecting, 169
  in renal failure, 679, 686
Gastric lavage, for drug overdose/poisoning, 991–992
Gastric pressure, elevation of, succinylcholine affecting, 186–187
Gastric ulcers, bleeding from, 986
Gastritis, erosive, upper gastrointestinal bleeding and, 986
Gastroesophageal reflux
  in pregnancy, 807
  surgical management of, 548
Gastroesophageal sphincter, pregnancy affecting, 807
Gastroesophageal varices, in cirrhosis, 723, 727
Gastrointestinal hemorrhage, **984–986**
Gastrointestinal motility
  anticholinergic drugs affecting, 209
  metoclopramide affecting, 242, 245, 251
  neuraxial anesthesia affecting, 261
  opioids affecting, 169
  pain affecting, 320
  in renal failure, 686
Gastrointestinal system
  age-related changes in, **878**
  antacids affecting, 245
  anticholinergic drugs affecting, 209
  cholinesterase inhibitors affecting, 202, 202*t*
  cirrhosis affecting, 727, 727*t*, 728*t*
  disorders of, hypokalemia and, 613–614
  in geriatric patient, **878**
  H₂-receptor antagonists affecting, 242, 244–245, 244*t*
  histamine affecting, 243
  5-HT₃-receptor antagonists affecting, 247
  hyperparathyroidism affecting, 744*t*
  metoclopramide affecting, 242, 245–246
  neuraxial anesthesia affecting, 261
  nitrous oxide affecting, 138
  obesity affecting, 748
  opioids affecting, 169
  pain affecting, 320

in pediatric patient, 851–852
pregnancy affecting, 807
proton pump inhibitors affecting, 246
in renal failure, 684t, 686
trimethaphan affecting, 229
Gastroschisis, 866
Gastrostomy tubes, for enteral feedings, 988
"Gate" theory, of pain processing, 318
GCS. See Glasgow Coma Scale
General anesthesia. See also specific type or agent used
awareness under, 897–899
bispectral index (BIS) monitoring in prevention of, 118
for cesarean section, 819, 829, 830–832, 831f, 832f
for cystoscopy, 692, 693
emergence from, 938–939, 943. See also Emergence
from anesthesia
for extracorporeal shock wave lithotripsy, 698
in geriatric patient, 875, 879, 880–881
for hip fracture repair, 880–881
with inhalational (volatile) agents, 127–150
during labor and vaginal delivery, 828, 828t
with nonvolatile agents, 151–177
for ophthalmic surgery, 765–766
for outpatient procedures, 884
for postpartum tubal ligation, 817, 818
for pregnant patient requiring surgery, 847
recall under, 897–899
regional anesthetic administration and, 263
for ophthalmic surgery, 767–768
routine recovery from, 939
slow recovery from, 197–198
Generalized seizures, 585, 585t
Genitourinary system
anesthesia for surgery on, 692–707. See also specific
procedure
anticholinergic drugs affecting, 209
cholinesterase inhibitors affecting, 202t
Gepirone, 592t
Geriatric anesthesia, 875–881
anatomic/physiologic changes and, 876–879, 876t,
877t
cardiovascular changes and, 876, 877t
endocrine changes and, 878
gastrointestinal changes and, 878
hip fracture and, 427–432, 783–784, 783f, 880–881
inhalational agents in, 879–880
metabolic changes and, 878
muscle relaxants in, 880
musculoskeletal changes and, 879
neurologic changes and, 878–879
nonvolatile agents in, 880
pharmacologic considerations and, 879–880
renal changes and, 877t, 878
respiratory changes and, 876–878, 877t, 878f
GH. See Growth hormone
Ginkgo, 7t
Ginseng, 7t
Glasgow Coma Scale (GCS), 576, 576t
Glaucoma, angle-closure, anticholinergic drugs and,
209
Glaucoma surgery, regional blocks for, 767
Gleason score, in prostate cancer, 700
Glenn shunt, bidirectional, for tricuspid atresia, 426
Global cerebral ischemia, 561
Glomerular capillaries, 663–664, 664f
Glomerular filtration pressure, 663–664
Glomerular filtration rate, 669–670
barbiturates affecting, 159
creatinine clearance in estimation of, 670, 680, 681
enflurane affecting, 138t, 142
fenoldopam affecting, 231
halothane affecting, 138t, 140
hyperkalemia and, 616
inhalational anesthetics affecting, 138t
inulin clearance in estimation of, 669–670
isoflurane affecting, 138t, 143
measurement of, 669–670
methoxyflurane affecting, 138t, 141
nitrous oxide affecting, 138, 138t
pregnancy affecting, 805t, 807
serum creatinine in estimation of, 680, 681f
in volume control, 611
Glomerulus, 663, 663t, 664f
Glossectomy, 776–777
Glossopharyngeal nerve, 60, 62f
blocking, 326, 327f
for awake intubation, 83, 83f
for pain management, 326

Glottic edema
airway obstruction in postanesthesia care unit caused by,
943
postintubation croup caused by, 863
Glucagon
myocardial contraction affected by, 364
pediatric dosing and, 854t
Glucocorticoids, 745. See also Corticosteroids
for asthma, 513, 514
deficiency of, 736, 746–747
excess of, 746
for pain management, 338–339, 338t
Gluconate, in crystalloid solutions, 629t
Gluconeogenesis
hepatic, 712
starvation and, 987
Glucose
blood/plasma levels of
in diabetes, 737, 738t
intraoperative monitoring of, 739–740
postoperative monitoring of, 740, 741t
insulin secretion regulated by, 737
in cardioplegia solutions, 438t, 439
in crystalloid solutions, 629t
metabolism of
aerobic, 476–477
in liver, 710–712, 711f
in pediatric patient, 852
for neonatal hypoglycemia, 846, 858
pediatric dosing and, 854t
Glucose tolerance, abnormal, in renal failure, 685–686
Glucose-6-phosphate dehydrogenase deficiency, 642–643,
643t
Glutamate, pain mediation/modulation and, 316, 316t
central sensitization and, 318
Glutamic-oxaloacetic transaminase. See Aspartate
aminotransferase
Glutamic pyruvic-transferase. See Alanine aminotransferase
γ-Glutamyl transpeptidase, in liver disease, 714t
Glycine, pain mediation/modulation and, 316t
central inhibition and, 318–319
Glycogen, hepatic stores of, 711–712
Glycogenolysis, starvation and, 987
Glycopyrrolate, 207, 208f, 208t, 210
for cesarean section in high risk patients, 830
cholinesterase inhibitor administration and, 202, 204t, 210
neostigmine, 204, 204t
pyridostigmine, 204, 204t
intraocular pressure and, 762
in oculocardiac reflex prevention, 763
pediatric dosing and, 854t
Glycosuria, 681
in pregnancy, 807
GM-CSF. See Granulocyte-macrophage colony-stimulating
factor
Goiter, 741
Gonadotropins, 581
Gorlin equation
for aortic valve area calculation, 416
for mitral valve area calculation, 410
Graft transplantation surgery, 782, 789–790
Graft-versus-host disease, blood transfusion causing, 637
Gram-molecular weight, 598
Grand mal (tonic-clonic) seizures, 585, 585t. See also Seizures
Granisetron, 247
in postanesthesia care unit, 940
Granulocyte colony-stimulating factor (G-CSF/filgrastim),
636
Granulocyte-macrophage colony-stimulating factor (GM-
CSF/sargramostim), 636
in immediate hypersensitivity reactions, 903
Granulocyte transfusions, 636
Graves' disease, 741. See also Hyperthyroidism; Thyroid
storm
Gravity
level of block after epidural anesthesia affected by, 271
level of block after spinal anesthesia affected by, 254, 267
Great arteries, transposition of, 426
Ground-leakage circuit breaker (ground-fault circuit
interrupter), in electrical shock prevention, 22
Grounding pad, for surgical diathermy unit, 23
Growth hormone (GH), 581
Guanadrel, for hypertension, 391t
Guanethidine, for intravenous regional sympathetic
blockade, 335
Guillain-Barré syndrome (acute demyelinating
polyneuropathy), 588
neuromuscular blocking agent response affected in, 190t

H-cylinders, 18t
for nitrous oxide, 17–19, 18t
for oxygen, 16, 16f, 18t
H$_1$-receptor antagonists, 243–244, 243t. See also specific
agent
H$_1$ receptors, 243
H$_2$-receptor antagonists, 242, 244–245, 244t
altered renal function and, 682
premedication for cesarean section and, 830
premedication for labor and delivery and, 820
premedication for obese patient and, 748
premedication for open eye surgery in full stomach
patient and, 769
H$_2$ receptors, 243
H$_3$ receptors, 243
Hageman factor, 718t, 720
Haldane effect, 505
Haldol. See Chlorpromazine
Halogenated anesthetics. See also Halothane
hepatic dysfunction and, 717
malignant hyperthermia caused by, 870, 870t
Haloperidol, 593
droperidol related to, 170f, 174
Halothane, 128, 135t, 139–141
alveolar concentration curve for, 131f
cardiovascular effects of, 138t, 139, 359, 363, 364, 378
cerebral effects of, 138t, 140, 557, 558, 558t
for closed-circuit anesthesia, 148, 149–150
electroencephalogram affected by, 563
evoked potentials affected by, 563t
for geriatric anesthesia, MAC value and, 879
hepatic effects of, 138t, 140, 716, 717
metabolism of, 138t
minimum alveolar concentration of, 135t
open drop administration of, 28–29
organ system effects of, 138t
partition coefficient of, 130t
for pediatric anesthesia, 860
for cardiac surgery, 461–462
MAC value for, 855t
renal effects of, 138t, 140, 672
uterine activity during labor affected by, 813
uteroplacental blood flow affected by, 811
vapor pressure/vaporization of, 47–48
Halothane hepatitis, 128, 140, 708, 717
Halothane hypoxic model, of liver damage, 140
Hamburger (chloride) shift, 505
Hamartomas, pulmonary, 534
Hanger-yoke assembly, on anesthesia machine, 42
Hanging (descending) bellows, for anesthesia ventilators,
52, 53f
Hanging drop technique, for epidural anesthesia, 270
Hb C disease. See Hemoglobin C disease
Hb E. See Hemoglobin E
Hb F. See Hemoglobin F
Hb S. See Hemoglobin S
Hb SC genotype, 642
Hb SS genotype, 640
HBsAg (hepatitis B surface antigen), 724
HCO$_3^-$. See Bicarbonate
Head drape, oxygen and air insufflation under, 28, 29f
Head and neck surgery. See also Otorhinolaryngologic
surgery
for cancer, 771, 776–777
Head-tilt chin-lift maneuver, for airway management, 915,
917f
in postanesthesia care unit, 942
Head trauma, 567, 575–578, 797–798
hypotension in, 577, 798
intraoperative management of, 577–578
intubation in patient with, 576–577, 798
preoperative management for, 576–577
Headache
post-dural puncture, 275–276, 281, 826
in outpatients, 885
postoperative, outpatient surgery and, 886
Health care workers, occupational hazards in anesthesiology
and, 889, 907–909
Heart, 360–372. See also under Cardiac and Myocardial
and Cardiovascular physiology
blood supply to, 376, 377f. See also Coronary
circulation/blood flow
herniation of in hemithorax, after pneumonectomy, 525,
540
innervation of, 366
Starling's law of, 368, 369f
Heart block
appearance of on electrocardiogram, 428

Heart block (*cont.*)
during carotid endarterectomy, 471
presentations of, 429
site of, 429
Heart disease
congenital. *See* Congenital heart disease
ischemic. *See* Ischemic heart disease
in pregnant patient, **839**
Heart failure
biventricular, in children, 460
cardiac transplant for, 463–464
after cardiopulmonary bypass, 455–456, 455*t*
in children, 460
compensatory mechanisms in, **380–381**
in congenital heart disease, 422
pathophysiology of, 360, **379–381**, 379*f*
potassium-sparing diuretics in management of, 676
renal failure and, 679, 685
as risk factor, 386, 388, 388*t*
Heart murmurs, in valvular heart disease. *See also specific lesion*
preoperative evaluation of, 406, 407*t*
Heart rate, **367–368**, 368*f*
adenosine affecting, 226*t*, 230
adrenergic agonists affecting, 217*t*
anticholinergic drugs affecting, 208, 208*t*
atracurium affecting, 191
barbiturates affecting, 158, 171*t*
benzodiazepines affecting, 161, 171*t*
β₁ adrenoceptor activation affecting, 215
cholinesterase inhibitors affecting, 202
coronary perfusion affected by, 376, 377*f*
desflurane affecting, 128, 138*t*, 144
dobutamine affecting, 217*t*, 219
dopamine affecting, 217*t*, 219
ephedrine affecting, 217*t*, 218
epinephrine affecting, 217*t*, 218
esmolol affecting, 221
fenoldopam affecting, 226*t*, 231
fetal
maternal opioids affecting, 821
monitoring, **840–842**, 841*f*
in geriatric patient, 876
histamine affecting, 243
hydralazine affecting, 226*t*, 229
hypotensive agents affecting, 226*t*
in hypovolemia evaluation, 627*t*
inhalational anesthetics affecting, 138*t*
intraoperative monitoring of, pulse oximetry for, 109
isoflurane affecting, 138*t*, 143
labetalol affecting, 220
neuraxial anesthesia affecting, 260
nonvolatile anesthetics affecting, 171*t*
opioids affecting, 167, 171*t*
pancuronium affecting, 195
in pediatric patient, 851, 851*t*
surgical incision affecting, 858–859
phentolamine affecting, 220
pregnancy affecting, 805*t*, 806
preload affected by, 368
propofol affecting, 171*t*, 174
propranolol affecting, 222
rapacuronium affecting, 197
succinylcholine affecting, 186
trimethaphan affecting, 226*t*, 229
tubocurarine affecting, 190
Heart transplant. *See* Cardiac transplant
Heart valves. *See also* Valve replacement; Valvular heart disease
transesophageal echocardiography for intraoperative assessment of, 444–446, 445*f*, 446*f*
Heat conservation
in circle system, 36
in Mapleson circuits, 32
Heat exchanger, for cardiopulmonary bypass machine, 435*f*, 436
Heat injury. *See also* Burns
of airway, smoke inhalation and, 801, 951, 974
Heat loss
in burn patient, 802
in pediatric patient, 851
Heat and moisture exchanger, in breathing circuit, 54
Heat therapy, in pain management, 339
Heat of vaporization, 47
Height (patient), level of block after epidural anesthesia affected by, 271
Heimlich maneuver, 917, 918*f*, 918*t*
Helium-oxygen therapy (heliox), 953, 958
airway resistance and, 486, 486*t*

HELLP syndrome, 838
Hematemesis, 985
Hematochezia, 985
Hematologic effects
of cirrhosis, 727–728, 727*t*
of local anesthetics, 240
of pain, 321
of pregnancy, 805*t*, 807
in renal failure, 684*t*, 685
in rheumatoid arthritis, 784*t*
Hematoma
airway compromise caused by, thyroidectomy and, 742
intra-arterial monitoring and, 93
Hemic hypoxia, 954*t*
Hemimandibulectomy, 776–777
Hemiplegia
neuromuscular blocking agent response affected in, 190*t*
postoperative, 564–566, 565*f*, 566*f*
Hemodialysis
continuous venovenous (CVVHD), 951, 979
for drug overdose/poisoning, 992
for renal failure, 979
Hemodilution, normovolemic, **639**
Hemodynamic pulmonary edema, **972**
Hemodynamic status
airway instrumentation affecting, 80
after cardiopulmonary bypass, 455–456, 455*t*
monitoring
in aortic regurgitation, 420
in carotid endarterectomy, 470–471
in descending aorta surgery, 468
hypovolemia evaluation and, **627–628**
in ischemic heart disease patient, 403–404
in mitral regurgitation, 414
in mitral stenosis, 411
pulmonary artery catheterization for, 105–106, 106*t*
in septic shock, 982
Hemofiltration, continuous venovenous (CVVHF), 951, 979
Hemoglobin, 501
abnormal forms of, 503
buffering action of, 644, 646, 648
carbon dioxide transport and, 505
oxygen transport and, 475, 476, 501–503, 501*f*, 502*f*
carbon monoxide affecting, 503, 974
in sickle cell anemia, 640
in thalassemia, 642
Hemoglobin C disease, 642
Hemoglobin dissociation curve, 501–502, 501*f*
in carbon monoxide poisoning, 503, 974
factors affecting, 502–503, 502*f*
Hemoglobin E, 642
Hemoglobin F (fetal hemoglobin), in sickle cell anemia, 640
Hemoglobin S (Hb S), 640
Hemoglobin saturation, 501–502
endobronchial intubation affecting, 510
Hemolytic transfusion reactions, 626, **636–637**
Hemophilia A, 722
Hemophilia B, 722
Hemoptysis, massive, lung resection and, 541
Hemorrhage/hemorrhagic shock. *See also* Bleeding; Blood loss
antepartum, **835–836**
gastrointestinal bleeding, **984–986**
postpartum, **839–840**
in trauma patient, 793, 795–796, 795*t*, 796*t*
fluid resuscitation and, 795–797
Hemorrhagic stroke, 584. *See also* Stroke
Hemostasis, 717. *See also* Coagulation
coagulation tests in evaluation of, 720–721, 721*t*, 722
intraoperative, for ear surgery, 779
mechanisms in, 718
Hemothorax, 799
Henderson-Hasselbalch equation, 646
for bicarbonate buffer, 647
Henle, loop of, 663*t*, 664*f*, 666–667, 666*f*, 667*f*
Henry's law, 501
Heparin-coated shunt, for descending aorta surgery, 469
Heparin concentration assays, anticoagulation for cardiopulmonary bypass and, 449
Heparin-induced thrombocytopenia, cardiopulmonary bypass anticoagulation in patients with, 450
Heparin rebound, after cardiopulmonary bypass, 458
Heparin therapy
for acute myocardial infarction, 976
for anticoagulation for cardiopulmonary bypass, 449–450

for anticoagulation during carotid endarterectomy, 471
coagulation tests in evaluation of, 721
neuraxial anesthesia in setting of, 280
for pulmonary embolism, 521
Hepatic artery, 708, 710, 710*f*
Hepatic blood flow, 709, 710*f*
anesthesia affecting, 708, 715–716, 723
barbiturates affecting, 159
control of, 710
enflurane affecting, 138*t*, 142
in geriatric patient, 878
halothane affecting, 138*t*, 140, 716
inhalational anesthetics affecting, 138*t*, 716
isoflurane affecting, 138*t*, 143, 716
methoxyflurane affecting, 138*t*, 141
neuraxial anesthesia affecting, 261
nitrous oxide affecting, 138, 138*t*
normal, 710
PEEP/CPAP affecting, 969
sevoflurane affecting, 138*t*, 145
Hepatic clearance, 154. *See also* Hepatic metabolism
Hepatic duct, 713, 713*f*
Hepatic dysfunction. *See also* Liver disorders
coagulopathy in patient with, 717–722, 718*t*, 719*f*, 721*t*
halogenated anesthetics and, **717**
in septic shock, 982
Hepatic encephalopathy, 723, 729
nutritional support in, 989
Hepatic enzyme induction, by barbiturates, 159
Hepatic extraction ratio, 154
of opioids, 165
Hepatic failure. *See also* Cirrhosis
fulminant, 724
nondepolarizing neuromuscular blocking agent metabolism affected by, 178, 187–189
opioid use and, 345
vecuronium metabolism affected by, 195–196
Hepatic lobules, 709, 709*f*
Hepatic metabolism, **710–713**
of amide local anesthetics, 238
anesthesia affecting, 716
of beta blockers, 220, 221*t*
of carbohydrates, 710–712
of cholinesterase inhibitors, 202
in cirrhosis, 729
first-pass, 152
in geriatric patient, 875, 878
of nondepolarizing neuromuscular blocking agents, 187–188
of pancuronium, 194–195
Hepatic physiology
anatomic considerations and, **708–709**, 708*f*, 710*f*
anesthesia affecting, **715–717**, 717*t*
barbiturates affecting, 159
bile formation/excretion and, **713–714**, 713*f*
desflurane affecting, 138*t*, 144
enflurane affecting, 138*t*, 142
halothane affecting, 138*t*, 140, 716, **717**
inhalational anesthetics affecting, 138*t*, 716
isoflurane affecting, 138*t*, 143, 716
liver transplant and, 734
metabolic functions and, **710–713**
methoxyflurane affecting, 138*t*, 141
nitrous oxide affecting, 138, 138*t*
pregnancy affecting, 807
sevoflurane affecting, 138*t*, 145
vascular functions and, **710**
Hepatic surgery, **731**
Hepatic veins, 709, 710*f*
Hepatitis, **724–726**
acute, **724–726**
chronic, 723, 726
drug-induced, 724, 725*t*
halothane, 128, 140, 708, 717
posttransfusion, 638
surgery in patient with, 723, 724–726
transmission of to health care worker, 907–908
viral, 724
Hepatitis A virus, 724
Hepatitis B surface antigen (HBsAg), 724
Hepatitis B virus, 724
chronic infection caused by, 726
transmission of to health care worker, 907, 908
Hepatitis C virus, 724
chronic infection caused by, 726
transmission of to health care worker, 907, 908
Hepatitis D virus (delta virus), 724
Hepatitis E virus, 724

Hepatobiliary disease, **730–731**
Hepatorenal syndrome, 729
Hepatotoxicity
    drug-induced hepatitis and, 724, 725*t*
    of halothane, 140
Heptamine, 989
Herbal medicines, perioperative effects of, 7*t*
Herbal remedies, for depression, 592*t*
Hering-Breuer reflex, 508
Hering's nerve, carotid baroreceptor signals carried by, 375
Hernia, diaphragmatic, congenital, **864–865**
Herniated disk, back pain caused by, 353–354, 353*t*
Herniation
    brain, elevated intracranial pressure and, 556–557, 557*f*
    heart, in hemithorax after pneumonectomy, 525, 540
Herpes zoster, **355–356**
Herpetic whitlow, 907
Hetastarch, for fluid management, 630
    for Jehovah's Witnesses, 790
Hexafluorenium, pseudocholinesterase affected by, 185
HFJV. *See* High-frequency jet ventilation
HFO. *See* High-frequency oscillation ventilation
HFPPV. *See* High-frequency positive pressure ventilation
HFV. *See* High-frequency ventilation
Hiatal hernia, aspiration risk and, 250
Hibernation, myocardial, 976
High airflow with oxygen-entrainment (HAFOE) system
    (Venturi mask), for oxygen therapy, 955*t*,
    957, 957*t*
High-dose opioids. *See also* Opioids
    for cardiac surgery
        in adults, 448–449
        in children, 461
High-dose thrombin time, anticoagulation for
    cardiopulmonary bypass and, 449
High-flow air/oxygen systems, 958
High-flow (fixed-performance) equipment, for oxygen
    therapy, 954, **956–958**
High-frequency jet ventilation (HFJV), 962*t*, 963*f*, 965
    for endoscopy, 773
    as one-lung ventilation alternative, 539
High-frequency oscillation ventilation (HFO), 965
High-frequency positive pressure ventilation (HFPPV), 965
    as one-lung ventilation alternative, 539
High-frequency ventilation (HFV), 965
    for endoscopy, 773
    for rigid bronchoscopy, 545
    tracheal resection using, 544
High-output heart failure, 380
High-output renal failure, methoxyflurane anesthesia and,
    141, 662, 672
High-pressure flush test, damping and natural frequency of
    transducer system determined by, 94, 98*f*
High-pressure jet nebulizers, for anesthesia machine, 55
High spinal anesthesia, 277
Hip. *See also* Lower extremity
    dislocation of, closed reduction of, **787**
    fracture, 427–432, **783–784**, 783*f*, 880–881
    replacement of, **784–787**, 784*t*, 785*f*
    somatic blockade of, **298–303**, 304*f*, 305*f*
Hip surgery, **783–787**
    for fracture repair, 427–432, **783–784**, 783*f*, 880–881
    total hip arthroplasty, **784–787**, 784*t*, 785*f*
Hirsutism, spironolactone for, 676
His, common bundle of, 362*f*, 363
Histamine
    in anaphylaxis, 904–905
    in carcinoid syndrome, 750*t*
    in pain modulation
        primary hyperalgesia and, 317
        secondary hyperalgesia and, 318
    physiology of, 242–243
    receptors for, 243
    release of, 243
        atracurium causing, 187, 188*t*, 191
        metocurine causing, 187, 188*t*, 191
        mivacurium causing, 187, 188*t*, 194
        nondepolarizing neuromuscular blocking agents
            causing, 187
        opioids affecting, 167, 345
        trimethaphan causing, 229
        tubocurarine causing, 187, 188*t*, 190, 191
Histamine-receptor antagonists, **242–245**, 243*t*, 244*t*
Histidine, 242
    in cardioplegia solutions, 439
History, preoperative, 6–7, 6*t*
    in asthma, 514

in hypertension, 392, 392*t*
in ischemic heart disease, 400
in valvular heart disease, 406, 406*t*
Histotoxic hypoxia, 954*t*
HIT. *See* Heparin-induced thrombocytopenia
HiTT. *See* High-dose thrombin time
HIV infection/AIDS
    transfusion-related, 626, 638
    transmission of to health care worker, 907–908
Hoarseness, postoperative, outpatient surgery and, 886
Hofmann elimination
    of atracurium, 179, 191
    of cisatracurium, 179, 192
Holter monitoring, preoperative, in ischemic heart disease,
    401
Home readiness, after outpatient surgery, 882, 886, 886*t*
Horizontal positioning, complications associated with, 898*t*
Hormones. *See specific type and* Endocrine system
5-HT₁ₐ-receptor antagonists, for depression, 592*t*
5-HT₂-receptor antagonists, for depression, 592*t*
5-HT₃-receptor antagonists, **247–248**, 247*t*
    for outpatients, 885
    in postanesthesia care unit, 940
Human error, anesthetic accidents and, 891, 891*t*
Human immunodeficiency virus
    transfusion-related transmission of, 626, 638
    transmission of to health care worker, 907–908
Humidifiers, for anesthesia machine, 41, **54–55**, 55*f*
Humidity, in operating room, **20**
Humidity conservation
    anesthesia machine and, 41, **54–55**, 55*f*
    in circle system, 36
    in Mapleson circuits, 32
Humoral systems, cardiopulmonary bypass and, 439
Hydralazine, 224, 225*f*, 226*t*, **228–229**, 394*t*, 395
    for pregnancy-induced hypertension, 838
    surgery in pregnant patient and, 847
Hydration and diuresis, for hypercalcemia, 597, 619
Hydrocephalus, obstructive, posterior fossa craniotomy
    and, 773
Hydrocodone, for postoperative pain management, 341*t*, 342
Hydrocortisone
    for pain management, 338*t*
    pediatric dosing and, 854*t*
Hydrogen fluoride, sevoflurane metabolism producing, 146
Hydrogen ion concentration, relationship of to pH,
    644–645, 645*f*, 647*t*
Hydrolysis, ester, of atracurium, 191
Hydromorphone
    for cancer pain, 348
    intraspinal, 347*t*
    for patient-controlled analgesia, 343*t*
    pediatric dosing and, 854*t*
    for postoperative pain management, 342*t*, 940
Hydromox. *See* Quinethazone
Hydrophilic group, of local anesthetic, 234
Hydroxocobalamin, for nitroprusside-induced cyanide
    toxicity, 226
5-Hydroxytryptamine (serotonin), 247*f*
    pain mediation/modulation and, 316*t*
    physiology of, 247
    receptors for, antagonists of, **247–248**, 247*f*
        for outpatients, 885
        in postanesthesia care unit, 940
Hydroxyzine, 243*t*
    for labor and delivery, 827
Hypalgesia (hypoalgesia), definition of, 311*t*
Hyperaldosteronism, 745, 745–746
    in renovascular hypertension, 690
    spironolactone for, 676, 746
Hyperalgesia
    definition of, 311*t*
    primary, 317–318, 317*f*
    secondary (neurogenic inflammation), 318
Hyperammonemia, absorption of irrigation solutions for
    transurethral resection of prostate (TURP)
    and, 696
Hyperbaric oxygen, 958
    for carbon monoxide poisoning, 802, 975
    toxicity and, 959
Hyperbaric solutions, for spinal anesthesia, 268–269
    level of block and, 254, 267, 268
Hyperbilirubinemia, 714–715
Hypercalcemia, 597, **619–620**, 619*t*, 744
    hyperparathyroidism and, 744
    minimum alveolar concentration affected by, 136*t*
    in multiple endocrine neoplasia, 750–751
    neuromuscular blocking agents affected by, 136*t*

Hypercalciuria, thiazide diuretics in management of, 675
Hypercapnia. *See also* Rebreathing
    during carotid endarterectomy, 471
    consequences of, 38–39
    electroencephalogram affected by, 563*t*
    during general anesthesia, 37–39
    in pediatric patient, 850
Hypercarbia, 970
Hyperchloremic metabolic acidosis, 654–655
    burn injuries and, 802
    urinary diversion and, 624–625
Hypercoagulability, pregnancy and, 807
Hyperdynamic circulatory state
    after cardiopulmonary bypass, 455, 455*t*
    in cirrhosis, 723, 728
    in hyperthyroidism, 742
Hyperdynamic septic shock, 982
Hyperesthesia
    definition of, 311*t*
    glycine and GABA inhibition producing, 318–319
Hyperextended supine position, for urologic surgery, 699,
    700*f*
Hyperglycemia
    intraoperative, in diabetics, 739
    in septic shock, 982
Hyperglycinemia, absorption of irrigation solutions for
    transurethral resection of prostate (TURP)
    and, 696
Hypericum (St. John's wort), for depression, 591, 592*t*
Hyperkalemia, 597, **615–618**, 616*t*, 617*f*
    aldosterone synthesis and, 616
    anesthesia in patient with, 618
    burn injuries and, 802
    diabetic ketoacidosis treatment and, 738
    hypoaldosteronism and, 616, 746
    massive transfusion and, 639
    in renal failure, 685
    renal transplant and, 692, 705
    succinylcholine-induced, 178, 186, 186*t*
Hyperkalemic periodic paralysis (sodium channelopathy),
    758–759
    anesthetic considerations in patients with, 759
Hypermagnesemia, 597, **623**
    neuromuscular blocking agents affected by, 136*t*, 623
    in renal failure, 685
Hypermetabolism, in burn injuries, 802
Hypernatremia, **604–606**, 604*t*, 606*f*
    anesthesia in patients with, 606
    minimum alveolar concentration affected by, 136*t*, 606
Hypernephroma, 703–704
Hyperosmolality, hypernatremia and, **604–606**, 604*t*,
    606*f*
Hyperosmolar nonketotic coma, 738
Hyperparathyroidism, **743–744**, 744*t*
    in renal failure, 686
Hyperpathia, definition of, 311*t*
Hyperphosphatemia, **621–622**
    hypocalcemia and, 620
Hyperreactivity, drug receptor, 155
Hyperreflexia, autonomic, 583, 590, 798
    trimethaphan in management of, 229
Hyperresonance, intra-arterial monitoring and, 93
Hypersensitivity, **902–907**, 903*t*, 904*f*, 905*t*, 906*t*. *See also*
    Allergic reactions
    anticholinergic drugs and, 209
    cytotoxic (type II), 903, 903*t*
    delayed/cell-mediated (type IV), 903, 903*t*
    histamine causing, 243
    immediate (type I), 902–903, **903**, 903*t*, 904*f*
    immune complex (type III), 903, 903*t*
    local anesthetics and, 240
    opioids causing, 345
Hypertension, **388–395**
    anesthesia recovery time and, 197
    borderline, 389
    after cardiac surgery, 459
    choice of anesthetic agent in patient with, 394–395
    definition of, 389
    drugs for management of, 389–390, 390–391*t*, 398*t*
        adverse effects of, 392, 392*t*
        loop diuretics, 390*t*, 674
        neuromuscular blocking agent interactions and, 185*t*
        potassium-sparing diuretics, 390*t*, 676
        thiazide diuretics, 390*t*, 675
    in head trauma, 577, 798
    intraoperative, 37–39, 394*t*, 395, 909–910
        barbiturate induction and, 158
        during carotid endarterectomy, 471

Hypertension (*cont.*)
  drugs for management of, **224–232**, 225*f*, 226*t*, 394*t*, 395
    inadequate level of anesthesia causing, 37
    medication errors causing, 909–910
    opioid anesthesia and, 167
  intraoperative management of patient with, **393–395**
  malignant, 389
  in multiple endocrine neoplasia, 750
  pancuronium causing, 179, 195
  pathophysiology of, 389
  pheochromocytoma causing, 747
  after pheochromocytoma surgery, 748
  portal, in cirrhosis, 726
  in postanesthesia care unit, 936, 946–947
  postoperative care of patient with, **395**
  pregnancy-induced, **837–839**, 838*t*
  preoperative considerations in patient with, 389
  preoperative management of patient with, **390–393**
  pulmonary, in septic shock, 982
  in renal failure, 685
  renovascular, 689–691
  as risk factor
    intraoperative complications and, 386, 391
    postoperative complications and, 388, 389, 390–391
  uncontrolled, 689–691
Hyperthermia
  drug-induced, malignant hyperthermia differentiated from, 873
  iatrogenic, malignant hyperthermia differentiated from, 873
  malignant, 38, 849, 869–870, 869*t*
    dantrolene in management of, 871
    differential diagnosis of, 872–873, 873*t*
    drugs causing, 870, 870*t*
    hereditary pattern of, 872
    masseter muscle (jaw muscle) spasm/rigidity in, 187, 869, 871
    in muscular dystrophies, 756
    in myotonic dystrophy, 757
    in pediatric patient, 849, 856, 869–873, 869*t*, 870*t*, 873*t*
      monitoring for, 849, 858
    risk factors for, 871–872
    safe anesthetics and, 873
    succinylcholine causing, 187, 870
    treatment of, 870–871, 874
  minimum alveolar concentration affected by, 136*t*
Hyperthyroidism, **741–742**. *See also* Thyroid storm
  hypokalemic periodic paralysis and, 758
  minimum alveolar concentration affected by, 136*t*
  perioperative fever and tachycardia caused by, 947–950, 948*t*
Hypertriglyceridemia, 686
Hypertrophic cardiomyopathy, **418–419**
  heart murmur in, preoperative evaluation of, 407*t*, 418
  transesophageal echocardiography for assessment of, 446
Hypertrophic pyloric stenosis, **866–867**
Hyperuricemia, in congenital heart disease, 422
Hyperventilation
  for craniotomy, 572
  for intracranial hypertension, 568
  intraoperative, anesthesia recovery time and, 198
  maternal, during labor, 812
Hyperviscosity, in congenital heart disease, 422
Hypervolemia, anesthesia in patients with, 611–612
Hypesthesia (hypoesthesia), definition of, 311*t*
Hypoalbuminemia
  hypocalcemia and, 745
  in renal failure, 685
Hypoaldosteronism, 746
  hyperkalemia and, 616, 746
Hypoalgesia (hypalgesia), definition of, 311*t*
Hypobaric solutions, for spinal anesthesia, level of block and, 254, 267
Hypocalcemia, 597, **620–621**, 620*t*, 744–745, 745*t*
  citrate toxicity from massive transfusion causing, 626, 638–639
  hypoparathyroidism and, 744–745, 745*t*
  in neonate, calcium gluconate for, 846
  neuromuscular blocking agents affected by, 136*t*
  in renal failure, 685
Hypocapnia
  during carotid endarterectomy, 471
  electroencephalogram affected by, 563*t*
  maternal, during labor, 812
  in systemic inflammatory response syndrome, 980*t*
Hypodynamic septic shock, 982

Hypoesthesia (hypesthesia), definition of, 311*t*
Hypofibrinogenemia, after cardiopulmonary bypass, 458
Hypogastric plexus block, for pain management, 334–335
Hypoglycemia
  in diabetic patient, 738
  intraoperative, prevention of, 739–740, 739*t*
  in neonates/infants, 852, 858
    glucose administration for, 846, 858
  during surgery, cardiovascular changes caused by, 38
  total parenteral nutrition withdrawal causing, 951, 990
Hypoglycemic agents, oral, preoperative, 740
Hypokalemia, **613–615**, 613*t*, 614*f*, 614*t*
  anesthesia in patients with, 615
  burn injuries and, 802
  diabetic ketoacidosis treatment and, 738
  in hypertension, 393
  massive transfusion and, 639
  neuromuscular blocking agents affected by, 136*t*
Hypokalemic periodic paralysis (voltage-gated calcium channelopathy), **758**
  anesthetic considerations in patients with, 759
Hypokinesis, 371, 433, 444, 444*f*
  transesophageal echocardiography for intraoperative assessment of, 444, 444*f*
Hypomagnesemia, 597, **623–624**, 623*t*
  in hypertension, 393
Hyponatremia, 597, **606–609**, 607*t*, 609*f*
  anesthesia in patient with, 609
  minimum alveolar concentration affected by, 136*t*
  urinary diversion and, 624
Hypo-osmolality, hyponatremia and, **606–609**, 607*t*, 609*f*
Hypoparathyroidism, **744–745**, 745*t*
  hypocalcemia and, 620, 744–745, 745*t*
  unintentional removal of parathyroids during thyroid surgery and, 742
Hypopharynx, 60, 60*f*
Hypophosphatemia, 597, **622**
  anesthetic management of TPN patient and, 990
Hypoplastic left heart syndrome, 426–427
Hyporeactivity, drug receptor, 155
Hypotension
  in abdominal trauma, 799
  atracurium causing, 191
  in autonomic dysfunction, 583, 589
  controlled, 231–232
    for cerebral aneurysm surgery, 579
    for hip replacement surgery, 786
    in pregnant patient, 847
  in drug overdose/poisoning, 991
  during epidural anesthesia for labor and delivery, 819, 825–826
  following transurethral resection of prostate, 705–707
  head trauma and, 577, 798
  in hypovolemic shock/trauma patient, 793, 797
  intraoperative, cardiopulmonary resuscitation for, 925–931
  in neonate, volume resuscitation and, 845
  neuraxial anesthesia causing, 253, 261
  in pheochromocytoma surgery, 747
  postoperative, 705–707
    in postanesthesia care unit, 936, 946
  postural
    patient positioning and, 896
    trimethaphan causing, 229
  propofol causing, 174
  supine, during pregnancy, 804, 806
  tubocurarine causing, 190
Hypotensive agents, **224–232**, 225*f*, 226*t*, 394*t*, 395. *See also specific type and* Antihypertensive therapy
  for controlled hypotension, 231–232
  organs system effects of, 226*t*
Hypothalamus
  in body temperature maintenance, anesthesia affecting, 117–118
  injury to, malignant hyperthermia differentiated from, 873
Hypothermia. *See also* Shivering
  atracurium duration of action and, 192
  cerebral blood flow affected by, 554
  definition of, 117
  delayed emergence and, 939
  deleterious effects of, 117, 117*t*
  in drowning/near drowning, 973
  intentional
    during cardiopulmonary bypass, 434, **437**, 452–453
    for cerebral protection, 552, 561–562

intraoperative, 20
  anesthesia recovery time affected by, 198
  electroencephalogram affected by, 563*t*
  monitoring/management of, 86, 117–120, 117*f*, 117*t*
    in pediatric patient, 849, 858
  massive transfusion and, 639
  minimum alveolar concentration affected by, 136*t*
  neuromuscular blocking agents affected by, 189
  in pediatric patient, 849, 851
  in postanesthesia care unit, 940–941
  potassium concentration affected by, 613
  succinylcholine hydrolysis affected by, 183
  transurethral resection of prostate and, 696
Hypothermic circulatory arrest, 462
  for aortic arch surgery, 468
Hypothyroidism, 736, **742–743**
  anesthesia recovery time affected by, 197
  minimum alveolar concentration affected by, 136*t*
Hypotonic fluid loss, hypernatremia and, 604–605
Hypoventilation
  obesity and (Pickwickian syndrome), 748
  oxygen therapy and, 959
  in postanesthesia care unit, 936, 943–945
Hypovolemia
  anesthesia in patients with, 611–612
  after cardiopulmonary bypass, 455, 455*t*
  hypernatremia and, 605
  hyponatremia and, 607
  hypotension in postanesthesia care unit caused by, 936, 946
  in neonate, volume resuscitation and, 845
  signs of, 627, 627*t*
Hypovolemic shock, in trauma patient, 795–797, 795*t*, 796*t*
Hypoxemia
  in ARDS, 973
  during one-lung ventilation, prevention/management of, 538–539
  oxygen therapy for, 953
  in postanesthesia care unit, 936, 945–946
  in pulmonary embolism, 520
  in respiratory failure, 970
  in septic shock, 982
  after thoracotomy, 539
Hypoxia, 954*t*
  agitation/restlessness in sedated patient and, 887
  classification of, 954*t*
  electroencephalogram affected by, 563*t*
  during general anesthesia, 37–39
  oxygen therapy for, 953
  in pediatric patient, 850
  pulmonary perfusion affected by, 475, 493
Hypoxic drive. *See also* Ventilation/ventilatory drive
  nitrous oxide affecting, 137
  opioids affecting, 167
Hypoxic hypoxia, 954*t*
Hypoxic pulmonary vasoconstriction
  nitroprusside affecting, 227
  one-lung ventilation and, 528
Hypoxic respiratory failure, 970

I cells (intercalated cells), **668**
IABP. *See* Intra-aortic balloon pump
Iatrogenic hyperthermia, malignant hyperthermia differentiated from, 873
Ibuprofen, for postoperative pain management, 341*t*
Ibutilide, in cardiopulmonary resuscitation, 929*t*
ICF. *See* Intracellular fluid
ICP. *See* Intracranial pressure
Idiopathic hypertrophic subaortic stenosis. *See* Hypertrophic cardiomyopathy
Idiosyncratic (intrinsic) asthma, 513. *See also* Asthma
IgE
  in asthma, 513
  in immediate hypersensitivity reactions, 903, 904*f*
Ileal fluid, electrolyte content of, 631*t*
Ileus
  pain causing, 320
  trimethaphan causing, 229
Iliohypogastric nerve block, 306–307, 306*f*
Ilioinguinal nerve block, 306–307, 306*f*
ILV. *See* Independent lung ventilation
Imipramine
  for depression, 591, 592*t*
  for pain management, 337*t*
Immediate (type I) hypersensitivity reactions, 902–903, **903**, 903*t*, 904*f*

Immobilization, head, for airway management in trauma patient, 793, 794
Immune complex (type III) hypersensitivity reactions, 903, 903t
Immunocompromised host
  infection in, 980–981, 981t
  septic shock in, 982–983, 984–985t
Immunoglobulin E (IgE)
  in asthma, 513
  in immediate hypersensitivity reactions, 903, 904f
Immunologic effects
  of barbiturates, 159
  of histamine, 243
  of local anesthetics, 240
  of pain, 321
Immunosuppreison, blood transfusion causing, 626, 637–638
Immunosuppressive therapy, for heart transplant, 427
IMV. See Intermittent mandatory ventilation
"In-line stabilization," for laryngoscopy in trauma patient, 794
Inapsine. See Droperidol
Incentive spirometry, 951, 970
Incisura, 366
Incremental dosing, for epidural anesthesia, 271
Indapamide, 675. See also Thiazide diuretics
Independent lung ventilation (ILV), 965. See also One-lung ventilation
Indirect Coombs test, for blood transfusion, 634
Indocin. See Indomethacin
Indocyanine green dye, in dye dilution cardiac output determination, 107
Indomethacin, for postoperative pain management, 341t
Induction
  airway obstruction and, 551
  for cardiac surgery
    in adults, 447–448
    in children, 460–462
  for craniotomy, 571–572
  of geriatric anesthesia, 881
  for hip fracture repair, 881
  in hypertensive patient, 393–394, 394
  in hypovolemic shock/trauma patient, 793, 797
  insufflation for, 28, 28f, 29f, 860
  intravenous agents for
    cerebral effects of, 559–560
    history of use of, 3
    in pediatric patient, 859
    in ischemic heart disease patient, 404, 404–405
  for lung resection, 537
  for lung transplant, 547
  for open eye surgery in full stomach patient, 761, 769
    in pediatric patient, 770
  for ophthalmic surgery, 765
  for outpatient procedures, 884
  of pediatric anesthesia, 858–860
    inhalational, 859–860
    intravenous, 859
  rapid-sequence, 251–252
  in renal failure patients, 687–688
  in renal insufficiency patients (mild to moderate renal impairment), 689
  steal, 860
  superior vena cava syndrome and, 551
Infant. See also Pediatric anesthesia
  respiratory system/physiology in, 850–851, 852f
Infection, 980f. See also Sepsis
  ARDS and, 972, 973
  bladder catheterization and, 120
  blood transfusion in transmission of, 638
  central venous catheterization and, 102
  chronic, neuromuscular blocking agent response affected in, 190t
  in diabetics, 739
  in ICU, 980–981, 981t
  intra-arterial monitoring and, 93
  nosocomial
    in critically ill patient, 980–981, 981t
    pneumonia, 981
    in ARDS, 973
  as occupational hazard, 889, 907–908
Inferior alveolar nerve block, 325–326, 325f
Inflammation
  ARDS and, 972
  cardiopulmonary bypass and
    in adults, 439
    in children, 462
  neurogenic (secondary hyperalgesia), 318

Informed consent, 1, 8
Infraclavicular brachial plexus block, 290, 291f
Infrared spectroscopy, for intraoperative anesthetic gas analysis, 114
Infusion anesthesia, 162–163, 162f, 163f, 887–888
Inguinal nerve block, 306–307, 306f
Inguinal orchiectomy, for testicular cancer, 702
Inhalation reflex, 508
Inhalational analgesia, for labor and delivery, 821–822. See also Inhalational (volatile) anesthesia/anesthetics
Inhalational (volatile) anesthesia/anesthetics, 127–150. See also specific agent
  absorbent granules causing degradation of, 27, 34, 144–145
  alveolar concentration (FA) of, 129–132, 130t, 131f, 132f
    in pediatric patient, 852
  arterial concentration (FA) of, 132
  for cardiac surgery
    in adults, 448
      postbypass, 458
    in children, 461–462, 462
  cardiovascular physiology affected by, 138t, 359, 363, 364
    indirect renal effects and, 672
  cerebral effects of, 138t, 557–559, 558f, 558t
  closed-loop system for administration of, 163, 163f
  electroencephalogram affected by, 563–564, 563t
  elimination of, 132–133
  emergence from, 938
  evoked potentials affected by, 564
  in geriatric anesthesia, 875, 879–880
  hepatic effects of, 138t, 716
  history of use of, 2–3
  for hypertensive patients, 394
  inspiratory concentration (FI) and, 128–129
  intracranial pressure affected by, 138t, 558t, 559
  intraocular pressure affected by, 762, 763t
  for ischemic heart disease patients, 405
  mechanism of action of, theories of, 133–135, 134f
  minimum alveolar concentration (MAC) of, 127, 135–137, 135f, 136t
    in geriatric anesthesia, 875, 879
    local anesthetics affecting, 239
    in pediatric patient, 849, 852–855, 855t
    during pregnancy, 804, 805, 805t
  neuromuscular blocking agent interactions and, 185t, 189
  neuronavigation and, 570, 571
  nondepolarizer dosage requirements affected by, 189
  for outpatient procedures, 884
  in pediatric anesthesia, 852–855, 855t
    for induction, 859–860
  pharmacodynamics of, 133–137
  pharmacokinetics of, 128–133, 129f
  placental transfer of, 810–811
  renal effects of, 138t, 672
    altered renal function and, 682
  uterine activity in labor affected by, 813
  uteroplacental blood flow affected by, 804, 811
Inhalational injury, burn injuries and, 801, 974–975
Inhibitory neurotransmitters. See also Neurotransmitters
  barbiturates affecting, 156
Inlet valve, in resuscitation breathing system, 37, 37f
Innovar. See Fentanyl/droperidol
Inotropic agents, 456t
  for cardiac transplantation, 464
    after cardiopulmonary bypass, 456–457, 456t
  for septic shock, 983, 986t
Inotropic support for β₁ adrenoceptor activation, 215
Inotropism, 370. See also Myocardial contraction/contractility
Inpatient, postoperative pain management in, 343–348
Inspiration, pulmonary pressure during, 480, 481f
Inspiratory capacity, 484f
Inspiratory concentration (FI), of inhalational anesthetic, 127, 128–129
  alveolar gas concentration (FA) affected by, 131–132
Inspiratory positive airway pressure (IPAP), 968
Inspiratory reserve volume (IRV), 484f, 484t
Inspiratory stridor, postoperative, 780
Inspiratory valve function, checking, 38, 39f
Inspired oxygen (FIO₂)
  with air-entrainment nebulizer, 957–958
  with air-entrainment Venturi mask, 957
  with bag-mask-valve system, 956–957
  with nasal cannula, 955
  with nonreservoir mask, 956
  with reservoir mask, 956

Insufflation, 15, 28, 28f, 29f, 33t, 860
  for endoscopy, 773
Insulin
  bioavailability characteristics of, 740, 741t
  deficiency of in diabetes, 737. See also Diabetes mellitus
  for diabetic ketoacidosis, 738
  endocrinologic effects of, 737, 737t
  intraoperative, 739–740, 739t
  pancreas producing, 737, 737t
  pediatric dosing and, 854t
  postoperative, 740, 741t
  potassium concentration affected by, 612
  pregnancy affecting, 807
  preoperative, 739t
  resistance to, in septic shock, 982
  total parenteral nutrition and, 951, 990
Intake valve, in resuscitation breathing system, 37, 37f
Intensive care unit. See also Critical care
  infections in, 980–981, 981t
Intercalated cells (I cells), 668
Intercostal blocks, 305, 305f
  for postoperative pain management, 357
    after thoracotomy, 540
Intercostal muscles, neuraxial anesthesia affecting, 261
Intercostal nerves, fixed anatomic relationships and, 285–286, 305, 305f, 306
Intercostobrachial nerve block, 286, 288f, 292
Interdigital nerve entrapment, 351t
Interleukins
  in immediate hypersensitivity reactions, 903
  in septic shock, 981
  in systemic inflammatory response syndrome, 980
Interlobar arteries, 669, 670f
Intermediolateral column, 314, 315t
Intermittent-apnea technique. See also Apneic oxygenation
  for endoscopy, 773
Intermittent mandatory ventilation (IMV), 961–962, 962t, 963f
  synchronized (SIMV), 52, 961–962, 962t, 963f
  weaning from ventilator with, 967
Internal jugular vein, for central venous pressure monitoring, 100, 100t, 101f
Internal (sensory) laryngeal nerve, 60, 62f
International units (SI), 598
Interneurons, in pain pathways, 313, 314
Interpleural analgesia, for postoperative pain management, 357–358, 540
Interscalene brachial plexus block, 283, 288–289, 289f
  dyspnea after, 308
Interstitial cerebral edema, 568
Interstitial fluid, 599, 599t
Interstitial hydrostatic pressure (Pi), in pulmonary edema, 971
Interstitial lung disease, 519–520
Interthreshold range, hypothalamic maintenance of, anesthesia affecting, 117–118
Intervertebral disk disease, 353–355, 353t
Intestinal motility
  anticholinergic drugs affecting, 209
  opioids affecting, 169
Intra-abdominal injury, 799–800
Intra-aortic balloon pump (IABP)
  for acute myocardial infarction, 976
  for pump failure after cardiopulmonary bypass, 456
Intra-arterial monitoring
  documentation of line placement for, 902
  intraoperative, 91–97
    in aortic stenosis, 417
    for cardiac surgery in children, 461
    for carotid endarterectomy, 470–471
    in cirrhosis, 730
    clinical considerations and, 93–97, 97f
    complications of, 93
    contraindications to, 91
    for craniotomy, 569
    for head and neck cancer surgery, 776
    indications for, 91
    in renal failure, 687
    selection of artery for, 91–93
    techniques and complications of, 91–93
Intracellular fluid (ICF), 598, 598t, 599, 599t
  osmolality of, plasma sodium concentration and, 503t, 602–604
Intracellular second messengers, in central pain modulation, 318
Intracerebral hemorrhage, arteriovenous malformation causing, 579–580
Intracerebral stimulation, for pain management, 340

Intracoronary steal
  adenosine causing, 230
  isoflurane causing, 128, 143
Intracranial compliance, 556–557, 556*f*, 557*f. See also*
      Intracranial hypertension; Intracranial
      pressure
Intracranial hemorrhage, **578–580**
  aneurysmal, **578–579**
  arteriovenous malformation causing, **579–580**
Intracranial hypertension, 567, **568–569**. *See also*
      Intracranial pressure
  head trauma and, 576, 577, 793, 798
  PEEP/CPAP and, 969–970
  perioperative ICP monitoring and, 569–570
  premedication contraindicated in, 569
  in ruptured aneurysm, 578
Intracranial masses, craniotomy for, 567, **569–573**
Intracranial pressure, 552, **556–557**, 556*f*, 557*f. See also*
      Intracranial hypertension
  barbiturates affecting, 158–159, 171*t*, 558*t*, 559
  benzodiazepines affecting, 164, 171*t*
  desflurane affecting, 138*t*, 144, 558*t*, 559
  droperidol affecting, 171*t*, 175
  enflurane affecting, 138*t*, 142
  etomidate affecting, 171*t*, 173, 558*t*, 560
  halothane affecting, 138*t*, 140, 558*t*
  hydralazine affecting, 226*t*, 229
  hypotensive agents affecting, 226*t*
  during induction, 571–572
  inhalational anesthetics affecting, 138*t*, 558*t*, 559
      neuronavigation and, 570, 571
  isoflurane affecting, 138*t*, 143, 558*t*, 559
  ketamine affecting, 151, 171*t*, 172, 558*t*, 560
  lidocaine affecting, 239
  methoxyflurane affecting, 138*t*, 141
  monitoring of
      during craniotomy, 569–570
      head trauma and, 576
      intracranial hypertension and, 569–570
  nitroglycerine affecting, 226*t*, 228
  nitroprusside affecting, 226*t*, 227
  nitrous oxide affecting, 137, 138*t*, 558*t*, 559
  nonvolatile anesthetics affecting, 171*t*
  opioids affecting, 167–168, 171*t*, 558*t*, 559
  PEEP/CPAP affecting, 969–970
  post-dural puncture headache and, 276, 826
  propofol affecting, 171*t*, 174, 558*t*, 560
  in ruptured aneurysm, 578
  sevoflurane affecting, 138*t*, 145
  succinylcholine affecting, 187
Intragastric pressure, elevation of, succinylcholine affecting,
      186–187
Intramuscular drug administration/absorption, 153
  for opioids, in pain management, 343
Intraocular gas expansion, 761, **763–764**
Intraocular pressure, 761, **761–763**, 762*t*, 763*t*
  anesthetic drugs affecting, 762–763, 763*t*
  fenoldopam affecting, 231
  normal, 762
  physiology of, 761–762, 762*t*
  prevention of increases in, 768, 768*t*
  reduction of, carbonic anhydrase inhibitors for, 676
  succinylcholine affecting, 187, 762–763,
      763*t*
Intraoperative anesthesia record, 1, 10, 11*f*
Intraoperative monitoring. *See* Patient monitoring
Intraosseous infusion, for pediatric patient, 861, 912,
      923–924, 923*f*
Intrapleural analgesia, for postoperative pain management,
      357–358, 540
Intrapleural pressure, during normal breathing, 475, 480,
      481*f*
Intrapulmonary shunt, 475, 493, **494–495**
  absolute, 494
  burn injuries and, 801
  in cirrhosis, 728
  closing capacity and, 485
  hypoxemia in postanesthesia care unit and, 936, 945
  PaO₂ affected by, 499, 499*f*
  physiologic (normal venous admixture), 495
  relative, 494
  venous admixture and, 494–495, 496*f*, 497*f*
Intraspinal opioids. *See also* Spinal anesthesia
  in pain management, **346–348**, 347*t*, 356
      cancer pain and, **349**
Intrathecal administration. *See also* Spinal anesthesia
  of opioids
      for cancer pain management, 349

  for labor and delivery, 823, 826
      with local anesthetics, 827, 827*t*
  unintentional, during epidural anesthesia/analgesia,
      270–271, 819, 825, 826
Intravascular administration, unintentional, during epidural
      anesthesia/analgesia, 270–271, 819, 825, 826
Intravascular fluid, 599–600, 599*t. See also* Plasma
Intravascular hemolysis, acute, blood transfusion causing,
      626, 636
Intravenous anesthesia/anesthetics. *See* Nonvolatile
      (intravenous) anesthesia/anesthetics
Intravenous drug administration/absorption, 153
  for opioids, in pain management, 343
Intravenous fluid therapy, **628–633**. *See also* Fluid
      replacement/management; Venous
      catheterization
  blood loss and, 630
  in cardiopulmonary resuscitation, 924
  colloid solutions for, 630
  crystalloid solutions for, **628–630**, 629*t*
  for extracorporeal shock wave lithotripsy, 699
  for hemorrhagic shock/trauma patient, 795, 796–797
  intraoperative, **632–633**, 632*t*, 633*t*
  during labor and delivery, 820
  normal maintenance requirements and, **630**, 631*t*
  perioperative, **630–633**
  preexisting deficits and, **631**, 631*t*
  in septic shock, 983
  surgical fluid losses and, **631–632**
Intravenous immunoglobulin, for myasthenia gravis, 753
Intravenous lines. *See* Venous catheterization
Intravenous regional anesthesia (Bier block), 283, 284
  of arm, **297–298**, 298*f*
  for pain management, 335
Intravitreal air injection, intraocular gas expansion and,
      761, 763–764
Intrinsic (idiosyncratic) asthma, 513. *See also* Asthma
Intrinsic pathway, of coagulation cascade, 718, 719*f*
Intrinsic PEEP, inverse I:E ratio ventilation and, 964
Intrinsic pulmonary disease
  acute, **518–519**
  chronic, **519–520**
Intubation, 67–69, 69*f*, 69*t*, **70–77**, 965–966. *See also*
      specific type and Airway management
  for airway obstruction in postanesthesia care unit, 943
  in asthma patient, 515
  atracurium for, 191
  in burn patient, 802
  for cardiac surgery
      in adults, 449
      in children, 461
  for cesarean section, 819, 830–831, 831*f*
  cisatracurium for, 192–193
  for craniotomy, 571–572
  difficult, 81, 81*t*, 82*f. See also* Difficult airway
  doxacurium for, 194
  for endoscopy, 772–773
  in head trauma, 576–577, 798
  in hypertensive patient, 393–394
  indications for, 70–71
  in ischemic heart disease patient, 404
  for laparoscopy, 523
  laryngeal mask airway compared with, 67*t*
  for lung resection, 537
  for mechanical ventilation in critical care unit, 965–966
  metocurine for, 191
  mivacurium for, 194
  of neonate, 844–845, 844*f*
  neuromuscular blocking agents for, 188–189
      for cardiac surgery
          in adults, 449
          in children, 461
      in pediatric patient, 856
  pancuronium for, 188, 195
  in pediatric patient, 860, 860*t*, 861
      muscle relaxants for, 856
  physiologic responses to, 80
  preparation for, 71–72, 71*f*
  rapacuronium for, 188, 197
  in renal failure patients, 687–688
  rocuronium for, 196
  for smoke inhalation, 975
  succinylcholine for, 185
  for tracheal resection, 543, 544*f*
  in trauma patient, 794
  tube position and
      errors associated with, 79–80
      verification of, 72–73, 74*f*, 118–119

  tubocurarine for, 190
  vecuronium for, 195
Inulin clearance, in glomerular filtration rate measurement,
      669–670
Inverse I:E ratio ventilation, 962*t*, 963*f*, 964
Iodide, for thyroid storm, 950
ION. *See* Ischemic optic neuropathy
Ion channels. *See also specific type*
  in cardiac muscle membrane, 361, 363*t*
  opening of, in neuromuscular blocking agent mechanism
      of action, 181
IOP. *See* Intraocular pressure
Iowa trumpet
  for paracervical plexus block, 822
  for pudendal nerve block, 822
IPAP. *See* Inspiratory positive airway pressure
Ipasirone, for depression, 592*t*
Ipecac, for drug overdose/poisoning, 991–992
Ipratropium, 207, 209
Irrigating solutions, for transurethral resection of prostate
      (TURP), 695
  absorption of, 692, 695, 696
IRV. *See* Inspiratory reserve volume; Inverse I:E ratio
      ventilation
Ischemic cardiomyopathy, 396
Ischemic cerebrovascular disease, **584–585**, 585*f. See also*
      Cerebrovascular disease
  carotid surgery for, 470–472
Ischemic heart disease, 386, **395–406**, 975–976. *See also*
      Angina; Myocardial infarction; Myocardial
      ischemia
  choice of anesthetic agent in patient with, 386,
      404–405
  intraoperative management of patient with, **402–405**,
      403*f*
  postoperative management of patient with, **405–406**
  preoperative considerations in patient with, 395–396
  preoperative management of patient with, **399–402**,
      401*t*
  treatment of, 396–399, 397*t*, 398*t*, 399*t*
      combination therapy for, 399
Ischemic optic neuropathy, as anesthetic complication, 900
Ischemic strokes, 470
Islets of Langerhans, insulin produced by, 737, 737*t*
Isobaric solutions, for spinal anesthesia, level of block and,
      254, 267
Isocarboxazid, for depression, 591
Isoetharine, for asthma, 514*t*
Isoflurane, 128, 135*t*, **143**
  alveolar concentration curve for, 131*f*
  cardiovascular effects of, 128, 138*t*, 143, 359, 363, 378
  cerebral effects of, 557, 558–559, 558*t*, 559
  for cerebral protection, 562
  electroencephalogram affected by, 563–564
  evoked potentials affected by, 563*t*, 564
  hepatic effects of, 138*t*, 143, 716
  for labor and delivery, 821–822
      uterine activity affected by, 813
      uteroplacental blood flow affected by, 811
  metabolism of, 138*t*
  minimum alveolar concentration of, 135*t*
  organ system effects of, 138*t*
  partition coefficient of, 130*t*
  for pediatric anesthesia, 860
      MAC value for, 855*t*
  renal effects of, 138*t*, 143, 672
Isolation transformer, protection from electrical shock and,
      15, 22, 22*f*, 23*f*, 24*f*
Isoproterenol, 217*t*, **219**, 456*t*
  for asthma, 514*t*
  during cardiac transplantation, 464
  after cardiopulmonary bypass, 456*t*
  organ system effects of, 217*t*
  pediatric dosing and, 854*t*
Isradipine, 398*t*
Isuprel. *See* Isoproterenol

Jackson-Rees' modification, of Mapleson circuit, 30*t*
Jaundice
  obstructive, 730
  postoperative, 717, 717*t*
  serum bilirubin and, 714–715
Jaw muscle (masseter muscle) spasm/rigidity, malignant
      hypothermia and, 187, 869, 871
Jaw-thrust maneuver, for airway management, 915, 917*f*
  in postanesthesia care unit, 942, 943
  in trauma patient, 794, 917*f*

Jehovah's Witnesses
 blood loss management in, 790–791
 postoperative pain management in, 791
Jejunostomy tubes, for enteral feedings, 988
Jet nebulizers, high pressure, for anesthesia machine, 55
Jet ventilation
 with cricothyrotomy, 914–915, 919–920, 920*f*
 high-frequency (HFJV), 962*t*, 963*f*, 965
  for endoscopy, 773
  as one-lung ventilation alternative, 539
 manual, for endoscopy, 773
 transtracheal, 912, 914–915, 919–920, 920*f*
Jugular vein, cannulation of for patient monitoring, 86
 external jugular, 100*t*
 right internal jugular, 100, 100*t*, 101*f*
Juxtaglomerular apparatus, 663*t*, 668–669, 669*f*

K⁺ channels. *See* **Potassium channels**
Kallikrein
 activation of, by cardiopulmonary bypass, 439
 in anaphylaxis, 904–905
 in carcinoid syndrome, 750*t*
 in immediate hypersensitivity reactions, 903
Kappa (κ) receptors, 164, 164*t*
 supraspinal pain inhibition and, 319
Kava, 7*t*
Kayexalate. *See* Sodium polystyrene sulfonate
Kent, bundle of, in preexcitation, 381
Ketamine, 151, **169–172**, 170*f*
 for asthma patients, 515
 for cardiac surgery
  in adults, 449
  in children, 461
 for cardiac tamponade drainage, 434, 465
 cerebral effects of, 171*t*, 172, 558*t*, 560
 contraindications to
  in hypertension, 394
  in ischemic heart disease, 404
 drug interactions and, 172
 electroencephalogram affected by, 564
 evoked potentials affected by, 563*t*, 564
 for induction
  history of use of, 3
  in pediatric patient, 858–859
 intraocular pressure affected by, 763*t*
 for labor and delivery, 821
 mechanisms of action of, 169
 minimum alveolar concentration affected by, 136*t*
 neuromuscular blocking agent interactions and, 185*t*
 organ system effects of, 171–172, 171*t*
 for outpatient procedures, 884
 in pediatric anesthesia, 855
  for induction, 858–859
 pediatric dosing and, 854*t*
 pharmacokinetics of, 169–171, 169*t*
 placental transfer of, 811, 821
 for postoperative pain management, 357
 preoperative, in pediatric patient, 857
 renal effects of, 673
  altered renal function and, 681
 seizure activity and, 586
 structure-activity relationships of, 169, 170*f*
 uses and doses of, 169*t*
 uteroplacental blood flow affected by, 811
Ketoacidosis, 654
 diabetic, 737–738
 treatment of, 655
Ketone bodies
 in diabetic ketoacidosis, 737, 738
 formation of in starvation, 987
Ketorolac, 242, **248**
 pediatric dosing and, 854*t*
 for postoperative pain management, 341*t*, 940
  with opioids, 344–345, 356
  in postanesthesia care unit, 940
 renal effects of, 673
Kidney rest position, 699
Kidney stones
 extracorporeal shock wave lithotripsy for, 697–699, 697*f*
 open procedures for, 699
Kidneys. *See also under* Renal
 anatomy of, **663–669**, 663*t*, 664*f*
 in blood pressure control, 375–376
 cancer of, surgery for, **703–704**
 drug excretion by, 154
 noncancer surgery on, **699**

revascularization of, in renovascular hypertension, 689–691
 transplantation of, **704–705**
Kinetics
 first-order, 155
 zero-order, 155
King-Denborough syndrome, malignant hyperthermia and, 871
Klonopin, *See* Clonazepam
Knee surgery, **787–788**
 arthroscopy, 787–788
 total knee replacement, **788**
Koback needle
 for paracervical plexus block, 822
 for pudendal nerve block, 822
Korotkoff sounds, 89
Kupffer cells, 709, 709*f*
 blood-cleansing function of, 710
Kussmaul's respiration, in metabolic acidosis, 653
Kussmaul's sign, in constrictive pericarditis, 466
Kyphoscoliosis, 520
 level of blockade after spinal anesthesia and, 267

L-type calcium channels, myocardial, 361, 363*t*
Labetalol, 207, **220–221**, 221*t*, 394*t*, 395, 399*t*
 pediatric dosing and, 854*t*
 for pheochromocytoma management, 223
 for pregnancy-induced hypertension, 838
 receptor selectivity of, 220, 220*t*, 221*t*, 399*t*
Labor and delivery. *See also* Obstetric anesthesia; Pregnancy
 anesthesia/analgesia for, 819, **820–828**, 828*t*
  caudal, 274
   with local anesthetics alone, 826
  effects of anesthetic agents and, 813
  epidural, 269, 819
   with local anesthetic and opioid mixtures, 819, 826–827, 827*t*
   with local anesthetics alone, 823–826
   maternal fever and, 277
   with opioids alone, 823
   with spinal anesthesia (CSE), 827
  inhalational agents in, **821–822**
  intrathecal
   with local anesthetic and opioid mixtures, 827, 827*t*
   with opioids alone, 823
  with local anesthetic and opioid mixtures, 819, **826–827**, 827*t*
  with local anesthetics alone, 823–826
  with opioids alone, **822–823**, 822*t*
  pain pathways and, 820
  paracervical plexus block in, **822**
  parenteral agents in, 821
  psychologic and nonpharmacologic techniques in, **820–821**
  pudendal nerve block in, 822
  regional techniques in, **822–827**
  spinal
   with epidural anesthesia/analgesia (CSE), 827
   with local anesthetics alone, 826
   with mixed local anesthetic and opioids, 827
   with opioids alone, **822–823**, 822*t*
  sympathetic nerve block in, 822
 difficult (dystocia/primary dysfunctional labor), **833–834**
 maternal physiology affected by, 812–813
 pain pathways during, 820
 physiology of, **811–813**, 812*f*
 preterm, **836–837**
  prevention of, 837
  β₂-agonists for, 813, 837
  magnesium for, 813
 stages of, 812, 812*f*
Laboratory tests/evaluation
 intraoperative, for cardiac surgery, 441
 in intravascular volume evaluation, **627**
 for outpatient procedures, **883–884**
 preoperative, 7, 7*t*
  in hypertension, 392–393
  in ischemic heart disease, 400
  in pediatric patient, 857
  in valvular heart disease, 406–407, 408*f*
Lactate, in crystalloid solutions, 629, 629*t*
Lactated Ringer's solution, 628, 629*t*
 for hemorrhagic shock/trauma patient, 796
Lactic acidosis, 654
 in septic shock, 982
 treatment of, 655

LAD. *See* Left anterior descending artery
Laennec's cirrhosis, 726
Laerdal resuscitator, 37, 37*f*
Lamaze technique, 821
Lambert-Beer law, in oximetry, 108
Lambert-Eaton myasthenic syndrome, 535, 752, **754**
 neuromuscular blocking agent response affected in, 190*t*, 754
Laminar air system, for operating room, 20
Laminar flow, airway resistance and, 485, 486
Laminectomy, for epidural abscess, 279
Lamotrigine
 for pain management, 337–338
 for seizures, 586*t*
Langerhans, islets of, insulin produced by, 737, 737*t*
Lansoprazole, 246
Laparoscopic cholecystectomy, 522–524, 731
Laparoscopic fulguration/tubal ligation, postpartum, 816–818
Laparoscopic pelvic lymph node dissection, in prostate cancer, 700
Laparoscopy, 522–524
 choice of anesthetic agent for, 523
 complications of, 523–524
Laparotomy, exploratory, in abdominal trauma, 799
Laplace's law, 369–370
Laryngeal mask airway, 59, 64–65, 65*t*, 66*f*, 67*t*
 for cardiopulmonary resuscitation, 918
 endotracheal intubation compared with, 67*t*
 face mask compared with, 67*t*
 for neonate/pediatric patient, 845, 860, 860*t*
Laryngeal nerve
 external (motor), 60
 internal (sensory), 60, 62*f*
 recurrent, 60, 62*f*, 63*t*
  paralysis of, 60
   thyroidectomy and, 742
  speech/voice disorders caused by damage to, 60, 63*t*
 superior, 60, 62*f*, 63*t*
  blocking, for awake intubation, 83, 84*f*
Laryngeal trauma, airway management and, 794
Laryngectomy, 776–777
Laryngoscope blades, 69, 70*f*
Laryngoscopy/laryngoscope, 772–773
 for neonatal intubation, 844–845, 844*f*
 rigid, 69, 70*f*, 72*f*
  airway trauma caused by, 78–79
  complications of, **77–84**, 77*t*
  difficult, 81, 81*t*, 82*f*. *See also* Difficult airway
  for double-lumen endobronchial tube placement, 531
  for orotracheal intubation, 72–73, 73*f*
  physiologic responses to, 80
  preparation for, 71–72
 in trauma patient, 794
Laryngospasm, 59, 78–79, 79*f*, 80, 942–943
 airway obstruction in postanesthesia care unit caused by, 942–943
 awake intubation and, 84
 barbiturate induction and, 158
 extubation and, 77
 in hypocalcemia, 620
 in pediatric patient, 850, 860, 863
 stridor caused by, 620, 780
Laryngospasm notch, 78, 79*f*
Larynx
 anatomy of, 59–61, 60*f*, 61*f*
 endotracheal tube placement in, 80
Laser airway surgery, 773–774, 774*t*
Laser ignition, endotracheal tube, 771, 773–774, 774*t*
Laser plume
 evacuation of, 773
 viral DNA in, 907
Lasers
 fires/explosions in operating room and, 25
 precautions for use of, 773–774, 774*t*
Lasix. *See* Furosemide
Late decelerations, in fetal heart rate monitoring, 841–842, 841*f*
Latent phase, of labor, 812, 812*f*
Lateral decubitus position
 complications associated with, 898*t*, 899*t*
 for neuraxial anesthesia, 254, 263–264, 264*f*
  level of blockade after epidural anesthesia and, 271
  level of blockade after spinal anesthesia and, 267
 for thoracic surgery, physiologic derangements and, **526–527**, 526*f*, 527*f*
Lateral femoral cutaneous nerve block, 300, 301*f*
Lateral femoral cutaneous nerve entrapment, 351*t*

Lateral flexed position, 699
Lateral phase separation theory, of anesthetic action, 133–134
Latex allergy, 889, **905–906**
Laudanosine toxicity, 191
Laughing gas. *See* Nitrous oxide
Law of Laplace, 369–370
LD₅₀. *See* Median lethal dose
Leakage current, electrocution risk in operating room and, 15, 21
Leaks, breathing circuit, 56–58, 891, 891*t*
  alarms signaling, 41, 53, 57
  inspection routine for prevention of, **55–56**, 56–57*t*
LeFort fractures, 777, 778*f*
LeFort osteotomies, 777–779
  repair of, 777–779
Left anterior descending artery, 376, 377*f*
Left bundle branch block, significance of, 429
Left coronary arteries, 376, 377*f*
Left heart, hypoplastic, 426–427
Left-to-right (simple) shunts, in congenital heart disease, 422, 423*f*, **423–425**. *See also causative lesion*
Left ventricle, underdevelopment of (hypoplastic left heart syndrome), 426–427
Left ventricular assist device, for pump failure after cardiopulmonary bypass, 456
Left ventricular end-diastolic pressure (LVEDP), 369
  in aortic stenosis, 416
  coronary perfusion pressure affected by, 376
Left ventricular failure. *See also* Heart failure
  after cardiopulmonary bypass, 455–456, 455*f*
Left ventricular hypertrophy. *See* Ventricular hypertrophy
Left ventricular outflow obstruction
  aortic stenosis causing, 416
  congenital lesions causing, **423**
  hypertrophic cardiomyopathy causing, 418
Left ventricular stroke-work index, monitoring, 106*t*
Left ventricular vent, for cardiopulmonary bypass machine, 437
Leg. *See also* Lower extremity
  somatic blockade of, **298–303**, 304*f*, 305*f*
Legal issues
  anesthesia documentation and, 10–13
  in critical care, **952–953**
LEMS. *See* Lambert-Eaton myasthenic syndrome
Leriche's syndrome, 467
Leukapheresis, 636
Leukocytosis
  in pregnancy, 807
  in septic shock, 982
  in systemic inflammatory response syndrome, 980*t*
Leukopenia
  in cirrhosis, 728
  in septic shock, 982
  in systemic inflammatory response syndrome, 980*t*
Leukotrienes
  in anaphylaxis, 904–905
  in immediate hypersensitivity reactions, 903
Levo-Dromoran. *See* Levorphanol
Levobupivacaine. *See also* Bupivacaine
  cardiovascular effects of, 239
  for epidural anesthesia, 271, 272
    for labor and delivery, 824
Levodopa, for Parkinson's disease, 583, 587
Levorphanol, for postoperative pain management, 341*t*
Levothyroxine, for myxedema coma, 743
Leyden-Mobius (pelvifemoral) muscular dystrophy, 756
LH. *See* Luteinizing hormone
Lidocaine, 236*t*
  for acute myocardial infarction, 976
  in cardiopulmonary resuscitation, 912, 926–927*t*
  cardiovascular effects of, 238
  for caudal anesthesia, 274
    in pediatric patient, 863
  cerebral effects of, 239, 558*t*, 560
  for differential neuraxial blockade, 335*t*
  for epidural anesthesia, 271, 272*t*
    for labor and delivery, 824
    test dose and, 270, 825
  epinephrine administered with, 238
  hematologic effects of, 240
  intravascular administration of, unintentional, 240–241
  for intravenous regional anesthesia of arm, 297
  for laryngospasm, 80
  neurologic effects of, 239, 239–240
  pediatric dosing and, 854*t*
  pK_a of, 234–235
  placental transfer of, 811

respiratory effects of, 239
specific gravity of, 267*t*
  for spinal anesthesia, 268, 268*t*
    for labor and delivery, 825
  systemic administration of, for pain management, 339
Life support, withholding/discontinuing, 952–953
Light, ambient, pulse oximetry artifacts caused by, 110
Light anesthesia, unexplained, 37–39, 39*f*
Limb-girdle dystrophy, 756
  anesthetic considerations in patients with, 757
Limb reimplantation surgery, 782, 789–790, 800–801
Lime (soda/barium hydroxide, as carbon dioxide absorbents, 27, 33–34, 33*t*
Limited-mobility joint syndrome, in diabetes, 736, 739
Line isolation monitor, 22, 22*f*, 24*f*
Linear skull fracture, 576
Lingual nerve (mandibular division of trigeminal nerve), 60, 62*f*, 323, 324*f*
  blocking, 325–326, 325*f*
    for awake intubation, 83, 83*f*
Linton tube, for upper gastrointestinal bleeding, 986
Lipolysis, in starvation, 987
Lipophilic group, of local anesthetic, 234
Lipopolysaccharides, in systemic inflammatory response syndrome, 980
Lipoxygenase pathway, in primary hyperalgesia, 317–318
Liquid oxygen, 15, 17, 17*f*
Lissauer's tract, 313
Lithium, 593
  minimum alveolar concentration affected by, 136*t*
  neuromuscular blocking agent interactions and, 185*t*
Lithotomy position, 692, 693, 694*f*
  complications associated with, 898*t*, 899*t*
  peripheral nerve injury and, 893
  for sciatic nerve block, 302
Lithotripsy
  extracorporeal shock wave, **697–699**, 697*f*
  neuraxial anesthesia for, 280–281
Liver. *See also under Hepatic*
  anatomy of, **708–709**, 708*f*, 710*f*
  drug biotransformation by, 154, 713. *See also* Hepatic metabolism
  as reservoir, 710
  surgery on, **731**
Liver disorders, **723–735**. *See also specific type*
  anesthesia recovery time and, 197
  coagulopathy in patient with, 717–722, 718*t*, 719*f*, 721*f*
  halogenated anesthetics and, **717**
  nutritional support in, 989
Liver failure. *See* Hepatic failure
Liver function tests, 708, **714–715**, 714*t*
  anesthesia affecting, 716–717
  preoperative, in valvular heart disease patient, 406
Liver transplant, 731, 732–735
"Living will," 952
LMA. *See* Laryngeal mask airway
LMWH. *See* Low molecular weight heparin
Local (regional) anesthesia/anesthetics, **233–241**. *See also specific type of block*
  absorption of, 235–238
  cardiovascular effects of, 233, 238–239, 363, 366
    indirect renal effects and, 672
  for carotid surgery, 471–472
  for cesarean section, 819, 828–829, **829–830**
  for COPD patients, 518
  for cystoscopy, 693–694
  distribution of, 238
  drug interactions and, 240
  duration of action of, 235
  for extracorporeal shock wave lithotripsy, 698
  for full stomach patient, 251
  in geriatric patient, 875, 879–881
  hematologic effects of, 240
  for hip fracture repair, 784, 880–881
  history of use of, **3**
  immunologic effects of, 240
  infiltration of, for postoperative pain management, **342–343**
  intravenous (Bier block), 283, 284
    of arm, **297–298**, 298*f*
    for pain management, 335
  in ischemic heart disease patient, 404
  for labor and delivery, **823–826**
    maternal heart disease and, 839
    with opioids, 819, **826–827**, 827*t*
    pregnancy-induced hypertension and, 838–839
    sensitivity/dose requirements and, 805
    uterine activity affected by, 813

mechanism of action of, theories of, **234**
metabolism and excretion of, 238
minimum alveolar concentration affected by, 136*t*
musculoskeletal effects of, 240
neuraxial (spinal/epidural/caudal) blocks, **253–282**
neurologic effects of, 239–240
neuromuscular blocking agent interactions and, 185*t*, 240
onset of action of, 234–235
for ophthalmic surgery, **766–768**, 767*f*, 768*f*
organ system effects of, 238–240
for outpatient procedures, **884–885**
overdose/toxicity of, 233, 238–240, 240–241, 278
in pain management, **323–336**, 342–343, 346–348, 347*t*
in pediatric patient, 862–863
peripheral nerve blocks, **283–308**
  in pain management, **323–336**, 346
pharmacokinetics of, **235–238**
physicochemical properties of, 236–237*t*
placental transfer of, 811
for postpartum tubal ligation, 817–818
potency of, 234
for pregnant patient requiring surgery, 847
respiratory effects of, 239
routine recovery from, 939
structure-activity relationships of, **234–235**, 236–237*t*
systemic administration of, for pain management, 339
systemic toxicity and, 278
uteroplacental blood flow affected by, 811
venous thromboembolism after hip surgery and, 787, 881
Local-general anesthesia, avoidance of for ophthalmic surgery, 765
Local standby. *See* Monitored anesthesia care
Loop diuretics, **674–675**. *See also specific agent*
  adverse effects of, 392*t*, 675
  for hypermagnesemia, 623
  for hypertension, 390*t*, 674
  for intracranial hypertension, 569
Loop of Henle, 663*t*, 664*f*, 666–667, 666*f*, 667*f*
Lorazepam, 160*f*. *See also* Benzodiazepines
  for cardiac surgery premedication, 440
  in geriatric anesthesia, 880
  for induction, history of use of, 3
  organ system effects of, 171*t*
  pharmacokinetics of, 161, 161*t*
  structure-activity relationships of, 160, 160*f*
  uses and doses of, 161*t*
Loss of resistance technique
  for caudal anesthesia in pediatric patient, 863
  for epidural anesthesia, 254, 270
Low back pain, **352–355**
Low-flow (variable-performance) equipment, for oxygen therapy, 954
Low molecular weight heparin. *See also* Heparin therapy
  neuraxial anesthesia in setting of therapy with, 280
  for pulmonary embolism, 521
Low pressure tamponade, 465
Lower extremity
  postoperative neuropathies involving, lithotomy position and, 893
  somatic blockade of, **298–303**, 304*f*, 305*f*. *See also* Epidural anesthesia; Spinal anesthesia
    ankle block for, 283, 303, 304*f*, 305*f*
    femoral nerve and "three-in-one" block for, 283, 298–299, 299*f*
    lateral femoral cutaneous nerve block for, 300, 301*f*
    obturator nerve block for, 299–300, 300*f*
    popliteal block for, 302–304, 303*f*
    sciatic nerve block for, 283, 301–302, 302*f*
Lower gastrointestinal bleeding, 986
Lozol. *See* Indapamide
LPLND. *See* Laparoscopic pelvic lymph node dissection
LPS. *See* Lipopolysaccharides
Ludiomil. *See* Maprotiline
Lumbar arachnoiditis, neuraxial anesthesia causing, 278
Lumbar disk radiculopathy, 353–354, 353*f*
Lumbar epidural blocks, 269. *See also* Epidural anesthesia
  for labor and delivery, 823–826
  after thoracotomy, 540
Lumbar medial branch and facet blocks, 330, 330*f*
Lumbar paravertebral blocks, 329–330, 330*f*
Lumbar puncture, for neuraxial anesthesia
  anatomic approach for, 264–266, 264*f*, 265*f*
  midline approach for, 254*f*, 265
  paramedian approach for, 265–266, 265*f*

patient positioning for, 263–264, 264f
surface anatomy and, 263
technical considerations and, 253, 263
Lumbar spinal nerves, 352
Lumbar sympathetic block, for pain management, 334, 334f
Lumbarization of S1, back pain caused by, 355
Lumbosacral joint sprain/strain, **352–353**
Lung. *See also under Pulmonary; Respiratory*
acute injury of (ALI), **972–973**
pressure control ventilation in, 964
fetal
changes at birth and, 816
maturation of, 804, 816
filtration function of, 508–509
intentional collapse of for thoracic surgery. *See also* One-lung ventilation
physiologic consequences of, 528
metabolism in, 509
nonrespiratory functions of, **508–509**
oxygen toxicity affecting, 959
as reservoir, 492
Lung abscess, lung resection and, 541
Lung cancer, 534, 535
resection for, 535–536, 535t
Lung capacities, 483–485, 484f, 484t, 485f, 486f. *See also* Lung volumes
total (TLC), 484f, 484t
Lung compliance, 482–483, 483f. *See also* Compliance
anesthesia affecting, 489–490, 492f
lateral decubitus position affecting, 526, 526f, 527, 527f
reduced, in restrictive lung disease, 518–519
Lung receptors, in breathing control, 507–508·
Lung resection, **534–543**
anesthetic management and, **536–541**
for bronchiectasis, **536**
bronchopleural fistula and, 541–543
complications of, 540–541
for infection, **536**
intraoperative management and, **537–539**
lung abscess and, 541
massive hemorrhage and, 541
postoperative management and, **539–541**
preoperative management and, **536–537**
pulmonary cysts and bullae and, 525, 541
for tumors, 534–536, 535t
Lung transplant, 525, **546–548**, 546t
Lung volume reduction surgery (LVRS), **549–550**
Lung volumes, **483–485**, 484f, 484t, 485f, 486f
anesthesia affecting, 489–490, 492f
in cirrhosis, 728
Lupus erythematosus, systemic, neuromuscular blocking agent response affected in, 190t
Luteinizing hormone (LH), 581
Luvox. *See* Fluvoxamine
Luxury perfusion, 558
LVEDP. *See* Left ventricular end-diastolic pressure
LVRS. *See* Lung volume reduction surgery
Lymph node dissection
laparoscopic pelvic, in prostate cancer, 700
retroperitoneal, in testicular cancer, 702, 702–703
Lymphokines, in immediate hypersensitivity reactions, 903

MAC. *See* **Minimum alveolar concentration**
Macintosh laryngoscope blade, 69, 70f
Macrodex. *See* Dextran
Macrophages, hepatic (Kupffer cells), 709, 709f
blood-cleansing function of, 710
Macula densa, 669, 669f
Mafenide, for burn injuries, acidosis caused by, 802
Magill attachment, in Mapleson circuits, 30t
Magnesium
balance of
disorders of, **622–624**. *See also* Hypermagnesemia; Hypomagnesemia
normal, **622**
in cardioplegia solutions, 438, 438t
in cardiopulmonary resuscitation, 929t
in crystalloid solutions, 629t
in fluid compartments, 599t
for hypomagnesemia, 624
pediatric dosing and, 854t
plasma concentration of, 622
uterine activity during labor affected by, 813
Magnesium sulfate
neuromuscular blocking agent interactions and, 185t
for seizures, 624
in eclampsia, 813, 838

Magnetic resonance imaging (MRI), patient monitoring during, 123–124
Mainstream (flow-through) capnographs, 110, 111f
in pediatric patient, 857–858
Maintenance-type crystalloid solutions, 628
Malignant hypertension, 389
Malignant hyperthermia, 38, 849, 869–873, 869t
dantrolene in management of, 871
differential diagnosis of, 872–873, 873t
drugs causing, 870, 870t
hereditary pattern of, 872
masseter muscle (jaw muscle) spasm/rigidity in, 187, 869, 871
in muscular dystrophies, 756
in myotonic dystrophy, 757
in pediatric patient, 849, 856, 869–873, 869t, 870t, 873t
monitoring for, 849, 858
risk factors for, 871–872
safe anesthetics and, 873
succinylcholine causing, 187, 870
treatment of, 870–871, 874
Mallaril. *See* Thioridazine
Malpractice, anesthesia documentation and, 10–13
Mandatory minute ventilation (MMV), 962, 962t
Mandibular division of trigeminal nerve (lingual nerve), 60, 62f, 323, 324f
blocking, 325–326, 325f
for awake intubation, 83, 83f
Mandibular (lingual) nerve block, 325–326, 325f
for awake intubation, 83, 83f
Mandibular osteotomies, 777–779
Mandibulectomy, 777–779
Mania, **593**
Mannitol, **673–674**
for drug overdose/poisoning, 992
for intracranial hypertension, 568
for oliguria/renal failure, 674, 979
pediatric dosing and, 854t
MAO inhibitors. *See* Monoamine oxidase inhibitors
MAP. *See* Mean arterial pressure
Mapleson A circuit, 15, 30t, 32
Mapleson circuits/systems, **29–32**, 30t, 31f, 32f, 33f, 33t
components of, 30t, 31–32, 31f, 32f
performance characteristics of, 32
Mapleson D circuit, 15, 30t, 32, 33f
for pediatric patient, 861
Maprotiline, for depression, 592t, 593
Marcaine. *See* Bupivacaine
Margin of safety, neuromuscular, 188
Marijuana use, anesthetic requirements affected by, 594t
Mask ventilation
for cardiopulmonary resuscitation, 918
face mask for, 59, 61–64, 64f
in geriatric patient, 877
laryngeal mask airway for, 59, 64–65, 65t, 66f, 67t
in pediatric patient, 62, 64f, 860, 860t
for resuscitation, 37
Masks
for CPAP, 968
for oxygen therapy, 955–956, 955t
Mass spectrometer, for intraoperative anesthetic gas analysis, 113–114, 113f
Masseter muscle (jaw muscle) spasm/rigidity (MMR), malignant hyperthermia and, 187, 869, 871
Masseter spasm (Chvostek's sign), in hypocalcemia, 620, 745
Massive blood transfusion, **638–639**
Mastoidectomy, 779
Maternal/fetal physiology, **804–818**. *See also* Fetal physiology; Pregnancy
Maternal fever, epidural analgesia and, 277
Maxair. *See* Pirbuterol
Maxillary artery, internal, ligation of in epistaxis control, 780
Maxillary division of trigeminal nerve (sphenopalatine nerves), 60, 62f, 323, 324f
blocking, 323–325, 325f
complications of, 326
Maxillary nerve block, 323–325, 325f
complications of, 326
Maxillary sinusotomy, 774–776, 775f
Maximum breathing capacity, pneumonectomy criteria and, 535t
Maximum oxygen consumption, pneumonectomy criteria and, 535t, 536
McGill Pain Questionnaire (MPQ), 321–322
MD. *See* Myotonic dystrophy

MEAC (minimum effective anesthetic concentration), of local anesthetic, 234
Mean arterial pressure (MAP), 87, 375. *See also* Arterial blood pressure
adrenergic agonists affecting, 217t
minimum alveolar concentration affected by, 136t
nonvolatile anesthetics affecting, 171t
oscillometric determination of, 90, 90f
Measured-flow vaporizer, copper kettle vaporizer as, 48
Mechanical ventilation, 41, **50–54**, 52f, 53f, 480, **959–970**, 960t. *See also specific type and* Positive pressure ventilation
for ARDS, 973
after cardiac surgery, 458–459
cardiopulmonary bypass and, 453
in cardiopulmonary resuscitation, 921
care of patient requiring, **965–966**
discontinuing, **967–968**, 967t
hepatic blood flow affected by, 716
for hypoventilation in postanesthesia care unit, 945
for hypoxemia in postanesthesia care unit, 945–946
initial ventilator settings for, 966
intraoperative monitoring standards and, 125
intubation for, 955–956
Mapleson D circuit and, 32
monitoring patient on, 966
for neonate/pediatric patient, 844–845, 844f, 845f, 861
noninvasive, 960. *See also* Positive pressure ventilation
physiologic effects of lateral decubitus position and, 527
positive pressure, **960–965**
for renal failure patients, 679, 688
sedation/paralysis for patient on, 966
for trauma patient, 795
Mechlorethamine, pseudocholinesterase affected by, 185
Meconium-stained neonate, **843–844**
Medial brachial cutaneous nerve block, 286, 288f, 292
Medial branch rhizotomy, for facet joint disease, 355
Medial cystic necrosis, aortic dissection and, 466
Median effective dose (ED$_{50}$), 155
Median lethal dose (LD$_{50}$), 155
Median nerve block, 295–297, 296f
Median nerve entrapment, 351t
Mediastinal adenopathy, 550–551
Mediastinal dissection, after thoracotomy, 540
Mediastinal shift, during thoracic surgery, 528, 528f
Mediastinoscopy, 545–546
Medical gas systems, **16–19**, 16f, 17f, 18f, 18t, 19f, 20f, 25–26. *See also specific gas*
characteristics of cylinders for, 17, 18t
delivery systems and, 18f, **19**, 19f, 20f
sources of gas in, **16–19**
testing/certification of, 25–26
Medical gas therapy, **953–959**, 954t. *See also* Oxygen therapy
Medical malpractice, anesthesia documentation and, 10–13
Medication errors
awareness/recall under anesthesia and, 897
intraoperative tachycardia and hypertension caused by, 909–910
Medication history, in preoperative patient evaluation, 6, 6t
Medullary chemoreceptor trigger zone, opioids affecting, 168
Medullary collecting tubule, 664f, 668
Medullary respiratory centers, 506–507
Medullary thyroid carcinoma, in multiple endocrine neoplasia, 750
Megaloblastic anemia, nitrous oxide causing, 127, 139
Melena, 985
Membrane potential, resting
local anesthetic action and, 234
potassium affecting, 612
MEN. *See* Multiple endocrine neoplasia
Mendelson's syndrome, 250. *See also* Aspiration
risk/prevention of, 242, 244t, 250–252
Meninges, spinal, 255, 258f
Meningitis, neuraxial anesthesia causing, 278
Mentum anterior presentation, 834
Mentum posterior presentation, 834
Meperidine, 166f, 940. *See also* Opioids
absorption of, 165
altered renal function and, 679, 682
biotransformation of, 165, 167t
cardiovascular effects of, 167, 171t
cerebral effects of, 168, 171t
distribution of, 167t
drug interactions and, 169
evoked potentials affected by, 564

Meperidine (*cont.*)
  excretion of, 165
  history of use of, 4
  intraspinal, 347*t*
  for labor and delivery, 821
    epidural, 823
    intrathecal, 823
    neonate affected by, 811, 821
  organ system effects of, 171*t*
  for patient-controlled analgesia, 343*t*
  pediatric dosing and, 854*t*
  for postoperative pain management, 940
  for postoperative shivering, 706
  seizure activity and, 586
  subarachnoid administration of, 168
  uses and doses of, 168*t*
Mepivacaine, 236*t*
  for epidural anesthesia, 271, 272*t*
MEPs. *See* Motor evoked potentials
Meralgia paresthetica, 351*t*
Mesangial cells, 663
Metabisulfite, allergic reactions to, 231
Metabolic acidosis, 646, 646*t*, **653–656**, 653*t*. *See also*
    Acidosis
  burn injuries and, 802
  definition of, 646, 646*t*
  in diabetes (diabetic ketoacidosis), 737–738
  high anion gap, 654
  hyperchloremic, 654–655
    urinary diversion and, 624–625
  massive transfusion causing, 639
  in mixed acid-base disorder, 660–661
  normal anion gap, 654–655
  pulmonary compensation during, 648
  in septic shock, 982
  treatment of, 655–656
Metabolic alkalosis, 646, 646*t*, **656–658**, 657*t*. *See also*
    Alkalosis
  carbonic anhydrase inhibitors in management of, 676
  chloride-insensitive, 656, 657–658, 657*t*
  chloride-sensitive, 656, 657, 657*t*
  definition of, 646, 646*t*
  massive transfusion causing, 626, 639
  pulmonary compensation during, 648
Metabolism
  aerobic, **476–477**
  age-related changes in, **878**
  anaerobic, **477**
  anesthesia affecting, **477**
  in burn injuries, 802
  cerebral. *See* Cerebral oxygen consumption/metabolic
    rate
  disorders of, in renal failure, 684*t*, 685
  drug. *See also specific agent and* Biotransformation
    in burn patient, 803
    hepatic, 713
      in cirrhosis, 729
    of inhalational anesthetics, 138*t*
    in obese patient, 749
  energy requirements and, 987
  in geriatric patient, **878**
  hepatic. *See* Hepatic metabolism
  in pediatric patient, 851
  pregnancy affecting, 807–808
Metaproterenol, for asthma, 514*t*
Metaraminol, 456*t*
  after cardiopulmonary bypass, 456*t*
Methadone
  for cancer pain, 348
  intraspinal, 347*t*
  for postoperative pain management, 341*t*
Methemoglobin, 503
Methemoglobinemia
  benzocaine causing, 238
  in burn injury, 802
  nitroglycerin causing, 228
  nitroprusside causing, 227
  oximetry in, 109
  prilocaine causing, 238
Methergine. *See* Methylergonovine
Methimazole, for thyroid storm, 949–950
Methionine synthetase, nitrous oxide affecting, 139
Methohexital, 157*f*. *See also* Barbiturates
  biotransformation of, 158
  cerebral effects of, 159, 171*t*
  distribution of, 157, 158
  for electroconvulsive therapy, 595
  excretion of, 158

for induction, history of use of, 3
organ system effects of, 171*t*
for outpatient procedures, 884
pediatric dosing and, 854*t*
preoperative, in pediatric patient, 857
respiratory effects of, 158, 171*t*
seizure activity and, 586
uses and doses of, 159*t*
Methoxamine, 456*t*
  after cardiopulmonary bypass, 456*t*
  uterine activity during labor affected by, 813
Methoxyflurane, 128, 135*t*, **141–142**
  alveolar concentration curve for, 131*f*
  metabolism of, 128, 138*t*
  minimum alveolar concentration of, 135*t*
  organ system effects of, 138*t*
  partition coefficient of, 130*t*
  renal effects of, 138*t*, 141, 662, 672, 682
N-Methyl-D-aspartate (NMDA) receptors
  in central pain modulation, 318
  ketamine as antagonist of, 169
Methyldopa, 217, 394*t*
  for intraoperative hypertension, 394*t*
  minimum alveolar concentration affected by, 136*t*
  for pregnancy-induced hypertension, 838
  receptor selectivity of, 216*t*, 217
Methylene blue
  for methemoglobinemia management, 227, 228, 238
  pulse oximetry artifacts caused by, 110
Methylergonovine, uterine activity during labor affected by,
    813
Methylmethacrylate cement, for total hip replacement, 786
Methylparaben, allergic reactions to, 240
Methylprednisolone
  for cerebral protection, 562
  epidural, for back pain, 354
  for pain management, 338*t*
  pediatric dosing and, 854*t*
Methylxanthines, for asthma, 513–514
Metoclopramide, 242, **245–246**
  antiemetic effects of, 246, 940
  for aspiration pneumonia prophylaxis, 242, 244*t*,
    245–246
    cesarean section and, 830
    labor and delivery and, 820
    obese patient and, 748
    open eye surgery in full stomach patient and, 769
  neuroleptic malignant syndrome caused by, 593
  for outpatients, 885
  pediatric dosing and, 854*t*
  renal effects of, 673
    altered renal function and, 682
Metocurine, 184*f*, 188*t*, **191**
  autonomic effects of, 187
  histamine release caused by, 187, 188*t*, 191
  renal excretion of, 188, 188*t*, 191
    altered renal function and, 683
Metolazone, 675. *See also* Thiazide diuretics
Metoprolol, 221*t*, 399*t*
  receptor selectivity of, 220*t*, 221*t*, 399*t*
Meyer-Overton rule, unitary hypothesis of anesthetic action
    and, 127, 133
MH. *See* Malignant hyperthermia
Microelectrocution (microshock fibrillation), 23
Microlaryngoscopy, 772–773
Microprocessor-controlled ventilators, 961
Microshock fibrillation (microelectrocution), 15, 23
Midamor. *See* Amiloride
Midazolam, 160*f*. *See also* Benzodiazepines
  for cardiac surgery
    with ketamine, 449
  for premedication
    in adults, 440
    in children, 460
  cardiovascular effects of, 161, 171*t*
  cerebral effects of, 560
  drug interactions and, 164
  in geriatric anesthesia, 880
  for induction, history of use of, 3
  for infusion anesthesia, 162
  organ system effects of, 171*t*
  pediatric dosing and, 854*t*
  pharmacokinetics of, 161, 161*t*
  preoperative
    in hypertensive patient, 393
    in pediatric patient, 857
  respiratory effects of, 161–164, 171*t*
  structure-activity relationships of, 160, 160*f*

uses and doses of, 161*t*
uteroplacental blood flow affected by, 811
Midline approach, for neuraxial anesthesia, 264*f*, 265
Miller laryngoscope blade, 69, 70*f*
  for neonatal intubation, 844
Milrinone, 456*t*
  after cardiopulmonary bypass, 456*t*, 457
  pediatric dosing and, 854*t*
Mimosa 2, as carbon dioxide absorbent indicator dye, 34*t*
Mineralocorticoids, 745. *See also* Aldosterone
  deficiency of, **746**
  excess of, **745–746**
Miniature end-plate potential, in neuromuscular
    transmission, 179
Minimum alveolar concentration (MAC), of inhalational
    anesthetic, 127, **135–137**, 135*f*, 136*t*
  in geriatric patient, 875, 879
  local anesthetics affecting, 239
  in pediatric patient, 849, 852–855, 855*t*
  during pregnancy, 804, 805, 805*t*
Minimum concentration (Cm), of local anesthetic, 233,
    234
  in geriatric patient, 875, 879
Minimum effective anesthetic concentration (MEAC)
  of local anesthetic, 234
  opioid management of postoperative pain and, 343
Minimum local analgesic concentration (MLAC), of local
  anesthetic, 233, 234
Minnesota Multiphasic Personality Inventory (MMPI), in
  pain evaluation, 322
Minnesota tube, for upper gastrointestinal bleeding, 986
Minute ventilation, 490
  labor and delivery affecting, 812
  $PaCO_2$ and, 476, 507, 507*f*
  pain affecting, 320
  PaO_2 and, 507, 508*f*
  pregnancy affecting, 805, 805*t*
Mirtazapine, for depression, 592*t*
Mishap chain, 889, 891
Mitral regurgitation, 387, **412–414**, 413*f*
  choice of anesthetic agent for patient with, 414
  heart murmur in, preoperative evaluation of, 407*t*
Mitral stenosis, 387, **409–412**, 410*f*
  choice of anesthetic agent for patient with, 411–412
  heart murmur in, preoperative evaluation of, 407*t*
Mitral valve area, calculation of, 410–411
Mitral valve flow, calculation of, 410–411
Mitral valve prolapse, 413*f*, **414–416**
  heart murmur in, preoperative evaluation of, 407*t*, 414
Mivacurium, 179, 184*f*, 188*t*, **193–194**
  altered renal function and, 683
  histamine release caused by, 187, 188*t*, 194
  history of use of, 4
  for outpatient procedures, 884
  pediatric dosing and, 854*t*
Mixed acid-base disorder, 660–661
  definition of, 646
Mixed adrenergic antagonists, **220–222**
Mixed venous blood oxygen saturation ($S_v O_2$)
  cardiac output indicated by, 359, 366
  intraoperative monitoring of, 110
Mixed venous carbon dioxide tension ($P\bar{v}CO_2$), 500
Mixed venous oxygen tension ($P\bar{v}O_2$), 498–499, 499, 500*t*
Mixing lesions (right-to-left/complex shunts), in congenital
    heart disease, 422, 422*t*, **425–427**. *See also*
    causative lesion
MLAC (minimum local analgesic concentration), of local
    anesthetic, 234
MMPI. *See* Minnesota Multiphasic Personality Inventory
MMR (masseter muscle rigidity). *See* Masseter muscle (jaw
    muscle) spasm/rigidity
MMV. *See* Mandatory minute ventilation
Moban. *See* Molindone
Moclobemide, for depression, 592*t*
Molality, **598**
Molarity, **598**
Mole, **598**
Molindone, 593
Monitored anesthesia care, 8, 124, **886–888**
  awareness and, 899
  choice of agent for, 887
  for extracorporeal shock wave lithotripsy, 698
  for ophthalmic surgery, 766, 886–888
    eye injury and, 899–900
  for outpatient procedures, **885**, 886–888
Monitoring, patient. *See* Patient monitoring
Monoamine oxidase inhibitors, 591–593, 592*t*
  opioid drug interaction and, 169, 583, 591

Monoamines, in pain inhibition, 319
Mononeuropathies, electromyography and nerve
    conduction studies in evaluation of, 322
Montage, for EEG electrode positioning, 114, 114f
Morphine, 151, 166f, 344–345, 940. *See also* Opioids
    absorption of, 165
    for acute myocardial infarction, 976
    altered renal function and, 679, 682
    biotransformation of, 151, 165, 167f
    for cancer pain, 348
    for cardiac surgery premedication
        in adults, 440
        in children, 460
    cardiovascular effects of, 167, 171t
    distribution of, 165, 167t
    excretion of, 165
    history of use of, 4
    inappropriate use of, 344
    intraspinal, 346, 347, 347t
    intrathecal, for labor and delivery, 823
    neonate affected by, 811, 821
    organ system effects of, 171t
    for patient-controlled analgesia, 343t
    in pediatric anesthesia, 855
    pediatric dosing and, 854t
    placental transfer of, 811, 821
    in postanesthesia care unit, 940
    respiratory effects of, 168f, 171t
    uses and doses of, 168t
Morton's neuroma, 351t
Motion, pulse oximetry artifacts caused by, 110
Motor end-plate, in neuromuscular transmission, 179, 180f
Motor evoked potentials (MEPs), for intraoperative
    monitoring, 115–116, 116t
Motor (anterior) horn, 314, 315t
Motrin. *See* Ibuprofen
Mouth-to-mask (mouth-to-barrier-device) rescue breathing,
    921
Mouth-to-mouth-and-nose rescue breathing, 921
Mouth-to-mouth rescue breathing, 921
MPQ. *See* McGill Pain Questionnaire
MRI. *See* Magnetic resonance imaging
MS Contin. *See* Morphine
Mu (μ) receptors, 164, 164t
    supraspinal pain inhibition and, 319
Mucociliary function
    halothane affecting, 140
    methoxyflurane affecting, 141
Mucomyst. *See* Acetylcysteine
Multiple endocrine neoplasia, 750–751
Multiple gestations, **834–835**
Multiple sclerosis, 583, **587–588**
Murphy eye endotracheal tube, 67, 69f
Muscarine, 200, 202f
Muscarinic effects
    of cholinesterase inhibitors, 202, 202t
        anticholinergic administration and, 202, 204t
    of neostigmine, 204
Muscarinic receptors, 200, 200t
    anticholinergic drugs affecting, 207
    cardiac, 366
    in heart failure, 380
    nondepolarizing neuromuscular blocking agents
        affecting, 187
    succinylcholine affecting, 186
Muscle biopsy, anesthesia for, 759–760
Muscle contractions
    generalized, succinylcholine causing, 187
    myocardial. *See* Myocardial contraction/contractility
Muscle grafts, autologous (free flaps), 789–790
Muscle groups, neuromuscular blocking agent selectivity
    and, 189–190
Muscle pain, succinylcholine causing, 186
Muscle relaxants. *See* Neuromuscular blocking agents
Muscle tissue, drug distribution and, 153, 153t
    absorption of nonvolatile anesthetics and, 153
    uptake of inhalational anesthetics and, 130–131, 130t,
        132f
Muscle weakness
    in Duchenne's muscular dystrophy, 755
    in facioscapulohumeral dystrophy, 756
    in hyperkalemia, 617
    in hypokalemia, 614, 614t
    in Lambert-Eaton myasthenic syndrome, 754
    muscle biopsy in evaluation of, 759–760
    in myasthenia gravis, 752
    in myotonic dystrophy, 755
    in periodic paralysis, 758, 759

Muscular denervation, neuromuscular blocking agent
    response affected in, 190t
Muscular disease, neuromuscular blocking agents affected
    by, 189, 190t
Muscular dystrophies, 752, **754–757**. *See also specific type*
    anesthetic considerations in patients with, 756–757
    Becker's, 755, 756
    Duchenne's, 754–756
    facioscapulohumeral, 756, 757
    limb-girdle, 756, 757
    malignant hyperthermia and, 871
    myotonic, 755–756, 756–757
    neuromuscular blocking agent response affected in, 190t,
        756–757
Muscular subaortic stenosis. *See* Hypertrophic
    cardiomyopathy
Musculocutaneous nerve, fixed anatomic relationships and,
    285
Musculocutaneous nerve block, 286, 288f, 292, 293f
Musculoskeletal system
    age-related changes in, **879**
    in hyperkalemia, 617
    hyperparathyroidism affecting, 744t
    in hypokalemia, 614, 614t
    hypoparathyroidism affecting, 745t
    local anesthetics affecting, 240
    pregnancy affecting, 808
Myasthenic crisis, 753
Myasthenia gravis, 752, **752–754**
    neuromuscular blocking agent response affected in, 190t,
        754
Myasthenic syndrome (Lambert-Eaton myasthenic
    syndrome), 535, 752, **754**
    neuromuscular blocking agent response affected in, 190t,
        754
Mydriasis, anticholinergic drugs causing, 209
Myocardial blood supply. *See* Coronary circulation/blood
    flow
Myocardial contraction/contractility, **364–366**
    antianginal agents affecting, 397t
    in aortic stenosis, 416
    β_1-adrenoceptor activation affecting, 215
    after cardiopulmonary bypass, 455–456, 455t
    dobutamine affecting, 219
    dopamine affecting, 219
    enflurane affecting, 142, 364
    epinephrine affecting, 218
    excitation-contraction coupling in, 364–366, 365f
    halothane affecting, 139, 364
    histamine affecting, 243
    hydralazine affecting, 229
    inhalational anesthetics affecting, 359, 364
    local anesthetics affecting, 238–239, 366
    mechanism of, **364–366**, 365f
    methoxyflurane affecting, 141
    in mitral regurgitation, 412
    neuraxial anesthesia affecting, 260
    nitrous oxide affecting, 137, 364
    norepinephrine affecting, 218–219, 366
    opioids affecting, 167
    propofol affecting, 174
    propranolol affecting, 222
    sevoflurane affecting, 145, 364
    stroke volume affected by, 370
    ventricular pressure change during systole (dP/dt) and,
        371–372
Myocardial contusion, 799
Myocardial hibernation, 976
Myocardial infarction
    acute, **975–976**
    as risk factor, 386, 388, 388t
    silent, in diabetics, 396, 738
Myocardial ischemia. *See also* Ischemic heart disease;
    Myocardial oxygen demand
    during cardiopulmonary bypass, prevention of,
        437–439, 438t
    in diabetics, 738
    intraoperative hypothermia associated with, 117
    postoperative, 406
    in prebypass period, 449
Myocardial oxygen demand. *See also* Ischemic heart disease;
    Myocardial ischemia
    in aortic stenosis, 416
    coronary blood flow regulated by, 376–378, **378–379**,
        379t
    dopamine affecting, 219
    epinephrine affecting, 218
    nitroglycerine affecting, 228

norepinephrine affecting, 219
    pain affecting, 320
    propranolol affecting, 222
Myocardial perfusion, halothane affecting, 139
Myocardial stunning, 975–976
Myocardium, preservation of during cardiopulmonary
    bypass, **437–439**, 438f
Myoclonus, succinylcholine causing, 187
Myofascial pain, **351–352**
Myoglobin, plasma levels of, in Duchenne's muscular
    dystrophy, 755
Myomectomy, transesophageal echocardiography for
    assessment of, 446
Myopathy, muscle biopsy in diagnosis of, 759–760
Myosin, in myocardial contraction, 364, 365f
Myotonias, **757**
    congenita, 757
    myotonic dystrophy causing, 755
    neuromuscular blocking agent response affected in, 190t,
        757
Myotonic dystrophy, 755–756
    anesthetic considerations in patients with, 756–757
Myotoxicity, of local anesthetics, 240
Myringotomy, with tympanostomy tube insertion, 779,
    868
Myxedema coma, 743

N₂O. *See* Nitrous oxide
N-methyl-D-aspartate (NMDA) receptors
    in central pain modulation, 318
    ketamine as antagonist of, 169
Na⁺ channels. *See* Sodium channels
Na⁺-K⁺-ATPase
    extracellular potassium concentration regulated by, 612
    intercompartmental potassium shifts and, 612
    in tubular reabsorption, 664–665, 666f
Nadbath's technique, for facial nerve block, 766
Nadolol, 399t
Nalbuphine
    neonate affected by, 811, 821
    in postanesthesia care unit, 940
Naloxone, 166f, 242, **249**
    for delayed emergence, 938
    for hypoventilation in postanesthesia care unit, 936, 945
    for neonatal resuscitation, 846
    for obtunded/comatose patient, 991
    pediatric dosing and, 854t
Naproxen, for postoperative pain management, 341t
Naproxen sodium, for postoperative pain management,
    341t
Naproxyn. *See* Naproxen
Narcosis, carbon dioxide, 650
Narcotics, 164–169. *See also* Opioids
    intraocular pressure affected by, 763t
Nardil. *See* Phenelzine
Nasal airways, 62, 63f
    for airway obstruction in postanesthesia care unit, 942,
        943
    for pediatric patient, 860
Nasal cannula, for oxygen therapy, 954–955, 955t
    in pediatric patient, 955
Nasal/nasotracheal intubation, 62, 63f, 73–74, 76f, 951
    "blind," 82–83, 83f
    flexible fiberoptic, 74–77, 76f
    inadvertent intracranial placement and, 74, 76f
    for mechanical ventilation in critical care unit, 965
    in trauma patient, 794
Nasal mask, for oxygen therapy, 955, 955t
Nasal polyps, removal of, 774–776, 775f
Nasal RAE tube, for craniofacial reconstruction and
    orthognathic surgery, 777, 777f
Nasal surgery, 771, **774–776**, 775f
    bleeding following, 779–780
Nasoduodenal tubes, for enteral feedings, 988
Nasogastric intubation, for enteral feedings, 988
Nasopharyngeal probes, for intraoperative temperature
    monitoring, 119
Nasopharynx, anatomy of, 59–60, 60f
Nasotracheal/nasal intubation. *See* Nasal/nasotracheal
    intubation
Natriuresis, pressure, in volume control, 610
Natriuretic peptide, atrial. *See* Atrial natriuretic peptide
Nausea and vomiting
    etomidate causing, 173
    5-HT₃-receptor antagonists in management of,
        247–248, 885, 940
    morphine causing, 348

Nausea and vomiting (*cont.*)
opioids causing, 168
postoperative, 882, 885–886, 885*t*, 940
ear surgery and, 779
ophthalmic surgery and, 765
outpatient procedures and, 885–886
Navane. *See* Thiothixene
NCF. *See* Neutrophil chemotactic factors
Near drowning, **973–974**
Nebulizers
air-entrainment, for oxygen therapy, 957–958
for anesthesia machine, 41, **54–55**
Neck, superficial cervical plexus block for procedures on, 288*f,* **304–305**
Neck dissection, 771, 776–777
Needle cricothyrotomy, 914–915, 919–920, 919*f,* 920*f*
Needles
epidural, 269, 270*f*
spinal, 266, 266*f*
Needlesticks, infection transmission and, 907–908
Nefazodone, for depression, 592*t,* 593
Negative-pressure pulmonary edema, postoperative laryngospasm and, 942–943
Negative pressure ventilation, 960
Negative resting potential, local anesthetic action and, 234
Neonatal circulation, 815*f,* 816
Neonatal resuscitation, **842–846**, 842*t,* 843*f,* 844*f,* 845*f*
chest compressions in, 845, 845*f,* 918*f*
drugs used in, 846
intubation for, 844–845, 844*f*
vascular access for, 845
ventilation in, 844–845
volume resuscitation and, 845
Neonate. *See also* Pediatric anesthesia
depressed, **844–846**, 844*f,* 845*f*
general care of, **842–843**, 843*f*
maternal anesthetics affecting, 810–811
opioids, 811, 821
naloxone administration and, 846
meconium-stained, **843–844**
neuromuscular blocking agent sensitivity in, 189
respiratory system/physiology in, 816, 850–851, 852*f*
resuscitation of, **842–846**, 842*t,* 843*f,* 844*f,* 845*f*
Neospinothalamic tract, 314
Neostigmine, **203–204**, 203*f,* 204*t*
altered renal function and, 683
mechanism of action of, 200–202
in pediatric patient, 856
dosing guidelines and, 854*t*
pseudocholinesterase affected by, 185
Nephrectomy
for nonmalignant disease, 699
radical, for renal cancer, 703
with excision of tumor thrombus, 704
Nephrogenic diabetes insipidus, 605
thiazide diuretics in management of, 675
Nephron, **663–669**, 663*t,* 664*f*
Nephrotoxins
enflurane as, 142
methoxyflurane as, 141
renal failure and, 978, 978*t*
Nerve blocks. *See* Peripheral nerve blocks
Nerve conduction studies, in pain evaluation, **322**
Nerve fibers, classification of, 258, 260*t*
Nerve stimulation technique, peripheral nerve blocks and, 286
axillary brachial plexus block and, 292
Nesacaine. *See* Chloroprocaine
Neuralgia, definition of, 311*t*
Neuraxial anesthesia, **253–282**. *See also* Caudal anesthesia; Epidural anesthesia; Spinal anesthesia
anatomic approaches for, 264–266, 264*f,* 265*f*
anatomic considerations and, **255–258**
surface anatomy and, 263
assessment of blockade level and, 266
autonomic blockade and, **260–262**
cardiovascular manifestations of, 260–261
clinical considerations and, **262–266**
complications of, **274–280**, 276*t*
contraindications to, 254, 262–263, 262*t*
differential blockade and, 253, 260, **335–336**
in pain evaluation/management, 309, 323, **335–336**, 335*t*
solutions for, 335, 335*t*
documentation and, 901–902
endocrine manifestations of, 262
gastrointestinal manifestations of, 261
general anesthesia and, 263

indications for, 262
metabolic manifestations of, 262
midline approach for, 254*f,* 265
nerve fiber classification and, 258, 260*t*
in pain management, 310, **346–348**, 347*t*
paramedian approach for, 265–266, 265*f*
patient positioning for, 263–264, 264*f*
physiologic considerations and, **258–262**
pulmonary manifestations of, 261
somatic blockade, **258–260**, 260*t*
spinal cord anatomy and, **255–258**, 258*f,* 259*f*
surface anatomy and, 263
technical considerations and, 253, 263
urinary tract manifestations of, 261
vertebral column anatomy and, **255**, 256*f,* 257*f*
Neurogenic inflammation (secondary hyperalgesia), 318
Neuroleptanalgesia, 175
Neuroleptanesthesia, 175
Neuroleptic malignant syndrome (NMS), **593–594**, 872–873
malignant hyperthermia differentiated from, 872–873
Neuroleptics (antipsychotics), 593
neuroleptic malignant syndrome and, **593–594**
in pain management, 338
Neurologic deficits
after cardiopulmonary bypass, 454
neuraxial anesthesia causing, 278
Neurologic system. *See also under* Cerebral *and* Neurophysiology
age-related changes in, 878–879
cirrhosis affecting, 727*t,* 729
disorders of, **583–596**
after cardiopulmonary bypass, 454
neuraxial anesthesia causing, 277, 278
neuromuscular blocking agents affected by, 189, 190*t*
renal failure and, 684*t,* 686
in geriatric patient, **878–879**
hyperparathyroidism affecting, 744*t*
hypoparathyroidism affecting, 745*t*
intraoperative monitoring of, **114–116**, 114*f*
anesthetic agents affecting, **562–564**, 563*t*
electroencephalography, **114–115**, 114*f,* 115*f,* 116*f*
evoked potentials, **115–116**, 116*t*
pregnancy affecting, 805, 805*t*
Neurolytic blocks, in pain management, **336**
for cancer pain, 336, **349–350**
Neuromuscular blocking agents (muscle relaxants), **178–198**. *See also specific agent*
altered renal function and, **682–683**
for cardiac surgery
in adults, 449
in children, 461
cerebral effects of, **561**
cost effectiveness/safety and, 192–193
for craniotomy, 572
delayed recovery and, 197–198
depolarizing, **183–187**, 184*f,* 185*t*
mechanism of action of, 181
response of to peripheral nerve stimulation, 181–182, 182*t*
reversal of block caused by, 182–183
versus nondepolarizing, **181–183**, 181*t*
for electroconvulsive therapy, 595
for endoscopy, 772
in geriatric anesthesia, **880**
history of use of, 3–4
for hypertensive patients, 395
inhalational anesthetics affecting, 138*t*
intraocular pressure affected by, 763*t,* 769–770
intraoperative monitoring of response to, 120–123, 121*f,* 122*f,* 181–182, 182*t*
during craniotomy, 569
in stroke patient, 583, 585
for ischemic heart disease patients, 405
in Lambert-Eaton myasthenic syndrome, 190*t,* 754
mechanism of action of, **181**
in muscular dystrophies, 190*t,* 756–757
in myasthenia gravis, 190*t,* 754
in myotonias, 190*t,* 757
neuromuscular transmission and, **179–181**, 180*f,* 199, 200
nondepolarizing, 184*f,* **187–197**, 188*t,* 190*t*
mechanism of action of, 181
response of to peripheral nerve stimulation, 181–182, 182*t*
reversal of block caused by, 182–183
versus depolarizing, **181–183**, 181*t*
for open eye surgery in full stomach patient, 769–770

for outpatient procedures, 884
in paramyotonia congenita, 190*t,* 757
in pediatric anesthesia, 856
in periodic paralysis, 190*t,* 759
peripheral nerve stimulation response and, **181–182**, 182*t*
respiratory failure in recovery room and, 205–206
reversal of block caused by, **182–183**
altered renal function and, 683
structures of, 184*f*
Neuromuscular disease, **752–760**. *See also specific disorder*
Neuromuscular function
blocking, **178–198**. *See also* Neuromuscular blocking agents
desflurane affecting, 138*t,* 144, 364
disorders of, 520
enflurane affecting, 138*t,* 142
halothane affecting, 138*t,* 140
hypokalemia affecting, 614, 614*t*
intraoperative monitoring of
during craniotomy, 569
peripheral nerve stimulators for, **120–123**, 121*f,* 122*f,* 181–182, 182*t*
in stroke patient, 583, 585
isoflurane affecting, 138*t,* 143
methoxyflurane affecting, 138*t,* 141
nitrous oxide affecting, 138, 138*t*
sevoflurane affecting, 138*t,* 145
Neuromuscular junction, 179, 180*f*
Neuromuscular margin of safety, 188
Neuromuscular transmission, **179–181**, 180*f,* 199, 200
Neuronal loss, in geriatric patient, 878
Neuronavigation, 570–571, 570*f,* 571*f*
Neurontin. *See* Gabapentin
Neuropathic pain, 309, 311
anticonvulsants in management of, 309, 337–338, 338*t*
antidepressants in management of, 309, 337, 337*t*
electromyography and nerve conduction studies in evaluation of, 322
neuroleptics in management of, 338
spinal cord stimulation for management of, 309, 340
systemic local anesthetics for, 229, 339
thermography in evaluation of, 322–323
Neuropathies. *See also specific type or nerve involved*
autonomic, in diabetics, 736, 738–739, 739*t*
entrapment, **351**, 351*t*
electromyography and nerve conduction studies in evaluation of, 322
nitrous oxide causing, 127, 139
postoperative, **893–897**, 897*f,* 899*t*
patient positioning and, 893, 897*f,* 899*t*
Neurophysiology, **552–566**. *See also* Cerebral physiology
anesthetic agents affecting, **557–561**
anesthetic effects on electrophysiologic monitoring and, **562–564**, 563*t*
brain protection and, **561–562**
doxapram affecting, 248–249
local anesthetics affecting, 233, 239–240
Neurosurgery, **567–582**
for arteriovenous malformation, **579–580**
for head trauma, **575–578**
for intracranial aneurysms, **578–579**
intracranial hypertension and, **568–569**
for mass lesions, **569–573**. *See also* Craniotomy
neuronavigation and, 570–571, 570*f,* 571*f*
for pituitary tumor, **581–582**
in posterior fossa, **573–575**
spinal surgery, **580–581**
stereotactic, **575**
Neurotoxins
local anesthetics as, 239–240
trichloroethylene degeneration to, absorbent granule exposure causing, 34
Neurotransmitters
barbiturates affecting, 156
droperidol affecting, 174
ketamine affecting, 169
opioids affecting, 166
pain mediation/modulation and, 316–317, 316*t*
central sensitization and, 318
Neutropenia, septic shock and, 982, 983*t,* 984*t*
Neutrophil chemotactic factors, in immediate hypersensitivity reactions, 903
Newborn. *See* Neonate
Nicardipine
for cerebral protection, 562
for intraoperative hypertension, 394*t,* 395
for ischemic heart disease, 397, 397*t,* 398*t*

Nicotine, 200, 202f
Nicotinic receptors, 200, 200t
  in neuromuscular transmission, 179, 180f
  nondepolarizing neuromuscular blocking agents
      affecting, 187
  succinylcholine affecting, 186
Nifedipine, 364, 397–398, 398t
  for intraoperative hypertension, 394t
  for ischemic heart disease, 397–398, 397t, 398t
Nimodipine
  for cerebral protection, 562
  for ischemic heart disease, 397, 397t, 398t
Nitrates
  for cyanide toxicity
      nitroprusside-induced, 226
      in smoke inhalation, 975
  for ischemic heart disease, 397, 397t
Nitric oxide, 224
  after cardiopulmonary bypass, 457
  in central pain modulation, 318
  circulation affected by, 373–374
  in nitroglycerin mechanism of action, 227
  in nitroprusside mechanism of action, 225
Nitrogen, storage of, 18t, 19
Nitroglycerin, 224, 225f, 226t, 227–228, 394t, 395
  for acute myocardial infarction, 976
  prophylactic, prebypass myocardial ischemia and, 449
  surgery in pregnant patient and, 847
Nitroprusside, 224, 225f, 225–227, 225f, 226t, 394t, 395
  cyanide toxicity and, 224, 226–227, 226f
  pediatric dosing and, 854t
  surgery in pregnant patient and, 847
Nitrous oxide, 127, 135t, 137–139
  adverse effects of, 127, 139
  altered renal function and, 682
  alveolar concentration curve for, 131f
  cardiovascular effects of, 137, 364
  cerebral effects of, 137, 138t, 558t, 559
  for craniotomy, 572
  ear surgery and, 771, 779
  electroencephalogram affected by, 563t, 564
  enflurane affecting, 149–150
  evoked potentials affected by, 563t, 564
  fires/explosions and, 24–25
  history of use of, 2–3
  intraocular gas expansion and, 761, 763–764
  intraocular pressure affected by, 763t
  metabolism of, 138t
  minimum alveolar concentration of, 135t
  organ system effects of, 138t
  partition coefficient of, 130, 130t
  for pediatric anesthesia, 860
      during cardiac surgery, 461–462
  storage of, 17–19, 18t
  uteroplacental blood flow affected by, 811
Nizatidine, 244, 244t
  for aspiration pneumonia prophylaxis, 244t
NMDA (N-methyl-D-aspartate) receptors
  in central pain modulation, 318
  ketamine as antagonist of, 169
NMS. See Neuroleptic malignant syndrome
Nociception. See also Pain
  anatomy and physiology of, 312–319
      chemical pain mediators, 316–317, 316t
      chronic pain and, 319–320, 319f, 320t
      nociceptors and, 315–316
      pain modulation and, 317–319, 317f
      pain pathways, 312–315, 313f, 314f, 315t
      systemic responses to pain and, 320–321
  central modulation of, 318–319
  definition of, 311
  peripheral modulation of, 317–318
  segmental modulation of, 318–319
  supraspinal inhibition of, 319
Nociceptive pain, 309, 311
  somatic, 311
  visceral, 311–312, 312t
Nociceptive-specific neurons, 313
Nociceptors, 315–316
  peripheral pain modulation and, 317–318, 317f
Noise, in operating room, 20
Noncardiogenic pulmonary edema, blood transfusion
    causing, 637
Noncompetitive antagonists (drug), 155–156
Nonconstant flow generators, 50–51, 52f, 960
Nondepolarizing neuromuscular blocking agents, 178,
    181t, 184f, 187–197, 188t, 190t. See also
    specific agent

acid-base balance and, 189
age and, 189
autonomic side effects of, 187
cholinesterase inhibitors for reversal of, 178, 199–206
combinations of, 189
concurrent disease and, 189, 190t
for craniotomy, 572
desflurane affecting, 138t, 145
drug interactions and, 189
electrolyte abnormalities and, 189
for endoscopy, 772
for fasciculation prevention, 189
  rocuronium, 189, 196
in geriatric anesthesia, 880
halothane affecting, 138t, 140
hepatic clearance of, 187–188
histamine release and, 187
inhalational anesthetics affecting, 138t
intraocular pressure affected by, 763t
for intubation, 188–189
in Lambert-Eaton myasthenic syndrome, 190t, 754
local anesthetic interactions and, 185t, 240
mechanism of action of, 181
muscle group selectivity and, 189–190
in muscular dystrophies, 190t, 756–757
in myasthenia gravis patients, 190t, 754
in myotonias, 190t, 757
for open eye surgery in full stomach patient, 770
in paramyotonia congenita, 190t, 757
in pediatric anesthesia, 856
for pediatric intubation, 461
in periodic paralysis, 190t, 759
pharmacology of, 187–190, 188t
  general characteristics, 189–190, 190t
  unique characteristics, 187–188
potentiation of
  by inhalational agents, 189
  by other nondepolarizers, 189
renal excretion of, 188
response to peripheral nerve stimulation and, 181–182,
    182t
reversal of block caused by, 178, 182–183
structure of, 184f
succinylcholine interactions and, 183–185
temperature affected by, 189
versus depolarizing agents, 181–183, 181t
Nonhemolytic immune transfusion reactions, 637–638
Noninvasive brain oximetry, for intraoperative monitoring,
    110
Non–Q wave infarction, 975, 976
Nonrebreathing anesthesia system, 146
Nonrebreathing oxygen mask, 955t, 956
Nonrebreathing valves, in resuscitation breathing systems,
    37
Nonreservoir (simple) oxygen mask, 955–956, 955t
Nonrestrictive shunt, left-to-right, 424
Nonseminomas, 702
Nonshivering thermogenesis, 851
Nonsteroidal anti-inflammatory drugs (NSAIDs)
  for arthritis, 785–786
  platelet function affected by, 721
  for postoperative pain management, 341–342, 341t
      with opioids, 344–345
Nonvolatile (intravenous) anesthesia/anesthetics, 151–177.
      See also General anesthesia
  absorption of, 152–153
  biotransformation of, 154
  for cardiac surgery
      in adults, 448–449
      in children, 461, 462
  cerebral effects of, 171t, 552, 558t, 559–560
  closed-loop system for administration of, 163, 163f
  continuous versus bolus administration of, 162–163,
      162f, 163f
  distribution of, 153–154, 153t
  dose-response curves of, 155, 156f
  electroencephalogram affected by, 563t, 564
  emergence from, 938
  evoked potentials affected by, 563t, 564
  excretion of, 154
  in geriatric anesthesia, 880
  history of use of, 3–4
  for hypertensive patients, 394–395
  intraocular pressure affected by, 762, 763t
  for labor and delivery, 821
      uterine activity affected by, 813
  for ophthalmic surgery, 767–768
  organ system effects of, 171t

for outpatient procedures, 884
in pediatric anesthesia, 855
pharmacodynamics of, 155–156, 156f
pharmacokinetics of, 152–155, 153t, 154f
  compartment models of, 154–155, 154f
placental transfer of, 810–811
receptors for, 155–156
renal effects of, 673
  altered renal function and, 681–682
  uteroplacental blood flow affected by, 811
Noradrenaline reuptake inhibitors, 592t
Norepinephrine, 217t, 218–219, 456t
  adrenergic activity and, 199, 212–213, 213f
  after cardiopulmonary bypass, 456t, 457
  cardiovascular effects of, 218–219, 366
      indirect renal effects and, 672
  in heart failure, 380
  with local anesthetics, 235–238
  metabolism of, 213, 215t
  organ system effects of, 217t
  pain mediation/modulation and, 316t
  pediatric dosing and, 854t
  pheochromocytoma secreting, 222
  receptor selectivity of, 216t, 218–219
  in renal blood flow regulation, 671
  in septic shock, 986t
  synthesis of, 212–213, 214f
Norepinephrine reuptake inhibitors, 592t
Normeperidine, toxic effects of, 165
Normokalemic periodic paralysis, 759
Normovolemic hemodilution, 639
Norpramin. See Desipramine
Nortriptyline
  for depression, 591, 592t
  for pain management, 337t
Norwood procedure, for hypoplastic left heart syndrome,
    427
Nose. See also under Nasal
  arterial supply of, 780
Nosocomial infections
  in critically ill patients, 980–981, 981t
  pneumonia, 981
      in ARDS, 973
Novocaine. See Procaine
NRM. See Nucleus raphe magnus
NSAIDs. See Nonsteroidal anti-inflammatory drugs
Nucleotidase, in liver disease, 714t
Nucleus pulposus, herniation of, back pain and, 353–354,
    353t
Nucleus raphe magnus (NRM), in central pain inhibition,
    319
Nupercaine. See Dibucaine
Nutrice. See AS-3 preservative
Nutrition
  assessment of patient status and, 987–988
  in critical illness, 987–988
  normal, 986–988
  organ-specific substrate utilization and, 987
  starvation and, 987
Nutritional support, 986–990
  enteral, 951, 988–989
  parenteral
      peripheral, 990
      total, 951, 989–990, 989t
  renal failure and, 979, 989–990

Obesity, 736, 748–749
  definition of, 748
Obesity-hypoventilation syndrome (Pickwickian
    syndrome), 748
O'Brien facial nerve block, 766, 768f
Obstetric anesthesia, 819–848
  abnormal vertex presentations and, 834
  abruptio placentae and, 835
  amniotic fluid embolism and, 839
  antepartum hemorrhage and, 835–836
  for appendicitis during pregnancy, 846–847
  approach to patient and, 820
  breech presentation and, 834
  for cesarean section, 828–833, 829t
      emergency, 833, 833t
  chorioamnionitis and, 836
  for complicated pregnancy, 833–840
  dystocia/dysfunctional labor and, 833–834
  fetal resuscitation and, 840–842, 841f
  general, 828, 828t, 829, 830–832, 831f, 832f
  for heart disease patient, 839

Obstetric anesthesia (*cont.*)
  inhalational agents in, **821–822**
  for labor and vaginal delivery, **820–828**, 828*t*. *See also* Labor and delivery
  psychologic and nonpharmacologic techniques in, **820–821**
  maternal and fetal physiology and, **804–818**
  multiple gestations and, **834–835**
  neonatal resuscitation and, **842–846**, 842*t*, 843*f*, 844*f*, 845*f*
  neuraxial anesthesia for, 254
    epidural, 269
      maternal fever and, 277
  pain pathways and, **820**
  parenteral agents in, **821**
  placenta previa and, 835
  postpartum hemorrhage and, **839–840**
  pregnancy-induced hypertension and, **837–839**, 838*t*
  premature rupture of membranes and, **836**
  preterm labor and, **836–837**
  pudendal nerve block in, **822**
  regional techniques in, **822–827**, 828–829, **829–830**
  sympathetic nerve block in, **822**
  umbilical cord prolapse and, **833**
  uterine activity affected by, 813
  uterine rupture and, **835–836**
Obstructive cardiomyopathy, hypertrophic. *See* Hypertrophic cardiomyopathy
Obstructive hydrocephalus, posterior fossa craniotomy and, 573
Obstructive cardiac lesions. *See also* Left ventricular outflow obstruction; Right ventricular outflow obstruction
  surgical correction of, induction of anesthesia for, 460
Obstructive pulmonary disease, 511, **512–518**
  asthma, 511, **513–516**
  chronic, 511, **516–518**, 516*t*
Obstructive shock, 795*t*
Obstructive sleep apnea, obesity and, 748
Obtunded patient, 990–992
Obturator nerve block, 299–300, 300*f*
Obturator nerve entrapment, 351*t*
Obturator reflex, blocking, for cystoscopy, 694
Occipital nerve block, in pain management, 326–327, 328*f*
Occiput posterior presentation, persistent, 834
Occupational hazards in anesthesiology, 889, **907–909**
Octopus retractor, for off-pump coronary artery bypass surgery, 459, 459*f*
Ocular muscles, in myasthenia gravis, 753
Oculocardiac reflex, 761, **763**
Oddi, sphincter of, 713*f*, 714
  opioids causing spasm of, 716
Off-pump coronary artery bypass surgery, **459–460**, 459*f*
Older patients. *See* Geriatric anesthesia
Oliguria, 683, 979
  furosemide in evaluation/management of, 674–675, 979
  intraoperative, 662, 677–678
  mannitol in evaluation/prevention/management of, 674, 979
  monitoring, 120
  in renal failure, 683, 979
    loop diuretics for, 675, 979
    mannitol for, 674, 979
  in septic shock, 982
Omentopexy, in lung transplant, 547
Omeprazole, 246
  for cesarean section in high risk patients, 830
Omphalocele, **866**
Ondansetron, 247, 247*f*
  for outpatients, 885
  pediatric dosing and, 854*t*
  in postanesthesia care unit, 940
One-lung ventilation, **529–534**, 538–539, 965
  alternatives to, 539
  double-lumen endobronchial tubes for, **529–533**, 529*t*, 530*f*, 531*f*, 532*f*, 533*f*, 533*t*
  indications for, 529*t*
  management of, 538–539
  physiologic consequences of, **528**
  single-lumen endobronchial tubes for, **534**
  single-lumen tracheal tubes with bronchial blocker for, **533–534**
  for thoracoscopic procedures, 544
Open drop anesthesia, **28–29**, 33*t*
Open-eye surgical procedures, 762*t*
  emergency/full-stomach, 761, 768–770, 768*t*, 769*t*
  intraocular pressure and, 762
Operant (behavior) therapy, for pain management, 339

Operating room, **15–26**
  electrical safety and, **20–24**, 21*f*, 22*f*, 23*f*, 24*f*, 25*f*
  environmental factors in, **20**
  fire/explosion dangers in, **24–25**
  medical gas systems for, **16–19**, 16*f*, 17*f*, 18*f*, 18*t*, 19*f*, 20*f*, 25–26
  transport to PACU from, **939**
Ophthalmic division of trigeminal nerve (anterior ethmoidal nerve), 60, 62*f*, 323, 324*f*
  blocking, 323, 324*f*
Ophthalmic drugs, systemic effects of, 210–211, 761, **764–765**, 764*t*
Ophthalmic/ophthalmologic effects
  of anticholinergic drugs, 209
  of cholinesterase inhibitors, 202*t*
  of fenoldopam, 231
Ophthalmic nerve block, 323, 324*f*
Ophthalmic surgery, **761–770**
  emergency/full stomach, 761, 768–770, 768*t*, 769*t*
  eye injury during, 899–900
  general anesthesia for, **765–766**
  intraocular gas expansion and, **763–764**
  intraocular pressure dynamics and, **761–763**, 762*t*, 763*t*
  monitored anesthesia care for, 766, 886–888
  oculocardiac reflex and, **763**
  postoperative care and, 766
  regional anesthesia for, **766–768**, 767*f*, 768*f*
  systemic effects of ophthalmic drugs and, 210–211, **764–765**, 764*t*
Ophthalmoscopy, preoperative, in hypertension, 392
Opioid antagonists, 166*f*, 249
Opioid receptors, 164, 164*t*
  supraspinal pain inhibition and, 319
Opioids/narcotics, 151, **164–169**, 166*f*, 342, 342*t*, **343–346**, 343*t*
  abuse of, anesthetic requirements affected by, 594*t*
  for cancer pain, 348–349
  for cardiac surgery
    in adults, 448–449
      postbypass, 458
      for premedication, 440
    in children, 461, 462
  with caudal anesthesia, 273
  cerebral effects of, 167–168, 168*t*, 171*t*, 558*t*, 559
  for craniotomy, 572
  drug interactions and, 169
  electroencephalogram affected by, 563*t*, 564
  with epidural anesthesia, 271
  evoked potentials affected by, 563*t*, 564
  in geriatric anesthesia, 875, 880
  history of use of, 4
  inappropriate use of, 344–345
  intramuscular administration of, 343
  intraocular pressure affected by, 763*t*
  intravenous administration of, 343
  for ischemic heart disease patient, 404–405
  for labor and delivery, 821
    epidural, 823
    intrathecal, 823
    with local anesthetics, 819, **826–827**, 827*t*
    neonatal depression caused by, 811, 819, 821
      naloxone for, 846
    spinal, **822–823**, 822*t*
    uterine activity affected by, 813
  mechanisms of action of, 164, 164*t*
  minimum alveolar concentration affected by, 136*t*
  monoamine oxidase inhibitor interaction and, 169, 583, 591
  oral
    for cancer pain, 348–349
    for postoperative pain, 342, 342*t*
  organ system effects of, 167–169, 167*f*, 168*f*, 168*t*, 171*t*
  parenteral administration of
    for cancer pain, 349
    for labor and delivery, 821
  patient-controlled analgesia and, 343–346, 343*t*
  in pediatric anesthesia, 855
  pharmacokinetics of, 165–167, 167*f*, 167*t*
  placental transfer of, 811, 819, 821
  for postoperative pain
    for inpatients, **343–346**, 343*t*, 940
    for outpatients (oral), 342, 342*t*
    in postanesthesia care unit, 940
  renal effects of, 673
    altered renal function and, 682
  sphincter of Oddi affected by, 716
  spinal
    for cancer pain, 349

  for labor and delivery, **822–823**, 822*t*
  for postoperative pain, **346–348**, 347*t*, 356
  structure-activity relationships of, 164–165, 166*f*
  subcutaneous administration of, 343
    for cancer pain, 349
  transdermal, for cancer pain, **349**
  uses and doses of, 168*t*
Optic neuropathy, ischemic, as anesthetic complication, 900
Optical fluorescence, in arterial blood gas monitoring, 97
Oral airways, 62, 63*f*
  for airway obstruction in postanesthesia care unit, 942, 943
  for pediatric patient, 860, 860*t*
Oral anticoagulants, neuraxial anesthesia in setting of therapy with, 280
Oral drug administration/absorption, 152
Oral hypoglycemic agents, preoperative, 740
Oral/orotracheal intubation, 72–73, 73*f*, 74*f*
  for mechanical ventilation in critical care unit, 965
Oral RAE tube, for nasal and sinus surgery, 775, 775*f*
Oralet. *See* Fentanyl lollipop
Oramorph SR. *See* Morphine
Orbit, proximity of to sinuses, 775, 775*f*
Orchiectomy
  for prostate cancer, 701
  for testicular cancer, 702
Organophosphates, mechanism of action of, 201
Oropharynx, anatomy of, 59–60, 60*f*
Orotracheal/oral intubation, 72–73, 73*f*, 74*f*
Orthognathic surgery, 771, **777–779**, 777*f*
Orthopedic surgery, **782–792**. *See also* specific type
  graft transplantation surgery, **789–790**
  hip surgery, **783–787**, 783*f*, 784*t*, 785*f*
  knee surgery, **787–788**
  limb reimplantation surgery, **789–790**
  spinal surgery, **788–789**
Oscillometry, for arterial blood pressure monitoring, 89–90, 90*f*
Osmolal gaps, 602–603
Osmolality, **598**
  plasma
    control of, **604**
    disorders of
      hyperosmolality/hypernatremia, **604–606**, 604*t*, 606*f*
      hypo-osmolality/hyponatremia, **606–609**, 607*t*, 609*f*
    normal, 602
    plasma sodium concentration and, 503*t*, **602–604**
    potassium concentration affected by, 612–613
  in pregnancy, 807
  urine, in azotemia, 977*t*
Osmolarity, **598**
Osmole, 598
Osmoreceptors, 604
  thirst and, 604
Osmoregulation, 611, 611*t*
Osmosis, 598
Osmotic diuretics, **673–674**. *See also* Mannitol
Osmotic pressure, 597, 598
Osteoarthritis, 784
Osteogenesis imperfecta, malignant hyperthermia and, 871
Ostium primum atrial septal defect, 424
Ostium secundum atrial septal defect, 424
Otorhinolaryngologic surgery, **771–781**. *See also* specific procedure
  craniofacial reconstruction, **777–779**, 777*f*, 778*f*
  ear surgery, **779**
  endoscopic/laser, **772–774**, 774*t*
  head and neck cancer surgery, **776–777**
  nasal and sinus surgery, **774–776**, 775*f*
    bleeding following, 779–780
  orthognathic surgery, **777–779**, 777*f*
Outflow obstruction. *See* Left ventricular outflow obstruction; Right ventricular outflow obstruction
Outlet valve, in resuscitation breathing system, 37, 37*f*
Outpatient anesthesia, **882–888**
  discharge criteria and, **886**, 886*t*, 937
  for eye surgery, 886–888
  general anesthesia and, **884**
  intraoperative considerations in, **884–885**
  laboratory testing and, 883–884
  monitored anesthesia care and, 885, 886–888
  patient evaluation for, **883–884**
  patient selection for, **883**
  postoperative complications and, **885–886**, 885*t*

postoperative pain management and, **341–343**
premedication for, **884**
preoperative considerations in, **882–884**
regional anesthesia and, **884–885**
site considerations and, **882–883**
surgical case selection and, 882, **883**
techniques in, **884–885**
Over-damping, of catheter-tubing-transducer system, 93, 98f
Overdose (drug), 990–992
Overfeeding, with total parenteral nutrition, 989
Overweight. See also Obesity
definition of, 748
Oxford infant laryngoscope blade, 70f
Oxidative phosphorylation, 476
Oximetry
brain, for intraoperative monitoring, 110
in carbon monoxide poisoning (cooximetry), 801, 974, 975
pulse
for intraoperative monitoring, **108–110**, 110f
during ophthalmic surgery, 765
in pediatric patient, 857
in postanesthesia care, 937
Oxprenolol, 399t
Oxycodone, for postoperative pain management, 341t, 342
Oxygen, 486t, **501–504**. See also Oxygen therapy
airway resistance and, 486t
blood content of, 503
cylinders for storage of, 16, 16f, 17, 18t
delivery of (total), 503–504
with helium (heliox), 953, 958
airway resistance and, 486, 486t
hemoglobin-bound, 475, 476, 501–503, 501f, 502f
carbon monoxide affecting, 503, 974
inspired (FiO₂)
with air-entrainment nebulizer, 957–958
with air-entrainment Venturi mask, 957
with bag-mask-valve system, 956–957
with nasal cannula, 955
with nonreservoir mask, 956
with reservoir mask, 956
inspired tension of (PiO₂), 496–497
liquid, 15, 17, 17f
partial pressures of, **496–499**, 498t, 499f. See also specific type
in acid-base disorder diagnosis, **660**
stores of, 504
transport of, 503–504
across placenta, 809–810
dissolved in blood, 501, 501f
in hemoglobin, 475, 476, 501–503, 501f, 502f
carbon monoxide affecting, 503, 974
use of in operating room, 16–17, 16f, 17f, 18t
fires/explosions and, 24–25
Oxygen administration. See Oxygen therapy
Oxygen analyzers, for anesthesia machine, 40, 41, **55**, 55t
Oxygen concentration, monitoring during anesthesia, 41, 55, 55t
Oxygen consumption (V̇O₂), 147
anesthesia affecting, 475, 477
carbon dioxide production and, 147
cerebral. See Cerebral oxygen consumption/metabolic rate
closed-circuit anesthesia and, 147
fetal, 809
in geriatric patient, 878
labor and delivery affecting, 812
maximum, pneumonectomy criteria and, 535t, 536
myocardial. See Myocardial oxygen demand
pain affecting, 320
pregnancy affecting, 805, 805t
ratio of to carbon dioxide consumption (respiratory quotient), 476–477
Oxygen content of blood, 503
carbon monoxide affecting, 503, 974
Oxygen flush valves, on anesthesia machine, 40, **42–43**
Oxygen hoods, 958
Oxygen-pressure-failure devices, on anesthesia machine, 40, 41, **42–43**, 44f
Oxygen requirements. See also Oxygen consumption
during closed-circuit anesthesia, 147
Oxygen saturation. See also Oxygen consumption
coronary sinus, 378
intraoperative monitoring of, oximetry for, 108–110, 110f
measurement of in neonate, 844–845
mixed venous (SvO₂)
cardiac output indicated by, 359, 366
intraoperative monitoring of, 110

Oxygen tension
alveolar, 496–498
arterial (PaO₂), 475, 498–499, 498t, 499f
cerebral blood flow affected by, 554, 554f
endobronchial intubation affecting, 510
of fetal blood, 809
in geriatric patient, 877, 878f
intraocular pressure and, 762, 762t
minimum alveolar concentration affected by, 136t
peripheral chemoreceptors in regulation of, 507, 508f
pneumonectomy criteria and, 535t
pregnancy affecting, 805, 805t
P₍tc₎O₂ (P₍t₎O₂) as measure of, 113
shunting affecting, 499, 499f
mixed venous (Pv̄O₂), 498–499, 499, 500t
pulmonary end-capillary, 498
Oxygen therapy, 953–954, **954–959**, 954t
absorption atelectasis and, 959
for acute myocardial infarction, 976
air-entrainment nebulizers for, 957–958
air-entrainment Venturi masks for, 955t, 957, 957t
air/oxygen systems for, 958
anesthesia bag for, 956–957
bag-mask-valve systems for, 955t, 956–957
for carbon monoxide poisoning, 802, 975
in cardiopulmonary resuscitation, 921
classification of equipment and, 954
in COPD, 511, 517
for drug overdose/poisoning, 991
extubation and, 77
fire hazard and, 959
fixed-performance (high-flow) equipment for, 954, **956–958**
hazards of, **958–959**
with helium (heliox), 953, 958
airway resistance and, 486, 486t
hoods for, 958
hyperbaric, 958
for carbon monoxide poisoning, 802
toxicity and, 959
hypoventilation and, 959
for hypoxemia in postanesthesia care unit, 945–946
before intubation, 71–72
for laryngospasm, 78, 80
methods of administration of, **954–956**, 955t
nasal cannula for, 955, 955t
nasal mask for, 955, 955t
nonreservoir (simple) mask for, 955–956, 955t
in postanesthesia care, 939
for postoperative shivering, 706
for pregnant patient, 806
pulmonary toxicity and, 959
reservoir mask for, 955t, 956
retrolental fibroplasia and, 959
for transport from operating room to PACU, 939
for trauma patient, 795
variable-performance (low-flow) equipment for, 954
Venturi masks for, 955t, 957, 957t
Oxygen toxicity, **958–959**
pulmonary, 959
Oxygenation
apneic
for endoscopy, 773
as one-lung ventilation alternative, 539
for rigid bronchoscopy, 544
during endoscopy, 772–773
inadequate, cardiopulmonary resuscitation for, 912
insufflation in maintenance of, 28
intraoperative monitoring of, 124
anesthesia machine oxygen analyzers for, 41, **55**, 55t
pulse oximetry for, **108–110**, 110f
transcutaneous, **112–113**
patient positioning affecting, 522
Oxygenator, for cardiopulmonary bypass machine, 435f, 436
Oxyhemoglobin, light absorption by, oximetry and, 108, 110f
Oxytocin, 581, 813
in labor initiation, 811
for primary dysfunctional labor, 834
uterine activity during labor affected by, 813, 834

P₅₀, 502
pregnancy affecting, 805t
P-450. See Cytochrome P-450
P-aminohippurate clearance, in renal plasma flow measurement, 669

P cells (principal cells), 668
P:F ratio
in ALI, 972
in ARDS, 972, 973
P–R interval, short, 381–385
significance of, 381
PAC. See Pulmonary artery catheterization
Pacemaker wires, electrocution risk in operating room and, 22
Pacemakers
choice of anesthetic agent in patient with, 432
classification of, 431, 431t
electroconvulsive therapy in patient with, 596
emergency, in cardiopulmonary resuscitation, 912, 924–925, 932f, 933f
evaluation of function of, 431, 432
extracorporeal shock wave lithotripsy in patients with, 692, 697–698
intraoperative malfunction of, 431–432
management of, 432
preoperative, electrophysiologic studies in determining need for, 430
temporary, 430–431
for acute myocardial infarction, 976
Packed red blood cells, transfusion of, 635
PaCO₂ (alveolar carbon dioxide tension), 500, 500f
PaCO₂ (arterial carbon dioxide tension), 500
bicarbonate buffering and, 647–648
central chemoreceptors in regulation of, 476, 507, 507f
cerebral blood flow affected by, 554, 554f
desflurane affecting, 138t, 144
enflurane affecting, 138t, 142
halothane affecting, 138t, 140
inhalational anesthetics affecting, 138t
intracranial compliance affected by, 556
intraocular pressure and, 762, 762t
labor and delivery affecting, 812
in metabolic acidosis, 646t, 648, 658–659, 658f, 659t
in metabolic alkalosis, 646t, 648
methoxyflurane affecting, 138t, 141
minimum alveolar concentration affected by, 136t
nitrous oxide affecting, 137, 138t
opioids affecting, 167, 168f, 344
pneumonectomy criteria and, 535t
pregnancy affecting, 805, 805t
P₍tc₎CO₂ (P₍t₎CO₂) as measure of, 113
pulmonary compensation and, 648
in respiratory acidosis, 646t, 650–653, 658–659, 658f, 659t
in respiratory alkalosis, 646t, 656, 658–659, 658f, 659t
PACU. See Postanesthesia care unit
PAH. See P-aminohippurate clearance
Pain. also type or cause and Nociception; Pain management; Pain pathways
acute, 311–312
systemic responses to, 320–321
anatomic considerations and, **312–315**
back, **352–355**
neuraxial anesthesia and, 275, 277
epidural abscess causing, 279
in cancer patient, **348–350**. See also Cancer pain
chronic, 309, 312
pathophysiology of, 319–320, 319t, 320t
systemic responses to, 321
definitions/classification of, 309, **310–312**, 311t
electromyography studies in, 322
entrapment syndromes causing, 351, 351t
evaluation of patient with, **321–323**
experience of, 311
during labor and delivery, 820. See also Labor and delivery; Obstetric anesthesia
measurement of severity of, **321–322**
modulation of, 309, **317–319**
central, 318–319
chemical mediators in, **316–317**, 316t
peripheral, 317–318, 317f
preemptive analgesia and, **319**
myofascial, **351–352**
nerve conduction studies in, 322
neuropathic, 309, 311
anticonvulsants in management of, 309, 337–338, 338t
antidepressants in management of, 309, 337, 337t
electromyography and nerve conduction studies in evaluation of, 322
neuroleptics in management of, 338
spinal cord stimulation for management of, 309, 340
systemic local anesthetics for, 229, 339
thermography in evaluation of, 322–323

Pain (*cont.*)
  nociceptive, 309, 311
  perception of, 310
    in geriatric patient, 878–879
  physiologic considerations and, **315–319**
  postoperative, **340–348**, 356–358. *See also specific type of surgery*
  psychologic evaluation of patient with, 322
  psychologic interventions and, **339**
  psychological/environmental factors in, 320, 320*t*, 322
  referred, 312, 312*t*
  somatic, 311
  sympathetically maintained, 310, 319–320, **350–351**, 350*t*
  systemic responses to, 309, **320–321**
  thermography in evaluation of, 322–323
  visceral, 311–312, 312*t*
    in failed epidural anesthesia, 273
Pain management, **309–358**. *See also* Pain
  acupuncture for, **339–340**
  adjuncts in, **339–340**
  alcohol blocks for, **336**
  brachial plexus blocks for, **335–336**
  for cancer patients, **348–350**
  cryoneurolysis for, **336**
  cyclooxygenase inhibitors for, 341–342, 341*t*
  definition of, 310
  differential neuraxial blocks for, 309, **335–336**, 335*t*
  electrical stimulation for, **340**
  intracerebral stimulation for, 340
  for Jehovah's Witnesses, 791
  local anesthesia for
    infiltration of, **342–343**
    intravenous administration of (Bier block), 335
  neural blockade for, **323–336**, 346–348, 347*t*
  neurolytic blocks for, **336**
  nonsteroidal anti-inflammatory agents for, 341–342, 341*t*
  opioids for, 168, 168*t*, 341–342, 342*f*
  oral analgesics for, **341–342**, 341*t*, 342*t*
  pharmacologic interventions for, **336–339**
  phenol blocks for, **336**
  physical therapy and, **339**
  postoperative, **340–348**, 356–358, 940
    in outpatient, 886
    in pediatric patient, 863
    in postanesthesia care unit, 940
  preemptive analgesia and, **319**
  psychologic interventions in, 339
  radiofrequency ablation for, 336
  somatic blocks for, **323–331**
  spinal cord (dorsal column) stimulation for, 340
  sympathetic blocks for, **331–335**
  transcutaneous electrical stimulation for, 340
Pain pathways, **312–315**, 313*f*, 314*f*, 315*t*
  during labor, **820**
Pain scales, **321–322**
Pain syndromes, **350–356**
Pain threshold, barbiturates affecting, antianalgesic effect and, 159
Palate, 60, 60*f*
Palatine nerves, 60
Paleospinothalamic tract, 314
Palpation, for arterial blood pressure monitoring, 88–89, 89*f*
Pamelor. *See* Nortriptyline
Pamidronate, for hypercalcemia, 619–620
Pancreas
  endocrine, **737–740**, 741*t*
    physiology of, 737, 737*t*. *See also* Insulin
  exocrine, electrolyte content of secretions of, 631*t*
Pancuronium, 179, 184*f*, 188*t*, **194–195**
  autonomic effects of, 187, 188*t*
  contraindications to, in hypertension, 395
  cost effectiveness/safety of, 192–193
  hepatic clearance of, 187–188, 194–195
  for intubation, 188, 195
    in children, 461
  for patients susceptible to malignant hyperthermia, 873
  renal excretion of, 188, 188*t*, 194
    altered renal function and, 683
  succinylcholine interaction and, 185
Pantoprazole, 246
PAO$_2$ (alveolar oxygen tension), 496–498
PaO$_2$ (arterial oxygen tension), 475, 498–499, 498*t*, 499*f*
  cerebral blood flow affected by, 554, 554*f*
  endobronchial intubation affecting, 510
  of fetal blood, 809
  in geriatric patient, 877, 878*f*

intraocular pressure and, 762, 762*t*
  minimum alveolar concentration affected by, 136*t*
  peripheral chemoreceptors in regulation of, 507, 508*f*
  pneumonectomy criteria and, 535*t*
  pregnancy affecting, 805, 805*t*
  P$_{tc}$O$_2$ (P$_s$O$_2$) as measure of, 113
  shunting affecting, 499, 499*f*
PAOP. *See* Pulmonary artery occlusion pressure
Paracervical plexus block, for labor and delivery, **822**
Paradoxic aciduria, in hypertrophic pyloric stenosis, 866
Paradoxic air embolism, 574
  liver transplant, 734
  in pediatric patient, 861
Paradoxic chest movement, in airway obstruction, 942
Paradoxic respirations, during thoracic surgery, 528, 529*f*
Paralysis
  awake, 897–899
  prolonged, succinylcholine causing, 187
Paralysis agitans (Parkinson's disease), **586–587**
Paralytic ileus, trimethaphan causing, 229
Paramagnetic sensor, for oxygen concentration monitoring, 55
Paramedian approach, for neuraxial anesthesia, 265–266, 265*f*
  level of blockade after spinal anesthesia and, 267
Paramyotonia congenita, 757
  neuromuscular blocking agent response affected in, 190*t*, 757
Paraneoplastic syndromes
  lung cancer and, 535
  renal cancer and, 703
Paraplegia, descending aorta surgery and, 468–469
Parasitic infections, blood transfusion in transmission of, 638
Parasympathetic nervous system, 201*f*
  acetylcholine as neurotransmitter for, 199, 200, 201*f*
  in asthma, 513
  in cerebral blood flow control, 555
  heart supplied by, 366
  liver supplied by, 709
  neuraxial anesthesia producing blockade of, 260–262
  pulmonary vasculature affected by, 480
Parathyroid glands, **743–745**
  physiology of, 743. *See also* Hyperparathyroidism; Hypoparathyroidism
Parathyroid hormone (PTH), 743, 744*t*. *See also* Hyperparathyroidism; Hypoparathyroidism
  calcium concentration affected by, 618–619, 620
Paratracheal technique, for stellate (cervicothoracic) block, 332–333, 332*f*
Paravertebral block
  cervical, for pain management, 328, 329*f*
  lumbar, for pain management, 329–330, 330*f*
  thoracic, 306, 306*f*, 328–329
    for pain management, 328–329
Paravertebral muscle sprain/strain, **352–353**
Parecoxib, for arthritis, 786
Parenteral drug administration/absorption, 153
Parenteral nutrition
  peripheral, **990**
  total, 951, **989–990**, 989*t*
Paresthesias
  definition of, 311*t*
  elicitation of, peripheral nerve block technique and, **286**
    axillary brachial plexus block and, 292
Parkinson's disease, **586–587**
Parnate. *See* Tranylcypromine
Parotidectomy, 776–777
Paroxetine
  for depression, 592*t*, 593
  for pain management, 337*t*
Paroxysmal supraventricular tachycardia (PSVT)
  adenosine for conversion of, 230, 385
  mechanisms of, 383
    in Wolff-Parkinson-White (WPW) syndrome, 382–383
    preexcitation causing, 382
Partial anomalous venous return, 425
Partial pressures. *See also specific type*
  cutaneous, transcutaneous sensors measuring, 113
Partial rebreathing anesthesia system, 146
Partial rebreathing oxygen mask, 955*t*, 956
Partial (focal) seizures, 585, 585*t*. *See also* Seizures
Partial thromboplastin time, 720, 721*t*
Partition coefficients
  of inhalational anesthetics
    closed-circuit anesthesia and, 148
    uptake affected by, 129–130, 130*t*
  of local anesthetics, distribution affected by, 238

Pass-over humidifier, in breathing circuit, 54–55
Patent ductus arteriosus, 425
Patient-controlled analgesia, 309, 343–346, 343*t*, 940
  in pediatric patient, 863
Patient evaluation, preoperative, 1, **5–8**, 6*t*, 7*t*, 8*t*
  difficult airway and, 80–81, 81*t*, 82
  documenting, 901
  fluid deficit evaluation and, **631**
  hypertension and, **390–393**
  ischemic heart disease and, **399–402**, 401*t*
  for outpatient procedures, **883–884**
  for pediatric patient, 856
Patient monitoring. *See also specific monitoring parameter*
  for burn excision/grafting procedures, 802
  for cardioversion, 473
  for electroconvulsive therapy, 595
  for extracorporeal shock wave lithotripsy, 698–699
  intraoperative, **86–126**
    airway obstruction and, 551
    anesthetic gas analysis, **113–114**
    in aortic regurgitation, 420
    in aortic stenosis, 417
    arterial blood pressure, **87–97**
    carbon dioxide, transcutaneous, **112–113**
    cardiac, **87–108**
    cardiac output, **106–108**
    during cardiac surgery
      in adults, 441–448, 451–452, 452*f*
      in children, 461
    during cardiopulmonary bypass, 451–452, 452*f*
    catheters for, electrocution risk in operating room and, 22
    central venous catheterization for, **100–102**
    in cirrhosis, 730
    controlled hypotension and, 232
    during craniotomy, 569–570
    electrocardiography, **97–100**
    electroencephalography, **114–115**
    end-tidal carbon dioxide analysis, **110–112**
    esophageal stethoscope for, **108**
    evoked potentials, **115–116**
    during head and neck cancer surgery, 776
    hemodynamic status (cardiac), **87–108**
    in hypertension, 393
    in hypertrophic cardiomyopathy, 418
    in ischemic heart disease, 402–404
    for Jehovah's Witnesses, 790
    during laparoscopy, 523
    during liver transplant, 733
    during lung transplant, 546–547
    minimum standards for, 94–95, 124–125
    in mitral regurgitation, 414
    in mitral stenosis, 411
    neurologic, **114–116**
    during ophthalmic surgery, **765**
    oxygen, transcutaneous, **112–113**
    peripheral nerve stimulation, **120–123**, 121*f*, 122*f*, 181–182, 182*t*
    physical examination and, 118–119
    precordial stethoscope for, **108**
    pulmonary artery catheterization for, **102–106**
    pulse oximetry, **108–110**
    in renal failure patients, 687
    in renal insufficiency patients (mild to moderate renal impairment), 689
    during renal transplant, 705
    respiratory, **108–114**
    during spinal surgery, 580–581, 789
    standards for, 94–95, 124–125
    superior vena cava syndrome and, 551
    temperature, **117–120**
    transcutaneous oxygen and carbon dioxide, **112–113**
    during transsphenoidal surgery, 582
    during transurethral resection of prostate (TURP), 697
    in tricuspid regurgitation, 421
    urinary output, **120**
    venous pressure, **100–102**
  for magnetic resonance imaging, 123–124
  for mechanical ventilation, 966
  for nutritional support, 990
  for pediatric anesthesia, 857–858
  for postanesthesia care, 937
  for pregnant patient requiring surgery, 847
  for total parenteral nutrition, 990
  for venous air embolism, 575

Patient positioning
  complications associated with, 893–897, 897f, 898t, 899t
  controlled hypotension and, 231
  for craniotomy, 572–574, 574f
  for gynecologic surgery, lithotomy position, 692, 693, 694f
  for intubation, 71, 72f
  for lung resection, 537–538, 538f
  for neuraxial anesthesia, 254, 263–264, 264f
    level of block after epidural anesthesia affected by, 271
    level of block after spinal anesthesia affected by, 267
  for ophthalmic surgery, 765
  oxygenation affected by, 522
  peripheral nerve injury and, 893, 897f, 899t
  for posterior fossa craniotomy, 573–574, 574f
  for spinal surgery, 580, 789
  for thoracic surgery, 537–538, 538f
    physiologic derangements and, **526–527**, 526f, 527f
  for tracheal resection, 543, 545f
  for transport from operating room to PACU, 939
  for urologic surgery
    hyperextended supine position, 699, 700f
    "kidney rest position" (lateral flexed position), 699
    lithotomy position, 692, 693, 694f
Patient valve, in resuscitation breathing system, 37, 37f
Patrick's sign, 352
Paxil. See Paroxetine
Pc. See Capillary hydrostatic pressure
PC-IRV. See Pressure-control/inverse ratio ventilation
PCA. See Patient-controlled analgesia
PCO_2 (partial pressure of carbon dioxide), **499–501**
  in acid-base disorder diagnosis, **660**
PCV. See Pressure control ventilation
PDA. See Posterior descending artery
PDPH. See Post-dural puncture headache
Peak amplitude, of evoked potential, 116
Peak flow diary, for asthma patients, 514
Peak inspiratory pressure, 40, 47, 47t
  graphic display of on anesthesia machine, 46f, 47
Pedi-lite sensors, for anesthesia machine, 45
Pediatric anesthesia, **849–874**, 851t. See also specific disorder
  anatomic development/characteristics and, **850–852**, 851t
  cardiac arrest and, 858–859
  for cardiovascular surgery, **460–463**
  cardiovascular system and, 851, 851t
  caudal block used in, 273
  drug dosing and, 852, 853–855t
  emergence/recovery and, 863
  fluid requirements and, 862
  gastrointestinal function and, 851–852
  glucose homeostasis and, 852
  heart rate response to incision and, 858–859
  induction of, 858–860
    inhalational, 859–860, 860t
      insufflation for, 28, 28f
    intravenous, 859
  inhalational agents in, 852–855, 855t
    for induction, 859–860, 860t
  intravenous access and, 860–861
  maintenance of, 861–862
  metabolism and, 851
  muscle relaxants in, 856
  nonvolatile agents in, 855
    for induction, 859
  overdose and, 858–859
  patient monitoring and, 857–858
  pharmacologic characteristics and, 851t, **852–856**, 853–855t
  physiologic development/characteristics and, **850–852**, 851t
  preoperative considerations and, 856–857
  regional, 862–863
  renal function and, 851–852
  respiratory system and, 850–851, 852f
  temperature regulation and, 851
  tracheal intubation for, 860, 860t, 861
  unique characteristics of neonates/infants and, 850, 851t
Pediatric face mask, 62, 64f, 860, 860t
PEEP. See Positive end-expiratory pressure
Pelvic lymph node dissection, in prostate cancer, 700
Pelvifemoral (Leyden-Mobius) muscular dystrophy, 756
Penbutolol, 399t
Penicillin allergy, 906–907
Penile block, 283, 307, 307f
Penthrane. See Methoxyflurane

Pentobarbital, 157f. See also Barbiturates
  for cardiac surgery premedication in children, 460
  pediatric dosing and, 854t
  uses and doses of, 157t
Penumothorax, central venous catheterization and, 102
Pepcid. See Famotidine
Peptic ulcers, bleeding from, 986
Percocet. See Oxycodone
Percodan. See Oxycodone
Percutaneous balloon valvuloplasty. See also Valvuloplasty
  for pulmonic stenosis, 423
Percutaneous transjugular intrahepatic portosystemic shunts (TIPS), 727
Perfusion. See also Circulation
  luxury, 558
  pulmonary, **492–494**, 494f, 495f
    distribution of, 493, 494f
  tissue
    intraoperative monitoring of, pulse oximetry for, 109
    local anesthetic distribution affected by, 238
Perfusion pressure, cerebral. See Cerebral perfusion pressure
Periaqueductal gray, in central pain inhibition, 319
Peribulbar anesthesia, for ophthalmic surgery, 767
Pericardial diseases, **464–466**. See also specific disorder
Pericardial effusions, 465
Pericardial pressure, in tamponade, 464
Pericardial tamponade, 434, **464–465**, 935
  central venous catheterization and, 102, 464
  traumatic, 799
Pericardiectomy, for constrictive pericarditis, 466
Pericardiocentesis, for tamponade, 465
Pericarditis
  constrictive, **465–466**
  uremic, 685
Periglottic edema, laryngoscopy causing, 79
Perineal prostatectomy, radical, 701
Periodic paralysis, 752, **757–759**
  anesthetic considerations in patients with, 759
  hyperkalemic (sodium channelopathy), **758–759**
  hypokalemic (voltage-gated calcium channelopathy), **758**
  neuromuscular blocking agent response affected in, 190t, 759
  normokalemic, 759
Peripheral chemoreceptors, in breathing control, 507, 508f
Peripheral compartment, in pharmacokinetic model, 154
Peripheral nerve blocks, **283–308**. See also specific type
  advantages and disadvantages of, 283, 284
  for awake intubation, 83–84, 83f, 84f
  contraindications to, **284–285**
  documentation and, 901–902
  field block and, 285
  fixed anatomic relationships and, 285–286
  indications for, **284**
  for lower extremity, **298–303**, 304f, 305f
  nerve stimulation technique for, 286
  in pain management, **323–336**, 346
  paresthesia elicitation technique for, 286
  premedication for, 285
  for surgical anesthesia, **283–308**
  technical considerations for, 285–286
  for trunk, **304–307**
  for upper extremity and shoulder, **286–298**
Peripheral nerve conduction studies, in pain evaluation, **322**
Peripheral nerve injury. See also Neuropathies
  neuromuscular blocking agent response affected in, 190t
  postoperative, **893–897**, 897f, 899t
Peripheral nerve stimulation
  intraoperative, **120–123**, 121f, 122f, 203
    depolarizing versus nondepolarizing blockade and, **181–182**, 182t
  peripheral nerve block technique and, 286
    axillary brachial plexus block and, 292
Peripheral pain modulation, 317–318, 317f
Peripheral parenteral nutrition, **990**
Peripheral sensors, in breathing control, **507–508**, 508f
Peripheral vascular resistance. See Vascular resistance, peripheral/systemic
Peristalsis. See also Gastrointestinal motility
  anticholinergic drugs affecting, 209
  cholinesterase inhibitors affecting, 202
  neuraxial anesthesia affecting, 261
Peritonitis, bacterial, cirrhosis and, 726
Permeability pulmonary edema, **972–973**. See also Acute lung injury (ALI); Acute respiratory distress syndrome (ARDS)
Pernicious anemia, nitrous oxide causing, 127, 139
Peroneal nerves

blockade of (ankle block), 303, 304f
entrapment of, 351t
postoperative neuropathy of, patient positioning and, 893, 899t
Perphenazine, 593
Persistent fetal circulation, 816, 817f
  meconium aspiration and, 843
Persistent occiput posterior presentation, 834
$PETCO_2$ (end-tidal carbon dioxide tension), 501
  monitoring, during laparoscopy, 523
Petit mal (absence) seizures, 585, 585t. See also Seizures
P:F ratio
  in ALI, 972
  in ARDS, 972, 973
pH
  in acid-base disorders, 658, 658f, **659–660**
    pulmonary compensation affecting, 648
    renal compensation affecting, 648–650, 649f, 650f
  atracurium duration of action and, 192
  calcium concentration affected by, 618
  hydrogen ion concentration relationship and, 644–645, 645f, 647t
  of local anesthetics, adjustment in for epidural anesthesia, 272
  potassium concentration affected by, 612
  transcutaneous carbon dioxide electrodes measuring, 113
  urine, 681
    renal excretion affected by, 154
pH indicator dyes, for carbon dioxide absorbents, 34, 34t
pH-stat management, during cardiopulmonary bypass
  in adults, 453
  in children, 462
Pharmacodynamics, 127, **155–156**, 156f. See also specific agent
  in geriatric anesthesia, 875, **879–880**
  of inhalational (volatile) agents, **133–137**
  of nonvolatile (intravenous) agents, **155–156**, 156f
Pharmacokinetics, 127, 152–155. See also specific agent
  cardiopulmonary bypass affecting, 439–440
  in geriatric anesthesia, 875, **879–880**
  of inhalational (volatile) agents, **128–133**, 129f
  of nonvolatile (intravenous) agents, **152–155**, 153t, 154f
Pharyngeal nerve, blocking, for awake intubation, 83, 83f
Pharyngectomy, 776–777
Pharyngoesophageal perforation, anesthesia-related, 892
Pharynx, 60
  suctioning, before extubation, 77, 942–943
Phase I block, depolarizing neuromuscular blocking agents causing, 181
Phase I metabolic reactions, 154, 713
Phase II block, depolarizing neuromuscular blocking agents causing, 182
Phase II metabolic reactions, 154, 713
Phencyclidine, 169, 170f. See also Ketamine
  abuse of, anesthetic requirements affected by, 594t
Phenelzine
  for depression, 591, 592t
  pseudocholinesterase affected by, 185
Phenergan. See Promethazine
Phenobarbital, 157f. See also Barbiturates
  excretion of, 158
  pediatric dosing and, 855t
Phenol blocks, in pain management, **336**
Phenolphthalein, as carbon dioxide absorbent indicator dye, 34t
Phenothiazines, altered renal function and, 682
Phenoxybenzamine
  for pheochromocytoma management, 222–223
  receptor selectivity of, 220t, 222
Phentolamine, **220**, 394t
  for intraoperative hypertension, 394t
  pediatric dosing and, 855t
  for pheochromocytoma management, 223
  receptor selectivity of, 220, 220t
Phenylalkylamines, for hypertension, 391t
Phenylephrine, 207, **216–217**, 217t, 456t
  after cardiopulmonary bypass, 456t
  with local anesthetics, 235–238
    for epidural anesthesia, 271
    for spinal anesthesia, 268
  ophthalmic, systemic effects of, 764, 764t
  organ system effects of, 217t
  pediatric dosing and, 855t
  receptor selectivity of, 216t, 217
  uterine activity during labor affected by, 813
  in Wolff-Parkinson-White (WPW) syndrome, 385

Phenytoin
  for pain management, 337, 338*t*
  pediatric dosing and, 855*t*
  for seizures, 586, 586*t*
Pheochromocytoma, 222–223, 747–748, 873
  droperidol contraindicated in, 175, 223
  malignant hyperthermia differentiated from, 873
Phlebotomy, for coagulopathy in congenital heart disease, 422
PHN. *See* Postherpetic neuralgia
Phonation, laryngeal nerve damage affecting, 60, 63*t*
Phosgene gas, trichloroethylene degradation to, absorbent granule exposure causing, 34
Phosphogluconate pathway, 711, 711*f*
Phosphorus
  balance of
    disorders of, **621–622**. *See also* Hyperphosphatemia; Hypophosphatemia
    normal, **621**
  in fluid compartments, 599*t*
  supplementary/replacement, for hypophosphatemia, 622
Phosphorylation, oxidative, 476
Phrenic nerve block, 327
  for pain management, 327
  pulmonary manifestations of neuraxial block and, 261
Phrenic nerves
  blockade of. *See* Phrenic nerve block
  diaphragm supplied by, 480
  injury to, 798
  liver supplied by, 709
Physical dependence, substance abuse and, 594
Physical examination
  intraoperative monitoring and, 118–119
  intravascular volume evaluation and, **627**, 627*t*
  preoperative patient evaluation and, 6*t*, 7
    in hypertension, 392–393
    in ischemic heart disease, 400
    in valvular heart disease, 406, 407*t*
Physical therapy, in pain management, 339
Physiologic dead space, 490. *See also* Dead space
Physiologic shunt, normal venous admixture and, 495
Physostigmine, 203*f*, 204*t*, **205**
  anticholinergic drug effects reversed by, 205, 209, 211
  for anticholinergic overdose/toxicity, 205, 211
  cerebral receptors affected by, 202, 205
  for delayed emergence, 938–939
  pediatric dosing and, 855*t*
Pi. *See* Interstitial hydrostatic pressure
Pia mater, spinal, 255, 258*f*
Pickwickian syndrome (obesity-hypoventilation syndrome), 748
PIH. *See* Pregnancy-induced hypertension
Pin index safety system, for medical gas delivery, 1, 19, 19*f*
Pindolol, 399*t*
Pinocytosis, placental exchange by, 808
PiO₂ (inspired tension of oxygen), 496–497
Pipecuronium, 184*f*, 188*t*, **196**
  in ischemic heart disease patients, 405
  renal excretion of, 188, 188*t*, 196
    altered renal function and, 683
Pipelines, for medical gas delivery, 18*f*, **19**, 20*f*
  alarm systems for, 19, 19*f*
  testing/certification of, 25–26
Pirbuterol, for asthma, 514*t*
Piriformis syndrome, 351*t*
Pitocin. *See* Oxytocin
Pituitary adenoma, 582
  thyroid-stimulating hormone-secreting, 741
Pituitary hormones, 581
Pituitary tumor resection, 581–582
pKₐ, 233, 234
  of local anesthetic, onset of action and, 233, 234–235
Placenta
  anatomy of, 808, 810*f*
  function of, 808, 814
  respiratory gas exchange across, 809–810
  retained, postpartum hemorrhage and, 839–840
  separation of, 835
Placenta accreta, 835
Placenta increta, 835
Placenta precreta, 835
Placenta previa, 835
Plasma, 599–600, 599*t*
  fresh frozen, transfusion of, 635
Plasma osmolality
  control of, **604**
  disorders of
    hyperosmolality/hypernatremia, **604–606**, 604*t*, 606*f*

hypo-osmolality/hyponatremia, **606–609**, 607*t*, 609*f*
  normal, 602
  plasma sodium concentration and, 503*t*, **602–604**
  potassium concentration affected by, 612–613
  in pregnancy, 807
Plasma protein-binding
  drug distribution affected by, 151, 153
  in geriatric patient, 879
  local anesthetic duration of action and, 235
Plasma protein fraction, in fluid management, 630
Plasma proteins, hepatic formation of, 712
Plasma thromboplastin antecedents, 718*t*
Plasma volume, pregnancy affecting, 805*t*, 806
Plasmalyte, for fluid management, 629*t*
Plasmapheresis, for myasthenia gravis, 753
Plasmin, 720
Plasminogen, 720
Plateau pressure, 40, 47, 47*t*
  graphic display of on anesthesia machine, 46*f*, 47
Platelet-activating factor
  in anaphylaxis, 904–905
  in immediate hypersensitivity reactions, 903
Platelet aggregation
  cyclooxygenase (COX) inhibitors affecting, 341, 342, 786
  lidocaine affecting, 240
  nitroglycerine affecting, 228
Platelet count, 721
  in pregnancy-induced hypertension, regional anesthesia for labor and delivery and, 838
Platelet transfusion, after cardiopulmonary bypass, 458
Plateletpheresis, 635
Platelets
  cardiopulmonary bypass affecting, 439
    persistent bleeding and, 458
  in coagulation, 718, 721
  evaluation of, 721
  pregnancy affecting, 805*t*, 807
  transfusion of, 635–636
    blood preparation for, 635
Plethysmography, for arterial blood pressure monitoring, 90
Pleural effusion, 520
Pneumatic anti-shock garment, 935
Pneumatic tourniquet, for knee arthroscopy, 782, 787–788
Pneumatochograph, for anesthesia machine, 44
Pneumocephalus, posterior fossa craniotomy and, 574
Pneumocytes, types I and II, 478
Pneumonectomy, 535
  operative criteria for, 535–536, 535*t*
  sleeve, 535
Pneumonia, 518–519
  aspiration. *See* Aspiration, pulmonary
  nosocomial, 981
    in ARDS, 973
  postoperative, risk factors for, 512
Pneumonitis, necrotizing, lung resection for, 536
Pneumopericardium, PEEP/CPAP and, 969
Pneumoperitoneum
  for laparoscopy, 522
  PEEP/CPAP and, 969
Pneumoretroperitoneum, PEEP/CPAP and, 969
Pneumotaxic center, 506–507
Pneumothorax, 520
  hypotension in postanesthesia care unit and, 936, 946
  hypoxemia in postanesthesia care unit and, 936, 945
  nitrous oxide contraindicated in, 139
  open, physiologic effects of thoracic surgery and, 527–528, 528*f*, 529*f*
  PEEP/CPAP and, 969
  tension, 798, 935
  thoracic paravertebral nerve block and, 329
  during thyroid surgery, 742
  traumatic, 798
PO₂ (partial pressure of oxygen), **496–499**, 498*t*, 499*f*
  in acid-base disorder diagnosis, **660**
Poisoning, 990–992
Polarographic cell (Clark electrode), for oxygen concentration monitoring, 55, 55*t*, 113
Polycitrate. *See* Sodium citrate
Polycythemia, neuromuscular blocking agent response affected in, 190*t*
Polymyositis, neuromuscular blocking agent response affected in, 190*t*
Polyneuropathies
  acute demyelinating (Guillain-Barré syndrome), **588**
    neuromuscular blocking agent response affected in, 190*t*
  electromyography and nerve conduction studies in evaluation of, 322

Polypectomy, 774–776, 775*f*
Polystyrene sulfonate, sodium, for hyperkalemia, 618
Polyuria, in head trauma, 577–578
Polyuric renal failure, methoxyflurane anesthesia and, 141, 662, 672
Pontine respiratory centers, 506–507
Pontocaine. *See* Tetracaine
Popliteal block, 302–304, 303*f*
Pop-off (pressure-relief/adjustable pressure-limiting) valve, 15
  in circle system, 35, 36*f*
  in Mapleson circuits, 30*t*, 31, 31*f*, 33*f*
  ventilator use and, 40, 53
Porphyria/porphyrin, barbiturate enzyme induction and, 159
Portal hypertension, in cirrhosis, 726, 727
Portal tracts, 709
Portal vein (porta hepatis), 708–709, 709*f*, 710, 710*f*
Portosystemic shunts, 727
  percutaneous transjugular intrahepatic (TIPS), 727
Positioning, patient. *See* Patient positioning
Positive airway pressure therapy, **968–970**. *See also* Continuous positive airway pressure (CPAP); Positive end-expiratory pressure (PEEP)
Positive end-expiratory pressure (PEEP), 968
  adverse nonpulmonary effects of, 969–970
  CPAP compared with, 968, 968*f*
  hepatic blood flow affected by, 716
  intrinsic, inverse I:E ratio ventilation and, 964
  optimum use of, 970
  "physiologic," 966
  pulmonary effects of, 969, 969*f*
  in testicular cancer surgery, 703
Positive pressure ventilation, 960, **960–965**. *See also specific type*
  classification of ventilators for, 960–961
  controlled hypotension and, 231
  cycling characteristics and, 961
  hepatic blood flow affected by, 716
  high-frequency (HFPPV), 965
    as one-lung ventilation alternative, 539
  inspiratory characteristics and, 960–961
  for laryngospasm, 78, 80
  microprocessor-controlled, 961
  modes for, 961–965, 962*t*, 963*t*
  for neonate, 844
  physiologic effects of lateral decubitus position and, 527
Postanesthesia care, **936–950**
  agitation and, 940
  airway obstruction and, 942–943
  arrhythmias and, 947
  circulatory complications and, **946–947**
  discharge criteria and, 941, 944*t*
  documentation of, 10
  emergence from anesthesia and, **938–939**, **943**
  fever and tachycardia and, 947–950, 948*t*
  after general anesthesia, 939
  hypertension and, 946–947
  hypotension and, 946
  hypoventilation and, 943–945
  hypoxemia and, 945–946
  nausea and vomiting and, 940
  pain control and, 940
  after regional anesthesia, 939
  respiratory complications and, **942–946**
  routine recovery and, **939–941**
  shivering and hypothermia and, 940–941
  suctioning and, 942–943
  transport from operating room to, **939**
Postanesthesia care unit (recovery room), **937–938**
  design of, 937
  discharge from, 941, 944*t*
  documentation of care in, 10
  equipment for, 937–938
  respiratory failure in, 205–206
  staffing of, 938
Post-dural puncture headache (PDPH), 275, 281, 826
  in outpatients, 885
Posterior descending artery, 376, 377*f*
Posterior fossa, craniotomy for lesion in, 567, **573–575**, 574*f*
Posterior spinal artery, 257, 259*f*
Posterior tibial artery catheterization, for arterial blood pressure monitoring, 93
Posterior tibial nerve
  blockade of (ankle block), 303, 304*f*
  entrapment of, 351*t*

Postganglionic blockers
  adverse effects of, 392*t*
  for hypertension, 391*t*
Postherpetic neuralgia (PHN), 356
Postintubation croup, 78, 850, 863, 886
Postnecrotic cirrhosis, 726
Postoperative bleeding/hemorrhage
  liver disease and, 717–722, 718*t*, 719*f*, 721*t*
  after nasal or sinus surgery, 779–780
  persistent, after cardiopulmonary bypass, 434, 458
  after thoracotomy, 525, 539
Postoperative note, 10, 12*f*
Postoperative pain. *See also specific type of surgery*
  management of, **340–348**, 356–358
    for inpatients, **343–348**
    for outpatients, **341–343**
Postpartum hemorrhage, **839–840**
Postpartum sterilization (tubal ligation/fulguration),
  816–818
Postrenal azotemia, 683, **977**, 977*t*. *See also* Renal failure
Post-retrobulbar apnea syndrome, 761, 766
Poststimulus latency, of evoked potential, 116
Postsynaptic adrenoceptors
  α₁, 214
  β₁, 215
  β₂, 215
Posttetanic potentiation, 182
Postural hypotension
  patient positioning and, 896
  trimethaphan causing, 229
Potassium
  balance of
    disorders of, **612–618**. *See also* Hyperkalemia;
    Hypokalemia
    normal, **612**
  in body fluid/fluid compartments, 599*t*, 631*t*
  in cardioplegia solutions, 438, 438*t*
  in crystalloid solutions, 629*t*
  for hypokalemia, 597, 615
  intake of
    decreased, hypokalemia caused by, 614
    increased, hyperkalemia caused by, 616–617
  intercompartmental shifts of, **612–613**
    hyperkalemia caused by, 615–617
    hypokalemia caused by, 613
  losses of, hypokalemia caused by, 613–614
  plasma concentration of, 612
    massive transfusion affecting, 639
  regulation of extracellular concentration of, **612**
  renal/urinary excretion of, 612, 613
    decreased, in hyperkalemia, 616
Potassium cardioplegia, 438–439, 438*t*, 452–453
  pump for delivery of, 437
Potassium channels
  adenosine affecting, 230
  myocardial, 361, 363*t*
    anesthetic-induced coronary vasodilation and, 378,
    379
Potassium chloride, for hypokalemia, 597, 615
Potassium-sparing diuretics, **675–676**
  adverse effects of, 392*t*, 676
  for hypertension, 390*t*, 676
  noncompetitive, **676**
Potency, drug, dose-response curve demonstrating, 155,
  156*f*
Prazosin, receptor selectivity of, 220*t*
Preanhepatic phase, of liver transplant, 733
Precordial stethoscope, for intraoperative monitoring, **108**,
  109*f*
  in pediatric patient, 857
Precurarization, for prevention of fasciculations, 189, 196
Prednisolone, for pain management, 338*t*
Prednisone, for pain management, 338*t*
Preeclampsia, **837–839**, 838*t*
Preemptive analgesia, **319**
Preexcitation, 381
  anesthetic agents for patients with, 383–384
  clinical significance of, 382
  P–R interval shortened by, 381–382
Pregnancy. *See also* Labor and delivery; Obstetric anesthesia
  "anaphylactoid syndrome of" (amniotic fluid embolism),
  839
  anesthesia sensitivity and, 804, 805
  appendicitis/appendectomy during, 846–847
  complicated, anesthesia and, **833–840**
  elective surgery and, 847
  ephedrine use during, 218
  hypertension during, **837–839**, 838*t*

  level of blockade after spinal anesthesia and, 268
  minimum alveolar concentration affected by, 136*t*
  neostigmine use in, atropine administration and, 204
  nitrous oxide use and, 139
  physiology of, **804–818**
    changes associated with, **805–808**, 805*t*
    uteroplacental circulation and, **808–811**, 809*f*, 810*f*
  surgery during, 846–847
Pregnancy-induced hypertension, **837–839**, 838*t*
Preload, 368–369, 369*f*, 369*t*, 370*f*
  antianginal agents affecting, 397*t*
  decreased, cardiac arrest during spinal anesthesia and,
  277
  hypotensive agents affecting, 226*t*
  increased, in heart failure, 380
  nitroglycerine affecting, 226*t*, 228
  nitroprusside affecting, 226*t*, 227
  stroke volume affected by, 368–369, 369*f*, 369*t*, 370*f*
Preload-dependence, of transplanted heart, 427
Premature labor, **836–837**
  prevention of, 837
    β₂-agonists for, 813, 837
    magnesium for, 813
Premature rupture of membranes (PROM), **836**
Prematurity, **864**
  retinopathy of, 850, 864
    oxygen toxicity and, 951, 959
Premedication, 175–176
  airway obstruction and, 551
  anesthesia recovery time affected by, 198
  in asthma patients, 514
  atropine as, 209
  for cardiac surgery
    in adults, 440
    in children, 460
  for craniotomy, 569
  for electroconvulsive therapy, 595–596
  for endoscopy, 772
  glycopyrrolate as, 210
  for hip fracture repair, 880
  in hypertensive patients, 393
  in ischemic heart disease patients, 402, 440
  for liver transplant, 733
  for lung resection, 536–537
  for open eye surgery in full stomach patient, 769
  for ophthalmic surgery, **765**
  for outpatient procedures, **884**
  in pediatric patient, 857
  peripheral nerve block and, 285
  in renal failure patients, 686–687
  scopolamine as, 210
  superior vena cava syndrome and, 551
  in valvular heart disease patients, **407–408**, 408–409*t*,
  440
Preoperative fasting. *See also* Full-stomach patient
  in pediatric patient, 857
  for cardiac surgery, 460
Preoperative history, 6–7, 6*t*
  in asthma, 514
  in hypertension, 392, 392*t*
  in ischemic heart disease, 400
  in valvular heart disease, 406, 406*t*
Preoperative medication. *See* Premedication
Preoperative note, 8–10, 9*f*
Preoperative patient evaluation, 1, **5–8**, 6*t*, 7*t*, 8*t*
  difficult airway and, 80–81, 81*t*, 82
  documenting, 901
  fluid deficit evaluation and, **631**
  hypertension and, **390–393**
  ischemic heart disease and, **399–402**, 401*t*
  for outpatient procedures, **883–884**
  for pediatric patient, 856
Preoperative risk factors, cardiac, 388
Preoxygenation, for intubation, 71–72
  in COPD patients, 518
  in pregnant patient, 806
Prerenal azotemia, 683, **976–977**, 977*t*. *See also* Renal
  failure
Pressure-broadening effect, end-tidal carbon dioxide
  analysis and, 111
Pressure control ventilation (PCV), 951, 962*t*, 964
Pressure-control/inverse ratio ventilation (PC-IRV), 946,
  962*t*, 964*f*
Pressure-cycled ventilators, 961
Pressure gauges
  Bourdon, 42, 43*f*
  breathing-circuit, for anesthesia machine, 41, **44–47**,
  46*f*, 47*t*

Pressure natriuresis, in volume control, 610
Pressure regulators, on anesthesia machine, 41, **42**, 43*f*
Pressure-relief (pop-off/adjustable pressure-limiting) valve,
  15
  in circle system, 35, 36*f*
  in Mapleson circuits, 30*t*, 31, 31*f*, 33*f*
  ventilator use and, 40, 53
Pressure support ventilation (PSV), 951, 962–964, 962*t*,
  963*f*, 964*f*
  weaning from ventilator with, 957
Pressure transducers, for intra-arterial monitoring, 93,
  94–95, 97*f*, 98*f*, 99*f*. *See also* Catheter-tubing-
  transducer system
  calibrating, 94–95
Presynaptic adrenoceptors, α₂, 215
Preterm labor, **836–837**
  prevention of, 837
    β₂-agonists for, 813, 837
    magnesium for, 813
Prilocaine, 237*t*
  for epidural anesthesia, 272*t*
  metabolites of, 238
Priming dose
  anesthesia uptake in closed-circuit and, 148
  of nondepolarizing neuromuscular blocking agent, for
  intubation, 188
Principal cells (P cells), 668
Prinzmetal's angina, 396. *See also* Angina
PRL. *See* Prolactin
Proaccelerin, 718*t*
Procainamide
  in cardiopulmonary resuscitation, 927*t*
  pediatric dosing and, 855*t*
  for ventricular tachycardia in acute myocardial
  infarction, 976
Procaine, 237*t*
  for differential neuraxial blockade, 335*t*
  history of use of, 284
  neurologic effects of, 239
  specific gravity of, 267*t*
  for spinal anesthesia, 268, 268*t*
  systemic administration of, for pain management, 339
Proconvertin, 718*t*
Prolactin (PRL), 581
Prolixin. *See* Fluphenazine
PROM. *See* Premature rupture of membranes
Promethazine, 243*t*
  altered renal function and, 682
  for labor and delivery, 821
Promit. *See* Dextran
Pronator syndrome, 351*t*
Prone position
  complications associated with, 898*t*, 899*t*
  for neuraxial anesthesia, 264
    level of blockade after spinal anesthesia and, 267
  for spinal surgery, 580, 782, 789
Propafenone, in cardiopulmonary resuscitation, 929*t*
Propofol, 152, 170*f*, **173–174**
  altered renal function and, 682
  cerebral effects of, 171*t*, 174, 558*t*, 560
  for cerebral protection, 562
  for electroconvulsive therapy, 595
  electroencephalogram affected by, 563*t*, 564
  evoked potentials affected by, 563*t*
  for induction, history of use of, 3
  for infusion anesthesia, 162
  for monitored anesthesia care, 887
  for neuronavigation, 571
  organ system effects of, 171*t*, 174
  for outpatient procedures, 884
  in pediatric anesthesia, 855
  pediatric dosing and, 855*t*
  placental transfer of, 811
  postoperative nausea and vomiting prevention and, 940
  uses and doses of, 169*t*
  uteroplacental blood flow affected by, 811
Propoxyphene, for postoperative pain management, 341*t*
Propranolol, 221*t*, **222**, 394*t*, 399*t*
  pediatric dosing and, 855*t*
  receptor selectivity of, 220*t*, 221*t*, 222, 399*t*
  for thyroid storm, 950
Propylthiouracil, for thyroid storm, 949–950
Prostacyclin, 718
  in pregnancy-induced hypertension, 837
Prostaglandin E₁
  after cardiopulmonary bypass
    in adults, 457
    in children, 462

Prostaglandin E₁ (cont.)

Prostaglandin E$_1$ (cont.)
  pediatric dosing and, 855t
  for tetralogy of Fallot, 425
  for transposition of great arteries, 426
Prostaglandin I$_2$ (prostacyclin), 718
Prostaglandins
  blockade of synthesis of, in pain management, 341
  in central pain modulation, 318
  in immediate hypersensitivity reactions, 903
  in primary hyperalgesia, 317–318, 317f
Prostate gland
  cancer of, **699–701**
  transurethral resection of (TURP), **694–697**, 695t
    choice of anesthetic agent for, 696–697
    hypotension after, 705–707
Prostatectomy
  radical perineal, 701
  radical retropubic, 700–701
Protamine, for heparin reversal after cardiopulmonary
    bypass, 434, 457–458
Protein
  dietary
    nutritional support in renal failure and, 979, 989–990
    requirements for in critical illness, 988
  in fluid compartments, 599t
  metabolism of
    in liver, 711f, 712
    pregnancy affecting, 807
Protein binding
  barbiturate excretion affected by, 158
  drug distribution affected by, 151, 153
  local anesthetic duration of action and, 235
Protein C, 720
Protein S, 720
Proteinuria, 681
  in pregnancy, 807
Prothrombin, 718t
Prothrombin time, 708, 720, 721t
  in liver disease, 714t, 715
Proton pump inhibitors, **246**
Protopathic sensation, 310
Protriptyline, for depression, 591
Proximal renal tubule, 663t, 664–666, 664f, 665f, 666f
Prozac. See Fluoxetine
Prune-belly syndrome, 866
Pruritus, propofol affecting, 174
P$_a$CO$_2$. See also PaCO$_2$
  intraoperative monitoring of, 113
Pseudoaneurysm, aortic, 467
Pseudocholinesterase, 182, 183
  abnormal, 183
  anesthesia recovery time and, 197–198
  drugs affecting, 185t
  ester local anesthetics metabolized by, 238
  hepatic production of, 712
  in mivacurium metabolism, 193–194
  serum levels of, pregnancy affecting, 807
  in succinylcholine metabolism, 183
Pseudoclaudication, in spinal stenosis, 354
Pseudohyponatremia, 607
P$_a$O$_2$. See also PaO$_2$
  intraoperative monitoring of, 113
PSV. See Pressure support ventilation
Psychiatric disease, **590–594**
Psychological considerations in pain, 320, 320t, 322
  interventions and, **339**
  patient evaluation and, 322
Psychological dependence, substance abuse and, 594
Psychological techniques for pain control, for labor and
    delivery, **820–821**
PT. See Prothrombin time
P$_{tc}$CO$_2$ (P$_s$CO$_2$). See also PaCO$_2$
  intraoperative monitoring of, 113
P$_{tc}$O$_2$ (P$_s$O$_2$). See also PaO$_2$
  intraoperative monitoring of, 113
PTH. See Parathyroid hormone
Pudendal nerve block
  for labor and delivery, **822**
  in pain management, 331, 331f
Pulmonary artery catheterization, **102–106**
  in aortic stenosis, 417
  for cardiac surgery, 433
    in adults, 461
    in children, 461
  clinical considerations and, 105–106, 106t
  contraindications to, 86, 103
  documentation of, 902
  indications for, 102, 103t

intraoperative temperature monitoring and, 119
  for lung resection, 537
  for lung transplant, 547
  in pediatric patient, 858
  techniques and complications of, 103–105, 103f, 104f,
    105
Pulmonary artery occlusion pressure (PAOP), 104, 104f,
    105–106, 106t
  in ARDS, 972–973
  in hypovolemia evaluation, 628
  in pulmonary edema, 972
Pulmonary artery pressure
  monitoring
    during bilateral hip arthroplasties, 782, 786
    during cardiac surgery, 441
    hypovolemia evaluation and, 628
    nitroprusside affecting, 227
    in tricuspid regurgitation, 421
Pulmonary artery rupture, pulmonary artery catheterization
    and, 104, 105
Pulmonary aspiration. See Aspiration, pulmonary
Pulmonary barotrauma
  mechanical ventilation and, 960
  PEEP/CPAP and, 951, 969
Pulmonary bullae, lung resection and, 525, 541
Pulmonary capillaries, 479–480
Pulmonary capillary wedge pressure, monitoring
  in aortic stenosis, 417
  in mitral regurgitation, 414, 415f
  in mitral stenosis, 411
Pulmonary carcinoids, 534
Pulmonary circulation/blood flow, **478–480**
  shunts in congenital heart disease affecting,
    422–424
Pulmonary compensation, in acid-base balance, **648**
Pulmonary contusion, 798–799
Pulmonary cysts, lung resection and, 525, 541
Pulmonary disease, **511–524**. See also specific disorder and
    Respiratory physiology; Thoracic surgery
  obstructive disease and, **512–518**
  restrictive disease and, **518–520**
  risk factors and, 512, 512t
Pulmonary dysfunction, postoperative, risk factors for, 512,
    512t
Pulmonary edema, **971–973**
  hemodynamic, **972**
  hypoxemia in postanesthesia care unit and, 945
  noncardiogenic, blood transfusion causing, 637
  pathophysiology of, 971
  permeability (ALI/ARDS), 972–973. See also Acute lung
    injury (ALI); Acute respiratory distress
    syndrome (ARDS)
  postoperative laryngospasm and, 942–943
  renal failure and, 679, 685
Pulmonary embolectomy, 521
Pulmonary embolism, 511, **520–522**, 520t
  anesthesia for patient with, 521–522
  intraoperative, 521–522
Pulmonary end-capillary oxygen tension, 498
Pulmonary function. See Respiratory physiology
Pulmonary function tests, pneumonectomy criteria and,
    535–536, 535t
Pulmonary gas exchange
  across placenta, 809–810
  across respiratory epithelium, 477
  anesthesia affecting, **495–496**
  cirrhosis affecting, 728
  in respiratory failure, 970, 971f
Pulmonary hemorrhage, massive, lung resection and, 541
Pulmonary hypertension, in septic shock, 982
Pulmonary hypoplasia, congenital diaphragmatic hernia
    and, 864–865
Pulmonary infarction, in pulmonary embolism, 520
Pulmonary infections, lung resection for, **536**
Pulmonary innervation, **480**
Pulmonary lymphatics, 480
Pulmonary mechanics, **482–490**
  airway resistance and, 485–488, 486t, 487f, 488f, 489f
    anesthesia affecting, 490
  anesthesia affecting, 489–490, 492f
  compliance and, 482–483, 483f
    anesthesia affecting, 489–490, 492f
  elastic resistance and, 483f
  lung volumes and, 483–485, 484f, 484t, 485f, 486f
    anesthesia affecting, 489–490, 492f
  nonelastic resistance and, 485–488, 486t, 487f, 488f,
    489f
  surface tension forces and, 482

tissue resistance and, 488
  work of breathing and, **488–489**, 490f, 491f
    anesthesia affecting, 490
Pulmonary perfusion, **492–494**, 494f, 495f
  distribution of, 493, 494f
Pulmonary physiology. See Respiratory physiology
Pulmonary resection. See Lung resection
Pulmonary toxicity, oxygen therapy and, **959**
Pulmonary tumors, lung resection for, **534–536**, 535t
Pulmonary valve regurgitation, heart murmur in,
    preoperative evaluation of, 407t
Pulmonary valve stenosis, 423
  heart murmur in, preoperative evaluation of, 407t
Pulmonary vascular resistance
  in left-to-right shunts, 424, 434
  in mitral stenosis, 410
  pulmonary artery catheterization monitoring of, 106t
Pulmonary vasoconstriction, hypoxic, 475, 493
  one-lung ventilation and, 528
Pulmonary ventilation, **490–492**. See also Ventilation
  distribution of, 491, 493f
  time constants and, 491–492
Pulmonic stenosis, 423
  heart murmur in, preoperative evaluation of, 407t
Pulsatile flow, for cardiopulmonary bypass, 436
Pulse oximetry
  for intraoperative monitoring, **108–110**, 110f
    during ophthalmic surgery, 765
    in pediatric patient, 857
    in postanesthesia care, 937
Pulse pressure, 87
  in hypovolemia evaluation, 627t
Pulse rate. See Heart rate
Pulsed Doppler, for intraoperative monitoring, 107
Pulseless electrical activity, algorithm for management of,
    931f
Pulsus paradoxus, in cardiac tamponade, 799
Pump failure, after cardiopulmonary bypass, 455–456,
    455t
Pumps, for cardiopulmonary bypass machine
  accessory, 435f, 437
  main, 435f, 436
Pupillary dilatation, anticholinergic drugs causing,
    209
Pure autonomic failure, 589
Pure ventilatory failure, 970
Purkinje fibers, 362f, 363
Purpura, posttransfusion, 637
P$\bar{v}$CO$_2$. See Mixed venous carbon dioxide tension
P$\bar{v}$O$_2$. See Mixed venous oxygen tension
PVR. See Pulmonary vascular resistance
Pyloric stenosis, hypertrophic, **866–867**
Pyrexia. See also Fever
  cerebral blood flow affected by, 554
Pyridostigmine, 203f, **204**, 204t
  altered renal function and, 683
  mechanism of action of, 200–202
  for myasthenia gravis, 753
  pseudocholinesterase affected by, 185

Qs. See Venous admixture
Quadrate lobe of liver, 708
Quincke needle, 266, 266f
Quinethazone, 675. See also Thiazide diuretics

Rabeprazole, 246
Radial artery cannulation, for arterial blood pressure
    monitoring, 87f, 92, 93, 96f
Radial nerve block, 293–295, 294f, 295f
Radial nerve injury, patient positioning and, 899t
Radiation exposure, occupational, 889, **908–909**
Radical cystectomy, for bladder cancer, 701–702
Radical neck dissection, 771, 776–777
Radical nephrectomy, 703
  with excision of tumor thrombus, 704
Radical orchiectomy, for testicular cancer, 702
Radical perineal prostatectomy, 701
Radical retropubic prostatectomy, 700–701
Radiculopathy
  definition of, 311t
  epidural steroids for management of, 354
  lumbar disk, 353–354, 353t
Radiocontrast media, renal failure caused by, acetylcysteine
    in prevention of, 673
Radiofrequency ablation, in pain management, **336**
Radioiodine, for hyperthyroidism, 741

RAE tube
  nasal, for craniofacial reconstruction and orthognathic surgery, 777, 777f
  oral, for nasal and sinus surgery, 775, 775f
Raman spectroscopy, for intraoperative anesthetic gas analysis, 114
Ranitidine, 244, 244t, 245
  for aspiration pneumonia prophylaxis, 244t
    cesarean section and, 830
    labor and delivery and, 820
    open eye surgery in full stomach patient and, 769
    pediatric dosing and, 855t
Rapacuronium, 178, 179, 184f, 188t, **196–197**
  hepatic clearance of, 187–188, 197
  for intubation, 188, 197
  in ischemic heart disease patients, 405
  for open eye surgery in full stomach patient, 770
  in pediatric anesthesia, 856
  renal excretion of, 188, 188t, 197
  withdrawal of from market, 4, 178, 188, 197, 770
Rapid-sequence induction, 251–252
  in renal failure patients, 687
Rapid shallow breathing index (RSBI), 967
Rastelli procedure/repair
  for transposition of great arteries, 426
  for truncus arteriosus, 426
RBF (renal blood flow). See Renal circulation/blood flow
RCA. See Right coronary artery
Reboxetine, for depression, 592t
Rebreathing, 33t. See also Hypercapnia
  circle system and, 33–35, 33t, 34f, 34t, 35f
  equipment malfunction and, 38, 39f
  humidifiers and, 197
  Mapleson circuits and, 32, 33t
  partial, 146
  total, in closed-circuit anesthesia, 146–150
Recall under general anesthesia, 897–899
Receptor binding, 155–156
  dose-response curve demonstrating characteristics of, 155, 156f
Receptor down-regulation
  in heart failure, 380
  response to neuromuscular blocking agents and, 181
Receptor up-regulation
  propranolol causing, 222
  response to neuromuscular blocking agents and, 181
Receptor field expansion, in central pain modulation, 318
Receptor hyperreactivity, 155
Receptor hyporeactivity, 155
Recoil, elastic resistance and, 482
Recovery room. See Postanesthesia care unit
Rectal drug administration/absorption, 152–153
Rectal temperature, intraoperative monitoring of, 119
Recurrent laryngeal nerve, 60, 62f
  paralysis of, 60
    thyroidectomy and, 742
  speech/voice disorders caused by damage to, 60, 63t
Red blood cell scan, in lower gastrointestinal tract bleeding, 986
"Red man syndrome," vancomycin causing, 907
Redistribution, 153
  of esmolol, 221
  of nondepolarizing neuromuscular blocking agents, 178, 182
  of nonvolatile anesthetics, 151, 153
    barbiturates, 157, 158f
    ketamine, 169–171
    opioids, 165
Redistributive fluid loss, during surgery, 631–632
  fluid replacement for, 633, 633t
  testicular cancer surgery and, 703
REE. See Resting energy expenditure
Reentry
  paroxysmal supraventricular tachycardia (PSVT) caused by, 383
  tachyarrhythmias caused by, 382, 383f
Referred pain, 312, 312t
Reflex sympathetic dystrophy (CRPS type I), 350, 350t
Refractory period, in myocardial cells, 361
Regional (local) anesthesia/anesthetics, **233–241**. See also specific type of block
  absorption of, 235–238
  cardiovascular effects of, 233, 238–239, 363, 366
    indirect renal effects and, 672
  for carotid surgery, 471–472
  for cesarean section, 819, 828–829, **829–830**
  for COPD patients, 518
  for cystoscopy, 693–694

distribution of, 238
drug interactions and, 240
duration of action of, 235
for extracorporeal shock wave lithotripsy, 698
for full stomach patient, 251
in geriatric patient, 875, 879, 880–881
hematologic effects of, 240
for hip fracture repair, 784, 880–881
history of use of, 3
immunologic effects of, 240
infiltration of, for postoperative pain management, **342–343**
intravenous (Bier block), 283, 284
  of arm, **297–298**, 298f
  for pain management, 335
in ischemic heart disease patient, 404
for labor and delivery, **823–826**
  maternal heart disease and, 839
  with opioids, 819, **826–827**, 827t
  pregnancy-induced hypertension and, 838–839
  sensitivity/dose requirements and, 805
  uterine activity affected by, 813
mechanism of action of, theories of, **234**
metabolism and excretion of, 238
minimum alveolar concentration affected by, 136t
musculoskeletal effects of, 240
neuraxial (spinal/epidural/caudal) blocks, **253–282**
neurologic effects of, 239–240
neuromuscular blocking agent interactions and, 185t, 240
onset of action of, 234–235
for ophthalmic surgery, **766–768**, 767f, 768f
organ system effects of, 238–240
for outpatient procedures, **884–885**
overdose/toxicity of, 233, 238–240, 240–241, 278
in pain management, **323–336**, 342–343, 346–348, 347t
in pediatric patient, 862–863
peripheral nerve blocks, **283–308**
  for pain management, **323–336**, 346
pharmacokinetics of, **235–238**
physicochemical properties of, 236–237t
placental transfer of, 811
for postpartum tubal ligation, 817–818
potency of, 234
for pregnant patient requiring surgery, 847
respiratory effects of, 239
routine recovery from, 939
structure-activity relationships of, **234–235**, 236–237t
systemic administration of, for pain management, 339
systemic toxicity of, 278
uteroplacental blood flow affected by, 811
venous thromboembolism after hip surgery and, 787, 881
Regional oxygen saturation in brain (rSO$_2$), intraoperative oximetry for monitoring of, 110
Reglan. See Metoclopramide
Regurgitant fraction, calculation of
  in aortic regurgitation, 419
  in mitral regurgitation, 412–414
Regurgitant stroke volume, calculation of
  in aortic regurgitation, 419
  in mitral regurgitation, 412–414
  in tricuspid regurgitation, 421
Reheparinization (heparin rebound), after cardiopulmonary bypass, 458
Rehydration and diuresis, for hypercalcemia, 597, 619
Reimplantation (limb) surgery, 782, 789–790, 800–801
Relative humidity, 54
Relative intrapulmonary shunt, 494
Relaxation techniques, for pain management, 339
Relaxin, pregnancy affecting levels of, 808
Release hypotension, 468
Remeron. See Mirtazapine
Remifentanil, 166f. See also Opioids
  biotransformation of, 165, 167f
  cardiovascular effects of, 167, 171t
  context-sensitive half time of, 165, 167f
  distribution of, 167f
  history of use of, 4
  for infusion anesthesia, 162
  organ system effects of, 171t
  for outpatient procedures, 884
  stress response affected by, 169
  uses and doses of, 168t
Renal artery, 669, 670f
  stenosis of, hypertension caused by (renovascular hypertension), 689–691

Renal azotemia, 683, 977, 977t. See also Renal failure
Renal calculi
  extracorporeal shock wave lithotripsy for, 697–699, 697f
  open procedures for, 699
Renal cancer, **703–704**
Renal cell carcinoma, 703–704
Renal circulation/blood flow, 662, **669–671**, 670f
  adrenergic agonists affecting, 217t
  barbiturates affecting, 159
  control of, 662, 670–671
  distribution of, 671
  dopamine affecting, 217t, 219
  enflurane affecting, 138t, 142, 672
  epinephrine affecting, 217t, 218
  fenoldopam affecting, 217t, 220, 231
  in geriatric patient, 877t, 878
  glomerular filtration and, **669–671**
  halothane affecting, 138t, 140, 672
  hydralazine affecting, 229
  inhalational anesthetics affecting, 138t, 672
  isoflurane affecting, 138t, 143, 672
  measurement of, 669
  methoxyflurane affecting, 138t, 141
  neuraxial anesthesia affecting, 261
  nitrous oxide affecting, 138, 138t
  norepinephrine affecting, 217t, 219
  PEEP/CPAP affecting, 969
  pregnancy affecting, 807
  sevoflurane affecting, 138t, 145
Renal clearance, 154, 669. See also Renal failure; Renal physiology
  of cholinesterase inhibitors, 202
  in geriatric patient, 875, 878
  of nondepolarizing neuromuscular blocking agents, 188
  of pancuronium, 188t, 194
  of vecuronium, 188t, 195
Renal compensation, in acid-base balance, 644, **648–650**, 649f, 650f, 651f
Renal disease, **679–691**. See also specific disorder and Renal failure; Renal function; Renal physiology
  in diabetics, 739
Renal failure, **683–688**, 976–979
  acute, 683, 951, **976–979**
  anesthesia in patient with, 687–688
  anesthesia recovery time and, 197
  cardiovascular abnormalities and, 684t, 685
  causes of, 978, 978t
  chronic, 683–685, 684t
  descending aorta surgery and, 469
  in diabetics, 739
  drug therapy adjustments/contraindications and, 686, 687t
  endocrine abnormalities and, 684t, 685–686
  fluid therapy and, 688
  gastrointestinal abnormalities and, 684t, 686
  hematologic abnormalities and, 684t, 685
  intraoperative considerations in patient with, **687–688**
  manifestations of, 685–686
  mannitol prophylaxis and, 674
  metabolic abnormalities and, 684t, 685
  methoxyflurane anesthesia and, 141, 662, 672
  morphine duration of action affected by, 165
  need for dialysis and, 686, 686t
  neurologic abnormalities and, 684t, 686
  nondepolarizing neuromuscular blocking agent excretion affected by, 178, 188, 189
  nonoliguric, 683, 979
  nutritional support in, 979, 989–990
  oliguric, 683, 979
    conversion of to nonoliguric
      loop diuretics for, 675, 979
      mannitol for, 674, 979
  opioid use and, 345
  pathogenesis of, 978
  pharmacokinetics affected by, 154
  premedication and, 686–687
  preoperative considerations in patient with, **683–687**, 686t, 687t
  preoperative evaluation of patient with, 686, 686t, 687t
  pulmonary abnormalities and, 684t, 685
  treatment of, 979
  vecuronium use in, 195
Renal failure index, 977t, 978
Renal function. See also Renal failure; Renal physiology
  age-related changes in, 877t, **878**
  altered
    anesthesia for patients with mild to moderate impairments and, **688–689**
    anesthetic effects and, **681–683**

Renal function (*cont.*)
anesthesia/surgery affecting, 662, **671–673**, 677–678
blood urea nitrogen:creatinine ratio in evaluation of, **680–681**
blood urea nitrogen in evaluation of, **680**
in cirrhosis, 727*t*, 728–729
creatinine clearance in evaluation of, 670, 679, 680, **681**
evaluation of, **679–681**, 680*t*
in geriatric patient, 875, 877*t*, **878**
hyperkalemia and, 616
hypokalemia and, 614–615, 614*t*
in pediatric patient, 851–852
preoperative evaluation of, in hypertension, 393
serum creatinine in evaluation of, **680**, 681*f*
urinalysis in evaluation of, **681**
Renal insufficiency (mild to moderate renal impairment), **688–689**
Renal medulla, hypertonicity of
collecting tubule in maintenance of, 668
urea and, 667, 668
Renal physiology, **662–678**
adenosine affecting, 230
age-related changes in, 877*t*, **878**
barbiturates affecting, 159, 673
cirrhosis affecting, 727*t*, 728–729
desflurane affecting, 138*t*, 144
enflurane affecting, 138*t*, 142, 672
fenoldopam affecting, 231
in geriatric patient, 875, 877*t*, **878**
halothane affecting, 138*t*, 140, 672
hydralazine affecting, 229
hyperparathyroidism affecting, 744*t*
inhalational anesthetics affecting, 138*t*
intravenous agents affecting, 673
isoflurane affecting, 138*t*, 143, 672
methoxyflurane affecting, 138*t*, 141, 662, 672
neuraxial anesthesia affecting, 261
nitroprusside affecting, 227
nitrous oxide affecting, 138, 138*t*
in pediatric patient, 851–852
pregnancy affecting, 805*t*, 807
sevoflurane affecting, 138*t*, 145, 672
solute reabsorption and, 664–666, 665*f*, 666*f*
surgery affecting, 662, **673**, 677–678
trimethaphan affecting, 229
Renal plasma flow, 669
Renal transplant, 692, **704–705**
Renal tubular acidosis, hyperchloremic metabolic acidosis and, 655
Renal tubules
collecting, 663*t*, 664*f*, 668, 668*f*
distal, 663*t*, 664*f*, 667–668
in potassium excretion, 613
proximal, 664–666, 664*f*, 665*f*, 666*f*
Rendell-Baker-Soucek pediatric face mask, 64*f*
Renin
in hyperaldosteronism, 746
release/secretion of
hydralazine affecting, 229
nitroprusside affecting, 227
propranolol affecting, 222
in renal blood flow regulation, 671
Renin-angiotensin-aldosterone system
in blood pressure control, 375–376
in volume regulation, 610
Renovascular hypertension, 689–691
Reperfusion, injury associated with, 439
Replacement-type crystalloid solutions, 628
Rescue breathing, 918*t*, **920–921**
Resectoscope, for transurethral resection of prostate, 695
Reserpine
for intravenous regional sympathetic blockade, 335
minimum alveolar concentration affected by, 136*t*
Reserve volume
expiratory (ERV), 484*f*, 484*t*
inspiratory (IRV), 484*f*, 484*t*
Reservoir
for cardiopulmonary bypass machine, 436
liver as, 710
lung as, 492
Reservoir masks, for oxygen therapy, 955*t*, 956
Reservoir valve assembly, in resuscitation breathing system, 37, 37*f*
Residual capacity, functional (FRC), 475, 483–484, 483*f*, 484*f*, 484*t*
anesthesia affecting, 475, 489–490
closing capacity and, 485, 485*f*, 486*f*
in geriatric patient, 875, 876–877

in pediatric patient, 849, 850
PEEP/CPAP affecting, 969
pregnancy affecting, 805*t*, 806
Residual volume (RV), 484*f*, 484*t*, 485*f*
in geriatric patient, 876
Resistance
to airflow, endotracheal tubes and, 67
in circle system, 36
vascular. *See* Vascular resistance
Respiration. *See also* Breathing; Respiratory physiology; Ventilation
anesthesia affecting, 482
at birth, 816
cellular, **476–477**
anesthesia affecting, **477**
muscles of, **477**
accessory, neuraxial anesthesia affecting, **477**
weakness of, in Duchenne's muscular dystrophy, 755
paradoxical, during thoracic surgery, 528, 529*f*
work of, **488–489**, 490*f*, 491*f*
anesthesia affecting, 490
Respiratory acidosis, 644, 646, 646*t*, **650–653**, 652*t*. *See also* Acidosis
definition of, 646, 646*t*
neuromuscular blocking agents affected by, 189
renal compensation during, 648, 649, 649*f*, 650*f*, 652
after thoracotomy, 539
treatment of, 652–653
Respiratory alkalosis, 644, 646, 646*t*, **656**, 657*t*. *See also* Alkalosis
definition of, 646, 646*t*
in mixed acid-base disorder, 660–661
in septic shock, 982
Respiratory anatomy, functional, **477–480**, 478*f*, 479*f*
Respiratory care/respiratory therapy, **953–970**. *See also* Mechanical ventilation; Oxygen therapy
medical gas therapy, **953–954**
Respiratory centers, central, 506–507
Respiratory disease, **511–524**. *See also specific disorder and* Respiratory physiology; Thoracic surgery
risk factors and, **512**, 512*t*
Respiratory distress/depression
after interscalene block, 308
laryngeal nerve damage causing, 60
in neonate, **844–846**, 844*f*, 845*f*
maternal anesthetics causing, 811
naloxone for, 846
opioids, 811, 821
meconium-staining and, 843
opioids causing, 167, 168*f*, 171*t*, 310, 344, 347–348, 356
intraspinal, 347–348
in postanesthesia care unit, 205–206, **942–946**
Respiratory epithelium, 478, 479*f*
gas exchange across, 477
Respiratory failure, **970–975**, 971*f*
drowning/near drowning and, **973–974**
hypoxic, 970
initial ventilator settings and, 966
pulmonary edema and, **971–973**
pure ventilatory, 970
in recovery room, 205–206
smoke inhalation and, **974–975**
treatment of, **970–971**
Respiratory gas exchange
across placenta, 809–810
across respiratory epithelium, 477
anesthesia affecting, **495–496**
cirrhosis affecting, 728
in respiratory failure, 970, 971*f*
Respiratory gas tensions, **496–501**
in acid-base disorder diagnosis, 658–659, 658*f*, **659**, 659*t*
cerebral blood flow affected by, 554, 554*f*
Respiratory muscles, **477**
accessory, neuraxial anesthesia affecting, 261
weakness of
in Duchenne's muscular dystrophy, 755
muscle biopsy and, 759
Respiratory physiology, **475–510**. *See also under Pulmonary and* Breathing; Respiration
adenosine affecting, 230
age-related changes in, **876–878**, 877*t*, 878*f*
anatomic considerations and, **477–480**, 478*f*, 479*f*
anticholinergic drugs affecting, 207, 208*t*, 209
barbiturates affecting, 158, 171*t*
benzodiazepines affecting, 151, 161–164, 171*t*
breathing control and, **505–508**

breathing mechanisms and, **480–482**
burn injuries affecting, 801–802, 974–975
cellular respiration and, **476–477**
cholinesterase inhibitors affecting, 202, 202*t*
cirrhosis affecting, 727*t*, 728
desflurane affecting, 138*t*, 139–140, 144
doxapram affecting, 248–249
droperidol affecting, 171*t*, 175
enflurane affecting, 138*t*, 142
etomidate affecting, 171*t*, 172
gas tensions (alveolar/arterial/venous) and, **496–501**
cerebral blood flow affected by, 554, 554*f*
gas transport and, **501–505**
in geriatric patient, **876–878**, 877*t*, 878*f*
histamine affecting, 243
inhalational anesthetics affecting, 138*t*
intraocular pressure affected by, 762, 762*t*
intraoperative monitoring of, **108–114**, 125
anesthetic gas analysis, **113–114**
end-tidal carbon dioxide analysis, **110–112**
esophageal stethoscope for, **108**
precordial stethoscope for, **108**
pulse oximetry, **108–110**
transcutaneous oxygen and carbon dioxide, **112–113**
isoflurane affecting, 138*t*, 143
ketamine affecting, 171*t*, 172
laparoscopy affecting, 522
local anesthetics affecting, 239
lung volumes and, **483–485**, 484*f*, 484*t*, 485*f*, 486*f*
methoxyflurane affecting, 138*t*, 141
neuraxial anesthesia affecting, 261
nitroglycerine affecting, 228
nitroprusside affecting, 227
nitrous oxide affecting, 137, 138*t*
nonvolatile anesthetics affecting, 171*t*
opioids affecting, 167, 168*f*, 171*t*, 310, 347–348, 356
pain affecting, 320
patient positioning affecting, 898*t*
in pediatric patient, 816, 850–851
pregnancy affecting, 805–806, 805*t*
propofol affecting, 171*t*, 174
renal failure affecting, 685
rheumatoid arthritis affecting, 784*t*
thoracic surgery affecting, **526–528**
lateral decubitus position and, **526–527**, 526*f*, 527*f*
one-lung ventilation and, **528**
open pneumothorax and, **527–528**, 528*f*, 529*f*
ventilation mechanisms and, **482–490**
ventilation/perfusion relationships and, **490–496**
Respiratory quotient (RQ), 476–477
Respiratory rate
desflurane affecting, 138*t*, 144
enflurane affecting, 138*t*, 142
halothane affecting, 138*t*, 139–140
inhalational anesthetics affecting, 138*t*
isoflurane affecting, 138*t*, 143
methoxyflurane affecting, 138*t*, 141
nitrous oxide affecting, 137, 138*t*
in pediatric patient, 850, 851*t*
sevoflurane affecting, 138*t*, 145
Respiratory work, **488–489**, 490*f*, 491*f*
anesthesia affecting, 490
Respirometers/spirometers, for anesthesia machine, 41, **44–47**, 45*f*, 46*f*, 47*t*
Resting energy expenditure (REE), calculating, 988
Resting membrane potential
cardiac, 361
local anesthetic action and, 234
potassium affecting, 612
Resting potential, negative, local anesthetic action and, 234
Restlessness, in postanesthesia care unit, 936, 940
Restrictive pulmonary disease, 511, **518–520**
acute intrinsic, **518–519**
chronic intrinsic, **519–520**
extrinsic, **520**
Restrictive shunt, left-to-right, 424
Resuscitation. *See* Cardiopulmonary resuscitation; Fetal resuscitation; Neonatal resuscitation
Resuscitation breathing systems, **37**, 37*f*
Reteplase, for acute myocardial infarction, 976
Reticular activating system
barbiturates affecting, 156
etomidate affecting, 172
Reticular formation, in central pain inhibition, 319
Retinal ischemia, patient positioning and, 899*t*
Retinopathy of prematurity (retrolental fibroplasia), 850, 864
oxygen toxicity and, 951, 959

Retrobulbar blockade, for ophthalmic surgery, **766**, 767*f*, 887
 apnea after, 761, 766
Retrolental fibroplasia (retinopathy of prematurity), 850, 864
 oxygen toxicity and, 951, 959
Retroperitoneal lymph node dissection, in testicular cancer, 692, 702–703
Retropubic prostatectomy, radical, 700–701
Return electrode, for surgical diathermy unit, 23–24
Revascularization, after liver transplant, 733
 problems associated with, 734–735
Reverse steal (Robin Hood) phenomenon, 559
Reverse Trendelenburg position, complications associated with, 898*t*, 899*t*
Rewarming, after cardiopulmonary bypass, 454
Rexed's spinal cord laminae, 313, 314*f*, 315*t*
Reye's syndrome, aspirin use and, 342
Reynolds number, 486
RF. *See* Regurgitant fraction
Rh system
 for blood typing, 633
  testing before blood transfusion and, 633–634
 transfusion reactions caused by incompatibility of, 636–637
Rheomacrodex. *See* Dextran
Rheumatic fever
 aortic stenosis and, 416
 mitral regurgitation and, 412
 mitral stenosis and, 409, 410
Rheumatoid arthritis, 782, 784–785, 784*t*, 785*f*
Rhinoplasty, 774–776, 775*f*
Rhizotomy, medial branch, for facet joint disease, 355
Rib cage, anatomy of, **477**
Rib fractures, in flail chest, 798
Right-angle endotracheal tube
 for craniofacial reconstruction and orthognathic surgery, 777, 777*f*
 for nasal and sinus surgery, 775, 775*f*
Right bundle branch block, significance of, 429
Right coronary artery, 376, 377*f*
Right internal jugular vein, for central venous pressure monitoring, 100, 100*t*, 101*f*
Right-to-left (complex) shunts, in congenital heart disease, 422, 422*t*, **425–427**. *See also causative lesion*
Right ventricular assist device, for pump failure after cardiopulmonary bypass, 456
Right ventricular failure. *See also* Heart failure
 after cardiopulmonary bypass, 455–456, 455*f*
 in mitral stenosis, 410
Right ventricular hypertrophy
 in pulmonic stenosis, 423
 in tetralogy of Fallot, 425
Right ventricular outflow obstruction
 in pulmonic stenosis, 423
 in tetralogy of Fallot, 425
Right ventricular stroke-work index, pulmonary artery catheterization monitoring of, 106*t*
Riley-Day syndrome (congenital/familial dysautonomia), 589
Ringer's lactate, 628, 629*t*
 for hemorrhagic shock/trauma patient, 796
Risk factors
 cardiac, 386, **387–388**, 388*t*
  for coronary artery disease, 395–396
 pulmonary, **512**, 512*t*
Risperdal. *See* Risperidone
Risperidone, 593
Ritanserin, for depression, 592*t*
Ritodrine, uterine activity affected by, 813, 837
Robert-Shaw double-lumen endobronchial tube, 529*t*, 530
Robin Hood (reverse steal) phenomenon, 559
Rocuronium, 179, 184*f*, 188*t*, **196**
 altered renal function and, 683
 history of use of, 4
 for intubation, in children, 461
 in ischemic heart disease patients, 405
 for open eye surgery in full stomach patient, 770
 for outpatient procedures, 884
 in pediatric anesthesia, 856
 pediatric dosing and, 855*t*
 for prevention of fasciculations, 189, 196
Rofecoxib
 for arthritis, 786
 for postoperative pain management, 341, 341*t*
Roller pumps, for cardiopulmonary bypass machine, 436
Ropivacaine, 237*t*
 cardiovascular effects of, 239, 363

for caudal anesthesia, 273
 in pediatric patient, 863
for epidural anesthesia, 271, 272, 272*t*
 for labor and delivery, 824, 827, 827*t*
 placental transfer of, 811
for spinal anesthesia, 268, 268*t*
 with opioids, 347, 827, 827*t*
RPF. *See* Renal plasma flow
RPLND. *See* Retroperitoneal lymph node dissection
RQ. *See* Respiratory quotient
rSO₂ (regional oxygen saturation in brain), intraoperative oximetry for monitoring of, 110
RSV. *See* Regurgitant stroke volume
Rule of nines, 801, 801*t*
Rupture of membranes, premature (PROM), **836**
RV. *See* Residual volume
Ryanodine receptor, in malignant hyperthermia, 870

SA node. *See* Sinoatrial (SA) node
Saccular aneurysms, cerebral, 578–579
Sacral cornuae, 273, 274*f*
Sacral hiatus, 273, 275*f*
Sacral nerves, blockade of, in pain management, 330–331, 331*f*
Sacral sparing, in failed epidural anesthesia, 273
Sacralization of L5, back pain caused by, 355
Sacroiliac joint injury, back pain and, 353
Saddle block, 826
Salicylates
 high anion gap acidosis caused by, 654
 for postoperative pain management, 341*t*
Saline
 for differential neuraxial blockade, 335, 335*t*
 for fluid management, 629*t*, 630
  in cardiopulmonary resuscitation, 924
  in hemorrhagic shock/trauma patient, 796
 for hyponatremia, 608–609, 609*f*
Saliva, electrolyte content of, 631*t*
Salivary secretions, anticholinergic drugs affecting, 208*t*, 209
Salmeterol, for asthma, 514*t*
SAM. *See* Systolic anterior motion
Sameridine, subarachnoid administration of, 168
SaO₂ (arterial oxygen saturation). *See also* Oxygen consumption
 coronary sinus, 378
 intraoperative monitoring of, oximetry for, 108–110, 110*f*
 measurement of in neonate, 844–845
Saphenous nerve
 blockade of (ankle block), 303, 304*f*
 entrapment of, 351*t*
Saphenous vein, for IV access in pediatric patient, 860–861
Sargramostim (granulocyte-macrophage colony-stimulating factor/GM-CSF), 636
SBP. *See* Systolic arterial blood pressure
Scalenus anticus syndrome, 351*t*
Scapulo-humeral (Erb's) muscular dystrophy, 756
SCARMD. *See* Severe childhood autosomal recessive muscular dystrophy
Scavenging, anesthetic-gas, 20
 active, 54
 by anesthesia machine, 41, **54**, 54*f*
 breathing circuits and, 33*t*
 passive, 54
Schimmelbusch mask, for open drop anesthesia, 29
Schizophrenia, **593**
Sciatic nerve block, 283, 301–302, 302*f*
Sciatic nerve entrapment, 351*t*
Scintigraphy, thallium, preoperative, in ischemic heart disease, 401
Scleroderma (systemic sclerosis), surgical management of, 548
Scoliosis, 850, **869**
 level of blockade after spinal anesthesia and, 267
Scopolamine, 207, 208*t*, 208*t*, **210**
 ophthalmic, systemic effects of, 764*t*
 for outpatients, 885–886
 overdose/toxicity of, physostigmine for, 205
Screening tests, 1
Seated position. *See* Sitting position
Secobarbital, 157*f*. *See also* Barbiturates
 uses and doses of, 159*t*
Second-degree block, 801
Second gas effect, 132
Second messengers, in central pain modulation, 318

Second-order neurons, in pain pathway, 313–315, 314*f*, 315*t*
 in central pain modulation, 318
 wind-up of, 313, 318
Sedation
 anticholinergic drugs causing, 208*t*
 for mechanical ventilation, 966
Sedative–hypnotics
 opioid use and, 345
 for pediatric patient, 857
Segmental pain inhibition, 318–319
Segmental sparing, in failed epidural anesthesia, 273
Seizures, 583, **585–586**, 585*t*, 586*t*
 classification of, 585, 585*t*
 drugs for management of, 586, 586*t*
  benzodiazepines, 164, 560
  neuromuscular blocking agent interactions and, 185*t*
  thiopental, 159
 eclamptic, 837
  magnesium for, 813, 838
 electroconvulsive therapy causing, 595
 enflurane and, 138*t*, 142, 559
 fentanyl and, 168
 inhalational anesthetics and, 138*t*, 559
 local-anesthetic induced, 239, 241
 magnesium sulfate for, 624
  in eclampsia, 813, 838
 propofol and, 174
Seldinger's technique
 for pulmonary artery catheterization, 103
 for right internal jugular cannulation, 100–102, 100*f*
Selective serotonin reuptake inhibitors, 592*t*, 593
Selegiline, for Parkinson's disease, 587
Sellick's maneuver, 251
Seminomas, 702
Sengstaken-Blakemore tube, for upper gastrointestinal bleeding, 986
Senning (atrial switch) procedure, for transposition of great arteries, 426
Sensitivity, of screening test, 1
Sensory blockade, neuraxial anesthesia producing, **258–260**, 260*t*
Sepsis, 951, **979–984**, 980*f*. *See also* Infection; Systemic inflammatory response syndrome
 ARDS and, 972, 973
 malignant hyperthermia differentiated from, 873
 shock associated with, **981–984**, 983*t*, 984–985*t*, 986*t*
Septal hypertrophy, asymmetric. *See* Hypertrophic cardiomyopathy
Septic shock, **981–984**, 983*t*, 984–985*t*, 986*t*
Septicemia, transurethral resection of prostate (TURP) and, 696
Septoplasty, 774–776, 775*f*
Serevent. *See* Salmeterol
Serotonin, 247*f*
 in asthma, 513
 in carcinoid syndrome, 750*t*
 pain mediation/modulation, 316*t*
 physiology of, 247
Serotonin receptor antagonists, **247–248**, 247*t*
 for depression, 592*t*
 for outpatients, 885
 in postanesthesia care unit, 940
Serotonin reuptake inhibitors, 592*t*
Serotonin syndrome, malignant hyperthermia differentiated from, 873
Sertraline
 for depression, 592*t*, 593
 for pain management, 337*t*
Serzone. *See* Nefazodone
Severe childhood autosomal recessive muscular dystrophy (SCARMD), 756
Sevoflurane, 3, 128, 135*t*, **145–146**
 alveolar concentration curve for, 131*f*
 cardiovascular effects of, 145, 364
 cerebral effects of, 557, 558*t*
 metabolism of, 138*t*
 minimum alveolar concentration of, 135*t*
 organ system effects of, 138*t*
 partition coefficient of, 130*t*
 for pediatric anesthesia, 860
  MAC value for, 855*t*
 renal effects of, 138*t*, 145, 662, 672, 682
 uterine activity during labor affected by, 813
SF₆. *See* Sulfur hexafluoride
SGOT (serum glutamic-oxaloacetic transaminase). *See* Aspartate aminotransferase

SGPT (serum glutamic pyruvic-transferase). *See* Alanine aminotransferase
Shivering, postoperative, 705, 706–707, 940–941
  in postanesthesia care unit, 936, 940–941
Shock
  classification of, 795, 795*t*, 796*t*
  dopamine in management of, 219
  hemorrhagic/hypovolemic, in trauma patient, 795–796, 795*f*, 796*f*
    fluid resuscitation and, 795, 796–797
  septic, **981–984**, 983*t*, 984–985*t*, 986*t*
  spinal, 590, 798
Short-axis (transgastric) view, for transesophageal echocardiography during cardiac surgery, 443, 443*f*, 444*f*
Shoulder. *See also* Upper extremity
  somatic blockade of, 283, **286–298**
Shoulder dystocia, 834
Shoulder presentation, 834
Shunting. *See also specific type or causative lesion*
  arteriovenous, in cirrhosis, 723, 728
  intrapulmonary, 475, 493, **494–495**
    A-a gradient affected by, 499
    burn injuries and, 801
    in cirrhosis, 728
    closing capacity and, 485
    hypoxemia in postanesthesia care unit and, 936, 945
    PaO₂ affected by, 499, 499*f*
    physiologic (normal venous admixture), 495
  left-to-right (simple), 387, 422, 422*t*, **423–425**
  right-to-left (complex), 387, 422, 422*t*, **425–427**
  surgical correction of, induction of anesthesia for, 461
  transesophageal echocardiography for assessment of, 446
SI. *See* Stroke index; System of international units
Sick sinus syndrome, 428
Sickle cell disease, 640–642, 641*t*
Sickle cell trait, 640
Sidestream (aspiration) capnographs, 111
  in pediatric patient, 857–858
Siggaard-Andersen nomogram, for base excess calculation, 650, 651*f*
Sigma (σ) receptors, 164, 164*t*
Silent ischemia/myocardial infarction, 396
  in diabetics, 396, 738
Silver chloride electrodes, for intraoperative electrocardiographic monitoring, 99, 99*f*
Silver nitrate, for burn injuries, methemoglobinemia caused by, 802
Simple (nonreservoir) oxygen mask, 955–956, 955*t*
SIMV. *See* Synchronized intermittent mandatory ventilation
Sinemet. *See* Carbidopa, with levodopa
Sinequan. *See* Doxepin
Single-lumen endobronchial tubes, **534**
Single-lumen endotracheal tubes. *See also* Endotracheal tubes
  with bronchial blockers
    for one-lung ventilation, **533–534**
    for pulmonary hemorrhage, 541
Single lung transplant, 547
Single twitch, in neuromuscular monitoring, 121, 122*t*
Sinoatrial (SA) nodal reentrant tachycardia, paroxysmal supraventricular tachycardia (PSVT) caused by, 383
Sinoatrial (SA) node, 361, 362*f*
  antianginal agents affecting, 397*t*
  blood supply to, 376
  inhalational anesthetics affecting, 359, 363
Sinoatrial (SA) reentrant tachycardia, paroxysmal supraventricular tachycardia (PSVT) caused by, 383
Sinus arrest, cholinesterase inhibitors causing, 202
Sinus node dysfunction, pathophysiology of, 428
Sinus surgery, 771, **774–776**, 775*f*
  bleeding following, 779–780
  proximity of sinuses to orbit and, 775, 775*f*
Sinus venosus defect, 424
Sinusoid channels, 709, 709*f*
Sinuvertebral nerve, 352
SIRS. *See* Systemic inflammatory response syndrome
Sitting position
  complications associated with, 894–896, 894*f*, 895*f*, 898*t*, 899*t*
  for neuraxial anesthesia, 254, 263
    level of block after epidural anesthesia affected by, 271
    level of blockade after spinal anesthesia and, 267
Skeletal muscle
  local anesthetics affecting, 240

relaxation of, neuromuscular blocking agents for, **178–198**. *See also* Neuromuscular blocking agents
Skin
  histamine affecting, 243
  postoperative necrosis of, patient positioning and, 899*t*
  rheumatoid arthritis affecting, 784*t*
Skull fracture, 576
Sleep apnea, obstructive, obesity and, 748
Sleep disorders
  acute pain and, 321
  chronic pain and, 321
Sleeve resection, 535
Smoke inhalation, 801, **974–975**
Smoking
  discontinuing, before surgery in COPD patient, 517
  emphysema and, 516
Smooth muscle
  α₁ agonists affecting, 214
  β₂ adrenoceptor activation affecting, 215
Sniffing position, for intubation, 71, 72*f*
Soda lime, as carbon dioxide absorbent, 27, 33–34, 33*t*
Sodium. *See also* Saline
  balance of
    disorders of, **609–612**. *See also* Hypernatremia; Hyponatremia
    anesthesia in patients with, 611–612
    minimum alveolar concentration affected by, 136*t*
    normal, **610**
    regulation of, **610–612**, 611*t*
  in body fluid/fluid compartments, 599*t*, 631
  in cardioplegia solutions, 438, 438*t*
  in crystalloid solutions, 629*t*
  extracellular fluid volume regulation and, **610–612**, 611*t*
  fractional excretion of, in azotemia/renal failure, 977*t*, 978
  plasma concentration of
    normal, 602
    plasma osmolality and, 503*t*, **602–604**
    volume control and, 611
  reabsorption of
    in loop of Henle, 666–667, 666*f*, 667*f*
    tubular, 664–665, 665*f*, 666*f*, 667
  urinary, in azotemia/renal failure, 977*t*, 978
Sodium bicarbonate. *See* Bicarbonate
Sodium channels
  abnormalities of
    in paramyotonia congenita, 757
    periodic paralysis and (sodium channelopathy/hyperkalemic periodic paralysis), **758–759**
    anesthetic considerations in patients with, 759
  local anesthetic action and, 234
  myocardial, 361, 363*t*
Sodium chloride, in metabolic alkalosis, 656–658, 657*t*
Sodium citrate, for aspiration pneumonia prophylaxis, 244*t*, 245
Sodium deficit, calculation of, 608
Sodium metabisulfite, allergic reactions to, 231
Sodium nitrate, for cyanide toxicity
  nitroprusside-induced, 226
  in smoke inhalation, 975
Sodium nitroprusside, 224, **225–227**, 225*f*, 226*t*
  cyanide toxicity and, 224, 226–227, 226*f*
Sodium overload
  loop diuretics in management of, 674
  thiazide diuretics in management of, 675
Sodium polystyrene sulfonate, for hyperkalemia, 618
Sodium thiosulfate, for cyanide toxicity
  nitroprusside-induced, 226
  in smoke inhalation, 975
Solu-Medrol. *See* Methylprednisolone
Solutions, nomenclature of, **598**
Somatic afferents, in pain pathway, 314
  integration of, 314–315
Somatic blockade
  neuraxial anesthesia producing, **258–260**, 260*t*
  in pain management, **323–331**
  peripheral nerve blocks producing. *See also specific type*
    of lower extremity, **298–303**, 304*f*, 305*f*
    of trunk, **304–307**
    of upper extremity, 283, **286–298**
Somatic pain, 311
Somatosensory evoked potentials (SSEPs), for intraoperative monitoring, 115–116, 116*t*
  anesthetic agents affecting, 563*t*, 564
  during spinal surgery, 782, 789

Somatostatin, pain mediation/modulation and, 316*t*
Somnolence, prolonged, outpatient surgery and, 886
Sore throat, postoperative, outpatient surgery and, 886
Sotalol, 399*t*
  in cardiopulmonary resuscitation, 929*t*
  for ventricular tachycardia in acute myocardial infarction, 976
sP. *See* Substance P
Space of Disse, 709, 709*f*
Specific gravity
  of anesthetic agent, neural blockade after spinal anesthesia affected by, 267, 267*t*
  urinary, 681
    in azotemia, 977*t*
Specific/true cholinesterase. *See* Acetylcholinesterase
Specificity, of screening test, 1
Spectrophotometers, for perioperative blood glucose monitoring, 740
Speech, laryngeal nerve damage affecting, 60, 63*t*
Sphenopalatine nerves (maxillary division of trigeminal nerve), 60, 62*f*, 323, 324*f*
  blocking, 323–325, 325*f*
  complications of, 326
Sphincter of Oddi, 713*f*, 714
  opioids causing spasm of, 716
Spinal anesthesia, 253–255, **266–269**. *See also* Neuraxial anesthesia
  agents used for, 268–269, 268*t*
  cardiac arrest during, 277, **900**
  catheters for, 266
  for cesarean section, 819, 828–829, **829–830**
  clinical considerations and, **262–266**
  complications of, **274–280**, 276*t*
  for cystoscopy, 692, 693–694
  differential blockade in pain evaluation and, 335–336, 335*t*
  with epidural anesthesia/analgesia (CSE)
    for cesarean section, **830**
    for labor and delivery, 827
  factors affecting level of block and, 267–268, 267*t*
  in geriatric patient, 875, 879
  high/total, 277
  for hip fracture repair, 784
  for labor and delivery
    with epidural anesthesia/analgesia (CSE), 827
    with local anesthetics, 826
    with mixed local anesthetic and opioids, 827
    with opioids alone, **822–823**, 822*t*
    uterine activity affected by, 813
  needles for, 266, 266*f*
  for outpatient procedures, 882, 885
  pheochromocytoma and, 223
  for postpartum tubal ligation, 817–818
  special techniques in, **274**
  for transurethral resection of prostate (TURP), 696–697
  uteroplacental blood flow affected by, 811
Spinal arteries, 257, 259*f*
Spinal canal, anatomy of, 255, 256*f*
  back pain and, 352
Spinal cord. *See also* Vertebral column
  anatomy of, neuraxial anesthesia and, **255–258**, 258*f*, 259*f*
  blood supply of, 257, 259*f*
  injury of, 583, **589–590**, **797–798**
Spinal cord ischemia, descending aorta surgery and, 468–469
Spinal cord laminae, 313, 314*f*, 315*t*
Spinal cord (dorsal column) stimulation, for pain management, 309, 340
Spinal cord transection, 583
  acute, 590
  chronic, 590
Spinal curvatures, level of blockade after spinal anesthesia and, 267
Spinal deformities, congenital, back pain caused by, 355
Spinal epidural abscess, neuraxial anesthesia and, 279
Spinal headache (post-dural puncture headache/PDPH), 275–276, 281, 885
  in outpatients, 885
Spinal hematoma, neuraxial anesthesia and, 279
Spinal infection, back pain caused by, 355
Spinal nerve roots, 255, 258*f*
  blood supply of, 257, 259*f*
Spinal nerves, 352
Spinal shock, 590, 798
Spinal stenosis, back pain caused by, 354–355
Spinal surgery, **580–581**, **788–789**
Spinal trauma, 583, **589–590**, **797–798**

Spinal tumors, back pain caused by, 355
Spinocervical tract, 314
Spinohypothalamic tract, 314
Spinomesencephalic tract, 314
Spinoreticular tract, 314
Spinotelencephalic tract, 314
Spinothalamic tract, 314
Spinous processes, 255, 256f, 352
  neuraxial anesthetic administration and, 263
Spirometers, for anesthesia machine, 41, **44–47**, 45f, 46f, 47t
Spirometry, incentive, 951, 970
Spironolactone, **676**, 746
Splanchnic nerve block, for pain management, 334
Splenic sequestration crises, in sickle cell anemia, 641
Splenomegaly, in cirrhosis, 728
SpO_2 (oxygen saturation of arterial pulsations), intraoperative monitoring of, pulse oximetry for, 108–110, 110f
Spondylitis, ankylosing, back pain caused by, 355
Spondylolisthesis, back pain caused by, 355
Spondylosis, back pain caused by, 354
Spontaneous awakening, **943**
Spontaneous bacterial peritonitis, cirrhosis and, 726
Spontaneous ventilation, 480, 481f
  in lateral decubitus position, 526, 526f
  Mapleson A circuit for, 27, 32
  open pneumothorax and, 528, 528f, 529f
  in pediatric patient, 861
Sprotte needle, 266, 266f
Square root of time model, for anesthesia uptake in closed-circuit, 148, 149
SSEPs. *See* Somatosensory evoked potentials
SSRIs. *See* Selective serotonin reuptake inhibitors
St. John's wort (hypericum), for depression, 7t, 591, 592t
ST segment changes, intraoperative monitoring of, 100
Stable angina. *See also* Angina
  chronic, 396
Standby anesthesia. *See* Monitored anesthesia care
Standing (ascending) bellows, for anesthesia ventilators, 52, 53f
Stapedectomy, 779
Starling's law of the heart, 368, 369f
Starvation, 987
Static compliance, plateau pressure and, 47
Static electricity, fires/explosions in operating room and, 25
  humidity in prevention of, 20, 25
Steal induction, 860
Stelazine. *See* Trifluoperazine
Stellate (cervicothoracic) block, for pain management, 332–333, 332f
Stellate ganglion, 332
Stereotactic neurosurgery, **575**
Sternotomy, for tamponade, 465
Steroid replacement therapy, in glucocorticoid deficiency, 736, 747. *See also* Corticosteroids
Stimulation (nervous system), anticholinergic drugs causing, 209
Storage vesicles, in neuromuscular transmission, 179, 180f
Straight leg-raising tests, in back pain, 353–354
Strain gauge principle, in transducer design, 94, 99f
Streptokinase, for acute myocardial infarction, 976
Stress response
  acute pain and, 320–321
  cardiopulmonary bypass and, 439
  chronic pain and, 321
  indirect renal effects and, 662, 672
  neuraxial anesthesia affecting, 262
  opioids affecting, 151, 169
Stress ulcers
  H_2-receptor antagonists in prevention of, 244
  in septic shock, 982
Stridor
  inspiratory, postoperative, 780
  laryngeal nerve damage causing, 60
    thyroidectomy and, 742
  laryngeal spasm causing, 780
    in hypocalcemia, 620
Stroke, 470, 584
  anesthesia after, 584–585, 585f
  after cardiopulmonary bypass/cardiac surgery, 454, 584
  postoperative, 584
Stroke in evolution, 470
Stroke index (SI), pulmonary artery catheterization monitoring of, 106t
Stroke volume, **368–371**, 368t
  adenosine affecting, 230
  afterload affecting, 369–370, 371f

in aortic regurgitation, 419
  contractility affecting, 370
  in mitral regurgitation, 412–414
  in pediatric patient, 849, 851
  pregnancy affecting, 805t, 806
  preload affecting, 368–369, 369f, 369t, 370f
  pulmonary artery catheterization monitoring of, 106t
  in tricuspid regurgitation, 421
  valvular dysfunction affecting, 371
  wall motion abnormalities affecting, 371
Stroke-work index, left and right ventricular, pulmonary artery catheterization monitoring of, 106t
Structure-activity relationship, 156. *See also specific agent*
Stuart factor, 718t
Stunning, myocardial, 975–976
Stylet, for endotracheal intubation, positioning, 71, 71f
Subaortic stenosis
  idiopathic hypertrophic. *See* Hypertrophic cardiomyopathy
  muscular. *See* Hypertrophic cardiomyopathy
Subarachnoid administration
  of meperidine/sameridine, 168
  of opioids, for cancer pain management, 349
Subarachnoid hemorrhage, ruptured aneurysm causing, 578–579
Subarachnoid space, 255, 255f
Subclavian (supraclavicular) brachial plexus block, 289–290, 290f
Subclavian vein, cannulation of, for central venous pressure monitoring, 100, 100t
Subcutaneous drug administration/absorption, 153
  for opioids, in pain management, 343
Subcutaneous emphysema, PEEP/CPAP and, 969
Subdural administration, of opioids, 168
Subdural bolt, for intracranial pressure monitoring, 570
Subdural hematoma, 576
Subdural space, spinal, 255, 258f
  inadvertent injection into during epidural anesthesia, 277
Sublimaze. *See* Fentanyl
Sublingual drug administration/absorption, 152
Substance abuse, **594**, 594t
  as occupational hazard, 889, **908**
  overdose and, 990–992
Substance P, pain mediation/modulation and, 316–317, 316t
  central sensitization and, 318
  secondary hyperalgesia and, 318
Substantia gelatinosa, 314, 315t
Substrate utilization, organ-specific, 987
Subxiphoid drainage, for tamponade, 465
Succinylcholine, 178, **183–187**, 184f. *See also* Depolarizing neuromuscular blocking agents
  altered renal function and, 679, 682–683
  contraindications to in burn patient, 803
  cost effectiveness/safety of, 192–193
  drug interactions and, 183–185, 185t
  for endoscopy, 772
  fasciculations caused by, 186
    nondepolarizing neuromuscular blocking agents for prevention of, 189
    rocuronium, 191, 196
    pheochromocytoma and, 223
  in geriatric anesthesia, 880
  history of use of, 4
  hyperkalemia caused by, 178, 186, 186t
  intraocular pressure affected by, 187, 761–763, 763t, 769–770
  for laryngospasm, 78, 80, 943
  malignant hyperthermia caused by, 187, 870
  metabolism/excretion of, 183, 185t
  for open eye surgery in full stomach patient, 769–770
  for outpatient procedures, 884
  in pediatric anesthesia, 849, 856
    pediatric dosing and, 855t
  for pediatric intubation, 461
  side effects/clinical considerations and, 186–187, 186t
  structure of, 183, 184f
  uses/doses of, 185–186
Succinylmonocholine, bradycardia caused by, 186
Suctioning
  before extubation, 77, 942–943
  postoperative, routine, 942–943
Sufenta. *See* Sufentanil
Sufentanil, 166f. *See also* Opioids
  altered renal function and, 682
  biotransformation of, 165, 167f
  for cardiac surgery

  in adults, 448–449
  in children, 461, 462
  cardiovascular effects of, 167, 171t
  context-sensitive half time of, 167f
  distribution of, 165, 167f
  history of use of, 4
  for hypertensive patients, 394–395
  intraspinal, 347, 347t
  for labor and delivery
    epidural, 823, 827, 827t
    intrathecal, 823, 827t
  organ system effects of, 171t
  for outpatient procedures, 884
  for patient-controlled analgesia, 343t
  in pediatric anesthesia, 855
    pediatric dosing and, 855t
  placental transfer of, 811
  in postanesthesia care unit, 940
  stress response affected by, 169
  uses and doses of, 168t
Sulfonamide allergy, 907
Sulfur hexafluoride, intravitreal injection of, intraocular gas expansion and, 763–764
Superficial cervical plexus block, 288f, 304–305
Superficial peroneal nerve
  blockade of (ankle block), 303, 304f
  entrapment of, 351t
Superior laryngeal nerve, 60, 62f
  blocking, for awake intubation, 83, 84f
  speech/voice disorders caused by damage to, 60, 63t
Superior vena cava syndrome, 550–551
Supine hypotension syndrome, 804, 806
Supine position
  complications associated with, 899t
  hyperextended, for urologic surgery, 699, 700f
  for spinal surgery, 789
Supraclavicular (subclavian) brachial plexus block, 289–290, 290f
Suprane. *See* Desflurane
Supraorbital (ophthalmic) nerve block, 323, 324f
Suprascapular nerve block, for pain management, 327, 328f
Suprascapular nerve entrapment, 351t
Supraspinal pain inhibition, 319
Suprasternal continuous-wave Doppler, for intraoperative monitoring, 107
Supraventricular tachycardia
  calcium channel blockers for, 398t
  paroxysmal (PSVT)
    adenosine for conversion of, 230
    mechanisms of, 383
     in Wolff-Parkinson-White (WPW) syndrome, 382–383
    preexcitation causing, 382
  in postanesthesia care unit, 947
Sural nerve, blockade of (ankle block), 303, 305f
Surface charge theory, of local anesthetic action, 234
Surface tension, ventilation and, 482
Surfactant
  alveolar surface tension affected by, 482
  fetal lung maturation and, 816
  in neonatal resuscitation, 846
Surgical airway, 914–915
Surgical diathermy
  electrical burns and, 15, **23–24**, 25f
  fires/explosions in operating room and, 25
Surmontil. *See* Trimipramine
S_vO_2 (mixed venous blood oxygen saturation)
  cardiac output indicated by, 359, 366
  intraoperative monitoring of, 110
SVR. *See* Vascular resistance, peripheral/systemic
SVRI. *See* Systemic vascular resistance index
Swan-Ganz catheter, 103, 103f
Sweat, electrolyte content of, 631t
Sympathetic dystrophy (CRPS type I), 350, 350t
Sympathetic nervous system, 213f
  activation of, in heart failure, 380
  anesthetics stimulating, 38
    indirect renal effects and, 672
  blockade of
    intravenous, 335
    for labor and delivery, **822**
    in pain management, 310, **331–335**, 350–351
  in cerebral blood flow control, 555
  in chronic pain, 310, 319–320, **350–351**, 350t
  heart supplied by, 366
  in hepatic blood flow regulation, 710
  liver supplied by, 709

Sympathetic nervous system (*cont.*)
in malignant hyperthermia, 869, 869*t*
myocardial contraction and, 364
neuraxial anesthesia producing blockade of, 253, 260–262
norepinephrine as neurotransmitter for, 212, 213*f*
potassium concentration affected by, 612
pulmonary vasculature affected by, 480
in renal blood flow regulation, 671
systemic vasculature controlled by, **374–375**
in volume control, 610–611
Sympatholytic agents
adverse effects of, 392*t*
clonidine as, 218
dexmedetomidine as, 218
for hypertension, 390*t*
methyldopa as, 218
minimum alveolar concentration affected by, 136*t*
Sympathomimetic activity, of beta blockers, 221, 221*t*
Sympathomimetic agents
for asthma, 513
minimum alveolar concentration affected by, 136*t*
Synaptic cleft, in neuromuscular transmission, 179, 180*f*
Synchronized intermittent mandatory ventilation (SIMV), 52, 961–962, 962*t*, 963*f*
Syncope
causes of, 428, 428*t*
in elderly patient, anesthetic concerns and, 428
vasodepressor (vasovagal), 374
Syringe pump, for intravenous infusion, 888
Syringe swap, 891
Syringobulbia, 589
Syringomyelia, **589**
Syrup of ipecac, for drug overdose/poisoning, 991–992
System of international units, 598
Systemic circulation. *See* Circulation
Systemic inflammatory response syndrome (SIRS), 979, 980*f*, 980*t*
ARDS and, 972
pathophysiology of, **979–980**
Systemic lupus erythematosus, neuromuscular blocking agent response affected in, 190*t*
Systemic sclerosis (scleroderma), surgical management of, 548
Systemic vascular resistance. *See* Vascular resistance, peripheral/systemic
Systemic vascular resistance index, 370
Systole, 366
ventricular pressure change during (dP/dt), contractility and, 371–372
Systolic anterior motion (SAM), in hypertrophic cardiomyopathy, 418
Systolic arterial blood pressure, 87. *See also* Arterial blood pressure
Systolic function
assessment of, 360, **371–372**
disorders of, in heart failure, 379, 379*f*

T₃. *See* Triiodothyronine
T₄. *See* Thyroxine
T lymphocytes, H₂-receptor affecting, 243
T-piece, weaning from ventilator with, 967–968
T-type calcium channels, myocardial, 361, 363*t*
Tachyarrhythmias. *See also* Tachycardia
antiarrhythmic selection for, 384*t*, 385
development of, 382, 383*f*
in valvular heart disease patient, management of, 412
Tachycardia. *See also* Heart rate
anticholinergic drugs causing, 208, 208*t*
atracurium causing, 191
barbiturates causing, 158
fenoldopam causing, 231
inadequate level of anesthesia causing, 37
intraoperative, 37–39, 909–910
medication errors causing, 909–910
pancuronium causing, 179, 195
paroxysmal supraventricular (PSVT)
adenosine for conversion of, 230
mechanisms of, 383
in Wolff-Parkinson-White (WPW) syndrome, 382–383
preexcitation causing, 382
perioperative causes of, 947–950, 948*t*
phentolamine causing, 220
in postanesthesia care unit, 947
in systemic inflammatory response syndrome, 980*t*
tubocurarine causing, 190

Tachyphylaxis
in local/regional anesthesia, 235
in nitroprusside-induced cyanide toxicity, 224, 226
Tagamet. *See* Cimetidine
Tamponade, 434, **464–465**, 935
central venous catheterization and, 102, 464
traumatic, 799
Tandospirone, for depression, 592*t*
"Target controlled infusion" (TCI), 162–163
Tarsal tunnel syndrome, 351*t*
Tau (τ≥ time constant, lung inflation and, 475, 491–492
TBW. *See* Total body water
TCI. *See* "Target controlled infusion"
TCP. *See* Transcutaneous cardiac pacing
Technetium-99 red blood cell scan, in lower gastrointestinal tract bleeding, 986
TEE. *See* Transesophageal echocardiography
Tegratol. *See* Carbamazepine
Telethermography, in pain evaluation, 322
Temperature (ambient), in operating room, **20**
Temperature (body). *See also* Hyperthermia; Hypothermia
acid-base disorder diagnosis and, 644, 659
anticholinergic drugs affecting, 209
atracurium duration of action and, 192
cerebral blood flow affected by, 554
intraoperative monitoring of, **117**, 117*f*, 125
for cardiac surgery, 441
in pediatric patient, 849, 858
minimum alveolar concentration affected by, 136*t*
neuromuscular blocking agents affected by, 189
in pediatric patient, 849, 851
in systemic inflammatory response syndrome, 980*t*
Temporary pacing, 430–431
for acute myocardial infarction, 976
Temporomandibular joint
anesthesia-related injuries of, 892
limited mobility of, in diabetes, 736, 739
Tenecteplase, for acute myocardial infarction, 976
TENS. *See* Transcutaneous electrical stimulation
Tension pneumothorax, 798, 935
Teratogenicity
maternal anesthetics and, 810–811, 846–847
of nitrous oxide, 139
Terbutaline
for asthma, 514*t*
receptor selectivity of, 216*t*, 514*t*
uterine activity affected by, 813, 837
Terminal membrane, storage vesicle, 179, 180*f*
Test dose, in epidural anesthesia, 270–271, 825
in parturients, 825
Testicular cancer, **702–703**
Tetanus, neuromuscular blocking agent response affected in, 190*t*
Tetany, at 50 Hz or 100 Hz, in neuromuscular monitoring, 121, 122*t*, 181, 182*t*
respiratory failure evaluation and, 199, 206
Tetracaine, 237*t*
neurologic effects of, 239–240
specific gravity of, 267*t*
for spinal anesthesia, 268, 268*t*
for labor and delivery, 825
Tetracyclic antidepressants, 592*t*
Tetralogy of Fallot, 387, 425–426
TGA. *See* Transposition of great arteries
Thalassemia
pathophysiology of, 642
sickle cell anemia and, 642
Thalitone. *See* Chlorthalidone
Thallium imaging (scintigraphy), preoperative, in ischemic heart disease, 401
THAM, in cardioplegia solutions, 439
Therapeutic index, 155
Thermistors, for intraoperative temperature monitoring, 117
Thermocouple, for intraoperative temperature monitoring, 117
Thermodilution curve, 106–107
Thermodilution technique, for cardiac output determination, 106–107
Thermogenesis, nonshivering, 851
Thermography, in pain evaluation, **322–323**
Thermoregulation
anticholinergic drugs affecting, 209
in pediatric patient, 851
Thiamine, for obtunded/comatose patient, 991
Thiamylal, 157*f*. *See also* Barbiturates
biotransformation of, 158
distribution of, 157, 158

organ system effects of, 171*t*
uses and doses of, 159*t*
Thiazide diuretics, **675**
adverse effects of, 392*t*, 675
for hypertension, 390*t*, 675
Thiocyanate, nitroprusside metabolized to, 226–227, 226*f*
Thiopental, 157*f*. *See also* Barbiturates
biotransformation of, 158
cerebral effects of, 159, 171*t*
distribution of, 157–158, 158*f*
drug interactions and, 159
in geriatric anesthesia, 880
organ system effects of, 171*t*
for outpatient procedures, 884
for patients susceptible to malignant hyperthermia, 873
pediatric dosing and, 855*t*
placental transfer of, 811
respiratory effects of, 158, 171*t*
for seizure management, 159
local anesthetic-induced, 239, 241
uses and doses of, 159*t*
Thioridazine, 593
Thiosulfate, for cyanide toxicity
nitroprusside-induced, 226
in smoke inhalation, 975
Thiothixene, 593
Third-degree burns, 801
Third-order neurons, in pain pathway, 315
"Third spacing"
fluid loss during surgery and, 631–632
replacement and, 633, 633*t*
testicular cancer surgery and, 703
in septic shock, 983
Thirst, in plasma osmolality control, 604
Thomsen's myotonia congenita, 757
Thoracic aorta, surgery on
ascending aorta and, 467–468
descending aorta and, 468–469
Thoracic bioimpedance, in intraoperative monitoring, 107
Thoracic epidural blocks, 269. *See also* Epidural anesthesia
Thoracic nerve injury, during surgery, 893
Thoracic paravertebral block, 306, 306*f*, 328–329
for pain management, 328–329
Thoracic surgery, **525–551**. *See also specific procedure*
diagnostic, **544–546**
esophageal surgery, 525, **548–549**
lateral decubitus position for, **526–527**, 526*f*, 527*f*
lung resection, **534–543**
lung transplant, 525, **546–548**, 546*t*
mediastinal adenopathy and, 550–551
one-lung ventilation and, **528**, 529–534, 529*t*, 530*f*, 531*f*, 532*f*, 533*f*, 533*t*
open pneumothorax and, **527–528**, 528*f*, 529*f*
physiologic considerations and, **526–528**, 526*f*, 527*f*, 528*f*, 529*f*
thoracoscopic, **543–544**
tracheal resection, 542*f*, **543**, 544*f*, 545*f*
volume reduction surgery, **549–550**
Thoracic sympathetic chain block, for pain management, 333
Thoracoabdominal surgery, analgesia following, 356–358
Thoracolumbar blockade, neuraxial anesthesia producing, 260–262
Thoracoscopy, **543–544**
for tamponade, 465
Thoracotomy. *See also* Thoracic surgery
for open-chest cardiac massage, 922
patient positioning for, 537–538, 538*f*
for single lung transplant, 547
tamponade after, 465
for tamponade drainage, 465
Thorazine. *See* Chlorpromazine
Thorpe type flowmeter, 43, 44*f*
THR (total hip replacement). *See* Total hip arthroplasty
Three-compartment model, 155
"Three-in-one" block, 283, 298–299, 299*f*
Threshold level, local anesthetic action and, 234
Thrombin, in coagulation, 718
Thrombin time, 720, 721, 721*t*
high-dose, anticoagulation for cardiopulmonary bypass and, 449
Thrombocytopenia, 721
in cirrhosis, 728
dilutional
bleeding after transfusion and, 626, 638
transurethral resection of prostate and, 696
heparin-induced, cardiopulmonary bypass anticoagulation in patients with, 450

persistent bleeding after cardiopulmonary bypass and, 458
in septic shock, 982
Thrombolytic therapy, neuraxial anesthesia in setting of, 280
Thromboplastin, tissue, 718*t*
Thrombosis
  aortic, 467
  hip surgery and, 787, 881
  intra-arterial monitoring and, 93
  lidocaine affecting, 240
  in mitral stenosis, 410
  pulmonary embolism and, **520–522**, 520*t*
  risk of in valvular heart disease patients, 407–408
Thrombotic stroke, 584. *See also* Stroke
Thromboxane A$_2$, in pregnancy-induced hypertension, 837
Thymectomy, 753
Thymic hyperplasia, in myasthenia gravis, 753
Thymidylate synthetase, nitrous oxide affecting, 139
Thymoma, in myasthenia gravis, 753
Thyroid adenoma, functioning, 741
Thyroid artery, larynx supplied by, 60–61
Thyroid cartilage, 60, 61*f*
Thyroid gland, **741–743**
  cancer of, in multiple endocrine neoplasia, 750
  disorders of. *See also* Hyperthyroidism; Hypothyroidism
    minimum alveolar concentration affected by, 136*t*
  physiology of, 741
  pregnancy affecting, 808
Thyroid hormone, 741. *See also* Hyperthyroidism;
    Hypothyroidism
  after cardiopulmonary bypass, 456*t*, 457
  for myxedema coma, 743
Thyroid iodine concentration, 741
Thyroid steal, 741–742
Thyroid-stimulating hormone (TSH), 581, 741
  in hypothyroidism, 742
Thyroid storm, 742, 873, 949–950
  malignant hyperthermia differentiated from, 873
Thyroidectomy, 741, 742
Thyroiditis, 741
Thyrotropin-releasing hormone, 741
Thyroxine (T$_4$), 741
  for myxedema coma, 743
Tiagabine, for seizures, 586*t*
TIAs. *See* Transient ischemic attacks
Tibial artery, posterior, catheterization of for arterial blood
    pressure monitoring, 93
Tibial nerve
  blockade of (ankle block), 303, 304*f*
  entrapment of, 351*t*
Tidal volume, 484*f*, 484*t*
  dead space and, 490–491
  delivery of by anesthesia ventilator, 52
  desflurane affecting, 138*t*, 144
  halothane affecting, 138*t*, 140
  inhalational anesthetics affecting, 138*t*
  methoxyflurane affecting, 138*t*, 141
  nitrous oxide affecting, 137, 138*t*
  in pediatric patient, 850
  pregnancy affecting, 805, 805*t*
Time constants (τ), lung inflation and, 475, 491–492
Timed-cycle ventilators, 961
Timolol, 399*t*
  ophthalmic, systemic effects of, 764, 764*t*
TIPS. *See* Percutaneous transjugular intrahepatic
    portosystemic shunts
Tirilazad, for cerebral protection, 562
Tissue/blood partition coefficients. *See* Partition coefficients
Tissue mass, local anesthetic distribution affected by, 238
Tissue perfusion
  intraoperative monitoring of, pulse oximetry for, 109
  local anesthetic distribution affected by, 238
Tissue plasminogen activator (tPA), 720
Tissue resistance, airway resistance and, 488
Tissue thromboplastin, 718*t*
Tissue uptake, of inhalational anesthetic, 130–131, 130*t*
TIVA. *See* Total intravenous anesthesia
TLC. *See* Total lung capacity
TNS. *See* Transient neurologic symptoms
Tocodynamometer, for surgery during pregnancy, 847
Tocolysis, 837
  β_2-agonists for, 813, 817
  magnesium for, 813
Tofranil. *See* Imipramine
Tolerance
  opioid, in cancer pain management, 348
    intraspinal administration and, 349
  substance abuse and, 594

Tonic-clonic (grand mal) seizures, 585, 585*t*. *See also*
    Seizures
Tonicity, **598**
Tonometry, arterial, for arterial blood pressure monitoring,
    91, 91*f*
Tonsillectomy, **867–868**
  as outpatient procedure, 883
Topical anesthesia. *See* Local (regional)
    anesthesia/anesthetics
Topiramate
  for pain management, 337–338
  for seizures, 586*t*
Toradol. *See* Ketorolac
Tornalate. *See* Bitolterol
Torsemide, 674–675. *See also* Loop diuretics
Torsion, pulmonary, after thoracotomy, 540
Total anomalous venous return, 426
Total body water, 598, 598*t*
Total hip arthroplasty (total hip replacement), **784–787**,
    784*t*, 785*f*
Total intravenous anesthesia (TIVA), 887–888
Total knee arthroplasty (total knee replacement), **788**
Total lung capacity (TLC), 484*f*, 484*t*, 485*f*
Total parenteral nutrition (TPN), 951, **989–990**, 989*t*
Total peripheral resistance, pulmonary artery
    catheterization monitoring of, 106*t*
Total rebreathing, in closed-circuit anesthesia, 146–150
Total spinal anesthesia, 277
Tourniquet, pneumatic, for knee arthroscopy, 782, 787–788
Tourniquet pain, 787
Toxemia of pregnancy (pregnancy-induced hypertension),
    837–839, 838*t*
Toxic multinodular goiter, 741
tPA. *See* Tissue plasminogen activator
TPN. *See* Total parenteral nutrition
Tracheal compression, in mediastinal adenopathy, 550
Tracheal edema, postintubation croup caused by, 863
Tracheal injuries, anesthesia-related, 892
Tracheal resection, 542*f*, **543**, 544*f*, 545*f*
Tracheal tubes/tracheal intubation, 67–69, 69*f*, 69*t*. *See also*
    Intubation
  in pediatric patient, 860, 860*t*, 861
Tracheobronchial tree, **477–478**, 478*f*
  anatomy of, **477–478**, 478*f*, 530, 530*f*
  double-lumen endobronchial tubes and, 530, 530*f*, 531*f*
  irritant receptors in, 508
  vagus nerve innervating, 480
Tracheoesophageal fistula, **865–866**, 865*f*
Tracheostomy
  for head and neck cancer surgery, 776
  for mechanical ventilation in critical care unit, 965–966
  for trauma patient, 794
Tracheotomy, 920
Train-of-four, in neuromuscular monitoring, 121, 122*t*,
    181, 182*t*
  respiratory failure evaluation and, 206
Tramadol, for postoperative pain management, 341*t*
Tranexamic acid
  for bleeding prophylaxis in cardiopulmonary bypass, 450
  for persistent bleeding after cardiopulmonary bypass, 458
Transaminases, serum levels of, 714*t*, 715
Transamination, hepatic, 712
Transcranial Doppler, during cardiac surgery, 447
Transcutaneous cardiac pacing, in cardiopulmonary
    resuscitation, 912, 924–925, 932*f*, 933*f*
Transcutaneous electrical stimulation (TENS), for pain
    management, 340
Transcutaneous gas monitors, **112–113**
Transcutaneous oxygen sensors, in neonate, 845
Transdermal drug administration/absorption, 153
Transdermal opioids, for cancer pain, **349**
Transducers, for intra-arterial monitoring, 93–95, 97*f*,
    98*f*, 99*f*. *See also* Catheter-tubing-transducer
    system
  calibrating, 94–95
Transesophageal Doppler color-flow mapping, for
    intraoperative monitoring, 107
  in mitral regurgitation, 414, 415*f*
Transesophageal echocardiography (TEE). *See also*
    Echocardiography
  documentation of probe placement and, 902
  intraoperative, 107
    during cardiac surgery, 433, 442–443*f*, 443–446,
      444*f*, 445*f*, 446*f*
    in children, 461
    in ischemic heart disease patient, 404
    venous air embolism monitoring and, 575
  in mitral regurgitation, 412

Transformer, isolation, protection from electrical shock
    and, 15, 22, 22*f*, 23*f*, 24*f*
Transfusion, **633–639**. *See also* Fluid
    replacement/management
  for abdominal trauma, 799
  alternatives to, **639–640**
  autologous, **639**
  blood bank practices and, **634–635**
  blood groups and, **633**, 633*t*
  blood salvage/reinfusion and, **639**
  compatibility testing for, **633–634**
  complications of, 626, **636–638**. *See also* Transfusion
    reactions
  determining need for, 626, 632
  disease transmission and, **638**
    screening in prevention of, 634
  donor-directed, **639–640**
  emergency, **634**
  for gastrointestinal hemorrhage, 985
  for hemorrhagic shock/trauma patient, 793, 795, 796
  intraoperative, 632–633, **635–636**
    during head and neck cancer surgery, 776–777
  intravascular volume evaluation and, 527*t*, **626–628**
  massive, **638–639**
Transfusion reactions, 626, **636–638**
  hemolytic, **636–637**
  nonhemolytic, **637–638**
Transgastric (short-axis) view, for transesophageal
    echocardiography during cardiac surgery, 443,
    443*f*, 444*f*
Transient ischemic attacks (TIAs), 470, 584
Transient neurologic symptoms (TNS), neuraxial
    anesthesia causing, 277
Transplantation. *See specific type or organ*
Transport ventilators, automatic, 921
Transportation
  of cardiac surgery patient, 458
  from operating room to postanesthesia care unit, **939**
Transposition of great arteries, 426
Transpulmonary pressure, 480
Trans-sacral nerve block, 330–331, 331*f*
Transsphenoidal approach, for pituitary surgery, 581–582
  monitoring for, 582
Transtracheal Doppler, for intraoperative monitoring, 107
Transtracheal jet ventilation, 912, 914–915, 919–920,
    920*f*
Transtracheal nerve block, for awake intubation, 83, 84*f*
Transurethral resection of prostate (TURP), **694–697**,
    695*f*
  choice of anesthetic agent for, 696–697
  hypotension and, 705–707
Transurethral resection of prostate (TURP) syndrome, 692,
    695–696, 695*t*
  monitoring patient for, 697
Transvalvular gradient, calculation of
  in aortic stenosis, 416–417
  in mitral stenosis, 410–411
Transverse four-chamber view, for transesophageal
    echocardiography during cardiac surgery,
    442*f*, 443, 444*f*
Tranylcypromine, for depression, 591, 592*t*
Trauma, **793–803**. *See also specific type*
  abdominal, **799–800**
  airway management and, 794
  ARDS and, 973
  breathing support and, 795
  burn injury, 800*f*, 801–803, 801*f*
  chest, **798–799**
  circulatory support and, 795–797
  classification of, 795, 795*t*, 796*t*
  extremity, **800–801**
  fluid resuscitation in, 796–797
  head, 567, **575–578**, 797–798
  hemorrhage and, 795–796, 795*f*, 796*f*
    fluid resuscitation and, 795, 796–797
  initial assessment of, 793, **794–797**
  primary survey in, 793, **794–797**
  secondary survey in, 793, **797**
  spinal cord, 589–590, **797–798**
Trazodone
  for depression, 592*t*, 593
  for pain management, 337*t*
Trendelenburg position
  breath sounds affected by, 510
  complications associated with, 898*t*, 899*t*
  functional residual capacity affected by, 490
  with lithotomy position, 693
  oxygenation affected by, 522

Trendelenburg position (cont.)
  pulmonary perfusion affected by, 492
  reverse, complications associated with, 898t, 899t
Triamcinolone
  epidural, for back pain, 354
  for pain management, 338t
Triamterene, 676
Triazolopyridine, for depression, 592t
Trichloroethylene, absorbent granules causing degradation
  of, 34
Tricuspid atresia, 426
Tricuspid regurgitation, **420–421**
  choice of anesthetic agent in patient with, 421
  heart murmur in, preoperative evaluation of, 407t
Tricuspid stenosis, heart murmur in, preoperative
  evaluation of, 407t
Tricyclic antidepressants, 583, 591, 592t. See also
  Antidepressants
Trifascicular block, presentation of, 429
Trifluoperazine, 593
Trifluoracetic acid, isoflurane metabolized to, 143
Trigeminal nerve
  blocking, 323–326, 324–325f
  mandibular division of (lingual nerve), 60, 62f, 323,
    324f
    blocking, 325–326, 325f
    for awake intubation, 83, 83f
  mask ventilation causing pressure injury of branches of,
    64
  maxillary division of (sphenopalatine nerves), 60, 62f,
    323, 324f
    blocking, 323–325, 325f
    complications of, 326
  ophthalmic division of (anterior ethmoidal nerve), 60,
    62f, 323, 324f
    blocking, 323, 324f
Trigeminal nerve block, in pain management, 323–326,
    324–325f
Trigeminal neuralgia, trigeminal nerve block in
    management of, 323–326, 324–325f
Trigger-point injection, of local anesthetics, 240
Trigger points, in myofascial pain, 310, 351–352
Triiodothyronine (T_3), 741
  for myxedema coma, 743
Trilafon. See Perphenazine
Trillisate. See Choline magnesium trisalicylate
Trimethaphan, 224, 225f, 226t, **229–230**, 394t
  pseudocholinesterase affected by, 185
Trimipramine, for depression, 592t
Trismus (masseter/jaw muscle spasm/rigidity), in malignant
  hyperthermia, 187, 869, 871
Trisomy 21 (Down syndrome), **868**
Tromethamine
  in cardioplegia solutions, 439
  for respiratory acidosis, 652–653
Tropisetron, 247
Tropomyosin, in myocardial contraction, 364, 365f
Troponin, in myocardial contraction, 364, 365f
Trousseau's sign (carpopedal spasm), in hypocalcemia, 620,
  745
True/specific cholinesterase. See Acetylcholinesterase
Truncus arteriosus, 426
Trunk, somatic blockade of, **304–307**
  inguinal nerve block for, 306–307, 306f
  intercostal block for, 305, 305f
  penile block for, 283, 307, 307f
  superficial cervical plexus block for, 288f, 304–305
  thoracic paravertebral block for, 306, 306f
TSH. See Thyroid-stimulating hormone
TT. See Thrombin time
Tubal ligation, postpartum, 816–818
Tube feedings (enteral nutrition), **988–989**
Tubocurarine, 184f, 188t, **190–191**
  autonomic effects of, 187
  histamine release caused by, 187, 188t, 190, 191
  for prevention of fasciculations, 189
  renal excretion of, 188, 188t, 190
Tubuloglomerular balance/feedback
  in renal blood flow regulation, 671
  volume control and, 611
Tumor necrosis factor
  in septic shock, 981
  in systemic inflammatory response syndrome, 980
Tumor thrombus, in renal cancer, radical nephrectomy
  with removal of, 704
Tuohy needle, 269, 270f
Turbulent flow, airway resistance and, 485–486
TURP. See Transurethral resection of prostate

TURP syndrome, 692, 695–696, 695t
  monitoring patient for, 697
Twins, delivery of, 834–835
Twitch, in neuromuscular monitoring, 121, 122t, 181
Two-compartment model, 154–155, 154f
Two-stage pressure regulators, on anesthesia machine, 42
Tylenol. See Acetaminophen
Tympanic membrane, for intraoperative temperature
  monitoring, 119
Tympanoplasty, 779
  nitrous oxide and, 771, 779
Tympanostomy tube insertion, myringotomy and, 779,
  868
Type and cross match, for blood transfusion, versus type
  and screen, 634
Tyrosine, 741

**UA/UV. See Umbilical artery/umbilical vein
  concentration**
Ulcers
  H_2-receptor antagonists in prevention of, 244
  peptic, bleeding from, 986
Ulnar artery catheterization, for arterial blood pressure
  monitoring, 93
Ulnar nerve block, 297, 297f
Ulnar nerve entrapment, 351t
Ulnar nerve stimulation, in neuromuscular monitoring,
  120, 121f
Ulnar neuropathy, postoperative, patient positioning and,
  893, 897f, 899t
Ultane. See Sevoflurane
Ultrafilter, for cardiopulmonary bypass machine, 437
Ultram. See Tramadol
Ultrasonic nebulizers, for anesthesia machine, 55
Ultrasonography, intraoperative, 107
Umbilical artery catheterization, for vascular access in
  neonatal resuscitation, 845
Umbilical artery/umbilical vein concentration (UA/UV),
  placental transfer of anesthetic agents affected
  by, 804, 810
Umbilical cord prolapse, **833**
Umbilical vein catheterization, for vascular access in
  neonatal resuscitation, 845
Umbilical vein/maternal venous concentration (UV/MV),
  placental transfer of anesthetic agents affected
  by, 804, 810
Under-damping, of catheter-tubing-transducer system, 93,
  98f
Unidirectional valves
  in circle system, 27, 35, 35f, 36f
  competence test of, 38, 39f
Unilateral block, in failed epidural anesthesia, 273
Unit dose, anesthesia uptake in closed-circuit and, 148, 149
Unitary hypothesis, of anesthetic action, 127, 133, 134f
Universal precautions, infection prevention and, 908
Unstable angina, 396, 976. See also Angina
Up-regulation, receptor
  propranolol causing, 222
  response to neuromuscular blocking agents and, 181
Upper arm, radial nerve block at, 294, 294f
Upper extremity, somatic blockade of, 283, **286–298**
  brachial plexus anatomy and, **286–288**, 287f, 288f
  brachial plexus block for, **288–292**
  intravenous regional anesthesia for, **297–298**, 298f
  peripheral nerve blocks for, **292–297**, 298f
Upper gastrointestinal bleeding, 986
Upper respiratory tract infection, in pediatric patient,
  preoperative evaluation of, 849, 856–857
Uptake, drug. See also Distribution
  of inhalational anesthetics
    alveolar gas concentration (F_A) and, 129–131, 130t,
    131f, 132f
    factors affecting, 127
Urea
  liver in formation of, 712
  renal medullary hypertonicity and, 667, 668
Urea nitrogen, **680**
  in azotemia/renal failure, 976, 977t
  in geriatric patient, 878
  in pregnancy, 807
Urea nitrogen:creatinine ratio, **680–681**
Uremia, 684, 684t. See also Renal failure
  need for dialysis and, 686, 686t
Uremic encephalopathy, 686
Uremic pericarditis, 685
Ureters, noncancer surgery on, **699**
Urinalysis, **681**

Urinary calculi
  extracorporeal shock wave lithotripsy for, 697–699, 697f
  open procedures for, 699
Urinary catheterization. See Bladder catheterization
Urinary diversion, 702
  electrolyte abnormalities after, 624–625
Urinary output
  decreased. See Oliguria
  enflurane affecting, 138t, 142
  halothane affecting, 138t, 140
  in hypovolemia evaluation, 627t
  inhalational anesthetics affecting, 138t
  intraoperative monitoring of, **120**, 677
    for cardiac surgery, 441
    controlled hypotension and, 232
    in hypertensive patient, 393
    during renal transplant, 705
  isoflurane affecting, 138t, 143
  nitrous oxide affecting, 138, 138t
  surgery affecting, 662, 677–678
Urinary retention
  anticholinergic drugs causing, 209
  neuraxial anesthesia and, 261, 276
  pain causing, 320
  postoperative, outpatient surgery and, 886
  trimethaphan causing, 229
Urinary sediment, microscopic analysis of, 681
Urinary tract
  neuraxial anesthesia affecting, 261, 276
  nosocomial infection of, 981
  obstruction of, postrenal azotemia caused by, 977
  pain affecting, 320
Urine
  alkalinization of, carbonic anhydrase inhibitors for, 676
  anion gap in, in hyperchloremic acidosis, 654
  concentration of, in medullary collecting tubule, 668
  osmolality of, in azotemia, 977t
  specific gravity of, 681
    in azotemia, 977t
Urine pH, 681
  renal excretion affected by, 154
Urokinase, 720
Urologic surgery. See also specific procedure
  anesthesia for, **692–707**
  noncancer, **699**
  radical, for malignancies, **699–704**, 700f
URTI. See Upper respiratory tract infection
Urticaria, 903
Urticarial reactions, blood transfusion causing, 637
Uterine atony, postpartum hemorrhage and, 839–840
Uterine blood flow, during pregnancy, 808
Uterine contractions
  Braxton Hicks, 811, 812
  fetal heart rate changes related to, 840–842, 841f
  in labor, 812
    anesthetic agents affecting, 813
Uterine muscle, nitroglycerine affecting, 228
Uterine rupture, 835–836
  vaginal birth after cesarean delivery (VBAC) and, 823,
    836
Uteroplacental circulation, **808–811**, 809f, 810f
  anesthetic agents affecting, 811
UV/MV. See Umbilical vein/maternal venous
  concentration

V̇/Q̇ ratio. See Ventilation/perfusion ratio
v wave, 102, 102f, 366, 367f
Vacuum system, central, 19
Vaginal bleeding, antepartum, **835–836**
Vaginal delivery. See also Labor and delivery
  after cesarean section (vaginal birth after cesarean
    delivery/VBAC), 820
    regional anesthesia and, 823
  general anesthesia for (emergency/surgical), **828**, 828t
  techniques for, 828
Vagus nerve, 60, 62f
  baroreceptor signals carried by, 375
  injury to, 60
    speech/voice disorders caused by, 60, 63t
  liver supplied by, 709
  tracheobronchial tree supplied by, 480
Valdecoxib, for arthritis, 786
Valerian, 7t
Valproate/valproic acid
  for pain management, 337, 338t
  for seizures, 586, 586t
Valve replacement, for mitral stenosis, 411

Valvular dysfunction
 stroke volume affected by, 371
 transesophageal echocardiography for intraoperative
  assessment of, 444–446, 445f, 446f
Valvular heart disease, **406–421**. *See also specific lesion*
 antibiotic prophylaxis in, 407, 408–409t
 anticoagulation management in, 407–408
 patient evaluation in, **406–407**, 406t, 407t, 408f
 pregnancy and, 839
 stroke volume affected in, 371
Valvuloplasty
 for mitral stenosis, 411
 for pulmonic stenosis, 423
Vancomycin, allergic reactions to, 907
van Lint facial nerve block, 766, 768f
Vaporization, heat of, 47
Vaporizers
 for anesthesia machine, 40, 41, **47–50**, 48f, 49f, 51f
 draw-over, for anesthesia administration, 29
Variable-bypass vaporizers, for anesthesia machine, 49–50,
  49f
Variable decelerations, in fetal heart rate monitoring, 841f,
  842
Variable-orifice flowmeters, constant-pressure, 43–44, 44f
Variable-performance (low-flow) equipment, for oxygen
  therapy, 954
Variable-threshold angina, 396. *See also* Angina
Variceal bleeding, in cirrhosis, 723, 727
Variegate porphyria, barbiturate enzyme induction causing,
  159
VAS. *See* Visual analog scale
Vasa recta, 667
Vascular resistance
 peripheral/systemic, 370
  adenosine affecting, 230
  adrenergic agonists affecting, 217t
  afterload and, 370
  barbiturates affecting, 158
  benzodiazepines affecting, 161
  desflurane affecting, 138t, 144
  dobutamine affecting, 217t, 219
  dopamine affecting, 217t, 219
  enflurane affecting, 138t, 142
  etomidate affecting, 172
  fenoldopam affecting, 217t, 220
  halothane affecting, 138t, 139
  hydralazine affecting, 228
  inhalational anesthetics affecting, 138t
  isoflurane affecting, 138t, 143
  labetalol affecting, 220
  mitral regurgitation and, 412
  nitroprusside affecting, 227
  phenylephrine affecting, 207, 216, 217t
  pregnancy affecting, 805t, 806
  propofol affecting, 174
  sevoflurane affecting, 138t, 145
 pulmonary
  in left-to-right shunts, 424, 434
  in mitral stenosis, 410
  pulmonary artery catheterization monitoring of, 106t
 renal, volatile agents affecting, 672
Vascular surgery, **466–472**. *See also specific type or vessel*
Vasculature, autonomic control of, 374–375
Vasoactive intestinal polypeptide (VIP), pain
  mediation/modulation and, central
  sensitization and, 318
Vasoconstriction
 autonomic control of, 374–375
 cocaine causing, 239
 hypoxia causing, 475, 493
 hypoxic pulmonary
  nitroprusside affecting, 227
  one-lung ventilation and, 528
  phenylephrine causing, 207, 216
Vasoconstrictors, with local anesthetics, 235–238
 for epidural anesthesia, 271
 for spinal anesthesia, 268
Vasodepressor (vasovagal) syncope, 374
Vasodilation
 adenosine causing, 230
 antianginal agents causing, 397t
 autonomic control of, 374–375
 calcium channel blockers causing, 397, 397t, 398
 after cardiopulmonary bypass (hyperdynamic patients),
  455, 455t
 coronary, myocardial oxygen demand and, 378
 dopamine causing, 219
 fenoldopam causing, 230–231

histamine causing, 243
hydralazine causing, 228
neuraxial anesthesia causing, 253, 260–261
nitrates causing, 397, 397t
nitroglycerine causing, 227
nitroprusside causing, 225, 227
phentolamine causing, 220
trimethaphan causing, 229
Vasodilators
 adverse effects of, 392t
 after cardiopulmonary bypass, 457, 457t
 cerebral effects of, **560**
 for hypertension, 391t
Vasogenic cerebral edema, 568
Vasomotor centers, vascular tone controlled by, 374–375
Vaso-occlusive crises, in sickle cell anemia, 640–641
Vasopressin, arginine (AVP/antidiuretic hormone), 456t,
  581
 in blood pressure control, 375–376
 after cardiopulmonary bypass, 456t, 457
 in cardiopulmonary resuscitation, 912, 912–914, 913f,
  916f, 927t, 930f, 931f
 in heart failure, 380
 medullary collecting tubule affected by, 668
 nonosmotic release of, 604
 in plasma osmolality control, 604
 for septic shock, 986t
 in urine concentration, 668
 in volume control, 611
Vasopressin-resistant high-output renal failure,
  methoxyflurane anesthesia and, 141
Vasopressors, 456t
 after cardiopulmonary bypass, 456–457, 456t
 cerebral effects of, 552, **560**
 in hypertensive patients, 395
 uterine activity during labor affected by, 813
Vasospasm
 cerebral
  calcium channel blockers for, 398t
  ruptured aneurysm and, 567, 578–579
 coronary, 396
Vasovagal (vasodepressor) syncope, 374
VBAC. *See* Vaginal delivery, after cesarean section
VC. *See* Vital capacity
V$_d$. *See* Volume of distribution
Vecuronium, 179, 184f, 188t, **195–196**
 hepatic clearance of, 187–188, 195
 in ischemic heart disease patients, 405
 for outpatient procedures, 884
 renal excretion of, 188, 188t, 195
 altered renal function and, 683
Vena cava filters, for pulmonary embolism, 521
Vena caval compression, during pregnancy, 804, 806–807
Venlafaxine
 for depression, 592t, 593
 for pain management, 337t
Venous access. *See* Venous catheterization
Venous admixture, 475, 494–495, 496f, 497f
 endobronchial intubation affecting, 510
 normal (physiologic shunt), 495
Venous air embolism, 567, 574–575
 liver transplant and, 734
 sitting position and, 894–895
Venous cannulas, for cardiopulmonary bypass, 450–451
Venous catheterization. *See also* Intravenous fluid therapy
 for cardiac surgery
  in adults, 440–441
  in children, 461
 in cardiopulmonary resuscitation, 922–924
 central. *See* Central venous catheterization
 for fluid replacement/management in trauma patient, 795
 for head and neck cancer surgery, 776
 for liver transplant, 732–733
 for lung resection, 537
 in pediatric patient, 860–861
Venous gas tensions, **496–501**. *See also specific type*
 in acid-base disorder diagnosis, 659
Venous pressure, central. *See* Central venous pressure
Venous reservoir, for cardiopulmonary bypass machine,
  435f, 436
Venous return
 partial anomalous, 425
 preload affected by, 368
 total anomalous, 426
 work of breathing and, anesthesia affecting, 490
Venous thrombosis. *See also* Thrombosis
 hip surgery and, 787, 881
 pulmonary embolism and, 520t

Venovenous hemodialysis, continuous (CVVHD), 951,
  979
Venovenous hemofiltration, continuous (CVVHF), 951,
  979
Ventilation/ventilatory drive, 490–492. *See also* Breathing;
  Respiration; Respiratory physiology
 airway resistance and, 485–488, 486t, 487f, 488f, 489f
  anesthesia affecting, 490
 alveolar gas concentration (FA) affected by, 131
 barbiturates affecting, 158, 171t
 benzodiazepines affecting, 151, 161–164, 171t
 in cardiopulmonary resuscitation, 917–918, 918t
 cirrhosis affecting, 728
 compliance and, 482–483, 483f
  anesthesia affecting, 489–490, 492f
 distribution of, 491, 493f
 droperidol affecting, 171t, 175
 elastic resistance and, **482–483**, 483f
 during endoscopy, 772–773
 etomidate affecting, 171t, 172
 intraocular pressure and, 762, 762t
 intraoperative monitoring of, **108–114**, 125
 ketamine affecting, 171t, 172
 lidocaine affecting, 239
 lung volumes and, **483–485**, 484f, 484t, 485f, 486f
  anesthesia affecting, 489–490, 492f
 Mapleson circuit selection and, 32
 mask. *See* Mask ventilation
 mechanical. *See* Mechanical ventilation
 mechanics of, **482–490**
  anesthesia affecting, **489–490**, 492f
 minute, 490
  PaCO$_2$ and, 476, 507, 507f
  pain affecting, 320
  PaO$_2$ and, 507, 508f
  pregnancy affecting, 805, 805t
 nonelastic resistance and, **485–488**, 486t, 487f, 488f,
  489f
 nonvolatile anesthetics affecting, 171t
 opioids affecting, 167, 168f, 171t, 344
  in pediatric patient, 850
 propofol affecting, 171t, 174
 spontaneous, 480, 481f
  in lateral decubitus position, 526, 526f
  Mapleson A circuit for, 27, 32
  open pneumothorax and, 528, 528f, 529f
 surface tension forces and, 482
 time constants and, 491–492
 tissue resistance and, 488
 trauma and, 795
 work of breathing and, **488–489**, 490f, 491f
Ventilation (airflow control), in operating room, **20**
Ventilation/perfusion mismatch, arterial concentration of
  inhalational anesthetic affected by, 132
Ventilation/perfusion ratio, 493–494, 495f, 496f
 absorption atelectasis and, 959
 in pulmonary embolism, 520
Ventilation/perfusion relationships, 475, **490–496**
 lateral decubitus position affecting, 526–527, 526f, 527f
Ventilator bellows, 52, 53f
 ventilator failure and, 52, 57
Ventilators, anesthesia, 40, 41, **50–54**, 52f, 53f. *See also*
  Mechanical ventilation
 disconnect alarms for, 41, 53, 57
 malfunction/leak in, 56–58, 891, 891t
  alarms signaling, 41, 53, 57
 inspection routine for prevention of, **55–56**, 56–57t
Ventilatory failure, pure, 970
Ventilatory mode, for mechanical ventilation, 961–965,
  962t, 963t
Ventolin. *See* Albuterol
Ventricular assist devices, for pump failure after
  cardiopulmonary bypass, 456
Ventricular compliance, 368–369, 370f
Ventricular ejection fraction, 360, 372
Ventricular fibrillation, emergency management of, 912,
  913f, 916f, **922**, 923t, 925t, 930f
Ventricular filling, determinants of, 368, 369t
Ventricular function. *See also* Cardiac output
 assessment of, **371–372**, 372f
 after cardiopulmonary bypass, 455–456, 455t
 determinants of, **366–371**
 pulmonary artery monitoring of, 105–106, 106t
 transesophageal echocardiography for intraoperative
  monitoring of, 444, 444f, 445f
Ventricular function curves, **371**, 372f, 373f
Ventricular hypertrophy
 in aortic regurgitation, 419

Ventricular hypertrophy (*cont.*)
  in aortic stenosis, 416
  in heart failure, 380–381
  in mitral regurgitation, 412
  in pulmonic stenosis, 423
  in renal failure, 685
  in tetralogy of Fallot, 425
Ventricular outflow obstruction
  aortic stenosis causing, 416
  congenital lesions causing, **423**
  hypertrophic cardiomyopathy causing, 418
  in pulmonic stenosis, 423
  in tetralogy of Fallot, 425
Ventricular pressure, change in during systole (dP/dt),
    contractility and, 371–372
Ventricular pressure-volume diagrams, 371, 373*f*
Ventricular septal defect, 424
  heart murmur in, preoperative evaluation of, 407*t*
  in tetralogy of Fallot, 425
Ventricular tachycardia, emergency management of, 913*f*,
    916*f*, 922, 923*t*, 930*f*, 934*f*
Ventriculostomy, for intracranial pressure monitoring, 570
Venturi masks, for oxygen therapy, 955*t*, 957, 957*t*
VER. *See* Visual evoked response/potentials
Verapamil, 364, 397–398, 397*t*, 398*t*
  in cardiopulmonary resuscitation, 928*t*
  for ischemic heart disease, 397–398, 397*t*, 398*t*
  minimum alveolar concentration affected by, 136*t*
  pediatric dosing and, 855*t*
Vertebral arteries, brain supplied by, 564, 565*f*
Vertebral body, 255, 256*f*, 352
Vertebral column. *See also under* Spinal
  anatomy of
    back pain and, 352
    neuraxial anesthesia and, **255**, 256*f*, 257*f*
      level of blockade after spinal anesthesia and, 267
    ligaments of, 255, 257*f*
Vertex presentations, abnormal, 834
Vessel-poor tissues, drug distribution and, 153, 153*t*
  absorption of nonvolatile anesthetics and, 153
  uptake of inhalational anesthetics and, 130*t*, 131, 132*f*
Vessel-rich tissues, drug distribution and, 153, 153*t*
  absorption of nonvolatile anesthetics and, 153
  uptake of inhalational anesthetics and, 130–131, 130*t*,
    132*f*
Vicodin. *See* Hydrocodone
Viloxazine, for depression, 592*t*
VIP. *See* Vasoactive intestinal polypeptide
Viral hepatitis, 724
Visceral afferents, in pain pathway, 314
  integration of, 314–315
Visceral nociceptors, 316
Visceral pain, 311–312, 312*t*
  in failed epidural anesthesia, 273
Viscosity, blood
  cerebral blood flow affected by, 554–555
  in congenital heart disease, 422
Vistaril. *See* Hydroxyzine
Visual analog scale (VAS), in pain evaluation, 321
Visual evoked response/potentials, for intraoperative
    monitoring, 115–116, 116*t*
  anesthetic agents affecting, 563*t*, 564
  during craniotomy, 569
Vital capacity (VC), 484*f*, 485
  forced (FVC), 475, 487–488, 489*f*
    pneumonectomy criteria and, 535*t*
  neuraxial anesthesia affecting, 261
Vital signs, age-related changes in, 851*t*

Vitamin B₁₂, nitrous oxide affecting, 138–139
Vitamin D, 744*t*
  calcium concentration affected by, 619, 744*t*
  deficiency of, hypocalcemia and, 620
Vitamin K
  in hepatic production of coagulation factors, 708, 712
    liver disease and, 720
  supplemental, in extrahepatic biliary obstruction, 731
Vitreous surgery, gas bubble injection during, expansion
    and, 761, **763–764**
Vivactil. *See* Protriptyline
VO₂. *See* Oxygen consumption
Vocal cord paralysis, recurrent laryngeal nerve damage and,
    60, 78–79
  thyroidectomy and, 742
Voiding, neuraxial anesthesia affecting, 261, 276
Volatile anesthetics. *See* Inhalational (volatile)
    anesthesia/anesthetics
Voltage-gated calcium channelopathy (hypokalemic
    periodic paralysis), **758**
  anesthetic considerations in patients with, 759
Volume-cycled ventilators, 961
Volume of distribution (Vd), 153–154
  in geriatric patient, 879
  of nonvolatile anesthetics, 153–154
Volume overload, in aortic regurgitation, 419
Volume resuscitation. *See also* Fluid
    replacement/management
  for neonate, 845
Volumetric pump, for intravenous infusion, 888
Volutrauma, mechanical ventilation and, 960
Vomiting. *See also* Nausea and vomiting
  chloride-sensitive metabolic alkalosis caused by, 644, 657
  induced, for drug overdose/poisoning, 991–992
  postoperative, 882, 885–886, 885*t*, 940
    ear surgery and, 779
    ophthalmic surgery and, 765
    outpatient procedures and, 885–886
von Willebrand factor
  deficiency/abnormalities of, 721–722
  persistent bleeding after cardiopulmonary bypass and,
    458
von Willebrand's disease, 721–722
VSDs. *See* Ventricular septal defect
Vₜ. *See* Tidal volume
vWF. *See* von Willebrand factor

Wall motion abnormalities, 371, 433, 444, 444*f*
  stroke volume affected by, 371
  transesophageal echocardiography for intraoperative
    assessment of, 444, 444*f*
Walther, ganglion of (ganglion impar), blockade of, for
    pain management, 335
Warfarin, for pulmonary embolism, 521
"Warm-up" phenomenon, 755
Waste-gas scavenging, 20
  active, 54
  by anesthesia machine, 41, **54**, 54*f*
  breathing circuits and, 33*t*
  passive, 54
Water, dissociation constant for, hydrogen ion/pH
    relationship and, 645
Water balance
  antidiuretic hormone in, 604
  disorders of, **602–609**, 603*t*. *See also specific disorder*
  normal, **602**

Water bath, for extracorporeal shock wave lithotripsy, 697,
    698
Water intoxication
  absorption of irrigation solutions for transurethral
    resection of prostate (TURP) and, 695
  cerebral edema caused by, 568
Waters' to-and-fro circuit, 30*t*
WDR neurons. *See* Wide dynamic range (WDR) neurons
Weak acids, 645
Weak bases, 645
Weaning/extubation, from mechanical ventilation,
    967–968, 967*t*
Wedging, in pulmonary artery catheterization, 104. *See also*
    Pulmonary artery catheterization
Weight, in nutritional assessment, 988
Weiss winged needle, 270*f*
Wellbutrin. *See* Bupropion
Wenger chestpiece (precordial stethoscope), for
    intraoperative monitoring, **108**, 109*f*
Wheal-and-flare response, to histamine, 243
Wheatstone bridge circuit, in pressure transducers, 94, 99*f*
Whitacre needle, 266, 266*f*
White double-lumen endobronchial tube, 529*t*, 530
Wide dynamic range (WDR) neurons, 313, 315*f*
  in central pain modulation
    facilitation and, 318
    inhibition and, 318
Wind-up, of second-order neurons, 313, 318
Wisconsin laryngoscope blade, 70*f*
Wolff-Parkinson-White (WPW) syndrome, 381
  adenosine in management of, 230, 385
  atrial fibrillation in, 383
  drugs in management of, 385
  mechanism of paroxysmal supraventricular tachycardia
    in, 382–383
Work of breathing, **488–489**, 490*f*, 491*f*
  anesthesia affecting, 490
  in pediatric patient, 850
Wound infections, 981
WPW syndrome. *See* Wolff-Parkinson-White (WPW)
    syndrome
Wright respirometer, 44–45, 45*f*
Wrist
  median nerve block at, 295, 296*f*
  radial nerve block at, 294–295, 295*f*
  ulnar nerve block at, 297, 298*f*

x descent, 102, 102*f*, 366
Xenon (Xe) anesthesia, advantages and disadvantages of,
    137*t*
Xylocaine. *See* Lidocaine

y descent, 102, 102*f*, 366
YAG laser, 773
Yoke assembly, on anesthesia machine, 42
Yttrium-aluminum-garnet (YAG) laser, 773

Zantac. *See* **Ranitidine**
Zaroxolyn. *See* Metolazone
Zero-order kinetics, 155
Zoloft. *See* Sertraline
Zyban. *See* Bupropion
Zygapophyseal joints, degeneration of, back pain caused by,
    355

DATE DUE

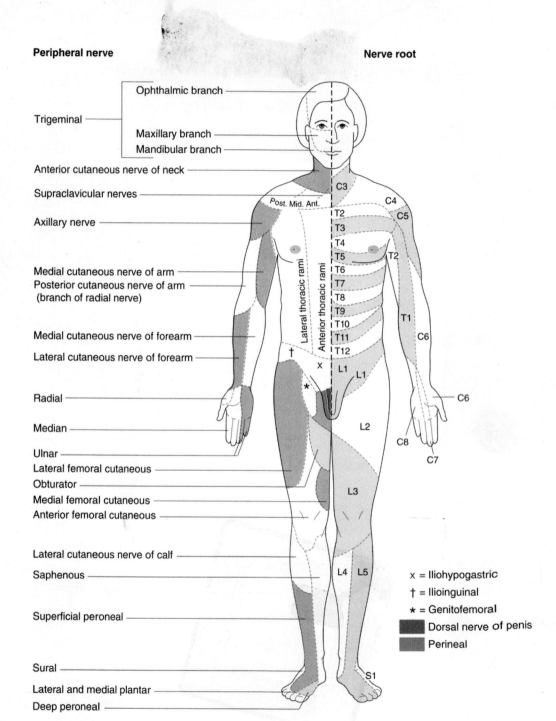

Peripheral nerve

Nerve root

Ophthalmic branch

Trigeminal

Maxillary branch

Mandibular branch

Anterior cutaneous nerve of neck

Supraclavicular nerves

Axillary nerve

Medial cutaneous nerve of arm

Posterior cutaneous nerve of arm
(branch of radial nerve)

Medial cutaneous nerve of forearm

Lateral cutaneous nerve of forearm

Radial

Median

Ulnar

Lateral femoral cutaneous

Obturator

Medial femoral cutaneous

Anterior femoral cutaneous

Lateral cutaneous nerve of calf

Saphenous

Superficial peroneal

Sural

Lateral and medial plantar

Deep peroneal

Post. Mid. Ant.

Lateral thoracic rami

Anterior thoracic rami

C3

C4

C5

T2

T3

T4

T5

T2

T6

T7

T8

T9

T1

T10

C6

T11

T12

L1

L1

†

x

C6

★

L2

C8

C7

L3

L4   L5

x = Iliohypogastric

† = Ilioinguinal

★ = Genitofemoral

Dorsal nerve of penis

Perineal

S1